HUMAN PHARMACOLOGY
MOLECULAR-TO-CLINICAL

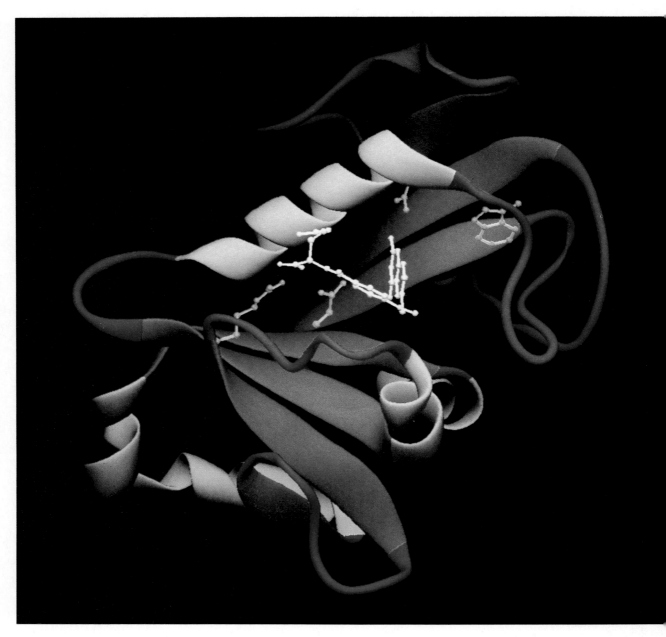

Ribbon representation of human dihydrofolate reductase with methotrexate modeled into the substrate cleft. (Courtesy Jay F. Davies II and Joseph Kraut, Ph.D.)

HUMAN PHARMACOLOGY
MOLECULAR-TO-CLINICAL

LEMUEL B. WINGARD JR, Ph.D.

Professor, Department of Pharmacology and
    Anesthesiology
University of Pittsburgh School of Medicine
Pittsburgh, Pennsylvania

THEODORE M. BRODY, Ph.D.

Professor, Department of Pharmacology and
    Toxicology
College of Human Medicine
Michigan State University
East Lansing, Michigan

JOSEPH LARNER, M.D., Ph.D.

Alumni Professor, Department of Pharmacology
University of Virginia School of Medicine
Charlottesville, Virginia

ARNOLD SCHWARTZ, Ph.D.

Edward Wendland Professor of Materia Medica and
    Therapeutics
Chairman, Department of Pharmacology and Cell
    Biophysics
University of Cincinnati College of Medicine
Cincinnati, Ohio

With 482 illustrations

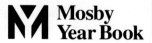

St. Louis Baltimore Boston Chicago London Philadelphia Sydney Toronto

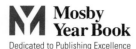
Mosby
Year Book
Dedicated to Publishing Excellence

Editor   Kim Kist
Senior Developmental Editor   Elaine Steinborn
Assistant Editor   Jo Salway
Project Manager   Carol Sullivan Wiseman
Manuscript Editors   Florence Achenbach, David Brown, Pat Joiner, Linda McKinley
Book Design   John Rokusek, Candace Conner, David Zielinski
Cover Design   David Zielinski
Production   Florence Achenbach, Linda McKinley

Cover Photo Courtesy of   Jay F. Davies II, Joseph Kraut, Ph.D.
Illustration Program   Donald O'Connor

Printed in the United States of America

Mosby–Year Book, Inc.
11830 Westline Industrial Drive
St. Louis, Missouri 63146

Library of Congress Cataloging in Publication Data

Human pharmacology: molecular-to-clinical / Lemuel B. Wingard, Jr.
. . . [et al.].
         p.   cm.
     Includes bibliographical references.
     Includes index.
     ISBN 0-8016-5632-X
     1. Pharmacology.   2.   Chemotherapy.   I. Wingard, Lemuel B.
     [DNLM: 1.   Drug Therapy.   2.   Pharmacology.   QV 4 H918]
     RM300.H86   1991
     615.5'8—dc20
     DNLM/DLC
     for Library of Congress   90-13668
                                                              CIP

GW/CD/VH   10   9   8   7   6   5   4   3   2

Contributors

TAI AKERA, M.D., Ph.D.
Director
National Children's Hospital Medical Research Center
Tokyo, Japan
Chapter 15 **Drugs affecting cardiac contractile force**

RICHARD L. ATKINSON, M.D.
Professor
Department of Medicine
Eastern Virginia Medical School
Associate Chief of Staff for Research
Veterans Administration Medical Center
Hampton, VA
Chapter 61 **Nutritional aspects of pharmacology**

ROBERT L. BALSTER, Ph.D.
Professor
Department of Pharmacology and Toxicology
Medical College of Virginia
Virginia Commonwealth University
Richmond, VA
Chapter 32 **Drug abuse**

LOUIS A. BARKER, Ph.D.
Professor
Department of Pharmacology
Louisiana State University Medical Center
New Orleans, LA
Chapter 58 **Histamine and antihistamines**

JAMES L. BENNETT, Ph.D.
Professor
Department of Pharmacology and Toxicology
College of Osteopathic Medicine
Michigan State University
East Lansing, MI
Chapter 54 **Drugs effective against parasitic helminthic infections**
Chapter 55 **Drugs effective against parasitic protozoal infections**

JAMES P. BENNETT, M.D., Ph.D.
Assistant Professor
Departments of Neurology, Behavioral Medicine and
   Psychiatry, and Pharmacology
University of Virginia Medical School and Children's
   Medical Center
Charlottesville, VA
Chapter 23 **Antipsychotic agents**
Chapter 24 **Drugs to treat affective (mood) disorders**
Chapter 27 **Drugs for the treatment of movement disorders and spasticity**

JEFFREY L. BLUMER, M.D., Ph.D.
Professor
Department of Pediatrics
Division of Pediatric Pharmacology and Critical Care
University of Virginia Medical school and Children's
   Medical Center
Charlottesville, VA
Chapter 63 **Perinatal/neonatal pharmacology**

BARBARA W. BRANDOM, M.D.
Associate Professor
Department of Anesthesiology
University of Pittsburgh School of Medicine
Children's Hospital
Pittsburgh, PA
Chapter 30 **Pain control with general and local anesthetics**

DAVID BRASE, Ph.D.
Postdoctoral Fellow
Department of Pharmacology and Toxicology
Medical College of Virginia
Virginia Commonwealth University
Richmond, VA
Chapter 28 **Pain control with narcotic analgesics**

MICHAEL J. BRODY, Ph.D.

Professor
Department of Pharmacology
Associate Director of Cardiovascular Center
University of Iowa College of Medicine
Iowa City, IA
Chapter 12 **Regulation of arterial blood pressure by central and peripheral autonomic nervous systems**
Chapter 13 **Antihypertensive drugs**

THEODORE M. BRODY, Ph.D.

Professor
Department of Pharmacology and Toxicology
College of Human Medicine
Michigan State University
East Lansing, MI
Chapter 15 **Drugs affecting cardiac contractile force**
Chapter 17 **Vasodilators**
Chapter 29 **Pain and inflammation control with nonnarcotic analgesics**
Chapter 31 **Alcohol**
Chapter 65 **Drugs to treat anemia**

THOMAS F. BURKS, Ph.D.

Professor and Head
Department of Pharmacology
Associate Dean of Research
College of Medicine
University of Arizona
Tucson, AZ
Chapter 58 **Histamine and antihistamines**
Chapter 59 **Gastrointestinal drugs**

EDWARD J. CAFRUNY, M.D., Ph.D.

Professor
Department of Pharmacology
University of Medicine and Dentistry of New Jersey
Newark, NJ
Chapter 19 **Diuretics: Drugs that increase excretion of water and electrolytes**

GEORGE P. CHROUSSOS, M.D.

Chief
Pediatric and Endocrinology Section
National Institute of Child Health and Human Development
Bethesda, MD
Chapter 35 **Glucocorticoids and other adrenal steroids**

D. RYAN COOK, M.D.

Professor
Departments of Anesthesiology and Pharmacology
University of Pittsburgh School of Medicine

Chief of Anesthesiology
Children's Hospital
Pittsburgh, PA
Chapter 30 **Pain control with general and local anesthetics**

RICHARD O. DART, M.D.

Associate Professor
Research Director
Section of Emergency Medicine
University of Arizona College of Medicine
Tucson, AZ
Chapter 62 **Toxicology**

RICHARD A. DEITRICH, Ph.D.

Professor
Department of Pharmacology
University of Colorado School of Medicine
Denver, CO
Chapter 31 **Alcohol**

WILLIAM L. DEWEY, Ph.D.

Professor
Department of Pharmacology
Medical College of Virginia
Associate Provost for Research and Graduate Affairs
Virginia Commonwealth University
Richmond, VA
Chapter 28 **Pain control with narcotic analgesics**

EDWARD F. DOMINO, M.D.

Professor
Department of Pharmacology
University of Michigan Medical School
Ann Arbor, MI
Chapter 33 **Drugs to treat sleep disorders**

PETER H. DOUKAS, Ph.D.

Professor
Department of Medicinal Chemistry
School of Pharmacy
Research Associate Professor of Pharmacology
School of Medicine
Temple University
Philadelphia, PA
Chapter 9 **Drugs affecting the parasympathetic nervous system**

ANN D. DUNN, Ph.D.

Research Associate Professor
Division of Endocrinology
Department of Medicine
University of Virginia Medical School
Charlottesville, VA
Chapter 38 **Thyroid and antithyroid drugs**

JOHN T. DUNN, M.D.

Professor
Department of Medicine
Division of Endocrinology
Medical School and University Hospital
University of Virginia
Charlottesville, VA
Chapter 38 **Thyroid and antithyroid drugs**

PAUL D. ELLNER, Ph.D.

Professor Emeritus
Department of Clinical Microbiology Services
Columbia University College of Physicians and Surgeons
Columbia-Presbyterian Medical Center
New York, NY
Chapter 56 **Antiseptics and disinfectants**

WILLIAM S. EVANS, M.D.

Associate Professor
Department of Medicine
Division of Endocrinology
Medical School and University Hospital
University of Virginia
Charlottesville, VA
Chapter 41 **Hypothalamic-pituitary hormones**

GREGORY D. FINK, Ph.D.

Professor
Department of Pharmacology and Toxicology
College of Osteopathic Medicine
Michigan State University
East Lansing, MI
Chapter 12 **Regulation of arterial blood pressure by central and peripheral autonomic nervous systems**
Chapter 13 **Antihypertensive drugs**

MICHAEL K. FRITSCH, M.D.

Physician Research Fellow
Department of Biochemistry
University of Wisconsin
Madison, WI
Chapter 36 **Estrogens, progestins, and oral contraceptives**

JACK GORSKI, Ph.D.

Professor
Department of Biochemistry
University of Wisconsin
Madison, WI
Chapter 36 **Estrogens, progestins, and oral contraceptives**

BRENDA J. GROSSMAN, M.D.

Medical Officer
American Red Cross
Washington, DC
Chapter 65 **Drugs to treat anemia**

JAYA HALDAR, Ph.D.

Professor
Department of Biological Sciences
St. John's University
Jamaica, NY
Chapter 40 **Drugs affecting uterine motility**

DANIEL H. HAVLICHEK, M.D.

Professor
Department of Medicine
Division of Infectious Diseases
College of Human Medicine
Michigan State University
East Lansing, MI
Chapter 53 **Antiviral drugs**

JOSEPH R. HUME, Ph.D.

Associate Professor
Department of Physiology
University of Nevada
School of Medicine
Reno, NV
Chapter 14 **Cardiac electrophysiology and antidysrhythmic agents**

STEVEN J. JACOBS, M.D.

Director
Division of Cell Biology
Burroughs Wellcome Co.
Research Triangle Park, NC
Chapter 34 **Hormone receptors and signaling mechanisms**

THOMAS T. KAWABATA, Ph.D.

Assistant Professor
Department of Pharmacology
Medical College of Virginia
Virginia Commonwealth University
Richmond, VA
Chapter 60 **Immunopharmacology**

CHARLES D. KOWAL, M.D.

Senior Director
Clinical Oncology Research Program
Warner Lambert Parke-Davis Co.
Ann Arbor, MI
Part VI **Neoplastic cells: Drugs affecting cell growth and viability**

JAMES M. LARNER, M.D.

Assistant Professor
Department of Radiology and Radiological therapy
Medical School
University of Virginia
Charlottesville, VA
Part VI **Neoplastic cells: Drugs affecting cell growth and viability**

JOSEPH LARNER, M.D., Ph.D.
Alumni Professor
Department of Pharmacology
University of Virginia Medical School
Charlottesville, VA
Part V **Endocrine systems: Hormones and related compounds (Introduction)**

THOMAS J. LAUTERIO, Ph.D.
Assistant Professor
Departments of Medicine and Physiology
Eastern Virginia Medical School
Veterans Administration Medical Center
Hampton, VA
Chapter 61 **Nutritional aspects of pharmacology**

JOHN C. LAWRENCE, Ph.D.
Associate Professor
Department of Pharmacology
Washington University School of Medicine
St. Louis, MO
Chapter 39 **Insulin and oral hypoglycemic agents**

ERIC W. LOTHMAN, M.D., Ph.D.
Professor
Department of Neurology and Comprehensive Epilepsy
    Program
Medical School and University Hospital
University of Virginia
Charlottesville, VA
Chapter 26 **Drugs to treat seizure disorders**

ANDREW N. MARGIORIS, M.D.
Associate Professor
Medical University of Crete
Crete, Greece
Chapter 35 **Glucocorticoids and other adrenal steroids**

ROBERT H. McDONALD JR, M.D.
Professor
Departments of Medicine, Pharmacology and
    Epidemiology
Chief
Division of Pharmacology and Hypertension
Department of Medicine
University of Pittsburgh School of Medicine
Pittsburgh, PA
Chapter 20 **Lipid-lowering drugs and atherosclerosis**

JOHN C. McGIFF, M.D.
Professor and Chairman
Department of Pharmacology
New York Medical College
Valhalla, NY
Chapter 18 **Prostaglandins and related autacoids**

CHRISTINE MIASKOWSKI, Ph.D.
Assistant Professor
Department of Physiological Nursing
University of California
San Francisco, CA
Chapter 40 **Drugs affecting uterine motility**

KENNETH P. MINNEMAN, Ph.D.
Professor
Department of Pharmacology
Emory University Medical School
Atlanta, GA
Chapter 22 **Pharmacological organization of the central nervous system**

KENNETH E. MOORE, Ph.D.
Professor and Chairman
Department of Pharmacology and Toxicology
Michigan State University
East Lansing, MI
Chapter 10 **Drugs affecting the sympathetic nervous system**

ALBERT E. MUNSON, Ph.D.
Professor
Department of Pharmacology
Medical College of Virginia
Virginia Commonweath University
Richmond, VA
Chapter 60 **Immunopharmacology**

FERN E. MURDOCH, Ph.D.
Research Associate
Department of Biochemistry
University of Wisconsin
Madison, WI
Chapter 36 **Estrogens, progestins, and oral contraceptives**

HAROLD C. NEU, M.D.
Professor
Departments of Medicine and Pharmacology
Chief Division of Infectious Diseases
Columbia University College of Physicians and Surgeons
Columbia-Presbyterian Medical Center
New York, NY
Part VII **Invading organisms: Agents that kill invaders**

JOHN J. O'NEILL, Ph.D.
Professor
Department of Pharmacology
Temple University School of Medicine
Philadelphia, PA
Chapter 9 **Drugs affecting the parasympathetic nervous system**

RICHARD H. RECH, Ph.D.
Professor
Department of Pharmacology and Toxicology
College of Human Medicine
Michigan State University
East Lansing, MI
Chapter 25 **Drugs to treat anxiety and related disorders**

ROBERT R. RUFFOLO JR, Ph.D.
Group Director
Department of Pharmacology and Molecular
    Pharmacology
Smith Kline and French Laboratories
King of Prussia, PA
Chapter 8 **Physiology and biochemistry of the peripheral autonomic nervous system**

ARNOLD SCHWARTZ, Ph.D.
Edward Wendland Professor of Materia Medica and
    Therapeutics
Chairman
Department of Pharmacology and Cell Biophysics
University of Cincinnati College of Medicine
Cincinnati, OH
Chapter 15 **Drugs affecting cardiac contractile force**
Chapter 16 **Calcium antagonists**

I. GLENN SIPES, Ph.D.
Professor and Head
Departments of Pharmacology and Toxicology and
    Anesthesiology
College of Pharmacy
University of Arizona
Tucson, AZ
Chapter 62 **Toxicology**

MICHAEL J. SOLLENBERGER, M.D.
Assistant Professor
Department of Medicine
Division of Endocrinology
Bowman Grey School of Medicine
Winston-Salem, NC
Chapter 41 **Hypothalamic-pituitary hormones**

GARY E. STEIN, Pharm.D.
Associate Professor
Departments of Medicine and Pharmacology and
    Toxicology
College of Human Medicine
Michigan State University
East Lansing, MI
Chapter 66 **Regulated drug development and usage**

PAULA H. STERN, Ph.D.
Professor
Department of Pharmacology

Northwestern University Medical School
Chicago, IL
Chapter 42 **Agents affecting calcium-regulating hormones**

RICHARD L. STILLER, Ph.D.
Assistant Professor
Departments of Anesthesiology and Pharmacology
University of Pittsburgh School of Medicine
Pittsburgh, PA
Chapter 11 **Neuromuscular blocking agents**

CONSTANTINE A. STRATAKIS, M.D.
Department of Pediatrics
Georgetown University Medical School
Washington, DC
Guest Scientist
Pediatric and Endocrinology Section
National Institute of Child Health and Human
    Development
Bethesda, MD
Chapter 35 **Glucocorticoids and other adrenal steroids**

JANET L. STRINGER, M.D., Ph.D.
Research Assistant Professor
Department of Neurology
Medical School and University Hospital
University of Virginia
Charlottesville, VA
Chapter 26 **Drugs to treat seizure disorders**

JOHN E. THORNBURG, D.O., Ph.D.
Professor
Departments of Pharmacology and Toxicology and Family
    Medicine
College of Osteopathic Medicine
Michigan State University
East Lansing, MI
Chapter 57 **Drugs affecting respiratory function**
Chapter 64 **Gerontological pharmacology**

PAL L. VAGHY, M.D.
Associate Professor
Department of Pharmacology and Cell Biophysics
University of Cincinnati
College of Medicine
Cincinnati, OH
Chapter 16 **Calcium antagonists**

MARY LEE VANCE, M.D.
Associate Professor
Department of Medicine
Medical School and University Hospital
University of Virginia
Charlottesville, VA
Chapter 41 **Hypothalamic-pituitary hormones**

ELIZABETH A. VANDEWAA, Ph.D.
Senior Research Associate
Department of Comparative Biosciences
University of Wisconsin
Madison, WI
Chapter 54 **Drugs effective against parasitic helminthic infections**
Chapter 55 **Drugs effective against parasitic protozoal infections**

LEMUEL B. WINGARD JR, Ph.D. (deceased)
Professor
Department of Pharmacology and Anesthesiology
University of Pittsburgh School of Medicine
Pittsburgh, PA
Part I **General principles**
Chapter 11 **Neuromuscular blocking agents**
Chapter 21 **Drugs affecting coagulation, fibrinolysis, and platelet aggregation**
Part VI **Neoplastic cells: Drugs affecting cell growth and viability**

STEPHEN J. WINTERS, M.D.
Associate Professor
Department of Medicine
University of Pittsburgh
School of Medicine and Montifiore Hospital
Pittsburgh, PA
Chapter 37 **Androgens and antiandrogens**

BEN G. ZIMMERMAN, Ph.D.
Professor
Department of Pharmacology
University of Minnesota Medical School
Minneapolis, MN
Chapter 12 **Regulation of arterial blood pressure by central and peripheral autonomic nervous systems**
Chapter 13 **Antihypertensive drugs**

This book is dedicated to the memory of Dr. Lemuel B. Wingard Jr, whose vision was largely responsible for the philosophy embodied herein. This book was his dream, and he invested countless hours converting that dream into reality. His death when the completion of the manuscript was within sight was especially tragic.

Preface

Although some excellent pharmacology texts already exist, the editors felt that a timely, readable, balanced text would fill a currently unmet need in this area. Pharmacology, a discipline bridging basic and clinical science, is now increasingly directed toward developing new drugs and therapeutic agents based on sound mechanistic principles. For example, coincident with the explosion of information in the molecular biology, biochemistry, and physiology of receptors and signaling mechanisms; the neurobiology of transmitters; and the immunochemistry of monoclonal antibodies and lymphokines, the aim of pharmacology is to develop new drugs and therapeutic agents of greater selectivity than previously thought possible. Classical physiological responses to drugs and fundamental studies of disease processes in clinical medicine also continue to contribute important insights for drug development. Accordingly, in this book, appropriate, balanced emphasis is placed on both basic and clinical mechanistic aspects with the goal of providing the student with a sound fundamental understanding of the discipline, within a text of reasonable size, to better prepare for future self-learning in pharmacology.

The text is unique in its overall organization, including the stressing of drug classes and prototypical drugs to treat disease, the use of boxes and tables to summarize factual data related to basic principles, and the emphasis on relevant fundamental clinical information. Illustrations stress current models of mechanisms. Chapter sections, boxes, tables, and figures can be used conveniently, either separately or in any order desired by the instructor or student. Chapters were invited from authoritative experts who are well-versed in both basic and clinical aspects of

the subject. Content was carefully selected to meet the immediate needs of medical and related professional students within the framework of either a standard or an innovative professional curriculum. This book was also designed to provide residents and practicing physicians with easy access to clinical information related to drug use.

A consistent chapter format was followed wherever feasible throughout the text. Each section of the book is introduced by an appropriate summary to focus and highlight the content of that section. Each chapter is subdivided into the following heads:

 THERAPEUTIC OVERVIEW

 MECHANISMS OF ACTION

 PHARMACOKINETICS

 RELATION OF MECHANISMS OF ACTION TO CLINICAL RESPONSE

 SIDE EFFECTS, CLINICAL PROBLEMS, AND TOXICITY

A list of tradenames is given at the end of each relevant chapter. Much of the information is presented in color-coded tables and boxes to provide easy access for the student. Pharmacological and therapeutic concepts are reinforced by the use of new, full-color illustrations; these were generated by the authors and editors to enable the student to visualize important mechanisms described in the text.

A number of features serves as guides to students. Major drugs or drug classes considered are presented at the beginning of each chapter. Abbreviations used in the chapter are highlighted. Tables and boxes indicating therapeutic summary, pharmacokinetics, clinical problems, and tradenames are color-coded throughout the text for ready access. Special topics, not ordinarily emphasized in standard pharmacology texts but currently important, include full chapters on nutritional aspects of pharmacology, perinatal/neonatal pharmacology, and gerontological pharmacology.

Finally, we were saddened by the sudden death in July 1990 of one of our principal editors and authors, Dr. Lemuel B. Wingard Jr. Lem's original ideas led to the conceptualization of this text. We hope that this book will serve as a living memorial to his dedication in moving it to completion.

Acknowledgments

The Editors are indebted to many of their colleagues for critically reviewing some of the chapters, including Drs. C. Asplin, W. Atchison, C. Ayers, R. Biltonen, J. Galligan, J. Garrison, J. Goodman, G. Grupp, I. Grupp, P. Guyenet, J. Harmony, R. Haynes, E. Hewlett, P. Isakson, D. Johns, K. Killam, L. Lane, D. Lathrop, K. Lookinglad, R. Millard, M. Peach, R. Pearson, G. Romero, and J. Veldhuis; and with special thanks to one of our contributors, Dr. Harold C. Neu.

Theodore M. Brody
Joseph Larner
Arnold Schwartz

Contents

GENERAL PRINCIPLES

I

Part I describes principles that apply to essentially all drugs. These principles pertain to administration, distribution to different body sites, general mechanisms by which drugs produce beneficial effects, and mechanisms for drug disappearance from the body. Because of differences in chemical structure, not all drugs undergo the same specific processes.

Examples of drug groups in some of the key processes are given. Examples in Chapter 4 explain how to determine specific pharmacokinetic parameter values based on realistic data, but actual drug names are omitted to emphasize principles rather than values for specific drugs.

1

Introduction and Definitions

ABBREVIATIONS	
ATP	adenosine triphosphate

THERAPEUTIC IMPORTANCE OF DRUGS

Both physicians and patients acknowledge the major role played by drugs in modern medical therapy. Many millions of prescriptions are written each year in the United States for dispensing over 700 active ingredients available in several thousand different combinations, pharmaceutical preparations, or delivery forms. Additionally, 100,000 over-the-counter nonprescription preparations are available. These nonprescription items vary from a single high purity active ingredient, such as aspirin mixed with tableting materials, to mixtures of several ingredients, many of which have questionable efficacy.

Despite the proliferation of active chemical compounds for the treatment of diseases, new and better drugs are still needed. The search is intense and yields excitement when a new chemical compound provides symptomatic relief or cures a previously untreatable disease. Similar responses arise with new drugs that provide as good or better relief compared to existing compounds but with fewer undesirable side effects. The excitement of discovery, however, is often blended with controversy. New drugs must be made available for clinical use as early as possible, but not before potentially damaging side effects can be ruled out. The controversy arises because the mechanism of action and therefore the safety of the drug may be poorly understood and the decision to allow clinical use of the agent may profoundly affect the lives of patients.

THE SCOPE OF PHARMACOLOGY

For hundreds of years most drugs were highly impure mixtures of only vaguely known composition and primarily of plant or animal origin. A physician was required to know only what effects to expect from a preparation. How the mixture produced such effects was beyond the knowledge of that day. Over the past 60 years the situation has changed markedly. Today a physician is required to know the expected effect, how the beneficial effect is brought about, and how the drug interacts with body components at the molecular level to initiate such an effect.

This broader knowledge of how drugs interact with body constituents to produce therapeutic effects is termed *pharmacology*. This term covers the spectrum from the molecular level to the whole body and relies heavily on knowledge of biochemistry, physiology, molecular biology, and organic chemistry. The elucidation of molecular mechanisms of drug response, the development of new drugs, and the formulation of clinical guidelines for the safe and effective use of drugs in the therapy or prevention of disease states and in the relief of symptoms are all part of pharmacology.

UNDERSTANDING DRUG ACTIONS AT THE MOLECULAR LEVEL

As recently as the 1920s, relatively few therapeutically beneficial active ingredients (by today's standards) existed. Most active ingredients were used in only partially purified forms. Since then, vastly improved tools and methods for the purification of chemical compounds have been developed and elucidation of chemical structures has taken place. It is possible to identify which compounds in the earlier crude mixtures produced the beneficial effects and which the undesirable responses. Techniques of synthetic organic chemistry are applied not only to work out the structure of each parent drug, but also to synthesize thousands of structural analogs and to test these analogs for pharmacological activity. These efforts resulted in the current research thrust to develop structure-activity relationships for different classes of drugs.

Another breakthrough in the 1940s resulted from the realization that microorganisms could produce compounds (antibiotics) capable of killing other microorganisms. This led to the discovery and subsequent fermentative production of thousands of potentially useful antibiotics. Chemical structures of these antibiotics were more complex than those of previous drugs. Therefore deciphering the structures required additional time and delayed the synthesis of analogs. Thus during the 1940s and 1950s, pharmacology depended heavily on organic chemistry to provide the information to synthesize new drugs and develop an understanding of the relationships between chemical structures and pharmacological activity.

Developments in biochemistry during the 1950s and continuing today also had a major influence in establishing the present molecular emphasis in pharmacology. Sophisticated purification techniques provide greatly improved insights into the qualitative and quantitative molecular mechanisms of cellular processes. It also is possible to identify, isolate, and characterize body fluid or tissue constituents where drugs initiate their beneficial effects. Therefore the processes of how drugs act can be approached from two directions: (1) drugs can be studied as chemical compounds of known structure and (2) tissue or body fluid sites where the drugs act can be studied as chemical compounds of known structure. The pace of defining the structures of drug sites of action has accelerated greatly in the 1980s as a result of advances in molecular biology and genetic engineering. Cellular or body fluid constituents that are present in too small a concentration to be isolated and characterized can now, in principle, be produced in milligram and even gram quantities through gene cloning and expression in foreign cell lines. Therefore the understanding of how drugs or other compounds act on body constituents at the molecular level is expected to increase markedly over the coming years. This understanding will provide a sound basis for rational drug use in successful medical therapy, as well as a foundation for development of improved drugs with minimal unwanted side effects.

CLINICAL USE OF DRUGS

Main Factors

Molecular drug action information to formulate practical therapeutic guidelines for clinical use is a valuable link between basic medical science and clinical medicine. As mentioned earlier, the information available through pharmacology depends on principles of biochemistry and physiology. Clinically, the initial molecular action of a drug in an individual patient cannot be detected. Instead, the initial molecular process sets off a cascade of events, which at some point produces a change that is detectable in one of the following ways:

1. With instruments
2. Laboratory tests on body fluid or tissue samples
3. Direct observation by the physician or the patient

This cascade concept is illustrated in Figure 1-1 for digitalis and its action on the heart and how this leads to reduced edema.

The dose of digitalis and the frequency of administration are influenced by numerous variables that control the distribution and disposition of the drug and are of high clinical relevancy (see Pharmacokinetic Variables, p. 7). One of the more difficult aspects of pharmacology is providing rational explanations that tie the initial drug-induced molecular events to the observable clinical effects.

In a given clinical situation the choice of drug to obtain a desired therapeutic effect may be easy or

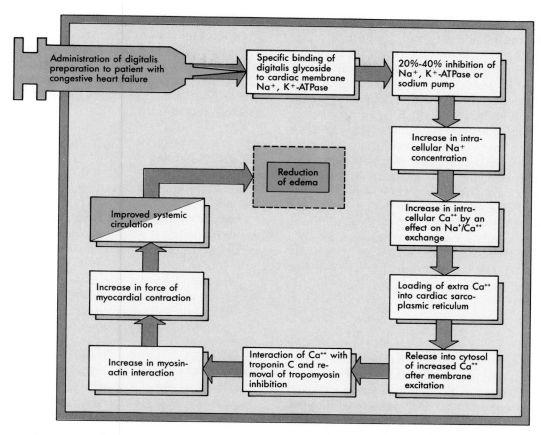

FIGURE 1-1   Initial molecular interaction of digitalis with a body constituent and the subsequent cascade of events that results in an observable pharmacological response. In 1785 the Scottish physician William Withering published his famous treatise on the effect of the foxglove, or digitalis plant, on the treatment of dropsy (edema). After 200 years of research, it is recognized that a series of events is initiated by the interaction of a digitalis glycoside with a protein embedded in the cardiac cell membrane. The red boxes indicate events that are readily detectable or observable.

complicated. In either case, numerous factors, including the following, should be taken into account:

1. Each patient is different. Many will respond adequately to the selected drugs, but not all will. The reason may be simple or complex, but a scientific explanation for each case often cannot be determined or the effort to do so justified clinically.
2. Therapy without all the data. In life-threatening situations or in disease states that prove difficult to diagnose, drug therapy often must be started before all of the laboratory results or consulting physician reports are received.
3. Patient status changes. The drug and the size

and frequency of the dose may need to be modified as the condition of the patient improves or declines.

4. Multiple drugs. Many hospitalized patients receive five to ten different drugs concurrently, outpatients may be taking two to four drugs, and elderly patients may be taking up to twelve drugs concurrently. The opportunity for drug interactions is high when the presence of a second drug influences the effect produced by the first drug.

All of these factors produce uncertainty; therefore the selection of a specific drug and a dosing schedule for an individual patient involves an element of experimentation. Individual patients may react differently. The drug may bring about the desired therapeutic result or various unwanted results, including lack of efficacy, toxicity, or altered disease state. Such occurrences may result from rapid or slow disposition of the drug by the patient, an inappropriate dosing schedule, a drug-drug interaction, incorrect diagnosis, or a change in disease state. In dealing with these uncertainties, the physician trained in molecular mechanisms of action, principal routes of disposition, and pharmacological and toxic effects of the drugs has an advantage. This physician assesses the patient's pharmacological response, as well as the validity of the diagnosis with each drug used. This aids in choosing a subsequent course of therapy. The course of the disease and the therapeutic intervention with drugs should be viewed as dynamic rather than static processes.

Therapeutic Index

Drugs must produce beneficial effects to qualify for government approval for clinical use (see Chapter 65). In addition, all drugs in high doses produce toxic responses. The range between the concentration of drug needed to produce the therapeutic response and that which produces a toxic response is a key factor in classifying a drug as easy or difficult to use. The ratio of these concentrations is called the *therapeutic index* (also called the *therapeutic ratio*) and is expressed as the minimum concentration (or dose) that produces toxicity divided by the minimum concentration (or dose) that gives the therapeutic response in a patient population. When this ratio is 2.0 or less,

the compound can be difficult to use in patients without encountering significant toxicity. Such is the case with the cardiac drug, digoxin, where the therapeutic index is close to 2.0. When the therapeutic index is considerably larger, there is less chance that toxicity will be encountered when the normal recommended dosage is used.

TERMINOLOGY

Basic Terms

General terms of the pharmacology literature are listed in Table 1-1 with their definitions. The terms *action, effect*, and *response* are used interchangeably in this book.

Pharmacodynamics is a general term often defined as the study of fundamental or molecular interactions between drug and body constituents, which through a subsequent series of events results in a pharmacological response. In many instances the basic molecular mechanism may be unknown; then the pharmacological response must be described at a higher level of biochemical or physiological complexity. Pharmacodynamics is used by some investigators to relate response to drug concentration.

Pharmacological Response

Pharmacological response is initiated by a drug at its site of action on its so-called receptor (see Chapter 2). For most drugs, the magnitude of the pharmacological response increases as the concentration of

Table 1-1	Definitions
Term	**Definition**
Action, effect, response	Used interchangeably to represent the molecular interaction between drug and a body constituent, or the observable output
Pharmacodynamics	Broad term, defined in several ways, including effects of drugs on the body and biochemical and physiological mechanisms of action of drugs
Pharmacokinetics	Drug concentrations in body fluids and tissues and variables that influence how the concentrations vary with time
Site of action	Specific enzyme, receptor, other protein, organ, cell type, membrane component, nucleic acid, etc., where the initial molecular event occurs between the drug and the constituent, leading to the therapeutic response
Pharmacogenetics	Area of pharmacology that examines relation of genetic factors to variations in response to drugs
Toxicology	Study of effects, antidotes, and detection of poisons

drug increases at the site. When the drug's action is reversible, the pharmacological response decreases as the concentration of drug decreases. But not all drugs act reversibly. The clinical use of drugs would be more precise if procedures existed to (1) measure the magnitude of the response and (2) monitor the magnitude in a specific patient. Unfortunately, these methods exist only for a few drugs. One of these drugs is the neuromuscular blocking agent, succinylcholine. Figure 1-2 shows an example of the pharmacological response and how it varies with time in a patient.

Figure 1-2 also offers a description of *magnitude of effect*. Specifically the magnitude of pharmacological effect is defined as the percentage of neuromuscular blockade achieved. Thus 0% blockade corresponds to the predrug condition, whereas 100% blockade represents complete paralysis. The blockade is calculated as

$$\% \text{ blockade} = (1.0 - \frac{F}{F_o}) 100 \qquad \textbf{(1)}$$

In this expression F_o and F are measured in millimeters. The results for various times and for an F_o of 53 mm are illustrated in Figure 1-2. Succinylcholine is a reversibly acting drug; thus the system returns to the predrug state after disappearance of the drug. The initial increased magnitude of effect results from a gradual buildup of drug at the neuromuscular junction (site of action) after a single bolus intravenous injection. Succinylcholine is rapidly hydrolyzed in plasma to essentially inactive compounds, thus accounting for the rapid disappearance of the drug at the site of action.

Pharmacokinetic Variables

As previously stated, for most drugs the magnitude of pharmacological effect depends on the concentration of drug at the site of action. The factors that influence the rates of delivery, distribution, and disappearance of drug to or from the site of action must be understood from a clinical standpoint. Factors in-

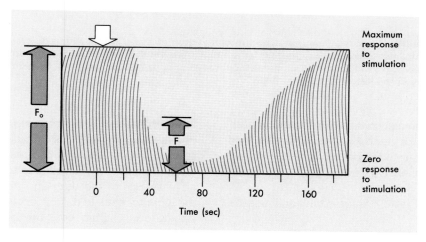

Time (sec)	Blockade (%)	Time (sec)	Blockade (%)
0	0	55	84
30	12	72.5	90
35	38	135	38
45	72	175	2

FIGURE 1-2   Pharmacological response of neuromuscular blocking agent succinylcholine in a 6-year-old patient undergoing surgery. Plot shows force exerted by thumb (attached to strip chart recorder pen) after repeated electrical stimulation of ulnar nerve. F_o is force before drug and F after drug. Succinylcholine administered IV (4 mg/m^2) at arrow. Magnitude of effect is defined in text. Blockade calculated from illustration and Equation 1.

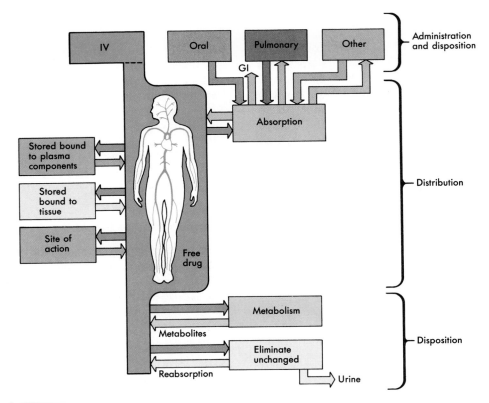

FIGURE 1-3   Factors influencing concentration of drug at site of action and at different times after administration. Free drug molecules are those that are not bound to blood constituents or to other body components. The circulatory system is shown as the major pathway for drug delivery to the site of action.

volved in how the concentration of drug varies with time in body fluids or tissues are the substance of pharmacokinetics. These factors are outlined in Figure 1-3, discussed extensively in Chapter 4, and listed as follows:

Input site, input rate, dosage form, and dosage schedule

Rate of adsorption, bioavailability

Location of site of action, ease of crossing membranes

Binding to plasma and tissue constituents

Pathways and rates of elimination or metabolism

Influence of disease states, other drugs, genetic factors

DRUG SHAPE

The three-dimensional structure of a drug molecule is a key factor that determines how well the drug can interact with tissue or body fluid molecules at the site of molecular action. Most drugs act by binding to a specific site on a body component, with the compatibility of the two structures influenced by the relative shapes of the drug and the binding site, (i.e., the receptor site). In describing the three-dimensional structure of a drug, both the *configuration* and the *conformation* of the molecule are important concepts.

The arrangement of the functional groups about a multibonded atom, especially carbon, is known as the configuration. This is exemplified by two types of atomic models (Figure 1-4) for the dextro (D) and levo (L) configurations of alanine. These configurations form mirror images of each other and are called *enantiomorphs,* a form of stereoisomers. The three-dimensional representation is characterized by the groups at the wide end of the filled triangle positioned above the plane of the page and those at the wide end of the open triangles positioned below the plane of the page.

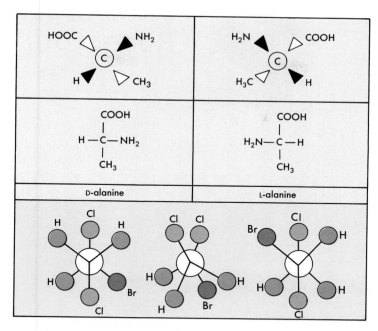

FIGURE 1-4   Configuration and conformation of molecules. Alanine is shown in D- and L-configurations as three-dimensional and planar models. The conformation of ClHBrC-CClH$_2$ is presented in three forms, viewed looking parallel to the C-C bond.

Conformation represents rotation of groups about a single bond; in Figure 1-4 the rotation is about the carbon-carbon bond.

Although in synthesizing a compound the configuration can be controlled, the conformation generally cannot. It represents the net response of the molecule to the relative sizes and energetic interactions of the different functional groups.

In pharmacology the scale of sizes ranges from molecular interactions of drugs and target receptors, through cellular and organ levels, to whole body responses. Most covalent bonds are 1 to 2 Å or 1 to 2×10^{-10} meters long, whereas erythrocytes have a diameter of about 7×10^{-6} meters (7μm).

CHAPTER

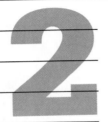

Sites of Action: Receptors

PHARMACOLOGICAL RESPONSE

In the previous chapter the point is made that pharmacological responses are initiated by molecular level interactions of drugs with cells, tissues, or other body constituents. The key phrase is "molecular level." What specific biological molecules must be present? How do the drugs and the biological molecules interact to produce molecular level changes? How are these changes converted into the next step toward generating observable responses? In this chapter these questions are addressed, especially for the large group of drugs that act through "receptors."

AXIOMS OF SITES OF ACTION

For most drugs the site of action is at a specific biological molecule, generally termed a *receptor*, which may be, for example, a membrane or a membrane protein, or a cytoplasmic or extracellular enzyme. In some cases a drug shows organ or tissue selectivity for the biological molecule; for example, selectivity may be more pronounced in cardiac as compared to pulmonary tissue. Although a few drug types such as osmotic diuretics (Chapter 19) and general anesthetic agents (Chapter 30) may not involve receptors, the concept of receptor sites of action is so important to understanding pharmacology that the remainder of this chapter is devoted to the description of receptor molecules and how they interact with drugs at the molecular level.

The first axiom of a molecular level drug-initiated response is that the drug molecule and the biological molecule must come together; they do not act at a distance. But if mere coming together is all that is required, then there is no way to build selectivity into the scheme. Therefore, the second axiom is that the coming together must result in selective binding of the drug to the biological molecule before the molecular level drug-initiated response can take place. This brings into focus the concept of *molecular level recognition*. The biological molecules to which drugs bind must have molecular locales that are both spatially and energetically favorable for binding of specific drug molecules. These locales are termed "receptors" in a general sense; although as is pointed out in the next section, a more restricted definition of receptors is usually applied in classical pharmacology.

Essentially all of the drug binding sites discovered so far are on proteins, glycoproteins, or proteolipids. This is not surprising because of the strong tendency of proteins to undergo folding to form unique three-dimensional structures. Thus it is logical to conclude that proteins can form special binding sites of the correct three-dimensional shape to accommodate drug molecules. Receptors, enzyme active sites, enzyme allosteric regulatory or binding sites, and antibody and antigen binding sites all possess similar molecular level recognition capabilities. Actually, enzymes constitute the site of action for many drugs, with selective binding of the drug usually resulting in inhibition of catalytic activity. However, from the standpoint of classical pharmacology, the drug binding sites on enzymes are *not* called receptors. Since drug binding sites are found predominantly on proteins, a discussion of protein folding as it relates to the three-dimensional structure and the formation of binding sites is included here before going on to describe receptors of the classical type.

PROTEIN FOLDING

The three-dimensional shape that a particular protein assumes is the net result of its primary, secondary, and tertiary structures. The primary structure is the sequence of amino acids, connected through amide bonds; the secondary structure consists of the spatial restrictions caused by sulfur bridges and ionic interactions; and the tertiary features result from steric factors and weak attraction and repulsion forces between atoms, including hydrogen bond formation. The denaturing process results in unfolded or random chains that are void of tertiary structure. Four features contribute to the tertiary structure of native proteins: (1) α helix, (2) β sheets, (3) β folds, and (4) random sections. Sequences of roughly 8 to 30 amino acids can form a spiral in the shape of an α helix, with 3.6 amino acid residues required per 360 degree angle turn and 5.4 Å in length per turn.

The enzyme dihydrofolate reductase (Figure 2-1) is the site of action for the antitumor drug methotrexate (see Chapter 43). When the drug binds to the

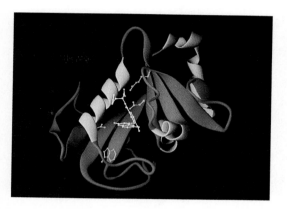

FIGURE 2-1   Ribbon representation of human dihydrofolate reductase with methotrexate (in white) modeled into the left substrate cleft. α Helices are yellow, β strands orange, and connecting loops blue. Also shown (in pale blue) are side chains of some key binding residues (Trp-24, Glu-30, Asn-64, Arg-70). (Courtesy Jay F. Davies, II and Joseph Kraut, Ph.D.)

enzyme, the latter is inactivated. The tertiary structure of this enzyme and how it binds to methotrexate have been established using enzyme from *Escherichia coli*. It was recently estimated for enzyme from humans (see Figure 2-1). With the *E. coli* enzyme, the amino acid residues involved in binding of the drug appear too far apart in the drug-free enzyme to accommodate multipoint drug binding. Yet, in spite of this spatial misalignment, enzyme-drug multipoint binding does occur. This problem can be resolved by employing the concept of *induced fit*, which assumes that binding to one or more of the residues causes a conformational change in the enzyme that modifies the tertiary structure to bring the other amino acid residues involved in binding closer to the drug. Induced fit is thought to apply to the binding of methotrexate to the human enzyme and also to the functioning of classical receptors and other enzymes.

A short discussion of the principal types of chemical bonds is included here. These bond types apply to the interactions between drugs and classical receptors and to those between drugs and enzymes. The main chemical bond types are summarized in Figure 2-2. Covalent bonds require considerable energy to break and are classified as irreversible when formed in drug-receptor binding. Ionic bonds also are strong but under some circumstances can be reversed by a change in pH. The other bond types are weak but can exert considerable influence when several bonds occur to the same drug molecule.

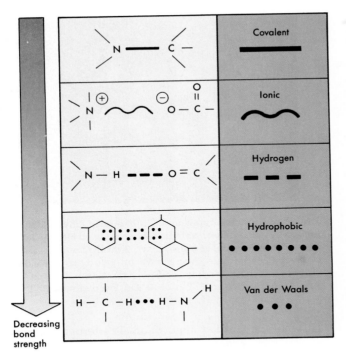

FIGURE 2-2   Types of chemical bonds and attractive forces between molecules that are pertinent to drugs binding to sites of action.

CLASSICAL RECEPTORS AND LIGAND BINDING

In the classical sense the term *receptor* is reserved for proteins, which usually are imbedded in a cellular or subcellular membrane and facilitate communication between the two sides of the membrane. This is shown schematically in Figure 2-3 for several proteins imbedded in cell membrane.

The membranes of cells are present as phospholipid bilayers. The bilayer forms because of the physical-chemical properties of the phospholipid constituents and their interaction with water. Phospholipid molecules have two distinct regions and are thus termed *amphipathic*. One region is nonpolar, consisting of the tails of the fatty acyl chains. The other region is very polar, consisting of charged phosphate, choline, and ethanolamine headgroups. It is the potential interaction of these distinct regions with the hydrogen bonds of water that determines the structural organization of a membrane. Disruption of hydrogen bonds of water by the nonpolar lipid region is energetically very unfavorable. Therefore, these

nonpolar regions tend to avoid contact with water by facing inward and self-associating. Disruption of the hydrogen bonds of water by the polar headgroups is energetically more than compensated for by the formation of new polar interactions between the water molecules and the headgroups. Therefore contact of the polar groups with water is favored. These types of interactions are optimized by the bilayer structure.

Protein constituents of the membrane are either peripheral proteins, associated with the external surfaces of the membrane, or integral proteins, deeply imbedded in the bilayer and sometimes spanning the membrane. As might be anticipated by their function of recognizing ligands of the external surface of the cell and transmitting information to the inside of the cell, membrane receptors span the membrane. Like phospholipids, membrane receptors are amphipathic. There are distinct domains that have polar hydrophilic surfaces and that are exposed to the aqueous solvent on either side of the membrane. These polar domains are separated by transmembrane regions of hydrophobic nonpolar components.

Characteristically, the transmembrane regions of receptors are formed by α helices that are composed of 19 to 24 sequential amino acids, having nonpolar side groups. Several basic amino acids are the cytoplasmic end of the transmembrane sequence. These are thought to interact with the phosphate headgroups of the bilayer and anchor the receptor so that it cannot slip into or out of the bilayer. This characteristic sequence of 19 to 24 nonpolar amino acids, flanked by several basic amino acids, is used to identify presumptive membrane-spanning domains within the amino acid sequences of membrane receptors.

Although the movement of membrane receptors into and out of the bilayer is restricted by the amphipathic nature of the receptor, lateral diffusion of the receptor within the plane of the membrane is free to occur, unless specifically restrained by interaction with the intracellular cytoskeletal elements. This lateral diffusion has been demonstrated experimentally by labeling receptors with fluorescent-tagged ligands and measuring the rates of diffusion of the fluorescent tags into membrane areas that have been rendered nonfluorescent by photobleaching. Lateral diffusion of receptors is an important concept because it means that membrane receptors can interact freely with other membrane components to which the receptors are not permanently attached. Indeed, many recep-

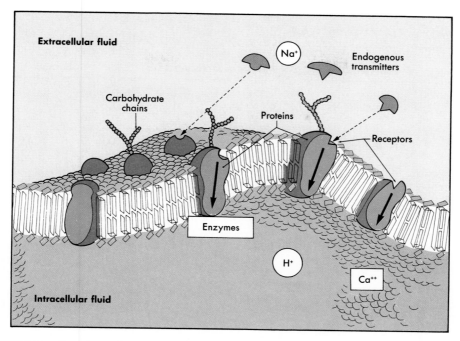

FIGURE 2-3   Proteins embedded in cell membranes, often extending further on the extracellular than on the intracellular sides. Attached to the proteins, primarily on the extracellular side, are carbohydrate (glycosylation) chains. Also shown on the extracellular side of some of the proteins are receptor sites to which endogenous transmitter compounds bind. Arrows indicate the direction of communication to the other side of the membrane.

tors depend on such interactions to trigger a response to receptor-ligand binding.

In the classical case, an endogenous compound is present on one side of the membrane only; and by binding to the proper "receptor" the endogenous compound transmits a molecular change to the other side of the membrane. Neurotransmitters, hormones, growth factors, and a host of other compounds are part of the growing list of endogenous materials for which classical receptors have been discovered. For the remainder of this chapter the term *receptor* is limited to this classical definition.

The idea that drugs might act by first binding to a receptive substance in the cell is attributed to Langley's work in the late 1800s and early 1900s and to Ehrlich's studies of a few years later. It was not until the 1920s and 1930s that drug-receptor interactions were approached from a quantitative standpoint by both Clark and Gaddum. By the 1960s, receptor proteins were isolated and purified by highly selective chromatography techniques; and by the 1970s receptor subunits were sequenced for their amino acid arrangement. The 1970s also saw early success in the isolation of receptor cDNAs for the cloning of subunit genes. As the 1990s begin, evidence is accumulating on the three-dimensional structure of several of the key receptors, with the result that our molecular understanding of receptors will increase greatly and introduce possibilities for improved drug design.

Table 2-1 contains a list of the main receptors that are relevant to the action of present therapeutic drugs. Additional receptors are known to exist in human tissues and may become pertinent to drug actions in the future. For some receptors, two or more subtypes have been identified. These subtypes may represent different variants of the receptor subunits, although for some cases the subtypes may turn out to be different receptors. Additional research will be needed to clarify these points.

Receptor identification and classification is based in large part on ligand-binding specificity. The experimental procedures to perform ligand-receptor binding measurements are highly important, and

Table 2-1   Examples of Classical Receptors

Type	Subtype*	Endogenous Transmitter	Ion Channel	Secondary Messenger
acetylcholine	nicotinic	acetylcholine	X	—
	muscarinic: M_1, M_2	acetylcholine	X	X
adrenergic	α_1, α_2	epinephrine and norepinephrine	X	X
	β_1, β_2	epinephrine and norepinephrine	—	X
GABA	A	GABA	X	—
	B	GABA	?	X
sodium channel	—	—	X	—
acidic amino acids	NMDA, kainate, quisqualate	glutamate or aspartate	X	?
calcium	L, N, T	—	X	X
opiate	μ, μ_1, κ, δ, ϵ, τ	enkephalins	X†	X
serotonin	5-HT_1, 5-HT_2, 5-HT_3	5-HT	—	X
dopamine	D_1, D_2	dopamine	—	X
adenosine	A_1, A_2	adenosine	—	X
glycine	—	glycine	X	—
histamine	H_1, H_2, H_3	histamine	—	X
insulin	—	insulin	—	X
glucagon	—	glucagon	—	X
ACTH	—	ACTH	—	X
steroids	—	several	—	special
LDL (lipid particle)	—	—	—	—

*Other subtypes in various stages of documentation have been proposed, especially where no endogenous transmitter is defined yet.
†Results not clear.

briefly described here. Using radiolabeled ligands, it is possible to obtain accurate measurements of the concentrations of bound, as well as free, drugs. Receptor preparations, with the receptor solubilized or still intact in the membrane, are mixed with radiolabeled ligand.

After equilibrium binding is established, the bound and free ligand must be separated rapidly (often in 1 second or less) to maintain the binding equilibrium. Then the concentration of bound ligand can be determined by measuring the amount of radioactivity associated with the high molecular weight residue obtained from the separation. For the reversible binding of ligand and receptor, the equilibrium expression can be written

$$L + R \; \frac{k_1}{k_{-1}} \; LR \qquad (1)$$

In this expression
L = free ligand
R = unoccupied receptor
LR = ligand-receptor complex

The association and dissociation rate constants are k_1 and k_{-1}, respectively. At equilibrium, the rates of association and dissociation are equal. Therefore the law of mass action can be employed to give

$$k_1 \, (L) \, (R) = k_{-1} \, (LR) \qquad (2)$$

In equation 2 the use of ( ) denotes concentration. Rearrangement gives

$$\frac{(L) \, (R)}{(LR)} = \frac{k_{-1}}{k_1} = K_d \qquad (3)$$

Here K_d is the equilibrium binding constant, or just the binding constant. Now, only *(L)* and *(LR)* can be determined experimentally for most systems. Therefore, *(R)* is defined in terms of the total receptor concentration *(R_T)* and that part which is bound *(LR)*, as

$$(R) = (R_T) - (LR) \qquad (4)$$

Substituting in equation 3 and rearranging gives

$$\frac{(LR)}{(L)} = \frac{(R_T)}{K_d} - \frac{(LR)}{K_d} \qquad (5)$$

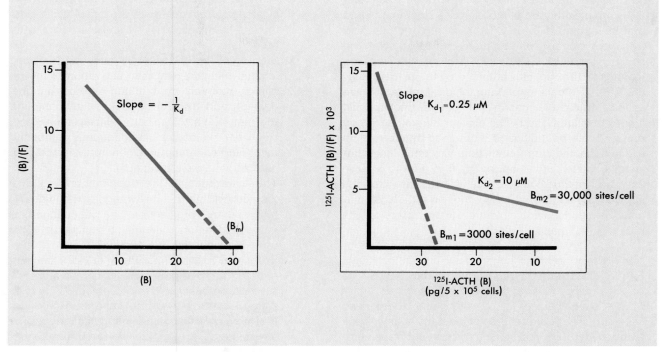

FIGURE 2-4   Scatchard plot of ligand-receptor binding to obtain values for K_d and B_m. **A,** Simple case of only one type of binding site. **B,** Case where ligand, shown here as ACTH, binds to two types of sites.

This can also be expressed as

$$\frac{(B)}{(F)} = \frac{(B_m)}{K_d} - \frac{(B)}{K_d} \qquad (6)$$

In equation 6

(B) = concentration of bound ligand

(F) = concentration of free ligand

(B_m) = maximum possible concentration of bound ligand, which is assumed to be the same as the concentration of total receptor

A plot of *(B)/(F)* versus *(B)* should be linear when a single subtype of binding site is involved. If ligand binding occurs at more than one subtype of binding site, the plot will be curved and the interpretation becomes more difficult. Scatchard plots (equation 6) are shown for the simple case of one subtype of binding site and for the more complex case of two subtypes (Figure 2-4). Typically, Scatchard plots are used to obtain values for K_d and (B_m).

When performing ligand-receptor binding measurements, take great care to differentiate between specific binding of ligand to receptor sites and non-

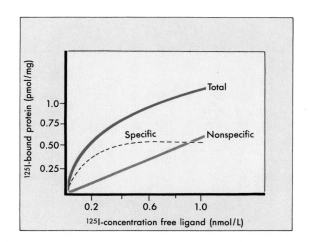

FIGURE 2-5   Determination of specific binding of ^{125}I-radiolabeled β-blocking drug to β-adrenergic receptors. "Total" data obtained with only radiolabeled drug added. "Nonspecific" data obtained with radiolabeled drug and also nonradiolabeled drug present (nonradiolabeled drug concentration at least 10 times K_d). "Specific" results obtained by taking difference.

specific binding of ligand to adsorption sites that likely are present on the protein or the membrane and that have nothing to do with the receptor of interest. Nonspecific ligand binding increases linearly with the concentration of ligand, whereas specific binding reaches saturation, as evidenced by the plateau (Figure 2-5). Separate experimental determinations are used to obtain the amounts of total and nonspecific ligand that are bound. The amount or concentration of specifically bound ligand is obtained by subtracting the nonspecific component from the total. The nonspecific values are obtained by first adding a large excess of nonradiolabeled ligand (that saturates the specific sites) followed by adding the radiolabeled ligand (the nonspecific sites are the only place for the radiolabeled ligand to bind).

RECEPTOR MECHANISTIC CONCEPTS

The main features of receptors are summarized schematically in Figure 2-6. The details of how these features are used, particularly to carry out transmembrane signal transmission, is a complex process with many of the details still not clear at the molecular level. Several key points are emphasized here before describing the mechanistic processes of specific ligand-receptor signal transmission systems and their modulation by drugs. The key points are as follows:

1. Receptors are membrane proteins having one or more subtypes of binding sites and glycosylated pendant chains on the extracellular side. Special lipids also may be associated with the protein.

2. Binding of the endogenous compound specific for that receptor results in activation of the receptor (probably by inducing a conformational change) and transmission of a signal through the membrane to the intracellular side. Sometimes two molecules of endogenous compound must bind per receptor to generate a signal. The binding is usually reversible.

3. The magnitude of the transmembrane signal may depend on the percentage of the available receptors that are occupied by the endogenous compound or on the rate of occupancy. This topic is discussed in Chapter 3.

4. Drugs can enhance, diminish, or block the generation, transmission, or receipt of the signal by several approaches. These approaches are classified according to whether the drug produces a signal (or enhances the signal produced by an endogenous ligand) or whether it diminishes the signal.

The terms *agonist* and *antagonist,* as introduced here, represent drugs that enhance or diminish a response. These terms are described in greater detail in Chapter 3. The approaches are as follows:

1. Agonist I: the drug binds to the same site as the endogenous compound and produces the

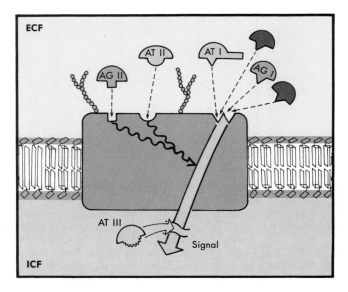

FIGURE 2-6   Major features of classical receptors. These include embedding in a membrane, glycosylated chains on the extracellular side, binding sites on the extracellular side for an endogenous transmitter *(dark green symbol)* with two molecules needing to be bound (as shown here) to activate transmembrane signal. Drugs can use many targets *(AG,* Agonist; *AT,* antagonist): (1) AG I and AT I compete with endogenous transmitter for activation sites, AG I to enhance and AT I to block signal; (2) AG II and AT II enhance or block signal, respectively, by binding to allosteric sites that influence *(wavy line)* signal transmission; and (3) AT III blocks signal within the membrane or at intracellular signal reception points.

same type of signal, usually of equal or greater magnitude than the endogenous agent.

2. Agonist II: the drug binds to a different site on the extracellular side than does agonist I, producing no signal by itself; however, an enhanced signal is generated when the endogenous agent also binds to its site. This is an *allosteric action*.

3. Antagonist I: the drug binds to the site used by the endogenous agent and diminishes or blocks the signal generated by the endogenous agent.

4. Antagonist II: the drug binds to an allosteric site on the extracellular side, similar to agonist II, but produces a diminished signal generated by the endogenous agent.

5. Antagonist III: the drug dissolves in the membrane or crosses the membrane and intercepts the signal generated by the endogenous agent within the membrane or on the intracellular side.

The approaches by which drugs interact with classical membrane receptor complexes are discussed in general terms later in this chapter and in Chapter 3. However, the discussions that relate these approaches to specific drugs are found in the chapters that deal with those drugs.

An important topic of ligand-receptor binding is that of transmembrane signal transmission. As the mechanisms for transmission of the ligand-receptor activated signal through the membrane and for activation of metabolic or other processes on the intracellular side become better understood at the molecular level, the opportunities for modulation by drugs become more apparent. The therapeutic use of existing drugs can be applied in a safer and more rational manner. So far, four mechanisms for signal transmission are known. Three specific examples are given later in this chapter. The mechanisms are listed as follows:

1. Direct receptor control of ion channels (ligand gated or voltage gated)
2. Receptor controlled generation of secondary messengers (G-protein/cAMP or G-protein/phosphoinositide systems)
3. Receptor internalization and recycling-polypeptide redistribution
4. Receptor initiated phosphorylation cascade (discussed in Chapter 34)

The remainder of this chapter contains descriptions of several key receptor systems that function to open or close channels to allow certain ions to pass through the cell membrane, plus a discussion of receptor-based secondary messenger systems. The chapter ends with an overview of some of the common features that are beginning to emerge for many of the key receptor systems.

SPECIFIC RECEPTOR EXAMPLES

Nicotinic Acetylcholine Receptor

The nicotinic acetylcholine receptor is a well-characterized, ligand-gated, ion channel type. This receptor is found on the muscle cell end plate of the neuromuscular junction in the peripheral autonomic nervous system and in the central nervous system. The role of the acetylcholine receptor is to convert the binding of the neurotransmitter, acetylcholine, into an electrical signal for stimulation of the receptor cell. It does this, for example, by depolarization of the postsynaptic muscle cell membrane in which the receptor resides; and it does it by means of opening the channel and letting Na^+ or K^+ pass through the membrane into the cell.

The acetylcholine receptor consists of five subunits of four different types. The subunits are all glycosylated. The protein subunit molecular weights are as follows:

alpha (α)	50,200 daltons
beta (β)	53,700 daltons
delta (δ)	57,600 daltons
gamma (γ)	56,300 daltons

Because the α subunit appears twice and the carbohydrate adds another 20,000 daltons, the receptor total molecular weight is approximately 288,000 daltons. The data presented here are for acetylcholine receptors from the electroplaque membrane of the *Torpedo california* electric eel. The quantities of this receptor in human tissues are minute; whereas the availability of receptor from the electric fish organ is much greater, and the differences in structure of the receptor from fish versus humans appear to be small.

The receptor view from the extracellular side shows a nearly pentameric symmetrical arrangement of the subunits in α, γ, α, β, δ order (clockwise) (Figure 2-7). About 10% of the acetylcholine gated channel activity is obtained with only an α, β, γ combination. All of the subunits appear necessary for hold-

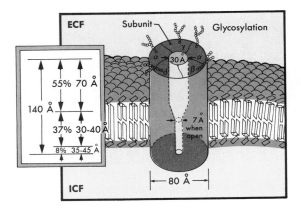

FIGURE 2-7 Schematic drawing of acetylcholine receptor showing nearly symmetrical pentameric arrangement of subunits, glycosylation of each subunit, water-filled ion channel, and approximate dimensions. The dimensions vary with methods used in determining the sizes. Percentages refer to the relative mass of the receptor protein found in each region. The acetylcholine binding site is on each α subunit, presumedly near the top of the 30 Å opening.

ing the acetylcholine and other binding sites in the proper conformation for normal binding and for full channel opening activity. Approximate dimensions of the receptor and the water-filled central channel also are included.

Channel opening occurs when two molecules of acetylcholine bind to the receptor. Because the binding sites for acetylcholine, agonists, competitive antagonists, and bungarotoxin (a channel blocking compound) all are on the α subunit, this means that both α subunit acetylcholine binding sites must be occupied for channel opening to occur. Normally the channel is closed. Binding of acetylcholine opens the narrow part to at least 7 Å, enough to allow the passage of partially hydrated cations, particularly sodium or potassium. Anions are blocked from passage through the channel. Protons appear to block the channel. The mechanism of channel opening is not known; although binding of acetylcholine causes the release of four to six calcium ions per receptor molecule. It is postulated that the calcium ions help stabilize the membrane-spanning portions. The calcium release may augment the conformational change brought about by acetylcholine binding, thus causing the channel to open. With acetylcholine binding, the mean channel open time is 2.4 ms. A subsequent influx of calcium ions may be the mechanism that causes the channel to close.

The amino acid sequence of the α subunit in relation to the cell membrane is shown in Figure 2-8. It is controversial whether four or five helical, hydrophobic transmembrane regions are present in the single, roughly 500 amino acid chain that constitutes each subunit.

Prolonged contact of the acetylcholine receptor with elevated concentrations of agonist results in inactivation (desensitization) of the receptor. The mechanism for this is only postulated and includes the concept of two conformational states (Figure 2-9). In a low affinity conformation the channel can be opened when two molecules of agonist bind; in a high affinity conformation the channel cannot be opened. Additional research is needed to clarify this aspect.

Sodium Channel Receptors

The sodium ion channel receptor system is subject to voltage-controlled channel opening, also termed *gating;* whereas the nicotinic acetylcholine ion channel system is controlled by ligand gating. Sodium channels are present in the membranes of excitable nerve, cardiac, and skeletal muscle cells. In their resting state, these cells maintain the intracellular sodium ion concentration much lower (more negative voltage) than that in the extracellular environment. This is accomplished by means of the Na^+, K^+-ATPase pump. The sodium channels can be opened by voltage gating, brought about by membrane depolarization. Channel opening allows a transient influx of Na^+ ions to take place before inactivation and return to the resting state can occur. Local anesthetic agents bind to sodium channels and block the transient increase in membrane sodium ion permeability, thereby blocking nerve conduction.

The structure of the sodium channel is shown schematically in Figure 2-10. The α subunit (molecular weight about 260,000) is heavily glycosylated and has four similar domains, each containing six hydrophobic α helix transmembrane regions. The β_1 and β_2 subunits (molecular weight 36,000 and 33,000 daltons, respectively) also are glycosylated.

Depolarization of the sodium channel membrane causes a voltage driven conformational change that moves about six positive charges into the extracellular space and an equivalent number of negative charges into the intracellular region. This may be explained

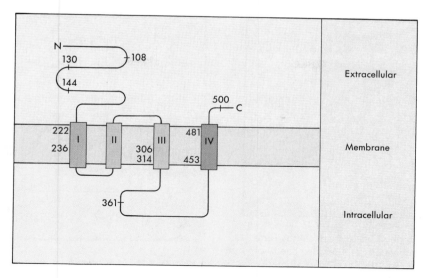

FIGURE 2-8   Proposed model for topology of amino acid chain in subunit of acetylcholine receptor, showing four (I, II, III, IV) helical, hydrophobic, transmembrane regions each 20 to 30 residues long. Numbers indicate approximate positions of amino acid residues starting from amino *(N)* end. Experimental data suggest *N* and *C* (carboxyl) ends are on extracellular side of membrane. (Developed from Claudio T: Molecular genetics of acetylcholine receptor-channels. In Molecular neurobiology, Glover DM and Hames BD, eds., Oxford, 1989, IRL Press.)

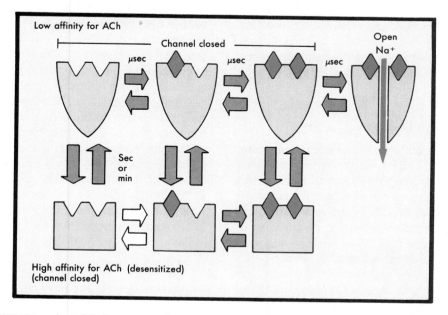

FIGURE 2-9   Acetylcholine receptor becomes desensitized in the presence of prolonged elevated concentrations of acetylcholine. The concept of two receptor conformational states has been suggested, but this still leaves some of the experimental observations only partially explained.

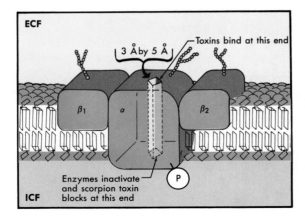

FIGURE 2-10   How voltage-gated sodium channel from human brain may be assembled in membrane. The α subunit is thought to have six helix transmembrane domains, with the channel roughly a 3 Å by 5 Å rectangular hole formed by four of the transmembrane helices within this subunit. The α subunit also is phosphorylated (P). At least one of the binding sites for inactivation of the increased sodium ion permeability is located on the intracellular side of the α subunit. The location of the binding site for local anesthetics is not known.

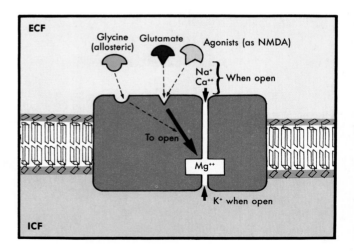

FIGURE 2-11   Suggested components of acidic amino acid receptors in CNS. Channel shown in resting stage. Depolarization by agonist binding or voltage gating releases blockade by magnesium ions and lets potassium ions pass outward and Na$^+$ and Ca^{++} pass into the nerve cell. Glycine acts to augment agonist effect.

by considering the transmembrane helical domains to have a sequence of positive charges paired with negative charges on nonhelix parts of the subunit. Sliding of each helix, to move one or two positive charges into the extracellular space, could be accomplished by a rotation of about 60 degrees and a linear displacement of about 5 Å. This explanation seems plausible; however, additional research is needed to clarify the details.

Acidic Amino Acid Receptors

It is now recognized that L-glutamate, L-aspartate, and possibly other acidic amino acids and peptides play a major role as excitatory neurotransmitters in the mammalian central nervous system. An ion channel is associated with their receptor, and both ligand gating and voltage gating appear to be involved in control of channel opening. The evidence suggests that this receptor system will be a target for development of new drugs for use as anticonvulsants, analgesics, and possibly for treating epilepsy and some neurodegenerative disorders.

The glutamate receptor system is characterized by three non-endogenous test compounds: N-methyl-D-aspartate (NMDA), kainate, and quisqualate (Quis).

Glutamate and aspartate can open the channel, but most of the studies have been done with the more potent test compounds. NMDA usually produces larger ion channel conductances than kainate or Quis. Amino acid or test compound–induced depolarization results in an ion current in which Na$^+$ and Ca^{++} flow into the cell and K$^+$ flows out. Magnesium ions block the channel in the resting state, but depolarization, by ligand or voltage gating, causes the magnesium ions to dislodge. Glycine, which is an inhibitory transmitter in the spinal cord, can also bind to the acidic amino acid receptor. Glycine binding enhances the ability of glutamate or NMDA to open the channel, presumably through an allosteric action. A schematic diagram of the receptor is shown in Figure 2-11. Psychoactive compounds, such as phencyclidine, also bind to the channel of this receptor and behave as noncompetitive antagonists.

GABA Type A Receptor

Another ligand-gated ion channel receptor of key interest in pharmacology is the type A γ-aminobutyric acid (GABA) receptor system. GABA is the main endogenous inhibitory transmitter in the vertebrate central nervous system (CNS), and its inhibitory actions

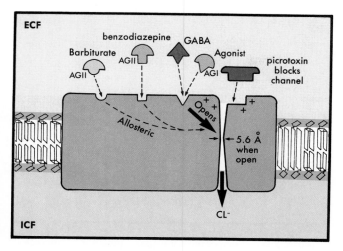

FIGURE 2-12   GABA type A receptor, showing four different binding sites. Only GABA or agonists that bind to the GABA site bring about channel opening. Benzodiazepines and barbiturates have strong allosteric actions. Picrotoxin binds to the channel opening and blocks the channel noncompetitively. Positive charges at channel ends filter out positive ions from passing through channel.

are enhanced by the presence of barbiturates or benzodiazepines (see Chapter 25 and Figure 2-12). The GABA type A receptor consists of α and β subunits and possibly γ and/or δ subunits, with four or five total subunits constituting a functional receptor assembly. The types and number of subunits in a receptor assembly may vary with the species and possibly with the anatomical location. Binding of GABA results in opening of a chloride ion channel. Benzodiazepines and barbiturates bind at other sites in allosteric fashion to augment the GABA channel opening. Sequence analysis shows that each subunit probably has four helix regions that are thought to span the membrane, with a long extracellular section on the amino end of each subunit that serves as the proposed sites for the binding domains.

G-PROTEIN BASED SECONDARY MESSENGER RECEPTORS

The receptors previously described in this chapter use ion channels as the primary mechanism for transmembrane signal transmission. These receptors modulate channel opening and closing directly through ligand or voltage gating. The ions that pass through

the channels serve as the signal for modification or initiation of intracellular processes.

A large group of other receptors uses second messenger systems for a major part of the transmembrane signaling. In these systems, ligand-receptor binding results in a sequence of reactions, usually within the membrane, that includes activation or inhibition of an enzyme that controls the formation of second messenger compounds. These messengers can move within the membrane or within the intracellular space and modify intracellular processes. Cyclic adenosine monophosphate (cAMP) and the phosphoinositides are the principal secondary messenger systems described here.

In cAMP secondary messenger ligand-receptor systems, binding of the ligand to the receptor results in activation or inhibition of adenylate cyclase. This is the enzyme that catalyzes the formation of cAMP. The mechanism involves intermediary G-proteins that are present in the receptor-membrane complex. Examples of receptors that produce adenylate cyclase activation are the β-adrenergic, histamine H_2, and dopamine D_1 subtypes. Adenylate cyclase inhibition occurs with the muscarinic M_2, α_2-adrenergic, dopamine D_2, opiate μ and δ, adenosine A_1, and GABA type B receptors.

G-proteins represent a group of membrane-associated compounds that serve three key roles in receptor based modification of adenylate cyclase activity. First, the G-proteins bind guanosine triphosphate (GTP) and guanosine diphosphate (GDP), of which GTP is required for activation of adenylate cyclase. The guanosine groups are the source of the "G" terminology. Second, the G-proteins provide the link between the ligand-activated receptor protein and the effector enzyme, adenylate cyclase.

Third, G-proteins exist in two states: an active form in which GTP is bound to the protein and an inactive form in which GDP is bound to the protein.

G-proteins have intrinsic GTPase activity, which spontaneously hydrolyzes bound GTP to bound GDP and thereby converts the G-protein from an active to an inactive form. The resulting GDP remains tightly bound to the protein and thereby locks the protein in its inactive state. When a ligand binds to a G-protein–associated receptor, the resulting complex interacts with the GDP form of the G-protein to facilitate the dissociation of the bound GDP. This allows nonbound GTP to bind to the protein and reactivate the complex. As the number of cycles of GTP binding and hydrolysis increases, the receptor complex paradoxically enhances the GTPase activity of the protein and promotes the active state in which the GTP is bound.

Based on their functional and biochemical properties, the G-proteins that couple ligand receptors to effectors, especially to adenylate cyclase, can be divided into the following three major classes:

1. G_s, couples stimulatory receptors to adenylate cyclase
2. G_i, couples inhibitory receptors to adenylate cyclase
3. G_o, thought to couple certain receptors to calcium channels in an inhibitory fashion

A fourth class of G-proteins in regard to a different secondary messenger system is described later, that is, one that couples the receptor to phospholipase C.

The G-proteins consist of the following three subunits:

1. 11,000 dalton molecular weight γ unit
2. 35,000 or 36,000 dalton molecular weight β unit
3. 39,000 to 52,000 dalton molecular weight α unit

The β and γ subunits from different G-protein sources are very similar and can be characterized as hydrophobic proteins that serve to anchor the α subunits in the cell membrane. The α subunits provide the major structural and functional differences between the various G-proteins. The α subunit interacts with the receptor and the effector enzyme (i.e., adenylate cyclase) and accounts for activation/deactivation of the G-protein through binding and hydrolysis of GTP. The α subunit from each type of G-protein has a unique region, which imparts the specificity. The interaction with the β and γ subunits and the hydrolysis of GTP are attributed to regions of the α subunit that are common for numerous types of G-proteins. The genes for the α subunits from several different G-proteins have been cloned and sequenced, and it is clear that the α subunits form a closely related family. There is particularly strong homology (i.e., commonality) among the GTP-binding regions of these subunits with respect to amino acid sequence and to location within the protein. Four noncontiguous regions of the α subunit are involved, with protein folding accounting for the positioning of the four regions in close proximity to one another. Through use of mutations, the C-terminal region of the subunit has been identified with receptor interaction, and this region thus has displayed considerable variation among α subunits from different G-proteins. Less is known about the regions involved in interaction with

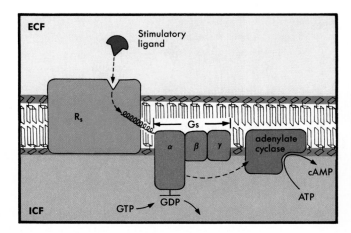

FIGURE 2-13   Components for ligand-receptor binding induced activation of adenylate cyclase. Binding of ligand to stimulatory receptor, R_s, produces conformation change that is coupled to carboxy terminus of α-helix domain of α subunit of G_s. This activates G_s by displacing bound GDP with GTP to give active α_s. G_s dissociates, with active α_s moving to adenylate cyclase location and activating this enzyme. Similar scheme can be shown for inhibition of adenylate cyclase using R_i and G_i.

the β and γ subunits and with the effector enzyme.

A surprising result from the cloning of the DNA for the α subunits is that there appear to be more types of α subunits than are needed to account for the known biochemical and functional classes of α subunits. This is an active area of research because of the importance of secondary messenger G-protein systems as possible targets for development of new drugs.

On activation of G_s or G_i, the α subunit dissociates from the β and γ subunits. In the common situation, the GTP-α_s or GTP-α_i forms interact with adenylate cyclase to produce enzyme activation or inhibition, respectively. Enzyme activation by the GTP-β-γ complex is much less common. The G-protein adenylate cyclase system is shown schematically in Figure 2-13 for G_s. Activated G_i can inhibit the enzyme directly, or it can work indirectly by inhibiting activated G_s.

The other system for ligand-receptor generation of a secondary messenger involves the enzyme phospholipase C. This phosphodiesterase-type enzyme catalyzes the hydrolysis of membrane phospholipids known as *phosphoinositides.* The hydrolysis releases two compounds, which appear to function as secondary messengers. Examples of receptor subtypes that use this secondary messenger approach are

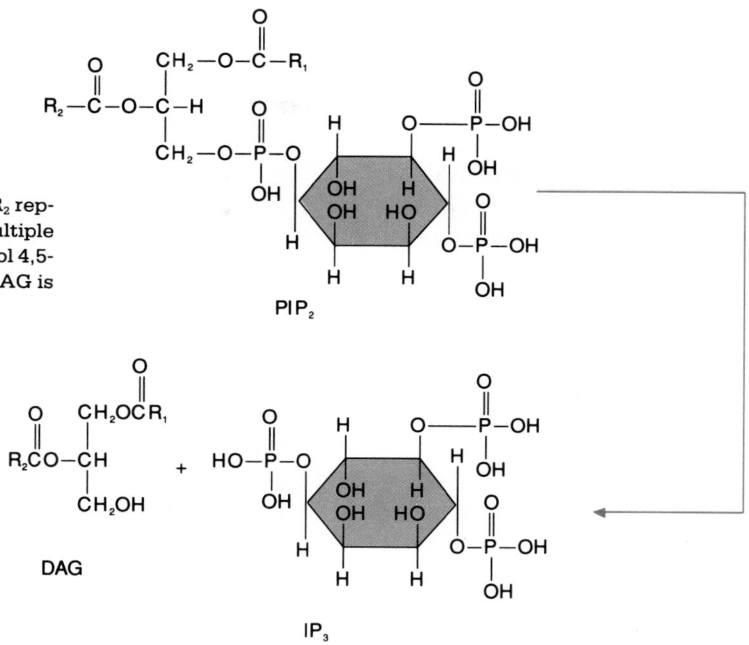

FIGURE 2-14   Chemistry of phosphoinositides. R_1 and R_2 represent lipids. R_1 is often a stearate derivative and R_2 a multiple double-bond long-chain lipid. PIP_2 is phosphatidylinositol 4,5-bisphosphate; IP_3 is inositol 1,4,5-trisphosphate; and DAG is 1,2-diacylglycerol.

α_1-adrenergic, muscarinic M_1 or M_2, serotonin $5\text{-}HT_2$, and thyrotropin releasing hormone.

In the phosphoinositide sequence, ligand-receptor binding again is coupled to activation of a G-protein. Inhibition studies with pertussis toxin show that there are at least two distinct G-proteins that can interact with phospholipase C, although neither has been identified biochemically or otherwise characterized. The activated G-protein converts phospholipase C into a catalytically active form that brings about the hydrolysis of phosphatidylinositol 4,5-bisphosphate (PIP_2). The two secondary messenger products are inositol 1,4,5-trisphosphate (IP_3) and 1,2-diacylglycerol (DAG). IP_3 is very water soluble and can migrate into the intracellular fluid where it binds to other receptors and causes the release of stored calcium ions. Further hydrolysis of IP_3 removes most of its activity. The degradation products probably undergo rephosphorylation eventually, to regenerate PIP_2. The chemistry of the PIP_2 secondary messenger system is summarized in Figure 2-14. The other secondary messenger, DAG, is highly lipid soluble and migrates within the membrane. DAG activates the enzyme protein kinase C, which in turn modulates many intracellular processes, including covalent phosphorylation of proteins, through control of Ca^{++} or by other means.

Many unexplained bits of evidence that relate to G-protein functions are available and obviously require additional research for a more complete understanding of their role in the mechanistic details of these ligand-receptor–generated secondary messenger systems. Several puzzling observations include the following:

1. Evidence for muscarinic receptor G-protein β-γ subunit activation of potassium ion channels
2. Direct activation of voltage-dependent calcium channels by GTP-activated G_s
3. Ability of glycosylated phosphatidylinositols to act as anchoring sites for connecting proteins to membranes

Modulation of localized intracellular Ca^{++} concentrations is one of the regulatory features attributed to all three of the secondary messengers (cAMP, IP_3, and DAG). Several types of transmembrane calcium ion channels also play key roles in the modulation of localized intracellular Ca^{++} concentrations. These calcium channels function primarily by voltage gating and possibly by ligand gating. The three types of voltage-gated calcium channels (L, N, and T) differ in the voltage needed for activation and in binding specificities. Whether these Ca^{++} channels operate by similar mechanisms as the ion channels described earlier in this chapter or whether secondary messengers are involved is not clear. A separate chapter on calcium channel drugs further describes Ca^{++} relevant to drug actions (see Chapter 16).

RECEPTOR TURNOVER

As mentioned earlier, membrane receptors are free to move laterally within the lipid membrane. There is also strong evidence that some hormone-receptor complexes such as those for insulin and glucagon undergo internalization into the intracellular fluid. The steroid hormones also undergo internalization, but into the nucleus compartment; are lipid soluble; and normally pass through the cell membrane into the intracellular fluid where they bind to receptors and are internalized into the nucleus. In either case the internalized hormone-receptor complex may be degraded by proteolytic and other enzymes or recycled back into the membrane for reuse. Possibly the internalization acts as a mode of transmembrane signal transmission; however, the mechanism of how this might work is not clear.

Concentrations of most membrane receptors are not constant with time. "Up" and "down" regulation (increase or decrease) of the number of cell surface receptors of a specific subtype is another way of modulation of the magnitude of transmembrane signal transmission. Densensitization may occur in which there is a decreased effectiveness of the same number of receptors. Where it is important to understand the magnitude and dynamics of action of specific drugs, up or down regulation of receptors is described in the chapters that deal with those drugs. Examples of the redistribution of polypeptides, such as the glucose transporters, coupled with insulin receptor activation are described in Chapter 39.

FAMILIES (HOMOLOGY) AND HETEROGENEITY OF RECEPTORS

Classification of receptors of relevance to pharmacology traditionally is based on ligand-binding specificity. There is no doubt that this is a very useful basis. However, the application of molecular biology and structural chemistry techniques to the study of receptors suggests that alternative classification schemes may emerge based on the structure or composition of receptors. Data on subunit amino acid sequences and on genetic coding indicate the existence of commonality among many receptors. For example, the nicotinic acetylcholine, glycine, GABA type A, and acidic amino acid (glutamate) receptors all show extensive homology in sequence, suggesting that these receptors belong to the same genetic family. Significant homology in sequences also is found between the β_1-adrenergic, β_2-adrenergic, and acetylcholine muscarinic receptors. Thus progress in grouping receptors into a few genetically distinct families is expected to increase.

Some of the apparent heterogeneity of receptor or channel subtypes, wherein a given receptor subtype appears to function differently depending on the type of tissue or anatomical location where it is found, may be attributable to genetic variations. For example, different genes are known to produce functional acetylcholine muscarinic receptors of the same subtype, and some ligands activate more than one G-protein through several receptor subtypes. The key example is norepinephrine, which activates adenylate cyclase through the β-adrenergic receptor, inhibits this same enzyme through the α_2-adrenergic receptor, and activates phospholipase C through the α_1-adrenergic receptor, all through G-protein intermediates.

REFERENCES

Bloom FE: Neurotransmitters: past, present, and future directions, FASEB J 2:32, 1988.

Hokin LE: Receptors and phosphoinositide-generated second messengers, Ann Rev Biochem 54:205, 1985.

Venter JC and Harrison LC, series eds: Receptor biochemistry and methodology, vols 1-10, New York, 1984-1987, Alan Liss Inc.

Worley PF, Baraban JM, and Snyder SH: Beyond receptors: multiple second-messenger systems in brain, Ann Neurol 21:217, 1987.

CHAPTER 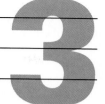 3 — Concentration-response Relationships

HOW MUCH DRUG IS NEEDED

The binding of drug molecules to receptors leads to enhancement, inhibition, or blockade of molecular signals. This applies to "classical" receptors, as well as enzyme inhibitors. The change in molecular signal is amplified through a sequence of biochemical and physiological processes to produce an "observable" pharmacological response. The question is how much drug is needed to obtain a desired magnitude and duration of response. This chapter provides part of the answer by defining the types of relationships between response and concentration. The other part of the answer is in Chapter 4 where the relationships between concentration and time are discussed.

Because the binding between drug and receptor molecules occurs according to the law of mass action, the concentrations of drug and receptor are the key variables. Therefore it is appropriate to address the question of how much drug is needed to produce a given response in terms of "concentration-response" relationships. When concentration data are not available, "dose-response" relationships are used.

GRADED AND QUANTAL RESPONSES

Multiple Magnitudes of Response

There can be more than one magnitude to the pharmacological response produced by a drug. Figure 3-1 illustrates the neuromuscular blocking agent succinylcholine, using data replotted from Figure 1-2. The response is defined as the *percentage blockade of neuromuscular transmission* and is determined by measuring the force of contraction of the thumb muscle on repeated electrical stimulation of the ulnar nerve. This is an example of a "graded" response. It is characterized by the magnitude of the response increasing continuously with greater concentration of unbound drug at the receptor site. Succinylcholine acts by binding to the acetylcholine receptor on the muscle cell surface and causing membrane depolarization, described in greater detail in Chapter 11. Succinylcholine undergoes such rapid hydrolysis that concentration data are not available, but the ease of quantifying the magnitude of pharmacological response makes this a good example for demonstrating the concept of a graded response. Actually, the outer membrane of each muscle cell contains several thousand nicotinic acetylcholine receptor sites. Each molecule of succinylcholine is assumed to elicit the same degree of membrane depolarization when a molecule of drug binds to an unoccupied receptor site. In other

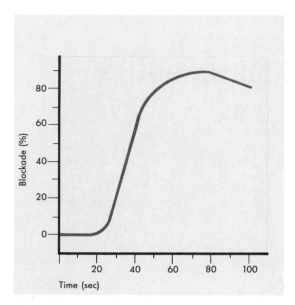

FIGURE 3-1   Magnitude of the pharmacological response for neuromuscular blockade by succinylcholine administered as a single IV injection and monitored by recording the force of thumb jerk on repeated electrical stimulation of the ulnar nerve. Results shown only for the first 100 sec after injection.

words each receptor molecule can be occupied or unoccupied; there are no intermediate degrees of occupancy for individual receptor molecules. Thus the increasing magnitude of neuromuscular blockade and the corresponding decreasing contraction of muscle fiber is the net result of many receptor sites on individual cells being occupied by drug and also of many muscle cells attempting to respond to the electrical stimulation.

A large number of drugs produce a graded pharmacological response; however, there are other drugs where the observable response can only be described in terms of an all-or-none event. This is called a *quantal* response. For example, the subject either does or does not respond to a pinprick pain stimulus in the presence of a particular concentration of pain suppressant. If the subject feels no pain, then the response to the drug is positive. Because of intersubject variations, not all persons show a positive quantal response at the same concentration of drug. Thus, the frequency of response to a given concentration of drug becomes the important variable in reporting quantal effects, whereas the magnitude of response is the comparable variable for a graded effect. This

distinction will become more evident after the two types of responses are described further. It is possible to convert a graded response to a quantal basis by defining some criterion, such as a 30% increase in blood clotting time, for a specific concentration of an anticoagulant drug and noting which subjects meet the criterion. However, it is not possible at present to convert many quantal responses to a graded basis.

Graded Response

Similar to the ligand-receptor binding equilibrium expression developed in the previous chapter, an expression for the fraction of receptors occupied, Y, at equilibrium is developed here (see equation 3). The symbols are

D = concentration of free (i.e., unbound) drug
R = concentration of unoccupied receptor
DR = concentration of drug-bound receptor
R_T = concentration of total receptor

The law of mass action is applied as

$$D + R \underset{k_{-1}}{\overset{k_1}{\rightleftharpoons}} DR \tag{1}$$

$$k - 1\,(D)\,(R) = k_{-1}\,(DR) = k_1\,(D)\,([R_T] - [DR]) \tag{2}$$

$$Y = \frac{(DR)}{(R_T)} = \frac{(D)}{K_d + (D)} \tag{3}$$

$$K_d = \frac{k_{-1}}{k_1}$$

In the classical theory for a graded response, the magnitude of effect (**E**) is assumed to be directly proportional to the fraction of the receptors occupied (receptor occupancy theory), and the maximum effect (**E_m**) is supposed to occur when all of a given subtype is occupied by drug. However, because some of the experimental results are not compatible with this theory, a modified theory has been introduced (1) to enable the maximum effect to occur without all of the receptors of a given subtype being occupied and (2) to relate the effect to the concentration of occupied receptors through a stimulus, (S), which in turn is governed by the fraction of receptor sites that are occupied. Modification number one uses the concept of "spare" receptors, discussed later in this chapter, to explain some of the experimental observations. Modification number two (see equation 4) adapts the theory to allow several different groups of compounds

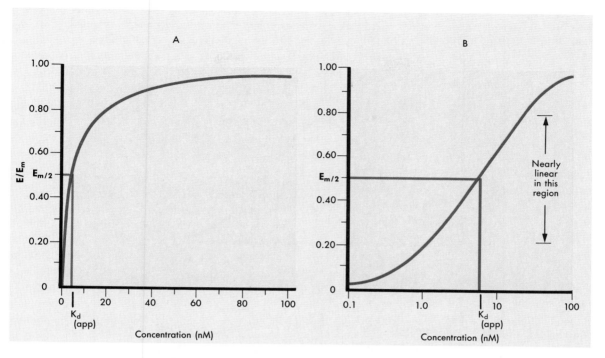

FIGURE 3-2   Concentration-response curve for graded response. **A,** Arithmetic scales; and **B,** log concentration scale. $K_d(app)$, arbitrarily taken to be 4.5 nM.

to act at the same receptor subtype without the need for spare receptors.

The modified theory can be expressed quantitatively as

$$\mathbf{E} = h\,S \quad \text{and} \quad S = \epsilon\,Y$$

$$\mathbf{E} = \frac{h\,\epsilon\,(D)}{K_d + (D)} \qquad \textbf{(4)}$$

In these expressions, h is an undefined function that relates $\boldsymbol{E}$ to the stimulus, S, and ϵ is the proportionality factor between S and the fraction of occupied receptors, Y. In Figure 3-2, equation 4 is plotted with h and ϵ both constant and with the product $h\epsilon$ equal to $\mathbf{E_m}$. In Figure 3-2, A the plot of equation 4 is shown with an arithmetic scale for concentration. The resulting curved line is difficult to fit to experimental data, particularly when appreciable scatter is present. Therefore, several alternative approaches have been developed in which the data are replotted and transform at least part of the curve into a nearly straight line. This is desirable because it is easier to fit the data to a linear expression, especially with the

natural variations often found in clinical studies. One of these transformations is used in Figure 3-2, B, where the concentration is plotted on a logarithmic, instead of an arithmetic, scale. This is an empirically based transformation, but it results in essentially a straight line between about 20% and 80% of the maximum response. More complex transformation techniques are available that linearize the curve from Figure 3-2, A over the entire range of concentrations, but such techniques are beyond the scope of this book. The log concentration-response curve in Figure 3-2, B is used later in this chapter to describe characteristics of agonist and antagonist drugs.

Graded log concentration-response curves, (see Figure 3-2, B) are obtained by administering different amounts of drug to a single subject. If a group of 50 subjects were given just enough drug to achieve a plasma concentration, (e.g., 10 nM) a variety of magnitudes of effect could be expected. In other words, interpatient variation results in a different magnitude of effect in individual patients, and mean values for $\mathbf{E_m}$ and for the concentration that produces $\mathbf{E_m}/2$ can be obtained for the general patient population. How-

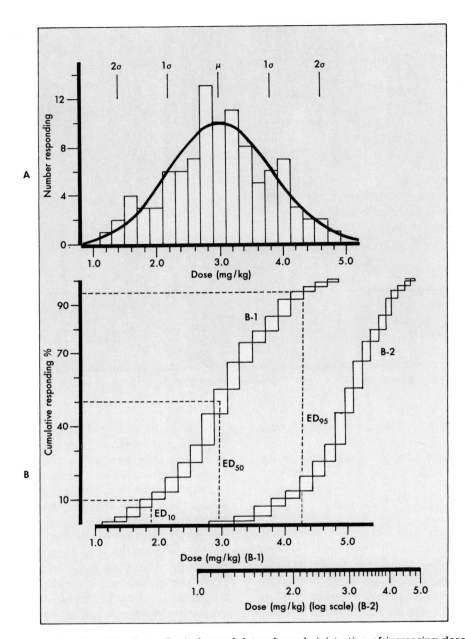

FIGURE 3-3   Quantal effects. Typical set of data after administration of increasing doses of drug to a group of subjects and noting minimum dose at which each subject responds. Data shown are for 100 subjects; dose increased in 0.2 mg/kg body weight increments. Mean (μ) (and median) dose is 3.0 mg/kg; standard deviation ($\bar{v}$) is 0.8 mg/kg. **A,** Results plotted as histogram *(bar graph)* showing number responding at each dose; smooth curve is normal distribution function calculated for μ of 3.0 and $\bar{v}$ of 0.8. **B,** Data of **A** replotted as cumulative percentage responding versus dose with dose shown in B-1 on arithmetic scale (as in **A**) and in B-2 on logarithmic scale. The reason for showing two dose scales is discussed in the text. ED (effective dose) values are shown for doses at which 10%, 50%, or 95% of subjects respond.

ever, the logarithmic concentration-graded response curve shown in Figure 3-2, *B* is for a single subject.

In defining the term *Y* in equation 3, the approach sometimes is called the *receptor occupancy theory*, which postulates that the net response from a cell, or more realistically from a mass of cells in a tissue bed, depends on the fraction of receptor molecules of a given subtype that are occupied by the drug. An alternative concept to the occupancy theory for explaining receptor concentration-response data is the rate theory. The rate theory postulates that the rate of drug-receptor binding, rather than the fraction of the sites occupied, is the controlling factor. So far no experiments have been devised to determine which theory is closer to the physical situation. The quantitative expressions have the same form for the occupancy and rate theories. However, the occupancy theory provides a more useful working concept and is thus the more widely cited of the two approaches.

Quantal Response

Mentioned earlier, the frequency of the response, that is, the number of subjects that respond to a given concentration or dose of drug, is the key factor in describing quantal responses. For a large group of subjects, the results can be organized by noting the minimum concentration of drug needed to obtain a response in each of the subjects. By plotting the number of subjects that respond versus the minimum concentration or dose required for the response, a distribution curve is obtained, with the majority of the subjects clustered about the median value (half of the subjects on either side).

It is usually not possible to know what type of statistical distribution the experimental data are likely to follow. However, the normal or Gaussian distribution often is encountered and is used here to explain several features of concentration-response or dose-response curves as applied to quantal effects. A set of typical quantal dose-response data is shown in Figure 3-3, *A*. One hundred subjects received increasing doses of a drug until all of the subjects responded. The number responding is plotted against the minimum dose needed to obtain the response, resulting in the histogram.

One of the first steps with a set of data such as this is to decide what statistical distribution can be used to represent the spread in the data. Because the results in the example have a mean of 3.0 mg drug/

kg body weight and a standard deviation of 0.8 mg drug/kg body weight, one approach is to calculate the normal distribution function for such a mean and standard deviation and compare the shape of the normal function with that of the histogram. The smooth curve is the calculated normal function, with the shape giving reasonably good agreement with the shape of the histogram. Thus, the statistical parameters of the normal distribution can be used with reasonably good reliability to predict the range of variability expected with this drug for use with the general population.

The histogram or normal distribution function is not a practical form in which to utilize dose-response data. A more linearized presentation of the data is desirous. Linearization can be accomplished in several ways; one of which is to replot the data as the *cumulative* percent responding versus the dose, as shown in Figure 3-3, *B-1*. This converts the bell-shaped curve of Figure 3-3, *A* into an S-shaped plot, with the region between, about 20% and 80%, forming essentially a straight line. This transformation from a histogram to an S-shaped cumulative response arithmetic plot has a firm theoretical basis.

Quantal response data often are presented in the literature as S-shaped dose-cumulative response curves with the dose plotted on a logarithmic, rather than an arithmetic, scale (see Figure 3-3, *B-2*). Note that the arithmetic *(B-1)* and logarithmic *(B-2)* dose scales give S-shaped cumulative plots that are essentially linear over the 20% to 80% region. The log transformation again has an empirical basis. The key factor in deciding whether the dose or the log dose gives the more accurate representation is based on the distribution function. The histogram, with the dose plotted on an arithmetic scale, agrees well with the shape of the normal distribution function, so the cumulative curve in *B-1* is the more accurate representation. If the histogram had been plotted with the dose on a logarithmic scale and the shape had agreed more closely with that for the normal distribution function, then the cumulative curve in *B-2* would be the more accurate.

There are numerous situations in which the response to a drug is skewed in one direction. For example, a drug that changes heart rate has a much larger range over which the rate can be increased than decreased without lethal consequences. Such a skewed response pattern is sometimes fitted better to a skewed distribution function, as is obtained by use of the logarithmic scale for the concentration or dose. The choice of the distribution function and whether to use an arithmetic or logarithmic scale must be determined empirically for each drug or type of drug.

The values labeled ED (see Figure 3-3) denote the effective dose (or effective concentration) at which 50% (ED$_{50}$), 95% (ED$_{95}$), or 10% (ED$_{10}$) of the subjects respond. With animal studies, a value for the lethal dose (LD$_{50}$) also may be obtained; this is the dose (or concentration) that causes death in 50% of the animals.

AGONISTS AND ANTAGONISTS

The term *agonist* is defined in the previous chapter as a compound that activates receptor-based processes. It is assumed that agonists bind reversibly to the receptor (see Chapter 2). The concentration-response curves for a series of agonist drugs, which bind to the same receptor subtype and produce the same maximum effect, are shown schematically in Figure 3-4. The term *potency* is used to differentiate between a series of such compounds. Drug A is the most potent of the four because it can produce 50% of the maximum effect with the smallest concentration of drug. Drug D is the least potent of the four. Apparent values of K$_d$ (dissociation constant) also are

shown for each of the drugs. The most potent agent has the smallest apparent K$_d$ and the least potent has the largest apparent K$_d$. Another term often associated with potency is that of *affinity* — the reciprocal of K$_d$.

Another parameter is *efficacy*. This term applies to a series of agonists, again that bind to the same receptor subtype. This is exemplified schematically in Figure 3-5, where the potency of the three drugs is essentially constant, with the most efficacious agonist defined as the one that can produce the greatest maximum effect. Thus, potency refers to the relative concentration required to produce a given magnitude of effect and efficacy refers to the magnitude of the maximum effect. An older term is *intrinsic activity*, which describes the relative maximum effects for a series of compounds.

The term *partial agonist* describes drugs of low efficacy that do not produce a very large maximum effect, yet where all of the receptors of a given subtype appear to be occupied. Further explanation of partial agonists depends on the development of a better molecular level understanding of the relationship between receptor occupancy and stimulus for such drugs.

Agonist drugs may compete with endogenous ligands, transmitters, or substrates for receptor binding sites. However, the concentrations of the endogenous compounds usually are not known or else they vary

FIGURE 3-4   Schematic representation of log concentration-response curves for a series of agonists (*A, B, C,* and *D*). Note that all of the drugs are shown having the same maximum response. The most potent drug produces **E$_m$/2** at the lowest concentration; thus drug A is the most potent. Concentration of each drug needed to produce 50% of maximum response also shown. Concentration values are arbitrary.

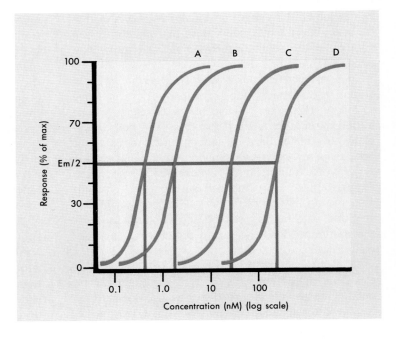

considerably at the receptor site, so that this type of competitive binding is addressed only qualitatively.

Antagonists are defined in the previous chapter as compounds that inhibit or block receptor activity. The main classifications of antagonists are competitive/ noncompetitive and reversible/irreversible. Other terminology is proposed to describe certain antagonist drugs, but only the main types are given here. In competitive antagonism the antagonist and an agonist compete for reversible binding to the same receptor sites. The log concentration-effect curve for the agonist is displaced to higher concentrations by the presence of the antagonist (Figure 3-6). The action of a competitive antagonist can be overcome by using an excess of agonist, essentially to displace the antagonist molecules from the vicinity of the receptor site.

Other forms of antagonism by drugs can be characterized as not capable of being reversed by excess agonist. With noncompetitive antagonists, the result is typically a decrease in the maximum effect obtainable by the agonist, although some shift to slightly higher agonist concentrations may also be needed to

obtain a given magnitude of effect in the presence of the antagonist. Noncompetitive or other forms of antagonism take place by the antagonist binding to other sites on the receptor from where the agonist binds. For example, certain toxins and drugs are thought to bind to the ion channel of the GABA receptor and to block the channel much as a cork plugs the opening of a bottle. The antagonist binding in such cases may be very strong but may eventually show reversibility. Other antagonists may bind irreversibly, especially those that produce irreversible inhibition of enzymes.

The potency of some antagonists, particularly those that act by inhibiting the activity of an enzyme, are often expressed as the I_{50} value. This is simply the concentration of antagonist needed to elicit 50% inhibition of enzyme activity.

SPARE RECEPTORS

Frequently, the measured biological response elicited by a compound binding to receptors is proportional to the fraction of receptors that are occupied.

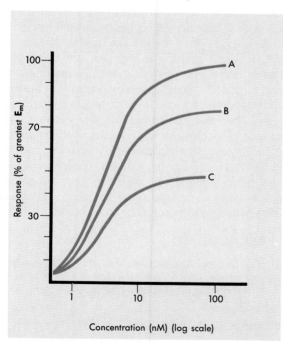

FIGURE 3-5   Series of agonists that vary in efficacy (E_m) at essentially constant potency. Drug A is the most efficacious and drug C the least. Concentrations are arbitrary but in therapeutic plasma concentration range for many drugs.

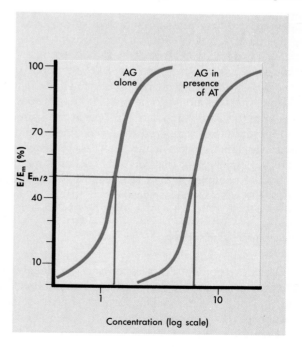

FIGURE 3-6   Competitive antagonism, where both the agonist *(AG)* and the antagonist *(AT)* compete to bind reversibly to the same subtype receptor sites.

Sometimes, however, a maximal biological response is achieved when only a small fraction of the receptors are occupied. This phenomenon is referred to as a situation involving "spare" receptors. It usually occurs when the measured biological response is separated from the initial receptor-triggering event by several intervening amplification steps, one of which becomes fully activated before all of the receptor molecules are occupied. For example, a receptor type produces a biological response by stimulating the production of cAMP. The cAMP in turn activates protein kinase, which initiates a cascade of events ultimately leading to the measured response. In this example, submaximal concentrations of cAMP maximally activate the kinase, so that further receptor occupancy leading to higher cAMP concentrations will not result in further kinase activity or to an increase in the measured response.

There are several interesting consequences of spare receptors. The concentration-response curve is shifted to smaller ligand concentrations, as compared to the curve location for saturation of the receptor sites. Small changes in the number of receptors have no effect on the maximal response but change the sensitivity to the ligand. In addition, partial agonists may still produce a maximal biological response but probably at a higher receptor occupancy than is required for a full agonist. This is exemplified by noting that a full agonist can produce 100% response with only 50% of the receptors occupied, if half of the total receptors are assumed to be present as spare receptors. For the partial agonist, 100% response (reduced in magnitude as compared to the maximum full agonist response) occurs when all of the receptors appear to be occupied; this can easily occur at a higher fractional occupancy than is needed for the full agonist-50% spare receptor case.

SPECIAL EFFECTS

The development of tolerance and the placebo effect are two experimentally observed conditions that do not fit into the receptor occupancy scheme of drug response.

Narcotic analgesics, opioids, and some other drugs that act primarily on the central nervous system may after one or more doses bring about a dampened response in which the magnitude of effect is decreased for subsequent doses of the same size as the initial dose. The dampened response is called *tolerance*. Some types of tolerance may be the result of changes in the concentration of drug at the receptor site and evolve from pharmacokinetic considerations, discussed in Chapter 4. Other types of tolerance may be caused by changes in some unknown aspect of receptor activity. A special type of acute tolerance that manifests by rapid repeated administration of catecholamines or other drugs is called *tachyphylaxis*. The forms of drug tolerance and their management are discussed further in the relevant drug chapters.

The *placebo effect* is a usually beneficial therapeutic result that apparently arises from psychological factors. If a patient is told that this new compound will bring marked beneficial changes—but unknown to the patient is an inert material instead of the new compound —beneficial effects will often be observed in as high as 35% of subjects. This placebo effect is not predictable, but it can be a contributing factor to changes in the clinical condition of a patient.

SUMMARY

Although an exact quantitative expression that relates drug response to drug concentration remains to be developed, the receptor occupancy theory provides a useful working model. For the types of response that vary continuously with the concentration of drug (graded response) the key variable is the magnitude of effect. For the all-or-none case (quantal response), frequency becomes the key variable. Classification of drugs as to whether they act as agonists, partial agonists, antagonists, or some other category and concepts of potency, efficacy, competitive/noncompetitive antagonists, tolerance, and the placebo effect all help to provide some organizational framework applicable to many classes of drugs.

REFERENCES

Ariens EJ, Simonis AM, and van Rossum JM: Drug-receptor interaction and relation between stimulus and effect. In Ariens EJ, ed., Molecular pharmacology, vol 1, 1964, Academic press.

Goldstein A: Biostatistics, New York, 1971, Macmillan Co.

Paton WDM: A theory of drug action based on the rate of drug-receptor combination, Proc Royal Soc 154B:21, 1961.

Stephenson RP: A modification of receptor theory, Brit J Pharmacol 11:379, 1956.

CHAPTER

4

Clinical Pharmacokinetics and Dosing Schedules

ABBREVIATIONS	
C_{ss}	steady state clearance
GI	gastrointestinal
IM	intramuscular, intramuscularly
IV	intravenous, intravenously
pH	logarithm of the reciprocal of the hydrogen ion concentration
SC	subcutaneous, subcutaneously
$t_{1/2}$	half-life
T	dosing interval

DRUG CONCENTRATIONS

Before using drugs for therapeutic intervention in individual patients, the decision to treat and the choice of drug must be made. Then, an observable pharmacological effect or end point may be selected and the rate of drug input manipulated until this effect, or end point, is achieved. With some drugs this approach works well. For example, blood pressure can be monitored in a hypertensive patient (Figure 4-1, drug *A*) and the rate of input for a drug modified until blood pressure is reduced to the desired level.

For other drugs this approach for selecting the rate of drug input does not work. This failure is usually caused by one or more of the following factors:

1. Observable effect or end point is not available
2. Therapeutic index of drug is small
3. Changes in condition of the patient require modification in rate of drug input

For example, an antibiotic with a narrow thera-

peutic index is being used to treat a severe infection (Figure 4-1, drug *B*). It is often difficult to obtain samples and quantify the progress of antibiotic therapy because an observable effect is not available. In addition, drug *B* is assumed to have a narrow therapeutic index, which affects the patient if the antibiotic concentration becomes excessive. Another example is shown in which the site of inflammation may be in a major organ and thus not accessible even for visual observation (Figure 4-1, drug *C*). Thus for drug *C* an observable effect again is not available.

Another factor that could necessitate adjustments to the rates of input of drugs *A*, *B*, or *C* is an appropriate change in the condition of the patient. If each drug is eliminated from the body through the kidneys, and the patient's kidney function changes for better or worse, then the rate of input of drugs *A*, *B*, or *C* will need modification. Reasons for this will be discussed later in this chapter. The point here is that the lack of an observable effect for drugs *B* and *C* could cause the adjustments in drug input rates to be implemented without knowing their adequacy for those patients.

An alternative approach, also listed in Figure 4-1, is to define a target concentration of drug rather than an observable effect as the desired end point. The *plasma* concentration of drug is usually selected because patient tissue samples cannot be justified, (see Figure 4-1, drug *C*) or the location of the specific site to be sampled may be unclear (see Figure 4-1, drug *B*). Thus for drugs where an observable effect is not available or where the therapeutic index (toxic: therapeutic concentration ratio) is less than about 2.5, a target plasma concentration of drug can be a useful

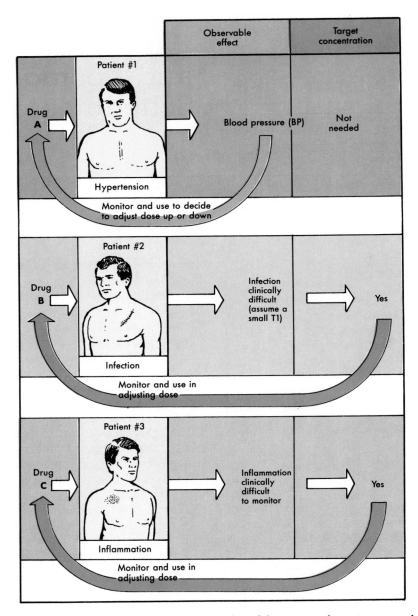

FIGURE 4-1 Concept of target plasma concentration of drug as an alternate approach to use of observable effect for determining if drug input rate is sufficient or needs to be modified. *TI,* Therapeutic index.

guideline for achieving the therapeutic response without incurring toxic side effects. Similarly, a target level drug concentration in patient plasma can be used to guide modifications in drug input rates needed to compensate for changes in patient conditions that bring about slower or faster rates of drug disappearance.

The major goals of this chapter are listed as follows:
1. Describe factors that control the plasma concentration of drug
2. Show how plasma concentration of drug changes with time for different routes and schedules of drug administration
3. Demonstrate how drug input rates and dosing

schedules can be developed or modified on a rational basis to achieve the plasma target concentration of drug

In most clinical situations, it is desirable to maintain the magnitude of pharmacological response at the target level for prolonged periods of time (often days or months). To accomplish this, the plasma concentration of drug must also be maintained near a target level over the same prolonged period of time. Multiple doses or continuous administration of drug is required, with dose size and frequency of administration constituting the *dosing schedule* or *dosing regimen*. In providing instructions for the treatment of a patient, the dosing schedule, the choice of drug, and the mode and route of administration must be specified. Pharmacokinetic considerations have a major role in establishing the dosing schedule, or in adjusting an existing schedule, to increase effectiveness of the drug or to reduce symptoms of toxicity.

Before addressing how to design or adjust a dosing schedule, several key pharmacokinetic parameters and principles must be described. For clarity, a single acute dose of drug is presented here and utilized in a later part of this chapter for the design or modification of multiple dosing regimens. The relevant pharmacokinetic concepts and parameters can be developed and used in the rational design of dosing schedules from one or two perspectives: physical or mathematical. The emphasis in this chapter is to stress the physical meaning of the principles and parameters but also to provide sufficient mathematical background for those readers who desire a somewhat greater in-depth coverage. The key equations are enclosed in boxes to highlight their importance.

ROUTES OF ADMINISTRATION

Major routes of drug administration are divided into (1) *enteral,* passing directly into the gastrointestinal (GI) tract and (2) *parenteral,* bypassing the GI tract. The main routes are given in Table 4-1. The oral route is the most widely prescribed because it can be easily used by the patient. However, poor absorption in the GI tract, first-pass destruction in the liver, delays in stomach emptying, degradation by stomach acidity, and complexation with food may preclude oral administration. Intramuscular (IM) and subcutaneous (SC) routes bypass the problems associated with the GI tract and do not give direct entry into the circulatory system. In many cases absorption

Table 4-1 Main Routes for Drug Administration	
ENTERAL (PER OS, BY MOUTH)	
Oral	(Swallowed)
Sublingual	(Under the tongue)
Buccal	(In the cheek pouch)
PARENTERAL (INJECTION)	
IV	(Intravenous)
IM	(Intramuscular)
SC	(Subcutaneous)
IA	(Intraarterial)
Intrathecal	(Into subarachnoid space)
PULMONARY	
RECTAL	
TOPICAL	

into the circulatory system is rapid for IM- and even for SC-administered compounds. The IV route advantage is a rapid onset of action plus a controlled rate of administration; however, this is countered by the disadvantages of possible infection, coagulation problems, and a greater incidence of anaphylactoid reactions. Most drugs given by injection, especially by IV, require administration by a trained person.

Because of the large number of drugs administered orally or by IV injection, these routes will be reviewed in terms of the relevant pharmacokinetic concepts and the time course of plasma concentration of drug. Chapter 6 describes approaches to drug delivery and targeting of drugs to specific organs or tissues.

DOSE ADJUSTMENT FOR SIZE OF PATIENT

The average adult weighs 70 kg and has a body surface area of 1.7 square meters. The dosage of drug often is scaled to give a constant mg/kg body weight for adults of different size. For some drugs the scaling works better when based on mg/m² body surface area; especially with children. Body surface area correlates with cardiac output and glomerular filtration rate better than body weight. However, body weight for scaling is still favored by many clinicians. Because the therapeutic plasma concentration can cover a considerable range without evidence of toxicity or ineffectiveness, many drugs require only gross scaling.

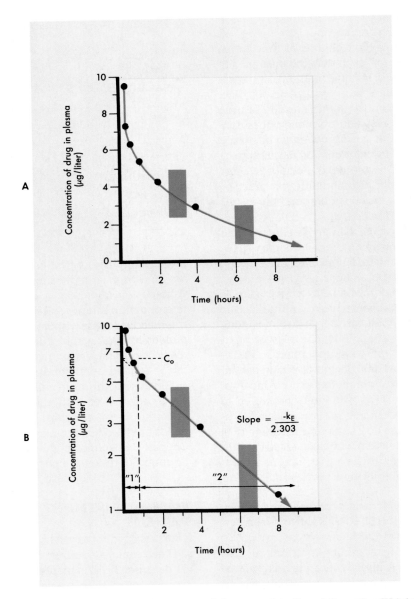

FIGURE 4-2   Plasma or serum concentration of drug as a function of time after IV injection of a single bolus over 5 to 30 seconds. **A,** Arithmetic plot. **B,** Same data with concentrations plotted on a logarithmic scale. The *1* represents the distribution (or alpha) phase and *2* the elimination-metabolism (or beta) phase. Fractional decrease in concentration is constant for a fixed time interval during the straight line portion of **B,** shown here as 18.6% decrease for any 1 hour period *(shaded areas).*

SINGLE DOSES

Single Dose IV Injection and Plasma Concentration of Drug

If a drug is injected as a single bolus over 5 to 30 seconds into a vein and then blood samples are taken periodically and analyzed for unchanged drug, the results should appear as in Figure 4-2, A. The concentration will be greatest a few minutes after injection, when the distribution of drug throughout the circulatory system has equilibrated. This initial mixing of drug and blood is essentially completed after several passes through the heart. Drug then disappears from the plasma by a variety of processes, listed as follows:

1. Slow distribution across membranes to tissue or other body fluids
2. Elimination of unchanged drug via renal or biliary routes
3. Exhalation through the pulmonary pathway if the drug is volatile
4. Metabolism to other active or inactive compounds

Some of the drug in the plasma is bound to plasma proteins or other plasma constituents, but this binding equilibrium is reached in a few seconds. Similarly, a considerable fraction of the injected dose may pass through capillary walls and bind to extravascular tissue. The tissue binding also reaches equilibrium within a few minutes. The values of drug concentration plotted on the vertical scale in Figure 4-2, A represent the sum of free drug and bound drug. In all but a few highly specialized research situations it is too difficult, and sometimes not possible with present assay techniques, to measure the concentrations of free (unbound) drug at therapeutic or below therapeutic concentrations.

The data in Figure 4-2, A can be presented in a more useful format if the concentrations are plotted on a logarithmic scale (Figure 4-2, B), resulting in data points on a straight line. The portion marked "1" represents the *distribution phase* (also called *alpha phase*), wherein the main process is redistribution of drug across membranes and into body regions that are *not* well perfused by capillary beds. In phase 2 (*beta phase* or *elimination/metabolism phase*) distribution is supplanted by elimination and metabolism as the principal influences governing the gradual de-

crease in the plasma concentration of drug. In many clinical situations the duration of time of the distribution phase is very short compared to that of the elimination and metabolism phase. Thus, the distribution phase can be ignored in many clinical situations.

If the distribution phase in Figures 4-2, A or B is neglected, then the equation of the line becomes

$$C(t) = C_o\, e^{-k_E t} \qquad \textbf{(1)}$$

where
$C(t)$ = Concentration of drug in the plasma as a function of time
C_o = Concentration at time zero
e = Base for natural logarithms
k_E = First order rate constant for the elimination/metabolism phase
t = Time

Equation 1 has the shape of a curve when plotted on an arithmetic scale (see Figure 4-2, A); however, equation 1 becomes a straight line when plotted on a semilogarithmic scale (see Figure 4-2, B). This is evident by taking the natural logarithm (ln, base e) of each side of equation 1 to give equation 2 and then converting from natural (ln, base e) to common (log, base 10) logarithms in equation 3, using the relationship that ln x equals (2.303) (log x) and noting the ln e is 1.0.

$$\ln C(t) = \ln C_o + (-k_E\, t)\ln e \qquad \textbf{(2)}$$

$$\log C(t) = \log C_o - \frac{k_E t}{2.303} \qquad \textbf{(3)}$$

Thus from equation 3, a plot of log C(t) versus t (see Figure 4-2, B) should be a straight line of slope $-k_E/2.303$ and concentration axis intercept log C_o. Both k_E and C_o can be obtained from such a plot, provided the data can be represented by a linear relationship. A characteristic of an equation 1 type of curve is that for a given duration time interval the *fractional change in concentration is fixed* and independent of the time at which the interval is begun. Thus, for a time interval of 4 hours, the fractional change in concentration is the same whether the interval is started at 1, 3, 5, 8, or some other number of hours after injection.

In situations where the elimination-metabolism is rapid, the error in describing C(t) becomes appreciable when the distribution phase is omitted. Therefore, the expression for C(t) with both the distribution and the elimination/metabolism phases included is given as

$$C(t) = C_o^d \, e^{-k_d t} + C_o \, e^{-k_e t} \qquad (4)$$

where k_d is the first-order rate constant for the distribution processes and C_o^d is the extrapolated time zero concentration component for the distribution phase. The actual concentration of drug at time zero is the sum of C_o^d and C_o. Equation 4 and each of the component terms are plotted in Figure 4-3. The meaning of each of the parameters can be understood more clearly (see Figure 4-3). It is an inherent assumption that the distribution occurs much more rapidly than the elimination-metabolism, so that k_d is much

greater than k_E. Therefore, the distribution term becomes zero after only a small portion of the dose is eliminated or metabolized and equation 4 reduces to equation 1 at these longer times. By back extrapolation of the linear postdistribution data, the value of C_o can be obtained, whereas k_E can be determined from the slope. The concentration component responsible for the distribution phase (shaded area in Figure 4-3) is obtained as the difference between the actual concentration and the extrapolated elimination-metabolism line, and this difference is plotted to give the line of slope $(-)k_d/2.303$ and intercept C_o^d. Because C(t) for many drugs can be described adequately in terms of the monoexponential of equation 1, the remainder of this chapter will deal only with the postdistribution phase and equation 1.

Rate Constants and Half-Lives

The monoexponential equation 1 for C(t) was given earlier but without any explanation of how such an expression is developed and what physical meaning is inherent in the derivation. Experimental data for many drugs show that the rates of drug elimination, metabolism, absorption, and distribution generally are directly proportional to concentration. Such a process follows first-order kinetics, because the rate varies with the first power of the concentration. This is shown quantitatively as

$$\frac{dC(t)}{dt} = -k_E \, C(t) \qquad (5)$$

where $dC(t)/dt$ is the rate of change of concentration, and k_E is the proportionality constant, also called *rate constant*. The negative sign denotes that the concentration is being decreased by elimination-metabolism.

Rate processes also can occur via zero-order kinetics where the rate is independent of the concentration. Two prominent examples are the metabolism of ethanol and the metabolism of aspirin at high doses. Under such conditions the process becomes saturated and the rate of metabolism becomes independent of the concentration of drug.

For readers who desire an in-depth explanation of the derivation of equation 1, note that equation 5 can be rearranged and integrated to obtain equation 1 as

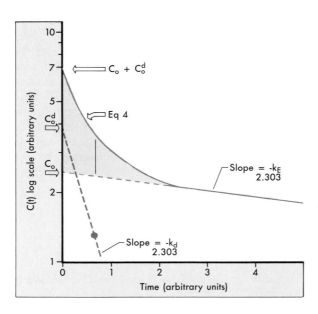

FIGURE 4-3 Semilogarithmic plot of plasma concentration of drug versus time where the distribution phase is included. Solid line represents equation 4 with terms for distribution and elimination-metabolism. The solid line can be obtained by nonlinear curve fitting of the data points (not shown) to equation 4 using one of the many available computer programs. Equation 4 can also be obtained by graphical means in which extrapolation of the linear portion of the data (elimination-metabolism phase) is used to get C_o and k_E. The differences between the data points and the extrapolated line in the distribution phase (*double arrow vertical line at 0.65 time units* and plotted as 1.3 concentration units) *(shaded area)* are plotted and extrapolated linearly to obtain C_o^d and k_d.

$$\frac{dC(t)}{C(t)} = -k_E \, dt \tag{6}$$

$$\int_{C_o}^{C(t)} \frac{dC(t)}{C(t)} = -k_E \int_0^t dt \tag{7}$$

$$\ln C(t) - \ln C_o = -k_E t \tag{8}$$

$$C(t) = C_o \, e^{-k_E t} \tag{1}$$

In the above expression k_E has the units of time^{-1}. Now any first-order rate constant is related to the half-life of the process by the following expression:

$$k = \frac{0.70^*}{t_{1/2}} \tag{9}$$

That equation 9 is correct is shown by expressing the time in equation 1 in terms of the number of half-lives $(n \, t_{1/2})$ to give:

$$\frac{C(t)}{C_o} = e^{-k_E n t_{1/2}} \tag{10}$$

Half-life is defined as the time it takes for the concentration to decrease to half the value it had at the start of the time interval. Thus, by definition $C(t)/C_o$ is 0.5 and n is 1.0 in equation 10. Taking the ln of each side gives $0.7 = -k_E \, t_{1/2}$, which can be rearranged to equation 9 for k_E. Note that the ln of 2 is

---

*Rounded off from 0.693.

0.693, but it is rounded off here to 0.7 and (2) that the half-life and k_E are constants that do not change with concentration as long as the plot of log $C(t)$ versus t is a straight line. The value of $t_{1/2}$ can be read directly from a graph of log $C(t)$ versus t as shown in the worked example with Figure 4-8. Values of $t_{1/2}$ for the elimination-metabolism phase range in practice from several minutes to days or longer for different drugs. In addition the $t_{1/2}$ may vary widely between patients receiving the same dose or in some cases can vary with dose in a given patient.

Single Oral Dose and Plasma Concentration of Drug

The plot of $C(t)$ versus time after oral administration is different from that following IV injection only during the drug absorption phase. The two plots become identical for the postabsorption or elimination-metabolism phase. A typical plot of the plasma concentration of drug versus time after oral administration is shown in Figure 4-4. Initially there is no drug in the plasma because the preparation must be swallowed, undergo dissolution if administered as a tablet, be absorbed in the stomach or small intestine, and await stomach emptying if absorption is mainly in the small intestine. As the plasma concentration of drug builds up due to rapid absorption, the rate of elimination-metabolism also increases because elimination and metabolism usually are first-order processes where

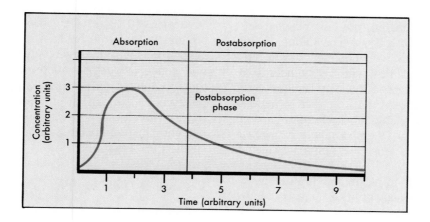

FIGURE 4-4   Typical profile for plasma concentration of drug versus time after oral administration and with the usual condition that the rate constant for drug absorption is at least ten times larger than that for drug elimination-metabolism.

the rates increase directly with increasing concentration of drug. The peak concentration is reached when the rates of absorption and disappearance are equal. The expression for the plasma concentration of drug and how the concentration changes with time is given in equation 11.

$$C(t) = \frac{C_o \, k_a \, F}{(k_a - k_E)} \, (e^{-k_E t} - e^{-k_a t}) \qquad (11)$$

In this expression k_a is the first-order rate constant for absorption of drug in the stomach or intestine and F is the fraction of the dose that is absorbed and gets past the liver and into the systemic circulation. For a drug to be useful, k_a must be at least 10 times larger than k_E; otherwise the drug will disappear as soon as it enters the systemic circulation and the concentration will not increase to therapeutically useful levels. The definition of F, the *bioavailability,* is discussed later in this chapter. The experimental determination of k_a is difficult and a knowledge of the absorption rate constant is usually of little value clinically. However, the half-life corresponding to k_E can still be obtained from data in the postabsorptive phase by plotting log C(t) versus t and getting the slope of the linear portion.

Binding of Drug to Plasma Constituents

The rates of drug disappearance and the concentration of free unbound drug available to the site of action are influenced markedly if a significant portion of the dose is bound to plasma constituents. In general, clinical laboratory assays for plasma drug concentrations are based on the total (bound plus unbound) concentration of drug. A knowledge of the concentration of free drug would be most useful clinically with those drugs that are highly bound to plasma components, because it is only the free drug that is available to interact with the site of action. However, the range of therapeutic concentrations of free drug for highly bound compounds is extremely low and often beyond the sensitivity limits of available assays.

The binding of drugs to plasma or serum constituents involves primarily albumin, α_1-acid glycoprotein, or lipoproteins (Table 4-2). Serum albumin is the most abundant protein in human plasma, with a normal concentration of about 4.0 g/100 ml. This material is synthesized in the liver at roughly 140 mg/kg body weight/day under normal conditions but of-

Bind Primarily to Albumin	Bind Primarily to α_1-Acid Glycoprotein	Bind Primarily to Lipoproteins
barbiturates	alprenolol	amitriptyline
benzodiazepines	bupivacaine	nortriptyline
bilirubin*	desmethyl-	
digitoxin	perazine	
diphenylhydantoin	dipyridamole	
fatty acids*	disopyramide	
penicillins	etidocaine	
probenecid	imipramine	
phenylbutazone	lidocaine	
streptomycin	methadone	
sulfonamides	perazine	
tetracycline	prazosin	
tolbutamide	propranolol	
valproic acid	quinidine	
warfarin	verapamil	

Table 4-2 Drugs That Bind Appreciably to Serum or Plasma Constituents

*May displace drugs in some disease states.

ten at markedly decreased rates in certain disease states. Albumin has a molecular weight of 68,000, no appreciable carbohydrate component, and a net electrical charge of 19 negative groups at pH 7.4. Many acidic drugs bind strongly to albumin but because of the normally high concentration of plasma albumin, the binding does not saturate the sites. Basic drugs bind primarily to α_1-acid glycoprotein, which has a molecular weight of 40,000 with 41% carbohydrate including sialic acid and present in plasma at a concentration of 0.08 g/100 ml. Less is known about drug binding to lipoproteins. Disease states often cause major changes in plasma albumin, α_1-acid glycoprotein concentrations, or in the binding affinities of these materials for specific drugs. Drugs that are highly bound to plasma proteins present a scenario for drug interactions; discussed in Chapter 7. The influence of protein binding on drug disposition is covered in Chapter 5.

Volume of Distribution

The actual volume in which drug molecules are distributed within a patient's body cannot be measured. However, an *apparent volume of distribution* (V_d) can be obtained, which in some cases may be of limited clinical usefulness. The easiest method for obtaining a value for V_d is to obtain the time zero concentration, C_o, after IV injection and by equation 12, knowing the dose (D) calculating V_d.

$$C_o = \frac{D}{V_d}$$

(12)

If C_o has the units of mg/L and D of mg, then V_d would be in liters. Another method for obtaining V_d is described later in this chapter (see equation 16). In some cases it is meaningful to compare the apparent volume of distribution with typical body water volumes. The following volumes in liters and percent of body weight apply to adult humans:

BODY WATER	BODY WEIGHT (%)	VOLUME (APPROX. LITERS)
Plasma	4	3
Extracellular	20	14
Total body	60	45

Experimental values of the volume of distribution vary from 5 to 10 liters for drugs such as warfarin and tolbutamide to 15,000 to 40,000 liters for chloroquine and quinacrine in a 70 kg adult. How can one calculate apparent volumes of distribution grossly in excess of the total body volume? This can occur as a result of protein binding of drug and of using plasma as the sole source of samples for determination of V_d (Figure 4-5). For a drug such as warfarin that is 97% bound to plasma albumin at therapeutic concentrations, nearly all of the dose initially is in the plasma, so that a plot of log plasma C(t) versus time, when extrapolated back to time zero, gives a large value for C_o (for bound plus unbound drug). Because from equation 12, $V_d = D/C_o$, the resulting value of V_d will be small and usually in the range of 2 to 10 liters. At the other extreme is a drug such as chloroquine, which is strongly bound to tissue sites and weakly bound to plasma proteins. Most of the dose initially will be at tissue sites, thereby resulting in quite small concentrations in the plasma samples. Thus, a plot of log plasma C(t) versus time will give a small value to C_o (for bound plus unbound drug), which in conjunction with equation 12 can result in apparent V_d values in great excess of the total body volume.

The volume of distribution can serve as a guide in noting whether a drug is bound primarily to plasma or tissue sites and possibly whether the drug is distributed primarily into plasma or into extracellular spaces.

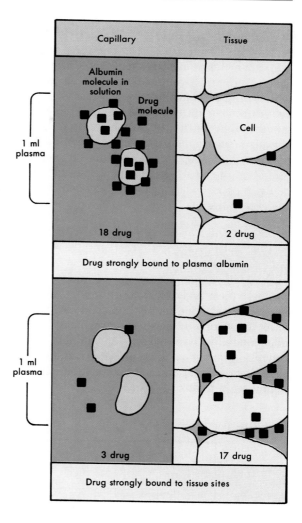

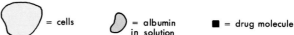

FIGURE 4-5   Influence of drug binding to plasma versus tissue sites on apparent volume of distribution. Numbers represent relative quantity of drug in 1 ml plasma as compared to adjacent tissue. Only the plasma is sampled to determine V_d and the albumin-bound drug is included in the sample.

Drug Clearance

Clearance is a pharmacokinetic parameter that is very useful clinically for describing the capability of the patient to dispose of a particular drug. The discussion in this chapter is limited to *total body clearance*. Chapter 5 includes descriptions of renal clearance, hepatic clearance, and other specific organ or specific mechanism modes of clearance that add up to total body clearance.

The plot of plasma C(t) versus time (see Figure 4-2) shows the concentration of drug decreasing with time. The corresponding rate (such as mg/min) at which drug is being removed from the plasma can be written as dX(t)/dt, where X(t) represents the quantity (mg) of drug. The rate of drug removal by various processes is assumed to follow first-order kinetics with respect to the plasma concentration of drug, and the total body clearance can be thought of as the proportionality constant between the rate and the concentration. Thus,

$$\frac{dX(t)}{dt} = (\text{clearance})_p \ C(t) = (Cl)_p \ C(t) \quad \textbf{(13)}$$

where p indicates "total body" removal from the *plasma*. Total body clearance thus has the units of volume/time, such as ml/min, and can be thought of as the volume of plasma from which all drug molecules need to be removed each minute to achieve the rate of removal (Figure 4-6). It is sometimes easier to rearrange equation 13 to obtain equation 14 for the definition of total body clearance.

$$(Cl)_p = \frac{dX(t)/dt}{C(t)} =$$
$$\frac{\text{rate of removal of drug (in mg/min)}}{\text{plasma concentration of drug (in mg/ml)}} \quad \textbf{(14)}$$

Two methods are available for obtaining values for $(C1)_p$ for a given drug in an individual patient. The first method requires that the half-life and the apparent volume of distribution be known and utilized as

$$(Cl)_p = \frac{0.7 \ V_d}{t_{1/2}} = k_E \ V_d \quad \textbf{(15)}$$

The second method is based on obtaining an empirical solution to equation 13, as follows:

$$\int_0^{X_o} dX = X_o = (Cl)_p \int_0^\infty C(t) \ dt \quad \textbf{(16)}$$

where X_o is the dose, or that part of the dose, that enters the systemic circulation. The integral of C(t) dt is the same as the area under the curve of concentration versus time. Thus the clearance is ob-

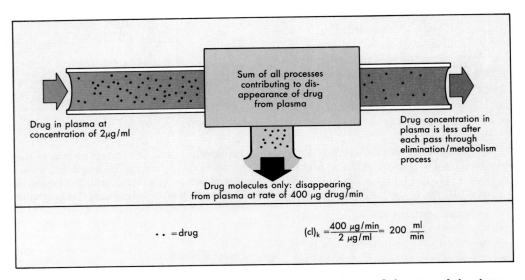

FIGURE 4-6   Concept of total body clearance of drug from plasma. Only *some* of the drug molecules disappear from the plasma on each pass of blood through kidneys, liver, or other sites that contribute to drug disappearance (elimination-metabolism). In this example, it required 200 ml of plasma to account for the amount of drug that disappears each minute (400 μg/min) at the concentration of 2 μg/ml. The total body clearance is thus 200 ml/min.

tained by dividing the dose that enters the systemic circulation by the area under the curve.

The area under the curve, the dose, and the value of k_E also can be used with equation 16 to obtain an alternate value for the apparent volume of distribution.

Bioavailability and First Pass Effect

When a drug is administered by IV injection, all of the dose enters the systemic circulation, but this may not be true for drugs administered by other routes, especially for drugs given orally. Dissolution of tablets can vary greatly between manufacturers of the same drug and is a major source of differences in drug bioavailability. The fraction of the dose that enters the systemic circulation when given orally, for example, compared to what enters when given by IV injection, is called the *bioavailability* or the *bioequivalence* (F). Physical or chemical processes that account for reduced bioavailability (F<1) include poor solubility of drug or incomplete absorption of drug in the GI tract and rapid metabolism of drug during its first pass through the liver (discussed later). Differences in bioavailability in oral preparations result from the inert ingredients present and the tableting process itself. Values of F are obtained by using equation 17, as follows:

$$F = \frac{X_{o_{(oral)}}}{X_{o_{(IV)}}} = \frac{(Cl)_{P(oral)} \int_0^\infty C(t)\ dt_{(oral)}}{(Cl)_{P(IV)} \int_0^\infty C(t)\ dt_{(IV)}}$$

(17)

$$\text{or } F = \frac{(AUC)_{(oral)}}{(AUC)_{(IV)}}$$

AUC is the area under the curve and the clearance is assumed to be independent of the route of administration. This assumption is valid for most drugs but is not followed in a few unexplained cases. The problem of bioavailability was first recognized in 1971 when unexplained low plasma concentrations of digoxin in several patients were traced to different fractions of the drug being absorbed from the GI tract. The digoxin was administered in tablet form as different lots from the same manufacturer or from different suppliers. Typical plots in Figure 4-7 show that the area under the curve can be markedly different.

Thus, for drugs where absorption from the GI tract is not always 100%, the pharmaceutical formulations must now pass a bioavailability test that verifies that the bioavailability is constant, within certain limits, between lots.

The potential problem of changes in bioavailability is one of the major considerations in choosing between free substitution of generic compounds and specifying a brand name. If substitution of a different brand or a generic product is made, and neither the physician nor the patient knows of the substitution, the bioavailability may be changed markedly without any compensating modification made in the size of the dose. This can have life-threatening consequences. No list of drugs having low bioavailability is included here because the values of F are subject to change with the compounding formulations used by the manufacturer.

A special case of low bioavailability can result when the drug is well absorbed from the GI tract, but subsequent metabolism of the drug is high during its transit from the splanchnic capillary beds through the

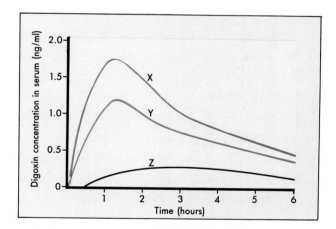

FIGURE 4-7   Before bioavailability regulations for pharmaceutical preparations, digoxin serum concentrations sometimes varied appreciably between brands and even between lot numbers of the same brand. The curves shown here are for a group of subjects receiving single 0.5 mg oral doses of each of the following digoxin tablets: X from company No 1; Y and Z, two different lots, from company No 2. The area under the curve differs markedly, thus showing that the bioavailabilities varied greatly, roughly from 0.8 to 0.4. For drugs in which the therapeutic index is less than about 2.5 and the bioavailability is less than about 0.95, arbitrary switching of brands or poor control of tableting operations by drug suppliers can result in serious situations in patients.

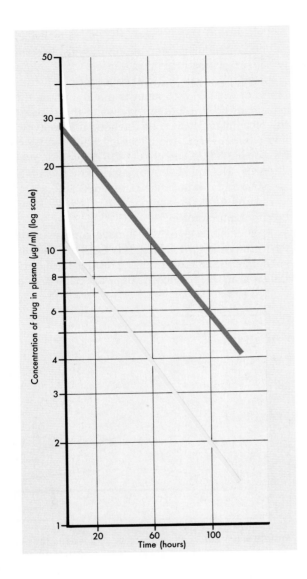

$$V_d = D/C_o = \frac{(100 \text{ mg}) (1000 \text{ μg/mg})}{(10.7 \text{ μg/ml})} = 9{,}300 \text{ ml}$$

To get the slope read two points from the line and solve text equation 3.

At t = 20 hr, C = 7.6 μg/ml

At t = 100 hr, C = 1.92 μg/ml

Thus: $\log 7.6 = \log C_o - \dfrac{k_E}{2.303} (20) = 0.8808$

$$\log 1.92 = \log C_o - \frac{k_E}{2.303} (100) = 0.2833$$
$$+ \frac{k_E}{2.303} (80) = 0.5975$$

$$- \text{slope} = \frac{k_E}{2.303} = 0.00746$$

$$k_E = 0.017 \text{ hr}^{-1}$$

$$t_{1/2} = \frac{0.7}{k_E} = 0.7/0.017 = 41 \text{ hr}$$

To check $t_{1/2}$ note from the plot that C is 10 μg/ml at 4 hr and 5 μg/ml at about 44 hr giving an estimate of 40 hr for $t_{1/2}$. This agrees well with the above value from the slope.

$$(Cl)_p = k_E V_d = (0.017 \text{ hr}^{-1}) (9{,}300 \text{ ml}) = 158 \text{ ml/hr}$$

Area Under Curve (AUC):

$$\text{AUC} = \int C(t) \, dt = C_o \int_o^{120} e^{-k_E t} \, dt = C_o \left. \frac{e^{-k_E t}}{-k_E} \right|_0^{120} =$$

$$- \frac{10.7}{0.017} (0.13 - 1.00) = 547 \frac{\text{μg, hr}}{\text{ml}} = \text{AUC}$$

Need to add an additional 15% to correct for the drug that disappears between 120 hours and infinite hours.

FIGURE 4-8   Use of plasma concentration versus time data to determine values for key pharmacokinetic parameters. Concentrations are plotted for drug administered by IV injection as single doses of 200 mg *(red line)* and 100 mg *(yellow line)* on two separate occasions. The yellow line was fitted by linear least squares on the semilogarithmic plot and extrapolated to time zero to get a C_o of 10.7 μg/ml. White line indicates distributive phase.

liver and on to the systemic circulation. The drug concentration in the plasma is at its highest level during this "first pass" through the liver. Therefore drugs that are subject to liver metabolism may encounter a very significant reduction in the level of active compound during the first pass through the liver. For example, with lidocaine the first pass effect is so large that this drug is not administered orally. Some drugs that show strong first pass effects are:

acetylsalicylic acid (aspirin): analgesic, arthritis agent
desipramine: antidepressant
hydralazine: antihypertensive
isoproterenol: bronchodilator
lidocaine: antiarrhythmic
methylphenidate: CNS stimulant
morphine: analgesic
pentazocine: analgesic
propoxyphene: analgesic
propranolol: antihypertensive

Sample Calculations of Pharmacokinetic Parameters

Figure 4-8 is a semilogarithmic plot of a highly plasma-protein–bound drug at two different doses. The slopes are parallel within the experimental error of the assays, demonstrating that the pharmacokinetics are the same at the two doses. The calculations of $t_{1/2}$, k_E, C_o, V_d, $C1_p$, (see equations 13 to 15) and the area under the curve are given for one of the sets of data in the figure legend.

MULTIPLE OR PROLONGED DOSING

As mentioned at the beginning of this chapter, most drugs require administration over a prolonged period of time to achieve the desired therapeutic effect. Two principal modes of administration are commonly employed to achieve the prolonged effectiveness: (1) *continuous IV infusion* and (2) discrete *multiple doses* on a designated dosing schedule. Special devices for prolonged drug delivery are discussed in Chapter 6. The basic objective with each mode is to increase the plasma concentration of drug until a steady state concentration is reached that will produce the desired therapeutic effect with little evidence of toxicity. This steady state concentration is then maintained for minutes, hours, days, or even

longer as required by the clinical situation. The steady state concentration must be maintained greater than the minimum concentration needed to produce a pharmacological response yet below the concentration that produces toxicity. The pharmacokinetic considerations for designing or adjusting a continuous infusion or a discrete multiple dosing schedule are described in the next two sections.

Continuous Intravenous Infusion

The continuous intravenous infusion mode of administration is used when it is necessary to obtain a rapid onset of drug action and to maintain the action for an extended period of time under controlled conditions. Continuous infusions normally are administered in a hospital or emergency setting.

In continuous infusion the drug is administered at a fixed rate. The plasma concentration of drug gradually rises and then plateaus at a concentration where the rate of infusion equals the total rate of elimination/metabolism. A typical plasma concentration profile is shown in Figure 4-9. The plateau (C_{ss}) is also called the *steady state* concentration (see equation 19). It should not be called the "infusion equilibrium" state.

The concentration curve in Figure 4-9 is described by equation 18 for simple cases in which the distribution phase is omitted and where k_o is the rate of infusion of drug in amount/time (that is, mg/min, mg/min/kg body weight, or mg/min/m^2 body surface area).

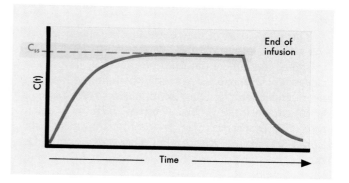

FIGURE 4-9   Typical profile showing how plasma concentration of drug varies with time for continuous IV injection at a constant rate and without a loading dose. C_{ss} is the concentration at the plateau or steady state, where the rate of drug input equals the rate of drug disappearance. At the end of the infusion the decay in the concentration will react as it would for any acute IV injection with C_o equal to C_{ss}.

$$C(t) = \frac{k_o}{k_E V_d} (1 - e^{-k_E t}) \tag{18}$$

From equation 18 it is apparent that the C_{ss} can be described by equation 19:

$$C_{ss} = \frac{k_o}{k_E V_d} = \frac{\text{infusion rate}}{\text{total body clearance}} \tag{19}$$

There is little point in memorizing equation 19, because a physical understanding of what is meant by the steady state and a realization of the units of each term enable the equation 19 expression to be developed as needed. Key points in this development are as follows:

1. At steady state the rate of drug input must equal the rate of drug disappearance.
2. The input rate is the infusion rate (mg/min).
3. What is needed to convert C_{ss} in mg/L to the disappearance rate in mg/min?
4. The answer is a term with units of L/min. Clearance has those units.
5. Thus at steady state:

$$k_o = C_{ss} (Cl)_p = C_{ss} \frac{V_d 0.7}{t_{1/2}}$$

This approach of determining the physical situation and making sure that the units are consistent is a much more useful approach to learning and applying pharmacokinetics than simply memorizing the pharmacokinetic equations.

The plateau level concentration is influenced by the infusion rate, the drug disappearance half life, the apparent volume of distribution, and the total body clearance. Of these factors, only the infusion rate can be modified as needed. For example, if the plateau level concentration is at 2.0 ng/ml with an infusion rate of 16 μg/hr and you decide that the concentration is too high and that about 1.5 ng/ml would be better, you can achieve the lower value by decreasing the infusion rate to 12 μg/hr. A 25% reduction in infusion rate should give a 25% decrease in the plateau concentration. How long it takes to get to the new plateau concentration is discussed later.

Dosing Schedule

Multiple dosing usually is specified so that the size of the dose and the dosing interval (i.e., the time between doses) are fixed. Two considerations are important in selecting the dosing interval (T). Smaller intervals result in minimal fluctuations in plasma concentration of drug; however, the interval must be a relatively standard number of hours to help ensure compliance by the patient or by the nursing staff. In addition, for oral dosing the mg per dose must be compatible with the size of the available tablets or other pharmaceutical preparations. Thus, an oral dosing schedule of 28 mg every 2.8 hours is impractical because the drug probably is not available as a 28 mg tablet. Also, a schedule of taking a tablet at 2.8 hour intervals is impractical. More practical dosing intervals, particularly for patient compliance, are every 6, 8, 12, or 24 hours.

The plasma concentration of drug versus time is shown in Figure 4-10 for multiple dosing by repeated IV injections. T is selected so that all of the drug from the previous dose disappears before the next dose is injected (see Figure 4-10, A). There is no accumula-

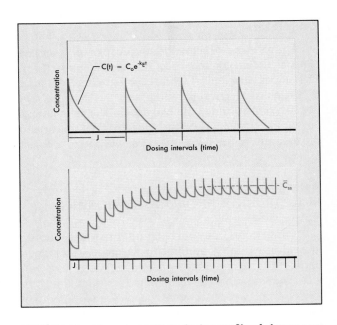

FIGURE 4-10   Discrete multiple dosing profile of plasma concentration of drug given by IV injections with the same size dose given each time. In part A, the dosing interval, T, is long enough so that each dose completely disappears before administration of the next dose. In part B, the dosing interval is much shorter so that drug from previous injection is still present when the next dose is administered. Accumulation results in part B, with $\overline{C}_{ss}$ representing the mean concentration of drug at the plateau level, where the mean rate of drug input equals the mean rate of drug disappearance for each dosing interval. No loading dose is shown in this profile.

tion of drug; therefore no plateau or steady state is reached.

If a plateau level is desired, then the dosing interval must be short enough so that drug from the previous dose is still present when the next dose is administered. In this way the plasma concentration gradually increases until the drug lost by elimination-metabolism during a dosing interval is equal to the dose of drug added at the start of the dosing interval. When this equality is achieved, then the mean concentration for a dosing interval, $\overline{C}_{ss}$ (the bar indicates *mean*) has plateaued. The stepwise accumulation is exemplified by the plot of plasma concentration of drug versus time for multiple IV injections with the dosing interval roughly equivalent to the half-life of drug disappearance (see Figure 4-10, *B*). The average rate (over a dose interval) of drug input is constant at D/T. The rate of drug disappearance is very small during the first dosing interval but increases with drug concentration during subsequent intervals until the average rate of disappearance and the average rate of input are equal. For significant accumulation, the dosing interval must be at least as short as the half-life and preferably shorter. However, this criterion cannot be used with very short half-life agents, such as some of the penicillins.

At the plateau, the mean concentration of drug, $\overline{C}_{ss}$, again is equal to the input rate divided by the clearance, just as for continuous infusion.

$$\overline{C}_{ss} = \frac{D/T}{(Cl)_p} \qquad \textbf{(20)}$$

From equation 20 it is evident that the size of the dose or the duration of the dosing interval can be changed to modify the mean plateau concentration of drug. The quantitative description of the entire curve (see Figure 4-10, *B*) for repetitive IV injections or for a modified curve for repetitive oral doses has been worked out, but the equations are complex and of use primarily in pharmacokinetic research studies.

Loading Dose

If all of the multiple doses are the same size, then the term *maintenance* dose can be used. In certain clinical situations, however, a more rapid onset of action is required. This can be achieved by giving a much larger "loading" dose just before the start of the

smaller maintenance dose regimen. An IV bolus loading dose is often used before starting a continuous IV infusion, or an IV or oral loading dose may be used at the start of discrete multiple dosing. Ideally, the loading dose is sized to raise the plasma drug concentration immediately to the plateau level and the maintenance doses are designed to maintain the same plateau concentration. Multiplying the plateau concentration by the apparent volume of distribution results in a value for the loading dose. However, the uncertainity in the V_d in individual patients usually leads to a more conservative loading dose to prevent overshooting the plateau by too much and encountering toxic concentrations. This is especially a problem with drugs that have a small therapeutic index.

Duration of Time to Steady State

For a continuous IV infusion or a series of discrete multiple doses, the time to get to the plateau concentration or from one plateau level to another depends only on the disappearance half-life of the drug. If a loading dose is given, then the time to get from the concentration produced by the loading dose to the plateau for the given drug input rate again depends only on the half-life. This principle can be shown using equation 18, which describes the time course of plasma concentration of drug for a continuous infusion. By replacing k_E with $0.7/t_{1/2}$ from equation 9 and describing the time as n number of half-lives ($n\, t_{1/2}$), the exponent becomes $-0.7n$ and equation 18 reduces to

$$\frac{c(t)}{C_{ss}} = 1 - e^{-0.7n} \qquad \textbf{(21)}$$

This is solved for several values for n, to give:

n	$C(t)/C_{ss}$
0	0
1	0.50
2	0.75
3	0.88
3.3	0.90
4	0.94
5	0.97

During each half-life, 50% of the change in concentration is achieved from the starting point to the new plateau. From a practical standpoint, 90% of the change to get to the plateau is usually taken as having reached the new plateau, so that the duration is simply 3 to 4 half-lives.

PRACTICAL PHARMACOKINETIC PRINCIPLES

EXAMPLE 1: Figure 4-11 is a plot of plasma concentration of a drug at different times during a continuous infusion at 3 mg/min for 70 minutes. Calculate k_E, $t_{1/2}$, $(Cl)_p$, V_d; the concentration 20 minutes after the infusion is stopped; and the infusion rate and loading dose to achieve a plateau of 7 mg/L.

From the plateau concentration of 5.0 mg/L and the infusion rate of 3 mg/min, a check of units, and knowing that input rate must equal disappearance rate, the $(Cl)_p$ must be (3 mg/min)/(5 mg/1000 ml), or 600 ml/min. Noting that the concentration gets 50% of the way to the plateau during the first half-life, the value of $0.50\ C_{ss}$ is 2.50 mg/L and from the graph this is reached at 11.5 minutes after the start of the infusion. Thus $t_{1/2}$ is 11.5 minutes (relatively fast) and k_E becomes 0.061 min^{-1} from the equality of k_E and $0.7/t_{1/2}$. Because $(Cl)_p$ is $k_E V_d$, the value for V_d is 9.8 liters (or 10 liters). After the infusion is stopped, the concentration is described by 5.0 exp(-0.061(20)), which solves to give 1.5 mg/liter. For a plateau concentration of 7 mg/liter, the infusion rate should be 40% greater or 4.2 mg/min. A loading dose of 68 mg will put the concentration at 7 mg/L; a practical loading dose might be 50 mg.

EXAMPLE 2: A patient has received a cardiac drug, digoxin, orally at 0.25 mg (one tablet/day) for several weeks and symptoms of appreciable toxicity appeared recently. A blood sample was taken and assayed to give a plasma concentration of 3.2 ng/ml. This is in the toxicity range for many patients. Because this drug has a low therapeutic index, you do not want to drop the plasma concentration too low but you decide to try cutting it to 1.6 ng/ml. What new dosing schedule should you use and how long will it take to reach the new plateau?

The once a day dosing interval is very convenient, so you continue that and specify 0.125 mg/day (one-half tablet/day); a 50% cut in the plateau level requires a 50% cut in the dose. There are two options for getting to the lower plateau: (1) immediately switch to the 0.125 mg/day dosing rate and reach the 1.6 ng/ml concentration in about 4 half-lives (you do not know what the half-life for digoxin is in your patient) or (2) stop all digoxin dosing for an unknown number of days until the concentration reaches 1.6 ng/ml and then start again at 0.125 mg/day. The

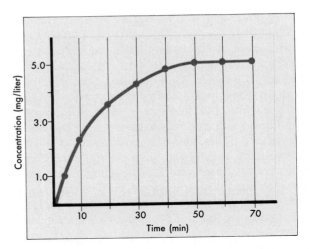

FIGURE 4-11   Data on plasma concentration of a drug at different times for an IV infusion at 3 mg/min for 70 minutes for use in example 1, for obtaining pharmacokinetic parameter values and for estimating the conditions to be used to accomplish other dosing goals.

second procedure undoubtedly will go faster, but you need to determine how many days to wait. You decide to stop all digoxin dosing, wait 24 hours from the previous 3.2 ng/ml sample, and get another blood sample. The concentration now has decreased to 2.7 ng/ml or by about one sixth in a day. From equation 1 the fractional decrease each day should remain constant. Therefore decrease of one sixth of the remaining concentration each day gives 2.25 ng/ml after day 2, 1.85 ng/ml after day 3, and 1.55 ng/ml after day 4. Therefore, by withholding drug for a total of 4 days, the plasma concentration could be reduced to 1.6 ng/ml. Because the half-life is calculated to be 3.8 days in this patient, merely switching to the 0.125 mg/day dosing rate without withholding drug would have required 12 to 15 days to reach the 1.6 ng/ml concentration.

An additional example is given in Chapter 5 under the section on modified renal function and drug elimination to show how to change the dosing schedule to compensate for decreased drug elimination capability by the patient.

SUMMARY

Pharmacokinetics provides a firm basis for the design of dosing regimens and for the characterization of the kinetics of drug disposition. The topic is approached here from a physical rather than a rigorous mathematical standpoint to show that pharmacokinetic considerations can be used readily in everyday clinical medicine without resort to a large number of equations. The major points include the following:

1. Half-life
2. Clearance
3. Bioavailability and first pass
4. Results of plasma-protein–binding of drugs
5. Concept of the apparent volume of distribution
6. Exponential disposition of drug (first order decline) in which the same fraction of drug is disposed of per unit time
7. Concept that the rates of drug input and disappearance are equal at the steady state or plateau concentrations
8. How to modify a dosing regimen to achieve a desired change in plateau level
9. Concept that the time to reach the plateau depends only on the disappearance half-life of the drug
10. The use of a loading dose to accelerate the onset of the desired therapeutic effect

REFERENCES

Notari RE: Biopharmaceutics and clinical pharmacokinetics, ed 4, (practical aspects, worked examples), Marcel Dekker, New York, 1987.

Roland M and Tozer TN: Clinical pharmacokinetics, Lea & Febiger, Philadelphia, 1980.

Wilkinson GR: Clearance approaches in pharmacology, Pharmacol Rev 39:1, 1987.

CHAPTER 5

Absorption, Distribution, Metabolism, and Elimination

WHAT HAPPENS TO DRUGS

In nearly all cases the site of drug action is located in a region that is on the other side of a membrane from the site of drug administration. Therefore the ease by which a compound crosses membranes is of key importance in assessing the rates and extent of absorption and distribution of the drug throughout different body compartments. One of the objectives of this chapter is to provide guidelines for assessing how well specific drugs will cross membranes and what variables will be most important.

Drugs are transported by blood flow throughout the circulatory system and, except for a few targeting techniques discussed in Chapter 6, end up at tissues and organs where their presence is beneficial, as well as at other tissues where their presence may be detrimental. Because of the potential seriousness of the problem, special mention is made in this chapter about drug distribution to the brain and to the fetus.

The principal routes by which drugs disappear from the body are by elimination of unchanged drug or by metabolism to other pharmacologically active or inactive compounds that are subject to further elimination or metabolism. The mechanisms of the elimination processes and the principal chemical pathways involved in drug metabolism also are described in this chapter. Some additional metabolic pathways that are of primary application in the detoxification of nontherapeutic compounds that may enter the body are discussed in Chapter 62 on toxicology.

ABSORPTION AND DISTRIBUTION

Transport of Drugs Across Membranes

Drugs that are administered orally (PO), intramuscularly (IM), or subcutaneously (SC) must cross membranes to be absorbed and to enter the systemic circulation. Not all agents need to enter the systemic circulation, but even those given orally to treat GI tract infections, stomach acidity, and other disease states centered within the GI tract often cross membranes and are absorbed into the general circulation. Drugs administered by intravenous (IV) injection also must cross capillary membranes to leave the systemic circulation and reach extracellular and intracellular sites of action. Even materials directed against platelets or other blood-borne elements must cross membranes to enter the particles. Discussed later in this chapter, the renal elimination of drugs also requires the traversing of membranes.

Membranes are highly lipid in chemical composition and thus strongly hydrophobic within the lipid bilayer. Most drugs, on the other hand, must have an affinity for water (i.e., hydrophilic) or they cannot dissolve and be transported by blood and other body fluids to their sites of action. The low water solubility of some active ingredients necessitates compounding the active ingredients with emulsifiers or complexing agents to prevent the drug from precipitating at the site of administration.

Several factors that favor the ability of a drug to cross membranes are listed in the box. Compounds that contain electrical charges or in which the electronic distribution is distorted toward one end of the molecule because of the nature of the atoms involved (imparts polarity to the compound) are not compatible with the uncharged nonpolar lipid environment. In addition the ordered structure of a lipid membrane does not allow many pores to exist; thus only small molecules of several hundred daltons in molecular weight normally can pass through the membrane. Large molecular weight proteins, for example, cannot pass through many membranes by simply dissolving in the membrane and diffusing to the other side. With proteins, active transport is often required, sometimes using carrier molecules to accomplish transmembrane transport. Most high molecular weight polypeptides and proteins cannot be administered orally because there are no mechanisms for their absorption from the GI tract, even if they could survive the high acidity of the stomach or the proteolytic enzymes of the GI tract.

As a general rule, drugs that have high lipid solubility cross membranes better than those with low lipid solubility. This is exemplified in Figure 5-1 for three different barbiturates. The oil/water equilibrium partition coefficient is a measure of the degree of lipid solubility. The drug is added to a mixture of equal volumes of oil and water and the mixture is agitated to promote solubilization of the compound

---

CHARACTERISTICS OF DRUG MOLECULES THAT FAVOR DRUG TRANSPORT ACROSS MEMBRANES

Uncharged	Low molecular weight
Nonpolar	High lipid solubility

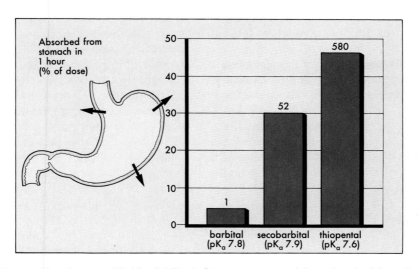

FIGURE 5-1   How increased lipid solubility influences amount of drug absorbed from the stomach for three barbiturate compounds. Number above each column is the oil/water equilibrium partition coefficient. The compounds have close pK_a values so that the degree of ionization will be the same in all three drugs.

in each phase. When equilibrium is attained, the phases are separated and assayed for drug. The ratio of the two concentrations becomes the partition coefficient. Therefore, larger numbers for the partition coefficient represent greater lipid solubility. Absorption across the stomach wall is greater for the barbiturate that has the largest lipid solubility (see Figure 5-1).

Many drugs, because of their chemical structure, behave as acids or bases in that they can take up or release a hydrogen ion. Within some ranges of pH, these drugs will carry an electrical charge, whereas in other pH ranges the compounds will be uncharged. It is the uncharged form of a drug that is lipid-soluble and therefore crosses biological membranes readily. In the barbiturate example, the compounds were selected so that the pK_a of each material was very similar. Otherwise, the differences in absorption could have been caused by variation in the degree of electrical charges on the three compounds. Further study of the pH influence will help predict the distribution of a drug between body compartments that differ in pH.

Influence on pH on Drug Distribution

The pH values of the major body fluids are shown in Table 5-1. The range is wide, from pH 1 to about pH 8. To predict how a drug will be distributed with gastric juice at pH 1.0 on one side of the membrane and blood at pH 7.4 on the other side, determine the degree of dissociation of the drug at each of these pH values.

An acid is defined as a compound that can dissociate and release a hydrogen ion; whereas a base can take up a hydrogen ion. By this definition,

RCOOH and RNH_3^+ are both acids and $RCOO^-$ and RNH_2 are bases. The equilibrium dissociation expression and the equilibrium dissociation constant (K_a) can be described for an acid HA or BH^+ and a base A^- or B as shown below. The convention for K_a requires that the acid appear on the left and the base on the right of the dissociation equation:

$$HA = A^- + H^+; \; K_a = \frac{(A^-)(H^+)}{(HA)} \qquad (1)$$

$$BH^+ = B + H^+; \; K_a = \frac{(B)(H^+)}{(BH^+)} \qquad (2)$$

The negative log of both sides gives

$$-\log K_a = -\log (H^+) -\log \frac{(A^-)}{(HA)} \qquad (3)$$

$$-\log K_a = -\log (H^+) -\log \frac{(B)}{(BH^+)} \qquad (4)$$

By definition the negative log of (H^+) is expressed as pH and the negative log of K_a is pK_a. Therefore equations 3 and 4 can be simplified and rearranged to give

$$pH = pK_a + \log \frac{(A^-)}{(HA)} \qquad (5)$$

$$pH = pK_a + \log \frac{(B)}{(BH^+)} \qquad (6)$$

Equations 5 and 6 are the acid and base forms, respectively, of the Henderson-Hasselbalch equation and can be used to calculate the pH of the solution when the pK_a and the ratios of $(A^-)/(HA)$ or $(B)/(BH^+)$ are known. In pharmacology it is often of interest to calculate the ratios of $(A^-)/(HA)$ or $(B)/(BH^+)$ when the pH and the pK_a are known. For this calculation equations 5 and 6 are rearranged to equations 7 and 8:

$$pH - pK_a = \log \frac{(A^-)}{(HA)} \qquad (7)$$

$$pH - pK_a = \log \frac{(B)}{(BH^+)} \qquad (8)$$

The results are plotted in Figure 5-2 to show the fraction of the nonionized (HA or B) forms. The pK_a is the pH when the drug is 50% dissociated. Applying equations 7 and 8 to an acidic drug with a pK_a of 6.0

Table 5-1 pH of Selected Body Fluids	
Fluids	**pH**
Gastric juice	1.0 to 3.0
Small intestine: duodenum	5.0 to 6.0
Small intestine: ileum	8
Large intestine	8
Plasma	7.4
Cerebrospinal fluid (CSF)	7.3
Urine	4.0 to 8.0

enables the degree of ionization to be calculated for this drug in the stomach or blood (assume the blood pH is 7.0 for ease of calculation) as follows:

Stomach: $1.0 - 6.0 = \log Y$; $\log Y = -5$, or $Y = 10^{-5}$; $Y = (A^-) / (HA) = 0.00001$; if [HA] is 1.0, then (A^-) is 0.00001 and the compound is ionized very little

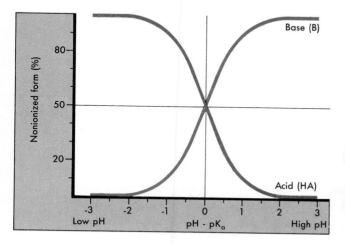

FIGURE 5-2   Degree of acidic or basic drug in nonionized (uncharged) form (*HA*, acid; *B*, base) at different pH values, with pH expressed relative to the drug pK_a.

Blood: $7.0 - 6.0 = \log Y$; $\log Y = +1$, or $Y = 10^{+1}$; $Y = (A^-) / (HA) = 10.0$; if [HA] is 1.0, then $[A^-]$ is 10.0 and the compound is ionized considerably

The drug is ionized very little in the stomach but appreciably in blood, so that the compound should cross readily in the stomach-to-plasma direction but hardly at all in the reverse direction.

Another example is shown in Figure 5-3 for a basic drug. This approach is particularly useful for predicting whether drugs can be absorbed in the stomach, upper intestine, or not at all. Figure 5-4 provides a summary of the pH effect on drug absorption in the GI tract for several acidic and several basic drugs. Another area of application is in predicting which drugs will undergo tubular reabsorption, which will be discussed later in this chapter.

Most drugs that cross membranes do so by simple passive diffusion. The concentration gradient across the membrane becomes the driving force that establishes the rate of diffusion, with the direction from the high towards the lower drug concentration. Other mechanisms of transmembrane drug transport such as active transport, facilitated diffusion, or pinocytosis occur, but trying to predict the type of transport expected for a specific drug and across a specific membrane type is difficult.

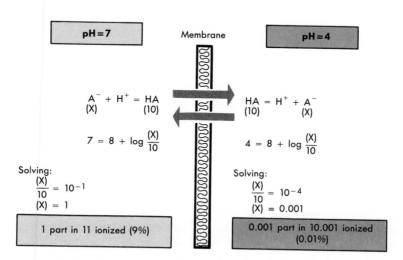

FIGURE 5-3   Equilibrium distribution of drug when pH is 4 on one side and 7 on the other side of membrane for an acid drug with a pK_a of 8.0. Nonionized form, HA, of the drug can readily cross the membrane. Thus, HA has the same concentration on both sides of the membrane. The concentration of nonionized drug is arbitrarily set at 10 µg/ml; and the expressions are solved to determine the concentration of ionized species at equilibrium.

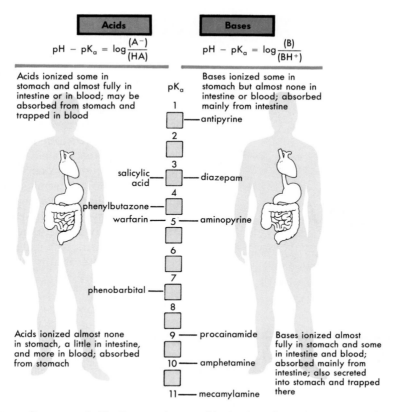

FIGURE 5-4   Summary of pH effect on degree of ionization of several acidic and basic drugs. Statements in corners refer to compounds with extremes of pK_a values and predict where drugs with the pK_as will be absorbed.

Distribution to Special Organs and Tissues

Blood flow rates set the maximum amount of drug per minute that can be delivered to specific organs and tissues at a given plasma concentration of drug. Tissues that are well perfused can receive a large quantity of drug, provided the drug can cross whatever membranes or other barriers are present between the plasma and the tissue. Similarly, tissues such as fat that are poorly perfused receive drug at a slow rate; so that the concentration of drug in fat may still be increasing long after the concentration in plasma has started to decrease.

Two areas of special importance are the brain and the fetus. Many drugs do not readily enter the brain. Capillaries in the brain differ structurally from those in other tissues, with the result that a barrier exists between blood within the brain capillaries and extra-cellular fluid in brain tissue. This "blood-brain barrier" hinders the transport of drugs and other materials from blood into brain tissue, or the reverse. The blood-brain barrier is found throughout the brain and spinal cord at all regions central to the arachnoid membrane, with the exception of the floor of the hypothalamus and the area postrema. The structural differences between brain and nonbrain capillaries and how these differences influence blood-brain transport of solutes are shown schematically in Figure 5-5. Nonbrain capillaries have fenestrations (openings) between the endothelial cells through which solutes move readily by passive diffusion, with compounds having molecular weights greater than about 25,000 daltons undergoing transport by pinocytosis. In brain capillaries tight junctions are present because there are no fenestrations, and pinocytosis appears to be markedly re-

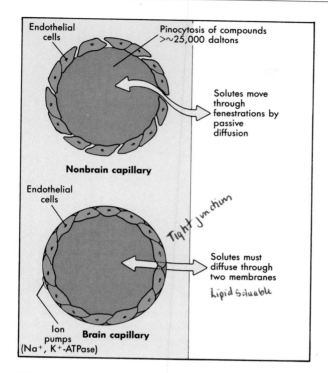

FIGURE 5-5 Structural differences between nonbrain and brain capillaries. In brain capillaries, lack of openings between endothelial cells in capillary wall requires drugs and other solutes to pass through two membranes to move from blood to tissue or the reverse. Ion pumps are mainly on the outer membrane of the brain endothelial cells and maintain a concentration difference between the two fluid regions.

duced. Special transport systems are available at brain capillaries for glucose, amino acids, amines, purines, nucleosides, and organic acids; all other materials apparently must cross the two endothelial membranes plus the endothelial cytoplasm to move from capillary blood to tissue extracellular fluid. Thus, the main route of drug entry into central nervous system (CNS) tissue appears to be by passive diffusion across membranes. This restricts the available compounds as potential drugs for treating brain disorders. At the same time, the potential effects of many compounds on the CNS are not known; for these compounds the blood-brain barrier acts as a safety buffer. The major problem arises from the lack of predictability — about whether or not a specific compound will readily enter brain tissue. Compounds such as salicylic acid or antipyrine (a base) follow the pH/pK_a relationship with only the un-ionized form crossing

into brain tissue. The only other generalization that can be made now is that most highly lipid soluble drugs cross the blood-brain barrier. In infants and the elderly, the blood-brain barrier may not be completely intact and drugs may diffuse into the brain.

An alternative approach for drug delivery to brain tissue is by intrathecal injection into the subarachnoid space and the cerebrospinal fluid (CSF). However, injection into the subarachnoid space can be difficult to perform safely because of the small volume of this region and the close proximity to easily damaged nerves. In addition, drug distribution within the CSF and across the CSF-brain barrier can be slow and show large interpatient variations; however, for some drugs there may not be another route.

One of the most difficult areas of pharmacology research is to assess the degree to which specific drugs cross the placenta and enter the fetal circulation and the potential pharmacologic, toxic, or teratogenic effects. There are a number of drugs that readily cross the placenta in humans at maternal therapeutic concentrations that have no known detrimental effects. For further discussion see Chapter 63.

METABOLISM AND ELIMINATION OF DRUGS

The term *elimination* refers to the removal of drug without any chemical changes being involved. For some drugs this is the only route of disappearance; for most drugs only some of the dose is removed unchanged. Elimination of drugs occurs mainly via renal mechanisms into the urine and to some extent via mixing with bile salts for solubilization followed by transport into the intestinal tract. The term *metabolism* and biotransformation refer to the disappearance of drug by chemically changing it to another compound, termed a *metabolite*. Some drugs are administered as inactive "prodrugs" that must metabolize into the pharamacologically active form. Although drug metabolism occurs largely in the liver, most other tissues and organs, especially the lung, carry out varying degrees of drug metabolism. A few drugs become essentially irreversibly bound to tissues and are metabolized or otherwise removed over long periods of time. Finally, drugs also may be excreted in feces, exhaled through lungs, or secreted through sweat or salivary glands.

Metabolism of Drugs

When drugs are metabolized, the change is usually an increase in water solubility often accompanied by a decrease in lipid solubility and/or an increase in the polarity of the products. The end result is the production of compounds that can more readily participate in renal elimination. Some drugs are administered as prodrugs in an inactive or less active form to promote absorption, to overcome potential destruction by stomach acidity, or to minimize exposure to highly reactive chemical species. Thus use is made of drug metabolizing systems to convert the prodrug into a more active species on entry into the systemic circulation. In other situations, drugs that are administered as the active species are metabolized to form products, which may be "active" and produce pharmacological effects similar to or different from those generated by the parent drug. An example is diazepam (Figure 5-6), an antianxiety compound that is metabolized to remove a methyl group and produce an active metabolite. The half-life of the parent drug is about 30 hours whereas that of the metabolite averages about 70 hours. Thus the effect of the metabolite is present long after the parent drug has disappeared. In this case the magnitude of the pharmacological effect is much less for the metabolite than for the parent drug, but in general the lingering presence of active metabolites makes the precise control of the magnitude of pharmacological effect harder to achieve. In the case of diazepam the therapeutic index is large enough so that precise control is not required.

Drug metabolism takes place primarily in the liver, through microsomal and in some cases nonmicrosomal enzyme systems. However, considerable drug metabolizing capability often is found in other body sites, including the placenta, GI tract bacteria, intestinal wall, pulmonary tissue, and cardiac cells.

Although a myriad of different types of chemical reactions are observed in drug metabolism, most of the reactions can be categorized into the following four groups:

Oxidation
Conjugation
Reduction
Hydrolysis

Oxidation and conjugation are most important and will be discussed further. Simple examples will be given for reduction and hydrolysis.

Oxidation can take place at many different sites

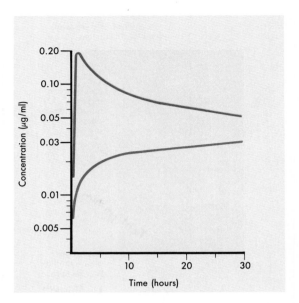

FIGURE 5-6   Plasma concentration of diazepam *(red line)* and its main metabolite *(blue line)* after a single oral dose of 10 mg of diazepam in humans. The metabolite is desmethyldiazepam.

on a drug molecule and can appear as one of several hundred different forms of reaction. Typically, an oxygen atom may be inserted to convert $-CH_2$ to $-CHOH-$ or $-CH(NH_2)-$ to $-C(=O)-$. By definition, an oxidation reaction requires the transfer of one or more electrons, and an important aspect is to define the group that acts as the final electron acceptor. A large fraction of drug oxidation reactions are thought to operate under the control of the cytochrome P-450 mixed function oxidase system. The overall net reaction can be summarized as

$$R + NAD(P)H + H^+ + O_2 = RO + NAD(P)^+ + H_2O$$

where

R = the drug

NADH or NADPH = reduced nicotinamide adeninedinucleotide cofactors

NAD or NADP = oxidized cofactors

In this reaction molecular oxygen serves as the final electron acceptor. Cytochrome P-450s are a family of iron-containing proteins that include flavin and NADP and NAD cofactor electron and proton transfer components. The iron undergoes a cycle that starts in the ferric oxidation state, when the drug binds to cytochrome P-450, and includes reduction to the ferrous state, activation of oxygen, and eventual regeneration of the ferric state. Free radical or ion-radical groups

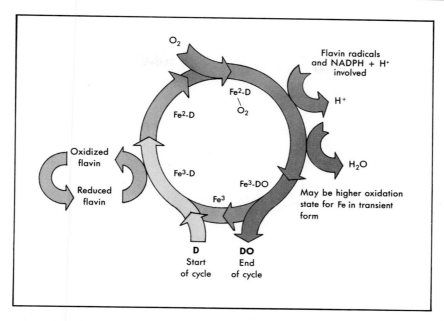

FIGURE 5-7   Simplified model of cytochrome P-450 mixed function oxidase reaction sequence. *D* is the drug undergoing oxidation to product *DO*. Molecular oxygen serves as the final electron acceptor. Flavin cofactor systems are involved at several sites. The iron of the cytochrome P-450 is involved in binding and electron transfer with changes in valance state.

are thought to be formed at one or more parts of the cycle. The subcellular site of this enzyme system is the endoplasmic reticulum. The reaction cycle is summarized in Figure 5-7. Cytochrome P-450s are very complex systems of enzymes in which the detailed molecular chemistry is still under investigation. Such detailed information will be helpful in the development of safer drugs. If drug metabolism via the cytochrome P-450 route leads to the generation of highly reactive free radical groups, then this must be taken into consideration in drug design to minimize the formation of reactive and potentially toxic drug metabolites.

Conjugation, the second major type of drug metabolism, involves coupling another group to the drug molecule so the resulting product will have greater water solubility or other features for enhanced renal or biliary elimination. Conjugation, just like other metabolism processes, requires the presence of drug metabolizing enzymes. In addition, the groups that are being coupled need to be "activated" through the participation of high energy phosphate compounds. For example, glucuronic acid can be conjugated, in the presence of the enzyme UDP-glucuronosyl transferase, to compounds of the general types ROH, RCOOH, RNH_2, or RSH, where R represents the remainder of the drug molecule. However, first the glucuronic acid must be activated. This occurs by reaction of glucose-1-phosphate with uridine triphosphate followed by oxidation of the resulting product to activated glucuronic acid. The reaction sequence is shown in Figure 5-8 for the formation of the ROH glucuronide of salicylic acid. Another glucuronide could be formed through conjugation with the RCOOH group. Several endogenous materials, including bilirubin, thyroxine, and steroids also undergo conjugation with activated glucuronic acid in the presence of UDP-glucuronosyl transferase. Conjugation occurs with activated glycine, acetate, sulfate, and other groups besides glucuronate.

Considerable research has been expended, with partial success, in an attempt to find a method for assessing the oxidative drug-metabolizing capability in individual patients. Antipyrine has given the most useful data so far. This compound is rapidly and completely absorbed from the GI tract, distributed in total body water, and removed completely by metabolism. Continuing research is needed to develop the practicality of this material for assessing hepatic drug metabolizing activity.

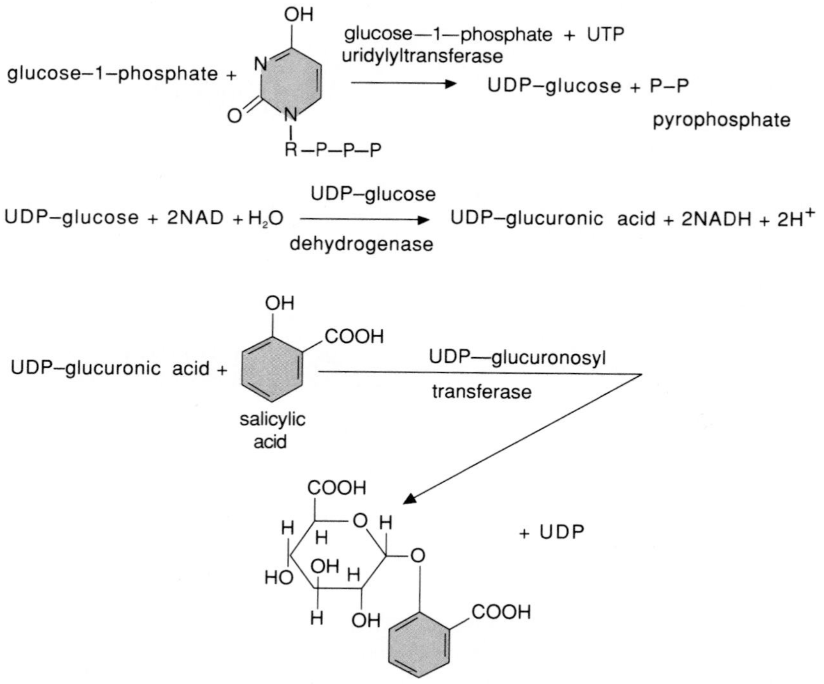

FIGURE 5-8   Sequence of reactions for conjugation of salicylic acid to form salicyl phenolic glucuronide. *P* is phosphate. Enzyme names are from IUB nomenclature listing. The glucuronic acid must first be activated, with glucose-1-phosphate coupling with high energy UTP to UDP-glucose, oxidation to UDP-glucuronic acid before conjugation can occur.

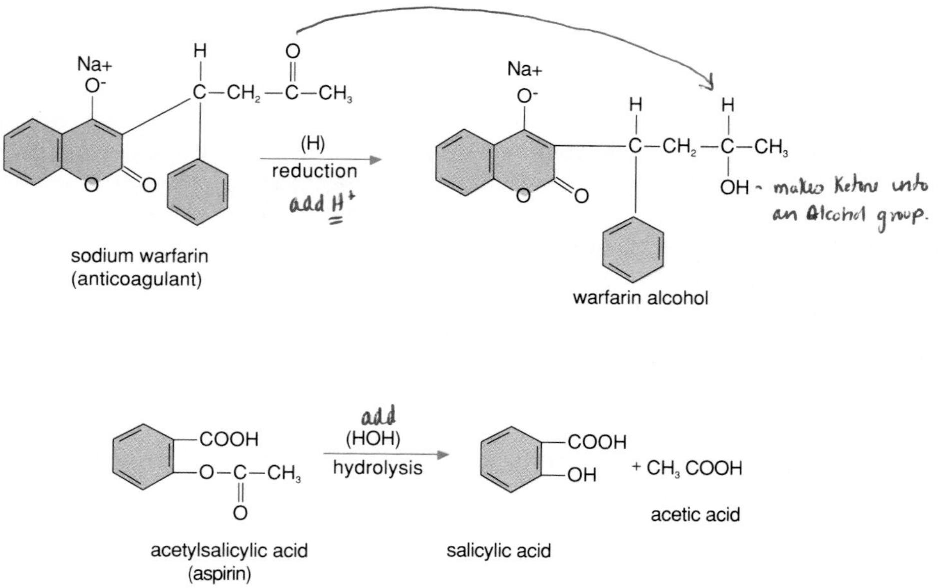

FIGURE 5-9   Representative reduction and hydrolysis reactions for metabolism of drugs.

Typical drug metabolism reduction and hydrolysis reactions are shown in Figure 5-9.

Drug Metabolizing Enzyme Kinetic Factors

Numerous chemical reactions that participate in the metabolism of drugs are governed by enzyme catalysts. Therefore, the kinetics of drug metabolism can be approximated by the single substrate relationship

$$v = \frac{V_{max}(S)}{K + (S)} \qquad (9)$$

In this expression

v = rate of reaction
V_{max} = maximum rate of reaction
(S) = concentration of drug
K = Michaelis constant

V_{max} is directly proportional to the concentration of enzyme. If a change occurs in the concentration of enzyme, there should be a proportional change in the rate of drug metabolism.

A wide variety of drugs, environmental chemicals, air pollutants, and components of cigarette smoke stimulate the synthesis of higher concentrations of drug-metabolizing enzymes. This process, termed *enzyme induction*, can be used clinically to elevate the level of hepatic drug-metabolizing enzymes. In the treatment of drug overdoses it is sometimes useful to stimulate enzyme induction to increase the rate of drug metabolism. Enzyme induction can be achieved clinically by the administration of barbiturates; however, the induction can be observed after about 24 hours in humans. An example is how phenobarbital and a highly reactive air pollutant, 3,4-benzo(a)pyrene, can increase the rate of oxidation of a CNS muscle relaxant, zoxazolamine, in an animal study (Figure 5-10). Chronic cigarette smokers have markedly higher levels of hepatic and lung drug-metabolizing enzymes, especially aryl hydroxylase.

Drug metabolism reactions typically follow first order kinetics in humans receiving therapeutic concentrations of drugs. Equation 9 reduces to a first order expression when the concentration of drug is much smaller than the Michaelis constant. Thus, for nearly all drugs within their normal therapeutic range of concentrations, the hepatic or other drug metabolizing systems operate far from saturation. An exception is the metabolism of salicylic acid in humans, in which saturation of the available enzymes can occur at elevated drug concentrations. Aspirin is used extensively for the treatment of inflammatory diseases, with the optimum therapeutic concentration only slightly below the concentration where signs of

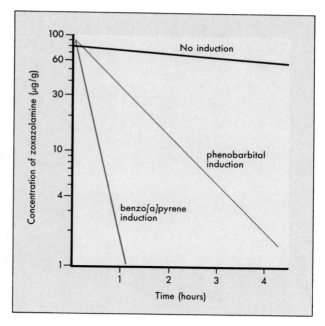

FIGURE 5-10   Example of enzyme induction. Zoxazolamine administered by intraperitoneal injection to rats. For induction studies phenobarbital or 3,4l-benzo[a]pyrene were injected twice daily for 4 days before injection of the zoxazolamine. Drug concentration is expressed as μg drug / gram of tissue.

toxicity begin to appear. Aspirin is hydrolyzed to salicylic acid, which in turn has several routes for elimination (Figure 5-11). Two salicylic acid metabolism pathways are subject to saturation in humans: (1) conjugation with glycine to form salicyuric acid and (2) conjugation with glucuronic acid to form salicyl phenolic glucuronide. For enzyme saturation, the kinetics change to zero order and the rate of reaction becomes constant at V_{max}. This is consistent with equation 9 when (S) is much larger than K. Saturation of drug-metabolizing enzymes has a marked influence on drug plateau concentrations.

Hepatic and Biliary Clearance

Hepatic clearance, $(Cl)_h$, can be defined as

$$\frac{\text{rate of hepatic removal of drug}}{\text{concentration of drug in portal vein}} \qquad (10)$$

Likewise, biliary clearance, $(Cl)_b$, can be defined in a similar manner with the bile flow rate times the drug concentration in the bile a measure of the rate of biliary removal of drug. Direct measurement of he-

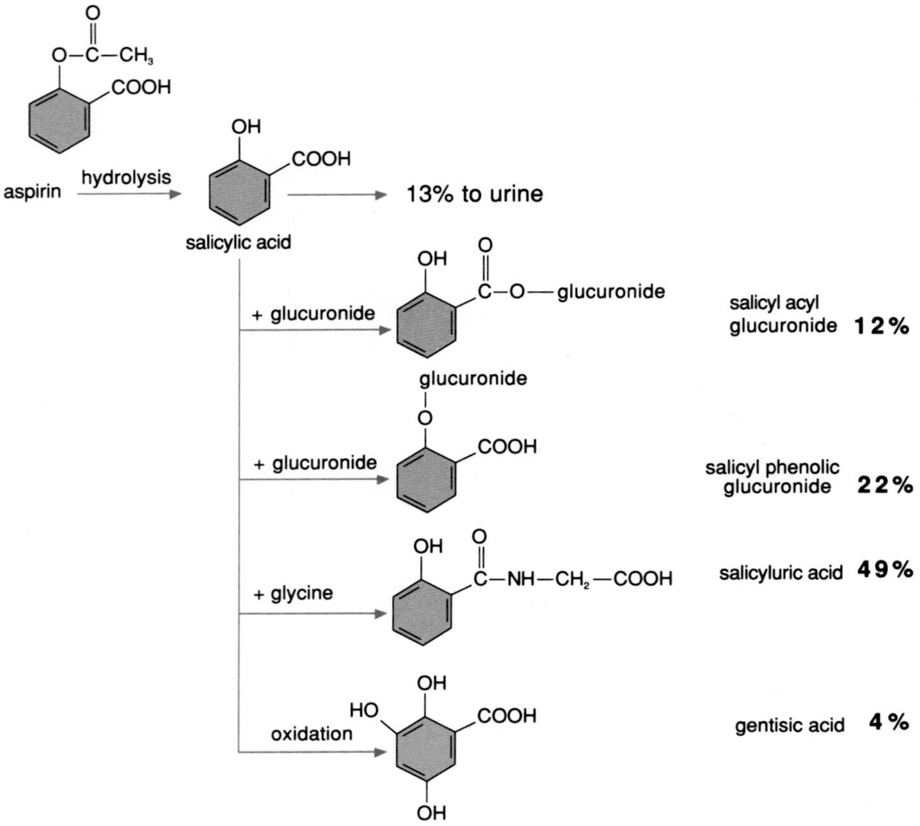

FIGURE 5-11   Disposition of main metabolite of aspirin, salicylic acid, at a single dose of 4 grams (54 mg/kg body weight) in a healthy adult. The % values refer to the dose. Oxidation produces a mixture of ortho and para (relative to original OH group) isomers.

patic or biliary clearance in humans is not practical because of the high risk in obtaining appropriate blood samples. The concept of hepatic and biliary clearance is included here to emphasize that the concept of clearance can be applied to any body region or organ system, as long as sample points can be designated.

A complicating result of biliary elimination of a drug sometimes occurs when the drug is reabsorbed from the GI tract and returned to the systemic circulation. This is termed *enterohepatic cycling,* and can result in a measurable increase in the plasma concentration of drug several half-lives after the drug originally was administered.

Renal Elimination of Drugs

The removal of unchanged drug via the renal route is one of the processes that is included in "total body

clearance," $(Cl)_p$, as defined in the previous chapter. The same general definition of clearance can also be applied to the renal route to define the *renal clearance,* $(Cl)_r$, as the volume of plasma that needs to be cleared per unit time to account for the rate of drug removal that takes place in the kidneys. This definition can be expressed in equation form as

$$(Cl)_r = \frac{\text{rate of drug removal by the kidneys}}{\text{plasma concentration of drug in renal artery}} \quad (11)$$

Renal clearance has the units of volume/time, the same as total body clearance. For a drug such as the antibiotic cephalexin that is removed entirely by renal elimination, the renal clearance and the total body clearance are equal. In this example the renal clearance can be determined from plasma data, by plotting log plasma concentration of cephalexin versus time after an IV injection. For other drugs, where only part of the dose is removed by renal elimination, data must be obtained for the appearance of unchanged drug in the urine to calculate the renal clearance. For example, the rate of drug removal via the renal route can be estimated by collecting urine volumes over known time intervals and assaying each urine volume for the concentration of unchanged drug. If the rates of drug removal are plotted against the mean plasma concentration of drug for each urine volume interval, the slope will be an estimate of the renal clearance of that drug. Other techniques are available for the determination of renal clearance, but their use is limited primarily to research studies. The interested reader is referred to pharmacokinetics texts for a discussion of these techniques.

The mechanisms by which the renal clearance of drugs takes place are the same as those responsible for the renal elimination of endogenous substances. Glomerular filtration, tubular secretion, and tubular reabsorption are the three mechanisms (Figure 5-12).

Molecules smaller than those of about 50,000 molecular weight pass through the glomeruli, with approximately 125 ml of plasma cleared each minute in a healthy adult. This figure of 125 ml/min is independent of the plasma concentration of drug, so that removal by glomerular filtration, expressed in mg/min, shows a linear increase with higher plasma concentration of drug in the renal artery. The glomerular filtration rate of 125 ml/min represents less than 10% of the total renal plasma flow of 650 to 750 ml/min, indicating that only a small fraction of the total renal plasma flow is cleared of drug by this mechanism on each pass through the kidneys. Because albumin and other plasma protein molecules do not pass through the glomeruli, any drug molecules that are bound to these plasma proteins also are retained. Inulin and creatinine are two compounds that can be used to assess the glomerular filtration capability of renal function in individual patients because these materials show very little binding to plasma proteins and do not undergo appreciable tubular secretion or reabsorption. These materials will be discussed later in regard to dosing schedules for patients who have impaired renal function.

Tubular secretion is the second mechanism for renal clearance of drugs. This is an active process that occurs in the proximal tubule, with different details pertinent to the secretion of acids and bases. Compounds that are secreted usually also undergo glomerular filtration, so that renal clearance is due to the sum of both routes. Because tubular secretion in-

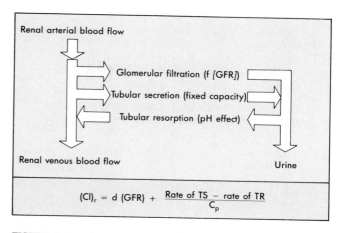

FIGURE 5-12 Summary of renal clearance mechanisms. *f,* Fraction of drug in plasma not bound; *GFR,* glomerular filtration rate of drug; *TS,* tubular secretion of drug; *TR,* tubular resorption of drug; C_p, renal arterial blood concentration of drug.

$$(Cl)_r = d\,(GFR) + \frac{\text{Rate of TS} - \text{rate of TR}}{C_p}$$

volves active transport by carrier groups and there are a limited number of carrier groups, the process can become saturated. The volume of plasma that can be cleared per unit time by tubular secretion varies with the concentration of drug in the plasma. This is in contrast to glomerular filtration where the *volume filtered per unit time* is independent of the plasma concentration of drug. At very low plasma concentrations of drug, tubular secretion can operate at its maximum rate of clearing 650 ml/min. If the concentration of drug in the arterial plasma is 4 ng/ml, then clearing 650 ml/min removes 2600 ng each minute. If the concentration of the same drug increases to 200 ng/ml and tubular secretion is saturated at the previous condition, the tubules will still only remove 2600 ng/min by secretion, so that the clearance by tubular secretion falls to 13 ml/min. If drug disappearance studies show that the renal clearance is considerably greater than 125 ml/min, the tubular secretion is involved because there is no other way to explain such a high clearance. In tubular secretion, both bound and free drug is removed. The transit time along the tubules is long enough so that binding dissociation can take place for those compounds in which the concentration change along the tubule is sufficient to shift the binding equilibrium and release additional drug.

The third mechanism in the renal clearance of drugs is reabsorption of filtered or secreted drug from the tubules back into the venous blood of the neph-

Table 5-2 Effect of Urine pH on Renal Clearance for Drugs that Undergo Tubular Resorption

Bases	Acids
CLEARED RAPIDLY BY MAKING URINE MORE ACIDIC	CLEARED RAPIDLY BY MAKING URINE MORE ALKALINE
amphetamine	acetazolamide
chloroquine	nitrofurantoin
imipramine	phenobarbital
levophanol	probenecid
mecamylamine	salicylates
quinine	sulfathiazole

rons. Although this process may be active or passive, for most drugs it occurs by simple passive diffusion. Drugs that are readily reabsorbed are characterized by high lipid solubility or by a significant fraction of the drug in a nonionized form at urine pH and in the ionized form at plasma pH. For example, salicylic acid with a pK_a of 3.0 is about 99.99% in the ionized form at pH 7.4 (per equation 5) but only about 90% ionized at pH 4.0. Thus, some reabsorption of salicylic acid could be expected from acidic urine. In drug overdose, the manipulation of urine pH is sometimes used to prevent reabsorption. Ammonium chloride administration leads to acidification of the urine and sodium bicarbonate administration to alkalinization. Some additional examples are given in Table 5-2.

Modified Renal Function and Drug Elimination The renal clearance of drugs may be less in neonates, geriatric patients, and those with improperly functioning kidneys. The effects of patient age on renal clearance of drugs are discussed in Chapter 7, 63, and 64. The modification of dosing regimens to compensate for changing renal function is discussed here.

The following situation is typical:

1. It is desired to use a particular drug in a patient
2. This drug usually is disposed of primarily through renal elimination
3. The patient's renal function is inadequate

The question is whether or not a safe dosing schedule can be worked out for the desired drug in this patient. In many cases the answer is yes. However, some measure of the degree of renal function is necessary. Creatinine clearance is a standard clinical determi-

nation that can be used to obtain an approximate measure of renal function. Creatinine is usually selected instead of the more accurate inulin clearance because endogenous creatinine can be used and because the assay and methodology with inulin are more difficult. Urine is collected over a known period of time (often 24 hours), pooled, the volume measured, and the urine assayed for creatinine. At the midpoint of the urine collection period, a plasma sample is obtained and assayed for creatinine. The creatinine clearance is calculated from equation 12 as follows:

$$(Cl)_{Cr} = \frac{\left(\text{Conc. Cr. } \frac{mg}{\text{in urine, } ml \text{ urine}}\right)(\text{Vol. urine, } ml)}{\left(\text{Urine collect time interval, } min\right)\left(\text{Conc. Cr } \frac{mg}{\text{in plasma, } ml \text{ plasma}}\right)} \quad (12)$$

$$= \frac{ml \text{ plasma}}{min}$$

Determination of the creatinine clearance for the patient gives a measure of glomerular filtration function. In addition it must be demonstrated what relationship exists between the rate constant for renal elimination of unchanged drug and creatinine clearance. For the usual case of first-order renal elimination the relationship is linear, so that a creatinine clearance of 50% of normal means that renal elimination of this drug would be expected to operate at 50% and the rate of drug input should be reduced accordingly. For example, a drug that is administered 100 mg every 6 hours (400 mg in 24 hours) to a patient with normal creatinine clearance could be given 40 mg every 12 hours (80 mg in 24 hours) if the creatinine clearance decreased to only 20% of normal. In this example any other pathways for disappearance of this drug retain their normal functionality.

Extraction Ratio

An alternative approach to the calculation of renal clearance or hepatic clearance is to multiply the blood flow rate to the organ by the extraction ratio. This ratio is the fraction of drug removed from each unit volume of blood per pass through the kidneys or liver, respectively. For drugs with a high extraction ratio, the limiting step in drug removal is the rate of delivery to the organ, (i.e., the blood flow rate). At the other extreme, (i.e., a low extraction ratio) the rate of removal of drugs is little influenced by blood flow rate but is strongly influenced by changes in the degree of plasma protein binding of the drug. The extraction ratio is a valid alternative approach for clearance concepts; however, few experimental results are available to apply this approach to humans other than as a research tool.

SUMMARY

The multiple routes for the disposition of aspirin and its hydrolysis product, salicylic acid (see Figure 5-11), represent the complexity of drug disappearance. Understanding the major routes of disposition of a drug and the factors that influence the functionality and capacity of each route can aid profoundly in the safe and effective use of drugs, especially in patients in which the state of the disease has compromised one or more of the main drug disposition routes.

REFERENCES

Baselt RC: Disposition of toxic drugs and chemicals in man, ed. 2, Davis, Calif, 1982, Biomedical Publications.

Guengerich FP and Macdonald TL: Chemical mechanisms of catalysis by cytochromes P-450: a unified view, Acc Chem Res 17:9, 1984.

LaDu, BN, Mandel HG, and Way EL, eds: Fundamentals of drug metabolism and drug disposition, Baltimore, 1971, Williams & Wilkins Co.

Lewis DVF: Physical methods in the study of the active site geometry of cytochromes P-450, Drug Metab Rev 17:1, 1986.

CHAPTER  6   Drug Delivery Approaches

---

ABBREVIATIONS

IM	intramuscular, intramuscularly
IV	intravenous, intravenously
pH	logarithm of the reciprocal of the hydrogen ion concentration
SC	subcutaneous, subcutaneously

DELIVERY GOALS

Direct placement of drugs into the oral or gastrointestinal (GI) cavities via discrete multiple doses for absorption is the major mode of drug administration for hospitalized and nonhospitalized patients. With this mode of administration, the plasma concentration of drug rises and falls during a dosing interval, even if the mean concentration has reached a plateau. Depending on the length of the dosing interval in relation to the disappearance half-life of the drug, the concentration may decrease below the minimum effective concentration for a significant portion of the dosing interval. In addition, the drug is distributed throughout the entire circulatory system and into many different tissue beds, even though the site of therapeutic action may be localized to a single organ or tissue type.

Clinically, it is therapeutically advantageous with some drug types (1) to minimize fluctuations in plasma drug concentration, (2) to be able to target drugs to the site of therapeutic action with minimal exposure of other body compartments to unwanted effects of the drug, and (3) for the rate of drug delivery to vary depending on the measured concentration of some constituent in blood or other body fluid. Some clinical progress has been made in achieving each of these delivery goals for certain drugs.

PROLONGED RELEASE PREPARATIONS

With drug administration by discrete multiple doses, there is rise and fall in drug concentration during the span of a dosing interval. Often this is not desirable. The disease may not be so threatening that the added hazards, patient discomfort, and cost of an IV infusion can be justified simply to diminish the amplitude of the concentration oscillations or to ensure that the concentration remains above the minimum effective concentration throughout the dosing interval. In a large number of these situations, added therapeutic benefit can be realized with fluctuations. One approach is to administer a larger dose but to extend the duration of drug absorption over a longer time interval. A wide variety of clinically available dosage forms with extended drug release–absorption have become available as "sustained-release" pharmaceutical preparations.

One approach involves coating drug tablets with materials that dissolve slowly in the GI tract or at IM or SC injection sites. Other approaches include administration of the drug as a drug-salt or as a drug-ion exchange resin complex, which undergo slow dissociation before absorption. Some sustained-release

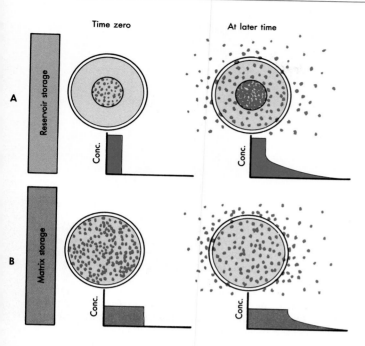

Time zero   At later time

A   Reservoir storage

B   Matrix storage

FIGURE 6-1   Diffusional release of drug from drug-polymer system in which drug is stored in a reservoir surrounded by the polymer or stored dispersed within the polymer matrix. See text for further discussion.

GENERAL CATEGORIES OF DRUG-POLYMER RELEASE MECHANISMS

Diffusional migration of drug
Chemical reaction of polymer or drug linkages with
    body constituents
Magnetic control of release rates
Solvent action on polymer release of drug

preparations prolong drug release and absorption for up to 15 to 20 hours; however, release rates may vary as a result of local fluctuations in pH.

Relatively constant drug release rates, not influenced by pH or other factors, can be obtained by the use of drug-polymer systems. These are designed to release drug at a relatively constant rate. The approaches employing polymer systems can be divided into the four categories listed in the box. Each is described; however, only the first category is widely used clinically.

Diffusional release of drug from an implanted polymer system is shown schematically in Figure 6-1. Two types of drug storage arrangements are available. In Figure 6-1, *A*, the drug is stored in a hollow reservoir within the polymer container, and the rate of drug release is dependent on the steepness of the concentration gradient between the reservoir and the fluid surrounding the delivery device. The steeper the gradient, the more rapid the rate of release for a given polymer system. The rate of release also is dependent on the diffusion coefficient for the random migration of drug molecules through the tangled polymer chains. In an alternative drug storage arrangement (see Figure 6-1, *B*), the drug is distributed uniformly throughout the polymer matrix, but the rate of release is dependent on the concentration gradient and the drug diffusion coefficient within the matrix.

The reservoir devices are expensive and have the inherent disadvantage of releasing a large quantity of drug if the device has a mechanical rupture or defects. However, mechanical damage to a matrix storage device would not cause the sudden release of drug. For very small molecular weight drugs (i.e., 100 to 200 daltons), diffusional control of the release rate is more difficult to maintain than with larger molecular weight compounds without resorting to thicker membranes of very tightly crosslinked polymers and thus larger devices. With either storage arrangement the stability of the drug for prolonged holding at 37° C without significant degradation is a factor that must be proven for each drug-polymer system.

A wide variety of alternatives exist for the anatomical placement of diffusional drug release devices. The controlled delivery of drugs to the eye and to the systemic circulation are two of the examples that are currently in clinical use. Pilocarpine is normally administered several times a day as eyedrops for the treatment of glaucoma. However, reservoir-type diffusional release devices (Figure 6-2) are available for insertion under the lower eyelid. These deliver pilocarpine at a constant rate for up to a week and thus give continuous, instead of intermittent, exposure of the eye to pilocarpine. In addition, transdermal matrix storage diffusional delivery devices are in clinical use, for example, for placement on the skin to deliver scopolamine for the prevention of motion sickness, nitroglycerin for the treatment of cardiac angina (Figure 6-3), estradiol for the treatment of menopausal problems, and clonidine for the systemic treatment of hypertension.

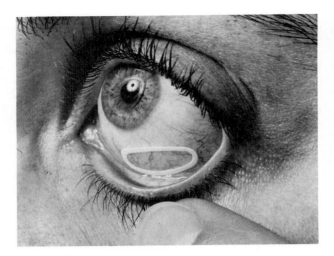

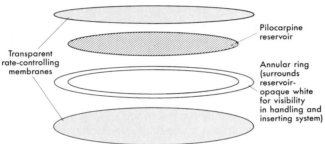

FIGURE 6-2   Ocusert ocular therapeutic system for delivery of pilocarpine (see Chapter 9) for treatment of glaucoma. Flexible wafer is placed under the eyelid and provides drug for a week. Eyelid is shown displaced to expose device. The expanded view denotes the purpose of each of the components. (Courtesy ALZA Corporation.)

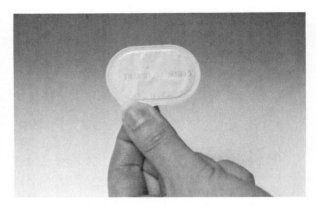

FIGURE 6-3   Transderm-Nitro delivery system for controlled release of nitroglycerin for prevention of angina (see Chapter 17). Patches are applied via an adhesive surface usually on the chest. Nitroglycerin diffuses from the matrix at a controlled rate of about 0.02 mg/cm²/hr and is absorbed through the skin into the systemic circulation. A typical intermittent dosage schedule of 12 to 14 hours with the patch on, followed by 10 to 12 hours off, provides drug delivery at 0.4 mg/hr. The intermittent schedule reduces development of tolerance. A new patch is used every day. (Courtesy Summit Pharmaceuticals, Division of CIBA-GEIGY Corporation.)

Transdermal diffusional drug delivery devices operate on the principle that diffusion through the polymer membrane is the slowest and therefore the rate controlling step. The skin location where the device is placed must be free of a hard epidermal layer so that transport through the skin does not become rate controlling. Transdermal delivery of drugs may be advantageous for certain compounds in that the liver first pass effect, transit through the highly acidic gastric region, and exposure to digestive enzymes all are bypassed. In addition, the duration of drug administration can be stopped or extended as needed, and the problem of patient compliance usually is less than with repeated oral dosing. However, a drug must have

enough lipid solubility to pass through the skin at an appreciable rate to be suitable for transdermal delivery.

The second category of drug-polymer release is release by chemical reaction. Two approaches appear promising: chemical erosion of the polymer matrix and chemical release of pendant drug molecules covalently attached to polymer chains (Figure 6-4). For the chemical erosion approach, the polymers undergoing clinical trials are selected such that endogenous hydrolytic enzymes catalyze polymer cleavage. As the polymer matrix disintegrates, drug is uniformly distributed throughout the matrix and is released into the surrounding body fluid. Likewise, hydrolytic enzymes present in body fluids catalyze the cleavage of pendant drug molecules from polymer chains in the second approach. Both approaches require the careful selection of polymers to ensure that the products of the polymer erosion are nontoxic. In addition, disposition of the polymer remaining after release of the pendant drug may require surgical removal, if the preparation initially was inserted via surgical implantation.

The third and fourth categories of drug-polymer release mechanisms have only research use (see box).

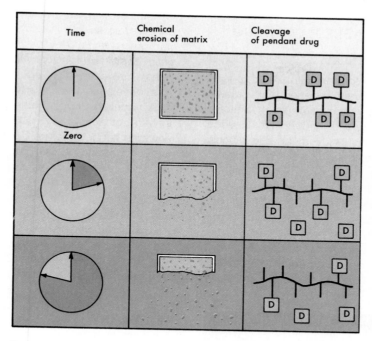

| Time | Chemical erosion of matrix | Cleavage of pendant drug |

FIGURE 6-4   Drug release by chemical reaction. One approach involves chemical erosion of the polymer matrix and co-release of drug distributed throughout the matrix. The other involves chemical cleavage of drug attached covalently to polymer chains.

One category uses magnetic materials dispersed throughout the drug-polymer matrix, with the diffusionally controlled rate of release of drug augmented by imposition of an oscillating magnetic field. The other category uses solvent action to raise the osmotic pressure in the space surrounding an implanted drug-filled container, with the increased pressure forcing drug solution out a small opening in the device. Routine clinical use of the latter two categories remain under investigation.

TARGETING OF DRUGS

Drugs that are administered for eradication of tumor cells will be most effective if delivered primarily to the tumor and minimally to other parts of the body. Likewise, a disorder within the central nervous system (CNS) or a severe infection within the pulmonary cavity may be more aggressively treated with drugs if the delivery can be targeted to the CNS or pulmonary spaces, respectively. Current extensive research examines cellular, physiological, and anatomical differences between diseased and normal tissues or between different body tissues for leads that may be exploited for purposes of targeting drugs to those cells or tissues. For example, drug-filled albumin microspheres 15 to 30 μm in diameter deposit nearly 99% in pulmonary capillary beds after IV injection but lodge about 90% in the liver if the microsphere diameter is reduced to 1 to 3 μm. The IV injection of drug-filled microspheres may become a clinically useful means of targeting drugs to these two organs, if the safety considerations caused by plugged capillary beds and scavenging of partially disintegrated albumin spheres from the circulatory system can be resolved favorably.

Another example is the use of carrier molecules, such as glycoproteins or antibodies with recognition sites on the surface of cells of the target organ or tissue. Cell surface glycoproteins, attached to liposomes, viral envelopes, and erythrocyte ghosts (empty red cell membranes) are under study as carriers. In particular, antibodies against tumor cell-surface antigens are under clinical study as carriers for targeting drugs to specific types of tumors.

CONTROLLED VARIABLE RATE DRUG DELIVERY

The delivery of insulin for control of blood glucose concentrations in type I insulin-dependent diabetes mellitus patients is the prime example in which a controlled yet variable rate of drug delivery is needed. Ideally, closed loop control with an in vivo glucose sensor continuously monitoring the level of blood glucose and directing the operation of an implanted, rechargeable insulin delivery pump is viewed as the needed device. Actually, all of the components for such a device are available and workable except that of the glucose sensor. As a result of the lack of a suitable sensor for in vivo measurement of glucose concentrations, insulin delivery pumps (Figure 6-5) have been used in patients on an open loop basis,

with blood sampling, and in vitro assay for glucose concentrations followed by manual correction of the pumping rate. Patient trials show therapeutic benefits with improved control of blood glucose concentrations; however, costs are high and some problems have developed, particularly with patient compliance.

A variety of implantable pumps are available for infusion of drug by IV, SC or IM modes. Pumps are powered by batteries or by vapor pressure of a fluorocarbon sealed within the pump unit. Pump reservoirs hold 25 to 35 ml of drug solution. Problems such as thermal stability of the drug for prolonged storage at body temperature, clogging of the outlet orifice, and refilling of the pump reservoir remain to be solved. A significant number of clinical applications are evident for open loop, as well as closed loop, delivery of drugs in the endocrine, CNS, anticancer, and immunosuppressant areas.

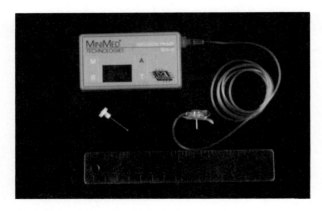

FIGURE 6-5 MiniMed pump, connecting tubing, and Sof-set infusion set for programmable subcutaneous delivery of drugs over several days. This system is used clinically to deliver insulin to ambulatory insulin-dependent diabetes mellitus patients (see Chapter 39). Wristwatch-sized batteries drive a motor that depresses a 3 ml syringe plunger to deliver insulin at a basal rate, programmable in 0.1 insulin units/hour increments, with bolus additions for meals added when and in amounts selected by the user. The syringe-tubing Sof-set unit and the infusion site are changed at 2 to 3 day intervals. The beeper-sized package contains the pump, computer, batteries, and syringe. The Sof-set unit is shown with the 26-gauge introducer needle removed (placed near the ruler) and with the flexible Teflon cannula (which remains subcutaneous) and adhesive patch (which goes directly on the skin) exposed. At a typical insulin supply concentration of 100 units/ml and a basal delivery rate of 1 unit/hr, the pump delivers 10 μl/hr. (Courtesy MiniMed Technologies.)

SUMMARY

Nontraditional methods of drug delivery are becoming more commonplace as the research in drug delivery techniques is reduced to clinical practice. Maintenance of constant drug concentrations at sites of drug action, targeting of highly toxic drugs to diminish deleterious side effects, and development of methods for feedback control of drug release rates all appear to be feasible, although the timing for practical development is difficult to predict because of the numerous safety, cost, and efficacy considerations that must be evaluated or surmounted.

REFERENCES

Juliano RL, ed.: Biological approaches to the controlled delivery of drugs, Ann NY Acad Sci 507:1, 1987.

Langer R: Implantable controlled release systems. In Ihler GM, ed.: Methods of drug delivery, New York, 1986, Pergamon Press.

Mecklenburg RS, Benson EA, Benson JW Jr et al.: Long-term metabolic control with insulin pump therapy, N Engl J Med 313:465, 1985.

Poste G: Drug targeting in cancer therapy. In: Gregoriadis G, Poste G, Senior J et al., eds.: Receptor mediated targeting of drugs, New York, 1985, Plenum Publishing Co.

7 Issues in Therapeutics

<table>
<tr><td colspan="2" align="center">ABBREVIATIONS</td></tr>
<tr><td>G6PD</td><td>glucose-6-phosphate dehydrogenase</td></tr>
<tr><td>NADPH</td><td>nicotinamide adenine dinucleotide
phosphate (reduced form)</td></tr>
<tr><td>$t_{1/2}$</td><td>half-life</td></tr>
</table>

CLINICAL PROBLEM AREAS

Several problem areas arise in the clinical use of drugs. These include drug interactions, genetic factors, dosage modifications required for the extremes of patient age (pediatric and geriatric), and drug reactions. The first three topics are discussed in this chapter, with more extensive coverage of the pharmacological considerations specific for pediatric or geriatric patients included in Chapters 63 and 64, respectively. This chapter also contains a list of drugs for which the therapeutic index is small and where the plasma concentration of drug is often monitored to assist in achieving the target concentration with minimal toxic side effects. Unexpected drug reactions caused by the release of histamine or by an allergic response are discussed in Chapter 58.

DRUG INTERACTIONS

One of the four factors mentioned (Chapter 1) for the individual clinical use of drugs is that patients often receive more than one drug. Hospitalized pa-tients, for example, receive an average of five to ten drugs, and outpatients may take two to four prepa-rations. Some geriatric patients receive as many as 12 drugs concurrently. With so many drugs admin-istered, especially in hospitalized patients, there are numerous opportunities for drug interactions to oc-cur.

In this context, a *drug interaction* refers to a change in the magnitude or duration of the phar-macological response of one drug because of the pres-ence of another drug. A classical example is the patient receiving chronic warfarin anticoagulant therapy, to which a 14-day regimen of the antiinflam-matory agent, phenylbutazone, is added. Warfarin and phenylbutazone are each about 97% bound to plasma albumin at therapeutic concentrations with both drugs competing for the same albumin binding sites. Introduction of phenylbutazone displaces some of the albumin-bound warfarin, thereby increasing the concentration of unbound warfarin, by as much as 50% to 100%. The magnitude of the anticoagulant effect of warfarin can become dangerously high. The dose of warfarin must therefore be reduced before the start of phenylbutazone administration.

The physician should know which drugs a patient is receiving and recognize the possibilities for drug interactions when adding new drug or discontinuing a currently used drug. Most pharmacies maintain rec-ords of drugs currently used by individual patients and can provide this information to other members of the health care team. Compendia are also available that list drug interactions.

In anticipation of changes in the pharmacological direction of therapy, steps sometimes need to be

Table 7-1 Drug Interactions

Site	Substance	Circumstances of Interaction
GI tract	tetracyclines	Complex with Al^{+3}, Ca^{+2}, or Mg^{+2} antacids or with aluminum hydroxide gels or milk; decrease absorption
	cholestyramine	Acts as ion exchange resin to complex with acidic compounds such as warfarin and prevents warfarin absorption
	propantheline	Slows gastric emptying, can have detrimental effect on penicillin G or erythromycin that are unstable at strong acid pH
	metoclopramide	Speeds up gastric emptying; increases absorption of acetaminophen
Protein binding in blood	salicylates	In each case, other drugs are present that bind to the same region on the protein and therefore displace some of the substance
	nonsteroidal antiinflam- matory agents	
	oral hypoglycemic agents	
	long-lasting sulfonamides	
Renal clearance	probenecid	Inhibits renal secretion of indomethacin; decreases clearance
	salicylates	Inhibit renal secretion of phenylbutazone, sulfinpyrazone, indomethacin, and probenecid; decrease clearance
	sulfinpyrazone	Inhibits renal secretion of salicylates; decreases clearance
	phenylbutazone	Inhibits renal secretion of acetoheximide; decreases clearance
	thiazide diuretics	Decrease lithium clearance
	tricyclic antidepressants	Interact with methylphenidate or guanethidine
Drug metabolism	ethanol	Speeds up metabolism of phenytoin, tolbutamide, and warfarin
	antihistamines	Speed up metabolism of phenobarbital or progesterone
	phenytoin	Speeds up metabolism of corticosteroids or warfarin
	barbiturates	Speed up metabolism of digitoxin, phenytoin, griseofulvin, phenylbuta- zone, warfarin, or testosterone
	glutethimide	Speeds up metabolism of warfarin
	phenylbutazone	Inhibits metabolism of tolbutamide or warfarin
	chloramphenicol	Inhibits metabolism of hexobarbital or tolbutamide
	allopurinol	Inhibits metabolism of 6-mercaptopurine or azathioprine
	cimetidine	Inhibits metabolism of benzodiazepines
	desipramine	Inhibits metabolism of amphetamine
	methylphenidate	Inhibits metabolism of warfarin, some anticonvulsants, and tricyclic anti- depressants

taken to modify existing dosing schedules to compensate for an anticipated interaction, or, where possible, to select another drug that does not participate in this interaction. Drug interactions can result in elevated concentrations of drug via displacement of protein-bound drug or reduced rates of drug disposition, including elevation to toxic concentrations. Drug interactions also can result in more rapid disappearance of drug, with the plasma concentration dropping below the minimum effective value. Both of these situations are undesirable. Being able to predict the direction and extent of the expected change in concentration or in magnitude of effect arises primarily from an understanding of the mechanisms by which the interaction occurs.

Drug interactions occur via several principal mech-

anisms. These include acceleration or inhibition of drug metabolism; displacement of plasma protein-bound drug; impaired uptake of drug from the gastrointestinal (GI) tract; altered renal clearance of drug; modifications in receptors or blockade of receptor channels; and changes in electrolyte balance, body fluid pH, or rates of protein synthesis. The more frequently encountered mechanisms are illustrated schematically in Figure 7-1. A partial listing of specific drug interactions is contained in Table 7-1. Some appreciation of the drug types that are most often associated with drug interactions can be obtained from Table 7-2. This empirical approach singles out the drug types in which the major interaction problems arise. A discussion of specific interactions with the oral anticoagulants is included in Chapter 21.

Table 7-2 Estimated Tendency of Drug Classes to Participate in Drug-Drug Interactions

Drug Class	Interactions/ Drug*
Anticoagulants, oral	43
Antidiabetics	16
Monoamine oxidase inhibitors	16
Phenothiazines	10
Anticonvulsants	10
Tricyclic antidepressants	6
Digitalis glycosides	6
Antiarrhythmics	5.9
Salicylates	4
Hormones	3
Diuretics	2.9
Antihypertensives	2.9
Antiinfective agents	2.2
Antineoplastic agents	1.7
Others	0.7

* Results obtained by counting the number of interactions of major clinical significance as listed in Hanston PD and Horn JR: Drug interactions, ed. 6, Philadelphia, 1989, Lea & Feibiger. For example, 26 combinations of antihypertensives and other drugs were reported to produce significant interactions. Twenty-six divided by the 9 different antihypertensive agents listed produces a frequency of 2.9 interactions for each type of antihypertensive drug.

Detailed descriptions of specific drug interactions are available in the pharmacology literature.*

GENETIC FACTORS

Variation in a patient's drug response can result from genetic differences. The drug response may be enhanced or reduced and the duration of action can be lengthened or shortened as a result of genetically based distinctions in specific patients. The study of the role of genetic factors in explaining unexpected responses to a given drug in an individual patient is termed *pharmacogenetics*. It is well known that genetic variations that relate to a given protein can be inherited and that the activity of an enzyme or the binding ability of a receptor may be diminished or enhanced in a genetically modified protein. Whether modifications result from predictable or random mutations is not important from a pharmacological stand-

*One journal that is particularly useful is *Clinical Pharmacology and Therapeutics*.

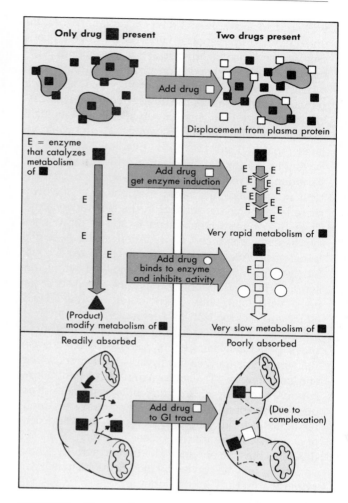

FIGURE 7-1 Frequently encountered mechanisms by which drug interactions occur.

point. Realizing that an abnormal genetically based response can occur in a given patient and being alert for such an occurrence is important. Several examples are included here to describe the more widely encountered pharmacogenetic variations and to demonstrate several of the pharmacological mechanisms through which genetic distinctions manifest. Omitted from the discussion are dysfunctions or conditions that are widely recognized and observable as genetically inherited traits (See Chapter 31 for alcohol and aldehyde dehydrogenase differences between races.)

Genetic modification of enzyme activity associated with the metabolism of specific drugs is a major mechanism encountered in pharmacogenetics. One well-studied example of a genetic explanation for an unexpected drug response involves the elevated concentrations of isoniazid that occur infrequently. Isoniazid undergoes disposition primarily through metabolism by N-acetylation. Population studies show a bimodal distribution for the ability of patients to acetylate isoniazid. One small group acetylates isoniazid slowly, whereas the larger population group acetylates rapidly. Thus the dose must be adjusted accordingly. A bimodal distribution indicates a genetic variation. The responsible enzyme appears to be identical in the slow and rapid metabolizers; however, there is less enzyme present in the slow acetylators. Thus the genetic mechanism is one of diminished synthesis or enhanced degradation of the N-acetyltransferase. Acetylation is also the pathway for metabolism of many other drugs, some of which are listed in Table 7-3, and thus may be involved in genetic variations with drugs other than isoniazid, which are metabolized by acetylation.

Another enzyme of drug metabolism that is sometimes genetically altered is plasma cholinesterase. This enzyme catalyzes the hydrolysis of succinylcholine (see Chapter 11), used as a muscle relaxant during surgical procedures. A significant proportion of patients does not hydrolyze this compound very rapidly, resulting in a duration of action for a standard dose of succinylcholine that is excessively long. Some individuals have an enhanced hydrolytic activity. These variations may be caused by modifications in isozyme primary structure or conformation.

Other genetic variations in drug metabolism in individual patients include decreased hydroxylation of diphenylhydantoin (phenytoin), impaired O-dealkylation of acetophenetidin, and diminished inactivation of fluorouracil by dihydropyrimidine dehydrogenase.

Many drugs are capable of inducing hemolytic anemia in patients genetically deficient in glucose-6-phosphate dehydrogenase (G6PD). Millions of people worldwide carry this genetic trait. Hemolysis is related to the cell's inability to maintain sufficient reduced glutathione. This results from the reduced availability of G6PD required to produce the NADPH necessary for maintaining cell membrane integrity. A list of some of the drugs capable of inducing hemolysis in G6PD-deficient patients is given in the box.

Another pharmacogenetic response is altered affinity of the drug-binding site. In the normal adult population a daily maintenance dose of 5 to 10 mg of

Table 7-3 Some Drugs that Undergo N-Acetylation
HYDRAZINE-TYPE DRUGS
hydralazine
isoniazid
phenelzine
ARYLAMINE-TYPE DRUGS
dapsone
p-aminobenzoic acid
p-aminosalicylic acid
procainamide

DRUGS CAPABLE OF INDUCING HEMOLYTIC ANEMIA IN G6PD-DEFICIENT PATIENTS	
acetophenetidin	p-aminosalicylic acid
chloramphenicol	primaquine
chloroquine	sulfonamides
nitrofuran derivatives	Vitamin K analogs

sodium warfarin produces a suitable anticoagulant response; however, members of one family required 10 to 30 times as much warfarin to obtain the same degree of anticoagulation. Possible explanations based on differences in plasma protein binding or in pharmacokinetics were rejected; the unexpected anticoagulant response was convincingly assigned to a variation in the affinity of the binding site for warfarin (see Chapter 21 for mechanism of action of warfarin).

DOSING MODIFICATIONS FOR PEDIATRIC AND GERIATRIC PATIENTS

Pharmacokinetic, as well as pharmacological, response differences exist between young adults and infants and between young adults and the elderly. The differences must be appreciated for safe and beneficial use of drugs in patients at the extremes of age. Some pharmacokinetic considerations are mentioned here, but an in-depth discussion is available in Chapters 63 and 64.

Numerous physiological changes take place during the life span, from infant, through young adult, to the

Table 7-4 Comparative Body Size and Renal Clearance Capacity Between Infants and Adults

Parameter	Infants	Adults
Body weight, kg	3.5	70
Body water, %	77	58
Inulin clearance		
ml/min/kg	0.85	1.85
ml/min	3	130
$t_{1/2}$, min	630	220
p-Aminohippuric acid clearance		
ml/min/kg	3.4	9.2
ml/min	12	650
$t_{1/2}$, min	160	43

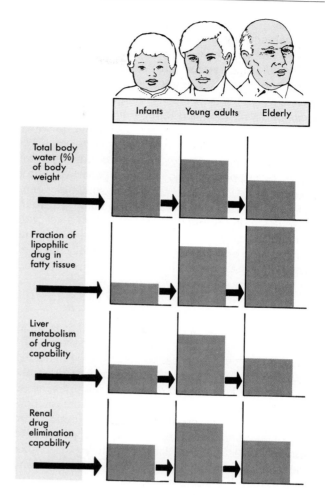

FIGURE 7-2   Areas of boxes indicate relative size or capability of function at each age.

geriatric years. These changes are important to drug pharmacokinetics and are discussed here—and include liver metabolic function, renal elimination capabilities, and body composition.

Liver metabolism and renal elimination of drugs are usually diminished at the extremes of age. The ability of the newborn infant to dispose of drugs is often limited. Liver drug metabolizing enzyme systems may be present at birth only in extremely low activities; renal elimination capabilities also may be depressed. Both hepatic and renal drug disposition is reduced in infants, as shown in Table 7-4. In infants, renal tubular secretion may not be well developed and renal blood flow may be less than expected. After age 40, liver mass decreases at a rate of about 1% per year, resulting in a diminished ability to metabolize drugs. What is not clearly defined is whether the intrinsic drug metabolizing activity of each molecule of enzyme also diminishes with increased age. Renal elimination in the elderly also shows diminished glomerular filtration and tubular secretion clearance mechanisms. Thus, it may be desirable to assess filtration capability in individual patients by determining creatinine clearance.

Changes in body composition also occur on aging. Infants contain the highest proportion of total body water in relation to body weight. The proportion of total body water decreases with aging and is accompanied by an increased proportion of body fat. Such changes in body composition can profoundly influence the distribution of a drug into the various body compartments, tissues, and fluids. The target plasma concentration of a drug, thus, may be different for the three age-groups as a result of the modified distribution pattern. These changes are shown schematically in Figure 7-2.

MONITORING PLASMA DRUG CONCENTRATIONS

Development of suitably sensitive assays for the quantitative determination of drug concentrations in small samples of patient blood and at therapeutic concentrations of drug has made it possible to monitor blood drug concentrations as a guide to the rapid achievement and maintenance of the desired target concentrations. Table 7-5 lists target concentration ranges for drugs that are most difficult to use without encountering toxic symptoms. A range of concentrations is given for each drug to compensate for differences in distribution and in the rates of drug absorption and disposition in individual patients, because values for pharmacokinetic and pharmacological response parameters are not known for individual patients. Monitoring of blood drug concentrations for the compounds in Table 7-5 may help in nonstandard situations to provide guidance in adjusting dosing schedules or obtaining a therapeutic drug level with a minimum of toxicity. However, the routine monitoring of drug blood concentrations is usually not warranted after the plateau concentration is reached and maintained for several dosing intervals.

SUMMARY

An unexpected response to the therapeutic dosing regimen of a drug occasionally occurs. The practitioner must quickly define the cause of the unexpected response and adjust if necessary to the situation. Possible causes include drug interaction, genetic variation, histamine release, immunological reaction, and incorrect adjustment of dose for patient age. Other unknown causes may also be responsible. In many cases dosing adjustment can be made so that the originally planned drug type can be used.

Table 7-5 Serum Concentrations of Drugs at Target Therapeutic and Estimated Toxic Levels

Drugs	Concentrations (μg/ml) Therapeutic	Toxic
carbamazepine	5-12	
digitoxin	0.013-0.025	>0.035
digoxin	0.0010-0.0022	>0.0025
diphenylhydantoin	10-20	>25
ethosuximide	50-100	
gentamicin	8-12	
lidocaine	1.5-5	>9
lithium	0.6-1.2*	
nortriptyline	0.050-0.080	
phenobarbital	15-30	>40
procainamide	4-8	>10
propranolol	0.030-0.120	
quinidine	2-4	>6
salicylate	150-300	>300
theophylline	10-20	>20

* Milliequivalents/liter.

REFERENCES

Goldstein A, Aronow L, and Kalman SM; Pharmacogenetics and drug idiosyncrasy, In Goldstein A, Aronow L, and Kalmah SM, eds: Principles of drug action, ed 2, New York, 1974, John Wiley & Sons, Inc.

Hansten PD and Horn JR: Drug Interactions, ed. 6, Philadelphia, 1989, Lea and Febiger.

Schmucker DL: Aging and drug disposition: an update, Pharmacol Rev 37:133, 1985.

Weber WW and Hein DW: N-acetylation pharmacogenetics, Pharmacol Rev 37:25, 1985.

PERIPHERAL AUTONOMIC NERVOUS SYSTEM: DRUGS AFFECTING TRANSMISSION AND FUNCTION

The autonomic nervous system controls key visceral processes including cardiac output, blood flow to specific organs, glandular secretions, waste elimination, sexual function, and other processes necessary for life. Many of the autonomic actions take place outside of the central nervous system (CNS), either at junctions along the nerve fibers that innervate specific organs or at the junction of the nerve with the organ innervated. Drugs developed to treat disease states that require modification of autonomically controlled functions can be divided into agents that act in the peripheral nervous system and those that act in the CNS. Part II pertains to drug actions that occur in the peripheral nervous system and specifically in the peripheral portion of the autonomic nervous system. Drug actions that occur in the CNS are described in Part III.

Chapter 8 describes the peripheral autonomic nervous system, with special emphasis on sites and biochemical or physiological processes in which clinically used drugs act. The approach is to treat the two main neurotransmitter systems of the peripheral autonomic nervous system separately. Thus Chapter 9 covers the parasympathetic nervous system in which acetylcholine is the endogenous transmitter, and Chapter 10 covers the sympathetic nervous system with norepinephrine as the endogenous transmitter. Because of the wide scope of actions of peripheral autonomic innervation, many of the drugs presented in Part II are mentioned in subsequent Parts as having therapeutic actions in other disease states not mentioned in this Part. Other therapeutic actions and the drugs involved are discussed in other appropriate chapters, with reference to Chapters 9 or 10.

Because the neuromuscular blocking agents act at peripheral sites, they also are included in this Part (Chapter 11).

CHAPTER 8

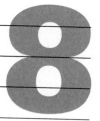

Physiology and Biochemistry of the Peripheral Autonomic Nervous System

The concept of neurochemical transmission is firmly established as the mechanism by which nerves interact with effector organs of the body. The basic premise is that a nerve releases a chemical mediator, termed a *neurotransmitter*, that diffuses across a small but defined area, the *neuroeffector junction*, to interact with a suitable receptor on the effector organ, thereby evoking a response in the effector organ. The nerve terminal contains all the necessary apparatus for the synthesis, storage, release, and subsequent inactivation of the neurotransmitter. The effector organ contains, on its cell surface membrane, the receptor with which the neurotransmitter interacts, the enzymes necessary for its degradation, and intracellularly the "signal transduction" mechanisms for information transfer from the receptor to the "cellular machinery," producing the end-organ response.

The release of the neurotransmitter by the nerve terminal is regulated by nerve impulses originating within the central nervous system (CNS). Nerves with cell bodies in the CNS that innervate the skeletal muscles are termed *somatic nerves*. In contrast, nerves originating within the CNS that innervate visceral organs of the body such as the heart, blood vessels, gastrointestinal (GI) tract, reproductive organs, and many others are termed *autonomic nerves*. Virtually all autonomic nerves have relay centers, *ganglia*, located outside the CNS, whereas neuronal connections for the somatic nervous system are located entirely within the CNS. Furthermore, most somatic nerves that control motor function are myelinated and transmit impulses rapidly; most autonomic nerves are nonmyelinated and conduct impulses at relatively slower rates. The function of peripheral autonomic nerves is to modulate the ongoing activity of the involuntary visceral organs by eliciting excitatory or inhibitory responses.

Because peripheral autonomic nerves have ganglia outside the CNS, autonomic nerves are actually composed of two parts, termed *preganglionic* and *postganglionic,* based on anatomical location relative to the ganglia. A preganglionic neuron has its cell body in the spinal cord and is modulated by higher centers in the brain and by spinal reflexes. The axon originating from the cell body of a preganglionic neuron exits the spinal cord from the cranial, thoracic, lumbar, or sacral regions and forms a synaptic connection in the autonomic ganglia with the cell body of the postganglionic autonomic nerve fiber. The postganglionic neurons send their axons directly to the effector organs to complete the pathway of autonomic innervation of the peripheral involuntary visceral organs.

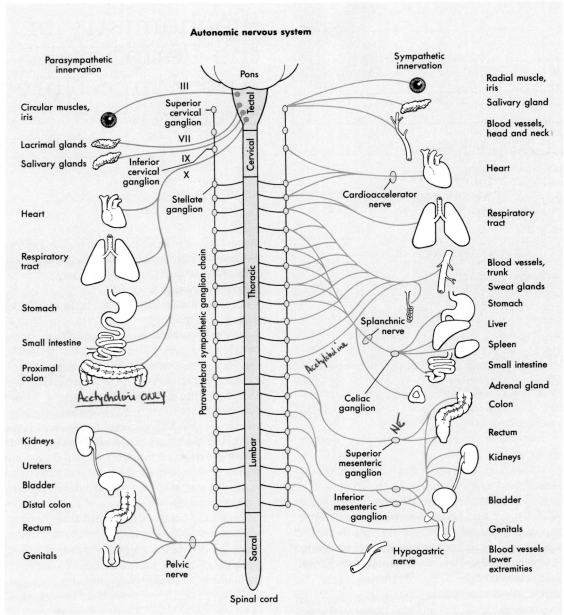

Autonomic nervous system

Parasympathetic innervation

Pons

III

Superior cervical ganglion

VII

IX

X

Inferior cervical ganglion

Stellate ganglion

Tectal

Cervical

Thoracic

Lumbar

Sacral

Paravertebral sympathetic ganglion chain

Sympathetic innervation

Circular muscles, iris

Lacrimal glands

Salivary glands

Heart

Respiratory tract

Stomach

Small intestine

Proximal colon

Acetylcholine ONLY

Kidneys

Ureters

Bladder

Distal colon

Rectum

Genitals

Pelvic nerve

Radial muscle, iris

Salivary gland

Blood vessels, head and neck

Heart

Cardioaccelerator nerve

Respiratory tract

Blood vessels, trunk

Sweat glands

Stomach

Liver

Spleen

Small intestine

Adrenal gland

Colon

Rectum

Kidneys

Bladder

Genitals

Blood vessels lower extremities

Splanchnic nerve

Acetylcholine

Celiac ganglion

NE

Superior mesenteric ganglion

Inferior mesenteric ganglion

Hypogastric nerve

Spinal cord

FIGURE 8-1   Schematic representation of the autonomic nervous system depicting the functional innervation of peripheral effector organs and the anatomical origin of peripheral autonomic nerves from the spinal cord. Although both paravertebral sympathetic ganglia chains are presented, the sympathetic innervation to the peripheral effector organs is shown only on the right part of the figure, whereas parasympathetic innervation of peripheral effector organs is depicted on the left. The roman numerals on nerves originating in the tectal region of the brain stem refer to the cranial nerves that provide parasympathetic outflow to the effector organs of the head, neck, and trunk.

DIVISIONS OF THE PERIPHERAL AUTONOMIC NERVOUS SYSTEM

There are two major divisions of the peripheral autonomic nervous system: *sympathetic* and *parasympathetic*. A number of anatomical and functional differences distinguish these two separate entities. An anatomical depiction of divisions is presented in Figure 8-1.

Sympathetic Nervous System

Cell bodies for preganglionic neurons of the sympathetic division of the autonomic nervous system originate in the intermediolateral cell column of the spinal cord at the thoracic and lumbar levels. Relatively short preganglionic neurons exit the spinal cord at the thoracic and lumbar levels, resulting in *thoracolumbar outflow*, which relates to the sympathetic division of the peripheral autonomic nervous system. These short preganglionic axons send projections to the sympathetic ganglia that consist of two chains of 22 segmentally arranged ganglia, located bilaterally with respect to the spinal cord, outside of the spinal vertebrae. Postganglionic neurons with their cell bodies located in the paravertebral sympathetic chain ganglia send relatively long postganglionic fibers to the effector organs innervated by the sympathetic nervous system. Although most preganglionic sympathetic neurons synapse in the paravertebral sympathetic ganglia, a few preganglionic sympathetic fibers pass through these vertebral ganglia without making synaptic connections and travel by way of the splanchnic nerves to the prevertebral ganglia located in front of the vertebral column. These ganglia are situated in the pelvis and abdomen and are named the *celiac, superior mesenteric,* and *inferior mesenteric (hypogastric)* ganglia (see Figure 8-1). Terminal ganglia lie close to the organs they innervate, namely the urinary bladder and rectum. The neurotransmitter that mediates synaptic transmission between preganglionic and postganglionic nerve fibers in the sympathetic pathway is acetylcholine. In contrast, the neurotransmitter liberated by the long postganglionic sympathetic nerves and which mediates the endorgan responses at the neuroeffector junctions is norepinephrine. Sites that use acetylcholine as the neurotransmitter are termed *cholinergic,* whereas those that use norepinephrine are called *adrenergic.* (See

Chapter 12 for additional comments on terminology.)

The adrenal medulla contains chromaffin cells, embryologically and anatomically homologous to the sympathetic ganglia in that they are derived from the neural crest. The adrenal medulla, unlike the postganglionic sympathetic nerve terminals, releases epinephrine as the primary catecholamine. The chromaffin cells of the adrenal medulla are innervated by typical preganglionic sympathetic nerve terminals, whose neurotransmitter is acetylcholine.

Parasympathetic Nervous System

The parasympathetic division of the autonomic nervous system differs markedly from the sympathetic division. Cell bodies giving rise to preganglionic parasympathetic nerves have their origins in the spinal cord. They exit the spinal cord at the cranial and sacral levels, giving rise to the term, *craniosacral outflow,* to describe the parasympathetic division of the autonomic nervous system. The cranial (tectobulbar) portion of the parasympathetic outflow innervates structures in the head, neck, thorax, and abdomen. These fibers travel in the oculomotor (III), facial (VII), glossopharyngeal (IX), and vagal (X) cranial nerves. The sacral division of the parasympathetic nervous system forms the pelvic nerve and innervates the remainder of the intestines and the pelvic viscera, including the bladder and reproductive organs. The preganglionic neurons of the parasympathetic division of the autonomic nervous system are extremely long, such that the parasympathetic ganglia are located in, or near, the effector organs. As such, the postganglionic parasympathetic neurons are short. The neurotransmitter mediating synaptic transmission in the parasympathetic ganglia is acetylcholine. Acetylcholine is also the neurotransmitter liberated by postganglionic parasympathetic nerves innervating the effector organs.

Autonomic Regulation of Peripheral Involuntary Organs

Most organs of the body receive dual innervation consisting of sympathetic and parasympathetic components of the autonomic nervous system. In general, the parasympathetic and sympathetic neurons mediate opposing responses in the effector organ, although some exceptions to this generalization exist. Because balance exists in most organs between the sympathetic and parasympathetic divisions of the autonomic nervous system, blockade or inhibition of one system leads to exaggeration in the response mediated by the other. Some organs of the body, such as the vasculature and the spleen, receive only one type of innervation, which in these cases is sympathetic.

Regarding thoracolumbar sympathetic outflow, one preganglionic neuron may ramify and ultimately synapse with many postganglionic sympathetic neurons, leading to diffusion of sympathetic responses. In contrast, the craniosacral parasympathetic preganglionic neurons form, in general, only single synaptic connections with postganglionic parasympathetic neurons, resulting in a more discrete and localized response (Auerbach's plexus in the small intestine is a notable exception). This anatomical distinction between the sympathetic and parasympathetic divisions of the autonomic nervous system has profound physiological significance in that *activation of sympathetic outflow,* resulting from anger, fear, or stress prepares the body for a ready state of activation characteristic of the "fight or flight" response. Thus, heart rate is accelerated, blood pressure is increased, perfusion to skeletal muscle is augmented as a result of the redirection of blood flow away from the skin and splanchnic region, blood glucose is elevated, bronchioles and pupils are dilated, and piloerection occurs. In contrast, because the parasympathetic system is organized in a more discrete and localized manner, *activation of parasympathetic outflow* is associated with conservation of energy and maintenance of organ function during periods of minimal activity. Activation of parasympathetic outflow produces a reduction in heart rate and blood pressure, activation of GI movements, and emptying of the urinary bladder and rectum. Furthermore, glandular cells such as lacrimal, salivary, and mucous cells are activated, and smooth muscle of the bronchial tree is constricted. Based on responses involved, it is clear that widespread activation of the parasympathetic nervous system is not beneficial.

Although the parasympathetic nervous system is essential for life, the sympathetic nervous system is not, and animals completely deprived of the sympathetic nervous system will survive, albeit with a lower level of efficiency. A deficiency in sympathetic innervation to visceral organs is apparent during times of stress, when activation of sympathetic outflow is essential.

NEUROTRANSMITTERS IN THE PERIPHERAL AUTONOMIC NERVOUS SYSTEM

Transmission Process

Transmission of information from preganglionic neurons to postganglionic neurons, or from postganglionic neurons to the effector organs, involves the chemical transmission of nerve impulses for the sympathetic and parasympathetic divisions of the autonomic nervous system. The sequence of events was studied in detail and is illustrated for the sympathetic and parasympathetic ganglia, as well as for the postganglionic sympathetic and parasympathetic neurons, in Figure 8-2. Electrical impulses, originating from within the CNS, result in local depolarization of the neuronal membrane as a result of the selective increase in the permeability of sodium ions that flow inwardly in the direction of their electrochemical gradient. Repolarization of the membrane follows immediately and results from the selective increase in permeability to potassium ions. These ionic flows are mediated by separate and distinct ion channels. The transmembrane ion fluxes, which lead to ion currents produced in a local circuit, result in the generation of an action potential that is propagated throughout the length of the axon. The arrival of the action potential at the preganglionic or postganglionic nerve terminal triggers the quantal release of neurotransmitter stored in intracellular vesicles. The synthesis of the neurotransmitter occurs in the nerve terminal where it is maintained in the storage vesicles until a sufficient action potential stimulus is received. The adrenergic storage vesicles in sympathetic nerve terminals and in adrenal chromaffin cells range in diameter from 400 to 1300 Å, whereas cholinergic storage vesicles in parasympathetic and ganglia terminals range in diameter from 200 to 400 Å.

The release of neurotransmitter after the arrival of a sufficient action potential occurs through a calcium-dependent process known as *exocytosis.* In this process the storage vesicle migrates to the nerve terminal membrane, fuses with the neuronal plasma membrane, opens to the extracellular space, and allows the contents of the storage vesicle, including the neurotransmitter, to be discharged into the synaptic cleft. The neurotransmitter diffuses across the synaptic cleft or the neuroeffector junction and interacts

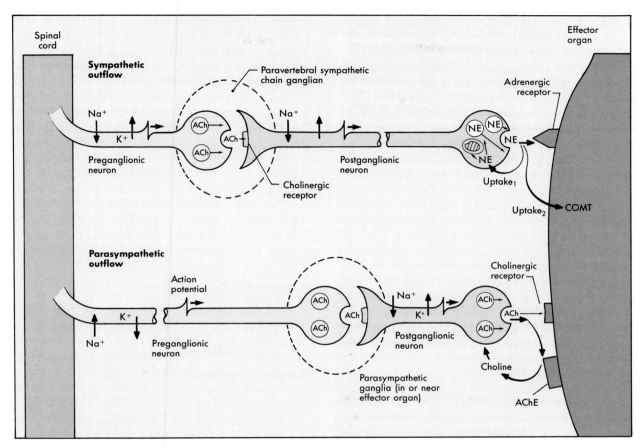

FIGURE 8-2   Schematic representation of neurochemical transmission in the sympathetic and parasympathetic divisions of the peripheral autonomic nervous system. Preganglionic neurons originate from the spinal cord and make synaptic connections in peripheral autonomic ganglia. The neurotransmitter liberated in both sympathetic and parasympathetic ganglia is acetylcholine *(ACh)*, which is liberated through an exocytotic process on the arrival of an action potential to the preganglionic nerve terminal. The electrochemical generation of these action potentials results from the influx of sodium ions and the efflux of potassium ions. ACh liberated from preganglionic neurons in the sympathetic and parasympathetic ganglia diffuses across the synaptic cleft to interact with cholinergic receptors on cell bodies of the postganglionic neurons. The interaction of ACh with ganglionic cholinergic receptors results in the generation and propagation of action potentials that elicit the release of neurotransmitter at the postganglionic nerve terminal (neuroeffector junction). The neurotransmitter liberated from postganglionic sympathetic nerves is norepinephrine *(NE)*, which diffuses across the neuroeffector junction to stimulate the adrenergic receptors and elicit the end-organ response. Most of the liberated NE is taken back up into the sympathetic nerve terminal by a process called *uptake$_1$* and is either stored in the adrenergic storage vesicles or is metabolized by monoamine oxidase *(MAO)* located in the mitochondria. A smaller amount of the liberated NE may diffuse away from the adrenergic receptors and be accumulated by extraneuronal cells by a process called *uptake$_2$*, after which it may be metabolized by the enzyme catechol-O-methyltransferase *(COMT)*. A similar process occurs at the postganglionic parasympathetic neuroeffector junction except that the neurotransmitter released is ACh, which diffuses across the synaptic cleft and activates cholinergic receptors on the effector organ. The liberated ACh is rapidly metabolized by acetylcholinesterase *(AChE)* and the product, choline, is taken up into the parasympathetic nerve terminal and used to synthesize additional ACh, which is subsequently stored in the cholinergic storage vesicles.

with a specific receptor located on the cell body of the postganglionic neuron or on the effector organ, respectively. In both sympathetic and parasympathetic ganglia, the neurotransmitter released by preganglionic neurons is acetylcholine. Activation of the postjunctional membrane receptors on the cell body of postganglionic neurons leads to an increase in ion permeability, and therefore to ionic conductance, in the postganglionic neuron (see Chapters 2 and 12). This increase in permeability of ions ultimately results in the generation of action potentials, which are propagated along the length of the postganglionic nerve. As at preganglionic nerve terminals, neurotransmitter is released when these action potentials reach the postganglionic sympathetic and parasympathetic nerve terminals. As indicated previously, the neurotransmitter liberated by postganglionic sympathetic nerve terminals is norepinephrine, whereas the neurotransmitter in the postganglionic parasympathetic neuron is acetylcholine. The response mediated in the effector organ subsequent to the release of the neurotransmitter is dependent on the neurotransmitter and the nature of the postjunctional receptor subtype present in the effector organ. These autonomic receptors are discussed in greater detail later in this chapter and in Chapters 2, 9, 10, and 12.

After release of the neurotransmitter, the effect of the neurotransmitter must be rapidly terminated to avoid excessive activation of the postjunctional elements. Most cholinergic synapses and neuroeffector junctions contain the highly selective enzyme, acetylcholinesterase, that rapidly hydrolyzes acetylcholine into the two inactive products, acetic acid and choline, thereby terminating the effect of the neurotransmitter. Choline is then rapidly taken up into the cholinergic nerve by an active neuronal membrane pump for use again in the synthesis of acetylcholine by the enzyme, choline acetyltransferase, present in the cytoplasm of the cholinergic nerves. Acetylcholine then accumulates in the storage vessels of the cholinergic nerve terminal until required for release, thereby conserving the neurotransmitter.

At adrenergic neuroeffector junctions, the response to norepinephrine is not terminated by enzymatic deactivation. Instead, termination occurs by a combination of neuronal re-uptake of the neurotransmitter into the sympathetic nerve by an energy-dependent amine uptake pump, called $uptake_1$, and by simple diffusion away from the region of the re-

ceptors through an extraneuronal uptake process referred to as $uptake_2$. Norepinephrine, accumulated in sympathetic nerves by $uptake_1$, has two fates (Figure 8-3). It may be oxidatively deaminated by the enzyme, monoamine oxidase, in the mitochondria of the sympathetic nerve terminal or sequestered in storage vessels for subsequent release. Norepinephrine diffusing away from the receptors to the extraneuronal site of $uptake_2$ may be inactivated by O-methylation through the enzyme, catechol-O-methyltransferase. The metabolism of the catecholamines, norepinephrine and epinephrine, by the catabolic enzymes, monoamine oxidase and catechol-O-methyltransferase, results in inactive degradation products that have been identified and quantitated in tissues, blood, and urine. The scheme for the metabolic breakdown of the catecholamines is well established (see Figure 8-3).

Biosynthesis of Neurotransmitters

Catecholamines The pathway for the biosynthesis of the catecholamines, epinephrine and norepinephrine, is well understood (Figure 8-4). The precursor for the synthesis of all catecholamines is the amino acid, tyrosine. Tyrosine is first hydroxylated in the *meta* position by the enzyme, tyrosine hydroxylase, to form the catechol derivative, 3,4-dihydroxyphenylalanine. Tyrosine hydroxylase is the rate-limiting enzyme in the biosynthesis of all catecholamines, and this step takes place in the cytoplasm of the postganglionic sympathetic nerve terminal. 3,4-Dihydroxyphenylalanine (DOPA) is subsequently decarboxylated by the enzyme, L-aromatic amino acid decarboxylase, to form dopamine, and this step also occurs in the cytoplasm. Dopamine is then actively accumulated by the storage vesicles in the sympathetic nerve terminals, and during this transport process, dopamine is β-hydroxylated by the enzyme, dopamine-β-hydroxylase, associated with the adrenergic storage vesicle. The product is norepinephrine, retained within the storage vesicle in association with adenosine triphosphate (ATP) until released on the arrival of an action potential at the sympathetic nerve terminal. Dopamine-β-hydroxylase represents the terminal enzyme in the biosynthesis of catecholamines in the postganglionic sympathetic neuron. As such, adrenergic nerves release only norepinephrine as the neurotransmitter.

In contrast, in the adrenal medulla, norepinephrine

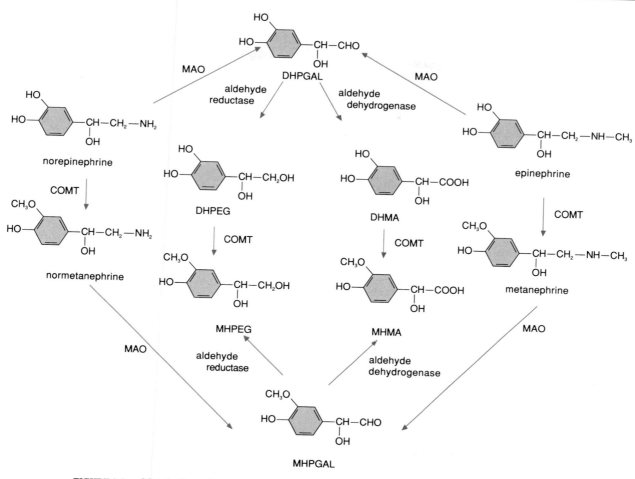

FIGURE 8-3   Metabolism of norepinephrine and epinephrine by monoamine oxidase (MAO) and catechol-O-methyltransferase *(COMT)*. The abbreviations for the individual metabolites are as follows: *DHPGAL*, 3,4-dihydroxyphenylglycol aldehyde; *DHPEG*, 3,4-dihydroxyphenylethylene glycol; *DHMA*, 3,4-dihydroxymandelic acid; *MHPEG*, 3-methoxy-4-hydroxphenylethylene glycol; *MHMA*, 3-methoxy-4-hydroxymandelic acid; *MHPGAL*, 3-methoxy-4-hydroxyphenylglycol aldehyde.

and epinephrine coexist. The synthesis of epinephrine in the adrenal gland occurs because of the presence of the enzyme, phenethanolamine-*N*-methyltransferase, which *N*-methylates norepinephrine to epinephrine in the cytoplasm. Cytoplasmic epinephrine is then accumulated in storage granules in the chromaffin cell and stored until released. In the adult human, epinephrine accounts for approximately 80% of the catecholamines in the adrenal medulla, with norepinephrine making up the remainder.

Acetylcholine The biosynthesis of acetylcholine

in cholinergic neurons occurs by the acetylation of choline, catalyzed by the enzyme, choline acetyltransferase, with acetyl coenzyme A serving as the acetyl donor (Figure 8-5). Choline is actively accumulated into the axoplasm of the neuron from extraneuronal sites by a high affinity choline uptake process. The synthesis of acetylcholine from choline occurs in the axoplasm with acetylcholine actively accumulated in storage vesicles in the cholinergic nerve terminal, releasing neurotransmitter on the arrival of sufficient action potential stimuli.

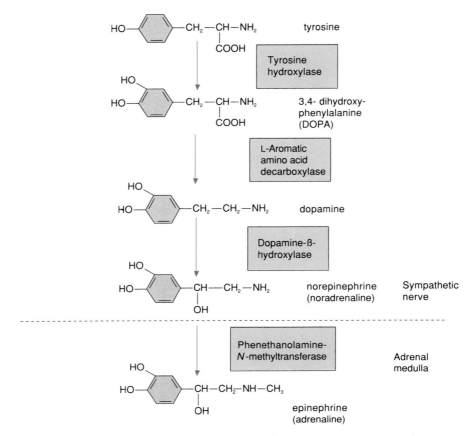

FIGURE 8-4   Steps in the enzymatic biosynthesis of the catecholamines, dopamine, norepinephrine (noradrenaline), and epinephrine (adrenaline). The enzymes involved in each catalytic step are enclosed in boxes. The first three enzymatic steps occur in postganglionic sympathetic nerve terminals leading to the synthesis of norepinephrine, and all four enzymatic steps occur in the adrenal medulla, resulting in the synthesis of epinephrine.

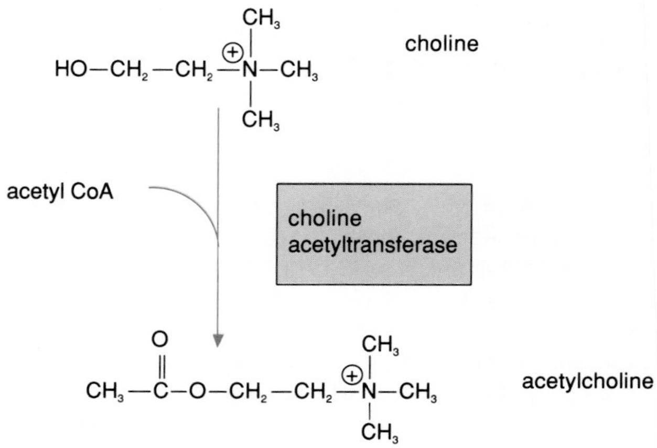

FIGURE 8-5   Enzymatic biosynthesis of acetylcholine, as catalyzed by the enzyme, choline acetyltransferase. The acetyl group is donated by the cofactor, acetyl coenzyme A.

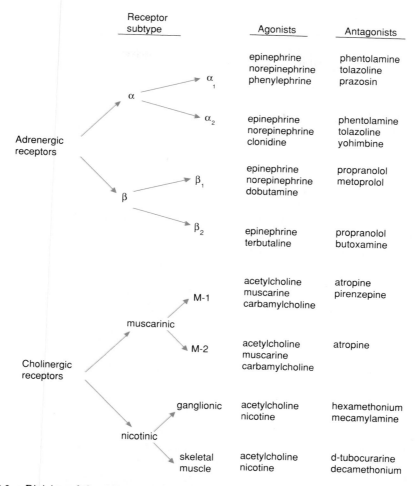

Receptor subtype		Agonists	Antagonists

Adrenergic receptors

α → α₁

epinephrine
norepinephrine
phenylephrine

phentolamine
tolazoline
prazosin

α → α₂

epinephrine
norepinephrine
clonidine

phentolamine
tolazoline
yohimbine

β → β₁

epinephrine
norepinephrine
dobutamine

propranolol
metoprolol

β → β₂

epinephrine
terbutaline

propranolol
butoxamine

Cholinergic receptors

muscarinic → M-1

acetylcholine
muscarine
carbamylcholine

atropine
pirenzepine

muscarinic → M-2

acetylcholine
muscarine
carbamylcholine

atropine

nicotinic → ganglionic

acetylcholine
nicotine

hexamethonium
mecamylamine

nicotinic → skeletal muscle

acetylcholine
nicotine

d-tubocurarine
decamethonium

FIGURE 8-6   Division of the adrenergic receptors and cholinergic receptors into individual receptor subtypes. Some of the drugs that stimulate (agonists) or block (antagonists) each of the individual adrenergic and cholinergic receptor subtypes are listed.

NEUROTRANSMITTER RECEPTORS IN THE PERIPHERAL AUTONOMIC NERVOUS SYSTEM

Acetylcholine and norepinephrine use different pharmacological receptors to mediate their end-organ responses, and each neurotransmitter may interact with a number of receptor subtypes (see Chapter 2). The classification of the numerous receptor subtypes is primarily based on pharmacological studies, but it is evident that the end-organ response is as much a function of the receptor mediating that response as it is of the neurotransmitter that elicits the response. A listing of the adrenergic and cholinergic receptor subtypes is presented in Figure 8-6, with examples of agents that stimulate (agonists) or block (antagonists) these receptor subtypes. Several compounds distinguish the M_1 and M_2 muscarinic subtypes, shown in Figure 8-7.

Adrenergic Receptors

In the classic study of Ahlquist, the graded actions of a series of sympathomimetic amines provided the first evidence that the neurotransmitter, norepinephrine, and the adrenal catecholamine, epinephrine, could activate more than one type of adrenergic receptor. For stimulation of smooth muscle in the vasculature, uterus, ureter, and dilator pupillae, and for the inhibition of intestinal smooth muscle, the following rank order of potency was obtained: epinephrine > norepinephrine > α-methylnorepinephrine > α-methylepinephrine > isoproterenol. In contrast, the rank order of potency for these same agonists for inhibition of vascular and uterine smooth muscle and for stimulation of the myocardium was: isoproterenol > epinephrine > α-methylepinephrine > α-methylnorepinephrine > norepinephrine. Based on these distinct potency orders, it was proposed that two types of adrenergic receptors existed, those being termed α, when the first potency order described above was obtained, and the other β, when the second order of potency was obtained. The existence of distinct α- and β-adrenergic receptors was confirmed shortly thereafter by the development of selective α- and β-adrenergic antagonists.

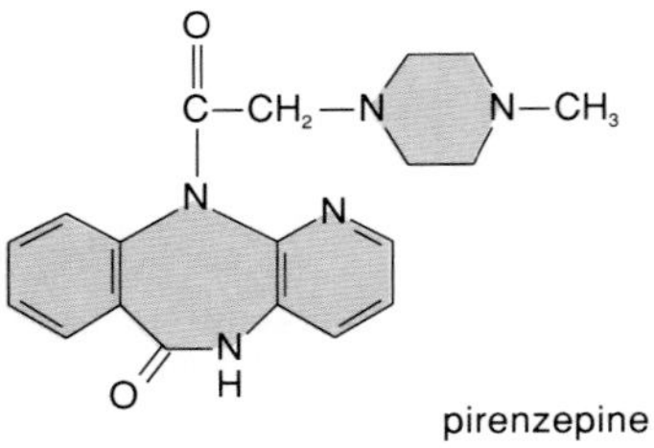

For many years, only two adrenergic receptors were known to exist, the α- and the β-types as defined. Subsequent studies later indicated that β-adrenergic receptors did not belong to one homogeneous population, but could be subdivided into β₁ and β₂ subtypes. Thus the β₁ subtypes are characterized by the following rank order of potency: isoproterenol > epinephrine = norepinephrine. In contrast, β₂ subtypes are characterized by the following order of potency: isoproterenol > epinephrine > > norepinephrine. The development of β-adrenergic receptor antagonists with high selectivities for either the β₁ or β₂ subtypes has confirmed this subclassification. In an analogous manner, studies have confirmed that α-adrenergic receptors do not represent one homogeneous population, but may be further subdivided into at least two subtypes, termed α₁ and α₂ (see also Chapter 12).

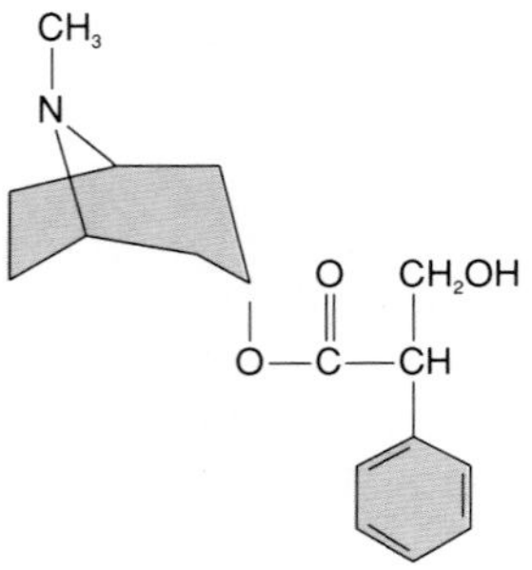

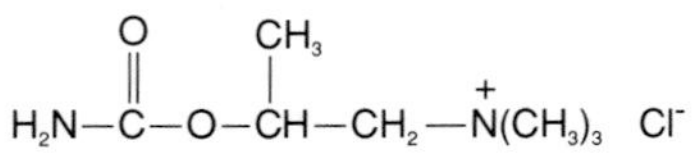

α₁-Adrenergic receptors are defined as those showing high potency to selective agonists, such as methoxamine and phenylephrine, and specific blockade by prazosin. α₂-Adrenergic receptors are characterized by high potency to specific agonists such as clonidine and α-methylnorepinephrine, and specific antagonism by yohimbine. Recent studies in which the genes for adrenergic receptors were cloned using molecular biology techniques have confirmed the existence of α₁, α₂, β₁ and β₂ subtypes as separate and distinct molecular entities (see Chapters 2 and 12).

Molecular biology DNA sequence results show the adrenergic receptor population to be more complex than expected. For example, at least five subtypes of β₁- and β₂-adrenergic receptors have been found in human tissues. Comparison of the amino acid sequences show a high degree of homology, but with some differences. All five types appear to possess seven hydrophobic regions, suggesting that the amino acid chain traverses the membrane seven times. Additional research will detemine what classification systems may be appropriate for the adrenergic receptors and other membrane receptors.

Cholinergic Receptors

As expected, differences in responses mediated by acetylcholine result from actual differences in cholinergic receptors (see Figure 8-6). The actions of acetylcholine can be mimicked in certain organs by the alkaloid, muscarine, whereas in other organs the response to acetylcholine is more closely mimicked by

FIGURE 8-7   Compounds helpful in defining M_1 and M_2 muscarinic receptor subtypes.

the alkaloid, nicotine. Thus, responses evoked by acetylcholine or by activation of the parasympathetic nervous system are described as being *nicotinic* or *muscarinic* and have led to the subclassification of cholinergic receptors as nicotinic cholinergic receptors or muscarinic cholinergic receptors. The response of most autonomic effector cells in peripheral visceral organs is typically muscarinic, whereas the response in parasympathetic and sympathetic ganglia, as well as responses of skeletal muscle, is nicotinic. The nicotinic receptors of autonomic ganglia and skeletal muscle are not homogeneous because they can be blocked by different antagonists. Thus, *d*-tubocurarine effectively blocks nicotinic responses in skeletal muscle, whereas hexamethonium is more effective in blocking nicotinic responses in autonomic ganglia, thereby confirming heterogeneity in nicotinic cholinergic receptors.

Muscarinic receptors may also be divided into at least two subtypes, M_1 and M_2, based on the phar-macologic specificities of certain agonists and antagonists. Atropine blocks both M_1 and M_2 muscarinic cholinergic receptors to nearly equivalent extents. However, the drug, pirenzepine, has proven a selective antagonist of the M_1 subtype. In general, muscarinic cholinergic receptors with the pharmacological profile characteristic of the M_1 subtype are found in autonomic ganglia and in the CNS, whereas M_2 muscarinic receptors exist at neuroeffector junctions of organs innervated by the parasympathetic system.

Molecular biology is currently used to explore the heterogeneity of cholinergic receptors and where they fit into the genetic classification scheme being developed for receptors. The cholinergic receptor population, similar to the adrenoceptor situation, is complex. For example, four different human genes have been identified that produce functional acetylcholine muscarinic receptors of the same subtype but with slight structural and mechanistic differences.

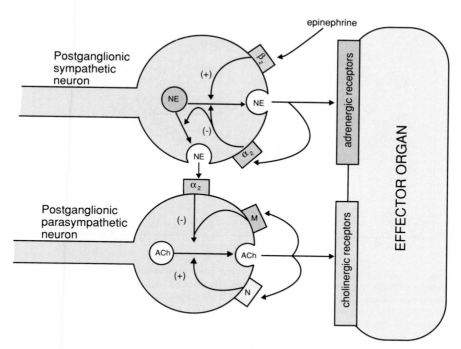

FIGURE 8-8   Schematic representation of the presynaptic autoreceptors that regulate neurotransmitter release in adrenergic and cholinergic neurons. Presynaptic α_2- and β_2-adrenoceptors exist on sympathetic nerve terminals and inhibit and facilitate, respectively, the release of the neurotransmitter, norepinephrine *(NE)*. Presynaptic muscarinic *(M)* and nicotinic *(N)* cholinergic receptors exist presynaptically on cholinergic neurons and inhibit and facilitate, respectively, the release of the neurotransmitter, acetylcholine *(ACh)*. Presynaptic α_2-adrenergic receptors also exist on cholinergic neurons and inhibit acetylcholine release.

Prejunctional Autoreceptors

In recent years, the functional significance of prejunctional autoreceptors has been established. Their distribution and function are illustrated schematically in Figure 8-8. On most adrenergic and cholinergic nerve terminals, the existence of prejunctional α-adrenergic receptors, belonging to the α_2 subtype, have been identified. Activation of these receptors by the released neurotransmitter, norepinephrine, or by exogenously administered α_2-adrenergic receptor ag-

onists, decreases the release of norepinephrine. This presynaptic inhibitory autoreceptor mechanism may be involved in the normal regulation of neurotransmitter release as evidenced by the fact that blockade of this prejunctional α_2-receptor leads to an enhanced overflow of the neurotransmitter, norepinephrine. Presynaptic α_2-receptors also exist on most cholinergic nerve terminals; and when these presynaptic α_2 subtype receptors are activated, the release of acetylcholine is inhibited. These prejunctional α_2-receptors

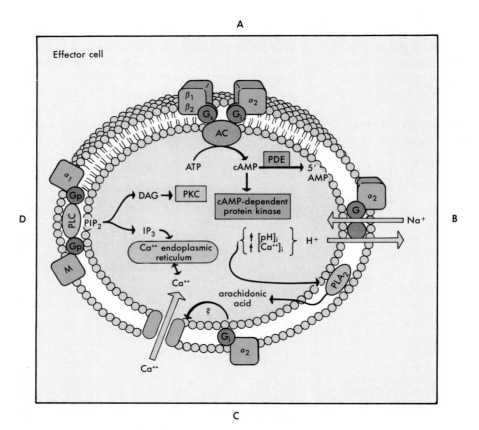

FIGURE 8-9   Mechanisms of signal transduction used by adrenergic and cholinergic receptors in eliciting cellular responses in a hypothetical effector cell. **A,** β_1- and β_2-receptors are coupled to adenylate cyclase *(AC)* through G_s-protein. AC mediates the conversion of ATP to cAMP. See Chapter 2 for discussion of cAMP activation of protein kinase, inactivation of cAMP by phosphodiesterase *(PDE)* and inhibition of cAMP formation by α_2-adrenergic receptors coupled through G_i-protein. **B,** In some cells, α_2-adrenergic receptors mediate responses through G-protein coupled to a sodium/hydrogen exchange system with activation raising intracellular pH. The resulting increase in the intracellular Ca^{++} concentration leads to the activation of membrane-bound phospholipase A_2 *(PLA$_2$)*. **C,** Activation of vascular smooth muscle α_2-adrenergic receptors coupled to G_i-protein leads to activation of membrane-associated calcium channels to produce an influx of calcium from extracellular sites. **D,** α_1-Adrenergic receptors and muscarinic cholinergic receptors are coupled to membrane-bound phospholipase C *(PLC)* through G_p-protein to act via phosphatidylinosotol bisphosphate *(PIP$_2$)*, diacylglycerol *(DAG)*, inositol trisphosphate (IP$_3$), and protein kinase C *(PKC)*. IP$_3$ releases calcium ions from the endoplasmic reticulum.

on cholinergic nerves may be activated by exogenously administered α_2-receptor agonists and may also play a physiological role in regulating the release of acetylcholine when activated by norepinephrine liberated from postganglionic sympathetic neurons that impinge on postganglionic cholinergic nerve terminals.

Presynaptic β-adrenergic receptors, belonging to the β_2 subtype, have also been identified on adrenergic nerve terminals. Activation of these receptors by β_2-receptor agonists, such as epinephrine, leads to facilitation of norepinephrine release, an effect that is opposite to that observed with presynaptic α_2-adrenergic receptor activation. The physiological role of the presynaptic β_2-subtype receptor is not known, but recent studies have suggested that presynaptic β_2-receptor activation by epinephrine may play an important role in the genesis of hypertension.

Presynaptic muscarinic cholinergic receptors have also been proposed to exist on postganglionic parasympathetic neurons, and when activated, these receptors mediate a decrease in the release of acetylcholine. Prejunctional nicotinic cholinergic receptors may also exist on cholinergic nerve terminals and facilitate the release of acetylcholine.

MECHANISMS OF SIGNAL TRANSDUCTION USED BY AUTONOMIC RECEPTORS

Detailed intracellular molecular events that are set into motion when a cell-surface receptor is stimulated by a neurotransmitter are beginning to be understood for the peripheral autonomic receptors. These mechanisms of signal transduction use ion channels and/or enzyme activation-inhibition with secondary messengers. A brief summary of signal transduction as used by autonomic receptors follows.

β-Adrenergic Receptors

The mechanism by which activation of β_1- and β_2-adrenergic receptors leads to generation of an observable pharmacological response is shown schematically in Figure 8-9. Stimulation of β_1- and β_2-receptors leads to the activation of the membrane-bound enzyme, adenylate cyclase, which catalyzes conversion of adenosine triphosphate (ATP) to cyclic adenosine monophosphate (cAMP). The activation of adenylate cyclase by β_1- and β_2-receptors involves

G proteins (see Chapter 2), which couple the β-receptor subtypes to the catalytic enzyme. These coupling proteins, or guanine nucleotide regulatory proteins (G-proteins; G_s, stimulation, G_i, inhibition) are essential for receptor-mediated activation of adenylate cyclase. The sequence of events is believed to be as follows:

1. β-Adrenergic receptor agonists bind to β_1- or β_2-receptors
2. Resulting receptor-agonist complex binds to the G_s-protein (the role of the α, β, and γ subunits of the G-proteins is discussed in Chapter 2)
3. Formation of the receptor-agonist-G_s-protein complex facilitates displacement of guanine diphosphate (GDP) by guanine triphosphate (GTP) on the G_s-protein
4. Complex between G_s-protein and GTP dissociates from the receptor-agonist complex and interacts with the catalytic subunit of adenylate cyclase, thereby promoting the conversion of ATP to cAMP
5. cAMP then activates an intracellular enzyme, cAMP-dependent protein kinase, which phosphorylates phosphorylase b kinase and a number of intracellular proteins leading to a pharmacological response.

α₂-Adrenergic Receptors

In many systems, α_2-receptors are coupled to the inhibition of adenylate cyclase and result in the opposite effect of that observed for β_1- and β_2-receptor activation. Thus, α_2-receptors are coupled to adenylate cyclase in an inhibitory manner through guanine nucleotide regulatory proteins termed G_i (see Chapter 2 for details). When α_2-receptors are activated, the G_i protein will ultimately inhibit the catalytic activity of adenylate cyclase, thereby leading to a reduction in intracellular concentrations of cAMP that decreases the activation of cAMP-dependent protein kinase (see Figure 8-9).

Although the inhibition of adenylate cyclase by α_2-receptor activation occurs in many systems, it is important to note that α_2-receptors may also use other mechanisms of signal transduction. For example, in the human platelet, activation of α_2-receptors leads to stimulation of a sodium-hydrogen exchange system that produces an influx of sodium and an efflux of hydrogen ions. The net effect is intracellular alkalinization leading to elevated intracellular calcium, activation of membrane-bound phospholipase A_2, release of arachidonic acid, and enzymatic conversion to thromboxane A_2 to produce platelet aggregation (see Chapters 18 and 21).

In blood vessels, a different mechanism for signal transduction is used by α_2-adrenergic receptors. Although details have not been fully elucidated, it appears that the activation of α_2-receptors is mediated via a G_i protein that leads to activation of a membrane calcium channel resulting in the influx of calcium from extracellular sites.

α_1-Adrenergic Receptors

α_1-Receptors produce their effects through increases in intracellular phosphatidylinositol turnover. That is, activation of the α_1-adrenergic receptor leads to stimulation of membrane-bound phospholipase C, the latter being coupled to the α_1-receptor by a guanine nucleotide regulatory protein termed G_p. The activation of phospholipase C results in the hydrolysis of phosphatidylinositol bisphosphate (PIP_2) to produce diacyglycerol (DAG) and inositol trisphosphate (IP_3). Diacyglycerol activates protein kinase C, in part by sensitizing it to Ca^{++}, which leads to phosphorylation of a set of intracellular proteins. Inositol trisphosphate acts to mobilize calcium from endoplasmic reticulum into the cytosol. Thus, diacyglycerol and inositol trisphosphate are intracellular messengers that lead to pharmacological responses mediated by α_1-receptor activation.

Muscarinic Cholinergic Receptors

Muscarinic cholinergic receptors are similar to α_1-adrenergic receptors in that they produce effects through increases in intracellular phosphatidylinositol turnover. Thus, activation of the muscarinic cholinergic receptor leads to association with a guanine nucleotide regulatory protein (G_p) and activation of phospholipase C. The subsequent generation of diacylglycerol and inositol trisphosphate from phosphatidylinositol bisphosphate after hydrolysis by phospholipase C ultimately mediates the muscarinic cholinergic effects (see Figure 8-9).

Nicotinic Cholinergic Receptor

Details of signal transduction for nicotinic cholinergic responses have not been fully elucidated. Activation of the nicotinic cholinergic receptor appears to require interaction with a guanine nucleotide regulatory protein that leads to the activation of specific membrane ion channels (see Chapter 2).

FUNCTIONAL RESPONSES MEDIATED BY PERIPHERAL AUTONOMIC NERVOUS SYSTEM

In Absence of Pharmacological Agents

Many organs of the body receive adrenergic and cholinergic innervation, and responses in these organs represent a complex interplay between two divisions of the autonomic nervous system. It is usual for one type of innervation to predominate over the other, so that an organ may be predominantly under the control of only one division of the autonomic nervous system, although both components are present and can modulate any given response. Organs receiving dual innervation from the sympathetic and parasympathetic divisions of the autonomic nervous system include the heart, eye, bronchial tree, GI tract, urinary bladder, and reproductive organs. Some organs receive only a single type of innervation, generally that of the sympathetic nervous system. Thus, blood vessels, spleen, and piloerector muscles receive predominantly an adrenergic innervation. As indicated earlier, the predominant cholinergic receptor located postjunctionally on the visceral effector organs and mediating the response to acetylcholine is the muscarinic cholinergic receptor of the M_2 subtype. In contrast, α_1-, α_2-, β_1-, or β_2-adrenergic receptors can mediate the adrenergic responses to nerve stimulation in the various visceral effector organs receiving adrenergic innervation. A detailed account of the adrenergic and cholinergic responses that occur in a number of important organs of the body is presented in Table 8-1. In most instances sympathetic and parasympathetic nerves mediate physiologically opposing effects. That is, if one system inhibits a certain function, the other system usually enhances that function. The responses presented in Table 8-1 represent only those mediated by stimulation of sympathetic or parasympathetic nerves, and therefore they represent responses mediated by the neurotransmitter interacting only with autonomic receptors located directly in the neuroeffector junction. However, autonomic receptors are also found at

Table 8-1 Responses Elicited in Effector Organs by Stimulation of Sympathetic and Parasympathetic Nerves

Effector Organ	Adrenergic Response	Receptor Involved	Cholinergic Response	Dominant Response* A or C
Heart				
Rate of contraction	Increase	β_1	Decrease	C
Force of contraction	Increase	β_1	Decrease	C
Blood vessels				
Arteries (most)	Vasoconstriction	α_1	—	A
Skeletal muscle	Vasodilation	β_2	—	A
Veins	Vasoconstriction	α_2	—	A
Bronchial tree	Bronchodilation	β_2	Bronchoconstriction	A
Splenic capsule	Contraction	α_1	—	C
Uterus	Contraction	α_1	Variable	A
Vas deferens	Contraction	α_1	—	A
Prostatic capsule	Contraction	α_1	—	A
GI tract	Relaxation	α_2	Contraction	A
Eye				C
Radial muscle, iris	Contraction (mydriasis)	α_1	—	A
Circular muscle, iris	—		Contraction (miosis)	C
Ciliary muscle	Relaxation	β	Contraction (accommodation)	C
Kidney	Renin secretion	β_1	—	A
Urinary Bladder				
Detrusor	Relaxation	β	Contraction	C
Trigone and sphincter	Contraction	α_1	Relaxation	A,C
Ureter	Contraction	α_1	Relaxation	A
Insulin release from pancreas	Decrease	α_2	—	A
Fat cells	Lipolysis	β_1	—	A
Liver glycogenolysis	Increase	α_1	—	A
Hair follicles, smooth muscle	Contraction (piloerection)	α_1	—	A
Nasal secretion	—		Increase	C
Salivary glands	Increase secretion	α_1	Increase secretion	C
Sweat glands	Increase secretion	α_1	Increase secretion	C

* A, Adrenergic; C, cholinergic.

sites away from the neuroeffector junction and these receptors may be different from the receptors or receptor subtypes located directly in the neuroeffector junction. For example, although vascular smooth muscle has no cholinergic innervation, it has a full complement of cholinergic receptors. Because these "extrajunctional" receptors are functional and may mediate responses to exogenously administered drugs, they probably play little or no physiological role in the normal autonomic response mediated by sympathetic or parasympathetic nerves and are therefore not listed in Table 8-1.

In Presence of Pharmacological Agents

Pharmacological agents that alter the adrenergic and cholinergic divisions of the autonomic nervous system are discussed in detail in Chapters 9 to 11. The purpose of this discussion is to present a brief overview of the points of pharmacological intervention (Table 8-2) that are possible in the peripheral autonomic nervous system and a few examples of the drugs that interfere at these points.

Ganglionic Blockers Drugs that block autonomic ganglia interfere with the transmission of nerve impulses from preganglionic nerve terminals to the cell

Table 8-2 Sites of Pharmacological Intervention in Peripheral Autonomic Nervous System

Site	Intervention
Ganglia	Block transmission
	Activate receptor
Synapse	Inhibit synthesis of neurotransmitter
	Inhibit release of neurotransmitter
	Promote release of neurotransmitter
	Reduce uptake or storage of neurotransmitter
	Inhibit metabolism of neurotransmitter
	Block receptor
	Activate receptor

bodies of postganglionic neurons. Because the neurotransmitters and receptors are identical in autonomic ganglia of both adrenergic and cholinergic nerves, ganglionic blockers appear to impede both divisions of the autonomic nervous system equally. However, the end-organ response may show a predominant adrenergic or cholinergic effect. The reason for this is that the degree of innervation by the adrenergic and cholinergic nervous system, and the extent of the adrenergic and cholinergic dominance in a given organ, may not be equivalent (see Table 8-1). Therefore, interruption of ganglionic transmission will have the overall effect of selectively eliminating that component of the autonomic nervous system that generally dominates, leading to a response that is characteristic of the less dominant component. For example, in the heart the cholinergic system generally dominates over the adrenergic component, and the administration of a ganglionic blocker will therefore have the greatest effect on the cholinergic component, resulting in an apparent adrenergic end-organ effect (i.e., tachycardia). The classic ganglionic blockers are hexamethonium and mecamylamine.

Drugs that Inhibit Synthesis of Neurotransmitter Several enzymes are necessary for the biosynthesis of norepinephrine and epinephrine from tyrosine (see Figure 8-4). Tyrosine hydroxylase, the rate-limiting enzyme, is inhibited by α-methyltyrosine. The next enzyme, L-aromatic amino acid decarboxylase, is inhibited by carbidopa and α-methyldopa. The latter also is a substrate for the decarboxylase, and converts to α-methylnorepinephrine, a potent and highly selective α_2-adrenergic receptor agonist.

Dopamine is synthesized in the cytoplasm and transported into storage vesicles. There the third enzyme, dopamine-β-hydroxylase, associated with the storage vesicle membrane, hydroxylates dopamine to norepinephrine, which is stored in the adrenergic vesicles in association with ATP. Fusaric acid is a selective inhibitor of dopamine-β-hydroxylase and produces a significant reduction in norepinephrine concentrations and a concomitant increase in dopamine concentrations.

Dopamine-β-hydroxylase is the terminal enzyme in the biosynthesis of catecholamines in postganglionic sympathetic nerve terminals, and norepinephrine is found in high concentrations in these neurons. However, in the adrenal medulla, a fourth enzyme exists that catalyzes the formation of epinephrine, the major catecholamine in the adrenal gland. The fourth enzyme, phenothanolamine-*N*-methyltransferase can be inhibited by agents such as 2,3-dichloro-α-methylbenzylamine.

As previously stated, synthesis of acetylcholine occurs by acetylation of choline through the enzyme, choline acetyltransferase, using acetyl coenzyme A (see Figure 8-5). Although there are no potent and specific inhibitors of choline acetyltransferase, the biosynthesis of acetylcholine can be indirectly inhibited with hemicholinium, which blocks the high affinity system that transports choline into the cholinergic nerve terminal. This results in marked depletion of acetylcholine in cholinergic neurons.

Drugs that Inhibit Release of Neurotransmitter Release of norepinephrine from postganglionic sympathetic nerve terminals involves an exocytotic process in which the storage vesicle membrane fuses with the neuronal membrane, allowing the storage vesicle to release its contents into the neuroeffector junction. Bretylium and guanethidine are two drugs that inhibit this process, and are classified as adrenergic neuronal blocking agents, which interfere with adrenergic neurotransmission.

The release of acetylcholine also occurs through exocytosis. Botulinus toxin prevents the release of acetylcholine from all types of cholinergic nerve fibers. Because the cholinergic nervous system is essential for survival, botulinus toxin is lethal.

Drugs that Promote Release of Neurotransmitter Two processes can promote the release of norepinephrine from postganglionic sympathetic nerve terminals. One is by activation of nicotinic ganglionic cholinergic receptors by 1,1-dimethylphenylpiperazinium (DMPP), which generates action potentials in the cell body of the postganglionic neuron. The action potentials are propagated to the nerve terminal and activate the calcium-dependent exocytotic release of norepinephrine from storage vesicles into the synaptic cleft. The second process is through tyramine, ephedrine, or amphetamine, which are indirectly-acting sympathomimetic amines evoking the release of cytoplasmic stores of norepinephrine. These drugs enter the sympathetic nerve terminal by an amine uptake$_1$ pump and displace cytoplasmic norepinephrine that passively diffuses through the neuronal membrane into the synaptic cleft by a process that does not involve calcium or exocytosis.

The release of acetylcholine from postganglionic cholinergic nerve terminals can be evoked by activation of ganglionic nicotinic cholinergic receptors by dimethylphenylpiperazinium (DMPP). As is the case for the release of norepinephrine, DMPP will elicit the generation of action potentials that ultimately produce the exotoxic release of acetylcholine. There are no known drugs that will displace acetylcholine from neuronal stores and thereby indirectly elicit release of this neurotransmitter. Because acetylcholine is a positively charged quaternary ammonium compound, it cannot readily penetrate the neuronal membrane, and therefore the ability of cholinergic agents to promote the release of acetylcholine is limited.

Drugs that Interfere with Storage of Neurotransmitter After its synthesis in the cytoplasm, norepinephrine is accumulated and stored in the cytoplasmic storage granules until subsequent release through exocytosis. There is an energy-dependent amine uptake pump in the storage vesicle membrane, which accumulates catecholamines. Reserpine blocks uptake of catecholamines into the storage vesicles, thereby decreasing the amount of norepinephrine available for release on nerve stimulation, leading to complete depletion of catecholamines from postganglionic sympathetic nerve terminals.

At present, no known drugs interfere with the accumulation of acetylcholine by the cholinergic storage vesicles. However, hemicholinium will lead to depletion of acetylcholine stores in cholinergic neurons by interfering with the accumulation of choline.

Drugs that Affect Neuronal Uptake After exocytotic release of norepinephrine from postganglionic sympathetic nerve terminals, most of the released catecholamine is actively reaccumulated in the sympathetic nerve terminal by uptake$_1$. Agents such as cocaine and imipramine block this amine uptake pump and thereby increase synaptic concentrations of norepinephrine, enhancing or facilitating adrenergic neurotransmission.

Acetylcholine is not taken up into cholinergic neurons after its release. As already discussed, high affinity uptake for choline is present, which is inhibited by hemicholinium.

Drugs that Inhibit Metabolism of Neurotransmitter Two enzymes involved in the metabolism of the catecholamines are monoamine oxidase and catechol-O-methyltransferase. Monoamine oxidase is inhibited by the drugs pargyline or tranylcypromine, and catechol-O-methyltransferase is inhibited by other catechols, such as pyrogallol. Inhibition of monoamine oxidase and catechol-O-methyltransferase results in higher concentrations of norepinephrine in peripheral tissues but does not enhance the effects of neuroeffector organs to sympathetic nerve stimulation (see Chapter 10).

Acetylcholinesterase is the major enzyme catalyzing the hydrolysis of acetylcholine and terminating the cholinergic effect. Acetylcholinesterase is inhibited by physostigmine, which enhances the magnitude and duration of effects elicited by stimulation of cholinergic neurons.

Drugs that Block Autonomic Receptors Older prototypic α-adrenergic blockers are phenoxybenzamine, phentolamine, and tolazoline, which block both α_1- and α_2-adrenergic receptors. Developed more recently, prazosin blocks α_1-receptors and yohimbine blocks α_2-receptors with relatively high selectivity.

The prototypic β-receptor blockers such as propranolol block both β_1- and β_2-adrenergic receptors with little selectivity. Newer and more selective β-receptor blockers include metoprolol, a relatively selective β_1-receptor antagonist, and butoxamine, a selective β_2-receptor antagonist.

Most effector organs of the autonomic nervous system contain muscarinic cholinergic receptors are blocked in a competitive manner by atropine. Nicotinic cholinergic receptors are of two types: those existing in skeletal muscle and those present in autonomic ganglia. Nicotinic cholinergic receptors in skeletal muscle are selectively antagonized by d-tubocurarine (Chapter 11) and ganglionic nicotinic receptors are selectively inhibited by hexamethonium or mecamylamine.

Drugs that Stimulate Autonomic Receptors

The neurotransmitter, norepinephrine, activates α_1-, α_2-, and β_1-adrenergic receptors with relatively weak activity at β_2-receptors. Epinephrine, on the other hand, activates all four adrenergic-receptor subtypes with similar potency. A number of drugs have been discovered that selectively activate each of the receptor subtypes. Phenylephrine is a potent and highly selective α_1-receptor agonist, and clonidine is a selective α_2-receptor agonist. Isoproterenol is equally effective at stimulating both β_1- and β_2-adrenergic receptors. However, dobutamine has been proposed as a selective β_1-receptor agonist, whereas terbutaline is a selective agonist of β_2-receptors.

Acetylcholine activates both muscarinic and nicotinic cholinergic receptors, as well as each of the individual subtypes of these cholinergic receptors. Muscarinic cholinergic receptors may be selectively stimulated by the alkaloid, muscarine, or by synthetic agonists, such as carbamylcholine. Nicotinic cholinergic receptors may be selectively stimulated by the alkaloid, nicotine, and selective stimulation of ganglionic nicotinic cholinergic receptors can be achieved with dimethylphenylpiperazinium.

REFERENCES

Berthelsen S and Pettinger WA: A functional basis for classification of α-adrenergic receptors, Life Sci 21:595, 1977.

Euler US von: Synthesis, uptake and storage of catecholamines in adrenergic nerves: the effects of drugs. In Blaschko H and Muscholl E, eds.: Catecholamines: handbook of experimental pharmacology, vol 33, Berlin, 1972, Springer-Verlag.

Gilman AG: Guanine nucleotide-binding regulatory proteins and dual control of the adenylate cyclase, J Clin Invest 73:1, 1984.

Langer SZ: Presynaptic regulation of the release of catecholamines, Pharmacol Rev 32:337, 1980.

Trendelenburg U: A kinetic analysis of the extraneuronal uptake and metabolism of catecholamines, Rev Physiol Biochem Pharmacol 87:33, 1980.

CHAPTER

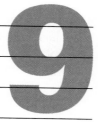

Drugs Affecting the Parasympathetic Nervous System

ABBREVIATIONS

Acetyl-CoA	acetylcoenzyme A
ATP	adenosine triphosphate
AV	atrioventricular
GI	gastrointestinal
IM	intramuscular, intramuscularly
IV	intravenous, intravenously

MAJOR DRUGS

cholinomimetic agonists
muscarinic blocking drugs
ganglionic blocking drugs
cholinesterase or enzyme inhibitors

 THERAPEUTIC OVERVIEW

The parasympathetic branch of the autonomic nervous system consists primarily of neural pathways that use acetylcholine as the neurochemical transmitter. The parasympathetic division innervates primarily the GI tract, eye, heart, respiratory tract, glandular secretion, and bladder (see Chapter 8). Although relatively few disease states are identifiable with dysfunctions of cholinergic sites of the peripheral autonomic nervous system, cholinergic sites are still key points for pharmacological intervention for restoration

of normal body functions. Because of the widespread accessibility and actions of the cholinergic system and the co-innervation of most organs and tissues by the parasympathetic and sympathetic divisions, two factors are of prime importance in pharmacological intervention: (1) the need for organ/tissue selectivity in the cholinergic-targeted drugs being used and (2) knowledge of the neuroeffector action of the sympathetic pathway when the input from the parasympathetic (cholinergic) division is blocked.

Knowing which cholinergic sites possess muscarinic and which have nicotinic subtype acetylcholine receptors allows one to select drug for the specific receptor subtype (see Chapter 8). Neuroeffector junctions of the parasympathetic division generally have muscarinic subtypes, whereas ganglionic synapses have nicotinic subtypes. Although the association of particular receptor subtypes with ganglia and with neuroeffector junctions provides a convenient operating classification, sophisticated research techniques demonstrate that the relationship is more complex. Some junctions and some synapses have only postjunctional or postsynaptic cholinergic receptors and others contain both postjunctional and prejunctional or postsynaptic and presynaptic receptors. These may be nicotinic or muscarinic subtype receptors, with the functions of the prejunctional or presynaptic control pathways not well understood.

In the previous chapter, sites and mechanisms of potential pharmacological intervention in the adrenergic or cholinergic portions of the peripheral autonomic nervous system are listed. The major mechanisms discussed in Chapter 8 by which drugs affect the cholinergic system are:

1. Stimulation of neuroeffector pathways by agonists
2. Blockade of neuroeffector receptors by antagonists
3. Inhibition of acetylcholine metabolism
4. Blockade (or stimulation) of ganglionic receptors

The therapeutic uses of cholinergic-targeted drugs are summarized in Table 9-1.

A special type of neuroeffector junction, which utilizes acetylcholine as a neurochemical transmitter but is not part of the cholinergic system, exists between skeletal muscles and the somatic nerves that innervate these muscles. The actions of the receptors at these junctions are very similar to the nicotinic receptors in the cholinergic system, and a group of drugs termed *neuromuscular blocking agents* disrupt somatic nerve-skeletal muscle signal transmission by blocking these receptors. These drugs are described in Chapter 11.

Several CNS problems are caused by cholinergic imbalance (see Chapter 27). A disease of central origin, but which bears directly on principles associated with the neuropharmacology of acetylcholine, is Alzheimer's disease. The hallmarks of this devastating illness appear to be a deficit of the enzyme choline acetyltransferase, a fall in sodium-dependent high-affinity choline uptake, and inadequate acetylcholine concentrations. Because the postsynaptic cholinergic receptor system remains intact, drug manipulations based on a knowledge of autonomic pharmacology may prove helpful in seeking therapeutic measures to treat this disease. Drugs that block dopamine receptors frequently cause extrapyramidal tremor with Parkinson's disease (Chapter 27) generally considered to result from a deficiency of dopamine. Perhaps the decline in dopamine concentration results in excessive release of acetylcholine, producing tremor, because clinically, atropine-related drugs that block cholinergic effects provide symptomatic relief from tremor.

Table 9-1   Tissue/Organ Effects and Therapeutic Applications of Cholinergic-Targeted Drugs

Tissue/Organ	Effect	Condition Treated or Use
MUSCARINIC AGONISTS		
Eye	Contraction of ciliary muscle and sphincter muscle of iris	Glaucoma
GI tract	Increased peristaltic movement, sphincter relaxation	Adynamic ileus
Urinary bladder	Increased contraction of detrusor muscle, sphincter relaxation	Urinary retention
Vascular smooth muscle	Dilation	—
Bronchial smooth muscle	Bronchoconstriction	—
All glands	Secretion	—
Heart	Negative inotropic, chronotropic, and dromotropic effect	—
ENZYME INHIBITORS*		
Skeletal muscle	Increased muscle activity	Myasthenia gravis
Eye	Similar to agonists	Glaucoma
MUSCARINIC ANTAGONISTS		
Eye	Mydriasis	Refraction studies
GI tract	Decreased muscle actions and secretions	Spasm
Urinary bladder	Relaxation, constriction of sphincter	Urinary incontinence
Bronchiolar smooth muscle	Decreased muscle action and secretions	Surgery, asthma
Brain	Blockade of central receptors	Parkinson's disease
Heart	Vagal blockade, tachycardia, increased AV nodal firing	—
Glands	Salivary secretion, sweat glands blocked	—
NICOTINIC ANTAGONISTS		
Ganglia	Decreased sympathetic activation	Hypertensive crisis (?)

*Blockade of acetylcholine metabolism.

MECHANISMS OF ACTION

The structure and molecular mechanisms of the nicotinic acetylcholine receptor are described in Chapter 2, and the biochemistry and physiology of the peripheral autonomic nervous system including cholinergic and adrenergic neurochemical transmission is discussed in Chapter 8. Some additional topics that pertain specifically to cholinergic neurochemical transmission are described in this section.

Synthesis and Release of Acetylcholine

Acetylcholine is synthesized at neuroeffector and ganglionic junctions from the immediate precursors acetyl-CoA and choline by action of choline acetyltransferase (Figure 9-1). This enzyme is present in the cytosol in soluble form with a small amount bound to membranes. Its activity is strongly dependent on ionic strength.

Neuronal cells depend on exogenous choline since they are deficient in the transmethylating system required to convert precursors such as ethanolamine to choline. It is estimated that the transmethylating enzyme is present in these cells in less than 1% of the concentration found in liver. Choline-containing phospholipids, lecithins, or lysolecithins are the usual precursors. They may arise from dietary sources or by synthesis in the liver from phosphatidyl ethanolamine and S-adenosylmethionine. Choline is transported via the blood in phospholipid form from the liver to nerve cells and is released through the action of a phospholipase. The choline is then taken up into cholinergic nerve terminals by a sodium-dependent high affinity choline uptake system. Although no therapeutically useful drugs act by blocking the uptake or synthesis of acetylcholine at nerve terminals, hemicholinium has been used experimentally to block choline uptake in animals.

While the source of choline for acetylcholine formation is well understood, the origin of the acetyl moiety is yet unclear. It is known that glucose carbon atoms are incorporated into the acetyl portion of acetylcholine with pyruvate as immediate precursor. Because pyruvate dehydrogenase, the required enzyme for producing acetyl-CoA from pyruvate, is localized exclusively in mitochondria, the acetyl-CoA formed requires translocation to the cytosol, the site of acetylcholine synthesis; but no mechanism has been discovered for transport of acetyl-CoA from the mitochondria to the cytosol. A possible indirect mechanism to accomplish this translocation may be the intramitochondrial condensation of acetyl-CoA and oxaloacetate to citrate catalyzed by citrate synthase, with citrate readily transported to the cytosol where

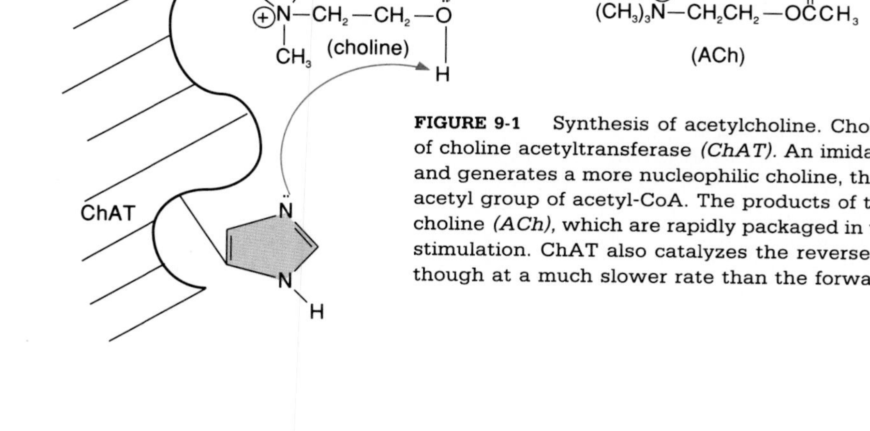

FIGURE 9-1 Synthesis of acetylcholine. Choline and acetyl-CoA bind to the surface of choline acetyltransferase *(ChAT)*. An imidazole on ChAT promotes proton removal and generates a more nucleophilic choline, thereby facilitating condensation with the acetyl group of acetyl-CoA. The products of the reaction are coenzyme-A and acetylcholine *(ACh)*, which are rapidly packaged in vesicles for immediate release on proper stimulation. ChAT also catalyzes the reverse reaction between ACh and CoASH, although at a much slower rate than the forward reaction.

it is cleaved to acetyl-CoA and oxaloacetate by ATP-citrate lyase. Finally, acetylcholine synthesis is tightly regulated, and the transmitter is packaged in small vesicles that protect acetyl choline from hydrolysis by intra- and extracellular cholinesterases.

Assuming that acetylcholine vesicles from humans are similar in composition to synaptic vesicles of the electric eel, vesicles from cerebral tissue are estimated to contain 100 nmol of acetylcholine per mg of protein. In contrast, the phrenic nerve contains only 1 nmol of acetylcholine/mg protein, requiring a very rapid turnover and making this tissue especially vulnerable to various neurotoxins that inhibit acetylcholine release.

The arrival of a sufficient action potential at the nerve terminal triggers the Ca^{++}-dependent release of acetylcholine from vesicles. The release is quantal and transient. An alternative mechanism to *vesicle* release is the *cytoplasmic* release theory in which acetylcholine is released from a cytoplasmic pool through "gates" in the presynaptic membrane. According to this theory, the function of the vesicles present at cholinergic endings is as a reserve for acetylcholine or as a sequestration site for free Ca^{++} ions. Without nerve stimulation, there is a small leakage of acetylcholine from nerve endings, which could come directly from the cytoplasm but this contributes little to the total fraction of acetylcholine released after nerve stimulation. Present data support the "vesicle release" theory following nerve stimulation. Although no therapeutic agents are available in the United States to block acetylcholine release, botulinus toxin is used in other countries by local injection to clinically ameliorate neuorological diseases with excessive muscle twitching.

Acetylcholine, after its release from nerve terminals, reacts with postsynaptic receptors or is hydrolyzed to terminate transmitter action. Unlike the catecholamines of the adrenergic system, the intact transmitter molecule is not taken back up into the prejunctional nerve cell; rather only its hydrolysis product, choline, is taken up and reused.

Stimulation of Muscarinic or Nicotinic Receptors (Agonists)

Terminology for muscarinic and nicotinic receptors resulted from the early use of the natural alkaloids muscarine and nicotine and the effects each produced in the presence of acetylcholine as transmitter. In keeping with this terminology, drugs that produce the same response as that obtained by stimulating the parasympathetic nervous system are termed *cholinomimetic*, and the effects produced are either *nicotinic* or *muscarinic* depending on the subtype of the receptor. A similar distinction is used to classify

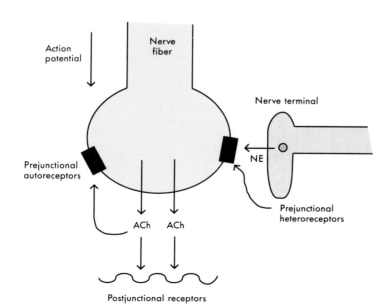

FIGURE 9-2   Prejunctional receptors. Receptors present on the membrane of the presynaptic nerve terminal can respond to acetylcholine *(ACh)* released from that particular terminal (autoreceptors) or to a different transmitter (in this case norepinephrine, *NE*) released from a terminal derived from another neuron (heteroreceptors). These prejunctional interactions modulate the release of ACh but are more important in the CNS than in the peripheral cholinergic system.

antagonists at cholinergic receptors as antimuscarinic, or antinicotinic, although *blocking agents* is the descriptive term often used.

Muscarinic receptors are linked to the G-protein adenylate or guanylate cyclase secondary messenger systems described in Chapters 2 and 8.

Some receptors exist postjunctionally and others exist also on prejunctional nerve terminals (Figure 9-2). This has led to the additional terminology of autoreceptors or heteroreceptors. If a neurotransmitter is released from a nerve terminal and reacts with a receptor on its own prejunctional nerve ending, that receptor is termed an *autoreceptor*. Such a mechanism has been invoked to explain feedback regulation of release; elevated junctional concentrations of neurotransmitter would react with these prejunctional autoreceptors to slow further release.

A heteroreceptor is present on prejunctional structures but responds to substances other than the neurotransmitter released at the terminal. For example, the α_2-adrenergic agonist, clonidine (Chapter 10), acts prejunctionally on cholinergic terminals to suppress acetylcholine outflow. Prejunctional α_2-adrenergic heteroreceptors are present on the splanchnic nerve and are stimulated by epinephrine and norepinephrine. This inhibits acetylcholine release from the nerve and decreases its interaction at adrenal nicotinic receptors, thus diminishing further release of catecholamines from the adrenal medulla.

Cholinergic agonists or cholinomimetic agents produce pharmacological effects by binding to muscarinic or nicotinic postjunctional receptors. The structures of pilocarpine, carbachol, bethanechol, methacholine (the latter compound used for diagnostic but not therapeutic purposes) and, as additional reference materials, acetylcholine, muscarine, and nicotine are shown in Figure 9-3.

Key elements of the acetylcholine structure are the cationic quaternary ammonium group and the ester function, which are separated by the short alkyl chain. The distance and the torsional angle between these two groups are identified as critical for association and subsequent stimulation of cholinergic receptor subtypes. The cationic head group is perceived as binding to an anionic site on the receptor surface while the carbonyl oxygen associates with a region of negative electrostatic potential a prescribed distance from the anionic site. It has been suggested that the conformations necessary for stimulation of muscarinic and nicotinic receptors differ.

Muscarinic Blocking Drugs

Naturally occurring alkaloid l-hyoscyamine undergoes racemization and on acid extraction yields atropine. Atropine and related compounds are classified as antimuscarinic or muscarinic blocking drugs because they competitively block the actions of acetylcholine at both central and peripheral muscarinic receptors. The structurally related l-hyoscine, or scopolamine, differs from atropine only in the presence of an epoxide ring on the tropane moiety. Numerous derivatives and analogs have been synthesized to provide a large number of antimuscarinic agents.

The muscarinic blocking agents, such as atropine, compete with acetylcholine for both M_1 and M_2 muscarinic receptors. There is discrimination for antagonists, with pirenzepine having high affinity for M_1 receptors and bethanecol for M_2. Yet both receptor subclasses are blocked by atropine. There is evidence that the muscarinic blocking agents are more effective in blocking exogenous acetylcholine, or injected agonists, than in inhibiting responses to postganglionic nerve stimulation. Under the latter circumstances a higher concentration of acetylcholine is achieved at or near the receptor, requiring a greater concentration for competitive blockade.

The majority of the muscarinic blocking drugs modeled on atropine are constructed so that an amine is present three to five atomic units from bulky constituents. Aminoalcohols and aminoalcohol esters and ethers also provide the essential structural requisites for muscarinic blocking activity. Structural features in tricyclic compounds analogous to those found in potent muscarinic blocking agents provide the molecular basis for antimuscarinic side effects observed with other classes of therapeutic agents. Examples include tricyclic antidepressants, such as amitriptyline and imipramine, certain phenothiazine neuroleptics such as thioridazine, and some of the antihistaminics. At normal therapeutic doses they elicit atropinelike effects, including urinary retention, adynamic ileus, dry mouth, and blurring of vision, especially in the elderly patient.

Ganglionic Blocking and Stimulating Drugs

Ganglionic transmission is modulated by the effects of released acetylcholine acting directly on nicotinic receptors and indirectly on small intensely fluorescent cells that contain and release dopamine. Dopamine acts on receptors on the ganglion cell

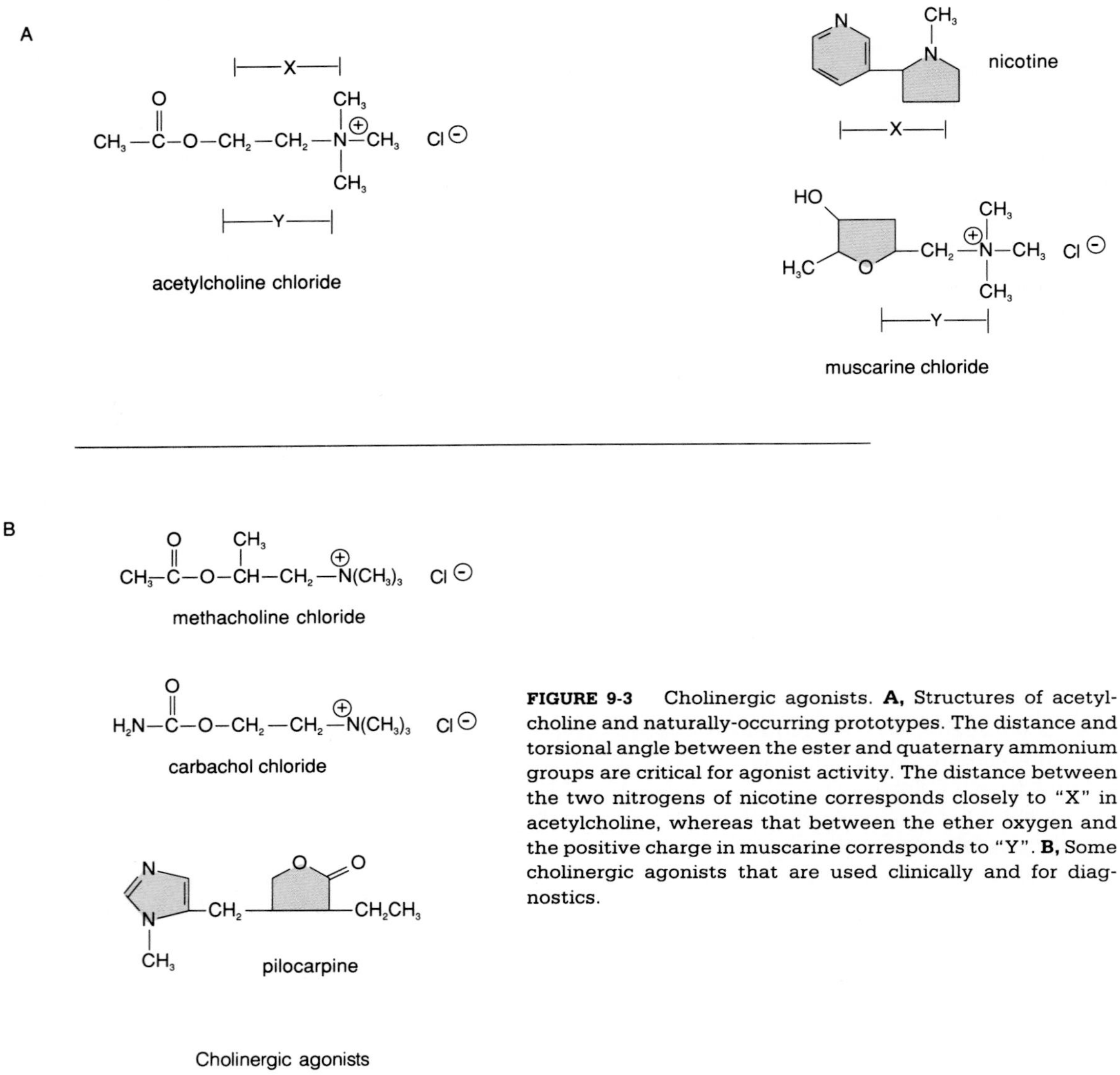

A

acetylcholine chloride

nicotine

muscarine chloride

B

methacholine chloride

carbachol chloride

pilocarpine

FIGURE 9-3 Cholinergic agonists. **A,** Structures of acetylcholine and naturally-occurring prototypes. The distance and torsional angle between the ester and quaternary ammonium groups are critical for agonist activity. The distance between the two nitrogens of nicotine corresponds closely to "X" in acetylcholine, whereas that between the ether oxygen and the positive charge in muscarine corresponds to "Y". **B,** Some cholinergic agonists that are used clinically and for diagnostics.

Cholinergic agonists

bodies to modulate ganglionic activity (Figure 9-4). In addition, there is evidence that peptides such as substance P further modulate electrical events associated with ganglionic transmission although the mechanism is still not clear. Substance P is present mainly in the CNS and is discussed further in Chapter 12. In the autonomic nervous system substance P is found at sympathetic ganglia and in the GI wall and appears to modulate cholinergic transmission. It appears to be selective for nicotinic receptors but not those present at the skeletal muscle end plate. Substance P may provide another site for the future development of more selective cholinergic drugs.

Because it is difficult to limit ganglionic blockade to either the parasympathetic or sympathetic division and further to specific organs, these agents are infrequently used clinically. Trimethaphan camsylate is available for injection and mecamylamine is used orally. Nicotine is important toxicologically and produces ganglionic stimulation followed by depression.

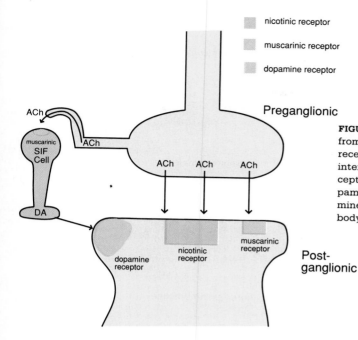

FIGURE 9-4 Ganglionic synapse. Acetylcholine *(ACh)* released from the preganglionic cell binds to nicotinic and muscarinic receptors postsynaptically on cell bodies. Also shown are small intensely fluorescent *(SIF)* cells, which possess muscarinic receptors on their outer membrane, and vesicles that contain dopamine. When released on appropriate stimulation, the dopamine interacts with dopamine receptors on the postsynaptic cell body and modulates the postsynaptic effect of ACh.

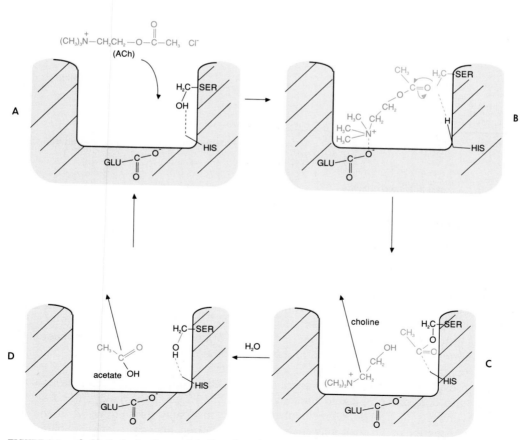

FIGURE 9-5 **A,** Hydrolysis of acetylcholine *(ACh)* by acetylcholinesterase. **B,** Activated serine -OH attacks the carbonyl of ACh, **C,** becomes acetylated, and **D,** is eventually hydrolyzed to acetate and the free enzyme (see text).

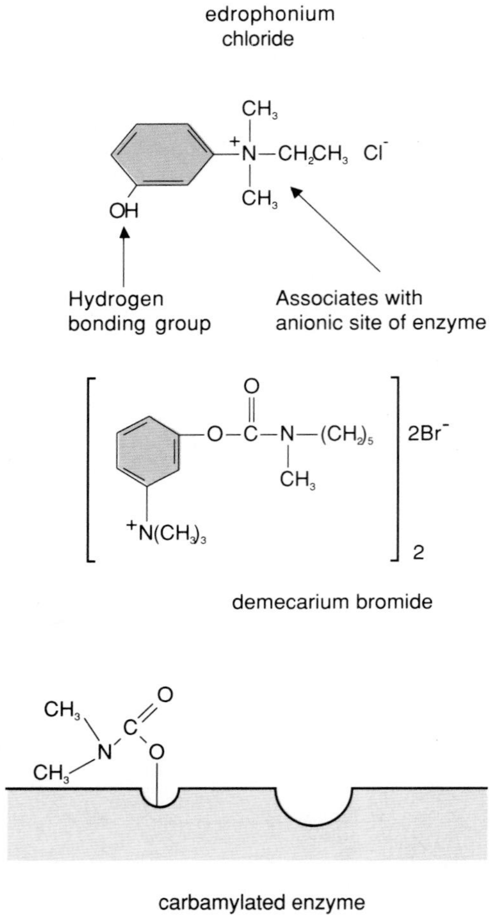

edrophonium
chloride

Hydrogen
bonding group

Associates with
anionic site of enzyme

demecarium bromide

carbamylated enzyme

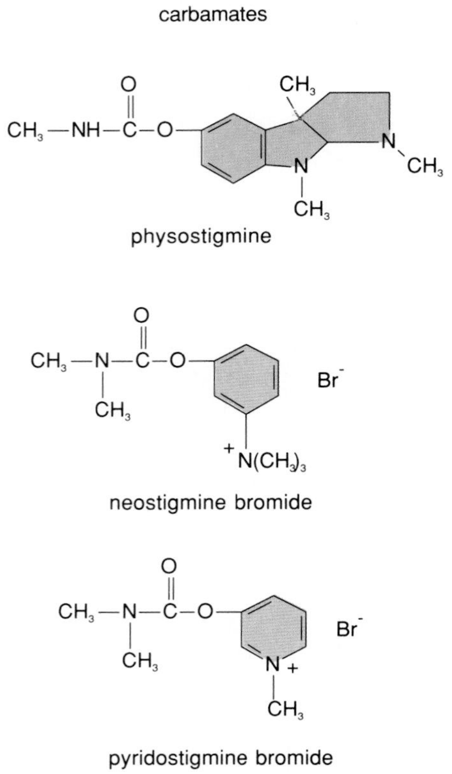

carbamates

physostigmine

neostigmine bromide

pyridostigmine bromide

FIGURE 9-6   Reversibly acting cholinesterase inhibitors.

Inhibition of Acetylcholine Metabolism

The indirect-acting cholinomimetics produce their pharmacological action by blocking the enzymatic hydrolysis of acetylcholine. Inhibitors of acetylcholinesterase and plasma pseudocholinesterase significantly increase local acetylcholine concentrations, which can be either therapeutic or life-threatening, depending on the extent of enzyme inhibition.

As shown in Figure 9-5, the active region of acetylcholinesterase contains the negative anionic site, namely, the γ-carboxyl of a glutamic acid residue, and an esteratic site containing a serine hydroxyl. The enzymatic hydrolysis of acetylcholine involves initial electrostatic attraction of the positively charged quaternary nitrogen to the anionic site and subsequent nucleophilic attack by the serine-OH (activated

by an adjacent histidine), leading to acetylation of the serine. The acetylated enzyme is rapidly hydrolyzed to acetate and free enzyme, enabling reuse of the enzyme and rapid turnover of acetylcholine. The deacetylation step is rate-limiting.

There are two types of cholinesterase inhibitors: reversible carbamates and related compounds (Figure 9-6) and irreversible organophosphates (Figure 9-7). Some of the latter are highly toxic and are not used clinically.

Simple quaternary compounds (i.e., tetraethylammonium ion) can weakly inhibit acetylcholinesterase by reversibly associating with the anionic site and hindering access to acetylcholine. More potent, although transient, inhibition is produced by the drug edrophonium, which in addition to associating with

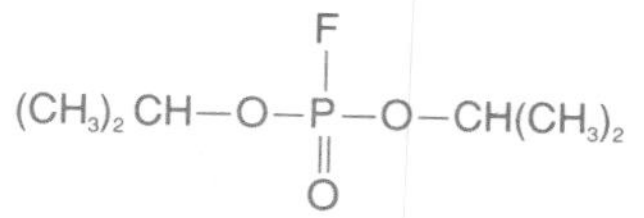

$(CH_3)_2 CH—O—\underset{\underset{O}{\|}}{\overset{\overset{F}{|}}{P}}—O—CH(CH_3)_2$

isoflurophate

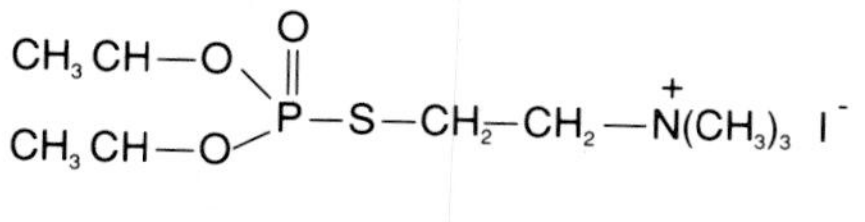

$CH_3 CH—O \diagdown \underset{CH_3 CH—O \diagup}{\overset{\overset{O}{\|}}{P}}—S—CH_2–CH_2—\overset{+}{N}(CH_3)_3 \quad I^-$

echothiophate iodide

serine   anionic site

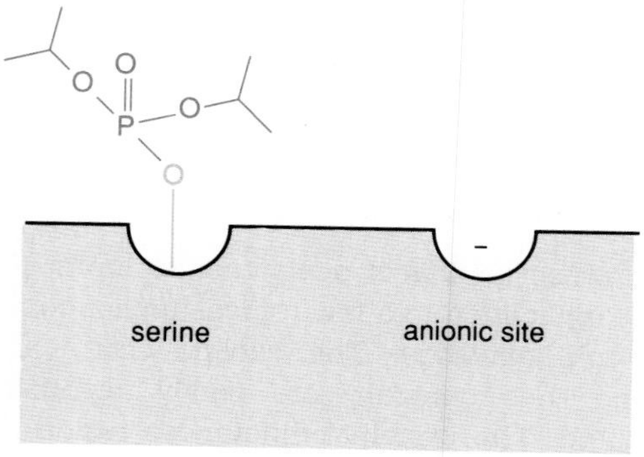

phosphorylated enzyme

FIGURE 9-7   Organophosphate inhibitors of acetylcholinesterase. Also shown is phosphorylation of the active site (serine -OH) after reaction with isoflurophate. Sarin, soman, and tabun are highly toxic and irreversible. Isoflurophate and echothiophate are used clinically for topical ophthalmology applications.

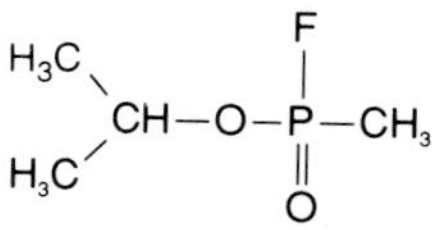

$\underset{H_3C \diagup}{\overset{H_3C \diagdown}{}} CH—O–\underset{\underset{O}{\|}}{\overset{\overset{F}{|}}{P}}—CH_3$

sarin

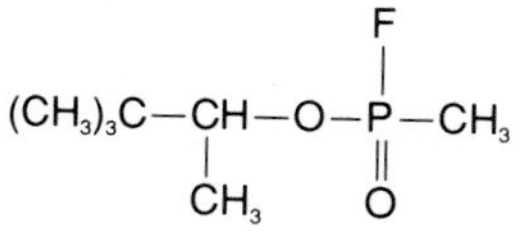

$(CH_3)_3C—\underset{\underset{CH_3}{|}}{CH}—O–\underset{\underset{O}{\|}}{\overset{\overset{F}{|}}{P}}—CH_3$

soman

$(CH_3)_2N—\underset{\underset{O}{\|}}{\overset{\overset{O—C_2H_5}{\diagup}}{P}}—CN$

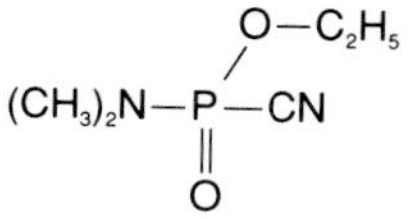

tabun

the anionic site also forms a hydrogen bond with the neighboring histidine. Prolonged inhibition is mediated by carbamate-containing molecules such as physostigmine and pyridostigmine, which behave as substrates, and carbamylate, the serine-OH at the esteratic site in a manner analogous to the previously described acetylation. Decarbamylation occurs much more slowly than does deacetylation. It is estimated that the half-life of acetylcholine hydrolysis via deacetylation is 40 microseconds, whereas that for decarbamylation is approximately 30 minutes or longer. Thus, in the presence of carbamylating drugs, acetylcholine accumulates, producing prolonged effects.

The carbamates also have agonist, desensitizing, and channel-blocking properties at sensitive nicotinic sites. The implications await further study, especially at the low concentrations that produce cholinesterase inhibition. At higher concentrations physostigmine exerts a blocking action at sympathetic ganglia. The quaternary amine-containing carbamates have nicotinic blocking and anticholinesterase activity. This

is expected in view of the actions of the bis-quaternary compounds hexamethonium, which blocks at ganglia, and decamethonium, which blocks at neuromuscular nicotinic sites.

Irreversible cholinesterase inhibitors act by covalently phosphorylating the hydroxyl group of serine on the enzyme (see Figure 9-7). The reaction is stoichiometric; one organophosphorus molecule reacts with a single serine in the active center. These irreversible binding organophosphorus compounds may be active in their native form, or they may require biotransformation to be effective. The structures of several of these compounds are shown in Figure 9-7. A few organophosphates, which show selective toxicity against insects but not against mammals, are used in agriculture mainly as pesticides. Some phosphorus compounds become active only after biotransformation. For example, parathion is converted by oxidation of the thiogroup to the very toxic oxygen analog, paraoxon, a potent anticholinesterase compound. It also undergoes acid-catalyzed rearrangement to form an equally toxic anticholinesterase. The time required for these changes to occur accounts for the delay before toxic signs appear. Malathion is a widely used pesticide that is much safer than others currently in use. It, too, must be bioactivated in vivo, but its oxidation product is rapidly metabolized by the plasma esterases.

The enzymes that hydrolyze acetylcholine are classified according to substrate specificity and distribution. The cholinesterase-type found distributed throughout the nervous system and present in the red blood cell membrane is specific for acetylcholine with much lower affinity for other choline esters. It is termed "true" or *erythrocyte cholinesterase*. The neuronal enzyme is synthesized in cell bodies throughout the central and peripheral nervous systems, secreted by the Golgi apparatus, and transported along the axon by "fast" axoplasmic flow to the nerve terminals. Its presence at somatic nerve muscle junctions, ganglia, parasympathetic neuroeffector junctions, and throughout the brain and spinal cord has been demonstrated histochemically. It is extensively distributed in the CNS and is found at synapses other than those containing acetylcholine. In dorsal root ganglia, there is a high concentration of this enzyme associated with various peptides such as substance P, without acetylcholine. It has been reported that in the dorsal horn, the enzyme acts as a peptidase, a possible explanation for its presence. Tissues highest in true cholinesterase activity include preganglionic fibers to sympathetic and parasympathetic ganglia, postganglionic parasympathetic and somatic motor fibers, and sympathetic axons, which innervate sweat glands. In noncholinergic cells the enzyme is absent or is present in substantially lower amounts. The enzyme may exist in monomeric, dimeric, and tetrameric forms and may contain a segment of collagen for attachment to membranes.

Plasma cholinesterase or pseudocholinesterase is more widely distributed than true cholinesterase. Plasma contains several forms of pseudocholinesterase. Unlike the erythrocyte enzyme, pseudocholinesterase has a very broad substrate specificity, with the following order of preference: benzoyl > butyryl > propionyl > acetyl esters of choline. It is sometimes referred to as *butyrylcholinesterase* because it has greater activity against this substrate, with the possible exception of benzoylcholine. Because of its liver origin, plasma concentrations of the enzyme in combination with glutamic-oxaloacetic and glutamic-pyruvic transaminases are useful as a measure of liver function. Its presence is important when the neuromuscular blocking agent succinylcholine is used, as discussed in Chapter 11. In addition to plasma, it is found in glial cells. Unlike true cholinesterase, the function of pseudocholinesterase in nerve tissue is unclear.

 ## PHARMACOKINETICS

The pharmacokinetics of many of the cholinergic drugs have not been well studied in humans. This is partly because of a lack of analytical methods and partly because of the rapid and intense actions that ensue with small drug concentrations. Available parameters are listed in Table 9-2.

Cholinomimetic Agonists

The hydrolytic lability of acetylcholine limits its therapeutic application to a few topical applications, chiefly in ophthalmology. The choline esters are charged and thus generally are poorly absorbed and distributed. The principal differences reside in their relative resistance to hydrolysis by acetylcholinesterase.

Pilocarpine is available for topical application as a solution or in an extended delivery device (see Chapter 6) placed into the conjunctival sac and providing continuous drug release for 7 days.

Muscarinic Blocking Drugs

In the muscarinic blockers, the tertiary amines cross membranes readily, whereas the quaternary ammonium compounds fail to traverse the membrane, or do so only poorly.

Atropine is rapidly absorbed after oral or parenteral administration. When applied topically to the eye, it is absorbed from the surrounding mucous membranes unless drainage from the conjunctiva is prevented by light pressure on the drainage canal. Atropine has a plasma half-life of about 2 hours and is well distributed throughout the body. Most of an administered dose is eliminated within 12 hours in the urine. Ten to fifty percent is unchanged and the remainder excreted as unidentified metabolites. The half-life in children below the age of 2 and in the elderly is considerably longer. The quaternary nitrogen derivatives are poorly absorbed, quantitatively, between 10% and 25% of the oral dose. A small fraction is excreted unchanged.

Table 9-2   Pharmacokinetic Parameters for Cholinergic Drugs

Drugs	Administration	Absorption	$t_{1/2}$ (hr)	Disposition
CHOLINOMIMETIC AGONISTS				
bethanechol	Oral, SC	—	—	—
MUSCARINIC BLOCKERS				
methscopolamine	Oral, topical	—	—	—
propantheline bromide	Oral	—	1.6	M (70%), R (30%)
clidinium bromide	Oral	—	—	—
glycopyrrolate	Oral	—	—	—
tridihexethyl chloride	Oral	—	—	—
dicyclomine HC1	Oral, IM	—	—	—
biperiden HC1	Oral, IV	Good	—	M
GANGLIONIC BLOCKERS				
mecamylamine		Good	—	R
CHOLINESTERASE INHIBITORS				
physostigmine	Oral, IV, IM	Good	1-3	—
neostigmine	Oral, IV		0.9-1.2* M	—
pyridostigmine	Oral, IV		1.9*	—
echothiophate	Topical	Poor	—	—
isoflurophate	Topical	Poor	—	—
demecarium bromide	Topical	Poor	—	—
edrophonium chloride	IV, IM	—	1.9*	—

M, metabolized; *R*, renal clearance as unchanged drug.
*$t_{1/2}$ increases by factor of 2 to 3 in renal failure.

Scopolamine, as the methyl analog, is available in a sustained delivery patch for topical skin application behind the ear, with a constant delivery rate over 3 days.

Other Drugs

Nicotine is available bound to an ion exchange resin as a chewing gum. The nicotine is released slowly for buccal absorption and is used as a possible aid in the cessation of smoking.

 ## RELATION OF MECHANISM OF ACTION TO CLINICAL RESPONSE

Cholinomimetic Agonists

Drugs can act by stimulating muscarinic receptors and thereby achieve organ or tissue selectivity because muscarinic sites are located predominately at neuroeffector junctions. The route of administration also can be used to achieve organ selectivity, (i.e.,

topical applications for the eye). Nicotinic receptors are present in autonomic ganglia, at skeletal muscle motor end plates (see Chapter 11), on adrenal medullary cells, and in the CNS. However, they are more limited in distribution than are muscarinic receptors.

In the eye, sustained increased intraocular pressure may result in glaucoma (described in anticholinesterase section). Some forms of this disease can be alleviated by administration of cholinomimetic drugs (e.g., pilocarpine) and anticholinesterases. But glaucoma can also be precipitated by the use of muscarinic receptor blocking drugs.

Pilocarpine acts on smooth muscles of the eye to constrict the pupil (miosis), causing a spasm of accommodation, and a transient rise in intraocular pressure followed by a fall that is longer lasting. Pilocarpine is a miotic of choice in initial maintenance therapy in primary open-angle glaucoma, and in conjunction with other drugs in the emergency treatment of acute angle-closure glaucoma. It penetrates the eye after topical application and miosis begins in 15 to 30 minutes, persisting for up to 8 hours. Reduction of intraocular pressure is maximal in 2 to 4 hours. Pilocarpine acts to increase aqueous outflow and possibly to reduce aqueous production. It is generally better tolerated than other miotics.

Carbachol, a carbamyl ester of choline, shares similar properties with bethanechol. In contrast to acetylcholine, carbachol stimulates the urinary and GI tracts fairly selectively. Its principal use, however, is in ophthalmology for cataract surgery or in other procedures in which rapid miosis is desired. For the chronic treatment of open-angle glaucoma, higher concentrations of carbachol are employed. Carbachol is often effective in reducing intraocular pressure when resistance to physostigmine or pilocarpine develops.

Bethanechol chloride is another choline ester that acts directly on effector cells. Its actions are like those of acetylcholine, but its effects are more persistent, again because of its resistance to hydrolysis by cholinesterases. It has no nicotinic effects and its actions on autonomic ganglia are minimal. However, its effects are much more pronounced on the urinary bladder and GI tract. It is used to facilitate emptying of the neurogenic bladder and is frequently administered to patients after surgery or parturition. In pa-

tients with spinal cord injury, it is sometimes used to enhance weak detrusor muscle contractions for bladder evacuation. The drug is also used in children with "lazy bladder" syndrome.

Muscarinic Blocking Drugs

Atropine, the prototype muscarinic blocking agent, is discussed in detail. Table 9-3 lists other drugs in this class with brief comments regarding their use.

Atropine acts on muscarinic receptors to block parasympathetic effects on smooth muscle, cardiac muscle, and glandular cells. By blocking vagal activity there is an increased firing rate of the sinoatrial node and facilitation of conduction at the atrioventricular (AV) node. In GI hypermotility and excessive gastric secretion, atropine is effective in blocking parasympathetic stimulation, diminishing these activities. A large number of atropine-like drugs with antimuscarinic actions have applicability in allaying symptoms associated with peptic ulcer (see Chapter 55). By blocking glandular secretions in the lung and mouth, atropine is useful as a preoperative medica-

---

Table 9-3 Muscarinic Blocking Drugs

Amines	Comments
TERTIARY	
atropine sulfate	Preoperative medication; treatment of anticholinesterase poisoning
scopolamine hydrobromide	Preoperative medication in childbirth
homatropine hydrobromide	Mydriatic and cycloplegic; used for mild anterior uveitis
adiphenine hydrobromide	To treat pyloric and biliary spasm, dysmenorrhea
dicyclomine	Alleviates GI spasm, dysmenorrhea: pylorospasm and biliary distention
oxyphencyclimine	Antisecretory compound in peptic ulcer
cyclopentolate	Mydriatic, cycloplegic; may cause severe CNS effects
tropicamide	Mydriatic, cycloplegic
benztropine methanesulfonate	Antagonizes extrapyramidal symptoms of antiparkinson drugs and the phenothiazines
trihexyphenidyl	Similar uses as benztropine methanesulfonate
QUATERNARY	
atropine methylbromide (and methylnitrate)	Mydriatic, cycloplegic, antispasmodic in pyloric stenosis
methscopolamine bromide	Decreases gastric hyperacidity and hypermotility; less CNS effects than scopolamine
homatropine methylbromide	Restricted to GI tract, diminish gastric acidity and spasm
ipratropium	Aerosol to diminish secretions in chronic emphysema
glycopyrrolate	Spasmolytic for ulcer therapy; preoperative drying of secretions
tridihexethyl chloride	Antispasmodic, preoperative to dry secretions
isopropamide iodide	May be used with cimetidine in Zollinger-Ellison syndrome
methantheline bromide	Spasmolytic to treat peptic ulcer; may precipitate exfoliative dermatitis
propantheline bromide	Spasmolytic in peptic ulcer; high doses may produce neuromuscular block
clidinium bromide	Spasmolytic in combination with librium in management of "psychogenic" ulcer

tion and as palliative treatment to decrease pulmonary edema and bronchoconstriction in anticholinesterase poisoning.

The primary uses of muscarinic blocking agents are in ophthalmology and gastroenterology. Atropine and the tertiary and quaternary amines (see Table 9-3) are used to relax GI smooth muscle and in various procedures involving the eye.

Atropine is applied topically for preoperative mydriasis (pupil dilation), frequently in combination with phenylephrine. It is also widely used for treating anterior uveitis adjunctively with topical corticosteroids or for postoperative mydriasis. The use of phenylephrine enhances mydriasis, with less atropine needed for the desired effect. Where a mydriatic-cycloplegic (paralysis of accommodation) of lesser duration is desired (atropine effects may persist from days to weeks), the shorter-acting agents such as cyclopentolate, homatropine, and tropicamide may be used. Mydriatic-cycloplegics are also used to break down adhesions (posterior synechiae) and in ciliary block glaucoma.

Atropine as an *antispasmodic* produces variable undesirable clinical responses. Some of the synthetic tertiary amines have more uniform bioavailability than most of the naturally-occurring alkaloids and their central effects are less prominent. Because quaternary compounds are permanently charged and unable to cross the blood-brain barrier, they remain in the periphery and seldom exhibit CNS effects. For example the tertiary amine, quinuclidine benzilate, readily distributes to the CNS and produces severe central effects, including short-term memory loss. It is no longer used. The quaternary amide clidinium bromide is characterized by the absence of any CNS actions and is widely prescribed as an antispasmodic. Despite the large number of synthetic agents available, preparations of the belladonna alkaloids are still used because few clear differences aid in the selection of an antispasmodic that may be used for GI disturbances.

Atropine is often administered preoperatively to diminish salivary secretions. It is also used with cholinesterase inhibitors to reverse the action of neuromuscular blocking agents, and to limit the effect of acetylcholine accumulation to the neuromuscular junction. In addition to its availability as a tertiary amine, atropine analogs are available as quaternary salts for more limited distribution.

Although there are few qualitative differences between atropine and scopolamine as muscarinic blocking drugs, quantitative differences limit the usefulness of the latter. Scopolamine is more potent centrally and even at relatively low doses can induce hallucinations and aberrant behavior in susceptible individuals. This is frequently observed in children premedicated with scopolamine before general anesthesia. Because of these actions, the drug is not widely used as an antisecretory or antispasmodic agent. Its action on the iris to produce mydriasis and on the ciliary muscle to produce cycloplegia is greater than the corresponding effects of atropine. It also produces xerostomia, or dry mouth, as does atropine. Atropine has less pronounced CNS effects. Atropine is more effective in promoting vagal slowing of the heart, in decreasing intestinal activity, in relaxing constricted bronchiolar smooth muscle, and in demonstrating a longer duration of action, particularly on the iris. Atropine is important as an antidote to treat poisoning by carbamate and organophosphate, agricultural insecticides that inhibit cholinesterases. Atropine also acts to reduce sphincter and bladder tone on the urinary tract and has a mild antispasmodic action on the biliary tract.

Ganglionic Blocking Drugs

Historically, ganglionic blocking drugs were used for their ability to lower systemic blood pressure in hypertensive patients, but, because of their broad actions resulting from inhibition of both sympathetic and parasympathetic systems, these agents now have only limited use. They have been supplanted by more selective and predictable antihypertensive drugs. Nevertheless, ganglionic blockers are important because they provide a basis for understanding the underlying principles of ganglionic function and reflex effects. Many of the prominent side effects of a wide variety of therapeutic agents result from actions on the autonomic system, although their major actions are elsewhere. Generalized ganglionic blockade leads to atony of the bladder and the GI tract. Actions on ciliary ganglion cause cycloplegia, and actions on superior cervical ganglion produce dry mouth and anhidrosis.

The greatest problem from ganglionic blockade is that of orthostatic hypotension, resulting from the loss of postural reflexes. The cardiovascular system depends on sympathetic innervation to maintain sympathetic activity. The effects of ganglionic blockade on blood pressure in the recumbent position may be small, but a precipitous drop in pressure can take place when the patient is sitting or standing. Thus postural hypotension poses a major problem to the ambulatory patient. This effect may become less pronounced with continued use of the drug. The action of ganglion blocking agents on cardiac rate depends on the relative importance of vagal tone, which is greater in well-conditioned patients and much less in sedentary patients. Usually, mild tachycardia with hypotension indicates fairly complete ganglionic blockade. As a result of the hypotension, the decrease in venous return after blockade of sympathetic ganglia can result in diminished cardiac output. In contrast to the systemic circulation, cerebral blood flow is less affected because circulation to the brain is under tight autoregulation. Only when a substantial fall in mean blood pressure occurs is there a significant fall in cerebral blood flow. In elderly patients, in which vessels may be sclerotic, a precipitous fall in blood pressure can produce a rebound rise that can result in cerebral vascular accident.

Trimethaphan camsylate is administered by IV in hypertensive crises. It is also used in surgical procedures involving highly vascularized tissues and has a short duration of action. Mecamylamine is administered orally.

Inhibitors of Acetylcholine Metabolism

The primary target organs in which the anticholinesterase drugs act are the eye; the skeletal muscle neuromuscular junctions; the GI, urinary, and respiratory tracts; and the heart and other tissues that receive parasympathetic innervation. In most respects the cholinesterase inhibitor drugs produce effects similar to those of direct-acting cholinergic agonists.

The major clinical use for the anticholinesterases is in the treatment of glaucoma. There are two types of primary glaucoma, open-angle and angle-closure, depending on the configuration of the angle of the anterior chamber of the eye at the point where reabsorption of the aqueous humor takes place. Open-angle glaucoma can be successfully managed with cholinesterase inhibitors, particularly the irreversible acting drugs, whereas angle-closure glaucoma may be treated initially with pilocarpine but generally requires surgery for correction. These agents relieve the elevated intraocular pressure of open-angle glaucoma by promoting outflow of the aqueous humor and perhaps also by diminishing secretion. This results from contraction of the ciliary muscle and the sphincter of

the iris. When this occurs, the trabecular meshwork at the base of the ciliary muscle is opened and the iris is pulled away, widening the angle at the anterior chamber and facilitating flow of the aqueous humor into the Schlemm canal. The intraocular pressure in the anterior chamber of the eye is thus reduced. This action is shown schematically in Figure 9-8.

Physostigmine is used to treat open-angle glaucoma and sometimes accommodative esotropia, a strabismus resulting from excessive accommodation. Physostigmine is a tertiary amine, extremely lipid soluble, but not well tolerated. Among the long-acting miotics used to treat open-angle glaucoma are the organophosphates, echothiophate and isoflurophate. Demecarium, a synthetic bis-quaternary compound, is also used in open-angle glaucoma and esotropia. These latter compounds are generally instilled into the conjunctival sac at 12 to 48 hour intervals. They reduce intraocular pressure maximally in 1 day, but tend to predispose to cataracts with prolonged use and are generally reserved for situations in which the shorter-acting cholinomimetics are not effective. The quaternary nitrogen in echothiophate essentially limits its distribution and does not allow ready systemic absorption after topical application. Isoflurophate, however, is lipophilic and can readily enter the systemic circulation after topical application to the eye.

Another important use of the anticholinesterases is in the treatment of myasthenia gravis. This disease is characterized by a progressive weakness of skeletal muscle resulting from an impairment in neuromuscular transmission. The disorder stems at least in part from a reduction in the number of postsynaptic acetylcholine receptors. Because myasthenia gravis is an autoimmune disease, it is proposed that the loss of receptors is brought about by antigenic modulation, so that the acetylcholine receptors are degraded and turned over at a more rapid rate than normal. Thus the rate of neurotransmitter-receptor binding is reduced and muscle fatigue results. Frequently used drugs to treat this disorder are the reversible, carbamate ester anticholinesterases, pyridostigmine and neostigmine.

The short-acting cholinesterase inhibitor, edrophonium chloride, as well as neostigmine and pyridostigmine also is used to reverse neuromuscular blockade (see Chapter 11), based on competitive antagonism between acetylcholine and the blocking drug. In this situation, the concentration of acetylcholine is permitted to increase by inhibiting acetylcholinesterase, thereby enhancing the ability of ace-

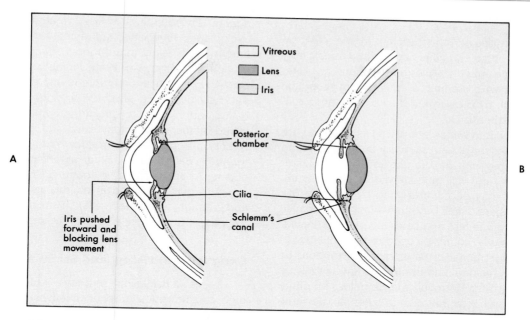

FIGURE 9-8   Treatment of glaucoma with cholinergic agonists or cholinesterase inhibitors. **A,** Before application of drug. **B,** After application of drug.

CLINICAL PROBLEMS

AGONISTS

Excessive parasympathetic activity: decreased blood pressure, bronchoconstriction, sweating, GI discomfort
At high concentrations, excess ganglionic activity
Mushroom toxicity

MUSCARINIC BLOCKERS

Lack of secretions, urinary retention, mydriasis, tachycardia, hypertension

GANGLIONIC BLOCKERS

Lack of selectivity makes drugs difficult to use

CHOLINESTERASE INHIBITORS

Side effects similar to those for agonists
Organophosphorus compound toxicity

tylcholine to compete with nicotinic receptors at the neuromuscular junction.

Edrophonium may also be used in the treatment of AV nodal reentrant tachycardia, particularly when carotid sinus massage is ineffective. The termination of the tachycardia is effected by the increase in acetylcholine released at the AV junction, thereby reducing AV conduction velocity. Edrophonium is the preferred anticholinesterase because of its rapid onset and short duration of action.

SIDE EFFECTS, CLINICAL PROBLEMS, AND TOXICITY

Clinical problems are summarized in the box.

Cholinomimetic Agonists

With pilocarpine administration, stinging and local irritation may occur and ciliary spasm and miosis may be troublesome initially. Allergic reactions are rare. In the patient with asthma, stimulation of bronchial smooth muscle by pilocarpine may precipitate a full-blown asthmatic attack.

Bethanechol may cause symptoms associated with excessive parasympathetic activity such as flushing of skin, sweating, nausea, cramps and diarrhea, asthmatic attacks, and fall in systemic blood pressure. These effects may be counteracted by atropine SC. Bethanechol should not be given IV or IM because acute circulatory failure and cardiac arrest can result. This drug should also not be used in the presence of anatomic or functional urinary tract obstruction. Its use should be avoided in patients who have problems associated with the detrusor muscle unless an effective external sphincter relaxant is given at the same time because of vesicoureteral reflux or other adverse effects. Because it increases intestinal motility, bethanechol should not be given to patients with peptic ulcer or patients who have had intestinal resection or anastomosis.

The major toxicity from muscarinic agonists results not from therapeutic use but from eating certain varieties of mushrooms, most commonly *Amanita muscaria* and other species, particularly the *Inocybes,* in which the muscarine content is high. After ingestion of these fungi, toxic signs develop rapidly and are maximal within 2 hours. The toxic signs include salivation, sweating, tearing, nausea, vomiting, diarrhea, visual disturbances, bradycardia, hypotension, and shock. In *Amanita muscaria* poisoning, typical CNS symptoms consist of irritability, confusion, restlessness, hallucinations, and convulsions. These symptoms contrast with those produced by *Amanita phalloides,* which contain nonmuscarinic substances highly toxic to the liver, resulting in hepatotoxicity that is sometimes fatal. Treatment of mushroom poisoning requires parenteral administration of atropine, specifically to counteract the cholinergic symptoms. Mild sedatives are also given to treat the central effects of other substances present in mushrooms, which appear to be indole related in structure. In some situations, other supportive therapy may also be indicated.

Muscarinic Blocking Drugs

There are several undesirable effects associated with therapeutic doses of the muscarinic blocking agents. These include urinary retention, dry mouth, cycloplegia, mydriasis, anhidrosis, and tachycardia. Larger doses result in additional effects such as photophobia, nausea, vomiting, flushing, and hypertension. CNS effects are prominent with overdoses of the naturally occurring alkaloids, including excitement, hallucinations, and convulsions, which may be followed by respiratory depression and death. The quaternary nitrogen drugs produce toxic effects characteristic of ganglionic blockade and do not include CNS effects. All anticholinergic agents are contraindicated in acute glaucoma and in conditions of the urinary and GI tracts where decreases in smooth muscle contractility and motility would have adverse results.

Ganglionic Blocking (and Stimulating) Drugs

The natural alkaloid nicotine, which is found in high concentration in tobacco leaves, stimulates the nicotinic receptor at ganglia. Nicotine has no therapeutic action but is medically important because of its potential toxicity.

Complex changes that occur after nicotine administration are both stimulant and depressant. The drug can cause an increased heart rate by stimulating sympathetic ganglia, or a decrease in heart rate by acting on parasympathetic ganglia. It stimulates adrenal release of epinephrine, accelerating heart rate and raising systemic blood pressure. Similar actions are produced by nicotine on the carotid and aortic bodies. Nicotine acts centrally to produce tremor and convulsions. Respiration is stimulated by nicotine at low doses by an indirect activation of reflex pathways and directly at high doses by stimulation of the medulla. It produces vomiting by stimulating the chemoreceptor trigger zone in the *area postrema*. Although this action may be life-saving, large doses of nicotine ultimately depress the CNS and death results from respiratory depression caused by skeletal muscle end plate depolarization blockade. Nicotine is rapidly absorbed percutaneously, orally through the buccal membranes, and via the respiratory tree. Treatment after oral ingestion includes gatric lavage and artificial respiration; oxygen should be used if respiratory function is markedly affected.

Acetylcholinesterase Inhibitors

The acute toxicity of organophosphorus compounds is the result of inhibiting the actions of cholinesterase enzymes, leading to accumulation of acetylcholine. These compounds are absorbed through the respiratory tract, conjunctiva, or skin. Exposure to high concentrations focuses on CNS effects. The accumulation of acetylcholine at nerve endings produces typical muscarinic and nicotinic actions. The duration of symptoms, if untreated, depends on the reversibility of the inhibition of the cholinesterase. With echothiophate this may be less than 24 hours. With soman or sarin the irreversible effects may persist for several days to months.

Mild exposure leads to pupillary constriction, tightness of the chest, watery discharge from the nose, and wheezing. In *severe* exposure, the symptoms become intensified and in addition to visual disturbances, muscle fasciculation becomes generalized. Excessive secretions lead to pulmonary edema after bronchoconstriction; there is subsequent marked muscle weakness and respiratory movements become shallow and intermittent. Central depression of respiratory control further intensifies the respiratory problems, which if untreated, can lead to respiratory failure and death. These symptoms are accompanied by CNS effects, beginning with anxiety, restlessness, and emotional instability often leading to seizures. Profound long-term effects are manifested as headache, tremor, loss of short-term memory, confusion, apathy, and depression. The irreversibly acting organophosphates are a highly toxic group of compounds that collectively are capable of inhibiting more than a hundred different enzymes including the pancreatic enzymes, chymotrypsin and trypsin, various kallikreins, thrombin and enzymes involved in clotting, and most importantly, the cholinesterases.

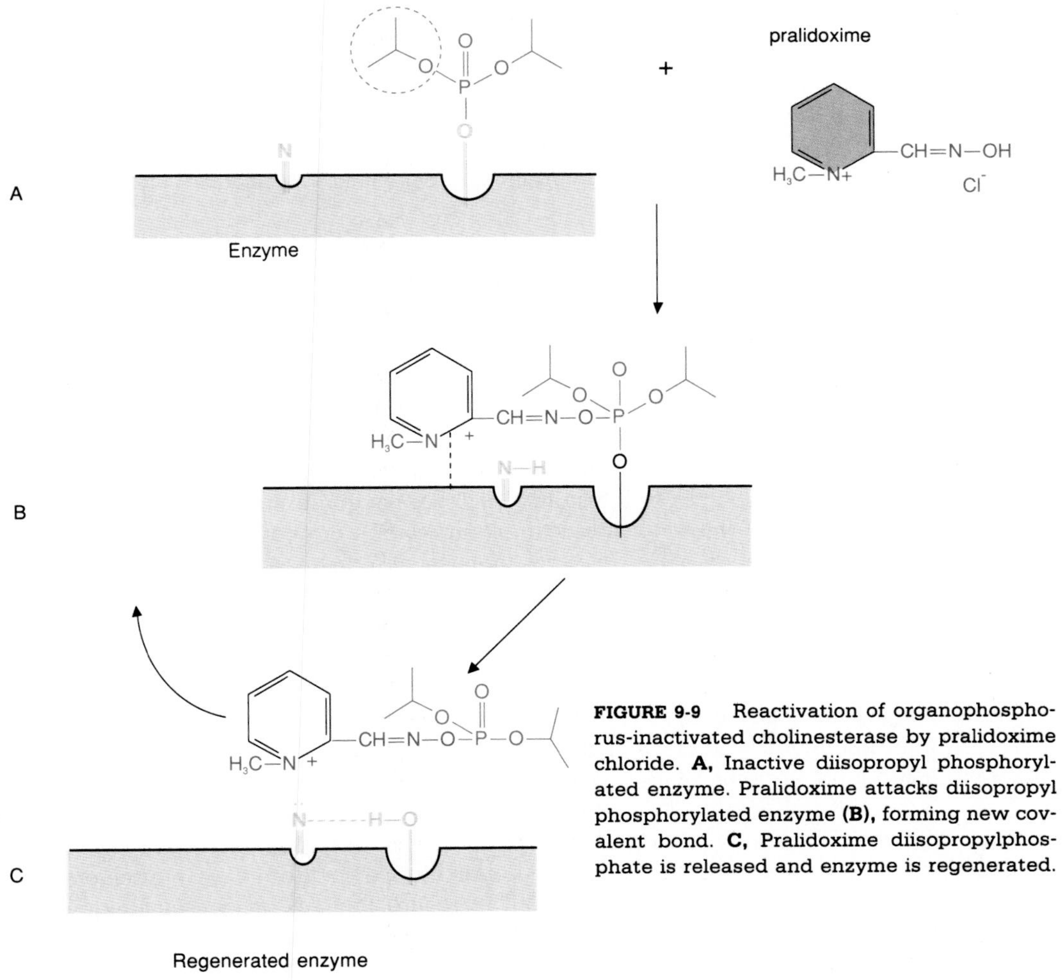

FIGURE 9-9   Reactivation of organophosphorus-inactivated cholinesterase by pralidoxime chloride. **A,** Inactive diisopropyl phosphorylated enzyme. Pralidoxime attacks diisopropyl phosphorylated enzyme **(B),** forming new covalent bond. **C,** Pralidoxime diisopropylphosphate is released and enzyme is regenerated.

Treatment of Toxicity In treating an individual exposed to an anticholinesterase, the first step is to remove the source to prevent further exposure. This may involve removal of clothing and possible lavage, or, if the environment is contaminated, evacuation to an uncontaminated area. The appearance of symptoms of poisoning requires prompt administration of atropine to block most sites of acetylcholine action except at neuromuscular junctions or other nicotinic sites. In mild cases, atropine can be administered over a 24 hour period. Eye symptoms, after local absorption of an anticholinesterase, are not relieved by systemic administration of atropine and require direct instillation of an ophthalmic solution of atropine or homatropine.

The use of atropine is palliative in nature; it relieves the symptoms of poisoning but does not reverse the inhibition of cholinesterases that results in neuromuscular activation and muscle paralysis. Reversal can be achieved by administration of pralidoxime (see Figure 9-9 for structure; the mechanism of reversal also is shown). With pralidoxime, regeneration of the enzyme occurs extremely rapidly compared to natural restoration. Other bis-quaternary compounds such as obidoxime, are even more potent reactivators. Pralidoxime acts as a site-directed nucleophile, which by virtue of possessing a quaternary nitrogen can interact with the negative subsite of the active center of cholinesterase. The oxime-phosphonate is split off, resulting in a regenerated enzyme. When a cholinesterase is phosphorylated, it can undergo a process in which an alkyl or alkoxy group is lost. This results in a phosphorylated enzyme that inherently is more stable and also more resistant to a reactivator such as pralidoxime. It is therefore important that pralidoxime treatment be instituted early after organophosphate exposure. Pralidoxime does not antagonize the toxicity produced by the carbamates.

REFERENCES

Dolly JO and Barnard EA: Nicotinic acetylcholine receptors: an overview, Biochem Pharm 33:841, 1984.

Donati F, Lahoud J, McCready D et al.: Neostigmine, pyridostigmine and edrophonium as antagonists of deep pancuronium blockade, Can J Anaesth 34:589, 1987.

Hartvig P, Wiklund L, and Lindstrom B: Pharmacokinetics of physostigmine after intravenous, intramuscular and subcunatenous administration in surgical patients, Acta Anaesth Scand 26:297, 1982.

Kerlavage AR, Fraser CM, and Venter JC: Muscarinic receptor structure: molecular biological support for subtypes, Trends Pharmacol Sci 8:426, 1987.

Levine RR, Birdsall NJM, Giachetti A et al., eds.: Subtypes of muscarinic receptors II, TIPS supplement, New York, February 1986, Elsevier Science Publishing Co, Inc.

Luyton WHML and Heinemann SF: Molecular cloning of the nicotinic acetylcholine receptor: new opportunities in drug design? In Bailey DM, ed.: Annual reports in medicinal chemistry, vol 22, San Diego, 1987, Academic Press.

Pernow B: Substance P, Pharmacol Rev 33:85-141, 1983.

Virtanen R, Kanto J, Iisalo E et al.: Pharmacokinetic studies on atropine with special reference to age, Acta Anaesth Scand 26:297, 1982.

CHAPTER 10

Drugs Affecting the Sympathetic Nervous System

 THERAPEUTIC OVERVIEW

The peripheral sympathetic neuronal system modulates the activity smooth muscle, cardiac muscle, and glandular cells by increasing or decreasing their activity. Transfer of information from terminals of most sympathetic neurons to the effector organs is mediated by norepinephrine. Exceptions are those few anatomically sympathetic neurons that project to sweat glands and to some blood vessels in the neck, face, and skeletal muscles that use acetylcholine as a transmitter (Chapter 8). The actions resulting from activation of sympathetic neurons are reinforced by epinephrine and norepinephrine secreted into the circulation from the adrenal medulla (sympathoadrenal discharge). Outside of the United States, epinephrine and norepinephrine are known as adrenaline and noradrenaline, respectively, from which the adjectives "adrenergic" and "noradrenergic" are derived.

Drugs that facilitate or mimic the actions of the sympathoadrenal system are termed *sympathomimetics;* drugs that block or reduce these actions are termed *sympatholytics.* Since the sympathetic nervous system modulates the activity of many organ systems throughout the body, drugs that modify the actions of these neurons produce a variety of responses, and many of these drugs are important clinically. However, because of their wide diversity of responses, these drugs also have a multiplicity of undesirable side effects.

By mimicking or facilitating the actions of norepinephrine on vascular smooth muscle, sympathomimetics constrict arterioles and veins and therefore can be administered locally to (1) reduce superficial bleeding, (2) prevent diffusion of locally administered drugs (e.g., local anesthetics), (3) decongest mucous membranes, and (4) reduce formation of aqueous humor so as to lower intraocular pressure in glaucoma. Systemic administration of sympathomimetics cause generalized constriction of blood vessels leading to increases in peripheral vascular resistance and mean arterial blood pressure. These drugs are used to increase blood pressure in some hypotensive states (e.g., neurogenic shock resulting from spinal anesthesia or spinal cord injury). By increasing blood pressure, sympathomimetics cause a reflex slowing of the heart rate and for this reason can be used therapeutically to treat paroxysmal atrial tachycardia.

Epinephrine and other adrenergic drugs have marked stimulatory effects on cardiac muscle and are used in the treatment of cardiogenic shock. These drugs also reduce the tone of various smooth muscles. By relaxing bronchial smooth muscle, adrenergic drugs are useful in treating bronchospasm resulting from allergies, and by reducing the tone of pregnant uterus smooth muscle cells, adrenergic drugs delay delivery in premature labor. Drugs that mimic epinephrine contract radial smooth muscle in the iris, causing dilation of the pupil, thereby facilitating eye examinations.

Drugs that reduce the actions of the sympathetic nervous system on vascular smooth muscle are used to treat essential hypertension and hypertensive emergencies. Drugs that reduce the actions of norepinephrine and epinephrine on cardiac muscle are used to treat cardiac dysrhythmias, angina pectoris, and other cardiac disorders (e.g., postmyocardial infarction). These drugs also have utility in treating migraine headaches, glaucoma, and some symptoms of anxiety.

The therapeutic uses of sympathomimetic and sympatholytic drugs are summarized in the box.

 ## MECHANISMS OF ACTION

Sympathetic Noradrenergic Processes

The molecular structures of receptors and second messenger signal systems are discussed in Chapter 2 and the biochemistry and physiology of the autonomic nervous system, including adrenergic and cholinergic neurochemical transmission, are discussed in Chapter 8. Some additional aspects specific to noradrenergic transmission and where the drugs act are described here.

Sympathetic noradrenergic neurons exhibit extensive branching. Fine preterminal axons at the end organs contain numerous beadlike enlargements called *varicosities* that may be the sites where norepinephrine is released into the neuroeffector junction. A schematic diagram of a varicosity and some of the chemical events that occur at the neuroeffector junction are depicted in Figure 10-1.

The chemical sequence in the synthesis of norepinephrine is illustrated in Figure 8-4 in Chapter 8, but several additional details are included here. Both dopamine and norepinephrine are synthesized within the neuronal varicosity. L-Tyrosine is transported into the neuron where it is converted to L-3, 4-dihydroxyphenylalanine (DOPA). This rate-limiting step in the synthesis of all catecholamines is catalyzed by tyrosine hydroxylase. The newly synthesized DOPA is rapidly decarboxylated to dopamine by L-amino acid decarboxylase, also known as DOPA decarboxylase. Peripheral sympathetic neurons contain dopamine-β-hydroxylase, which catalyzes the conversion of dopamine to norepinephrine. Because this enzyme is located within synaptic vesicles, dopamine must be actively transported into these vesicles before it can be converted to norepinephrine. When synthesized, norepinephrine is bound to ATP and stored within the vesicle until released.

When the nerve action potential arrives at the varicosity, calcium channels open, allowing Ca^{++} to enter the neuron. The norepinephrine-containing vesicles migrate and fuse with the neuronal membrane. Through *exocytosis*, the vesicles expel their contents into the neuroeffector junction, where norepinephrine is free to bind to receptor sites on the pre- and postsynaptic membranes. Depending on the organ innervated, the surface membranes of the cells contain β_1- or α_1-receptors. Receptors on smooth muscle and on gland cells are α_1, whereas receptors on cardiac cells are β_1. β_2-receptors respond primarily to epinephrine and are not discussed here because they respond only weakly to norepinephrine. Norepinephrine also binds to α_2-receptors on the presynaptic neuronal membrane. Activation of the α_2-"autoreceptor" inhibits the further release of norepinephrine. The biochemical events that occur in the postjunctional cells subsequent to the binding of norephinephrine to the various receptors are presented in Chapters 2, 8, and 12.

After norepinephrine reacts with the presynaptic or postsynaptic receptors, it is removed by the high affinity, uptake$_1$ system, which transports the amine back into the varicosity. Here the norepinephrine can be transported into the protective environment of the synaptic vesicle for eventual re-release or can be oxidatively deaminated by monoamine oxidase (MAO) located on the external membrane of mitochondria. The biologically inactive deaminated metabolites (3,4-dihydroxyphenylethylene glycol and 3,4-dihydroxymandelic acid) are then lost from the neuron, circulate in the bloodstream, and eventually are excreted in the urine. Norepinephrine can also be trans-

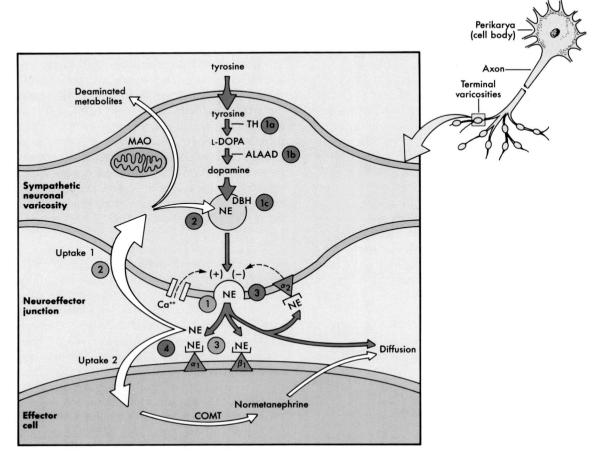

FIGURE 10-1   Prejunctional and postjunctional sites of action of drugs that modify noradrenergic transmission at a sympathetic neuroeffector junction. L-Tyrosine is actively transported into the axoplasm of the neuron, where it is converted first to L-DOPA by tyrosine hydroxylase *(TH)*, and then to dopamine by aromatic L-amino acid decarboxylase *(ALAAD)*. Dopamine is actively transported into synaptic vesicles, where it is converted by dopamine β-hydroxylase *(DBH)* to norepinephrine *(NE)*. The arrival of a nerve action potential at the varicosity causes the influx of calcium ions, which promotes the exocytotic release of NE into the neuroeffector junction where NE can activate receptors on postjunctional smooth muscle or glandular cells *(α_1)* or cardiac cells *(β_1)*, or on the prejunctional neuronal membrane *(α_2)*. Activation of the latter receptor inhibits the further release of NE. The action of NE is terminated by transport back into the varicosity, uptake 1. In the varicosity, NE can be stored in the synaptic vesicle or metabolized by monoamine oxidase *(MAO)* to inactive deaminated products. NE is also lost from the neuroeffector junction by diffusion and by transport into the postjunctional cell, uptake 2, where it is metabolized to normetanephrine by catechol-O-methyltransferase *(COMT)*. Sites at which drugs *enhance* or *mimic* this noradrenergic transmission process are identified by *green numbers; red numbers* identify sites where drugs *block* or *reduce* this process.

Drugs that enhance or mimic noradrenergic transmission
1. Facilitate release (e.g., amphetamine)
2. Block reuptake (e.g., cocaine)
3. Receptor agonists (e.g., phenylephrine)

Drugs that reduce noradrenergic transmission
1. *Inhibit synthesis (e.g., 1a, α-methyltyrosine; 1b, carbidopa; 1c, disulfiram)*
2. Disrupt vesicular storage (e.g., reserpine)
3. Inhibit release (e.g., guanethidine)
4. Receptor antagonists (e.g., tolazoline)

ported into the postjunctional cell by the uptake$_2$ system, where it is O-methylated by catechol-O-methyltransferase to normetanephrine. The transport of norepinephrine via the uptake$_1$ transporter is the major mechanism that terminates the actions of this amine at receptor sites. Preventing the metabolism of norepinephrine by the administration of inhibitors of catechol-O-methyltransferase and MAO does not enhance the transmission process at the sympathetic neuron terminals. Catechol-O-methyltransferase and MAO, however, play important roles in metabolizing circulating catecholamines (norepinephrine and epinephrine) and some exogenously administered sympathomimetic amines.

Norepinephrine is also synthesized in, and released from, chromaffin cells in the adrenal medulla. In addition, however, many cells in the adrenal medulla contain phenylethanolamine N-methyltransferase, which catalyzes the conversion of norepineph-

rine to epinephrine. Chromaffin cells of the adrenal medulla are innervated by sympathetic preganglionic cholinergic neurons and release catecholamines into the blood rather than into a neuroeffector junction. The released epinephrine is transported via the blood to various organs where it activates α- and β-receptors on the surface of glandular, smooth muscle, and cardiac muscle cells. Like norepinephrine, epinephrine binds to α$_1$-, α$_2$-, and β$_1$-receptors, but also activates β$_2$-adrenergic receptors on smooth muscle. Circulating catecholamines, whether given as drugs or released from the adrenal medulla, are taken up by the uptake$_1$ process in sympathetic nerves or are metabolized by the enzymes in the liver.

Sympathomimetics

Agonists Receptor agonists mimic the effects of sympathoadrenal discharge by combining directly

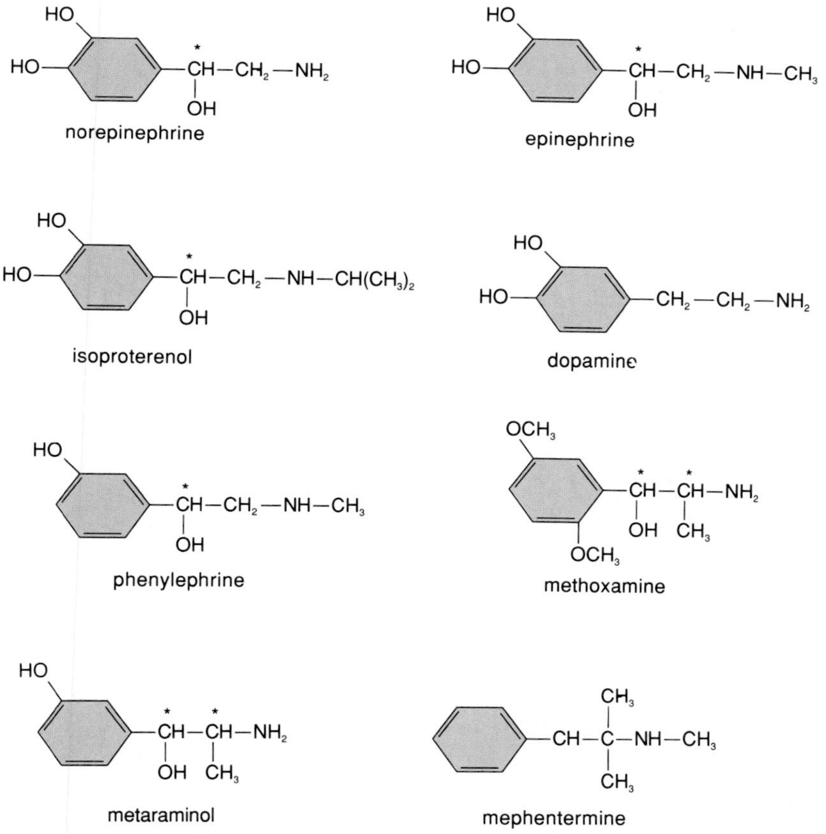

FIGURE 10-2 Sympathomimetic agonists; direct-acting. Asterisk indicates asymmetric carbon.

Continued.

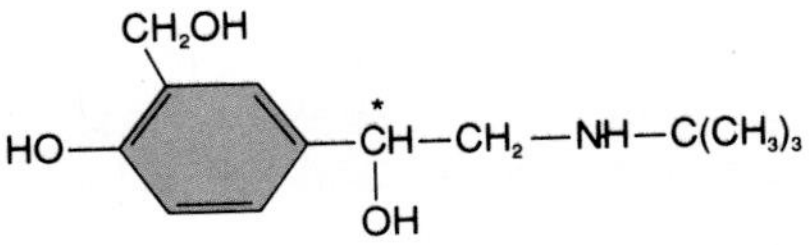

albuterol

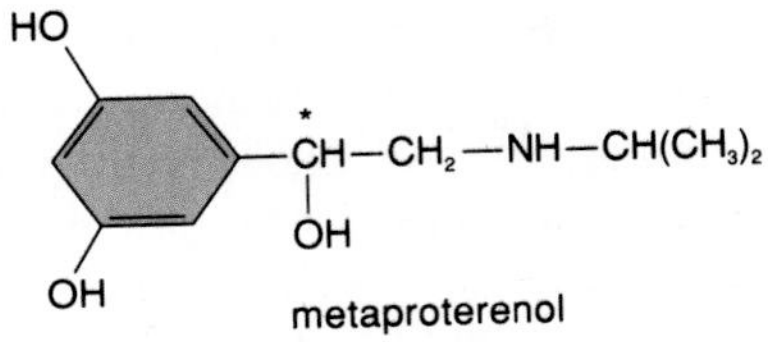

metaproterenol

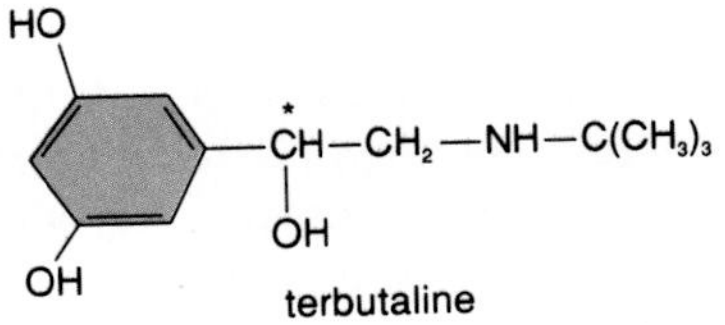

terbutaline

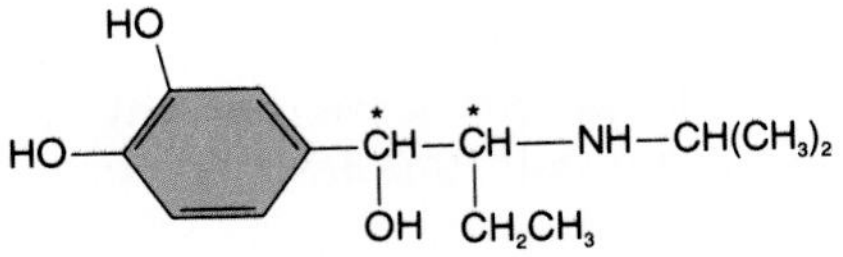

isoetharine

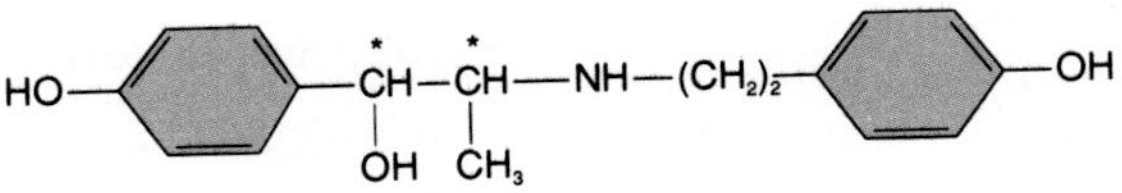

ß$_2$ agonist

ritodrine

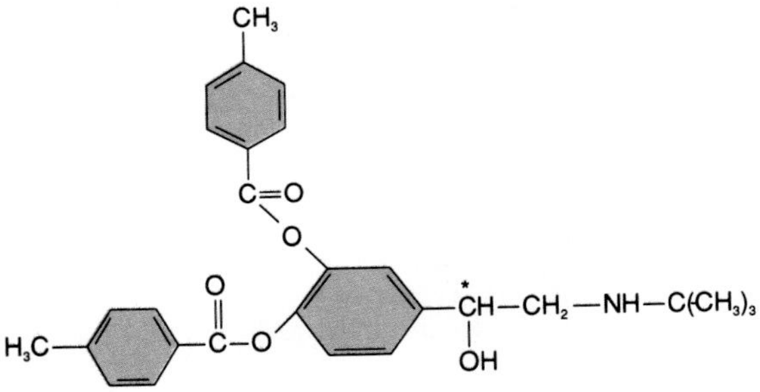

bitolterol

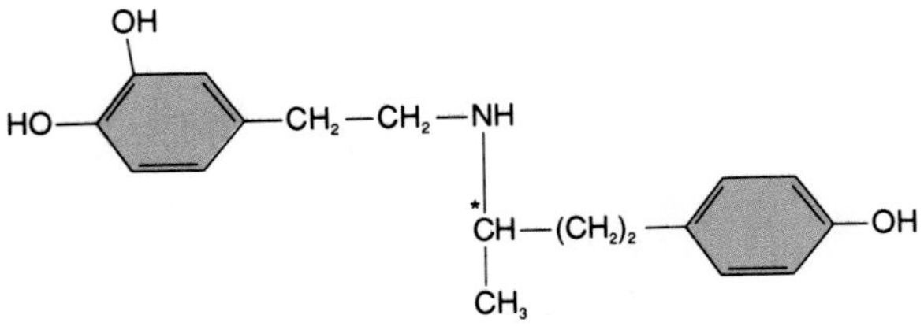

ß$_1$ agonist

dobutamine

FIGURE 10-2 cont'd   Sympathomimetic agonists; direct-acting. Asterisk indicates asymmetric carbon.

with postjunctional receptors (see site 3 [green] in Figure 10-1). Some drugs combine selectively with specific adrenergic receptors and mimic the effects of the endogenous ligands, epinephrine and norepinephrine. Each endogenous catecholamine activates several different receptors (norepinephrine binds to α_1-, α_2-, and β_1-receptors and epinephrine binds to α_1-, α_2-, β_1-, and β_2-receptors), but some sympathomimetic amines selectively activate a single receptor type. For example, phenylephrine preferentially activates α_1-receptors, and clonidine activates α_2-receptors. Similarly, dobutamine and terbutaline are relatively specific agonists at β_1- and β_2-receptors, respectively. The structures for many of the clinically important adrenergic agonists are shown in Figure 10-2. These are also known as *direct-acting sympathomimetics.*

Facilitation of Release or Inhibition of Reuptake or Metabolism of Norepinephrine These drugs also are known as indirect-acting sympathomimetics because the effects do not result from direct action of the drugs on the receptors.

Amphetamine and other drugs produce their sympathomimetic action by facilitating the release of norepinephrine from the sympathetic nerve terminal (see site *1* [green] in Figure 10-1). The structures of amphetamine and other indirect-acting sympathomimetics are shown in Figure 10-3, but the effects of amphetamine are described primarily in Chapter 32.

Because norepinephrine is removed from sympathetic neuroeffector junctional receptor sites by active transport back into the nerve terminal, sympathomimetic responses can be obtained by administering drugs that block the uptake$_1$ amine transporter in the neuronal membrane (see site *2* [green] in Figure 10-1). Cocaine and tricyclic antidepressants such as

imipramine exert sympathomimetic effects in this manner. The structure and discussion of cocaine is presented in Chapter 32, with similar information for the tricyclic antidepressants in Chapter 24.

Because neuronal reuptake and not metabolism is the primary mechanism by which norepinephrine and epinephrine disappear from the neuroeffector junction, it is not surprising that drugs that inhibit the metabolism of these amines have little or no sympathomimetic actions. On the other hand, inhibitors of MAO (e.g., pargyline) or catechol-O-methyltransferase (e.g., tropolone) can enhance the actions of exogenously administered sympathomimetic amines that are substrates for these enzymes (see Figure 10-1). This has some important toxicological implications. For example, the actions of tyramine, a sympathomimetic amine present in various foods, are greatly enhanced in patients treated with a MAO inhibitor (see Chapter 13).

Indirect-acting sympathomimetics can be recognized from the reduction in their actions if the effector organ is denervated (i.e., when there are no noradrenergic neurons innervating the cells) or if reserpine is administered to deplete norepinephrine stores in sympathetic nerve terminals (Figure 10-4). An indirect sympathomimetic amine that releases norepinephrine must gain access to the noradrenergic neuron before effecting the release of the transmitter. Nonpolar, lipid-soluble drugs (e.g., amphetamine) can diffuse across the neuronal membrane, whereas polar, water-soluble compounds (e.g., tyramine) achieve access to the varicosity only by the uptake$_1$ transporter. The sympathomimetic actions of tyramine can be prevented if the transporter is blocked, as by cocaine, which blocks the amine transport system.

As noted in Figure 10-4, treatments that reduce or

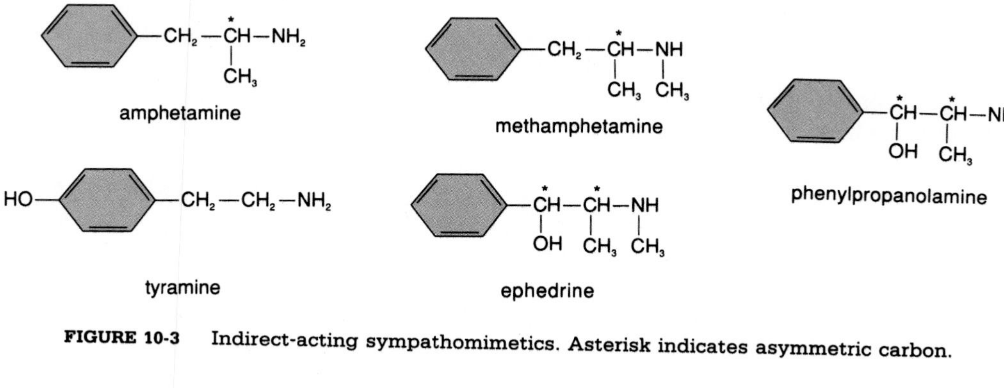

FIGURE 10-3   Indirect-acting sympathomimetics. Asterisk indicates asymmetric carbon.

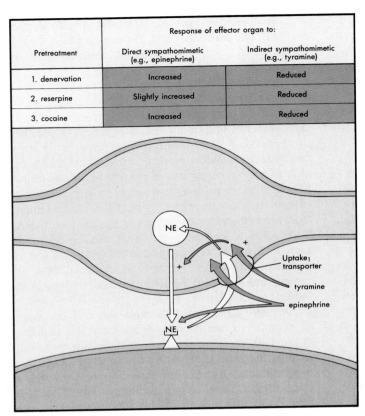

Pretreatment	Response of effector organ to:	
	Direct sympathomimetic (e.g., epinephrine)	Indirect sympathomimetic (e.g., tyramine)
1. denervation	Increased	Reduced
2. reserpine	Slightly increased	Reduced
3. cocaine	Increased	Reduced

FIGURE 10-4   Comparison of direct- and indirect-acting sympathomimetics (see text). *NE*, Norepinephrine.

block the effects of the indirect-acting sympathomimetic amine tyramine enhance the effects of epinephrine, which acts directly on the adrenergic receptors. The enhanced effects of a direct-acting sympathomimetic in denervated tissues result from two temporally distinguishable effects. An early (2 to 3 days) increase in response to epinephrine results from the loss of uptake$_1$ sites in the neuronal membrane. As the neuron degenerates, the transporter sites, which are primarily responsible for terminating the actions of epinephrine at the receptor sites, are lost. Later augmentation of epinephrine action occurs several days/weeks after denervation and is secondary to an increase (up-regulation) in postjunctional receptors. Cocaine causes a prompt increase in the response to epinephrine by blocking the uptake$_1$ system. Reserpine, however, disrupts amine transport in the synaptic vesicle membrane but not in the neuronal membrane; it does not therefore alter the transport of amine from the neuroeffector junction into the varicosity. By reducing the release of norepinephrine and thus the tonic activation of the postjunctional adrenergic receptors, reserpine may cause a slight increase in the number of postsynaptic receptors.

Sympatholytics

Inhibition of Synthesis, Storage, or Release of Norepinephrine

The synthesis of catecholamines can be disrupted in several ways, but effective in vivo blockade is obtained only when tyrosine hydroxylase, the enzyme catalyzing the first and rate-limiting step, is inhibited (see site *1a* in Figure 10-1). This can be effected clinically with α-methyltyrosine (metyrosine). A number of compounds can inhibit the other biosynthetic enzymes, (e.g., aromatic-L-amino acid decarboxylase is inhibited by carbidopa and dopamine β-hydroxylase is inhibited by disulfiram [see *1b* and *1c* in Figure 10-1]). These drugs have some experimental utility, but they do not effectively block endogenous catecholamine synthesis when administered clinically. On the other hand, carbidopa is clinically important because, by blocking peripheral decarboxylase activity, it reduces the side effects resulting from the formation of dopamine in the peripheral tissues of patients with Parkinson's disease treated with L-DOPA (i.e., carbidopa blocks the conversion of exogenously administered DOPA to dopamine).

Disruption of vesicular storage also modifies nor-

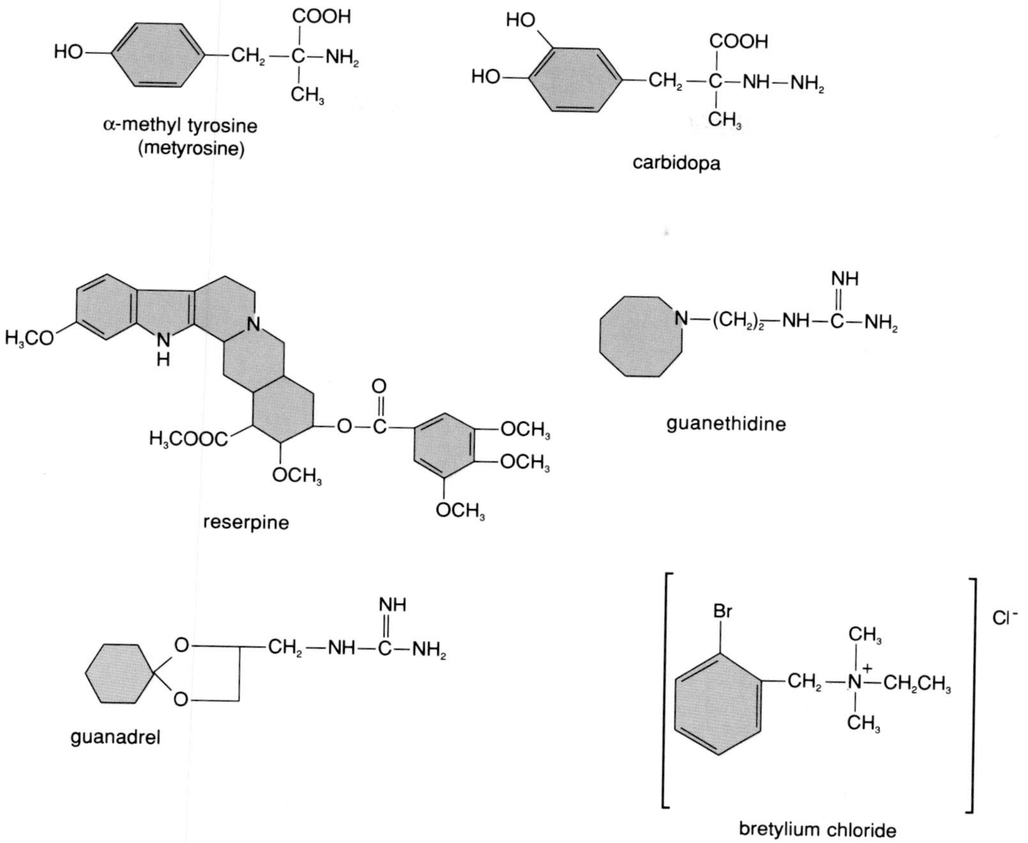

FIGURE 10-5   Sympatholytics: inhibitors of synthesis, storage, or release of norepinephrine.

adrenergic transmission (see *site 2* [red] in Figure 10-1). Reserpine, for example, disrupts the ability of the synaptic vesicles to transport and store dopamine and norepinephrine, so that the intraneuronal amines are not protected from MAO. In reserpine-treated patients therefore sympathetic neurons are depleted of norepinephrine and transmission at their terminals is reduced. Inhibition of release is also a mechanism for modulation of the adrenergic response (see site 3 [red] in Figure 10-1). Drugs such as bretylium and guanethidine are transported into, and become incorporated in, the membranes of noradrenergic nerve terminals and, possibly by a local anesthetic action at this site, prevent the release of norepinephrine in response to drugs and nerve action potentials (see Figure 10-5 for structures of sympatholytics).

Antagonists The antagonists have a high affinity for adrenergic receptors but lack intrinsic activity and thus effectively block the receptors (see *site 4* [red]

in Figure 10-1). The early antagonists blocked α-receptors (phenoxybenzamine) or β-receptors (propranolol). Now drugs are available that specifically block α_1- (prazosin), α_2- (idazoxan), or β_1- (metaprolol) receptors. These selective antagonists have valuable therapeutic advantages over the original, broad-spectrum adrenergic blockers. Experimentally, sympathetic transmission can be reduced by activating α_2-presynaptic receptors on terminals of peripheral sympathetic neurons with clonidine, which reduces the release of norepinephrine. The therapeutically useful antihypertensive action of this partial α_2 agonist, however, is secondary to a reduction in sympathetic tone resulting from an action of the drug in the brain. The structures of the above drugs and other clinically used adrenergic antagonists, with important CNS actions, are shown in Figure 10-6. Many of these antagonists are discussed further in Chapters 12 and 13.

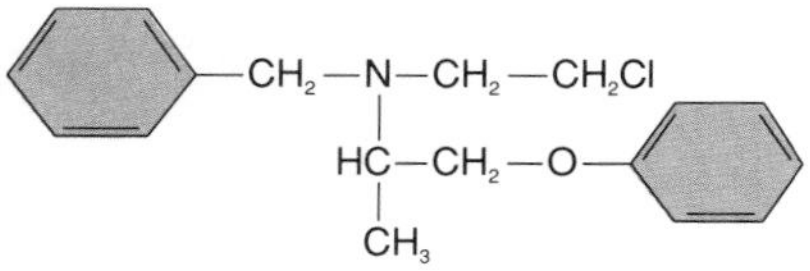

phenoxybenzamine

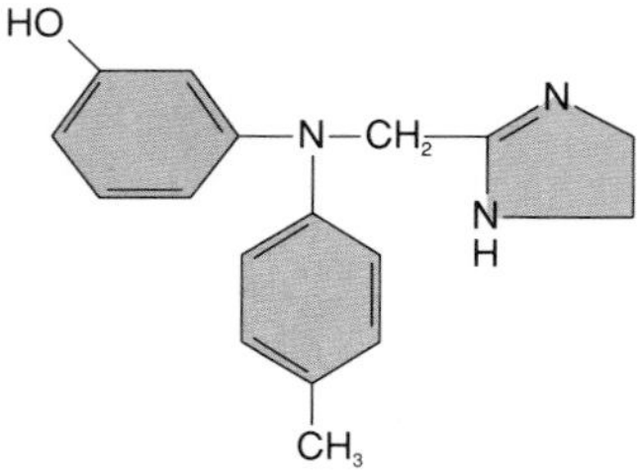

phentolamine

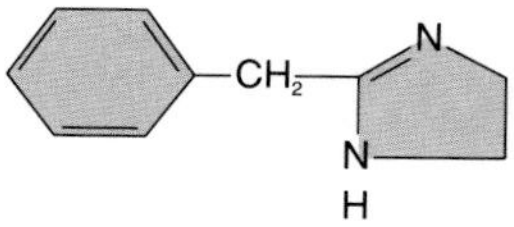

tolazoline

α_1 and α_2 antagonists

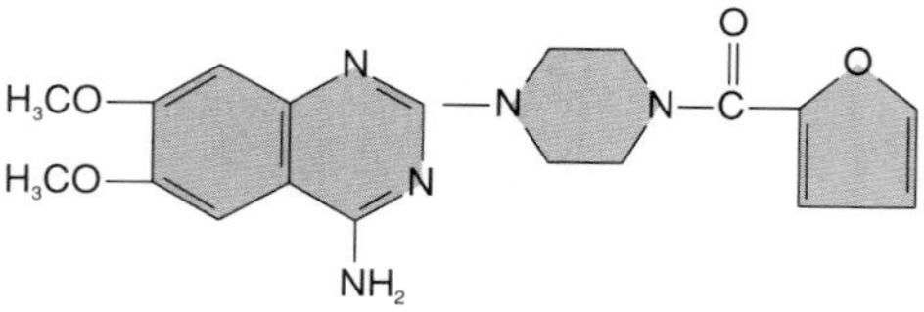

prazosin

α_1 antagonists

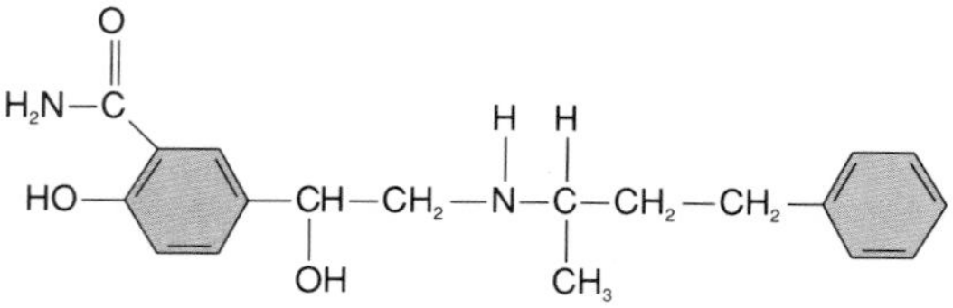

labetalol

α_1, β_1, and β_2
antagonists

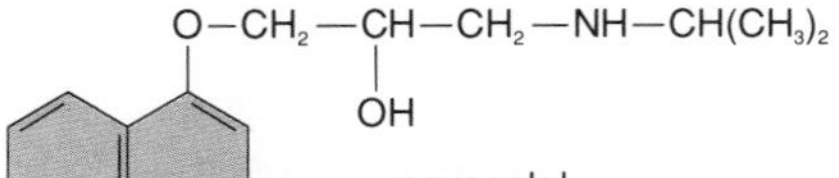

propranolol

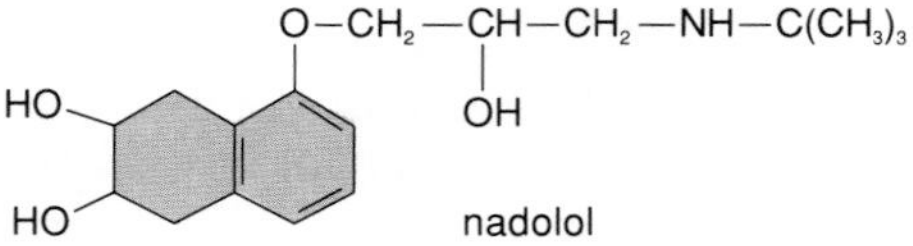

nadolol

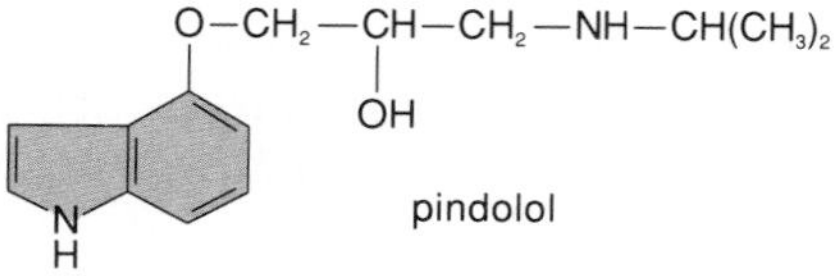

pindolol

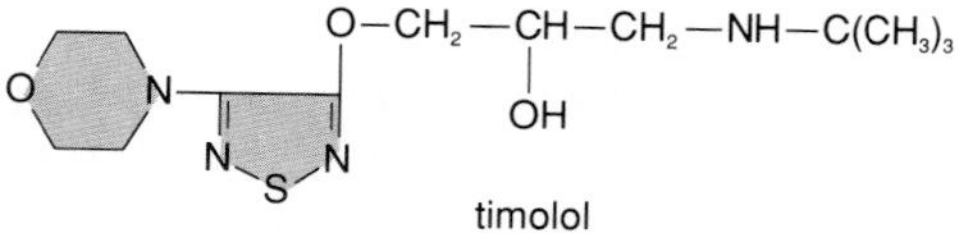

timolol

β_1 and β_2
antagonists

FIGURE 10-6   Sympatholytics: antagonists and reducers of CNS sympathetic outflow.

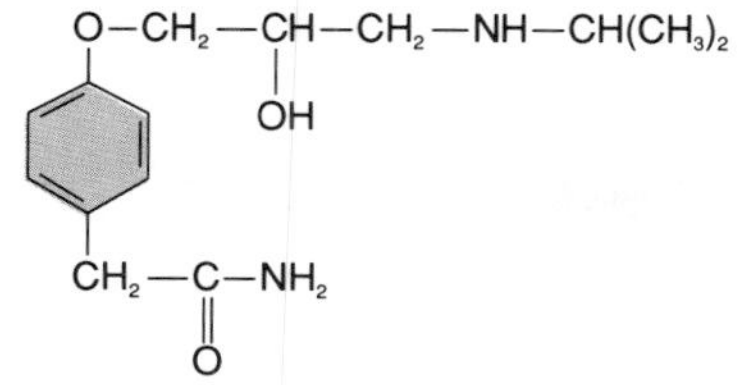

atenolol

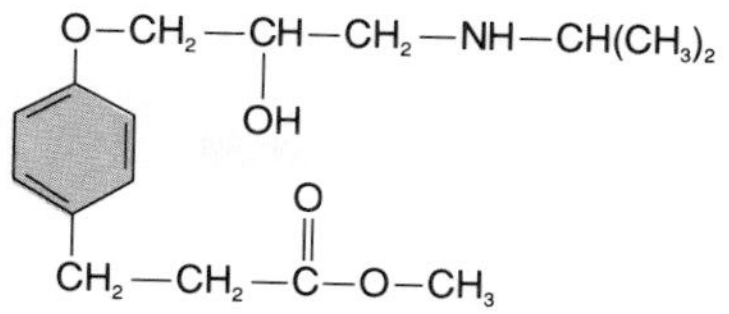

esmolol

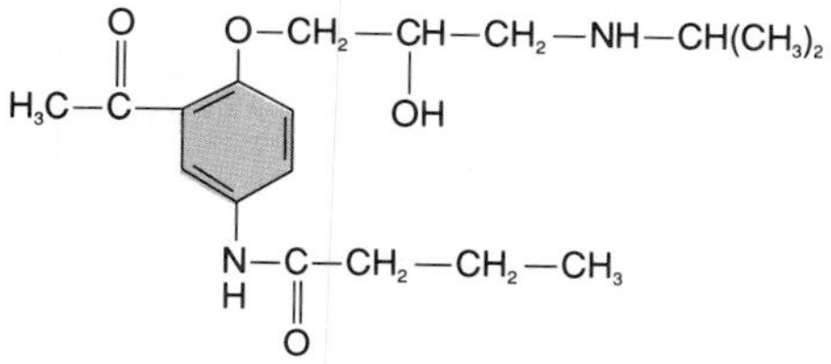

acebutolol

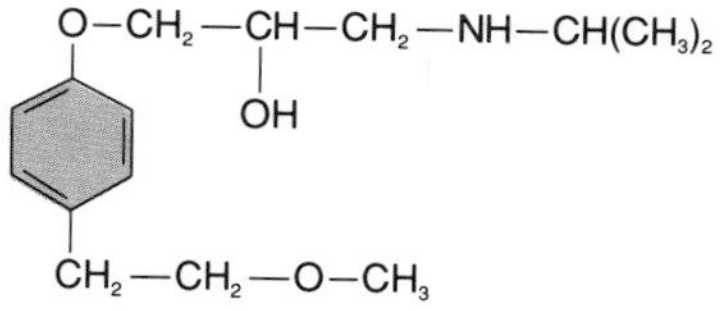

metoprolol

β_1 antagonists

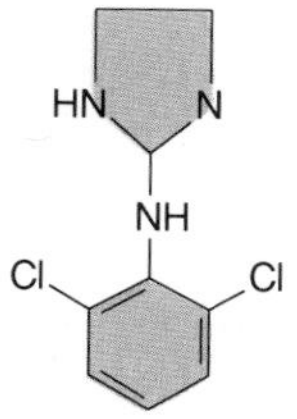

clonidine

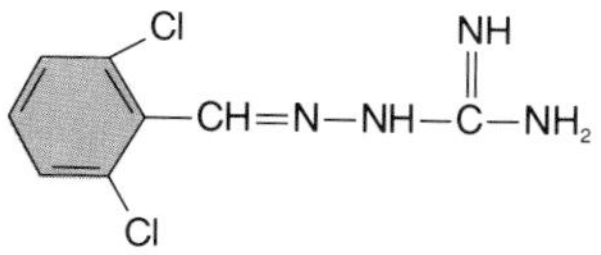

guanabenz

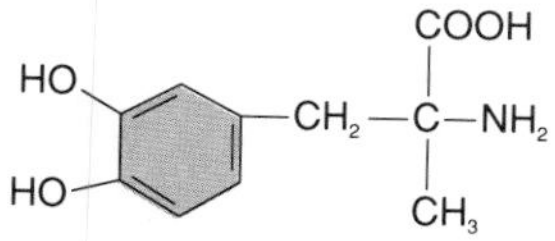

L-methyldopa

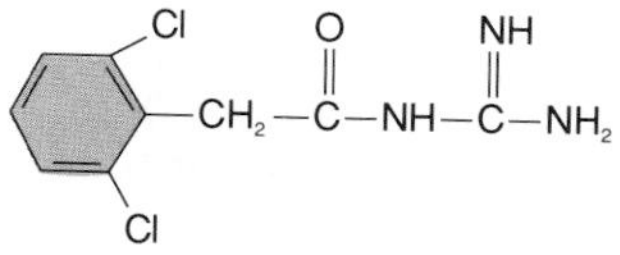

guanfacine

Miscellaneous antagonists (see text).

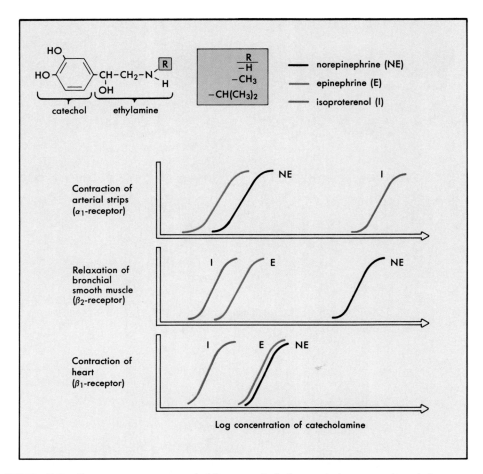

FIGURE 10-7   Dose-response curves (arbitrary scales) show relative potencies of three cate-cholamines on experimental muscle preparations. Changes in forces of contraction or relaxation for each muscle tissue hung in separate tissue baths after addition of progressively increasing concentrations of each catecholamine.

Summary of Catecholamine Activation of Adrenergic Receptors

There are multiple subtypes of both α- and β-adrenergic receptors. In Chapter 8 and earlier in this chapter, the relative potencies of norepinephrine, epinephrine, and isoproterenol on the activation of the receptor subtypes are described. Norepinephrine and epinephrine are endogenous catecholamines released from the adrenal medulla and in neurons in brain and at peripheral sympathetic neuroeffector junctions. Isoproterenol is a synthetic catecholamine congener.

These amines stimulate cardiac muscle to con-tract and smooth muscle to either contract or relax, depending on the receptor subtype. These receptor subtypes are revealed by dose-response curves to three catecholamines on tissues from arteriolar smooth muscle (α_1-receptor), bronchiolar smooth muscle (β_2-receptor), and cardiac muscle (β_1-receptor) preparations (Figure 10-7). The relative potencies are listed in rank order in Table 10-1.

Confirming evidence is shown in Figure 10-8 using dose-response curves with a catecholamine that activates the receptor subtype and a competitive blocking agent. Phentolamine is a competitive antagonist

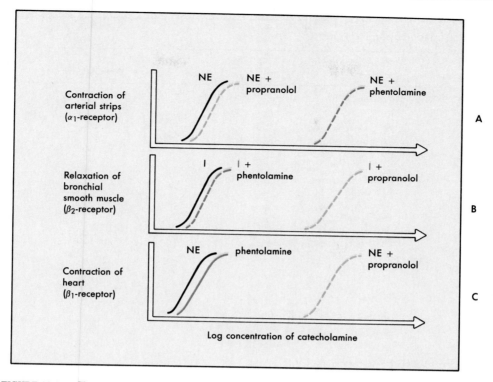

FIGURE 10-8   Change in force of contraction or relaxation (arbitrary scale) of different tissues hung in separate tissue baths after addition of increasing concentrations of catecholamine in absence and presence of a fixed concentration of an α_1-adrenergic (phentolamine), or β-adrenergic (propranolol) receptor blocking drug. *NE*, Norepinephrine; *I*, isoproterenol.

Table 10-1 Rank Order of Activation of Adrenergic Receptors by Catecholamines*

| Catecholamine | Receptor Type | | |
	α_1	β_1	β_2
epinephrine	1	2	2
norepinephrine	2	2	10
isoproterenol	10	1	1

*Ranking is based on potencies from Figure 10-7. Compounds are ranked in descending order with 1 most potent and 10 least potent (arbitrary scale).

at α_1-receptors. It demonstrates a competitive displacement only with α_1-receptors in the presence of a catecholamine that activates this subtype (Figure 10-8, *A*) and causes a parallel shift to the right of NE-induced contraction of arterial strips. Propranolol is a competitive antagonist at both β_1- and β_2-receptors and shows the expected parallel right shift in the dose-response curves (see Figure 10-8, *B* and *C*).

α_2-Subtype receptors are located on the terminal of sympathetic neurons where they modulate the release of norepinephrine. α_2-Receptors are also located presynaptically and postsynaptically on neurons in the brain; the activation of these receptors reduces central sympathetic outflow (discussed in Chapter 12).

PHARMACOKINETICS

Detailed pharmacokinetics for many of these drugs have not been studied in humans because of the short duration of action, intense nature of the effects, or limited clinical use of the preparations. Available pharmacokinetic parameters are summarized in Table 10-2.

Table 10-2   Pharmacokinetic Parameters

Drug	Route of Administration	$t_{1/2}$	Disposition	Remarks
DIRECT-ACTING SYMPATHOMIMETICS				
norepinephrine	IV			
epinephrine	IV, inhalation			
isoproterenol	IV, oral, inhalation			
dopamine	IV			
phenylephrine				
methoxamine	IV, IM			
metaraminol	IV, IM, SC			
mephentermine	Slow IV, IM			
albuterol	Oral, inhalation	3.8 hr	R (30%) M (50%)	
metaproterenol	Oral, inhalation		M (main)	
terbutaline	IV, oral, inhalation		M (60%) first pass; crosses placenta	
isoetharine	Inhalation			
ritodrine	IV, oral	12 hr oral	R (90%)	bioavailability 30% (oral)
bitolterol	Inhalation		M (main)	
dobutamine	IV	2 min	M (main)	
INDIRECT-ACTING SYMPATHOMIMETICS				
amphetamine	Oral, exchange resin			
ephedrine	Oral, SC, IM, IV			
phenylpropanolamine	Oral			
SYMPATHOLYTICS: BLOCKERS				
phenoxybenzamine	IV, oral	24 hr oral		25% absorbed
phentolamine	IV, IM	19 min	R (13%) M	
tolazoline	IV	3-10 hr (neonates)		
prazosin	Oral	2.5 hr	M (main) B	>90% pb
propranolol	Oral	4 hr	M	
nadolol	Oral	22 hr	R (90%)	
timolol	Oral	4 hr	M 50% first pass R	10% pb
pindolol	Oral	3.5 hr	M (60%) no first pass	40% pb
		7 hr (elderly)	R (40%)	
acebutolol	Oral	3.5 hr	M (main, active met (AM)	
		10 hr (am)	R, B	
atenolol	Oral	6.5 hr	R (90%)	50% absorbed, 10% pb
metoprolol	IV, oral, inhalation	5 hr	M (90%), 50% first pass R (50%)	12% pb

M, Metabolism; *R* renal, unchanged drug; *B*, biliary; *met*, metabolite; *first pass*, liver first pass effect; *inh*, inhalation as an aerosol; *pb*, plasma protein bound.
*Ester hydrolysis, gives weakly active metabolite.
†Terminal elimination phase.
‡Transdermal adhesive patch, 1 week.

Table 10-2 Pharmacokinetic Parameters—cont'd

Drug	Route of Administration	$t_{1/2}$	Disposition	Remarks
SYMPATHOLYTICS: BLOCKERS—cont'd				
esmolol	IV	9 min	M (98%), weak met* R	
labetolol	IV, oral	5.5 hr	M (65%), first pass	50% pb
OTHER SYMPATHOLYTICS				
α-methyl tyrosine (metyrosine)	Oral	3.5 hr	R (85%)	
reserpine	Oral	33 hr		96% pb, 50% bioavailability
bretylium	IV	7.8 hr	R (90%)	
guanethidine	Oral	1.5 da 4-8 da†	R M	
granadrel	Oral	10 hr	R (85%)	
REDUCTION OF CENTRAL SYMPATHETIC OUTFLOW				
clonidine	Oral‡			
methyldopa	Oral	105 min	M R	
guanabenz	Oral	6 hr	M (90%)	
guanfacine	Oral	17 hr	M (50%) R (50%)	70% pb
carbidopa	Oral			

RELATION OF MECHANISM OF ACTION TO CLINICAL RESPONSE

Direct and Reflex Cardiovascular Actions of Adrenergic Agents

The sympathetic nervous system has an important role in regulating the cardiovascular system; thus adrenergic drugs have marked effects on this system. These drugs alter the rate and force of contraction of the heart and the tone of blood vessels (and consequently blood pressure) by interacting directly with receptors located on cardiac and vascular smooth muscle cells. As a consequence of these direct actions, compensatory reflex adjustments take place. To understand the overall actions of adrenergic drugs on the heart and blood vessels, the cardiovascular reflexes must be considered.

Blood pressure is established as the value needed to deliver blood to all organs. It does not fluctuate widely because of feedback mechanisms that evoke compensatory secondary responses designed to maintain homeostasis. Homeostatic control of blood pressure is exerted primarily by baroreceptor reflexes (Figure 10-9). Baroreceptors are stretch receptors located in the walls of the heart and blood vessels, primarily in the carotid sinus and aortic arch, that are activated by distension of the blood vessels. Increased blood pressure augments the impulse traffic in the afferent neurons (baroreceptor neurons) that project to vasomotor centers in the medulla. Impulses generated in the baroreceptors inhibit the tonic discharge of sympathetic neurons projecting to the heart and blood vessels, and activate vagal fibers projecting to the heart. When a drug such as phenylephrine, which contracts vascular smooth muscle, is administered, the peripheral resistance, and consequently the blood pressure, increases (Figure 10-10). The resulting increase in pressure within the carotid sinus and aortic

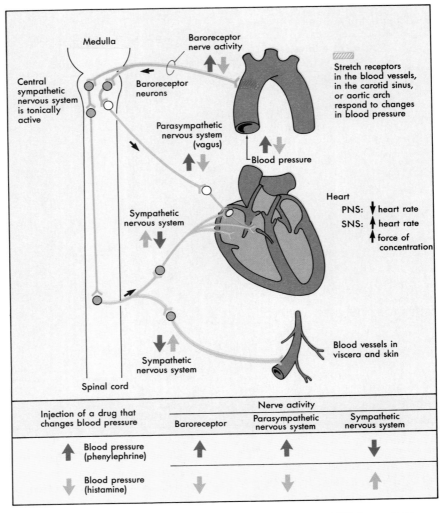

FIGURE 10-9   Baroreceptor control of blood pressure and heart rate. *SNS*, Sympathetic nervous system; *PNS*, parasympathetic nervous system (see text).

arch raises impulse traffic in the afferent baroreceptor neurons, and thereby reduces sympathetic, but increases vagal, nerve activity. As a consequence, the heart rate decreases (bradycardia). If a drug such as histamine, which relaxes vascular smooth muscle, is administered, the blood pressure decreases, reducing impulse traffic in the afferent buffer neurons. Consequently, sympathetic nerve activity increases and vagal nerve activity decreases, resulting in increased heart rate (tachycardia).

In summary, drugs that cause vasoconstriction (e.g., α_1 agonists) will secondarily cause a reflex slowing of the heart. On the other hand, drugs that cause vasodilation (e.g., α_1-receptor blocking drugs) produce tachycardia via the baroreceptor reflex mechanism. Thus when considering the actions of adrenergic drugs on the cardiovascular system, the direct actions of the drug on appropriate effector organs and compensatory reflex actions secondary to the direct actions must be considered.

Direct-acting Sympathomimetics

Epinephrine Epinephrine is a prototype of direct-acting sympathomimetic drugs because it activates α_1-, β_1- and β_2-receptors. The effects of the direct-

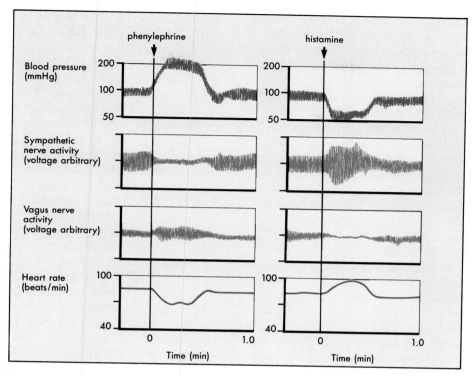

FIGURE 10-10   Responses to IV injections of drugs that cause vasoconstriction (phenylephrine) or vasodilation (histamine) by acting directly on vascular smooth muscle.

acting sympathomimetic drugs on selected tissues and organ systems are discussed here. Epinephrine is discussed first, and the properties of the more selective sympathomimetics are then compared with the prototype.

Cardiac Actions   By activating cardiac β_1-receptors epinephrine alters the strength, the rate, and the rhythm of cardiac contractions; these actions may be desirable or dangerous. Epinephrine increases the force of contraction (positive inotropic effect) by activating β_1-receptors on myocardial cells and increases the rate of contraction (positive chronotropic effect) by activating β_1-receptors on pacemaker cells in the sinoatrial (SA) node. Epinephrine also accelerates the rate of myocardial relaxation so that systole is shortened to a relatively greater extent than diastole. Thus, with epinephrine action, the fraction of time spent in diastole is increased, which allows for increased filling of the heart. The combination of increased diastolic filling time, more forceful ejection of blood, and increased rates of contraction and relaxation of the heart results in increased cardiac output.

The initial increase in heart rate after administration of epinephrine may be followed by reflex slowing of the heart (bradycardia) as a result of activation of the vagus. The reflex bradycardia is blocked by muscarinic antagonists such as atropine. Reflex slowing of the heart is more pronounced after the administration of norepinephrine because it causes a greater increase in the total peripheral resistance than epinephrine.

In addition to activating β_1-receptors on pacemaker cells in the SA node, epinephrine also activates conducting tissues, increasing conduction velocity and reducing the refractory period in the atrioventricular (AV) node, the bundle of His, Purkinje fibers, and ventricular muscle. These changes and the activation of latent pacemaker cells may lead to alterations in the rhythm of the heart. Large doses of epinephrine may cause tachycardia, premature ventricular systoles, and possibly fibrillation; these effects are more likely to occur in hearts that are diseased or have been sensitized to halogenated hydrocarbons, (e.g., certain anesthetic agents).

Vascular Smooth Muscle Effects The responses to epinephrine of smooth muscle cells in different organs depend on the type of adrenergic receptors present. Vascular smooth muscle is regulated by α_1- or β_2-receptor-containing cells, depending on the location of the vascular bed. Epinephrine is a powerful vasoconstrictor in some vascular beds; it activates α_1-receptors to constrict smooth muscle cells in precapillary resistance vessels (arterioles) in skin, mucosa, kidney, and in veins. Conversely, epinephrine relaxes vascular smooth muscle in skeletal muscle, liver, and gut as a result of the activation of β_2-receptors. Thus, epinephrine increases blood flow in skeletal muscle and some splanchnic beds but reduces flow in the skin and kidney. As a result of its opposing actions in different vascular beds, epinephrine does not have a marked effect on total peripheral resistance. After IV infusion of epinephrine, systolic blood pressure markedly increases, whereas there is little change of diastolic arterial pressure. Epinephrine increases arterial and venous pulmonary pressures primarily as a result of a redistribution of blood from the systemic to the pulmonary circulation. The overall action of epinephrine on blood flow varies with the dose; β_2-receptors appear to be more sensitive to epinephrine, so at low doses vasodilation predominates. At higher doses, vasoconstriction and increased diastolic pressure generally occur.

Systemic administration of epinephrine alters cerebral and coronary blood flow, but the changes are not due to the direct actions of the amine on α- or β_2-receptors on vascular smooth muscle in the brain and heart. Epinephrine-induced changes in cerebral blood flow primarily reflect changes in systemic blood pressure. Epinephrine increases coronary blood flow as a result of a relatively greater duration of diastole and metabolic changes (increased production of vasodilatory metabolites and the release of adenosine) secondary to increased work of the heart.

Other Smooth Muscle Effects Epinephrine is a potent bronchodilator. It relaxes bronchial smooth muscle by activating β_2-receptors. Epinephrine is a physiological antagonist to endogenous bronchoconstrictors (e.g., histamine, 5-hydroxytryptamine) and can be life-saving in the treatment of acute asthmatic attacks. This drug also relaxes smooth muscle in various organs by activating β_2-receptors, reduces the frequency and amplitude of gastrointestinal (GI) contractions, inhibits the tone and contractions of the pregnant uterus, and relaxes the detrusor muscle of the urinary bladder. Epinephrine, however, contracts smooth muscle of the splenic capsule and of GI and urinary sphincters by activating α_1-receptors. Epinephrine relaxes GI smooth muscle and contracts the pyloric and ileocecal sphincters, reducing motility in the gut, although at therapeutic doses this response is fleeting and has little clinical significance. Epinephrine can contribute to urinary retention by relaxing the detrusor muscle and contracting the trigone and sphincter of the urinary bladder.

The radial pupillary dilator muscle of the iris contains α_1-receptors and contracts in response to activation of sympathetic neurons, causing mydriasis. Because epinephrine is a highly polar molecule, it does not readily penetrate the cornea when instilled into the conjunctival sac. Application of the less polar, more lipid-soluble α-adrenergic agonists causes mydriasis (e.g., phenylephrine). Instillation of epinephrine, however, lowers intraocular pressure, possibly by reducing formation of aqueous humor by the ciliary bodies, the latter involving a mechanism that is not well understood.

Because polar epinephrine and other catecholamines such as norepinephrine, isoproterenol, and dopamine cannot penetrate the blood-brain barrier, systemic administration of this amine has no direct cerebral action. Nevertheless, possibly via a secondary reflex action, systemic administration of epinephrine can cause anxiety, restlessness, and headache.

Metabolic Effects Epinephrine exerts a number of metabolic effects, some of which are secondary to an action of epinephrine on the secretion of insulin and glucagon. The predominant action of epinephrine on islet cells of the pancreas is the inhibition of insulin secretion via activation of α_2-receptors and the stimulation of glucagon secretion via β_2-receptors.

The major metabolic effects of epinephrine are increased circulating concentrations of glucose, lactic acid, and free fatty acids. In humans, these effects are due to the activation of β-receptors on the surface of liver, skeletal muscle, heart, and adipose cells (Figure 10-11). Subsequent to binding to β-receptors, the G-proteins and adenylate cyclase are activated by epinephrine. The increase in cyclic adenosine monophosphate (cAMP) activates the cAMP-dependent protein kinase. This leads to phosphorylation and activation of other kinases, including phosphorylase b kinase, with subsequent additional phosphorylations of enzymes, including phosphorylase and lipase, both of which become activated. In fat, lipase catalyzes

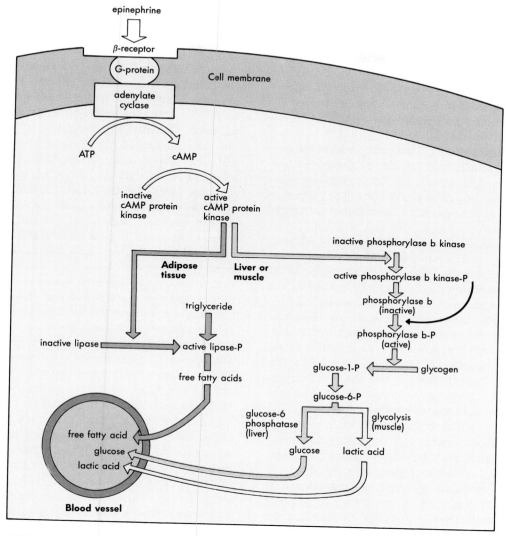

FIGURE 10-11   Mechanisms by which epinephrine (and other adrenergic agonists) exert metabolic effects in adipose, liver, heart, and skeletal muscle cells.

the breakdown of triglycerides to free fatty acids. The characteristic "calorigenic action" of epinephrine, which is reflected in a 20% to 30% increase in oxygen consumption may be due, in part, to the breakdown of triglycerides in brown adipose tissue. In liver, phosphorylase catalyzes the breakdown of glycogen to glucose. In muscle, glycogenolysis and glycolysis produce lactic acid, which is released into the blood. The release of glucose from the liver is accompanied by the efflux of potassium, so that epinephrine induces hyperglycemia and a brief period of hyperkalemia.

The hyperkalemia is followed by a more pronounced hypokalemia, as the potassium released from the liver is taken up by skeletal muscle.

Miscellaneous Actions Secretion of sweat from glands located on the palms of the hands and forehead is increased during psychological stress. This effect is mediated by α_1-receptors. Systemic administration of epinephrine does not activate these glands, but secretion of sweat in these areas can be induced by local injection of epinephrine. Epinephrine modulates the secretion of a number of hormones, although usually the physiological relevance and pharmacological effects are not marked. On the other hand, as noted previously, the secretion of insulin is inhibited by activation of α_2-receptors and slightly stimulated by activation of β_2-receptors. The secretion of glucagon is also stimulated by β-receptor activation. Epinephrine, by acting on β-receptors, also causes the release of renin from the juxtaglomerular apparatus in the kidney.

Other Direct-acting Sympathomimetics Several clinically useful, directly acting sympathomimetics differ from epinephrine in that they are more selective in activating α- or β-receptors. The properties of some of these compounds are compared with those of epinephrine.

Norepinephrine does not activate β_2-receptors, thus the actions of norepinephrine can be predicted, because it stimulates only α- and cardiac β_1-receptors. Norepinephrine produces only vasoconstriction in vascular beds and therefore increases diastolic blood pressure. Because total peripheral resistance increases, the reflex slowing of the heart rate is more pronounced with norepinephrine than with epinephrine. Unlike epinephrine, norepinephrine does not relax bronchial smooth muscle, and the metabolic responses (e.g., hyperglycemia) are much less pronounced than they are with epinephrine.

Phenylephrine and methoxamine are synthetic selective α-receptor agonists. They differ from norepinephrine in that they do not stimulate the heart. These drugs increase total peripheral resistance by causing vasoconstriction in most vascular beds. Consequently they produce a reflex slowing of the heart, which can be blocked by atropine. These drugs are less potent but longer-acting than norepinephrine.

Isoproterenol is a potent β agonist; it differs from epinephrine in that it does not have α-adrenergic receptor agonist properties. It reduces total peripheral resistance, resulting in a marked reduction in diastolic blood pressure. Further, it has a marked stimulatory effect on the heart; tachycardia results from a combined direct action on β_1-receptors and a reflex action secondary to the hypotension. Like epinephrine it relaxes bronchial smooth muscle and induces metabolic effects. Clinically, isoproterenol may be inhaled as an aerosol or injected subcutaneously to relieve bronchoconstriction resulting from allergies, drugs, or asthma. However when used for this purpose the side actions of isoproterenol on the heart, resulting from its β_1-agonist property, can be trou-

blesome. Accordingly, efforts are being made to develop β agonists that are relatively specific for the β_2-receptors and have less effect on the β_1-cardiac receptors.

Metaproterenol, terbutaline, albuteral, bitolterol, and ritodrine are relatively specific agonists at β_2-adrenergic receptors. Because they have little effect on β_1-receptors they have less tendency to stimulate the heart. Nevertheless, selectivity for β_2-receptors is not absolute, and at higher doses these drugs stimulate the heart directly. These drugs also differ from isoproterenol in that they are effective after oral administration and have a longer duration of action. The selective β_2-receptor agonists also relax vascular smooth muscle, supplying skeletal muscle and smooth muscle in bronchi and the uterus. Because of their relative selectivity for β_2-receptors these drugs provide a therapeutic advantage over isoproterenol in that they are less likely to stimulate the heart. Although the pharmacological properties of all the β_2 agonists are similar, ritodrine is marketed as a tocolytic agent; that is, it relaxes uterine smooth muscle and thereby arrests premature labor. Ritodrine can be administered intravenously in emergency situations and orally for maintenance therapy. All other drugs are marketed as bronchodilators for the treatment of bronchospasm and bronchial asthma. They can be administered by inhalation, parenterally, or orally. When used orally, the selective β_2 agonists have an advantage over ephedrine (see below) because they do not penetrate the blood-brain barrier and thus lack CNS stimulant properties.

In contrast to the drugs previously discussed, which are relatively specific agonists at the β_2-receptor, dopamine and dobutamine are relatively specific for β_1-receptors and are used to stimulate the heart. Dopamine is an endogenous catecholamine with important actions as a neurotransmitter in the brain (see Chapter 12). In peripheral sympathetic neurons and in the adrenal medulla dopamine serves as a precursor for the synthesis of norepinephrine and epinephrine; the endogenous amine, however, does not have marked sympathomimetic actions. The circulating concentrations of dopamine are low and the compound has a short half-life. When administered by intravenous (IV) infusion, the drug has a characteristic action on the cardiac muscle and vascular smooth muscle in the kidney and gut. It produces a positive inotropic action on the heart directly by stimulating β_1-receptors and indirectly by releasing nor-

Table 10-3 Actions of Selected Sympathomimetics on Heart Rate

Sympathomimetic Amine	Activated Receptors	Blood Pressure (Total Peripheral Resistance)	Heart Rate Effect		
			Reflex	Direct	Reflex and Direct
norepinephrine	α, β₁	↑	↓*	↑	↓ or ↑
phenylephrine	α	↑	↓*	0	↓
isoproterenol	β₁,β₂	↓	↑	↑	↑↑
dobutamine	β₁	0	0	↑	↑

*Blocked by atropine.

epinephrine. Dopamine relaxes smooth muscle in some vascular beds, specifically in the kidney and mesenteric arteries, by activating dopamine receptors on the smooth muscle cells (this effect is blocked by dopamine receptor antagonists, such as haloperidol [see Chapter 13], and not by β-adrenergic receptor antagonists, such as propranolol). Because it can dilate the renal vascular bed, dopamine increases glomerular filtration rate, sodium excretion, and urinary output. Dopamine is administered by IV infusion for treatment of shock as a result of myocardial infarction, trauma, or renal failure. High doses of dopamine have α-agonist effects. For example, local ischemia results if during IV infusion dopamine leaks into the region surrounding the vein. If such an accident occurs, the ischemia can be treated by infiltrating the region with an α-receptor antagonist such as phentolamine.

Dobutamine is a relatively specific β₁-receptor agonist which, like dopamine, increases myocardial contractility without markedly altering total peripheral resistance. It has less effect on heart rate than isoproterenol because it does not produce reflex tachycardia. Like dopamine, dobutamine is administered by IV infusion to treat acute cardiac failure. Dobutamine differs from dopamine in that it does not increase blood flow in the renal vascular bed.

Table 10-3 contains a comparison of the direct and reflex actions of selected sympathomimetics on heart rate.

Indirectly Acting Sympathomimetics

A number of drugs that do not interact directly with adrenergic receptors have sympathomimetic actions as a result of their ability to cause the release of norepinephrine from sympathetic neurons and/or block the neuronal reuptake of released norepineph-

rine. Some of these drugs (e.g., amphetamine, ephedrine, cocaine) have marked effects on the brain and heart. These effects are discussed in Chapter 32; the following sections focus on the sympathomimetic properties of these drugs.

Tyramine is not employed therapeutically, but it has pharmacological and toxicological importance because (1) it is widely used as an experimental tool to study mechanisms of norepinephrine release, (2) it is present in a variety of foods (e.g., ripened cheese, fermented sausage, wines), and (3) it is formed in the liver and GI tract as a result of the decarboxylation of tyrosine (Figure 10-12).

Tyramine does not have an intrinsic action on adrenergic receptors (e.g., it does not affect denervated organs) but enters the norepinephrine nerve terminal via the amine transporter and causes the release of norepinephrine (see Figure 10-4). The released norepinephrine causes the sympathomimetic actions of tyramine. If the norepinephrine transporter is blocked (e.g., with a tricyclic antidepressant such as imipramine), tyramine lacks sympathomimetic actions. Tachyphylaxis, a form of tolerance that manifests by repeated administration of drug, develops from the sympathomimetic actions of injected tyramine, presumably because of conversion to octopamine. After tyramine enters the noradrenergic neuron it is transported into the synaptic vesicle where it is converted to octopamine by dopamine β-hydroxylase (reaction 3, Figure 10-12). Octopamine then displaces norepinephrine, fills the synaptic vesicles and is subsequently released as a "false transmitter." With repeated injections, tachyphylaxis develops as tyramine releases progressively more and more octopamine, which does not activate α- or β-adrenergic receptors, and less norepinephrine (compare Figure 10-13, A and B).

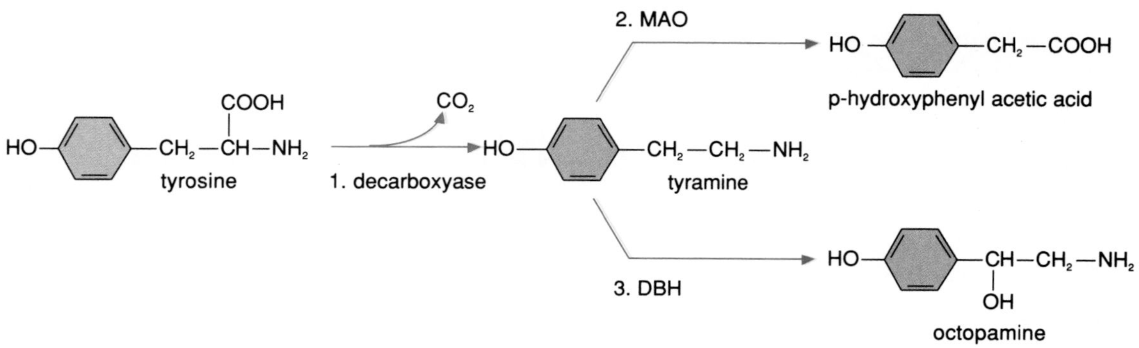

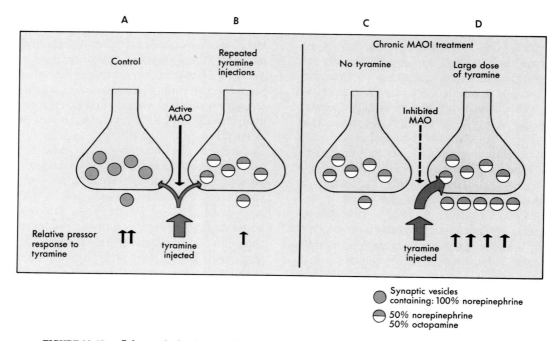

FIGURE 10-12   Synthesis and metabolism of tyramine. Reaction 1: decarboxylation of tyrosine in liver and GI tract. Reaction 2: oxidative deamination of tyramine by monoamine oxidase *(MAO)* in liver, kidney, and other tissues. Reaction 3: β-oxidation of tyramine by dopamine-β-hydroxylase *(DBH)* located in synaptic vesicles within terminal of sympathetic neurons.

FIGURE 10-13   Schematic depiction of **A,** acute response to an injection of tyramine; **B,** tolerance to repeated injections of tyramine; **C,** chronic treatment with a monoamine oxidase inhibitor *(MAOI);* **D,** effects of tyramine after chronic MAOI pretreatment. The relative increase in blood pressure is denoted by the number of arrows.

Even though tyramine is continually synthesized from dietary tyrosine, significant quantities of the amine are not found in blood or tissues because it is rapidly metabolized by MAO (reaction 2, Figure 10-12). In patients receiving repeated doses of an MAO inhibitor the circulating concentration of tyramine in-creases, and it is taken up by sympathetic nerve ter-minals (Figure 10-13, *C-D*). Here tyramine is con-verted to octopamine, which partially displaces nor-epinephrine. As a consequence, less norepinephrine (and the "false" transmitter, octopamine) is released when the sympathetic nervous system is activated;

this leads to a drop in blood pressure (see Figure 10-13, *C*). Patients receiving repeated doses of MAO inhibitors experience postural hypotension.

A more serious adverse effect that accompanies therapy with MAO inhibitors occurs if a patient consumes food containing tyramine. Normally there is no pharmacological response to tyramine-containing foods since the amine is rapidly destroyed by MAO. When this enzyme is inhibited, however, the consumed tyramine exerts a marked pharmacological action by releasing amine stores from terminals of sympathetic neurons (Figure 10-13, *D*). Although the tyramine releases active norepinephrine and inactive octopamine, the amount of norepinephrine released is sufficient to produce a severe hypertensive response. Patients treated with MAO inhibitors are cautioned to avoid foods containing tyramine, but if such foods are accidentally consumed, the hypertensive crisis can be treated by the administration of an α-adrenergic receptor antagonist.

Amphetamine and ephedrine are related chemically and exert their sympathomimetic effects primarily by facilitating the release and blocking the neuronal reuptake of norepinephrine. Ephedrine is not a substrate for either catechol-O-methyltransferase or MAO, and thus has a longer duration of action than exogenously administered epinephrine. The lack of ring hydroxyl groups also makes ephedrine less polar and more lipid soluble than epinephrine so that it readily traverses cell membranes and the blood-brain barrier. Consequently, in contrast to epinephrine, ephedrine is effective orally and has a stimulant action in the brain. Ephedrine has two asymmetric carbons and thus there are four isomers of the compound: *d*- and *l*-ephedrine and *d*- and *l*-pseudoephedrine. *l*-Ephedrine is the most potent sympathomimetic isomer, but the racemic mixture of ephedrine is also available for clinical use, as is *d*-pseudoephedrine.

Ephedrine exerts sympathomimetic effects by acting directly on β_2-receptors and by releasing norepinephrine, which activates α- and β_1-receptors. Ephedrine is used therapeutically to treat mild cases of asthma. Because of its central stimulant actions, it is no longer recommended for chronic treatment of asthma and has been largely replaced by the newer, more selective β_2 agonists.

Methamphetamine and amphetamine exist as *d*- and *l*-optical isomers. Acting on peripheral sympathetic neurons, *d*- and *l*-amphetamine are equi-

potent, but in the CNS the *d*-isomer is 3 to 4 times more potent than the *l*-isomer. Amphetamine is used therapeutically only for its central stimulant action (see Chapter 32), and to minimize peripheral sympathomimetic actions only the *d*-isomer is employed. Unlike ephedrine, amphetamine does not directly activate β_2-receptors but exerts its sympathomimetic actions by facilitating the release and blocking the reuptake of norepinephrine. Amphetamine has relatively more central stimulant and less peripheral sympathomimetic effects than ephedrine. The central stimulant actions of amphetamine appear to result from its ability to release and block reuptake of released dopamine in limbic forebrain regions.

Pseudoephedrine has little β_2-agonist activity and consequently is not effective in treating asthma. It has less central stimulant actions than ephedrine and is widely used in over-the-counter nasal decongestant oral preparations.

A racemic mixture of phenylpropanolamine, also referred to as norephedrine, is available for clinical use. The weak sympathomimetic actions of phenylpropanolamine result from its ability to release norepinephrine from sympathetic nerve terminals. It also has weak actions on α_1- and β_1-receptors, but unlike ephedrine it lacks β_2-agonist properties and is therefore not useful in treating bronchial asthma. Phenylpropanolamine is administered topically and orally to relieve nasal congestion. It is widely available as a component of over-the-counter drug preparations for the relief of discomforts of upper respiratory conditions that accompany the common cold. In these preparations phenylpropanolamine is often combined with analgesics, anticholinergics, antihistaminics, and caffeine. Phenylpropanolamine has less central stimulant actions than ephedrine but is widely used, with limited success, as an anorectic in the treatment of obesity.

Cocaine has central stimulant and peripheral sympathomimetic actions similar to those of amphetamine. It blocks the neuronal uptake of norepinephrine; unlike amphetamine it does not facilitate amine release. The local anesthetic properties of cocaine were recognized in the 1880s and it was widely used for this purpose in ophthalmology. Topical application of cocaine produces mydriasis and blanching as a result of its potent sympathomimetic effects. Also, cocaine causes sloughing of cells from the cornea and for this reason has been replaced in ophthalmology by other local anesthetics. This drug was formerly widely used by otolaryngologists to achieve local anesthetic and potent vasoconstrictor effects because it provided a dry area when operating in the upper respiratory passages. The abuse of cocaine (see Chapter 32) is currently at epidemic proportions, and the toxicity of the compound is of great concern. Repeated application of the drug via the nasal mucosa causes intense vasoconstriction that can lead to local ischemic damage. Acute toxicity is characterized by a wide spectrum of peripheral and central effects, including convulsions, myocardial infarction, and cardiac dysrhythmias that can result in death.

Drugs that Block α-Adrenergic Receptors

Compounds that bind covalently to the α-receptor, such as phenoxybenzamine, produce an irreversible blockade; compounds such as phentolamine and tolazoline bind reversibly and produce a competitive blockade. The characteristics of the effects of reversible and irreversible α-adrenergic blocking drugs are illustrated in Figure 10-14. Blockade produced by the reversible antagonist, tolazoline, is surmountable; as more agonist (i.e., norepinephrine) is administered, it effectively competes with tolazoline for the α-receptor. If more tolazoline is administered the dose-response curve shifts in a parallel manner to the right. Blockade produced by the irreversible blocker,

phenoxybenzamine, cannot be overcome by adding more norepinephrine. After the administration of phenoxybenzamine the response to norepinephrine depends on the number of receptors that are not covalently bound to phenoxybenzamine. If more phenoxybenzamine is administered, the dose-response curve for norepinephrine becomes shallow.

Phenoxybenzamine, phentolamine, and tolazoline block both α_1- and α_2-receptors, differing primarily in their potency and duration of action. These drugs are effective in blocking the actions of α-adrenergic agonists and the actions of the sympathetic nervous system on smooth muscle. By blocking sympathetic tone to blood vessels they cause vasodilation; the effect is proportional to the degree of sympathetic tone. α-Receptor blocking drugs cause only a small decrease in recumbent blood pressure but produce a marked fall during the compensatory vasoconstriction that occurs on standing, since the reflex sympathetic control of capacitance vessels (veins) is blocked. This results in "postural" or "orthostatic" hypotension, which is accompanied by reflex tachycardia. (Sympathetic control of heart rate is mediated by β_1-adrenergic receptors; phenoxybenzamine, phentolamine, and tolazoline do not block these receptors.)

The effects of α-adrenergic receptor blockade on mean blood pressure and heart rate to IV norepinephrine and epinephrine are illustrated in Figure 10-

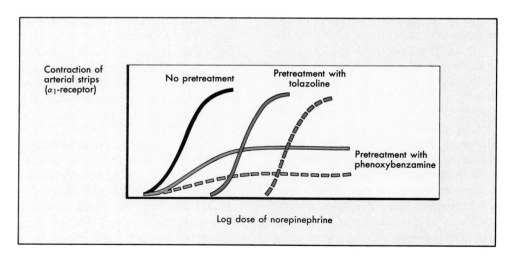

FIGURE 10-14   Comparison of effects of a reversible (tolazoline) and an irreversible (phenoxybenzamine) inhibitor of α-adrenergic receptors. Changes in the force of contraction of arterial strips were recorded after addition of increasing concentrations of norepinephrine in the absence and in the presence of low and high concentrations of tolazoline and low and high concentrations of phenoxybenzamine. The broken lines are larger doses.

15. The IV injection of large doses of norepinephrine and epinephrine increase peripheral resistance and produce a brief increase in mean blood pressure by activating α-adrenergic receptors on vascular smooth muscle. In response to the increased blood pressure, a reflex decrease in sympathetic tone and an increase in vagal tone to the heart occur; these are mediated via the baroreceptor reflex (see Figure 10-9). Although this should result in a slower heart rate, the reflex bradycardia is masked by the cardiac stimulatory actions of norepinephrine and epinephrine mediated by direct activation of β_1-receptors. Because of these opposing actions it is difficult to predict the effects of these two catecholamines on heart rate (see Table 10-3). After the administration of phenoxybenzamine, the α-receptors are blocked, thereby reducing sympathetic tone on blood vessels and slightly lowering blood pressure. This is accompanied by a reflex increase in heart rate. With α-receptors now blocked, the administration of norepinephrine has little effect on blood pressure, whereas the heart rate is increased due to the direct action of the drug on cardiac β_1-receptors. Because the blood pressure does not markedly increase, no opposing reflex bradycardia occurs. When epinephrine is administered, the former pressor response is converted to a marked depressor response (epinephrine "reversal"). This results because, with α-receptors blocked, the activation of β_2-receptors by epinephrine is unmasked. Epinephrine now causes a marked tachycardia as a result of the direct activation of cardiac β_1-receptors and the reflex tachycardia in response to the drop in blood pressure. Thus, when α-adrenoceptors are blocked, epinephrine (an agonist at α_1-, β_1-, and β_2- receptors) resembles isoproterenol (an agonist at β_1- and β_2-receptors).

Phenoxybenzamine, tolazoline, and phentolamine block α_1- and α_2-adrenergic receptors. The tachycardia that occurs after administration of these drugs is due, in part, to the blockade of α_2-receptors located on terminals of sympathetic noradrenergic neurons (Figure 10-16). Activation of these receptors inhibits the release of norepinephrine; this feedback inhibition is disrupted when α_2-receptors are blocked so that the release of norepinephrine is increased. This has little consequence when the postsynaptic receptors are α_1, since the α-receptor antagonists mentioned above block these receptors. However, in the heart, where the postsynaptic adrenergic receptors are β_1, the effects of sympathetic nerve activation are enhanced when the α_2-receptors are blocked. Thus by blocking α_2-receptors, phenoxybenzamine, tolazoline, and phentolamine increase norepinephrine release and thereby enhance reflex tachycardia.

Prazosin is a relatively specific α_1-adrenergic receptor antagonist. It causes less tachycardia than the nonselective α-receptor antagonists because the α_2-adrenoceptors, which when activated reduce norepinephrine release, are not blocked by this drug (see Figure 10-16).

The major side effects of α-adrenergic receptor antagonists are related to a reduced sympathetic tone at α-receptors. These effects include postural hypotension, tachycardia (not marked with prazosin), inhibition of ejaculation, and nasal stuffiness. Some ad-

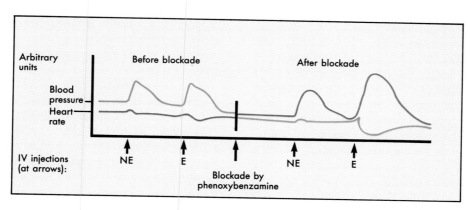

FIGURE 10-15   Schematic representation of effects of the IV injections of norepinephrine *(NE)* and epinephrine *(E)* on mean blood pressure and heart rate before and after blockade of α-adrenergic receptors by phenoxybenzamine (see Figure 10-10).

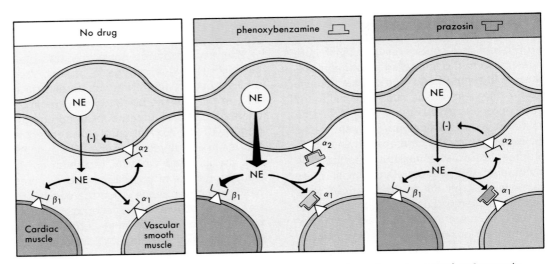

FIGURE 10-16   Comparison of actions of phenoxybenzamine (α_1 and α_2 antagonists) and prazosin (α_1 antagonist) at noradrenergic neuroeffector junctions in cardiac muscle (β_1-adrenergic receptors) and vascular smooth muscle (α_1-adrenergic receptors). (⊏⊐, antagonist).

verse effects of these drugs are not related to their α-blocking properties; for example, phenoxybenzamine acts centrally to cause nausea, vomiting, sedation, and weakness whereas phentolamine and tolazoline stimulate the GI tract, causing abdominal pain and diarrhea.

Drugs that Block β-Adrenergic Receptors

The prototype of nonselective β-adrenergic blocking drugs is propranolol. Compounds introduced more recently differ from propranolol in duration of action and selectivity for β_1-adrenergic receptors. Propranolol is a potent reversible antagonist at both β_1- and β_2-adrenergic receptors. As with all adrenergic receptor blocking drugs, the pharmacological effects depend on the activity of the sympathoadrenal system. When impulse traffic in the sympathetic neurons and circulating concentrations of norepinephrine and epinephrine are high (e.g., during exercise), the effects of these drugs are more pronounced, with the most profound effects on the cardiovascular system. Propranolol blocks the positive chronotropic and inotropic effects resulting from administration of β-adrenergic agonists and from activation of the sympathetic nervous system. It reduces the rate and contractility of the heart at rest, but the effects are more dramatic during physical exercise. The drug may pre-

cipitate acute failure in an uncompensated heart. Propranolol, but not other β blockers, has a direct membrane stabilizing action (local anesthetic effect) independent of its β-receptor blocking properties that may contribute to its antiarrhythmic cardiac effect.

The acute administration of propranolol does not markedly affect blood flow because vascular smooth muscle is not tonically activated by circulating concentrations of epinephrine. As a result of compensatory reflexes, the drug causes slightly increased peripheral resistance. Propranolol administered chronically is an effective antihypertensive agent. How it lowers blood pressure is not completely clear but this effect results from several actions, including reduced cardiac output and reduced release of renin from the juxtaglomerular apparatus.

Propranolol blocks the metabolic actions of β-adrenergic drugs and the sympathoadrenal system. It inhibits the rise in plasma free fatty acid and glucose resulting from lipolysis in fat and glycogenolysis in liver, heart, and skeletal muscle, which can present a problem to patients with diabetes. Insulin-induced hypoglycemia is augmented by propranolol, because the drug disrupts the compensatory glycogenolysis and glucose release resulting from increased sympathoadrenal activity. The β_1-selective blockers are less likely to delay recovery from hypoglycemia and to cause hypertension when the hypoglycemia releases epinephrine. These drugs also block the premonitory tachycardia associated with insulin-induced hypoglycemia. Patients must learn to recognize sweating (induced by activation of cholinergic sympathetic neurons) as well as weakness, hunger, and tachycardia as symptoms of low blood glucose concentrations.

Propranolol has few serious side actions in healthy individuals but can produce adverse effects in patients suffering from various disease states; heart failure may develop. Propanolol is usually contraindicated in patients with sinus bradycardia, partial heart block, and compensated congestive heart failure. Sudden withdrawal of propranolol from long-term patients can cause "withdrawal symptoms" such as angina, tachycardia, and arrhythmias. Rebound hypertension may occur in patients taking propranolol to control blood pressure. These withdrawal symptoms probably result from the development of supersensitive β-receptors (disuse supersensitivity) and can be minimized by reducing dosage of the drug gradually.

Propranolol increases airway resistance, which has little clinical importance in normal individuals but can be dangerous in patients with obstructive pulmonary disease or asthma, who may experience life-threatening increases in airway resistance. The new cardioselective (β_1) receptor antagonists should be used in these patients, but even these drugs should be used with caution or not at all because they are not completely devoid of β_2-receptor blocking properties.

Nadolol is a nonselective β-receptor blocking drug that is less lipid soluble than propranolol and less likely to cause central effects. It has a significantly longer duration of action than most other β blockers. Timolol is another nonselective β-adrenergic blocker that is administered orally for treatment of hypertension and angina pectoris or as an ophthalmic preparation for treatment of glaucoma.

Carteolol, pindolol, and penbutalol are nonselective β-adrenergic receptor blocking drugs that have partial agonist properties. As a result of their modest intrinsic sympathomimetic properties, these drugs cause less slowing of the resting heart rate and fewer abnormalities of serum lipids than do other β blockers. Pindolol is relatively short-acting; the others have longer durations of action. All are used to treat hypertension.

Labetalol is a reversible antagonist of α_1-, β_1-, and β_2-adrenergic receptors. Consequently it has hemodynamic effects similar to a combination of propran-olol (β_1- and β_2-blockade) and prazosin (α_1-blockade). Unfortunately, it also has similar side effects to both drugs (e.g., postural hypotension, nasal congestion, bronchospasm). It is a potent hypotensive agent and is used in the treatment of hypertension.

Nonselective β-adrenergic receptor antagonists, by blocking β_2-receptors, can precipitate bronchospasm in patients with obstructive pulmonary disease. At low doses, acebutolol, atenolol, metoprolol and esmolol are more selective in blocking β_1-receptors on cardiac muscle than in blocking β_2-receptors on bronchiolar and vascular smooth muscle, and are less likely to increase bronchoconstriction in patients with asthma than are the nonselective β blockers. Presumably because they block cardiac stimulation and renin release induced by sympathoadrenal activation, these β_1 blockers are useful in treatment of hypertension and angina pectoris. Esmolol is a β_1 antagonist that is rapidly metabolized by esterases in red blood cells and has a very short half-life. It is used for emergency treatment of sinus tachycardia and atrial flutter or fibrillation.

Drugs that Interfere with Sympathetic Neuronal Function

Drugs that disrupt the synthesis, storage, or release of norepinephrine or that act in the brain to reduce sympathetic neuronal activity have been used primarily in the treatment of hypertension.

Guanethidine is the prototype of a class of drugs that impair the release of norepinephrine from post-synaptic sympathetic neurons. Guanethidine and related drugs (bretylium, guanadrel) are polar compounds that do not penetrate the blood-brain barrier but are selectively taken up by the norepinephrine transporter in terminals of sympathetic neurons and stored within synaptic vesicles. Guanethidine depletes norepinephrine stores within these neurons, and the drug can be subsequently released as a "false transmitter." The pharmacological properties of guanethidine, however, relate to its ability to prevent the release of norepinephrine in response to nerve action potentials and indirect-acting sympathomimetics (e.g., tyramine, amphetamine).

The pharmacological consequences of the action of guanethidine are less specific than the receptor antagonists, previously discussed, because the drug depresses the response of α- and β_1-adrenergic receptors about equally. Chronic oral administration of guanethidine reduces sympathetic tone to all organs.

In the cardiovascular system guanethidine reduces blood pressure, heart rate, and cardiac output. In the GI system it increases motility and causes diarrhea. Because of its side effects, guanethidine is reserved for the treatment of moderate to severe hypertension. Because the drug is highly ionized, it is poorly and irregularly absorbed from the GI tract. Because it does not penetrate the blood-brain barrier, it has no central effects. After it accumulates in sympathetic noradrenergic neurons, its effects persist, generally causing cumulative responses that last for several days after termination of the drug. The troublesome side effects of the drug are due to disruption of sympathetic tone to various organs; these include postural hypotension, nasal stuffiness, impaired ejaculation, and diarrhea (the parasympathetic neuronal influence on GI smooth muscle is unopposed by the sympathetic nervous system).

Guanadrel mimics the action of guanethidine, differing only in its pharmacokinetic profile. When compared with guanethidine, guanadrel has a more rapid onset and a shorter duration of action. Bretylium also acts similarly to guanethidine in that it accumulates in noradrenergic sympathetic neurons and prevents the neurogenic release of norepinephrine; it is administered only by IV injection for emergency treatment of ventricular arrhythmias. Although guanethidine and related compounds block neurogenically released norepinephrine and the actions of indirectly acting sympathomimetics, they do not reduce the pharmacological effects of circulating catecholamines released from the adrenal medulla or the actions of administered "directly acting" sympathomimetics. Indeed, the responses of the latter compounds may be enhanced because of the up-regulation of α- and β_1- adrenergic receptors.

Reserpine depletes neurons of norepinephrine and thereby reduces sympathetic nervous system tone. The drug is the major active ingredient in *rauwolfia serpentina,* a plant indigenous to India, used in Hindu medicine to treat various diseases, including hypertension. Reserpine has two major sites of action. In the brain, reserpine depletes stores of several amine neurotransmitters, including 5-hydroxytryptamine, histamine, dopamine, norepinephrine, and epinephrine. It also causes a unique type of sedation (tranquilization) that appears to result from the depletion of dopamine. The central actions of reserpine are discussed in Chapter 13. Peripherally, reserpine reduces sympathetic tone by depleting norepinephrine

stores in the postsynaptic sympathetic neurons. It disrupts the ability of synaptic vesicles to bind norepinephrine so that the amine leaks from these vesicles and is oxidatively deaminated by monoamine oxidase (MAO) within the sympathetic neuron. After a single dose of reserpine, loss of sympathetic tone occurs progressively over several hours and becomes maximal by 24 hours. Depending on the dose administered, recovery of tissue concentrations of norepinephrine and sympathetic nerve function may take several days. Repeated doses have cumulative effects.

Loss of sympathetic tone after reserpine administration results in reduced peripheral resistance, cardiac output, and blood pressure. Only low doses of reserpine are used to treat hypertension, usually with other agents (e.g., thiazide diuretics) and it takes several weeks for the antihypertensive effects to become maximal. Because of its long duration of action, reserpine maintains good control of blood pressure in patients with mild hypertension who have poor drug compliance.

Untoward effects of reserpine result from its actions in the brain and GI tract. Disruption of the sympathetic tone to the gut results in a preponderance of parasympathetic tone, which is manifested as increased GI motility, cramps, and diarrhea. The drug also increases gastric acid secretion and is therefore contraindicated in patients with peptic or intestinal ulcers. Decreased sympathetic tone also results in nasal congestion. The central sedative actions of reserpine may be desirable in some hypertensive patients, but the drug can produce severe nightmares, depression, and psychotic-like episodes and should not be administered to patients with a preexisting depression or psychotic illness.

Drugs that Reduce Central Sympathetic Outflow

The activity of peripheral sympathetic neurons is regulated in a complex manner by neuronal systems located in the hypothalamus and medulla. These central neurons, in turn, are regulated, in part, by α_2-adrenergic receptors. Drugs such as clonidine that activate these receptors reduce the outflow of impulse traffic in peripheral sympathetic neurons without interfering with baroreceptor reflex control. Accordingly, these drugs lower blood pressure in patients with moderate to severe hypertension and produce

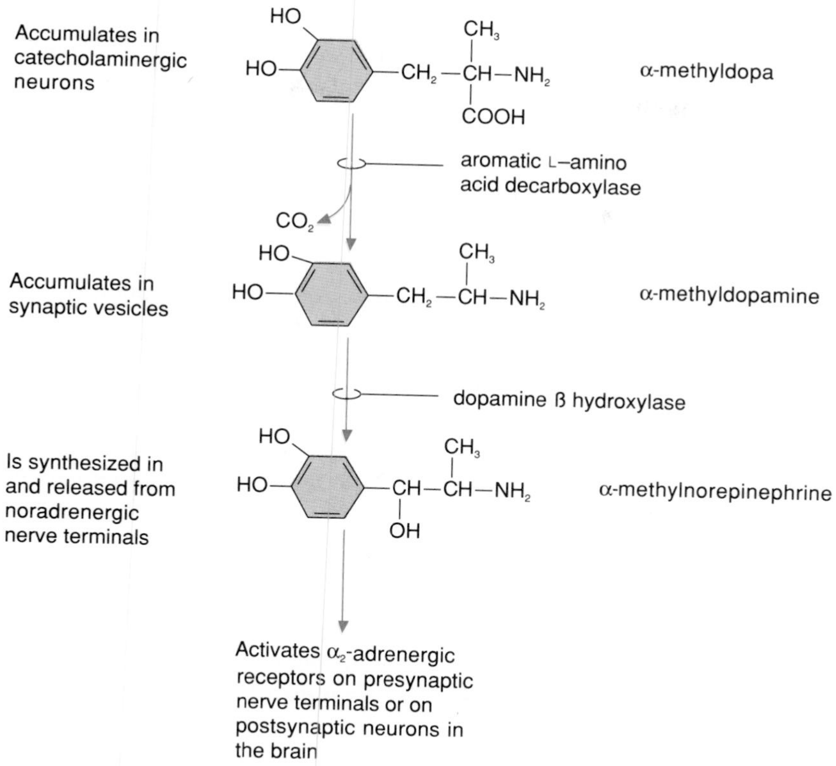

Accumulates in
catecholaminergic
neurons

α-methyldopa

aromatic L–amino
acid decarboxylase

CO_2

Accumulates in
synaptic vesicles

α-methyldopamine

dopamine β hydroxylase

Is synthesized in
and released from
noradrenergic
nerve terminals

α-methylnorepinephrine

Activates α_2-adrenergic
receptors on presynaptic
nerve terminals or on
postsynaptic neurons in
the brain

FIGURE 10-17   Metabolism of methyldopa in central noradrenergic nerve terminals.

less postural hypotension than drugs that act directly on peripheral sympathetic neurons.

Methyldopa is an analog of the catecholamine precursor L-DOPA that has hypotensive action resulting from its conversion to the false transmitter, α-methylnorepinephrine. Methyldopa is transported into noradrenergic neurons where it is decarboxylated by aromatic L-amino acid decarboxylase to α-methyldopamine; which in turn is transported into the synaptic vesicles and converted to α-methylnorepinephrine by dopamine β-hydroxylase (Figure 10-17). The α-methylnorepinephrine partially displaces norepinephrine in synaptic vesicles so that when these neurons are activated α-methylnorepinephrine is released instead of the normal transmitter. Because α-methylnorepinephrine is not a substrate for MAO it accumulates in noradrenergic neurons and produces its pharmacological effects long after methyldopa has disappeared from the tissues. It was initially believed that methyldopa reduced blood pressure by acting as a false transmitter in peripheral sympathetic neurons.

Based on the following observations it now appears that the hypotensive property of methyldopa is due to the action of the metabolite α-methylnorepinephrine in the brain, not in the periphery:

1. α-Methylnorepinephrine has actions similar to norepinephrine on peripheral α_1-adrenergic receptors so that as a false transmitter it does not markedly alter the signal received by the α_1-adrenergic receptors on vascular smooth muscle

2. Systemic administration of α-methyldopamine, which does not penetrate the blood-brain barrier, fills peripheral sympathetic neurons with α-methylnorepinephrine but fails to have a hypotensive action

3. Pretreatment with carbidopa, a peripheral decarboxylase inhibitor (see p. 142), blocks the conversion of methyldopa to α-methylnorepinephrine in sympathetic neurons, but not in the brain, and carbidopa does not prevent the hypotensive action of methyldopa

4. Pretreatment with a drug that blocks peripheral and central decarboxylase activity (benserazide) prevents the conversion of methyldopa to α-methylnorepinephrine in brain and peripheral sympathetic neurons and blocks the hypotensive actions of methyldopa

5. Hypotensive action of methyldopa is prevented by pretreatment with yohimbine, a centrally active antagonist of α_2-adrenergic receptors

It is believed therefore that α-methylnorepinephrine formed with methyldopa in central noradrenergic neurons is released as a false transmitter to act on pre- or postsynaptic α_2-receptors. Activation of the α_2-adrenergic receptors reduces sympathetic neuronal impulse. Methyldopa therefore reduces total peripheral resistance and blood pressure but has little effect on heart rate, cardiac output, or baroreceptor reflexes. The drug is less likely to cause postural hypotension than other drugs that disrupt sympathetic neuronal function. Major side effects of methyldopa are related to its central actions, primarily sedation, sleep disturbances, and depression; tolerance to these effects usually develops. More serious but relatively rare toxic actions of methyldopa include blood dyscrasias (hemolytic anemia, leukopenia, thrombocytopenia) and hepatitis.

Clonidine, like α-methylnorepinephrine, is a potent agonist at α_1- and α_2-adrenergic receptors. Unlike α-methylnorepinephrine, which must be delivered to the brain as a precursor, clonidine is lipid soluble and penetrates the blood-brain barrier to activate α_2-adrenergic receptors in the hypothalamus and medulla, resulting in diminished sympathetic outflow. Clonidine lowers blood pressure by reducing total peripheral resistance, heart rate, and cardiac output. Like methyldopa, clonidine does not interfere with baroreceptor reflexes and therefore does not produce marked postural hypotension. Hypotensive actions of clonidine are also blocked by yohimbine. Side effects of clonidine may include dry mouth, sedation, dizziness, nightmares, anxiety, and mental depression. Various symptoms related to sympathetic nervous system overactivity (hypertension, tachycardia, sweating) may occur with withdrawal of long-term clonidine therapy. As a precaution, the dosage of clonidine should be reduced gradually.

Guanabenz and guanfacine are recently developed α_2-adrenergic receptor agonists. Like clonidine, they cause a central inhibition of sypathetic tone with a relative sparing of cardiovascular reflexes. Guanfacine is longer acting and is reported to cause less reduction in cardiac output and less sedation than clonidine.

Drugs that Inhibit Catecholamine Synthesis

Only drugs that inhibit the rate-limiting step in the synthesis of catecholamines, catalyzed by tyrosine hydroxylase, can effectively slow the rate of endogenous synthesis of norepinephrine in peripheral sympathetic neurons. Metyrosine (α-methyltyrosine) inhibits tyrosine hydroxylase in catecholaminergic neurons in the brain and the periphery, and in the adrenal medulla, thereby reducing tissue stores of dopamine, norepinephrine, and epinephrine. Metyrosine is used in the management of patients with pheochromocytoma not amenable to surgery. The prevalent side effect of metyrosine is sedation. The drug is primarily excreted unchanged in the urine and, because of its limited solubility, adequate water intake is recommended.

Carbidopa, a hydrazine derivative of methyldopa, acts like methyldopa to inhibit aromatic L-amino acid decarboxylase. Unlike methyldopa, carbidopa does not penetrate the blood-brain barrier and therefore has no effect on the CNS. Because aromatic L-amino acid decarboxylase is ubiquitous, is present in excess, and does not control the rate-limiting step in catecholamine synthesis, carbidopa has no appreciable effect on endogenous synthesis of norepinephrine in sympathetic neurons. It does, however, reduce the conversion of exogenously administered L-DOPA to dopamine outside of the brain. Relatively large doses of L-DOPA are employed to replace dopamine in the caudate/putamen of patients with Parkinson's disease and thereby reduce some of the motor symptoms (bradykinesis) in these patients. By administering L-DOPA in combination with carbidopa, the dose of L-DOPA and the peripheral side effects (nausea, vomiting, tachycardia, arrhythmias) resulting from the actions of its decarboxylated product, dopamine, are reduced.

Clinical applications of the sympathomimetic and sympatholytic agents are listed in the box.

SIDE EFFECTS, CLINICAL PROBLEMS, AND TOXICITY

Major clinical problems are summarized in the box.

TRADENAMES

In addition to generic and fixed combination preparations, the following tradenamed materials are available in the United States.

SYMPATHOMIMETICS

Nonselective Directly Acting Agonists
Adrenalin, epinephrine chloride
Intropin and Dopastat, dopamine hydrochloride
Isuprel, isoproterenol hydrochloride
Levophed, norepinephrine
Medihaler, Vaponefrin; epinephrine

α Agonists
Vasoxyl, methoxamine HC1

β₁ Agonists
Dobutrex, dobutamine HCl

β₂ Agonists
Brethine, Bricanyl; terbutaline sulfate
Bronkosol, isoetharine HCl
Metaprel, Alupent; metaproterenol sulfate
Proventil, Ventolin; albuterol sulfate
Tornalate, bitolterol mesylate
Yutopar, ritodrine HCl

Nonselective Indirectly Acting
Biphetamine, amphetamine exchange resin
Dexedrine, *d*-amphetamine sulfate
Propagest, phenylpropanolamine

α Agonists Not Discussed in Text
Aramine, metaraminol bitartrate
Wyamine, mephenteramine

SYMPATHOLYTICS

α Blockers, Nonselective
Dibenzyline, phenoxybenzamine HCl
Regitine, phentolamine mesylate
Priscoline, tolazoline HCl

α₁ Blockers
Minipress, prazosin HCl

β Blockers, Nonselective
Blocadren, timolol maleate
Corgard, nadolol
Inderal, propranolol HCl
Visken, pindolol

β₁ Blockers
Brevibloc, esmolol HCl
Lopressor, metoprolol tartrate
Sectral, acebutolol HCl
Tenormin, atenolol

Combined α-β Blockers
Trandate, Normodyne; labetalol HC1

Reduce Central Sympathetic Outflow
Aldomet, methyldopa
Catapres, clonidine HCl
Tenex, guanfacine HCl
Wytensin, guanabenz acetate

Blockers of Norepinephrine Release
Bretylol, bretylium sulfate
Hylorel, guanadrel sulfate
Ismelin, guanethidine sulfate

CLINICAL PROBLEMS

DRUGS THAT INTERFERE WITH SYMPATHETIC NERVOUS SYSTEM NEURONAL FUNCTION

Block norepinephrine release and storage
Postural hypotension
Nasal stuffiness
Impairment of ejaculation
GI activity increased
Extrapyramidal effects (reserpine)
Interfere with central sympathetic outflow
Sedation
Endocrine problems
Mild postural hypotension
Sodium and water retention
Rebound hypertension on drug withdrawal

DRUGS THAT BLOCK ADRENERGIC RECEPTORS

α-Adrenergic blockers
Postural hypotension
Tachycardia
Nasal stuffiness
Impairment of ejaculation
Sodium and water retention
β-Receptor blockers
Heart failure in patients with cardiac disease
Increase in airway resistance
Fatigue and depression
Rebound hypertension
Augmentation of hypoglycemia

REFERENCES

Choice of a beta-blocker, Med Lett Drugs Ther 28:20, 1986.

A symposium: beta blockage, cardioselectivity and intrinsicsympathomimetic activity, Am J Cardiol 59:1F, 1987.

Drugs for hypertension, Med Lett Drugs Ther 29:1, 1987.

Foods interacting with MAO inhibitors, Med Lett Drugs Ther 31:11, 1989.

Frederickson MC: Tocolytic therapy with β-adrenergic agonists, Ration Drug Ther 17:1, 1983.

Frishman WH, Furberg CD and Friedewald WT: β-Adrenergic blockade for survivors of acute myocardial infarction, N Engl J Med 310:830 ,1984.

Kopin IJ, Fischer JE, Musacchio JM, et al.: "False neurochemical transmitters" and the mechanism of sympathetic blockade by monoamine oxidase inhibitors, J Pharmacol Exp Ther 147:186, 1965.

Labetalol for hypertension, The Medical Letter 26:83, 1984.

Lasagna L: Phenylpropanolamine: a review, New York, 1988, John Wiley & Sons.

CHAPTER

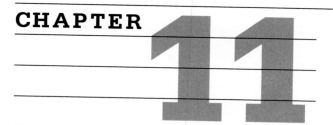

Neuromuscular Blocking Agents

ABBREVIATIONS

ACh   acetylcholine
AChE   acetylcholinesterase

MAJOR DRUGS

nondepolarizing drugs
depolarizing agents

THERAPEUTIC OVERVIEW

Many surgical procedures are performed more safely and rapidly with the aid of drugs that bring about skeletal muscle relaxation. Certain anesthetic agents can produce such relaxation only at high concentrations and therefore are too dangerous to use. Specific skeletal muscle relaxant drugs are available that reduce the amount of anesthetic agent required during surgery and improve the margin of safety and speed of recovery of the patient from anesthesia.

The muscle relaxant drugs widely used act by interrupting transmission at the junction between skeletal muscle fibers and somatic nerves that innervate these fibers. Signal transmission at these junctions occurs by endogenous acetylcholine (ACh) binding to nicotinic subtype receptors on the muscle cell. Although the mechanism of these drugs does not involve the autonomic nervous system, some of the side effects do include cholinergic autonomic blockade or stimulation, so there is a functional, as well as neu-

rotransmitter, commonality between these drugs and autonomic nervous system drugs.

The neuromuscular blocking agents find widespread use for (1) endotracheal intubation, (2) maintaining controlled ventilation during surgical procedures, and (3) reduction of muscle contraction in the region undergoing surgery. The neuromuscular blocking agents have the advantage of functioning without producing either analgesia or anesthesia, and for most agents, rapid and effective reversal of the blocking action is accomplished by drugs. However, the side effects of the blocking agents can be significant, especially at higher concentrations, so their clinical use is not without problems. Newer blocking agents, expected to be approved soon for clinical use, are reputed to have fewer side effects.

Additional nonsurgical applications of neuromuscular blocking agents include reduction of laryngeal or general muscle spasms, reduction of spasticity from tetanus in neurological diseases and multiple sclerosis, and prevention of bone fractures during electroconvulsive therapy. These drugs also are used as diagnostic agents for myasthenia gravis and for detecting neurological differences that sometimes develop between spinal and central control of muscle tone.

There are two main classes of neuromuscular blocking agents: nondepolarizing drugs such as d-tubocurarine, atracurium, and vecuronium, and depolarizing agents such as succinylcholine. Therapeutic uses of the neuromuscular blocking agents are summarized in the box on p. 146.

An additional group of muscle relaxant drugs that act by different mechanisms and are used primarily for central nervous system (CNS) disorders is discussed in Chapter 27.

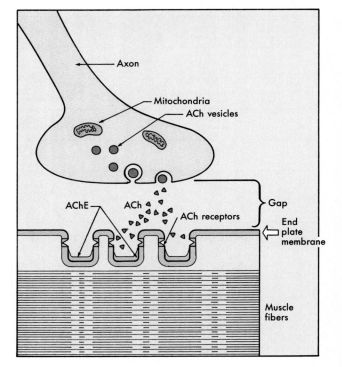

THERAPEUTIC USE OF NEUROMUSCULAR BLOCKING AGENTS

MUSCLE RELAXATION DURING SURGERY

Inhalational anesthetic agent
    Undesirable side effects (prominent hypotension, cardiac arrhythmias, myocardial depression, nausea at high concentrations)
Neuromuscular blocking agents
    Allow reduction of anesthetic agent concentration
    Have short (minutes) to long (hour) actions
    Allow endotracheal intubation (surgery)
    Needed for maintaining controlled ventilation (surgery)
    Reduce muscle fasciculations at surgical site
    Side effects must be considered in agent selection
    Action in some cases can be reversed by antagonists

NONSURGICAL USES

Reduce muscle spasms
Myasthenia gravis diagnosis
Adjunct relaxation during maximal electroshock therapy

FIGURE 11-1   Acetylcholine *(ACh)* release, diffusion across the synaptic cleft, binding to receptors on end plate membrane, and hydrolysis by acetylcholine esterase *(AChE)* in the absence of blocking drugs.

MECHANISMS OF ACTION

Skeletal muscles are innervated by somatic nerves that originate in the CNS and terminate at the muscle cell with cholinergic-type neurochemical transmission (Chapters 8 and 9). ACh is the neurotransmitter, and the receptor on the muscle cell end plate is the nicotinic subtype (different from that at ganglionic sites). At the concentrations of neuromuscular blocking agents used clinically, signal transmission is interrupted at the nicotinic neuroeffector junction. Because cholinergic transmission also occurs at sympathetic and parasympathetic ganglia (Chapters 8 and 9) the ganglionic sites are sources of side effects when the neuromuscular blocking agent concentrations reach higher values than those needed for neuromuscular blockade. This is discussed in a later section.

In the absence of drug, propagation of an action potential along the somatic nerve fiber results in opening of calcium channels at the nerve terminal. The resulting flux of calcium ions into the nerve cell triggers the release of ACh into the neuromuscular gap. Diffusion of ACh across the gap and binding to the nicotinic receptors on the muscle cell end plate causes the receptor-associated ion channels to open and the end plate membrane ion permeability to increase. This allows a transient flux of Na^+ and K^+ ions, thereby reducing the potential difference across the membrane until a critical value needed to activate muscle contraction is reached. AChE in the vicinity of the muscle end plate membrane acts quickly to catalyze the hydrolysis and inactivation of unbound ACh. This is described further in Chapters 8 and 9 and is summarized schematically in Figure 11-1. The ACh receptor is described in greater detail in Chapter 2.

Blockade of this process, (1) to exclude ACh from the receptor site (nondepolarizing) or (2) maintain end plate membrane depolarization and thus prevent transmission of another action potential, is the basis

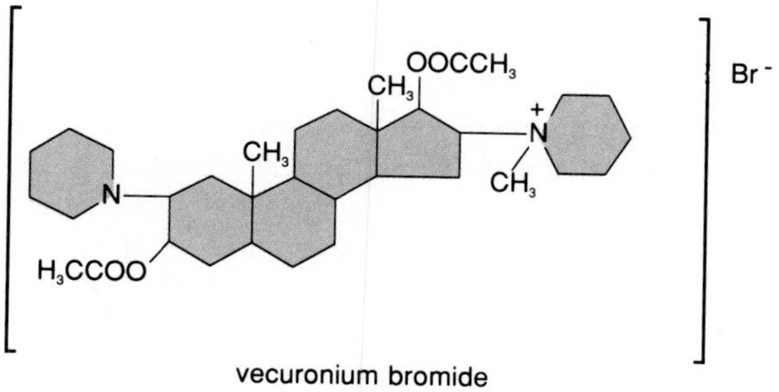

vecuronium bromide

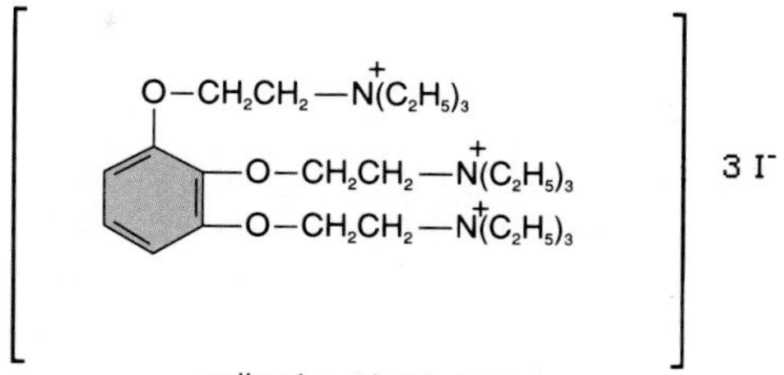

gallamine triethiodide

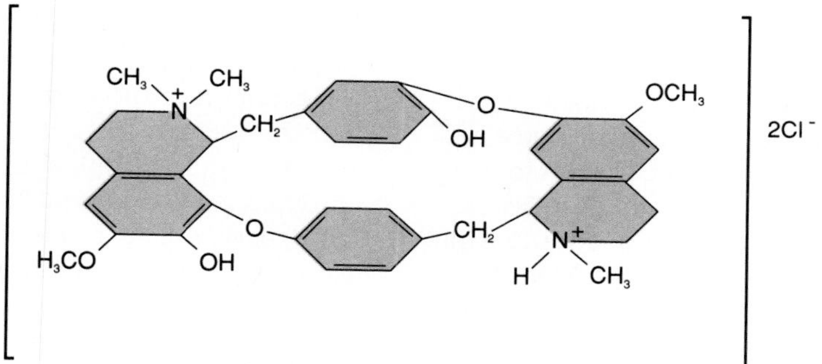

d-(+) tubocurarine chloride

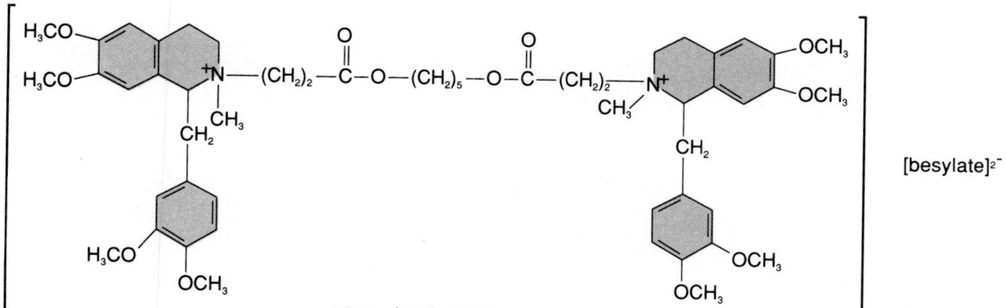

atracurium besylate

FIGURE 11-2   Competitive nondepolarizing blocking agents.

by which neuromuscular blocking drugs function. The nondepolarizing and depolarizing agents act by binding to the nicotinic receptor on the muscle cell; however, the detailed mechanisms that cause blockade are different.

The nondepolarizing or competitive blocking agents compete with ACh for unoccupied end plate receptor sites. The binding of these nondepolarizing agents is reversible and they occupy the receptor sites without activating the associated cation channel. The structures of the nondepolarizing blocking drugs are shown in Figure 11-2. Doxacurium, mivacurium, and pipecuronium are new agents expected to be approved soon for clinical use in the United States. Pancuronium, pipecuronium, and vecuronium have similar structures, as do atracurium, doxacurium, and mivacurium. Gallamine is used only occasionally because of the availability of agents with fewer side effects.

Interference with muscle contraction does not occur until 75% to 80% of the receptors on a muscle cell are occupied by the blocking agent, and complete interruption of contraction requires 90% to 95% occupancy of the receptors. The actual quantities and concentrations of drug required to induce block vary with the agent, the muscle location, and the individual patient. The ion channel actions of the blocking agents are summarized in Figure 11-3.

There also may be a prejunctional effect by which the blocking agent exerts a direct action on the nerve terminal to reduce the amount of ACh released in response to nerve stimulation. This mechanism could contribute to reduced muscle contraction through lack of ACh to bind to the receptors, but the mechanism is not well understood. Nor is it likely to be important for therapeutic actions.

The blockade caused by the competitive (nondepolarizing) agents can be reversed by increasing the concentration of ACh at the end plate membrane. The usual method is to inhibit the enzymes that catalyze the hydrolysis of ACh because this endogenous transmitter is still being released and is present in the gap between the nerve terminal and the muscle end plate. Neostigmine, pyridostigmine, and edrophonium are used clinically to reverse the blockade. The chemical structures are shown in Figure 9-10; the pharmacology of these drugs is discussed in Chapter 9. As with any competitive antagonist, an increase in the concentration of the agonist (in this case ACh) leads to displacement of the antagonist (the blocking agent) from the receptor. It is also possible, but not demonstrated, that edrophonium and the other enzyme inhibitors may additionally stimulate the prejunctional release of ACh, but this appears to be a secondary effect that is important only with excess edrophonium. When the concentration of the competitive blocking agent in the vicinity of the receptors is greater than the concentration needed for 95% blockade, edrophonium and the other enzyme inhibitors cannot reverse the blockade because the local con-

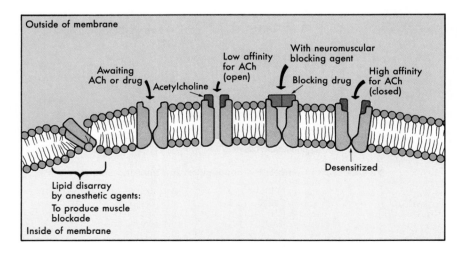

FIGURE 11-3   Summary of ion channel states relevant to neuromuscular blocking agents. *ACh, Acetylcholine.* See Figure 2-11 and Chapter 2 discussion on low and high affinity conformations and desensitized states.

centration of ACh is not adequate to overcome the high concentration of the blocking drug.

The mechanism by which depolarizing agents act is different. Among these agents, succinylcholine is the prototype agent in clinical use; decamethonium is still available, but side effects make it much less desirable. Succinylcholine is composed of two molecules of ACh coupled together (Figure 11-4). The binding of succinylcholine to ACh receptors causes opening of ion channels, Na$^+$ influx, and depolarization of the muscle cell end plate membrane in the same manner as ACh. However, with succinylcholine, the duration of the depolarization is longer than with ACh, since the rate of enzyme-catalyzed hydrolysis (inactivation) is slower for succinylcholine (0.1 to 2 min) than for ACh (turnover time about 100 μsec). The end plate membrane remains depolarized, with the channel presumably remaining open. This occurs at low concentrations of succinylcholine and is termed *phase I block*. Electrical stimulation and muscle twitch recordings fail to show any drop off in amplitude (termed *fading*) as the frequency of stimulation is increased. Controlled reversal of a phase I block with drugs such as edrophonium is not necessary, because the disappearance of the drug is still quite rapid. Edrophonium and the other reversal agents inhibit acetylcholinesterase (AChE) and pseudocholinesterase, but to different degrees, and succinylcholine is metabolized almost entirely by pseudocholinesterase. With repeated dosing of succinylcholine and the concentration increased, a more complicated form of blockade, called a *phase II block*, occurs. This type of block behaves similarly to that of nondepolarizing agents but shows fading at higher stimulation frequencies. The details on the state of the ion channels during phase II block (also called *desensitization block*) are controversial; further understanding must await additional research.

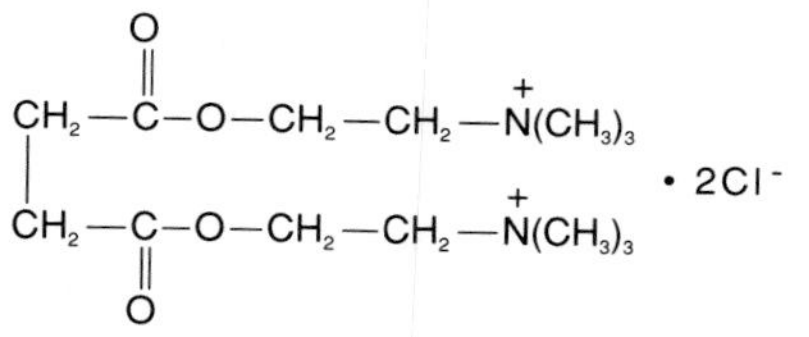

PHARMACOKINETICS

The clinically used and anticipated new neuromuscular blocking drugs differ in pharmacokinetic properties. This is important when choosing an agent for a particular patient. The pharmacokinetic values for the individual drugs are summarized in Table 11-1.

$$CH_2 - \overset{\displaystyle O}{\overset{\|}{C}} - O - CH_2 - CH_2 - \overset{+}{N}(CH_3)_3$$
$$CH_2 - \underset{\displaystyle O}{\underset{\|}{C}} - O - CH_2 - CH_2 - \overset{+}{N}(CH_3)_3$$

$\cdot \ 2Cl^-$

succinylcholine chloride

FIGURE 11-4   Succinylcholine.

Table 11-1	Pharmacokinetic Parameters		
Agent	**t$_{1/2}$ (min)**	**Elimination Route**	**Protein Binding (%)**
succinylcholine	3 (est)	M (100%)	—
mivacurium	9	M (100%)	—
atracurium	20	M (100%)	—
vecuronium	54	R (30%)	82
pancuronium	120	M (40%) R (60%)	27 15
gallamine	134	R (95%)	16
tubocurarine	234	R (60%) B	48*
pipecuronium	~200	N/A	N/A
doxacurium	~200	N/A	N/A
metocurine	280	R (55%) B	55*

M, Metabolism; *R*, renal; *B*, biliary.

* Additional drug binds to cartilage and to connecting tissue; figures are for plasma binding (to albumin, acid glycoproteins, and globulins).

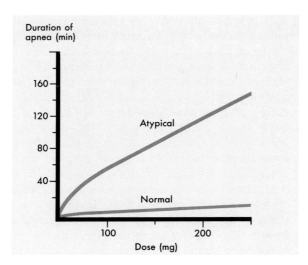

FIGURE 11-5   Length of time patients display apnea after IV dose of succinylcholine. Normal and atypical refer to the plasma pseudocholinesterase of each patient group.

These drugs contain two or three quaternary ammonium nitrogens and therefore are positively charged at all pH values. As a result, they traverse membranes poorly and are limited in distribution to the extracellular space. However, the steroidal structures of pancuronium, vecuronium, and pipecuronium enable small amounts of these agents to cross membranes. For example, small amounts of pancuronium cross the placenta, but not in sufficient amounts to cause problems in the fetus when used during a caesarean section.

Pancuronium, metocurine, tubocurarine, and gallamine use is influenced by impaired renal function, because appreciable fractions of these drugs are cleared by renal filtration. Atracurium is degraded almost entirely by metabolism, two thirds by enzymatic and one third by spontaneous nonenzymatic elimination. Vecuronium and pancuronium undergo significant metabolism and the 3-hydroxy metabolite of each has 25% or less neuromuscular blocking activity compared to the parent drugs. Succinylcholine and mivacurium are also metabolized via hydrolysis catalyzed by plasma pseudocholinesterase, with minimal hydrolysis by AChE.

The activity of pseudocholinesterase may be abnormal in some patients. This enzyme is synthesized in the liver, so that neuromuscular blockade by succinylcholine may be prolonged in patients with liver dysfunction, decreased hepatic blood flow, or genetic abnormalities. There are two explanations for the genetically abnormal pseudocholinesterase activity: lower concentrations of normal enzyme (heterozygous) or an abnormal enzyme (homozygous, 1:2500 frequency; or heterozygous). A clinical dose of 1 to 2 mg/kg succinylcholine in normal patients gives a blockade of <15 minutes. In an atypical patient the duration may be >2 hours. This is shown over a dosage range in Figure 11-5 with blockade defined as the duration of apnea. Trauma, alcoholism, pregnancy, use of oral contraceptives, and other conditions that can elevate or depress cholinesterase synthesis also can cause prolonged or shortened blockade.

The pharmacokinetics for the reversal drugs, edrophonium, neostigmine, and pyridostigmine are discussed in Chapter 9. Edrophonium is the most rapid-acting of the three.

 RELATION OF MECHANISMS OF ACTION TO RESPONSE

The choice of neuromuscular blocking agent is based primarily on the duration of the required blockade and tolerable side effects, although this may become less of a factor with the newer blocking agents expected to receive approval for clinical use. The duration of blockade required is influenced by the anatomical location of the surgery, the condition of the patient, and the patient's toleration of side effects. The relative potency of the agent is not a principal consideration, despite a 100-fold variation in dose needed to attain 95% blockade for the clinically used agents.

In terms of duration of action, the following rank order for IV administration of a typical clinically used dose is as follows:

Ultrashort acting (5 to 10 min):
    succinylcholine
Short acting (10 to 15 min):
    mivacurium
Medium acting (15 to 30 min):
    atracurium and vecuronium
Long acting (30 to 120 min):
    d-tubocurarine, metocurine, pancuronium,
    pipecuronium, doxacurium, gallamine

Atracurium and vecuronium have the advantage of minimal side effects; mivacurium, pipecuronium,

Table 11-2   Cardiac and Histamine Release Side Effects

| Agent | Cardiac Changes | | Histamine Release |
	Blood Pressure	Heart Rate	
succinylcholine	Increased	Increased	High
mivacurium	Slight	Slight	Slight
atracurium	Slight	Slight	Slight
vecuronium	None	None	None
pancuronium	Increased	Increased	Slight
gallamine	Increased	Increased	High dose only
tubocurarine	Decreased	Decreased	High
pipecuronium	None (?)	None (?)	Slight (?)
doxacurium	None (?)	None (?)	Slight (?)
metocurine	Decreased	Decreased (?)	Moderate

and doxacurium are emerging from clinical trials and should be approved for clinical use soon. The side effects of these experimental drugs must await more extensive use. Gallamine produces a serious tachycardia. Succinylcholine has the most rapid onset of action and shortest duration of effect. It is still used for intubation despite side effects at higher concentrations. One of the goals of neuromuscular blocking agent research is the development of a nondepolarizing, ultrashort-acting reversible agent with minimal side effects. Mivacurium may meet this goal.

The major side effects with the neuromuscular blocking drugs are cardiovascular actions and histamine release. The extent to which each agent exhibits these side effects is listed in Table 11-2. Vecuronium is essentially free of cardiac and histamine effects, and the newer mivacurium, pipecuronium, and doxacurium appear to have only minor cardiac effects. Mivacurium has some histamine-like effects. These are discussed in a later section.

Several additional factors such as patient age, the presence of anesthetic agents, and the electrolyte content of body fluids can influence the degree of blockade achievable with a given dose. The actions of tubocurarine and atracurium, for example, are potentiated in neonates as compared to children and adults, but succinylcholine is less potent in neonates and requires a dose two to three times greater on a weight basis than that used for children. Pharmacokinetic considerations can explain some of the differences in effectiveness of these drugs between children and elderly adults. The nondepolarizing blocking agents often are potentiated by inhalational anesthetic agents such as halothane, isoflurane, enflurane, or nitrous oxide and also by low concentrations of extracellular potassium or calcium, as may occur after the use of diuretic agents or in renal dysfunction or disease. Elevated potassium or calcium and reduced magnesium concentrations, on the other hand, may counter the action of the blocking agents through changes in sensitivity at the muscle end plate.

In most surgical procedures in which neuromuscular blocking agents are used, the drugs enter the systemic circulation and are distributed to all accessible tissues. Therefore, respiratory support capabilities must be available when these drugs are used. In addition, the fraction of receptors that must be free of blocking agent before recovery occurs varies with different muscles. Typically, muscles recover from blockade in the following order:

1. Respiratory and diaphragm
2. Eyeblink
3. Abdomen, arms, and legs
4. Neck, head, face, hands, and feet
5. Extraocular

It is not practical to attempt selective blockade of one anatomical area for prolonged periods of time.

In cases of burns, denervated muscles, spinal cord injury. or other trauma, the sensitivity to neuromuscular blocking drugs may vary. In some burn patients, for example, the doses of atracurium or metocurine may need to be two to three times normal to achieve blockade. The reason for this may be the presence of extra receptors that are normally not available until trauma brings about their activation, although this is somewhat speculative.

The primary precaution in the use of edrophonium and other enzyme inhibitors for reversal of blockade is to monitor carefully the dose of the reversal drug. Too much leads to excessive ACh and prolongation of channel opening, similar to the action of a depolarizing-type blocker. To avoid this problem, the degree of neuromuscular blockade should be assessed through electrical stimulation and determination of muscle activity and the patient titrated with the monitor output to determine the appropriate end point.

SIDE EFFECTS, CLINICAL PROBLEMS, AND TOXICITY

The strategy in the development of the newer neuromuscular blocking agents is to expand the margin of safety between the concentrations of blocker needed to produce 95% blockade and those that block transmission at ganglia or at cardiac muscarinic receptors. Parasympathetic and sympathetic ganglia and cardiac parasympathetic neuroeffector junctions are innervated by cholinergic neurons. These junctions are all subject to antagonism by the neuromuscular blocking agents if the concentration of the agent is sufficient. Tubocurarine gives a significant degree of ganglionic blockade, with less by metocurine, and essentially none by the other agents at neuromuscular blocking doses. Succinylcholine, because of its similarity in structure to ACh, binds to ganglionic nicotinic and cardiac muscarinic receptors and stimulates cholinergic transmission. Pancuronium exerts a direct blocking effect on muscarinic receptors, but tubocurarine, metocurine, and atracurium show muscarinic blockade only at much higher concentrations than are needed for neuromuscular blockade. Pancuronium, succinylcholine, and gallamine also produce direct muscarinic effects that result in cardiac arrhythmias. The lack of cardiac effects with the newer agents, if true, will greatly increase the safety in the use of neuromuscular blocking drugs.

Histamine release is a problem with tubocurarine, and to a lesser extent with succinylcholine, metocurine, and probably mivacurium. Histamine contributes markedly to the cardiovascular side effects of tubocurarine. The release of histamine and the cardiac, respiratory, vascular, and other responses to histamine together with the use of histamine antagonists to offset anticipated histamine response to neuromuscular blocking drugs is discussed in Chapter 58.

Some of the newer neuromuscular blocking drugs appear to have little or no histamine releasing potential, thus minimizing this side effect.

Primary problems in the clinical use of neuromuscular blocking agents are summarized in the box.

With succinylcholine, K^+ efflux is dangerous in patients with extensive soft-tissue damage as in burns. In addition a succinylcholine-halothane combination may potentiate a malignant hyperthermia syndrome in patients predisposed to this condition.

Drug interactions occur with anesthetics, calcium-channel blockers, and some antibiotics. Many anesthetic agents enhance the action of the nondepolarizing neuromuscular blockers. Isoflurane potentiates the effects of succinylcholine. The local anesthetic, bupivacaine, potentiates the blockade of both nondepolarizing and depolarizing agents, and both lidocaine and procaine prolong the duration of succinylcholine action through inhibition of pseudocholinesterase.

Calcium-channel blockade, and to a lesser extent β-adrenergic blockers, potentiate neuromuscular blocking drugs. Antibiotics that contribute to drug interactions with the neuromuscular blocking agents are the aminoglycosides, tetracyclines, polymyxin, and clindamycin.

Neuromuscular blocking agents must be used with caution in patients with underlying neuromuscular or renal disease or electrolyte imbalance.

CLINICAL PROBLEMS

OLDER DRUGS

Blood pressure and heart rate changes
Histamine release
Ganglionic effects
Muscarinic effects
Difficulty with controlled reversal (some drugs)
Succinylcholine: hyperkalemia, elevated intraocular or intragastric pressures, muscle pain, induced cardiac dysrhythmias, stimulation of ganglia, block muscarinic receptors

NEWER DRUGS

Minimal to no cardiac effects (?)
Slight to no histamine release (?)
Easier reversal (?)

TRADENAMES

In addition to generic and fixed combination preparations, the following tradenamed materials are available in the United States.

Anectine, succinylcholine
Arduan, pipecuronium bromide
Flaxedil, gallamine triethiodide
Metubine, metocurine iodide
Normuron, vecuronium bromide
Pavulon, pancuronium bromide
Quelicin, succinylcholine
Tracrium, atracurium besylate

REFERENCES

Bevan DR, Bevan JC, and Donati F: Muscle relaxants in clinical anesthesia, Chicago, 1988, Year Book Medical Publishers.

Savarese JJ and Wastila WB: Current research in relaxant development, Seminars in Anesthesia V 304-311, 1986.

CARDIOVASCULAR SYSTEM: DRUGS AFFECTING CARDIAC FUNCTION, BLOOD PRESSURE, RENAL FUNCTION, AND BLOOD COAGULATION

PART III

For persons living in industrialized nations, dysfunction of the cardiovascular system is the major cause of mortality. In the United States, about 50% of deaths are attributed to cardiovascular problems.

Included within the functions of the cardiovascular system are:

1. Cardiac pumping ability, including the rhythmic nature of the electrical signals, force of contraction, and magnitude of the discharge pressure.
2. Integrity of the vasculature, including presence of flow-restricting deposits in the arterial lumen, muscular tone and structural integrity of vessel walls, and pressure drops required to pump blood through vascular beds at rates needed to provide nutrients and remove wastes.
3. Blood volume and composition, including water and electrolyte balances, lipid composition, and capabilities for clot formation and lysis.

Many of these functions can be modified therapeutically or prophylactically with drugs. This section describes such drugs, how they act at the molecular level, and their clinical application.

In addressing drug use to modify the pumping ability of the heart, it is necessary to understand physiological and biochemical processes that govern cardiac pacing, the force of cardiac and smooth muscle contraction, and blood pressure. The nervous system plays such a large role in the control of blood pressure that the physiology (Chapter 12) and pharmacology (Chapter 13) of blood pressure control are discussed in separate chapters. For discussions of cardiac pacing (Chapter 14) and cardiac contractile force (Chapter 15) the physiology and pharmacology are described within the same chapters. Another topic that relates to the heart as a pump is that of calcium channel blocking drugs (Chapter 16), that can act at several points of the pump-pacing-pressure control cycle, as well as provide relief in angina pectoris—as can nitrates (Chapter 17).

Pharmacological intervention to assure the integrity of the vasculature is discussed in Chapter 20 in relation to the reduction of deposits that narrow the arterial lumen and cause atherosclerosis. Pharmacological intervention is also included to a lesser extent in Chapter 18, where the prostaglandins are discussed.

Control of water volume and electrolyte content of the blood, primarily through renal mechanisms, is discussed in Chapter 19. The section closes with a discussion of the pharmacological approaches for reduced blood clotting or for stimulation of clot dissolution, especially in conjunction with postmyocardial infarction of a lodged microembolus (Chapter 21).

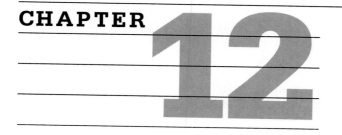

CHAPTER 12.

Regulation of Arterial Blood Pressure by Central and Peripheral Autonomic Nervous Systems

The first reviews the integrated control of arterial pressure provided by the central nervous system (CNS). Central control of both sympathetic and parasympathetic influences on cardiovascular function is discussed with CNS influences on humoral (endogenous chemicals) control of the circulation. The regulation of release of humoral factors by the brain is considered along with central actions of agents that reach the brain from the blood.

The second portion of the chapter reviews the peripheral autonomic and humoral factors that control vascular smooth muscle tone and cardiac function. These discussions include consideration of prejunctional receptors that inhibit and facilitate the release of neurotransmitters and the actions of a variety of hormonal factors that act directly on cardiovascular tissues and indirectly by exerting neural influences to modulate arterial pressure.

CONTROL OF ARTERIAL PRESSURE

Anatomical Organization of Central Autonomic Control

The anatomical organization of cerebral sites that regulate outflow from the sympathetic and parasympathetic branches of the autonomic nervous system provides the foundation for their understanding. These sites form a complex, highly integrated system that involves every major division of the CNS. Each division contains one or more integrative sites in which sensory input is linked to other CNS regions.

To understand how contemporary drugs effectively treat hypertension, an understanding of the integration and regulation of the central and peripheral autonomic nervous systems is essential. This chapter describes some of the more important features of blood pressure control and forms the basis for discussion (in Chapter 13) of the pharmacology of drugs used to treat high blood pressure or to reduce elevated vascular resistance.

This chapter is organized into two major sections.

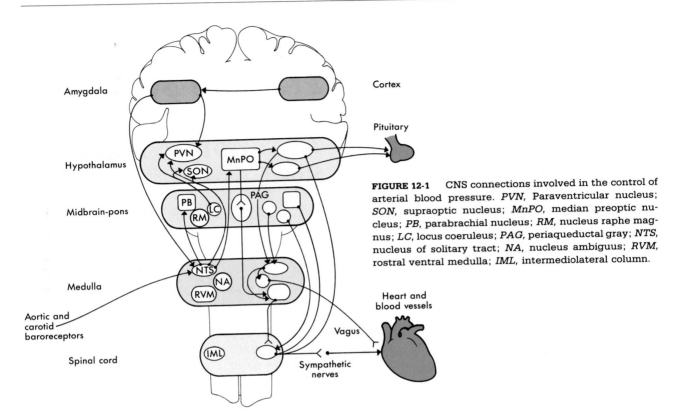

FIGURE 12-1   CNS connections involved in the control of arterial blood pressure. *PVN*, Paraventricular nucleus; *SON*, supraoptic nucleus; *MnPO*, median preoptic nucleus; *PB*, parabrachial nucleus; *RM*, nucleus raphe magnus; *LC*, locus coeruleus; *PAG*, periaqueductal gray; *NTS*, nucleus of solitary tract; *NA*, nucleus ambiguus; *RVM*, rostral ventral medulla; *IML*, intermediolateral column.

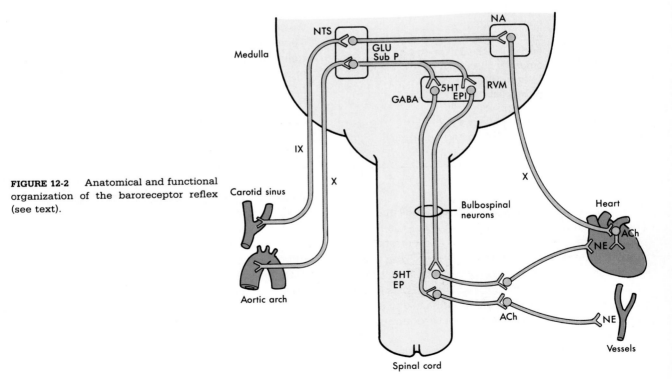

FIGURE 12-2   Anatomical and functional organization of the baroreceptor reflex (see text).

These regions ultimately regulate sympathetic and parasympathetic discharge to cardiovascular effectors. Figure 12-1 is a schematic representation of some major interconnections between CNS areas that are vital for autonomic control of arterial pressure.

Although the sites of origin for neural activity over the two branches of the autonomic nervous system can generate intrinsic discharge to cardiovascular effectors, their activity is carefully regulated by the organizational structure depicted in Figure 12-2, which shows the anatomical organization of the baroreceptor reflex. Stretch receptors located in the arch of the aorta and carotid sinus send projections over the tenth and ninth cranial nerves, respectively, to terminal fields in the nucleus of the solitary tract (NTS). Secondary interneurons from the NTS to the nucleus ambiguus (NA) and to vasomotor centers in rostral ventral medulla (RVM) complete the reflex arc.

Integrated Functions

Baroreceptor Reflex (see Figure 12-2). The minute to minute control of arterial pressure is achieved through reflex action that detects and corrects minor changes in pressure. Increased arterial pressure, detected as stretching at the aortic and carotoid sinus baroreceptors, leads to vagal activation and inhibition of sympathetic discharge. These produce slowing of heart rate and peripheral vasodilation, respectively. Excitation of interneurons between the NTS and NA increases vagal discharge to the heart and slows heart rate. In contrast, excitation of interneurons leading to vasomotor centers in the rostral ventral medulla inhibits the discharge of bulbospinal neurons leading to the intermediolateral cell column. These changes rapidly offset any tendency of arteral pressure to increase (see also Figure 10-9).

Conversely, when arterial pressure begins to fall, for example, in response to hemorrhage, stretch on the baroreceptors is reduced and less discharge is transmitted to the interneuronal connections. With less inhibition, the sympathetic system discharge rises and the heart rate and arterial pressure increase. The heart rate also increases in part as a result of the reduced activity of the vagal fibers leading to the heart.

Connections from higher centers can modulate baroreflex activity. For example, defense reactions impair the baroreflex via connections between the hypothalamus, the amygdala, and the NTS. Inhibition of baroreflex function allows enough increased arterial pressure and cardiac output to provide blood flow to the muscles needed to escape or defend against the threat.

Control of Vasopressin Secretion The peptide vasopressin participates in cardiovascular regulation through its direct actions on blood vessels and through its ability to regulate water homeostasis. Conditions that increase vasopressin secretion include hypotensive and nonhypotensive hemorrhage, dehydration, high sodium intake, surgical anesthesia, trauma, and stress. The hormone is released by nerve terminals projecting into the neural lobe of the pituitary gland from the paraventricular and supraoptic nuclei (see Figure 12-2). The neuroendocrine mechanisms providing stimulation for vasopressin release involve several systems that ultimately increase the neural activity of vasopressin-containing cells in these nuclei. Increased vasopressin secretion in response to lowered arterial pressure or lowered blood volume is mediated by altered baroreceptor input to the NTS, with relays to the vasopressin-containing hypothalamic nuclei. Dehydration and related stimuli increase vasopressin secretion by activating hypothalamic osmoreceptors that are connected neuronally to the paraventricular and supraoptic nuclei. Stress-induced vasopressin secretion is mediated by the amygdala's influence on vasopressin-containing hypothalamic nuclei. A final stimulus for vasopressin release is high circulating concentrations of angiotensin II.

Central Actions of Angiotensin II Stimuli for vasopressin secretion also increases circulating concentrations of angiotensin II. This peptide is produced via the biosynthetic cascade involving renin secretion from the juxtaglomerular cells in the kidney and the actions of angiotensin-converting enzyme (described in Chapter 13). Angiotensin II is a potent direct vasoconstrictor; however, it also acts directly on the CNS to amplify its hypertensive properties. The peptide does not penetrate into the CNS but reaches receptor regions located in or close to several circumventricular organs that lack a blood-brain barrier. The major receptor regions for angiotensin associated with circumventricular organs are located in the forebrain in the organum vasculosum of the lamina terminalis (OVLT) and the subfornical organ (SFO) and in the brain stem's area postrema, located close to the NTS. Through appropriate neuronal connections, activation of receptors for angiotensin II in these circumventricular organs produces increased sympathetic discharge and vasopressin release. Other centrally mediated effects of angiotensin II include thirst, increased drinking behavior, and the release of adrenocorticotropic hormone (ACTH).

Central Actions of Other Humoral Factors
Other substances exert effects on cardiovascular function after penetrating the circumventricular organs. Vasopressin (AVP) produces profound activation of the baroreflex, leading to sympathoinhibition and bradycardia. Such effects can occur even at blood concentrations that fail to raise arterial pressure. These actions appear to be mediated by receptors for AVP located within the area postrema.

Increased serum sodium concentration, like elevated blood concentrations of angiotensin II, produce sympathoexcitation and AVP release. These responses elevate arterial pressure and contribute to the body's defense against dehydration, among other influences.

The mineralocorticoid aldosterone plays a critical role in fluid electrolyte and cardiovascular homeostasis. This sodium-retaining steroid is released from the adrenal cortex in response to any situation that raises blood concentrations of angiotensin II. The peptide interacts with receptors for angiotensin directly on cells in the zona glomerulosa to stimulate aldosterone release. Excessive blood concentrations of aldosterone and related steroids associated, for example, with tumors of the adrenal cortex produce a surgically reversible form of hypertension. Because aldosterone is highly lipophilic, it easily gains access to the CNS, where it interacts with mineralocorticoid binding sites. Recent evidence suggests that central actions of aldosterone contribute to mineralocorticoid-induced hypertension.

PERIPHERAL NEUROHUMORAL REGULATION OF BLOOD PRESSURE

Systemic arterial blood pressure is regulated primarily through adrenergic innervation of the regional vascular beds and by influence of various hormonal substances and autacoids present in the circulating blood or produced in or near the blood vessels (Figure 12-3 and Table 12-1). Norepinephrine released during depolarization of the adrenergic nerves acts on α_1- or β_1-adrenergic receptors located within the synaptic cleft of blood vessels and heart muscle, respectively. Circulating and locally released substances act on receptor sites extrasynaptically on the vascular or cardiac cell membrane. These circulating substances also affect receptor sites on the adrenergic nerve terminal. Although tonic sympathetic nerve impulses that reach the adrenergic innervation originate in vasomotor areas of the CNS, adrenergic cardiovascular control is modulated at peripheral loci. This may occur at the sympathetic ganglion, at the postganglionic adrenergic nerve terminal, or even at the adrenergic receptor level. Adrenergic function at postganglionic adrenergic nerve terminals is modulated by activation of receptors on the nerve terminal that are responsive to the substances listed in Table 12-2. Inhibition and facilitation can be achieved, depending on the receptor(s) activated.

Table 12-1 Hormones and Autacoids Affecting Blood Pressure

Hormone, Autacoid	Circulating	Locally Released
Angiotensin II	X	X
Arginine vasopressin	X	—
Atrial natriuretic peptide	X	—
Kinins	*	X
Eicosanoids	*	X
Acetylcholine	*	X
Catecholamines	X	X
Serotonin	*	X

* Ultrashort plasma $t_{1/2}$.

Table 12-2 Receptors on Postganglionic Adrenergic Nerve Terminal

Receptor	Agonist	Response
α_2-Adrenergic	epinephrine or norepinephrine	Inhibition
Muscarinic (M_2?)	ACh	Inhibition
Prostaglandin E_2	PGE_2	Inhibition
Serotonergic	5-HT	Inhibition
Dopaminergic (D_2)	dopamine	Inhibition
Histaminergic (H_2)	histamine	Inhibition
Atrial natriuretic peptide	ANP	Inhibition
Angiotensin II	angiotensin II	Facilitation
β_2-Adrenergic	epinephrine, isoproterenol	Facilitation
Prostaglandin $F_{2\alpha}$	$PGF_{2\alpha}$	Facilitation
Neuropeptide Y	NPY	Facilitation

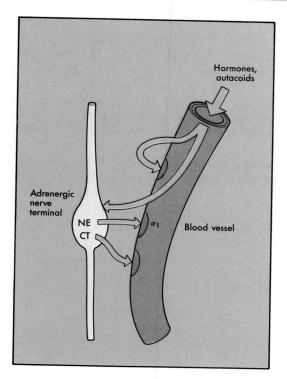

FIGURE 12-3   Adrenergic neuroeffector junction at a vascular site. Norepinephrine *(NE)* released from the postganglionic nerve terminal acts on α_1-adrenergic receptors of vascular smooth muscle. Circulating and locally released hormones and autacoids act directly on receptors of vascular smooth muscle and also on nerve terminals. Cotransmitters *(CT)* such as epinephrine, dopamine, opioids, and neuropeptide γ are released along with the transmitter, norepinephrine.

Biogenic Amines

Adrenergic Receptors and Catecholamines

Receptors for biogenic amines and other agents are present on postganglionic nerve terminals (Table 12-2). Muscarinic, cholinergic, dopaminergic, and histaminergic receptors, when stimulated by their respective agonists, mediate inhibition of adrenergic neurotransmission. Stimulation of presynaptic α_2- and β_2-adrenergic receptors causes a decrease and an increase, respectively, in the neurotransmitter (norepinephrine) released from the adrenergic nerve terminal (see Chapters 8 and 10). Norepinephrine inhibits transmission by stimulating α_2-adrenergic receptors, whereas isoproterenol facilitates transmission via β_2-adrenergic receptors. Endogenous circulating epinephrine can activate both α_2- and β_2-presynaptic

adrenergic receptors. Negative feedback from adrenergic transmitter release occurs through activation of α_2-adrenergic receptors on the presynaptic nerve terminal; positive feedback can be shown when α_2-adrenergic receptors are blocked. It is proposed that circulating epinephrine serves as a physiologic enhancer of adrenergic transmitter release by presynaptic β_2-adrenergic receptor stimulation. Presynaptic α_2-adrenergic receptors inhibit transmitter release.

When the presynaptic α_2-adrenergic receptors are stimulated (e.g., by an α_2-adrenergic receptor agonist such as clonidine), endogenous norepinephrine release and neurally mediated vasoconstriction diminish. Conversely, blockade of presynaptic α_2-adrenergic receptors enhances adrenergic neurotransmitter release. Administration of adrenergic antagonists such as phentolamine with α_2-adrenergic receptor blocking properties evokes the common side effect of tachycardia, attributable to greater activation of unblocked cardiac β_1-adrenergic receptors. Blockade of β_2-adrenergic receptors with β-adrenergic receptor antagonists should inhibit sympathetically mediated responses; however, this seems to occur only when the presynaptic α_2-adrenergic receptors are first blocked by treatment with an α_2-adrenergic receptor antagonist.

Abnormal presynaptic modulation of α_2-adrenergic receptors is believed to contribute to arterial hypertension. The α_2-adrenergic receptors in the tail artery of young spontaneously hypertensive rats were found to be subsensitive compared to their Wistar-Kyoto normotensive controls; a hypersensitivity of the presynaptic β_2-adrenergic receptors in mesenteric arteries was also observed. These changes would be expected to enhance adrenergic activity in hypertension. Increased adrenergic transmitter release and vascular responsiveness to adrenergic nerve stimulation in spontaneously hypertensive rats is commonly found. Changes in the sensitivity of presynaptic adrenergic receptors and increased numbers of vascular adrenergic nerve terminals account in part for the enhanced responsiveness and enhanced transmitter release seen in the spontaneously hypertensive rat.

There is no well-defined cellular mechanism by which adrenergic modulation is governed by presynaptic α_2-adrenergic receptors; however, Na, K-ATPase in the nerve terminal may be stimulated, resulting in reduced intracellular calcium concentrations and neurotransmitter release.

Ganglionic Sites Adrenergic neurotransmission can be modulated at the level of the sympathetic ganglia. These ganglia possess receptors for the biogenic amines; however, depending on the particular receptor stimulated, inhibition or facilitation may result. No modification of ganglionic modulation has been shown in hypertension or other pathophysiological processes.

Direct Actions Norepinephrine and epinephrine exert direct vasoconstrictor or vasodilator effects to control blood pressure. Circulating concentrations of these catecholamines can reflect the degree of sympathetic nervous activity and adrenergic neurotransmitter release. Extremely low catecholamine concentrations can be present in the plasma of normotensive and hypertensive people; the concentration in hypertensive individuals is reportedly elevated compared to that in normal individuals. Debate has centered on whether there are increased plasma catecholamine concentrations in subjects with essential hypertension. Epinephrine in plasma may be taken up by adrenergic nerve terminals and released as a cotransmitter. Direct vasoconstrictor effects and facilitation of the release of norepinephrine by stimulation of presynaptic β_2-adrenergic receptors may contribute to enhanced pressor activity. Relatively small doses of exogenous epinephrine appear to accentuate vasoconstrictor responses induced reflexively by lower-body negative-pressure maneuvers in humans. This effect may be due to the presynaptic action of epinephrine. Epinephrine also increases peripheral sympathetic nerve activity in humans, seemingly as a result of the catecholamine's effect on the CNS. Hypertensive individuals appear to have an exaggerated vascular response to exogenous epinephrine, not just resulting from the vascular hypertrophy of essential hypertension. Thus, circulating epinephrine may contribute by several mechanisms to elevated blood pressure.

Circulating norephinephrine is also involved in the pathophysiology of hypertension. It is well-established that plasma norepinephrine concentrations are very high in pheochromocytoma (a tumor of the adrenal medulla) and that the cardiovascular effect of norepinephrine contributes to the hypertension in this condition.

Peptides

Various vasoactive peptides act directly to stimulate or inhibit the contractility of vascular smooth muscle and in some cases to modulate adrenergic neurotransmission (Figures 12-1 and 12-4 and Table 12-1). Angiotensin II and neuropeptide Y (NPY) are peptides that cause vasoconstriction by direct receptor-mediated action, but also interact with their respective presynaptic peptidergic receptors to enhance release of norepinephrine.

Angiotensin II Angiotensin II apparently acts on the adrenergic nerve terminal via a calcium-mediated mechanism; however, the second messenger(s) responsible for triggering this event has not been identified. Much more is known about the mechanism by which activation of the angiotensin receptor leads to contraction of vascular smooth muscle.

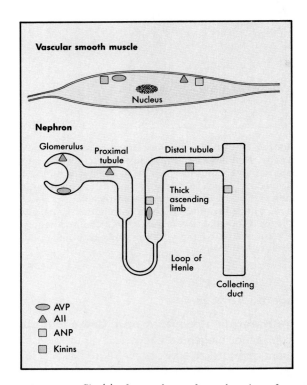

FIGURE 12-4   Site(s) of vascular and renal action of vasoactive peptides important in blood pressure control. Angiotensin II and arginine vasopressin *(AVP)* are vasoconstrictors, whereas atrial natriuretic peptide (ANP) and kinins are vasodilators, as a result of release of endothelium-derived relaxing factor (EDRF) from endothelial cells. Angiotensin II and AVP contract the mesangial cells in the glomerulus, decreasing glomerular filtration rate. Angiotensin II and AVP increase sodium reabsorption at the sites indicated, whereas ANP decreases sodium reabsorption at several sites. Kinins inhibit sodium reabsorption at distal sites and possibly in deep proximal tubules. Both ANP and kinins may also inhibit sodium reabsorption by washing out the medullary osmotic gradient through their vasodilator action.

Occupation of the angiotensin II receptor activates phospholipase C in the plasma membrane, leading to hydrolysis of the phospholipid, phosphatidylinositol 4,5 bisphosphate, into the second messengers, inositol trisphosphate (IP$_3$) and diacylglycerol. IP$_3$ diffuses into the cytoplasm where it acts on the endoplasmic reticulum to release Ca^{++}, and diacylglycerol remains in the membrane where it can activate protein kinase C. Initial rise in intracellular Ca^{++} mediates the contraction of smooth muscle by stimulating myosin light chain kinase to phosphorylate certain regulatory proteins of the actin-myosin complex, the 20 Kda myosin light chains. When these proteins are phosphorylated, actomyosin ATPase activity is stimulated, leading to cross-bridge cycling and contraction of the muscle cells. The initial change in contraction induced by the elevation in intracellular Ca^{++} concentration is transitory; however, with continued presence of agonist, a longer term contraction of smooth muscle ensues. Mechanisms to account for this phase of the contraction include continued presence of slightly elevated cytoplasmic concentrations of Ca^{++} and/or activation of protein kinase C, but exact molecular events are unknown.

Other calcium-mobilizing peptides such as arginine vasopressin (AVP) share this mechanism of stimulation of vascular smooth muscle.

The presynaptic facilitating action of angiotensin II may play a physiological role in amplifying the vasoconstrictor function of the sympathetic nervous system. Angiotensin II also acts at other sites (e.g., sympathetic ganglia, adrenal medulla, and CNS) in fulfilling this role. A major research effort was made to determine whether the adrenergic facilitating action of angiotensin II is involved in conditions of increased renin release. The concept that these two powerful blood pressure regulating systems—the renin-angiotensin and sympathetic nervous systems—interact to increase vascular resistance in hypertension and in low sodium and volume states is appealing. Possible mechanisms involved in angiotensin-dependent hypertension are illustrated in Figure 12-5.

Subjects with essential hypertension can be divided into low, normal, and high renin groups, depending on the relationship between the plasma renin activity and the sodium intake of the patient. When the plasma renin activity is high, the direct vasocon-

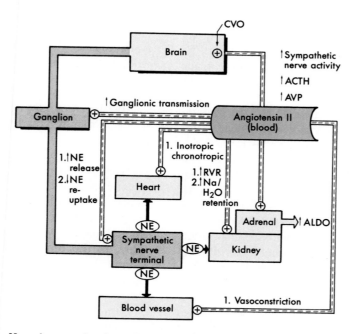

FIGURE 12-5   Neurohormonal actions of angiotensin II affecting arterial blood pressure. *Dashed lines* indicate effects of blood-borne angiotensin II. Red dashed lines indicate organs possessing localized tissue renin-angiotensin systems (e.g., capable of synthesizing angiotensin II independent of blood constituents). *CVO*, Circumventricular organs; *ACTH*, adrenocorticotrophic hormone; *AVP*, arginine vasopressin; *ALDO*, aldosterone; *RVR*, renal vascular resistance; *NE*, norepinephrine.

strictor actions of angiotensin II may predominate. When plasma renin is low, only the central and presynaptic mechanisms may be activated.

Another concept of blood pressure regulation developed recently involves the participation of angiotensin II produced locally in the vasculature. The enzymes and substrate of the renin-angiotensin system—renin, angiotensinogen, and angiotensin-converting enzyme—are present in the vasculature. Antiogensin I and angiotensin II can be generated in isolated blood vessels and in the intact vascular bed. Enhanced by β-adrenergic stimuli, antiotensin II is released from isolated blood vessels. It then has access to the adrenergic nerve terminal and can enhance norepinephrine release during nerve depolarization. Possibly, adrenergic facilitation by locally produced antiotensin II contributes to increased vascular resistance in low renin hypertension. The participation of the vascular renin-angiotensin system and adrenergic facilitation may help explain why agents that interrupt the function of the renin-angiotensin system are still effective when plasma renin concentrations are normal to low. Angiotensin converting enzyme inhibitors, used to treat essential hypertension, may depend for their antihypertensive efficacy in part on blocking the biosynthesis of tissue angiotensin II. Basic and clinical studies of angiotensin converting enzyme inhibitors, receptor antagonists, and renin inhibitors provide a better understanding of the participation of the renin-angiotensin system in the control of blood pressure.

Vasopressin Vasopressin (AVP) has an integral role in renal tubular reabsorption of water and sodium, and is also believed to serve a vasoconstrictor function in certain pathophysiological conditions. The sites of action of AVP and other peptides on the vasculature and kidney are illustrated in Figure 12-4. An increased plasma concentration of AVP is found in low volume states and in several forms of experimental hypertension. Although the plasma concentration of AVP increases in hypertensive conditions, the increase is slight and is not considered to be within the vasoconstrictor range. However, in some hypertension models, increased vascular sensitivity to AVP may assist in the blood pressure rise. AVP causes retention of sodium and water, and this factor, too, may be involved in hypertension. AVP contributes to the support of normal blood pressure when the compensatory function of the sympathetic and renin-angiotensin systems is interfered with or blocked pharmacologically. The introduction of specific an-

Table 12-3 Vasopressin Antagonists

AVP Receptors	Peptide Antagonist	Peptide Agonist
V_1	d(CH_2)5Tyr(CH_3)AVP dDVDAVP	
V_1, V_2	d(CH_2)5-D-Tyr(ET)VAVP	
V_2		VDAVP DDAVP

tagonists to the actions of AVP has made possible an analysis of the contributions of AVP to blood pressure regulation.

Peptides have been synthesized that block AVP receptors. These are designated V_1 for those that mediate smooth muscle contraction and V_2 for those controlling the renal tubular actions of the peptide (Table 12-3). The administration of V_1 antagonists has demonstrated that AVP, present in the circulation as a consequence of hypertension or low blood volume, exerts a vasoconstrictor action. A decrease in blood pressure is seen with the antagonist, reflecting a vasoconstrictor effect of AVP. However, caution is necessary when using these compounds because V_1 antagonists also may provoke a vasodilator effect via stimulation of V_2 receptors. It is uncertain therefore whether the absence of V_1-receptor stimulation or the activation of V_2 receptors actually accounts for the hypotensive response to the antagonist.

Another important action of AVP that appears to affect its role in hypertension is its effect on the arterial baroreflex. As described earlier, AVP acts on the CNS to sensitize the baroreceptor reflex, and the pressor response to AVP is markedly attenuated. For a given increase in blood pressure, AVP slows heart rate more than do the other pressor agents. In fact, subpressor quantities of AVP can reduce heart rate through centrally mediated mechanisms. Interestingly, in the Brattleboro rat (a genetically derived strain that is totally lacking AVP and that exhibits a depressed baroreflex), AVP is effective in restoring the reflex.

Stimulation of V_1 receptors by AVP results in the activation of phospholipase C and the hydrolysis of phosphoinositides, leading to increased intracellular calcium concentrations. Occupation of V_2 receptors causes increases in cAMP mediated through the action of a G_s-protein. One second messenger (calcium ion) causes contraction of smooth muscle and the other (cAMP) produces changes in renal tubular cell permeability.

Atrial Natriuretic Peptide The discovery of a potent natriuretic and hypotensive substance in the atria of the rat, and later in other species, including humans, opened new possibilities for blood pressure regulation. Atrial natriuretic peptide (ANP) consists of several related peptides derived from a 126 amino acid precursor, *prepro ANP*. A 28 amino acid, peptide, ANP 99-126 that has been sequenced and cloned is the chief product of prepro ANP processing, formed in the myocardium and released into the circulation by several stimuli, primarily by increased atrial pressure or atrial stretch. The physiological stimulus is increased plasma volume; however, ANP can also be released through the action of vasopressin and possibly by increased arterial blood pressure.

A large complement of physiological activities makes ANP extremely appealing in terms of its role in blood pressure control. ANP relaxes vascular smooth muscle, causes natriuresis and diuresis without loss of potassium, inhibits release of renin and vasopressin, and antagonizes the sodium retention caused by aldosterone. These properties are ideal for an antihypertensive hormone. Originally, it was thought that a deficiency of ANP was one cause of hypertension, but it was later found that the plasma concentration of ANP is actually increased in several forms of experimental hypertension and in essential hypertension. Like the eicosanoids (see below and Chapter 18), ANP release is probably expressed to compensate for an increase in systemic blood pressure.

ANP or pharmacological agents similar to ANP may be useful in the treatment of essential hypertension. However, because of the expense of synthesizing ANP and the relative ineffectiveness of peptides given orally, they are not practical. Effective use of the antihypertensive properties can still be made through inhibition of peptide breakdown to allow accumulation of plasma ANP. A neutral endopeptidase is one of the enzymes responsible for the degradation and inactivation of ANP. Inhibitors of neutral endopeptidase are effective in slowing ANP metabolism. Administration of these inhibitors increases the ANP plasma concentration, potentiates the hypotensive and renal effect of ANP, and produces reduction of blood pressure in steroid-induced hypertension in the rat.

ANP activates guanylate cyclase and increases cGMP in various tissues. By these mechanisms it also exerts at least some of its actions. Thus, vascular smooth muscle relaxation induced by ANP is mediated by an increase in cGMP. ANP causes a direct relaxant effect on vascular smooth muscle and it antagonizes the vasoconstrictor action of other agonists.

Kinins It is well accepted that the urinary excretion of kallikrein, the enzyme responsible for the generation of kinins from kininogen, is reduced in some forms of experimental hypertension and in essential hypertension. Because kinins are extremely potent vasodilators, it is assumed that the circulating or tissue concentration of kinin is also reduced, and that this results in elevated systemic arterial blood pressure. Besides their vasodilator action, kinins' action on the kidney may participate in a hypotensive effect. However, proof that kinins are important substances in the regulation of blood pressure is lacking. Previous pharmacological approaches to determine the role of kinins were unsuccessful because the pharmacological tools available were inferior to those used to study the sympathetic nervous system, the renin-angiotensin system, and AVP. The introduction of peptide antagonists to bradykinin provides clarification of the role of kinins in normal physiology, as well as in hypertension. The peptides studied are competitive antagonists of bradykinin and were employed successfully to demonstrate several important aspects of the kallikrein-kinin system. There are definite indications that the kinins are involved in normal renal function. The autoregulation of glomerular filtration and blood flow to the renal papilla appears to depend on the kallikrein-kinin system, with experimental evidence indicating the abolition of glomerular filtration autoregulation and decreased papillary blood flow produced by kinin antagonists. During sodium restriction, a condition in which the kallikrein-kinin system is activated, the hypotensive and renal vasodilator effects of an angiotensin-converting enzyme inhibitor are attenuated by the kinin antagonists. In animal models of severe hypertension, kinins may contribute to the hypotensive effects of the angiotensin-converting enzyme inhibitors. However, in other models such as the spontaneously hypertensive rat, or in renin-dependent hypertension, the kinin antagonists are ineffective. Thus, the kallikrein-kinin system may be involved only in the most severe forms of hypertension.

Eicosanoids Products of arachidonic acid (see Chapter 18) exert potent actions on the cardiovascular system, and many investigators seek to demonstrate a role for these substances in the regulation of blood pressure. Although the cyclooxygenase products, prostaglandin E_2 (PGE_2) and prostacyclin, which are potent vasodilators, were originally perceived as being important for the maintenance of normal blood pressure and renal blood flow, this did not prove to be the case. However, these substances are generated in greater amounts during traumatic events (e.g., laporotomy, hypotensive crisis, and organ damage). They are also increased in some forms of hypertension, probably to compensate for increased blood pressure. PGE_2 is produced in abundance in the kidney and is hypersecreted during renal ischemia. In contrast, prostacyclin is produced in blood vessels and in the kidney, but its role in hypertension is questionable. Thromboxane A_2, a vasoconstrictor product of arachidonic acid via cyclooxygenase, is thought to contribute to the rise of blood pressure in renovascular hypertension and in the spontaneously hypertensive rat. The role of eicosanoids in hypertension has been pursued using cyclooxygenase inhibitors, thromboxane synthesis inhibitors, and thromboxane antagonists as pharmacological tools, and through the measurement of circulating or renally derived eicosanoids and their metabolic or hydrolysis products. Besides their vasodilator action, the E prostaglandins also exert profound effects on renal function.

REFERENCES

1. Brody MJ, Alper RH, O'Neill TP et al.: Central neural control of the cardiovascular system. In Zanchetti A and Tarazi RC, eds.: Handbook of hypertension: cardiovascular regulation mechanisms in hypertension; pathophysiology of hypertension—regulatory mechanisms, vol 8, The Netherlands, 1986, Elsevier Science Publishers, BV.

2. Gebber GL: Brainstem mechanisms involved in cardiovascular regulation. In Randall WC, ed.: Nervous control of cardiovascular function, Oxford, 1984, Oxford University Press.

3. Langer SZ: Presynaptic regulation of the release of catecholamines, Pharmacol Rev 32:337, 1980.

4. Zimmerman BG: Peripheral neurogenic factors in acute and chronic alterations of arterial pressure, Circ Res 53:121, 1983.

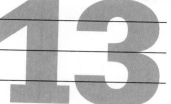

Antihypertensive Drugs

 ## THERAPEUTIC OVERVIEW

Hypertension is defined as an elevation of arterial blood pressure above an arbitrarily defined normal value. This normal value for blood pressure differs according to gender and age; men have higher average pressures than women, and in most populations older individuals have higher pressures than younger subjects. The American Heart Association defines hypertension as arterial blood pressure higher than 140/90 mm Hg whereas The World Health Organization uses the value 160/95 mm Hg. The prevalence of hypertension varies in different subgroups of the population but the overall rate in the United States is estimated at approximately 20% of all adults. A physician in general practice can expect to see 20 to 40 patients with hypertension each week.

A small number (<10%) of individuals with hypertension have identifiable causes such as renal disease or endocrine tumors; these are often managed by surgical means. The majority of patients diagnosed as hypertensive, however, are simply at the upper end of the normal distribution of blood pressure values for their population group. No single mechanism has been identified to explain the higher blood pressure values in such individuals, but it may result from genetic factors, because blood pressure is strongly influenced by inheritance in a polygenetic fashion. This type of hypertension is designated *essential* hypertension, and although usually first diagnosed in middle-aged individuals, it can be found in children and young adults as well.

Hypertension, unless rapid in onset and severe, does not produce noticeable symptoms. However, several cardiovascular diseases are common or more severe in humans with high blood pressure, including atherosclerosis, coronary artery disease, aortic aneurysm, congestive heart failure, stroke, diabetes, and renal and retinal disease. The presence of diabetes increases the frequency and severity of end-organ damage. The purpose of treatment of hypertension is to prevent these significant cardiovascular complications. Most importantly, effective drug therapy has been shown through controlled clinical trails to reduce the morbidity and mortality associated with high arterial pressure.

The choice of therapy for a patient with hypertension depends on a variety of factors: age, gender, race, body build, and lifestyle of the patient; etiology of the disease; other coexisting diseases; rapidity of onset and severity of the hypertension; and the presence or absence of other risk factors for cardiovascular disease, (e.g., smoking, alcohol consumption, obesity, and personality type).

A number of nonpharmacological approaches to therapy of hypertension are available. These are listed in the box. Patients differ in their sensitivity to these techniques, but on the average, only modest reduc-

---

NONPHARMACOLOGICAL THERAPY OF HYPERTENSION

Low sodium chloride diet
Weight reduction
Exercise
Cessation of smoking
Decrease in excessive (>30 ml ethanol per day) alcohol consumption
Psychological methods (relaxation, biofeedback, meditation)
Dietary increase in polyunsaturated fat intake

---

tions (5 to 10 mm Hg) in blood pressure can be achieved. Despite the modest effect of nonpharmacological interventions, when viewed across large populations, specific individuals may be classified based on their sensitivity to these interventions. For example, the "salt sensitive" individual will have a marked fall in blood pressure when placed on a low sodium diet. The major advantage of nonpharmacological therapies is the relative safety and freedom from side effects, compared with drug therapy. However, most patients with hypertension require drug treatment to achieve an adequate sustained reduction of blood pressure.

Arterial blood pressure is the product of cardiac output (CO) and total peripheral resistance (TPR). Patients with recent onset essential hypertension tend to have an elevated CO. With chronic sustained hypertension, most patients develop normal or low CO and a fixed elevated peripheral resistance. Drugs currently available act either by decreasing CO or TPR. However, CO and TPR are not independent variables, and changes in one can indirectly affect the other.

Reduction of blood pressure by any means may activate one or more of the physiological mechanisms discussed here and thereby oppose a drug-induced decrease in blood pressure (Figure 13-1).

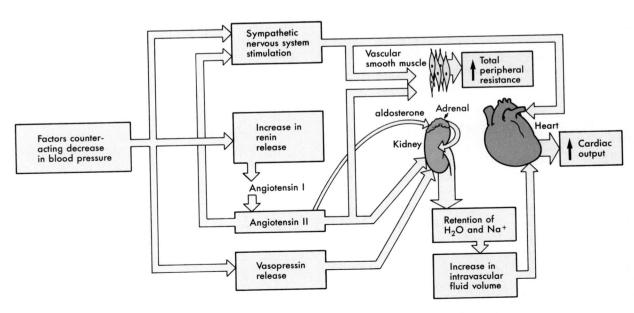

FIGURE 13-1   Processes that occur to counteract a decrease in blood pressure.

Renin-Angiotensin-Aldosterone System

A decrease in arterial pressure causes release of the enzyme renin from the kidney into the blood. Renin generates angiotensin I from a circulating substrate, angiotensinogen, synthesized in the liver and other tissues. Angiotensin I is converted to angiotensin II by "converting enzyme," found in the endothelial cell membrane, especially in the lung. Angiotensin II directly constricts blood vessels, enhances sympathetic nervous system activity, and causes renal salt and water retention by direct intrarenal actions, and by stimulating the adrenal gland to release the potent mineralocorticoid aldosterone.

Sympathetic Nervous System

A decrease in blood pressure activates the baroreflex, producing increases in sympathetic nervous system activity and leading to (1) increased force and rate of cardiac contraction and enhanced cardiac filling, which combine to elevate CO, (2) constriction of most blood vessels leading to a rise in TPR, and (3) renal retention of sodium chloride and water (via renal sympathetic nerves innervating renal blood vessels and tubules).

THERAPEUTIC OVERVIEW

Hypertension is defined as:

Arterial pressure
American Heart Association
> 140/90 mm Hg
World Health Organization
> 160/95 mm Hg

Exacerbates:
Atherosclerosis
Coronary artery diseases
Congestive heart failure
Diabetes
Stroke
Renal disease
Retinal disease
Therapy
Nonpharmacological
Dietary: ↓ Na, ↓ alcohol, ↓ weight, ↓ smoking
Pharmacological: Several drug classes
Physiological counter effects to ↓ blood pressure
Fluid retention
Release of renin
Sympathetic response ↑
Baroflex release of vasopressin

Vasopressin System

A decrease in arterial pressure causes baroreflex-mediated release of vasopressin (antidiuretic hormone), which acts on the renal collecting duct to enhance retention of water.

Fluid Retention by the Kidney

A decrease in arterial pressure causes decreased sodium chloride and water excretion by the kidney. This results in part from the direct intrarenal hydraulic effect of reduced renal perfusion pressure and in part from the other mechanisms just listed. The resultant expansion of extracellular fluid and plasma volumes tends to increase CO and arterial pressure and thus reduces the antihypertensive action of the drug.

The most effective and best tolerated antihypertensive drug regimens impair the operation of one or more of these physiological mechanisms. In addition, drug therapy for hypertension must usually be continued for the lifetime of the patient. Thus, it is imperative that the cost of therapy to the patient be minimized and that the minimum effective dose of drug (or drugs) be employed to reduce the incidence of undesirable side effects.

A summary of therapeutic approaches is given in the box.

MECHANISMS OF ACTION AND RELATION OF MECHANISMS OF ACTION TO CLINICAL RESPONSE

Antihypertensive drugs can be divided into seven classes, based on mechanisms of action (see box, p. 171, and Figure 13-2). Each of these classes is discussed in terms of (1) molecular mechanisms of action and (2) relationship of molecular mechanism to clinical effects. A summary of the physiological responses by drug class is given in Table 13-1. Whenever possible monotherapy is advisable, but if the blood pressure is not controlled by a single drug, the administration of additional drugs in a step-wise manner is frequently employed. The step-care approach is still endorsed by the Council of High Blood Pressure of the American Heart Association (Figure 13-3). The pharmacokinetic considerations and clinical problems are discussed in subsequent sections in which the seven classes of drug are considered together.

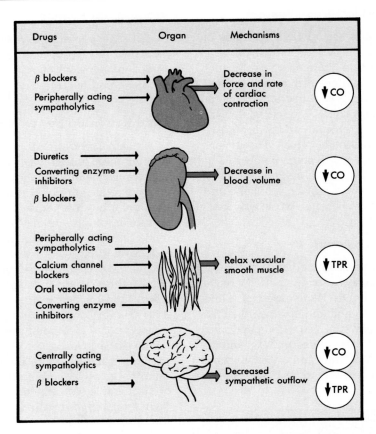

FIGURE 13-2   Summary of sites and mechanisms by which antihypertensive drugs bring about a reduction in blood pressure. *CO*, Cardiac output; *TPR*, total peripheral resistance.

Table 13-1   Physiological Responses to Antihypertensive Drugs

	Plasma Volume	CO	Heart Rate	TPR	Plasma Renin Activity	Sympathetic Nervous System Activity
Diuretics	↓	↓	↔ ↑	↓	↑	↔ ↑
β blockers	↔	↓	↓	↑ ↔	↓	↔ ↓
Centrally acting sympatholytics	↑ ↔	↓	↓	↓	↓ ↔	↓
Peripherally acting sympatholytics	↔ ↑	↔ ↓	↔ ↓	↓	↔	↑
Channel calcium blockers*	↔	↔	↔ ↑	↓	↑ ↔	↔ ↑
Orally active vaso-dilators	↑	↔ ↑	↑	↓	↑	↑
Converting en-zyme inhibitors	↔	↑ ↔	↔	↓	↑	↔ ↓

↑ Increase; ↓ decrease; ↔ no change.
*Some have diuretic effects also.

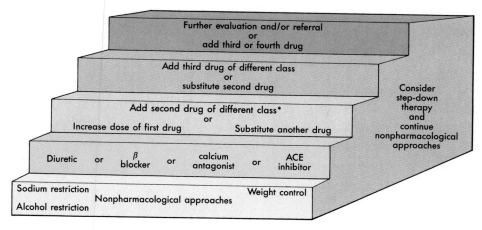

FIGURE 13-3   Individualized step-care therapy for hypertension. For some patients, nonpharmacological therapy should be tried first. If blood pressure reduction goal is not achieved, add pharmacological therapy. Other patients may require pharmacological therapy initially. In these instances, nonpharmacological therapy may be a helpful adjunct. *ACE,* Angiotensin converting enzymes; *asterisk,* drugs such as diuretics: *β blockers,* calcium antagonists, ACE inhibitors or blockers, centrally acting α_1-agonists, *Rauwolfia serpentina,* and vasodilators. (From 1988 Joint National Committee on Detection, Evaluation and Treatment of High Blood Pressure: The 1988 Report of the Joint National Committee on Detection, Evaluation, and Treatment of High Blood Pressure, Arch Intern Med 148:1023, 1988.)

DIURETIC DRUGS USED TO TREAT HYPERTENSION*	
amiloride†	indapamide
benzothiadiazides	metolazone
(thiazides)	spironolactone
bumetanide	triamterene†
chlorthalidone	
furosemide	

* See Chapter 19.
† Primarily used as adjunctive therapy to prevent potassium loss caused by other diuretics.

Diuretics

Diuretics reduce fluid volume by inhibiting electrolyte transport in the renal tubules. Their mechanisms of action on the renal tubule are discussed in Chapter 19.

Various diuretic drugs are used in the therapy of hypertension (see box). Chemical structures are shown in Figure 13-4 and in Chapter 19. However, the complete molecular mechanism of the antihypertensive action of diuretics is not known. Initial administration of a diuretic produces a marked increase in urinary water and electrolyte excretion and a reduction in extracellular and plasma volumes. These changes result in a decrease in CO that is primarily responsible for the fall in arterial pressure. Some investigators suggest that this initial decrease in extracellular water volume and in plasma sodium concentration is the full explanation for the antihypertensive effect and the mechanisms involved are those responsible for the diuretic effect. After several days the urinary excretion returns to normal, but blood pressure remains at the reduced level. Subsequently, plasma volume and CO also return to, or approximately to, pretreatment values and the TPR falls, whereas blood pressure remains lowered. The decline in TPR may initially involve autoregulatory vascular adjustments of various tissues to decreased perfusion, but this mechanism would not be expected to remain operative after CO is normalized.

Other possible mechanisms include decreased vascular reactivity to norepinephrine and other endogenous pressor substances, or decreased "structural" vascular resistance secondary to removal of sodium chloride and water from the blood vessel wall. These changes could result directly from the tissue

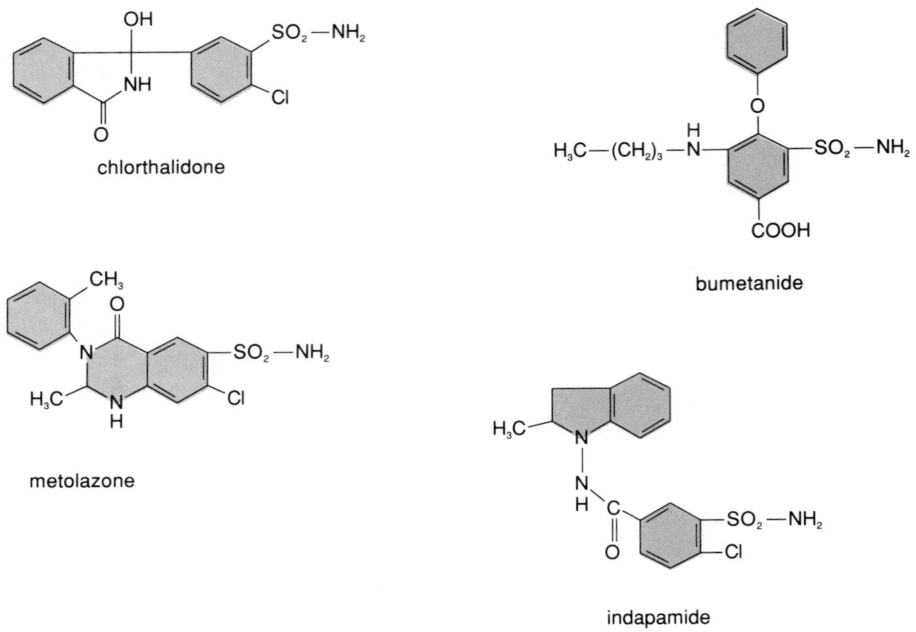

FIGURE 13-4   Some of the diuretics used in the treatment of hypertension. See Chapter 19 for structures of additional compounds listed in Table 13-5.

actions of diuretic drugs or indirectly from the generalized loss of sodium chloride and water from the body. The latter possibility seems probable in light of the observation that diuretics fail to lower blood pressure in patients who do not exhibit salt and water loss (i.e., patients on hemodialysis who have had a nephrectomy). On the other hand, the antihypertensive actions of diurectics do not parallel their efficacy in causing fluid loss, except in patients with renal insufficiency.

Finally, some diuretics relax vascular smooth muscle directly, but for most agents in this class vasodilation occurs only at doses well above the effective diuretic range. An exception is indapamide, which is a vasodilator at normal therapeutic doses, an action probably producing a major portion of its antihypertensive effect.

β-Adrenergic Receptor Blockers (β Blockers)

The common characteristic of β blockers is their ability to antagonize competitively the effects of the sympathetic effectors norepinephrine and epinephrine on cardiac β-adrenergic receptors. Although many β-adrenergic antagonists have other pharma-

cological effects, it is clear that blockade of cardiac β-adrenergic receptors is partially responsible for their ability to lower blood pressure. Compounds that exhibit selectivity for the β_1-subtype adrenergic receptors are effective antihypertensives; thus, one hypothesis is that all drugs in this class exert their effects on blood pressure via β_1-adrenergic receptor blockade.

The chemical structures of the β-blocking drugs used as antihypertensive agents are given in Figure 13-5 and in Chapter 10.

The details of secondary messenger systems of β-adrenergic receptors are given in Chapters 2 and 10.

Numerous reasons have been proposed to explain the antihypertensive response to administration of β blockers; none has achieved universal acceptance. In patients with "renin-dependent" hypertension (e.g., renovascular hypertension), a major portion of the blood pressure reduction caused by β blockers is due to inhibition of renin release secondary to blockade of β_1-adrenergic receptors present on renin-secreting juxtaglomerular cells in the kidney innervated by sympathetic nerves. Many hypertensive patients with low or normal plasma renin activity, however, also respond to β-blocker therapy. Thus therapeutic re-

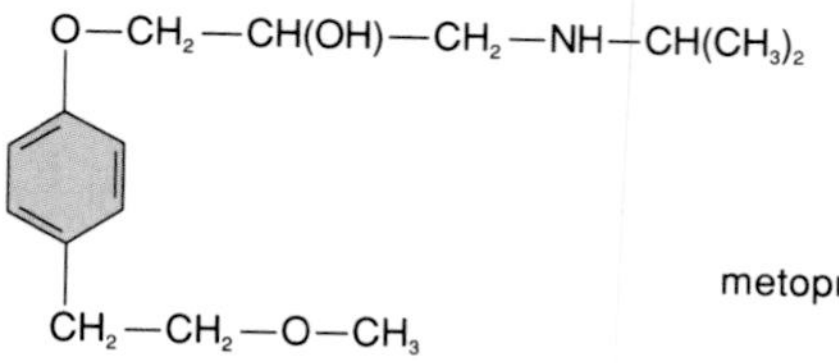

O—CH_2—CH(OH)—CH_2—NH—CH(CH_3)$_2$

CH_2—CH_2—O—CH_3

metoprolol

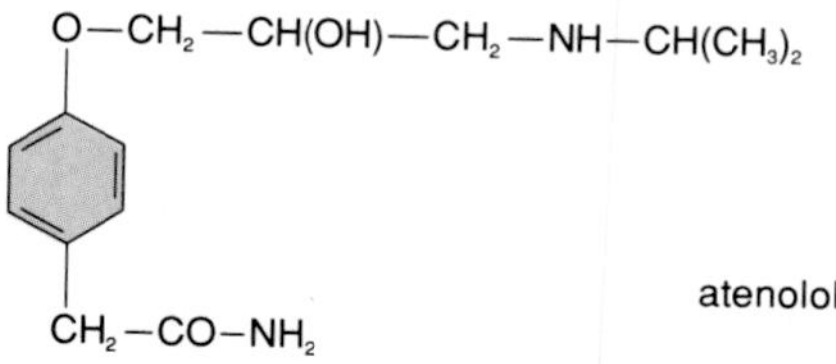

O—CH_2—CH(OH)—CH_2—NH—CH(CH_3)$_2$

CH_2—CO—NH_2

atenolol

CH(OH)—CH_2—NH—CH(CH_3)—CH_2—CH_2

—CO—NH_2

OH

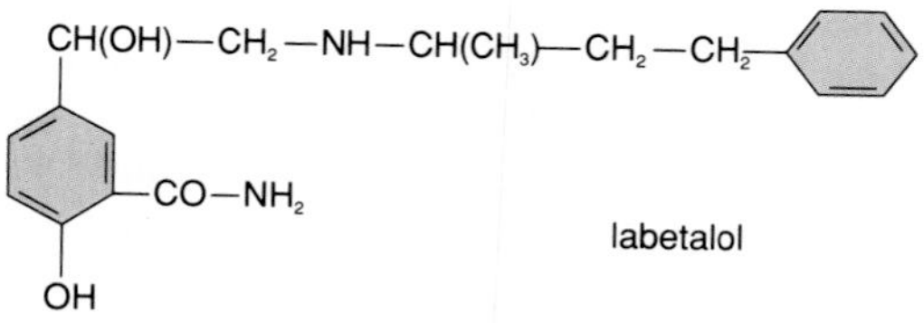

labetalol

FIGURE 13-5 Metoprolol and atenolol are highly selective blockers for β_1-adrenergic receptors. Other β blockers used in hypertension are not as selective for β_1-receptors; their structures are shown in Chapter 10. Labetalol also acts by blocking α-receptors. Propranolol is not selective for β_1-receptors but is the prototype β blocker.

sponse cannot be predicted based on pretreatment plasma renin values. Furthermore, β blockers such as pindolol, which have strong intrinsic sympathomimetic agonist activity, decrease blood pressure without affecting plasma renin activity.

Acute and chronic decreases in CO are observed in most studies employing β blockers in hypertensive patients, but in some studies CO is reported to return to normal over a period of days to weeks, while TPR also declines over the same time course. The decrease in TPR may be the result of long-term autoregulatory response to decreased tissue blood flow or to other effects of the drugs. However, some patients exhibit a rise in TPR after β-blockade, which has led to speculation that vascular α-receptors are activated (unopposed). For this reason β blockers are contraindicated in patients with peripheral vascular disease. An initial decrease in CO may therefore be necessary for the antihypertensive action of β blockers, but

alone it is not sufficient because CO declines similarly in patients whose blood pressure does not fall with administered β blockers.

The acute fall in blood pressure (hours) following β-blockade causes a reflex increase in plasma catecholamines, which is less than that produced by directly acting vasodilators. This fact may reflect an ability of β blockers to interfere with cardiovascular reflexes, or to inhibit release of norepinehrine from sympathetic nerve terminals by blocking a facilitatory prejunctional β_2-adrenergic receptor. However, not all β blockers inhibit baroreflexes or sympathetic neurotransmission; yet all lower blood pressure.

Some evidence such as reduced excretion of catecholomines suggests a CNS mediated sympathoinhibitory action for β blockers. Several of these drugs (e.g., propranolol) readily penetrate into the brain, and side effects attributable to perturbation of CNS processes are common with such agents. Studies in experimental animals also indicate that selective administration of β blockers into the cerebral ventricles lowers blood pressure at doses that are ineffective peripherally. Evidence against the hypothesis is that some drugs in this class do not readily penetrate into the brain after oral administration but retain antihypertensive efficacy. Furthermore, sympathetic neural activity is not reliably reduced by β blockers at clinically effective doses. It must be understood, however, that although brain penetration is minimal overall, selective access to the CNS at the loci of the circumventricular organs that lack a blood-brain barrier could contribute to the putative central antihypertensive action.

Labetalol is unique among β blockers in also possessing substantial α-adrenergic receptor blocking properties. This accounts for the greater blood pressure lowering ability of labetalol compared with other β blockers.

Centrally Acting Sympatholytics

Sympatholytics with central actions are thought to decrease blood pressure by causing a reduced sympathetic nerve firing rate; the locus of their action is within the CNS. The reduced sympathetic discharge is functionally selective because a hypotensive effect is obtained with only minimal impairment of baroreflexes. Drugs in this class include methyldopa, clonidine, and guanabenz. Reserpine also may act in part by this mechanism, but it will be discussed with the peripherally acting sympatholytics. The chemical structures and mechanism of action of the sympatholytics are discussed further in Chapter 10.

Clonidine and guanabenz are relatively selective agonists at α_2-adrenergic receptors (i.e., their interaction with α_1-adrenergic receptors is minimal, especially in the CNS). Both agents readily enter the brain after systemic administration. Evidence that blood pressure reduction occurs as a result of an effect of these substances on α_2-adrenergic receptors in the CNS includes findings that (1) pressure is lowered in experimental animals by low doses injected directly into the cerebral ventricles, into specific brain regions, or selectively into the arterial blood supply of the brain, and (2) the depressor response to peripherally and centrally administered clonidine or guanabenz can be attenuated by intracerebral injection of α_2-adrenergic receptor antagonists. The precise brain site (or sites) where α_2 agonists act to lower blood pressure is controversial but current evidence favors the ventrolateral medulla.

An endogenous clonidine-like material (clonidine-displacing substance) has been isolated from the brain of experimental animals. The clonidine-displacing substance appears to act in the ventrolateral medulla in a manner similar to clonidine, but at receptors that have high affinity for the imidazole moiety of clonidine. Guanabenz would not be expected to act at these receptors because it lacks an imidazole structure. The relative role of imidazole versus α_2-adrenergic receptors in the antihypertensive response to clonidine is thus unclear. Some studies indicate that the antihypertensive effect of clonidine may involve the release of endogenous opiate peptides. Clonidine has reasonable analgesic potency, and the depressor response to clonidine can be inhibited by the opioid antagonist naloxone. Finally, it is possible that under some circumstances activation of α_2-adrenergic receptors located on sympathetic nerve terminals may lead to inhibition of the release of norepinephrine during nerve activity.

Methyldopa is the drug in this class commonly employed clinically for reductions of blood pressure. Methyldopa (L-isomer) is a prodrug and must be converted in the CNS by dopa decarboxylase and dopamine-β-hydroxylase to active α-methylnorepinephrine (Figure 13-6) to exert an effect on blood pressure. Since α-methylnorepinephrine is a strong agonist at α_2-adrenergic receptors, it may act in a manner similar to clonidine and guanabenz. Similar

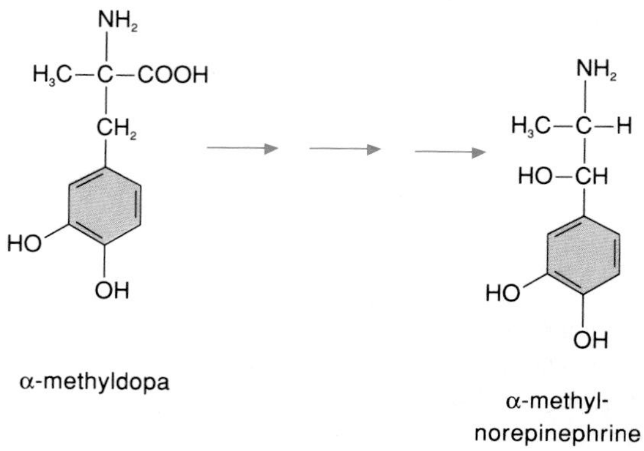

FIGURE 13-6   Activation of methyldopa to α-methylnorepinephrine. Detailed enzymatic systems are described in Chapter 10.

actions are found with the related metabolites α-methylepinephrine and α-methyldopamine. A peripheral action of methyldopa is unlikely because selective blockade of dopa decarboxylase in peripheral noradrenergic nerves does not influence the hypotensive response to methyldopa. As with clonidine, a potential site of action for methyldopa is within the nucleus of the solitary tract (NTS). This region contains interneurons that relay inhibitory information from baroreceptor terminals to excitatory vasomotor regions in the rostral ventral medulla. Activation of presynaptic α_2-adrenergic receptors in these interneurons inhibits sympathetic discharge. Noradrenergic innervation of the NTS provides the neural substrate for local synthesis and release of α-methylnorepinephrine and related amines.

Peripherally Acting Sympatholytics

Sympatholytics with peripheral action lower blood pressure by interfering with sympathetic neural control of cardiac and peripheral vascular function through effects produced on the sympathetic neuroeffector junction. Reserpine (Figure 13-7) blocks the uptake of dopamine and norepinephrine into storage granules of the sympathetic nerve terminal and subsequently depletes the terminal of neurotransmitter. Thus, a reduced release of transmitter occurs during terminal depolarization. Reserpine also acts centrally to decrease sympathetic outflow by an unknown mechanism. This could be related to depletion of norepinephrine or serotonin in the brain. Guanethidine and guanadrel inhibit exocytotic release of norepi-

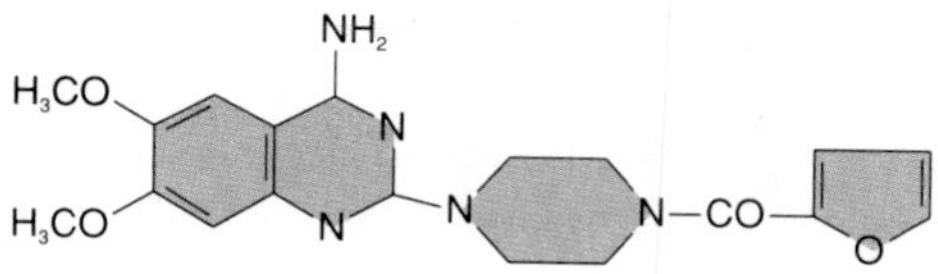

FIGURE 13-7   A peripherally acting sympatholytic (see Chapter 10 for structures of others).

FIGURE 13-8   Structures of antihypertensive drugs that act as direct vasodilators.

nephrine by a local anesthetic-like action on the nerve terminal. This requires uptake of the drugs by the nerve terminal catecholamine pump. Long-term treatment also results in depletion of transmitter from storage granules in peripheral sympathetic nerves. Guanethidine and guanadrel do not enter the brain.

Unlike the other agents in this class, prazosin (see Figure 13-7) acts at the postjunctional side of the sympathetic neuroeffector junction. It occupies α_1-adrenergic receptors selectively and blocks the effects mediated through this receptor of norepinephrine released from sympathetic nerves. Experimental data suggest that prazosin and other α_1 antagonists also can inhibit sympathetic nerve activity via a central mechanism.

The sympatholytic mechanisms are discussed in Chapter 10.

Calcium Channel Blocking Agents

The calcium channel blocking drugs decrease calcium entry into cells by binding to proteins of calcium channels in the cell membrane and thereby inhibit transmembrane calcium movement (see Chapter 16).

Orally Active Direct Vasodilators

Agents in this class (hydralazine and minoxidil) lower blood pressure by direct relaxation of arterial smooth muscle (see Figure 13-8 for structures). They differ from calcium channel blockers by different presumed cellular mechanisms of action, and by greater selectivity for arterial smooth muscles. Calcium channel antagonists do not show selectivity and affect both arterial and venous smooth muscle.

The cellular mechanism of vascular relaxation caused by hydralazine is not known, but may involve intracellular accumulation of cGMP. Administration of hydralazine to experimental animals also causes release of vasodilator prostaglandins and results in a decreased responsiveness to sympathetic nerve stimulation. It is not known if these effects contribute to

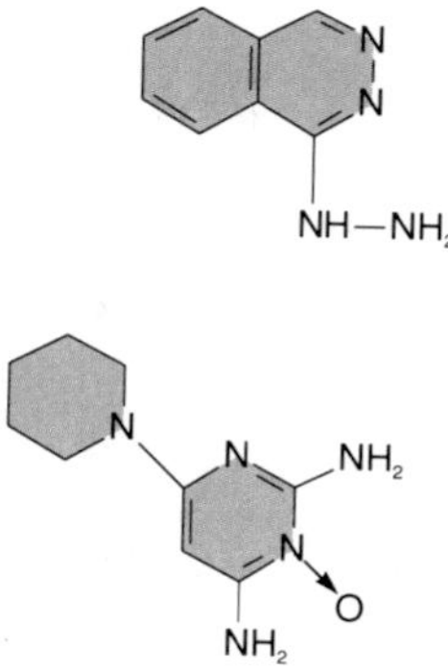

the hypotensive action of the drug clinically.

Minoxidil appears to cause vascular relaxation by increasing cellular potassium permeability, thus leading to potassium efflux from the cell, membrane hyperpolarization, and inhibition of stimulated calcium influx through receptor-operated calcium channels.

Angiotensin Converting Enzyme Inhibitors

The active component of the renin-angiotensin system, angiotensin II, is generated by the enzymatic conversion from the decapeptide angiotensin I, described earlier in this chapter. The enzyme catalyzing this reaction, converting enzyme (or kininase II) has a wide distribution in the body, but is found in highest activity in the endothelium of the pulmonary vasculature, probably because of the large length of the pulmonary capillaries. The converting enzyme inhibitors captopril, enalapril, and lisinopril (Figure 13-9) reversibly inhibit this enzyme. Although converting enzyme has a substantial number of physiological substrates that possess cardiovascular activity (or where the enzymatic products have cardiovascular activity) the hypotensive response to angiotensin converting enzyme inhibitors is the result of inhibition of angiotensin II formation, especially in hypertensive patients in whom circulating blood concentrations of this peptide are elevated.

When angiotensin II concentration in the plasma is relatively high (i.e., about 100 pg/ml) the peptide causes direct arterial constriction. Inhibition of angiotensin II formation reduces vasoconstriction and blood pressure falls. However, hypertensive subjects with lower, or even normal, plasma concentrations of

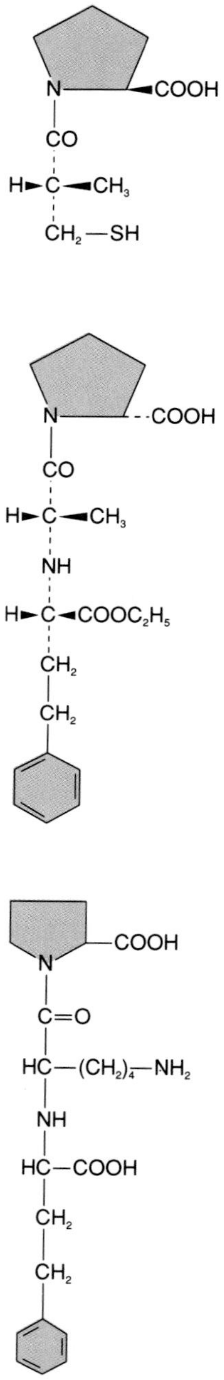

FIGURE 13-9   Converting enzyme inhibitors.

angiotensin II also exhibit a depressor response to converting enzyme inhibition. The mechanism of this effect is less clear. One possibility is that the converting enzyme inhibitors act by blocking local tissue generation of angiotensin II, and some evidence suggests that inhibition of vascular converting enzyme activity correlates temporally with the hypotensive response to converting enzyme inhibitors. Angiotensin II also can be produced by intrarenal renin-angiotensin, where the peptide exerts an antinatriurectic and antidiuretic effect. Inhibition of intrarenal angiotensin II formation by converting enzyme inhibitors could lower blood pressure by promoting salt and water excretion in a manner similar to that of the diuretic agents. A third possibility is that the converting enzyme inhibitors act through inhibition of brain converting enzyme. Brain tissue can generate angiotensin peptides independently, and in experimental animals an increase in intracerebral concentrations of angiotensin II causes an elevation in arterial pressure mediated through activation of the sympathetic nervous system. The converting enzyme inhibitors could decrease blood pressure by reducing the activity of the sympathetic nervous system in a manner similar to that of the centrally acting sympatholytic agents.

A final possibility to explain the depressor response to converting enzyme inhibitors in hypertensive subjects with normal circulating concentrations of angiotensin II is that such individuals are hyperresponsive to circulating angiotensin II. The blood-borne peptide is capable of increasing blood pressure by numerous mechanisms. These include direct vasoconstriction, renal sodium and water retention, release of aldosterone, and peripheral and central augmentation of sympathetic neural input to the cardiovascular system. Although hypertensive patients do not generally exhibit an increased sensitivity to the systemic vasoconstrictor effects of angiotensin II, heightened sensitivity of one or more of the indirect pressor mechanisms previously listed could lead to activation even by normal circulating amounts of angiotensin II.

Drugs for Hypertensive Emergencies

Under some clinical circumstances, blood pressure must be reduced rapidly but in a controlled fashion for a relatively short period of time (see box). Several of the antihypertensive agents already discussed are given parenterally for this purpose. Other drugs are used exclusively to achieve rapid blood pressure reduction, including the direct-acting vasodilators nitroprusside and diazoxide (Figure 13-10) and the short-acting ganglionic blocker trimethaphan.

CONDITIONS REQUIRING RAPID BLOOD PRESSURE REDUCTION
"Malignant" hypertension Pheochromocytoma Hypertensive encephalopathy Refractory hypertension of pregnancy Acute left ventricular failure Aortic dissection Coronary insufficiency Intracranial hemorrhage

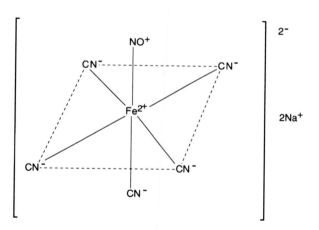

sodium nitroprusside

$$\left[Na_2(Fe(NO)(CN)_5) \right]$$

diazoxide

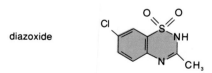

FIGURE 13-10 Rapid-acting antihypertensive drugs for emergency reduction of blood pressure.

Nitroprusside acts by increasing cGMP concentrations in vascular smooth muscle cells and thereby reducing intracellular calcium ion concentrations. Diazoxide, although related chemically to the thiazide diuretics, produces vasodilation by an unknown cellular mechanism of action. Trimethaphan is a reversible nicotinic receptor antagonist that blocks neurotransmission through all autonomic ganglia. Diazoxide is primarily an arterial vasodilator, whereas nitroprusside and trimethaphan produce equivalent relaxation of both arteries and veins.

 ## PHARMACOKINETICS

The pharmacokinetic parameters for most of the antihypertensive drugs are summarized in Table 13-2.

The diuretics are generally given orally. The onset of antihypertensive action occurs in 2 to 3 days with a plateau of action within 2 to 3 weeks. The β blockers also are administered orally, with labetalol also available for IV use. The antihypertensive effect usually is observed within a few hours.

Dosing schedules typically require more than one dose per day; although the long half-life of nadolol and a long-acting propranolol preparation enable these drugs to be used at a single dose per day.

The sympatholytic agents are administered orally with a rapid onset of action (few hours) for clonidine, guanabenz, guanadral, guanethidine, and prazosin. Methyldopa, a prodrug, requires several hours for onset of action because of the need for conversion to the active species; and reserpine takes 2 to 3 weeks for the full antihypertensive effect to develop.

The oral direct vasodilators, hydralazine and minoxidil, show a rapid onset of action. Minoxidil, a prodrug, is metabolized to the active form, minoxidil sulfate. The rate of metabolism of hydralazine to form the acetylated amine depends on the patient acetylator phenotype; there being basically two groups, fast and slow acetylators.

With the oral converting enzyme inhibitors the onset of action is rapid (minutes for captopril and hours for the prodrug enalapril).

Of the drugs used for emergency reduction of hypertensive conditions, diazoxide is usually given in repeated low dose IV injections to achieve the desired reduction in blood pressure. An effect occurs 1 to 5 minutes after dosing. The duration of effect varies

Table 13-2   Pharmacokinetic Parameters

Agent	Plasma $t_{1/2}$ (hour)	Disposition	Selectivity	Remarks
β BLOCKERS				
propranolol	2-3	M (100%)	$\beta_1\ \beta_2$	
metoprolol (oral and IV)	3-7	M (90%)	β_1 (first pass)	
nadolol	20-24	R (100%)	$\beta_1\ \beta_2$	
atenolol	6-7	R (100%)	β_1 (first pass)	
pindolol	3-4	M (60%-65%)	$\beta_1\ \beta_2$	
timolol	4	M (80%)	$\beta_1\ \beta_2$	
labetalol (oral and IV)	6-8	M (90%)	$\beta_1\ \beta_2\ \alpha_1\ \alpha_2$ (50% plasma protein bound, first pass)	
SYMPATHOLYTICS				
clonidine	12-16	M (45%)		
methyldopa	2-3	M (30%)		Given as prodrug
guanabenz	4-6	M (98%)		
reserpine	33	M		96% bound to plasma protein
prazosin	3-4	M (95%)		Highly bound to plasma protein
guanadrel	12	M (60%), R (40%)		
guanethidine	5 days	M (50%), R (50%)		High tissue binding
DIRECT VASODILATORS				
hydralazine	2-4	M (100%)		Acetylators vary
minoxidil	4-5	M (90%)		Active, eliminated via kidney; given as prodrug
CONVERTING ENZYME INHIBITORS				
captopril	1-2	M (5%), R (50%)		Absorption reduced by food
enalapril*	11	Active metabolite eliminated via kidney		Given as prodrug
lisinopril†	12-24	R (mainly)		

M, metabolism (% of drug disposed of via this route); *R*, renal elimination as unchanged drug (% via this route).
* Metabolized by deesterification to more active diacid enalaprilat (absorbed too slowly for direct use).
† Lysine derivative of enalapril.

considerably from hours to a day. Nitroprusside is given by continuous IV infusion; full effects occur in seconds and recovery takes place within a few minutes of terminating the infusion. Trimethaphan must be administered by continuous IV infusion; full response occurs in seconds and is greater in magnitude when the patient is upright. Recovery of blood pressure after trimethaphan infusion requires 10 to 60 minutes.

SIDE EFFECTS, CLINICAL PROBLEMS, AND TOXICITY

Diuretics are often used as adjuncts to other antihypertensive agents to prevent fluid retention, and diuretics potentiate the hypotensive effect of most other drugs. They are more effective in black than in white patients, perhaps because there is a high incidence of low renin hypertension among blacks.

Lower doses of diuretics are required to treat hypertension than to treat edema. Larger doses will not result in a greater blood pressure reduction but will simply increase the incidence and severity of side effects. There is concern that the hypokalemia frequently associated with diuretics may increase the incidence of ventricular arrhythmias. Monitoring of serum potassium concentration and the use of potassium supplements is often recommended. Additional details on the side effects of diuretics are found in Chapter 19.

β blockers are particularly effective in younger patients and in individuals with high plasma renin activity. White patients respond somewhat better to β blockers than do black patients. Side effects often observed with β-blocker therapy include nausea, anorexia, fatigue, dizziness, and bradycardia. Selective β₁ antagonists are preferable for use in patients with asthma, but any β blocker should be used with caution. Abrupt cessation of β blockers has been associated with tachycardia, angina pectoris, and (rarely) myocardial infarction. This may result from upregulation of β-adrenergic receptors with chronic β-blocker therapy.

Central acting sympatholytics (clonidine, guanabenz, or methyldopa) can be used alone in the treatment of hypertension, but are often used in combination with a diuretic. These drugs are notable for causing less orthostatic hypotension than many other antihypertensive agents. They do not impair renal function, and thus are suitable for hypertensive patients with renal insufficiency. Methyldopa is commonly used in pregnant women, in which long-term successful use has been documented. Side effects common to all three drugs are sedation, dry mouth, and dizziness. Methyldopa causes a positive direct Coombs test in 20% to 30% of patients and frank hemolytic anemia in 1%. The latter, but not the former, requires drug withdrawal. A special problem associated with clonidine (or with any centrally acting α₂-agonist) is a marked hypertensive response occurring in some patients after abrupt withdrawal of therapy. It can be counteracted or prevented with the use of peripherally acting sympatholytic agents.

Of the peripheral acting drugs, prazosin is used to treat mild to moderate hypertension, usually in conjunction with a diuretic. Guanadrel, and especially guanethidine and reserpine, are seldom used because of the frequent incidence of severe side effects.

Common side effects of reserpine are depression (including suicide), increased appetite, weight gain, sedation, and nasal congestion. Dizziness and weakness are side effects of prazosin and guanadrel. Side effects of guanethidine limit it to only occasional use in patients and include fluid retention, dizziness, weakness, retrograde ejaculation, impotence, and diarrhea.

The direct vasodilators hydralazine and minoxidil are used in combination with other drugs for the treatment of severe or resistant hypertension. Minoxidil is often effective in patients who do not respond to hydralazine. Relatively strong renal vasodilator activity makes these drugs particularly useful in patients with renal insufficiency.

The common side effects with hydralazine are headache, palpitations, dizziness, fatigue, tachycardia, and flushing. The incidence and severity of side effects with hydralazine use are greater in slow acetylators (see Chapter 5). A lupus-like syndrome has been observed in some patients taking hydralazine, mostly in slow acetylators taking high doses for long periods. The condition is reversible and necessitates discontinuation of the drug.

Common side effects of minoxidil are fluid retention, edema, palpitations, and abnormal hair growth. The latter effect limits compliance in patients and is being exploited to treat male-pattern baldness with topical application of the drug.

Angiotensin converting enzyme inhibitors. Captopril, enalapril, and lisinopril are effective for the treatment of hypertension in patients with normal or high plasma renin. Black subjects thus respond less predictably than white subjects. Combining converting enzyme inhibitors with diuretics, however, will lower blood pressure in the majority of patients and also reduce the incidence of diuretic-induced hypokalemia.

Common side effects observed in patients taking captopril are maculopapular rash, angioedema, cough, granulocytopenia, and diminished taste sensation. Similar side effects are observed with enalapril, although at a lower rate of incidence. Administration of converting enzyme inhibitors to patients with significant renal artery stenosis will occasionally precipitate acute renal failure.

With drugs used for hypertensive emergencies, side effects can be significant. The usual side effects of diazoxide are fluid retention, tachycardia, and hyperglycemia. Nitroprusside reacts with blood and tissue to release cyanide ion, which is converted to thiocyanate by the liver. Thiocyanate concentrations in blood should be monitored during chronic nitroprusside infusions because this metabolite can cause hypothyroidism or acute toxic psychosis. If liver disease is present, cyanide concentrations should be monitored. Other reversible side effects of nitroprusside include nausea, headache, abdominal cramping, and dizziness. Side effects of trimethaphan are those expected from ganglionic blockade, including mydriasis, cycloplegia, constipation, and urinary retention. Tachyphylaxis occurs within a day or two of the development of the hypotensive action of trimethaphan.

Although the goal of antihypertensive therapy is to reduce end-organ damage associated with chronically elevated blood pressure, the effects on other cardiovascular risk factors must be considered. The end-organ damage is not related exclusively to blood pressure level. If an antihypertensive drug effectively lowers blood pressure but increases the impact of other risk factors for cardiovascular disease, the benefit of therapy will be reduced accordingly. This scenario may explain the apparent failure of thiazide diuretics to decrease coronary artery disease in large hypertensive populations, despite their ability to effect a significant reduction in blood pressure. Specifically, potassium-losing diuretics caused increments in total low density and very low density lipoprotein cholesterol, and in total triglyceride content of blood of patients receiving these drugs long-term. Although a causal relationship between blood lipid changes and the failure of diuretics to decrease coronary artery disease is not established, it would seem prudent to consider the influence of antihypertensive agents on the blood lipid profile and other risk factors when choosing a drug for the individual patient.

Other cardiovascular risk factors that can be affected by antihypertensive drugs include plasma glucose, potassium, and uric acid concentrations. There is interpatient variability in the response of these metabolites to antihypertensive drugs, so that therapeutic generalizations are difficult. Nonetheless, thiazide diuretics appear most likely to cause pressure-independent changes in cardiovascular risk, whereas calcium channel antagonists and converting enzyme inhibitors may actually improve the metabolic risk profile. Nonselective β-adrenergic receptor blockers have been shown to reduce the risk of sudden death during

---

CLINICAL PROBLEMS

METHYLDOPA

Gives positive direct Coombs test (usually but not always false)

Accumulates in patients with impaired renal function

β BLOCKERS

Must be used with caution in patients with bronchial asthma

Abrupt stoppage can cause cardiovascular problems

CLONIDINE

Sudden withdrawal of drug produces rebound hypertension

Causes CNS side effects

RESERPINE

Interacts with MAO inhibitors

Must be used with caution in patients with peptic ulcers

CAPTOPRIL

Accumulates in patients with impaired renal function

GUANADREL

Interacts with tricyclic antidepressants

THIAZIDE DIURETICS

Causes potassium and magnesium loss

Increases cholesterol concentrations

Can cause dysrhythmias

---

or after myocardial infarction in hypertensive patients. The mechanism is presumed to be protection against catecholamine-induced ventricular fibrillation. The problems are summarized in the box.

REFERENCES

Bauer JH: Role of angiotensin converting enzyme inhibitions in essential and renal hypertension, Am J Med 75:43, 1984.

Frolich ED: Essential hypertension, Med Clin North Am 5:785, 1987.

McMahon FG: Management of essential hypertension: the new low dose era, ed. 2, Mount Kisco, New York, 1984, Futura Publishing Co.

TRADENAMES

In addition to generic and fixed combination preparations, the following tradenamed materials are available in the United States. (See Chapter 19 for diuretics, Chapter 10 for additional β blockers, and Chapter 16 for calcium channel blockers.)

SOME β BLOCKERS

Inderal, propranolol
Lopressor, metoprolol
Normodyne, labetalol
Tenormin, atenolol
Trandate, labetalol

SYMPATHOLYTICS

Aldomet, methyldopa
Catapres, clonidine
Hylorel, guanadrel
Ismelin, guanethidine
Minipres, prazosin
Serpasil, reserpine
Wytensin, guanabenz

CONVERTING ENZYME INHIBITOR

Capoten, captopril
Prinivil, Zestril, Lisinopril
Vasotec, enalapril

DIRECT VASODILATORS

Apresoline, hydralazine
Loniten, minoxidil

EMERGENCY TYPES

Arfonad, trimethaphan
Hyperstat, diazoxide

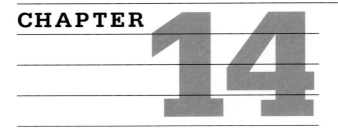

CHAPTER 14

Cardiac Electrophysiology and Antidysrhythmic Agents

<table>
<tr><td colspan="2" align="center">ABBREVIATIONS</td></tr>
<tr><td>AV</td><td>atrioventricular</td></tr>
<tr><td>GI</td><td>gastrointestinal</td></tr>
<tr><td>IV</td><td>intravenous, intravenously</td></tr>
<tr><td>pH</td><td>logarithm of the reciprocal of the hydrogen ion concentration</td></tr>
<tr><td>SA</td><td>sinoatrial</td></tr>
<tr><td>$t_{1/2}$</td><td>half-life</td></tr>
<tr><td>$\dot{V}_{max}$</td><td>maximum rate of depolarization</td></tr>
</table>

MAJOR DRUGS

antidysrhythmics that block myocardial Na^+ channels
sympatholytic antidysrhythmic agents
β-adrenergic blockers

 ## THERAPEUTIC OVERVIEW

Cardiac dysrhythmias are disorders of rate, rhythm, impulse generation, or conduction of electrical impulses within the heart. They often are associated with coronary artery disease, including myocardial infarction and atherosclerotic heart disease. Dysrhythmias disrupt the normal sequence of myocardial activation and can seriously compromise the mechanical efficiency of the heart, reducing cardiac output. As a result, dysrhythmias can be life-threatening events that require immediate intervention.

In the past 40 years, experimental techniques have allowed investigators to better understand the cellular basis of the electrocardiogram, as well as the basic electrical properties of cardiac cells. These kinds of studies have provided an understanding of the many ionic currents and membrane channels that regulate cell behavior. Studies of the effects of clinically effective antidysrhythmic drugs on these specific membrane channels have led to an understanding of the mechanism of action of antidysrhythmic agents with individual ionic channels at a molecular level. At a higher organizational level, comprehension of the electrical properties of the different types of cardiac cells that compose the specialized electrical conduction system of the heart and how these are modified by a variety of therapeutic agents is the basis for understanding the normal electrocardiogram and its alterations in disease states or during drug therapy.

The electrical activity of individual cardiac cells depends on the region of the heart from which cells are derived (i.e., SA node, atrium, AV node, His-Purkinje system, ventricle). In addition, electrical activity may be modified by changes in extracellular pH and ion concentration, as occur during ischemia. Electrical activity arises as a result of differences in ion (Na^+, K^+, Ca^{++}) concentrations across the cell membrane caused by metabolism-dependent processes (e.g., the Na^+-K^+ pump). The membrane potential thus established is modulated by ion-selective membrane channels that open and close in a voltage- and time-dependent manner to allow ions to flow

Electrically active cardiac cells
  Nonpacemaker
  Pacemaker
  Na^+, K^+, and Ca^{++} ion gradients and intra-
    cellular/extracellular potential difference
  Electrocardiogram
Therapy with drugs
  Modify ion fluxes: block Na^+, K^+, Ca^{++} chan-
    nels while possibly modifying β-adrener-
    gic receptor activated processes

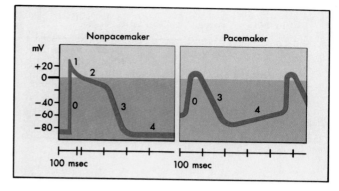

FIGURE 14-1   Phases of action potential (with respect to potential on extracellular side of cell membrane) in a nonpacemaker cell (NP) and in a pacemaker cell (P). Numbers
refer to phases. NP cell: *0*, rapid depolarization; *1*, initial
repolarization; *2*, action potential plateau; *3*, repolarization;
4, resting potential. P cell: *0*, rapid depolarization; *3*, plateau
and repolarization; *4*, slow diastolic depolarization (pacemaker potential).

through them down their respective electrochemical
gradients. As in the other excitable tissues, the action
potential thus generated is propagated throughout
the myocardium. Dysrhythmias result from disorders
in impulse formation, its conduction, or both. Many
antidysrhythmic drugs act by blocking myocardial
Na^+ or Ca^{++} ion channels or by prolonging the time
for these channels to recover from activation. Other
antidysrhythmic compounds act by modulating the
magnitude and time course of potassium currents
responsible for action potential repolarization and
maintenance of the diastolic membrane potential.
These concepts are summarized in the box.

MECHANISMS OF ACTION

Cardiac Electrophysiology

Membrane Potentials An understanding of the
molecular mechanisms requires knowledge of cardiac
electrophysiology. To accomplish this goal, ionic currents from nonpacemaker-type cardiac cells (ventricular myocardium) and pacemaker-type cardiac cells
(sinus node) are considered. Although the sinus node
constitutes a dominant pacemaker region of the heart
under normal conditions, many other regions (e.g.,
the His-Purkinje system, which comprises the specialized ventricular conducting system) are also capable of spontaneous rhythmic activity. Action potentials and ionic currents in these cells can range
from similarity to sinus nodal cells to showing distinctly different properties.

Figure 14-1 illustrates action potentials recorded
from a typical nonpacemaker cell (NP) and a typical
pacemaker cell (P) using glass microelectrodes. In the
nonpacemaker cell, the resting membrane potential
is usually in the range of -80 to -90 mV with respect
to the extracellular medium. There is no spontaneous
electrical discharge because the resting potential is
stable. Excitation of this cell by intracellular current
injection or by local current flow from an adjoining
cell can elicit a propagating action potential. This
action potential is described as having the five following distinct phases:
  1. Phase 0, rapid depolarization
  2. Phase 1, initial repolarization
  3. Phase 2, action potential plateau
  4. Phase 3, final repolarization
  5. Phase 4, return to a stable diastolic potential
In the pacemaker cell, only three distinct periods are
usually described: phase 0, rapid depolarization;
phase 3, plateau and repolarization; and phase 4, slow
diastolic depolarization (often called the *pacemaker
potential*), which culminates in initiation of another
spontaneous depolarization.

**Ionic Basis of the Cardiac Resting Membrane
Potential** The membrane potential of a cardiac cell
at any given time is determined by the activity of the
electrogenic Na^+, K^+-pump and the permeability of
the membrane to various ions (Table 14-1). The permeability involves the diffusion of ions across the

Table 14-1 Typical Ion Concentrations			
Ion	**Extracellular**	**Intracellular**	**Approximate Equilibrium Potential (mV)***
Na$^+$	145 mM	10 mM	+50
K$^+$	4 mM	150 mM	−90
Ca^{++}	2 mM	10^{-7} M	+140

*As calculated from Nernst equation.

membrane through various ion-selective channels. The reader is referred to an appropriate physiology text for the genesis of the resting membrane potential.

Ionic Basis of the Action Potential

Phase 0   Injection of current into a cardiac cell or local current flow from an adjoining cell can cause the membrane potential to depolarize. If the amplitude of depolarization is sufficient, the threshold potential for initiation of an action potential may be achieved. This threshold potential is related to the opening of active membrane channels, which may contribute to further depolarization and initiation of an action potential. This period of rapid depolarization in which the membrane potential changes from negative inside to positive inside relative to the outside is termed *phase 0* of the action potential. Which membrane channels are involved in mediating the depolarization depends on the type of cardiac cell and the level of diastolic potential. In a nonpacemaker cell, an increase in conductance of Na$^+$ ions results in phase 0 depolarization. (The opening of membrane channels and the flow of ions through these channels can be described as a *conductance change*.) Because conductance is the reciprocal of resistance, an increase in membrane conductance is equivalent to a decrease in membrane resistance. The magnitude of the increase in conductance to Na$^+$ is related to the maximum rate of depolarization (dV/dT_{max} or $\dot{V}_{max}$) during phase 0. As the membrane is depolarized, there is also Ca^{++} conductance, which in nonpacemaker cells occurs during phase 0, normally contributing a few percent to $\dot{V}_{max}$. These types of action potentials are often referred to as *fast responses*, because $\dot{V}_{max}$ can be on the order of several hundred volts per second.

In pacemaker cells, such as those found in the sinus node, conductance to Na$^+$ increases very little during phase 0. In these cells, phase 0 is mediated almost entirely by increased conductance of Ca^{++}

ions. These types of action potential are often referred to as *slow responses*, with $\dot{V}_{max}$ in the range of 1 to 20 V/sec.

Ion channels may operate as a function of membrane voltage and time. The voltage and time dependence of membrane currents through specific populations of ion channels is characteristic. Na$^+$ channels open at different membrane voltages than Ca^{++} channels, and the kinetics of the currents through these two channels are quite different. It is currently believed that there are physical structures that comprise portions of the channel protein that act as molecular gates to regulate the opening and closing of the channel, as discussed in Chapter 2. In the case of Na$^+$ channels, an activation gate and an inactivation gate exist to regulate the flow of Na$^+$ through the channel. As a result of the operation of these gates, Na$^+$ channels are thought to exist in at least three distinct states during the cardiac action potential, as shown in Figure 14-2. At the resting potential, the majority of the Na$^+$ channels are in a resting state, available for activation. On depolarization of the membrane potential to a level near the activation threshold for Na$^+$ channels, most channels become activated (gate I open), allowing Na$^+$ ions to flow into the cell to cause a rapid depolarization during phase 0. Very quickly, Na$^+$ channels become inactivated (gate II closes), limiting the time for Na$^+$ entry to a few milliseconds or less.

Phase 1   Near the end of phase 0, the action potential overshoot occurs. This is the most positive potential achieved during the action potential and represents an abrupt transition between the end of depolarization and the onset of repolarization. This phase of initial repolarization is due to two factors: the inactivation of the inward Na$^+$ current and the activation of a transient outward current. The transient outward current was thought to involve activation of a chloride current; however, recent evidence has shown that this is at least partially carried by K$^+$.

Phase 2   The plateau phase of the cardiac action potential is perhaps one of its most distinguishing features. In marked contrast to action potentials recorded in nerves and other types of cells, the cardiac action potential has a relatively long duration of 200 to 500 msec, depending on the type of cell (see Figure 14-1). The plateau results from a voltage-dependent decrease in potassium conductance (the inward rectifier) and is maintained by the influx of Ca^{++} through Ca^{++} channels that inactivate slowly at positive membrane potentials. During this phase there also is a

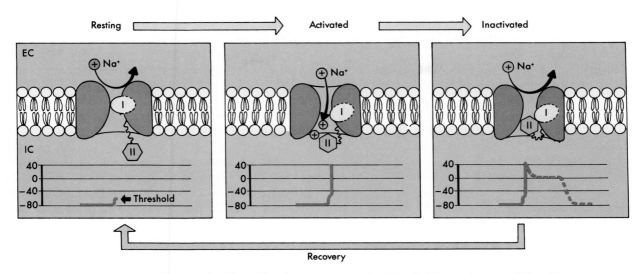

FIGURE 14-2   Postulated conformational arrangements of cardiac Na^+ channels compatible with concept of resting, activated, and inactivated states. Transitions between resting, activated, and inactivated states is dependent on membrane potential and time. Activation gate is shown as I and inactivation gate as II. Potentials typical for each state are shown under each channel schematic as a function of time. *EC*, Extracellular; *IC*, intracellular.

slow activation of another outward K^+ current, the delayed rectifier, which nearly balances the maintained influx of Ca^{++}. As a result of the offsetting effect of these two currents, there is only a small change in potential during the plateau, since the net conductance change is small. With time, the slowly increasing magnitude of K^+ current begins to dominate and this triggers repolarization, or phase 3.

Phase 3   The repolarization phase results from a combination of two factors: inactivation of the plateau Ca^{++} current and increase in the magnitude of the plateau-delayed rectifier K^+ current.

Phase 4   In a nonpacemaker cell, phase 4 is characterized by return of the membrane potential to the resting potential of the cell. It depends on an increase in the conductance of the potassium channels. At this time during diastole, the potential is relatively stable. In a pacemaker cell, however, there is a slow depolarization during diastole that brings the membrane potential into the threshold range for activation of a regenerative inward current, which will initiate a new action potential (see Figure 14-1). This period of diastolic depolarization is often called *phase 4 depolarization* or simply the *pacemaker potential*. In a cell in the sinus node region, phase 4 depolarization brings the membrane potential to a level near the threshold for activation of the inward Ca^{++} current.

Phase 4 depolarization is the result of the time-dependent recovery and activation of several ion selective channels. The final repolarization phase of the action potential results from activation of the outward plateau K^+ current. This current is activated at positive membrane potentials. As repolarization proceeds, this current begins to decline or deactivate. Decline of this outward current is thought to occur during phase 4 and to significantly influence the time course of the pacemaker potential. A declining K^+ current in the presence of a background leakage current of Na^+ may account for diastolic depolarization. Activation of the Ca^{++} and a nonselective inward current may also play a role.

Mechanisms Underlying Cardiac Dysrhythmias

Most arrhythmias are thought to result from disorders of impulse formation, impulse conduction, or a combination of both. A number of factors are believed to be involved in precipitating cardiac dysrhythmias: ischemia with resulting pH and electrolyte abnormalities, excessive myocardial fiber stretch, excessive discharge of or sensitivity to autonomic transmitters, or exposure to foreign chemicals or toxic substances. There is a 80% to 90% occurrence of dysrhythmias associated with myocardial infarction, 20% to 50% with general anesthesia, and 10% to 20% with digitalis therapy.

Disorders of impulse formation can involve (1) no change in pacemaker site (e.g., sinus bradycardia or tachycardia) or (2) a change in pacemaker site involving the development of an ectopic pacemaker. Several factors might lead to the development of an ectopic pacemaker. Ectopic activity might arise due to the emergence of a latent pacemaker. Many cells of the specialized conduction system are capable of rhythmic spontaneous activity. Normally these latent pacemakers are prevented from spontaneously discharging as a result of the dominance of the SA nodal pacemaker cells. Under some conditions, a latent pacemaker might become dominant due to abnormal slowing of the SA rate, or due to abnormal acceleration of the latent pacemaker rate. Ectopic pacemaker activity might result from a current of injury. Myocardial cells that are damaged by ischemia or hypoxia become depolarized and may be located proximal to normally polarized tissue. Two areas of cells with different membrane potentials may cause current to flow between adjacent regions, which might depolarize normally quiescent tissue into a range of potentials where spontaneous activity is initiated. Finally the

development of oscillatory after-depolarizations can initiate spontaneous activity in normally quiescent tissue. These after-depolarizations can occur at the end of phase 3 (Figure 14-3) and, if large enough in amplitude, reach threshold and initiate a burst of triggered spontaneous activity. Toxic concentrations of digitalis or norepinephrine can initiate this type of activity.

Disorders of impulse conduction can be grouped into those not involving reentry and those involving a reentrant circuit. Differing degrees of nodal block involve slowed conduction, usually without reentry. Slowed conduction with reentry can lead to the development of circus movement within some regions of the heart. Figure 14-4 shows an example of a hypothetical reentry circuit. For circus activity to develop, a region of unidirectional block must exist and the conduction time around the alternative pathway must exceed the effective refractory period of the tissue adjacent to the site of block. Before the development of unidirectional block (Figure 14-4, *A*), im-

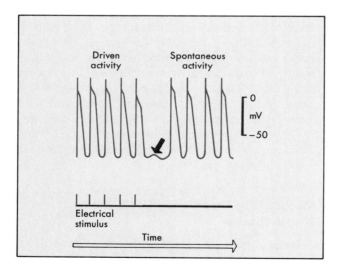

FIGURE 14-3 Development of oscillatory delayed after-depolarization *(arrow)* that leads to spontaneous activity, as observed with cardiac glycosides. First five action potentials were elicited by electrical stimuli *(bottom trace)*, followed by an after-depolarization, which was subthreshold initially, but attained threshold subsequently, leading to spontaneous discharges.

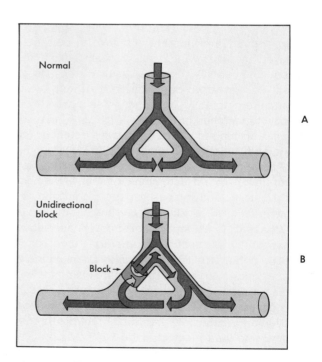

FIGURE 14-4 Hypothetical reentry circuit. **A,** Normally electrical excitation branches around the circuit and becomes extinguished due to collision. **B,** An area of unidirectional block develops in one of the branches, allowing excitation of the blocked area by an impulse travelling from the opposite direction. This can lead to reexcitation and reentry.

pulse propagation initially branches as a result of the anatomical properties of the circuit. Some of these impulses collide and extinguish around the other side of the branch point. If an area of unidirectional block develops, impulses around the branch do not collide and extinguish but may reexcite tissue proximal to the site of block, establishing a circular pathway for continuous reentry (Figure 14-4, B). A long reentry pathway, slow conduction, and a short effective refractory period are factors that will favor the development of reentry circuits.

Specific Drugs

General Antidysrhythmic Drugs In the normal heart, antidysrhythmic agents have minimal effects on automaticity and conduction velocity at therapeutic concentrations; however, at toxic concentrations, they can depress automaticity and conduction velocity and even be arrhythmogenic. Because dysrhythmias usually involve abnormal automaticity or conduction, most antidysrhythmic agents seem to selectively depress areas exhibiting abnormal pacemaker activity or conduction, while having minimal effects on normal healthy tissue. Conditions such as hypoxia, metabolic poisoning, ischemia, or elevated extracellular K^+ are known to precipitate dysrhythmias. All of these conditions depolarize myocardial cells. Therefore one possible mechanism for the selectivity of antidysrhythmic agents is that they cause a greater degree of depression in cells that are depolarized, compared to normally polarized cells.

Most antidysrhythmic agents block myocardial Na^+ or Ca^{++} channels in a state-dependent manner. That is, they bind with a higher affinity to activated or inactivated channels than to resting channels. In addition, they prolong the time required for channels to recover from inactivation and cycle back into the resting state. This is shown schematically in Figure 14-5. As a result, cells that become depolarized will have more channels in the inactivated state and will bind antidysrhythmic compounds with a higher affinity. This provides an explanation for their ability to selectively depress depolarized cells.

In normally polarized cells, they may also exhibit some selectivity for cells that are firing at abnormally fast rates. The basis for this selectivity might be due to the prolongation of the recovery of inactivated channels. This is believed to account for the phenomenon of "frequency-dependent block." Cells discharg-

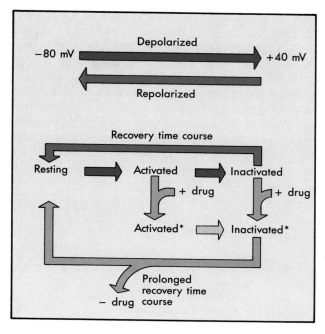

FIGURE 14-5   State-dependent binding of antidysrhythmic drugs to cardiac Na^+ channels. Preferential binding occurs to the activated and inactivated states of the sodium channel, and recovery from inactivation is prolonged in the presence of these drugs.

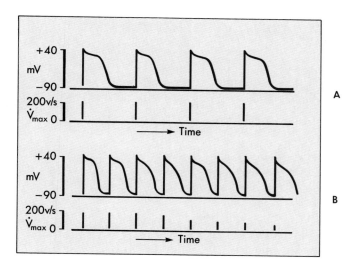

FIGURE 14-6   Frequency-dependent block of $\dot{V}_{max}$ by an antidysrhythmic drug. **A,** Cell is stimulated at relatively low frequency in presence of antidysrhythmic drug and $\dot{V}_{max}$ is not affected (*second trace from top*). **B,** At faster stimulation frequency, there is a progressive reduction of $\dot{V}_{max}$.

ing at normal rates will be little affected by an antidysrhythmic agent if the diastolic interval between action potentials is longer than the drug-modified recovery time course of inactivated channels (Figure 14-6, *A*). However, for an ectopic pacemaker discharging at an abnormally high rate, channels will be selectively blocked, as evidenced by a reduction of $\dot{V}_{max}$, if the diastolic interval between action potentials is shorter than the drug-modified recovery time course of inactivated channels (Figure 14-6, *B*).

There is no universally accepted classification scheme for antidysrhythmic agents. One scheme widely used by clinicians classifies agents that depress myocardial Na^+ channels and hence reduce $\dot{V}_{max}$ into class I, those that have sympathetic blocking actions into class II, agents that prolong action potential duration and refractoriness into class III, and agents with Ca^{++} channel blocking properties into class IV. Unfortunately, depending on dose, a number of agents exhibit multiple classes of action. A slight variation of this scheme is to classify agents according to their major actions on ionic currents underlying the cardiac action potential. The classification used here includes class III with class II drugs.

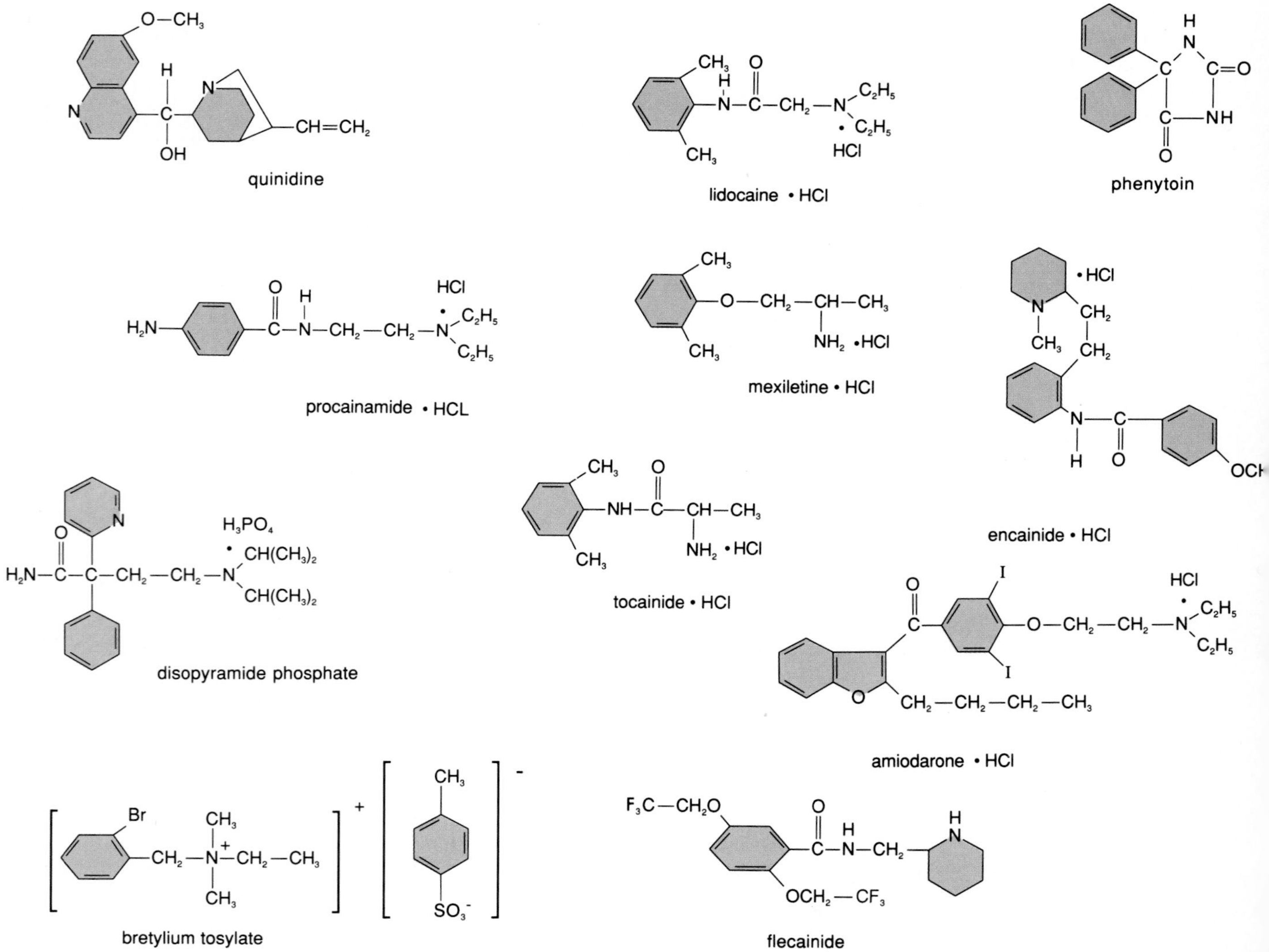

FIGURE 14-7   Structures of Na^+ channel-blocking antidysrhythmic drugs.

Antidysrhythmics that Block Myocardial Na⁺ Channels The structures of these drugs are shown in Figure 14-7.

Quinidine Quinidine is an optical isomer of quinine and is commonly used as an orally active antidysrhythmic agent. It will reduce $\dot{V}_{max}$ of cardiac action potentials in a frequency dependent manner by its ability to preferentially block activated Na⁺ channels. This effect can occur for Na⁺-dependent action potentials in the atrium, ventricle, and His-Purkinje system. These actions are often described as "local anesthetic properties" of the drug and often manifest as a reduction in membrane responsiveness, which is an alteration in the relationship between $\dot{V}_{max}$ of the action potential and the resting membrane potential. Many other antidysrhythmic agents that block Na⁺ channels produce a similar hyperpolarizing shift in the membrane responsiveness relation (Figure 14-8).

Quinidine also slows pacemaker activity by depressing the rate of phase 4 depolarization in SA nodal cells and especially in ectopic pacemakers. In addition, repolarization is prolonged and the effective refractory period lengthened in the atrium, ventricle, and His-Purkinje system. The effect on action potential duration is probably related to blockade of K⁺ channels involved in mediating repolarization. The lengthening of the effective refractory period is due to a combination of effects on myocardial Na⁺ and K⁺ channels.

Procainamide and disopyramide The electrophysiological effects of procainamide and disopyramide are nearly identical to those of quinidine. These agents depress membrane responsiveness of Na⁺-dependent action potentials by specifically blocking activated myocardial Na⁺ channels.

Lidocaine Lidocaine is a local anesthetic agent that has been used as an antidysrhythmic agent since the late 1940s. It depresses membrane responsiveness primarily in cells in the ventricular myocardium and the His-Purkinje system. Unlike quinidine, lidocaine blocks activated and inactivated Na⁺ channels. This additional interaction with the inactivated state of Na⁺ channels might explain the relative selectivity of this agent for cells with longer action potential durations, which are depolarized for longer periods of time or depolarized due to ischemia or digitalis toxicity. As a result, atrial cells seem less sensitive to concentrations of lidocaine, which reduce $\dot{V}_{max}$ in ventricular cells or depolarized cells. At therapeutic concentrations, lidocaine has minimal effects on normal ventricular myocardial cells or cells in the specialized conduction system but significantly depresses damaged or depolarized cells.

Mexiletine and tocainide are chemically related derivatives of lidocaine that are orally active. Their electrophysiological effects, antidysrhythmic spectrum, and side effects are similar to lidocaine. They are resistant to the first-pass hepatic metabolism that occurs with lidocaine.

Phenytoin Phenytoin (diphenylhydantoin) was introduced in the 1930s as an anticonvulsive agent and has been used as an antidysrhythmic agent since the 1950s. Many of the electrophysiological actions are similar to those of lidocaine. It depresses membrane responsiveness to a greater extent in ventricular myocardium and the His-Purkinje system than in the atrium. In addition to blocking myocardial Na⁺ channels there is evidence that phenytoin may also block myocardial Ca⁺⁺ channels.

Encainide and flecainide Encainide depresses membrane responsiveness in Purkinje and ventricular cells and produces a slight shortening of action potential duration without significant alterations in refractory period. With flecainide the conduction velocity is slowed as a result of its ability to depress membrane responsiveness.

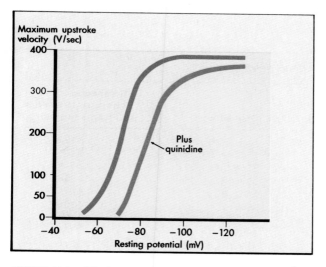

FIGURE 14-8 Maximum upstroke velocity (dV/dt_{max} or $\dot{V}_{max}$) of action potential during phase 0 as influenced by resting membrane potential. This relationship is called *membrane responsiveness*. Plot to the left is in the absence of drugs. Addition of many antidysrhythmic agents such as quinidine shifts the curve to more negative resting potentials (hyperpolarizing direction).

Amiodarone Like lidocaine, amiodarone preferentially blocks inactivated myocardial Na^+ channels and therefore is more effective in depressing conduction in cells that are depolarized or have a longer action potential duration. In addition, it prolongs the action potential duration, presumably because of its ability to also block myocardial K^+ channels. It has been reported that amiodarone blocks myocardial Ca^{++} channels and has α- and β-adrenergic blocking activity. It is unclear which action is responsible for its antiarrhythmic activity.

Other investigational drugs Other drugs that have myocardial Na^+ channel blocking properties and are under investigation as potential antidysrhythmics include: ajmaline, aprindine, cibenzoline, ethacizin, lorcainide, propafenone, and recainam.

Sympatholytic Antidysrhythmic Agents

Propranolol and Other β-Adrenergic Blockers
The antidysrhythmic properties of β-adrenergic antagonists such as propranolol are due to two major effects: (1) blockade of myocardial β-adrenergic receptors (β_1-receptors), thereby preventing or antagonizing the actions of endogenous catecholamines, and (2) direct membrane effects, which relate to the ability to block at higher concentrations myocardial Na^+ channels and depress membrane responsiveness "quinidine-like effect." Propranolol exhibits direct membrane effects in atrium, ventricles, and the His-Purkinje system. In addition, it slows SA nodal and ectopic pacemaker automaticity and slows AV nodal conduction velocity by virtue of its ability to block intrinsic sympathetic activity. However, some of these effects may also be due to direct membrane actions of the drug. Propranolol produces a small prolongation of the action potential duration and refractoriness that is greater in the atrium than in ventricular tissue. The structures of these drugs are described in Chapters 10 and 13.

Bretylium Bretylium has indirect and direct effects on the heart; it is concentrated in adrenergic nerve terminals and interferes with the release of catecholamines. Initially, release occurs but then is decreased. Part of bretylium's action in the heart is mediated by this release and subsequent block. These are the indirect effects of the drug.

The major direct effect of bretylium is prolongation of action potential duration and refractoriness in atrium, ventricle, and the His-Purkinje system.

Calcium Channel Blocking Drugs These drugs are discussed in Chapter 16.

PHARMACOKINETICS

The pharmacokinetic parameters of antidysrhythmic drugs are summarized in Table 14-2. Additional β-blocker pharmacokinetic considerations are discussed in Chapters 10 and 13. Similarly, the

Table 14-2   Pharmacokinetic Parameters of Antidysrhythmic Agents

Drugs	Plasma Protein Bound (%)	$t_{1/2}$ (hour unless otherwise noted)	Disposition	Therapeutic Concentration Range in Plasma (μg/ml)
quinidine (O, I)	80	5-7	M/R (50%)	2-5
procainamide (O, I)	15	2.5-5	M (20%)/R (50%)	4-10
disopyramide (O)	35-65	4.5	M (30%)/R (50%)	2-5
lidocaine (I)	60	1-2	M (90%)/R (10%)	10-20
mexiletine (O)	50-60	9-11	M/R (20%)	0.5-2
tocainide (O)	50	11-17	M/R (40%)	4-10
phenytoin (O, I)	70-95	22	M (90%)/R	10-20
encainide (O)	70	—	M/R	
flecainide (O)	40	13	M (60%)/R (30%)	0.2-1
amiodarone (O, I)	96	20-100 days	M/bile	1-2.5
propranolol (O, I)	90-96	4-6	M	40-100
metoprolol (O, I)	12	3-7	M	
acebutolol (O)	26	8-13	M/R	
bretylium (I)	0	8-13	R (100%)	
verapamil (O, I)	90	3-7	M/R	

O, Oral; *I*, IV; *M*, hepatic metabolism; *R*, renal elimination as unchanged drug (percent by this pathway, if known).

pharmacokinetics of calcium channel blocking drugs are found in Chapter 16.

Quinidine is readily absorbed from the gut. Both hepatic and renal functions need to be assessed to prevent the accumulation of toxic concentrations (above 8 μg/ml) in the plasma.

Lidocaine is inactive when administered orally because of the large first pass metabolism, and therefore is usually given only IV for acute treatment of cardiac dysrhythmias. Because the majority of the drug is metabolized, liver function is important. The main route of metabolism is by N-dealkylation to produce metabolites that show only mild antidysrhythmic activity.

The large first pass effect seen with lidocaine is not observed with mexiletine or tocainide, which have similar structures and modes of action. Although mexiletine and tocainamide demonstrate bioavailabilities in the range of 90% to 100%, the half-life of mexiletine is about 35% less for smokers than for non-smokers. This difference probably results from induction of hepatic enzymes in smokers. Other hepatic enzyme inducers, such as barbiturates, phenytoin, and rifampin, increase the rate of mexiletine metabolism; and antacids, cimetidine or narcotic analgesics interact with mexiletine to slow its absorption from the gastrointestinal (GI) tract.

The metabolism of procainamide produces the N-acetyl derivative, which shows mild antidysrhythmic activity and has a long plasma half-life.

The long plasma half-life (22 hours mean) of phenytoin shows considerable interpatient variation. Drugs that influence liver microsomal drug metabolism can significantly alter plasma concentrations and thus change the half-life of phenytoin. Considerable interpatient diversity in half-life also is observed with the newer drug flecainide, where metabolism is the major pathway for drug disposition and where one of the metabolites is slightly active.

A more complex situation is found with encainide. Metabolism is the primary route for drug disappearance but (1) two genetic phenotypes exist within the normal population and (2) the phenotypes differ in rate and pathway of metabolic degradation and in the antidysrhythmic activity of the metabolites. The metabolic pathways are summarized schematically in Figure 14-9.

Pathway 1 predominates in 93% of the U.S. and European populations and results in extensive metabolism, with a half-life of 0.5 to 4 hours and low bioavailability (30%) because of first pass metabolism. A metabolite ODE (see Figure 14-9) that is 80% protein bound and has greater efficacy than encainide is produced. A second product MODE (see Figure 14-9) (92% bound to plasma proteins) of similar activity to encainide also is formed.

Pathway 2 occurs in the other 7% of the population and takes place at a much slower rate to give an inactive product; therefore the encainide half-life and bioavailability are greater, 8 to 22 hours and 85%.

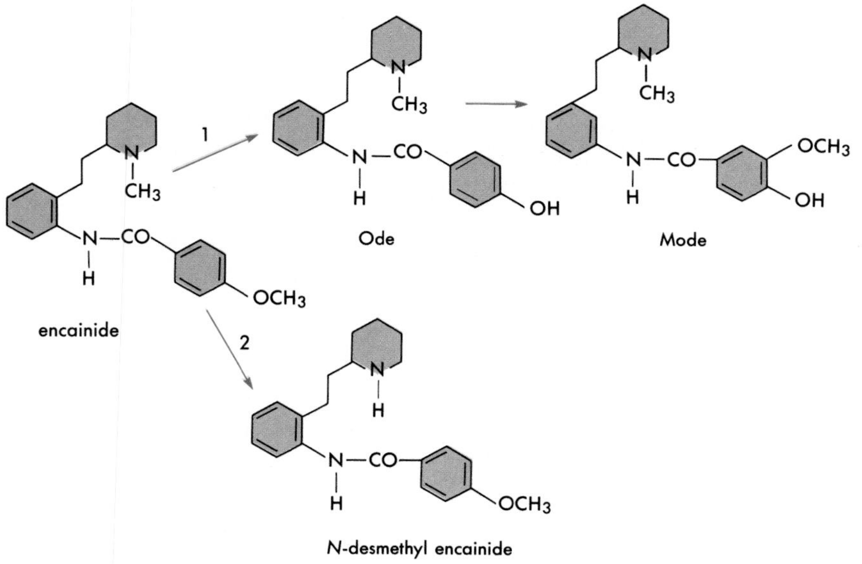

FIGURE 14-9   Bimodal metabolism of encainide. Pathway 1 is more general. ODE, O-desmethyl encainide, MODE, 3-methoxy analog.

Table 14-3   Summary of Antidysrhythmic Therapy

Dysrhythmia	Drug of Choice	Alternatives
Atrial flutter or fibrillation*	digoxin	verapamil, β blockers to control rate; quinidine disopyramide, procainamide for long term suppression
Supraventricular tachycardia	verapamil	β blockers, digoxin
Premature ventricular complexes (PVCs)	lidocaine	β blockers, procainamide, quinidine, disopyramide, mexiletine
Ventricular tachycardia*	lidocaine	procainamide, bretylium
Ventricular fibrillation*	lidocaine	bretylium, procainamide, amiodarone
Digitalis-induced dysrhythmias	lidocaine	phenytoin, procainamide, β blockers, digoxin antibody fragments, elevated serum K^+

Modified from Med Lett Drugs Ther 31:40, 1989.
* Cardioversion is treatment of choice.
† Used to control ventricular rate resulting from vagal enhancing properties.

 ## RELATION OF MECHANISMS OF ACTION TO CLINICAL RESPONSE

Antidysrhythmic Agents

A summary of antidysrhythmic drug choices is shown in Table 14-3.

Quinidine Quinidine has potent anticholinergic properties that are usually manifest at low doses in areas of the heart that are richly innervated, namely, the SA and AV nodes. These indirect effects are the opposite of the direct effects of this agent in these areas. After initial administration, there may be a small SA nodal tachycardia and an increase in AV nodal conduction velocity (decrease in PR interval) as a result of the indirect, anticholinergic effects of the drug. These initial effects are usually followed by the direct effects of the drug, including a decrease in heart rate and a slowing of AV nodal conduction velocity (increase in PR interval). At therapeutic concentrations, the QRS complex often shows widening as a result of a decrease in ventricular conduction velocity. The QT interval may be lengthened due to the prolonged action potential in the ventricular myocardium.

Quinidine is a broad-spectrum antidysrhythmic agent that is effective for nearly all types of cardiac dysrhythmias. It is administered for cases of premature atrial contractions, atrial flutter or fibrillation, AV nodal reentry dysrhythmias, premature ventricular contractions, and ventricular tachycardias. It also is effective in the treatment of digitalis-induced dysrhythmias, but is not the drug of first choice. Quinidine should be administered with caution in patients experiencing atrial flutter or fibrillation, because the indirect anticholinergic effects of the drug might exacerbate these conditions by increasing AV nodal conduction velocity. Often quinidine is given with digitalis for treatment of atrial flutter or fibrillation because the vagal enhancing effects of the glycosides tend to offset the anticholinergic properties of quinidine. Because quinidine produces a negative inotropic effect, it should be used cautiously in patients with congestive heart failure or severe hypotension.

Procainamide and Disopyramide Procainamide and disopyramide depress automaticity in SA nodal cells, as well as automaticity of ectopic pacemakers. Procainamide, in contrast to quinidine, has much less anticholinergic effect. Therefore the effects on heart rate and AV nodal conduction velocity are more direct and are usually characterized by a decrease in heart rate and a prolongation of the PR interval. Disopyramide, on the other hand, has similar if not more potent anticholinergic properties than quinidine. Therefore the same indirect and direct effects on heart rate and AV conduction velocity are observed after administration of this agent. When given for the treatment of atrial flutter or fibrillation, a digitalis glycoside will very often be coadministered to minimize the anticholinergic properties of disopyramide. Both procainamide and disopyramide prolong action potential duration and effective refractory period in the atrium, ventricle, and the His-Purkinje system. Therefore, a widening of the QRS complex and a lengthening of the QT interval are also observed after administration of these agents. Both compounds are broad-spectrum antidysrhythmics used to treat supraventricular as well as ventricular dysrhythmias.

Lidocaine Over a relatively large concentration range, lidocaine has little effect on automaticity of the SA node, and hence heart rate remains relatively normal. Despite this, lidocaine does suppress automaticity of both ectopic ventricular pacemakers and Purkinje fibers. Some shortening of the action potential duration and effective refractory period also is possible; this is more prominent in Purkinje fibers compared to ventricular myocardium. Lidocaine has little effect on AV nodal conduction. At therapeutic concentrations, lidocaine produces minimal changes in the electrocardiogram.

Lidocaine has a narrow antidysrhythmic spectrum compared to quinidine. It is primarily effective in the treatment of ventricular dysrhythmias, especially those associated with acute myocardial infarction. It has little efficacy for the treatment of supraventricular dysrhythmias such as atrial flutter or fibrillation. Lidocaine is the drug of choice for the treatment of digitalis-induced dysrhythmias, of either atrial or ventricular origin. This may be due to its apparent selectivity for depolarized myocardium.

Phenytoin Unlike lidocaine, phenytoin depresses automaticity of SA nodal cells and ectopic pacemakers. Phenytoin, although devoid of the anticholinergic properties of quinidine and disopyramide, increases AV nodal conduction velocity through some unknown mechanism. The only significant changes observed in the electrocardiogram after administration of phenytoin are a small decrease in the PR and QT intervals. Its antidysrhythmic spectrum is similar to that of lidocaine. It is a second-level drug for the treatment of ventricular dysrhythmias or dysrhythmias induced by cardiac glycosides and is often used in conjunction with other agents.

Encainide and Flecainide Encainide is a new agent that is effective in the treatment of some ventricular dysrhythmias, in particular premature ventricular complexes. At therapeutic concentrations, encainide can prolong the PR interval and widen the QRS complex. Preliminary reports indicate that it has minimal effects on myocardial contractility or cardiac output at therapeutic doses and can be used in patients with congestive heart failure. It may aggravate existing dysrhythmias, especially in patients with sustained ventricular tachycardia and underlying heart disease.

Flecainide may depress sinus node automaticity and slow AV nodal conduction. In patients with preexisting AV nodal conduction disturbances, it may produce conduction block. At therapeutic concentrations, flecainide may prolong the PR interval and widen the QRS complex. In contrast to encainide, it

should not be used in patients in heart failure or with drugs that depress cardiac contractility such as β blockers or Ca^{++} channel antagonists. Flecainide is effective in the treatment of premature ventricular complexes, but may aggravate dysrhythmias in patients with sustained ventricular tachycardia.

Amiodarone In some antidysrhythmic classifications, amiodarone is considered a class III agent because of its ability to prolong action potential duration and refractoriness. It depresses SA nodal automaticity and automaticity of ectopic pacemakers. Effects on the electrocardiogram include prolongation of the PR and QT intervals and a widening of the QRS complex. It is effective in suppressing ventricular dysrhythmias that are refractory to other agents, but its toxicity and long half-life limit its utility.

β-Adrenergic Blockers At therapeutic doses, the only significant change in the electrocardiogram produced by β blockers is a prolongation of the PR interval with occasional shortening of the QT interval.

In general, β-adrenergic antagonists have a low efficacy for suppressing ventricular ectopic pacemakers and are not useful for treating most ventricular dysrhythmias. They are useful in the treatment of many supraventricular dysrhythmias because of their ability to slow AV nodal conduction and SA nodal rate, and thereby allow stabilization of the ventricular rate. They also are used on a prophylactic basis to prevent or reduce the incidence of recurrent myocardial infarction in patients.

β-Adrenergic antagonists such as metoprolol or acebutolol (but not propranolol) have a greater selectivity for β_1-receptors than for β_2-receptors. There also are differences between these compounds with regard to their direct effects on cardiac membrane channels and their intrinsic sympathomimetic activity. Another β-adrenergic antagonist, esmolol, has recently been approved for emergency control of ventricular rate in patients with atrial flutter or fibrillation. In contrast to other β blockers, esmolol has a short duration of action (approximately 10 minutes) when given IV.

Bretylium Bretylium is used in the emergency treatment of ventricular fibrillation.

Calcium Channel Blockers Calcium channel blockers are most effective in treating supraventricular dysrhythmias, which often involve reentry. Their ability to slow AV nodal conduction velocity and refractoriness makes them useful for controlling ventricular rate. They often convert atrial tachycardia to normal sinus rhythm. Calcium channel blockers have little efficacy in the treatment of most ventricular dysrhythmias. They will suppress the development of oscillatory after-depolarizations induced by cardiac glycosides, but here they are not the drug of first choice (see Chapter 16).

Diltiazem, bepridil, lidoflazine, and flunarizine are other calcium channel blocking drugs currently under investigation as potential antidysrhythmic agents. The chemical structures, toxicity, and side effects of calcium channel blockers are described in Chapter 16. These agents' cardiotoxic effects relate to their negative inotropic properties and cardiac depressant effects produced on SA nodal automaticity and AV nodal conduction. They are contraindicated in patients with sick sinus syndrome, AV nodal conduction disturbances, or congestive heart failure. Caution should be exercised when they are administered in conjunction with other drugs such as digitalis glycosides or β-adrenergic blockers, which also slow AV nodal conduction.

SIDE EFFECTS, CLINICAL PROBLEMS, AND TOXICITY

Major problems associated with use of antidysrhythmic agents are summarized in the box, although information for the β blockers and calcium channel blockers are found in Chapters 10 and 16, respectively.

Quinidine is rarely given IV, due to its tendency to depress cardiac output and produce hypotension. Side effects observed after oral administration include diarrhea, nausea, and vomiting, as well as a condition known as *cinchonism,* characterized by headaches, dizziness, and tinnitus. In some patients, quinidine syncope may develop where the patient experiences fainting or lightheadedness. Syncope is likely the result of drug-induced ventricular tachycardia, which often subsides spontaneously. Quinidine overdosage can cause severe cardiac depression and precipitate dysrhythmias such as ventricular tachycardia, fibrillation, or asystole. Quinidine interacts with a wide range of other drugs.

Lidocaine has minimal toxic effects on the heart. At very high doses it may cause asystole. Most of the toxic side effects associated with lidocaine administration are due to its local anesthetic effects on the CNS. These include drowsiness, tremor, nausea,

hearing disturbances, slurred speech, and, at high doses, psychosis, respiratory depression, and convulsions.

The electrophysiological effects, antidysrhythmic spectrum, and side effects of mexiletine and tocainide are similar to those of lidocaine, but pharmacokinetic differences allow their oral use.

Procainamide overdose may produce cardiotoxic effects similar to those observed with quinidine. These include severe cardiac depression and the development of dysrhythmias. In addition, severe hypotension, due to procainamide peripheral actions, may also occur at high doses. Side effects observed with therapeutic doses include GI disturbances such as diarrhea, nausea, and vomiting. Chronic use of procainamide results in the development of a syndrome similar to systemic lupus erythematosus. Symptoms include arthralgia, skin rash, fever, and hepatomegaly. The development of this syndrome appears to be dose-dependent and is readily reversed on cessation of procainamide therapy. These lupus-like effects limit the chronic use of the compound, because approximately one third of all patients will exhibit lupus-like symptoms. Granulocytopenia also is observed in some patients.

Toxic concentrations of disopyramide may produce electrophysiological disturbances similar to those produced by high doses of quinidine. Disopyramide, in addition, appears to be more cardiodepressant than quinidine, requiring careful monitoring to ensure that cardiac failure does not develop. It should be used with extreme caution in patients with congestive heart failure. Many of the side effects of

---

CLINICAL PROBLEMS

Production of hypotension
New or worse dysrhythmias
Cardiac depression
Anticholinergic effects
Caution required with congestive heart failure patients
Lupus-like syndrome with procainamide
Interpatient variation in rates of drug metabolism
Dual genetic phenotypes for encainide metabolism associated with a potent metabolite (in some patients)

disopyramide are associated with its anticholinergic properties and include dry mouth, blurred vision, nausea, urinary retention, and constipation.

Oral overdose of phenytoin produces effects related to its interaction with the CNS, including vertigo, nystagmus, ataxia, tremors, slurring of speech, and sedation. Due to its relatively long plasma half-life, and the ability of other drugs that influence microsomal metabolism to significantly alter plasma concentrations of phenytoin, considerable patient-to-patient variations in response to a given oral dose typically occur.

Both encainide and flecainide can potentiate dysrhythmias in patients with a history of sustained ventricular tachycardia and severe ventricular dysfunction. The polymorphic hepatic metabolism of encainide and formation of a potent metabolite can pose pharmacokinetic problems in achieving a satisfactory dosing schedule. However, the relatively minor side effects normally associated with encainide administration make it easier to use in some patients. With flecainide, side effects include dizziness, blurred vision, headache, nausea, and abdominal pain. The compound is orally active but, as noted above, reserved for the treatment of life-threatening ventricular dysrhythmias, especially ones that are refractory to more traditional drugs, and is now approved only for the management of life-threatening dysrhythmias.

Adverse cardiac effects of amiodarone are significant and include sinus bradycardia and AV conduction block. Other effects observed are anorexia, nausea, vomiting, and clinical hepatitis and cirrhosis. CNS effects include dizziness, ataxia, tremor, and postural instability.

Because of its toxicity and side effects, bretylium is not considered a first-choice antidysrhythmic agent. It is primarily used to stabilize cardiac rhythm in patients with ventricular fibrillation or recurrent tachycardia resistant to other treatment. Its most severe side effect is persistent hypotension due to peripheral vasodilation as a result of blockade of peripheral adrenergic nerves. In addition, catecholamine release can transiently enhance ectopic pacemaker activity and cause increases in myocardial oxygen consumption in patients with ischemic heart disease. Nausea and vomiting are also common side effects of bretylium administration.

Caution is indicated when administering β-adrenergic antagonists in conjunction with other drugs that also slow AV nodal conduction velocity because the

---

TRADENAMES

In addition to generic and fixed combination preparations, the following tradenamed materials are available in the United States. (See Chapter 26 for calcium channel blockers and Chapters 10 and 23 for β blockers.)

Bretylol, bretylium
Cordarone, amiodarone
Dilantin, phenytoin
Enkaid, encainide
Mexitil, mexiletine
Norpace, disopyramide
Procan SR, procainamide
Pronestyl, procainamide
Quinidex Extentabs, quinidine
Quinora, quinidine
Tambocor, flecainide
Tonocard, tocainide
Xylocaine, lidocaine

---

effects may be synergistic. β-adrenergic antagonists are generally contraindicated in patients with existing AV nodal conduction disturbances, congestive heart failure, or bronchial asthma. The toxicity and side effects of these drugs are described elsewhere in this book.

REFERENCES

Arnsdorf MF and Wasserstrom JA: Mechanisms of action of antiarrhythmic drugs: a matrical approach. In Fozzard HA, Haber E, Jennings RB et al., eds.: The heart and cardiovascular system; scientific foundations, vol. 2, New York, 1986, Raven Press.

Mudge GH Jr.: Manual of electrocardiography, Boston, 1981, Little, Brown & Co.

Noble D: Initiation of the heartbeat, Oxford, England, 1979, Oxford University Press.

Reiser HJ and Sullivan ME: Antiarrhythmic drug therapy: new drugs and changing concepts, Fed Proc 45:2206, 1986.

Rosen MR and Wit AL: Electropharmacology of antiarrhythmic drugs, Am Heart J 106:829, 1983.

Singh BN, Collett JT, and Chew CYC: New perspectives in the pharmacological therapy of cardiac arrhythmias, Prog Cardiovasc Dis 22 (no. 4):243, 1980.

Smith WB and Wallace AG: Drugs used to treat cardiac arrhythmias. In Hurst JW, ed.: The heart, ed. 6, New York, 1986, McGraw-Hill, Inc.

CHAPTER 15

Drugs Affecting Cardiac Contractile Force

THERAPEUTIC OVERVIEW

The function of the heart is to pump blood to provide adequate flow to the various organs in the body and to furnish oxygen and substrates while removing metabolites and other materials. Compared with other organs, skeletal muscle requires a large blood flow, especially during exercise. The heart itself also requires an ample blood supply via the coronary arteries and, unlike skeletal muscle, operates with little or no reserve, so that the coronary vasculature must respond instantly to meet demand. The need for oxygen and substrates and the removal of waste materials,

and therefore the demands for blood, vary widely depending on the activity of each organ. When the cardiac force of contraction is compromised and the heart cannot meet the prevailing demand for blood, "heart failure" develops.

Several conditions reduce the cardiac force of contraction, including myocardial ischemia (diminished blood supply) and subsequent injury to heart muscle, toxic injury caused by chemical agents, infections of the heart, and congenital or genetically linked abnormalities. If the cardiac force of contraction is reduced only minimally, the heart can meet the demand when the patient is not subjected to stress or exercise. This condition is called *compensated failure*. Patients may appear normal; however, their exercise tolerance is reduced. It should be realized that it is the heart's ability to pump blood *relative* to its demand that is important. When the force of cardiac contraction is decreased further, exercise tolerance is reduced. Moreover, the pressures in the systemic and pulmonary veins increase, although the pressure on the arterial side rarely decreases until the terminal stage of the illness. Congestion of blood in the venous system causes edema, especially of the lower extremities. Congestion of blood in the pulmonary veins and capillaries may cause pulmonary edema (i.e., fluid leaves the capillaries and enters the extracellular space and alveoli). This condition occurs frequently when the patient is recumbent during sleep and the edematous fluid of lower extremities returns to the circulating blood pool. In extreme cases of pulmonary edema, large amounts of fluid accumulate in the alveoli and the patient may "drown" in his or her own body fluid. In less severe cases, the patient experiences shortness of breath or difficulties in breathing. These are typical signs of *congestive heart failure.*

Arterial blood pressure is maintained in congestive heart failure partly because sympathetic tone increases and the renin-angiotensin-vasopressin system is activated. These homeostatic mechanisms are brought into play to maintain blood pressure; however, they also increase the total peripheral resistance against which the heart has to pump blood and therefore add an additional burden on the compromised heart. Moreover, increases in peripheral resistance decrease tissue perfusion for a given blood pressure. Because tissue perfusion is more important than the blood pressure itself, maintenance of the blood pressure by the above mechanisms may not be advantageous. The maintenance of adequate blood flow to various organs, rather than heart rate and blood pressure, is the ultimate function of the heart, although rate and pressure are apparently influenced by cardiac function and are frequently taken as vital signs.

Among the pathophysiological changes associated with congestive heart failure are increases in end-systolic volume, end-diastolic pressure, end-diastolic volume, and dilation of the ventricle. These changes occur because the heart cannot remove the blood that returns to it when the force of contraction is reduced. The increase in end-diastolic volume, however, increases the force of contraction because developed tension is a function of the preload or stretching of the muscle fibers before contraction as described by the Frank-Starling ventricular function curve (Figure 15-1, *A, arrow*). Thus an adequate increase in end-diastolic volume causes the compromised heart muscle to develop a greater force. It is, however, an increase in intraventricular pressure and not the increase in wall tension itself that causes ejection of blood into the aorta.

The relationship between wall tension and intraventricular pressure can be described by the law of LaPlace: assuming that the cross section of the ven-

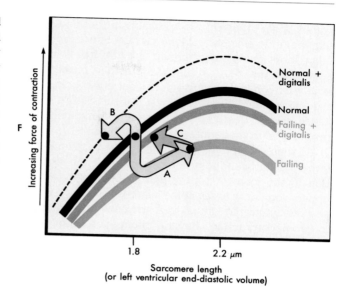

FIGURE 15-1   Frank-Starling ventricular function curve. Force of contraction, expressed as left ventricular dP/dt (rate of pressure development during early systolic phase), is a function of (1) left ventricular volume immediately before the onset of contraction or (2) sarcomere length. The sarcomere, the unit length between two Z lines of a myofibril, in the normal heart is 1.7 to 1.8 μm at the endocardial and epicardial layers and 2.0 μm in the middle layer. Reduced force of contraction in a failing heart is partly compensated by stretching of the muscle, which increases the force of contraction (**A,** *arrow*). Positive inotropic interventions in the normal heart are cancelled by shortening of the muscle (**B,** *arrow*). The digitalis glycosides shift the ventricular function curve and reduce the end-diastolic volume that is required for the muscle to develop the necessary force of contraction (**C,** *arrow*). *F,* Force required for normal pumping function.

tricle is a circle, pressure is proportional to tension/ diameter of the ventricle. This means that a greater wall tension is required in the dilated heart to develop a pressure that is greater than the aortic pressure and to move blood from the left ventricle into the aorta. Therefore the energetic efficiency is reduced in the dilated heart because (1) a greater wall tension is required to develop the necessary intraventricular pressure, and (2) the peripheral resistance is increased. The energetic efficiency decreases further when the heart rate is increased by activation of the sympathetic nervous system and the stroke volume is decreased.

Chronic stress on the heart causes hypertrophy of the cardiac muscle. The number of myocardial cells does not increase (hyperplasia); instead, each cell becomes larger (hypertrophy), probably further decreasing energetic efficiency. Moreover, the hypertrophied heart loses compliance, preventing the free flow of blood into the heart during the diastolic phase. Inability for complete relaxation is a serious problem of the failing heart. Continued severe heart failure may cause cellular death and other severe complications resulting from inadequate tissue perfusion.

All these symptoms of congestive heart failure are either direct or indirect consequences of the reduction in the force of contraction. Therefore it would appear logical to treat some of these patients with *positive inotropic* drugs that increase the cardiac force of contraction. Several groups of drugs are known to have this pharmacological property. Among them, the digitalis glycosides have been used most extensively and for the longest time. The glycosides, however, are not ideal drugs because of their tendency to produce toxicity. Moreover, the glycosides are incapable of reversing basic processes that make the heart fail and stopping the progress of pathological changes. In fact, some investigators feel that the glycosides may actually augment the deterioration of the heart in advanced congestive heart failure. Recent evidence suggests that an alternative and more palliative treatment to minimize deficiencies of the failing heart by reducing its work load may be a better choice (see Chapter 17 on vasodilators).

The basic problem and therapeutic approaches are summarized in the box.

THERAPEUTIC OVERVIEW

PROBLEM: CONGESTIVE HEART FAILURE

Contractile force ↓
 Exercise tolerance ↓
 Venous pressure ↑
 Edema ↑
 Total peripheral resistance ↑
 Tissue perfusion ↓
 Arterial pressure initially maintained
 Congestive heart failure occurs

THERAPY

Pharmacological intervention
 Contractile force ↑
Work load reduction
 Decrease tissue need

 MECHANISMS OF ACTION

Drug Types

Among drugs that affect the cardiac force of contraction, only those that increase the force are clinically useful. Four groups of drugs are currently used to increase the cardiac force of contraction. These are (1) digitalis glycosides and related drugs, (2) catecholamines, (3) xanthine derivatives, and (4) newer experimental drugs. Each group has a different mechanism of action. In addition, many cardiotonic drugs with known and unknown mechanisms of action have been developed in recent years. Except for a few, all cardiotonic drugs increase the force of contraction by ultimately modifying Ca^{++} movement. Ca^{++} ions have positive inotropic effects; however, Ca^{++} is not useful in treating chronic heart failure because it is not practical to try to maintain Ca^{++} in plasma at an elevated concentration without seriously affecting the functions of other organs and because homeostatic mechanisms make it extremely difficult to maintain a stable elevation of Ca^{++} in the plasma.

Excitation-contraction Coupling

In cardiac muscle cells, the resting state is one of high-energy, characterized by steep Na^+, K^+, and Ca^{++} gradients and transmembrane potentials. Among these, the K^+ and Na^+ gradients are important for the maintenance of the transmembrane potential and excitability, whereas the low intracellular Ca^{++} concentration is important for maintaining the diastolic state of resting muscle. The first event in membrane excitation is a sudden opening of the Na^+ channels, which causes Na^+ ions, driven by chemical and electrical gradients, to rush into the cell (Figure 15-2). Although the Na^+ channels are open for a very short period (typically, 1 to 2 msec), Na^+ ions crossing the sarcolemma during this period are sufficient to depolarize the cell membrane. During the depolarization phase, Ca^{++} channels open and Ca^{++} ions enter the cell driven by the steep Ca^{++} gradient. The inward flow of positively charged Ca^{++} ions keeps the membrane potential depolarized, maintains Ca^{++} channels open and raises the cytoplasmic Ca^{++} concentrations. The latter triggers the release of Ca^{++} stored in the cisternal area of the sarcoplasmic reticulum, and the cytoplasmic Ca^{++} concentration rises transiently (Ca^{++} transients). The intracellular concentration of calcium varies, diastole to systole, from about 5×10^{-8} M to 5×10^{-7} M.

Typical myocardial cells have mitochondria, contractile proteins, and sarcoplasmic reticulum; this leaves only approximately 10% of the total cell volume as cytoplasmic fluid. Therefore the movement of Ca^{++} into this compartment across the cell membrane and from the sarcoplasmic reticulum has a significant effect on the free Ca^{++} ion concentration. The sudden and transient increase of cytoplasmic Ca^{++} activates the contractile proteins, causing the muscle to contract (Figure 15-2). Subsequently, K$^+$ channels open and K$^+$ efflux occurs. The outward movement of positively charged K$^+$ ions reestablishes the membrane potential (repolarization), which in turn closes the Ca^{++} channels. During membrane depolarization, each Ca^{++} channel may open and close several times; however, a certain percentage of the channels are open at a given moment, allowing Ca^{++} to enter the cell.

All Ca^{++} channels close after repolarization. When the transmembrane Ca^{++} influx and Ca^{++} release

from the sarcoplasmic reticulum are terminated, Ca^{++} ions in the cytoplasm are rapidly taken up into the sarcoplasmic reticulum by the Ca^{++} pump, terminating the Ca^{++} transients. A fraction of the increased cytoplasmic Ca^{++} is extruded from the cell by the sarcolemmal Ca^{++} pump and also by the Na$^+$/Ca^{++} exchange mechanism. The initial rate of Ca^{++} influx (the so-called trigger calcium) and the amount of Ca^{++} released from the sarcoplasmic reticulum determine the magnitude of the Ca^{++} transients and hence myocardial contraction.

The relative contributions of "trigger calcium" and the Ca^{++} released from the sarcoplasmic reticulum to contractile force activation vary, depending on the type of muscle. In skeletal muscle, most of the Ca^{++} that participates in contractile activation is released from the sarcoplasmic reticulum, whereas transmembrane Ca^{++} influx plays the predominant role in vascular smooth muscle. In cardiac muscle, as described above, trigger calcium derived from the extracellular space is vital.

Mechanism of Positive Inotropic Effect of Digitalis Glycosides

Of the many cardiac glycosides and related drugs, digoxin and digitoxin (Figure 15-3) are almost exclusively used clinically even though several other preparations are available. These glycosides selectively bind to and inhibit the sarcolemmal sodium pump, also known as Na$^+$, K$^+$-ATPase. This leads to an increase in intracellular Na$^+$, which in turn affects Na$^+$/Ca^{++} exchange, leading to an increase in Ca^{++} and the force of contraction.

One of the primary functions of the sodium pump is to exchange three intracellular Na$^+$ ions for two extracellular K$^+$ ions (Figure 15-4). Both Na$^+$ and K$^+$ ions are moved against their concentration gradients. Moreover, one net positive charge is moved from the inside of the cell membrane to the outside against an electrical potential. This chemical and electrical work is accomplished at the expense of ATP; one molecule of ATP is hydrolyzed to ADP and inorganic phosphate during each cycle of the sodium pump to furnish energy for the active transport of these ions.

The current hypothesis on the mechanism of action of the cardiac glycosides is that a slight, but significant increase in the intracellular Na$^+$ concentration (e.g., a change from 8 to 10 mM) during diastole inhibits Ca^{++} efflux and thereby increases

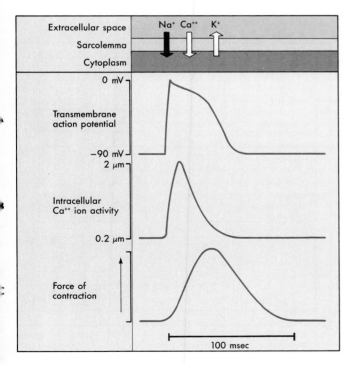

FIGURE 15-2   Time course of events of a single contraction. **A,** Transmembrane potential. **B,** Intracellular ion activity (Ca^{++} transients). **C,** Developed tension.

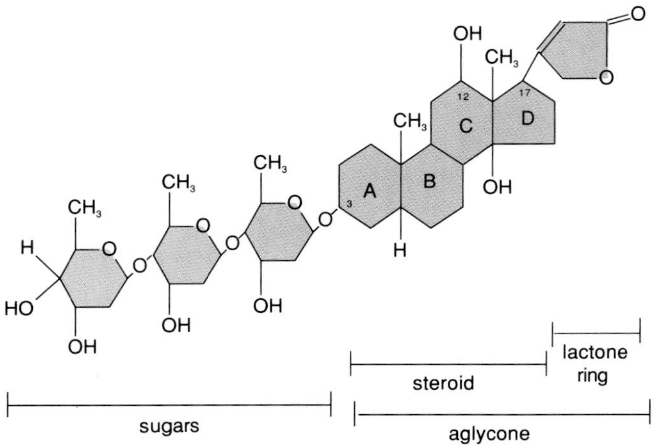

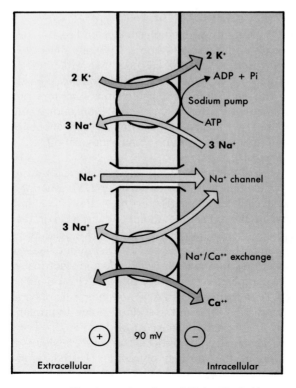

FIGURE 15-3   Structure of digoxin. This molecule consists of an unsaturated lactone ring, a steroid nucleus, and three digitoxose (sugar) groups. The unsaturated lactone ring and the steroid nucleus with the trans C-D ring fusion are essential for cardiotonic activity, whereas the sugar moiety is not an absolute requirement. Drugs that lack sugars are called aglycones. Digitoxin lacks the hydroxyl group at the C-12 position and has a higher lipid solubility.

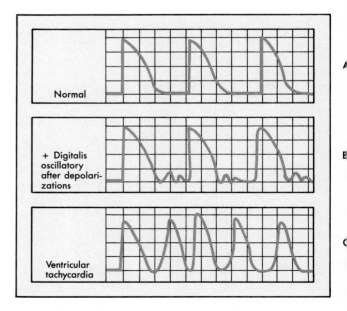

FIGURE 15-4   Membrane ion flux of Na^+, K^+, Ca^{++} in the heart.

FIGURE 15-5   Normal action potential **(A)** and changes in cardiac action potentials caused by toxic doses of the cardiac glycosides. **A,** Typical normal action potential recording from a cardiac Purkinje fiber cell. Toxic doses produce oscillatory after depolarizations **(B)** and ventricular tachycardia **(C).**

Ca^{++} loading of the sarcoplasmic reticulum. The inhibition of Ca^{++} efflux is the result of an effect on the cardiac sarcolemmal Na^+/Ca^{++} exchange system, which mediates the coupled exchange of three Na^+ ions for one Ca^{++} (Figure 15-4). Unlike the active transport mechanism of the Na^+ pump that moves Na^+ and K^+ ions against their chemical and electrical gradients at the expense of ATP, the Na^{++} exchange mechanism moves Na^+ and Ca^{++} via their respective transmembrane gradients and the transmembrane potential.

The relationship of intracellular Na^+ to intracellular Ca^{++} is such that a very small increase in Na^+ leads to a large increase in Ca^{++}. Because the sarcoplasmic reticulum has an active Ca^{++} pump, an inhibition of Ca^{++} extrusion from the cell results in a larger fraction of Ca^{++} ions that can be taken up by the sarcoplasmic reticulum rather than being extruded. An increase in Ca^{++} uptake by the sarcoplasmic reticulum increases the amount of Ca^{++} to be released from the cisternal area of the sarcoplasmic reticulum and thereby augments the Ca^{++} transients, which leads to an enhancement of contractile force.

Thus the cardiac glycosides produce their positive inotropic effects by essentially augmenting Ca^{++} transients. It is also possible that inhibition of the sodium pump augments Ca^{++} transients by enhancing Ca^{++} influx coupled with Na^+ efflux, which occurs during membrane excitation. In any case it is apparent that sodium pump inhibition and the ensuing increase in intracellular Na^+ enhances Ca^{++} transients and hence the force of cardiac contraction. This is the mechanism of the cardiotonic action of digitalis glycosides observed with therapeutic doses. It should be noted that the specific receptor for the digitalis glycosides is the α-subunit of the Na^+, K^+-ATPase.

Mechanism of Direct Toxic Effects of Digitalis Glycosides

When the cardiac muscle is exposed to toxic concentrations of a glycoside and sodium pump inhibition and cellular Ca^{++} overload become alarmingly high, the cytoplasmic membrane becomes "unstable" during the time immediately following membrane repolarization. In normal ventricular muscle cells membrane depolarization is followed by repolarization; the membrane potential attains approximately $-90mV$ and then remains at that level until the next membrane excitation (Figure 15-5). In digitalis toxicity,

however, the permeability of the cell membrane to Na^+, Ca^{++}, and K^+ increases immediately following repolarization; ions flow according to their concentration and electrical gradients, causing the membrane potential to move toward 0 mV. The movements of Na^+ and Ca^{++} are particularly prominent because these ions are driven by both chemical and electrical gradients whereas the movement of K^+ is minimal because the chemical and electrical gradients cancel each other. Therefore the net movement is the transient inward movement of cations, causing transient inward currents.

In mild toxicity, the transient inward current subsides, causing the transmembrane potential to return to its resting level. This process may be repeated a few times causing oscillatory afterpotentials (see Figure 15-5). These small oscillatory afterpotentials are most easily observed in cardiac Purkinje fibers and do not propagate beyond each individual cell. When the magnitude of the oscillatory afterpotentials increases in advanced digitalis toxicity and reaches a threshold potential, however, it causes the cell to fire (i.e., to trigger action potentials). Such triggered action potentials propagate from Purkinje fiber cells to ventricular muscle proper causing that muscle to contract in rapid repetition no longer under control of the SA node. This leads to dysrhythmogenesis.

Thus, toxicity resulting from direct actions of the glycoside on cardiac muscle are caused by Ca^{++} overload of myocardial cells. Because the therapeutic positive inotropic effect of the drugs is also caused by an enhanced Ca^{++} loading of the cells and the sarcoplasmic reticulum in particular, it appears that the therapeutic and toxic effects are inseparable with this class of cardiotonic drugs and the small therapeutic ratio (i.e., narrow margin of safety) is therefore an inherent property of digitalis.

Mechanisms of Extra-cardiac Effects of Digitalis Glycosides

Most cells in the body have low Na^+ and high K^+ intracellular concentrations, deemed necessary for the functions of many intracellular organelles and enzymes, including mitochondrial oxidative phosphorylation. Such intracellular ionic environments are maintained because these cells have Na^+, K^+-ATPase present in their cell membrane and actively pump Na^+ out and K^+ in. The Na^+, K^+-ATPases of various human tissues have a high affinity for cardiac glycosides and are inhibited at therapeutic or toxic concentrations of glycoside. Therefore the glycoside can and does influence the activities of many cells and tissue types.

Several factors determine whether inhibition of a Na^+, K^+-ATPase by the cardiac glycoside will influence cellular functions. The immediate consequence of sodium pump inhibition is an increase in intracellular Na^+ concentration. Because such an increase in Na^+ concentration stimulates the activity of the noninhibited pump sites, the net rate of Na^+ ejection increases to match the prevailing new rate of Na^+ influx, and equilibrium is reestablished. Therefore the impact of sodium pump inhibition by therapeutic or toxic concentrations of the glycoside on intracellular Na^+ ion concentration may be relatively small for most tissues. In cardiac muscle, however, such a slight increase in Na^+ concentration drastically alters Ca^{++} movement, producing therapeutic and toxic effects of the glycoside. In other tissues, the reserve capacity of the sodium pump, the possible presence of an effective Na^+/Ca^{++} exchanger, the relative importance of transmembrane Ca^{++} movements on intracellular Ca^{++} ion concentrations (rather than extracellular calcium as is the case with heart muscle), and the role of Ca^{++} on cellular functions determine whether the glycoside will alter the function of a particular cell type.

Mechanisms of Action of the Catecholamines and Xanthines

These drugs have marked cardiac inotropic and chronotropic effects and generally dilate blood vessels, although they may also produce constriction. Therefore systemic administration of these drugs has profound effects on hemodynamics and the cardiac force of contraction.

Cardiac muscle cells have some α_1 and β_2 in addition to β_1-adrenergic receptors, all of which can be stimulated by catecholamines. The most prominent effects of catecholamines on heart muscle are mediated via stimulation of β_1-adrenergic receptors, with the mechanisms by which stimulation activates adenylate cyclase, increases tissue cAMP concentrations, and thereby promotes phosporylation by protein kinase described in Chapters 2, 8, and 10. In cardiac muscle, substrates for cAMP-dependent protein kinase include Ca^{++} channels, the Ca^{++} pump polypeptide (phospholamban) in the sarcoplasmic re-

ticulum, troponin I, myosin light chain, and phosphorylase kinase. Because these proteins have diverse functions, direct effects of catecholamines on cardiac muscle functions are complex.

Phosphorylation of Ca^{++} channels is necessary for channel opening. Therefore catecholamines increase the number of Ca^{++} channels that open in response to membrane depolarization and increase Ca^{++} influx. The enhanced Ca^{++} influx elevates the plateau phase of the action potential. The initial rate of Ca^{++} influx, which is important in determining the size of Ca^{++} transients, and hence the cardiac force of contraction, is markedly increased by catecholamines.

Phosphorylation of the Ca^{++} pump in the sarcoplasmic reticulum stimulates pump activity and enhances the removal of Ca^{++} from the cytoplasm. This is the mechanism by which catecholamines enhance relaxation and shorten the duration of contraction. The duration of muscle contraction is further shortened by the phosphorylation of troponin I. The amino N-terminal of troponin I from cardiac muscle is longer than that from skeletal muscle and contains a serine residue that can be phosphorylated by cAMP-dependent protein kinase. Phosphorylation of this serine residue of troponin I decreases the affinity of troponin C for Ca^{++}, and thereby enhances relaxation of cardiac muscle. Therefore, both the sarcoplasmic reticulum and troponin I work in concert to regulate relaxation. The significance of the phosphorylation of myosin light chain in cardiac muscle is unknown in contrast to the significance of light chain phosphorylation in vascular smooth muscle. Phosphorylation of phosphorylase kinase activates this enzyme and enhances glycogenolysis via phosphorylation and activation of phosphorylase and thereby increases availability of substrates for metabolism.

Energetic efficiency of cardiac muscle is reduced by the direct effect of catecholamines on the SA node to produce positive chronotropic effects (increased heart rate). Catecholamines enhance phase 4 depolarization of the SA nodal cells, thereby increasing heart rate. When the heart rate is increased, contraction occurs with smaller amounts of blood in the ventricle, since blood flows in the coronaries only during ventricular diastole. Since increasing heart rate shortens diastole the energetic efficiency of overall blood pumping decreases.

Catecholamines also stimulate α_1-adrenergic receptors. This should increase Ca^{++} release from the sarcoplasmic reticulum via the phosphotidylinositol breakdown product, IP_3. In addition, catecholamines can stimulate β_2-adrenergic receptors. The significance of α_1- and β_2-adrenergic receptor stimulation by catecholamines on the overall effects of catecholamines on cardiac muscle is still being actively debated.

Similarly to the action of cardiac glycosides, toxic doses of catecholamines cause dysrhythmias. Both classes of drugs *increase* Ca^{++} *loading of the sarcoplasmic reticulum, although by different mechanisms*. The glycosides inhibit Ca^{++} extrusion and increase cytoplasmic Ca^{++} that is subsequently taken up by the sarcoplasmic reticulum. Catecholamines stimulate the Ca^{++} pump and enhance Ca^{++} uptake through the membrane. During the diastolic phase, *cytoplasmic* Ca^{++} *is lowered as the* Ca^{++} *is sequestered into the sarcoplasmic reticulum (SR). Thus* Ca^{++} *overload of the SR is a common feature of the action of both classes of drugs.* Common to both classes of drugs is Ca^{++} overload of the sarcoplasmic reticulum.

Xanthine derivatives have even more complex mechanisms of action. These drugs (1) inhibit phosphodiesterase, (2) directly inhibit Ca^{++} uptake by the sarcoplasmic reticulum, and (3) act as antagonists at adenosine receptors. In cardiac muscle, cAMP turns over rapidly. Therefore inhibition of phosphodiesterase increases tissue cAMP concentrations, which in turn causes effects similar to those of catecholamines. These actions are observed with lower doses of caffeine and theophylline ethylenediamine. At higher doses, inhibition of the Ca^{++} uptake mechanism becomes prominent, with the inhibition of muscle relaxation. Adenosine has a negative inotropic effect. Therefore blockade of adenosine receptors may increase the cardiac force of contraction. However, the importance of this mechanism is presently unknown.

New and Experimental Positive Inotropic Drugs

In recent years, many compounds have been investigated as cardiac positive inotropic drugs in attempts to find a replacement for the cardiac glycosides. New mechanisms of action have been proposed for these compounds with better therapeutic indices than the cardiac glycosides. In addition, some have been reported to be effective in patients who are refractory to the cardiac glycosides.

Bipyridine derivatives (e.g., amrinone), imidazolone derivatives (enoximone and piroximone), and benzimidazole derivatives (sulmazole, pimobendan) inhibit cAMP phosphodiesterase. The profile of cardiac effects of these compounds, however, is different from that of classical phosphodiesterase inhibitors such as caffeine and theophylline ethylenediamine. The reason for the difference is thought to be that the new positive inotropic drugs are relatively selective inhibitors of a subclass of phosphodiesterase, (i.e., phosphodiesterase III), whereas the classical inhibitors nonselectively affect all types of phosphodiesterases.

The cardiac actions of catecholamines, caffeine, or theophylline ethylenediamine are mediated by an increase in tissue cAMP concentration. These drugs, however, influence the metabolism of both cAMP and cGMP; catecholamines stimulate adenylate cyclases that enhance production of cAMP and cGMP, whereas xanthine derivatives inhibit various phosphodiesterases and thereby cause accumulation of both cyclic cAMP and cGMP. Selective inhibition of phosphodiesterase III, however, causes an increase in tissue cAMP concentration without presumably affecting the cGMP concentration because this subtype of phosphodiesterase hydrolyzes cAMP but not cGMP. Whether the inotropic action of the newer cardiotonic drugs can be totally accounted for by an inhibition of phosphodiesterase or whether there are other mechanisms of action is still controversial. A remarkable feature of the newer cardiotonic drugs is that they produce smaller positive chronotropic effects compared to catecholamines or xanthine derivatives, and therefore probably a lower potential to produce dysrhythmias. It is important for positive inotropic drugs used in chronic heart failure that they not have positive chronotropic effects, because these effects lower energetic efficiency of the failing heart and add an additional burden. The difference between classical and newer phosphodiesterase inhibitors may be a result of the latter selectively influencing cAMP. Alternatively, differences in subcellular distribution of the phosphodiesterases affected by these drugs may also be important.

Ca^{++} channel agonists (e.g., Bay k 8644), chemically related to Ca^{++} channel antagonists, increase force of contraction by increasing the probability of Ca^{++} channel opening and thereby augmenting Ca^{++} influx through Ca^{++} channels during membrane depolarization. Bay k 8644 appears to have a larger therapeutic index than cardiac glycosides; however, since it also constricts blood vessels, it cannot be used to treat patients with chronic heart failure. Several drugs (sulmazole, pimobendan, DPI 201-106) have been reported to increase Ca^{++} sensitivity of contractile proteins. This mechanism of action should have the advantage of not causing cellular Ca^{++} overload. They may interfere with rapid and complete relaxation, probably as important therapeutically as increased force of contraction in the patient with chronic heart failure. Another very important potential site for therapeutic intervention is the potassium channel.

PHARMACOKINETICS

The principal pharmacokinetic parameters of the cardiotropic drugs are given in Table 15-1. Avid tissue binding and the ensuing large apparent volume of distribution for digitoxin contribute to its long half-life. Although more than 90% of digitoxin in plasma is albumin bound, avid binding to many tissue proteins results in an apparent volume of distribution as large as 1000 liters, when the calculation is based on the free drug concentration in plasma.

The absorption of digoxin varies from 45% to 85% when the drug is given as tablets. Digoxin tablets are subjected to a dissolution test to reduce variations in bioavailability (see Chapter 4); however, even slight differences in dissolution rate and bioavailability may pose serious problems because of the narrow margin of safety inherent with cardiac glycoside therapy. Therefore the patient should probably be maintained on a specific brand of the drug. Bioavailability is approximately 85% when digoxin is given as an elixir or in a stable solution in capsules.

Skeletal muscle is an important tissue binding site for glycosides. Therefore changes in the mass of skeletal muscle affect the apparent volume of distribution, requiring some adjustment of the dosage. The most important factor determining total body elimination of digoxin is renal function, with clearance of digoxin proportional to creatinine clearance. Digitoxin is largely metabolized by the liver, and renal function does not significantly affect its half-life. Large interpatient variations exist in the metabolism of digitoxin, partly because intestinal flora play a significant role in its overall metabolism. The major pathway of metabolic disposition is a complex hydrolysis of the carbohydrate moiety, catalyzed by the mixed function oxidase system, followed by conjugation with glycuronic acid or sulfate. Conversion of digitoxin to digoxin is a minor pathway in humans.

Binding of cardiac glycosides to the receptor site, Na^+, K^+-ATPase, is slow with the rate dependent on intracellular Na^+ and extracellular K^+ concentrations. Thus glycoside binding rate and the subsequent phar-

Table 15-1 Pharmacokinetic Parameters

Agent	Route of Adminis-tration	Bioavailability (Oral, %)	Peak Effect*	Plasma Protein Binding (% Bound)	Disposition	$t_{1/2}$	Concentration in Plasma (ng/ml)
digoxin	Oral, IV	45-85	6 hr	25	R (40%-90%)	35 hr	0.5-1.4
digitoxin	Oral, IV	90	12 hr	90	M (liver†)	5-6 days	9-30‡
amrinone	Oral, IV	—	—	15-40	R, M	3.6 hr; 5.8 hr in congestive heart failure	—
milrinone	Oral, IV	92	—	—	R, M	0.8 hr (normal patient); 2.3 hr in congestive heart failure	—

M, Metabolized; *R*, renal clearance as unchanged drug.
* After a single oral dose.
† Large individual variation.
‡ Total (free plus bound) drug.

macological effects are greater in hypokalemic patients. Larger doses of cardiac glycoside, expressed as mg/kg body weight, are used in newborn and young infants compared with adults. This is not based on pharmacokinetic considerations but is due to differences in the sensitivity of the heart muscle to the glycoside. Variations in pharmacokinetics may be compensated for by using target concentration strategy, (i.e., maintaining a predetermined digoxin or digitoxin concentration in plasma using feedback from assays of serum or plasma glycoside concentrations). This approach, however, does not entirely solve the problem, since a given plasma concentration of the glycoside may be therapeutic in some patients but toxic in others. Since it is impractical to monitor directly the positive inotropic effect of the glycoside, clinical evaluation of the effects of the cardiac glycoside, including analysis of the ECG (Table 15-2), is important.

Because digitoxin has a long half-life, it takes more than 20 days for the serum digitoxin concentration to reach a steady state, when treatment is begun without giving a loading dose. Therefore digitoxin treatment should be started with a digitalizing (loading) dose. Digoxin, which has a shorter half-life, may be given without a loading dose; a steady state serum concentration being obtained in 3 to 4 days. Special pharmacokinetic considerations are required when the glycosides are switched during chronic treatment. For a patient maintained on digoxin, termination of digoxin treatment and substitution of main-

tenance doses of digitoxin result in temporary loss of pharmacological effects, since digoxin is excreted from the body rapidly, whereas the accumulation of digitoxin is slow. Switching from maintenance doses of digitoxin to maintenance doses of digoxin causes a transient overdose because the effect of the rapidly increasing digoxin concentration is superimposed on the effect of a slowly declining digitoxin concentration.

Because digitoxin has a longer half-life, fluctuation of drug concentration in plasma is smaller with digitoxin than with digoxin.

Pharmacokinetic parameters for amrinone and milrinone also are included in Table 15-2. Milrinone competes for the same albumin binding sites as iodothyronine and may be a potential source of drug interactions with iodinated compounds.

Pharmacokinetic data for catecholamines and xanthines are in Chapters 10 and 32, respectively.

 ## RELATION OF MECHANISMS OF ACTION TO CLINICAL RESPONSE

Digitalis Glycosides

Effect on Heart Rate While the cardiac glycosides are capable of increasing the myocardial force of contraction, it has long been debated whether the positive inotropic effect of the glycosides is truly the basis for the therapeutic efficacy of these drugs in patients. The glycoside has two clinically useful effects; one is to increase the force of cardiac contraction and the other is to slow the beating of the ventricle in patients with atrial fibrillation or flutter or in patients with chronic heart failure. The negative chronotropic effects of the glycoside result from stimulation of the cardiac parasympathetic (vagus) nerve, suppression of the sympathetic discharge to the heart, and a direct depressant action of the drug on conduction through the AV node. The cardiac glycosides do not have significant direct effects on the SA node. The direct and indirect actions of the glycoside on the AV node prolong its effective refractory period. When the glycosides are used to reduce the frequency of the beating of the ventricle in patients with atrial fibrillation or flutter, the therapeutic end point can be clearly defined and the effects are easily evaluated. In this type of dysrhythmia, the cardiac

Table 15-2 Effects of the Cardiac Glycosides on the ECG	
ECG Features	**Glycoside-induced Changes**
P wave	Size and shape may change with large doses
PR interval	Prolongation and various degrees of AV block
QRS complex	Widening of abnormal complex in Wolff-Parkinson-White syndrome; however, no widening in normal QRS complex
QT interval	Shortened
ST segment	Depression when QRS complex is upward
	Elevation when QRS complex is downward
T wave	Diminished amplitude or inversion

glycosides are highly effective in reducing the ventricular rate and restoring pumping efficiency. Therefore the cardiac glycosides can be used as an efficacious means of treating a patient with certain types of dysrhythmias despite the fact that the glycosides are dysrhythmogenic and their overdose may cause various types of dysrhythmias. The cardiac glycosides, however, are incapable of reversing an atrial fibrillation or flutter to a normal sinus rhythm and simply reduce the number of depolarizations that pass through the AV node and reach ventricular muscle. The result is a reduction of the frequency of ventricular beats in the patient with tachydysrhythmias of supraventricular origin.

Effect on the Cardiac Autonomic Nervous System The primary mechanism for stimulation of the cardiac parasympathetic nerve and inhibition of the sympathetic nerve is glycoside-induced inhibition of the sodium pump in neuronal cells, especially in the pressure-sensitive cells of the baroreceptor. Discharge of the cardiac sympathetic nerve is normally synchronized with systemic blood pressure; during cardiac systole, blood pressure in the carotid artery increases, resulting in suppression of sympathetic outflow. Frequency of the cardiac sympathetic discharge is markedly higher during the diastolic phase when the pressure in the carotid artery is low. This pattern of fluctuating sympathetic discharge is markedly enhanced in patients treated with the cardiac glycosides because these drugs sensitize the baroreceptors to changes in blood pressure. Animal experiments indicate that activity of the cardiac sympathetic nerves may be totally inhibited during systole when a dose of the glycoside approaching toxicity is given. Overall sympathetic discharge is also reduced unless a toxic dose of the glycoside causes dysrhythmias and thereby markedly decreases the systemic blood pressure.

Indirect effects of the glycosides mediated by the parasympathetic system may be eliminated by the administration of the cholinergic muscarinic antagonist, atropine. In fact, atropine is quite effective in eliminating many electrophysiological effects of the glycoside. The glycoside, however, has a direct action of the AV node in addition to indirect actions via parasympathetic stimulation and sympathetic inhibition. When the cardiac glycosides are given to patients with atrial fibrillation or flutter, the net effect to slow the ventricular rate is probably caused by the combination of all three actions of the glycoside. Ef-

fects of the glycosides on the electrocardiogram are summarized in Table 15-2.

Because the glycosides do not have significant direct effects on the SA node, they do not alter heart rate in normal subjects; however, the glycosides do reduce the heart rate in patients with chronic heart failure because they decrease the elevated sympathetic influence on the heart, secondary to the improvement of hemodynamics.

Inotropic Action and Hemodynamic Effects When glycosides are used in patients with a normal sinus rhythm to increase force of contraction, the therapeutic end point cannot be easily monitored because of the difficulty in estimating the force of cardiac contraction in patients. This is further complicated because the binding of glycoside to its pharmacological receptor is extremely slow, ordinarily taking several hours to reach equilibrium even when the drug is administered intravenously. Therefore an immediate change in the force of cardiac contraction or improvement of the patients' condition does not occur. Moreover, an overdose of the glycoside decreases force, making it difficult to determine if the desired effect is not obtained because of an insufficient dose or because too much drug was administered. Finally, the cardiovascular system has multiple regulatory mechanisms that maintain homeostasis, and drug interventions for the purpose of altering cardiac function may be counteracted by a homeostatic mechanism.

Because the cardiac glycosides modify basic biochemical mechanisms for excitation-contraction coupling, these drugs are capable of increasing the force of cardiac contraction in either the normal or the failing heart. For a long time, however, the glycosides have been thought capable of increasing force only in patients with failing hearts. This was because the positive inotropic effect could be counterbalanced by normal physiological homeostatic mechanisms. For example, the administration of glycoside to a normal heart would initially increase the force of contraction and reduce end-diastolic volume. Reduced end-diastolic volume decreases the force of contraction to cancel the positive inotropic effect of the cardiac glycoside (Figure 15-1, *B, arrow*). In the failing dilated heart, however, the glycoside-induced increase in the force of contraction, and the associated decrease in end-diastolic volume, makes the heart's operation more nearly normal (Figure 15-1, *C, arrow*). Therefore hemodynamic improvements can be obtained only in the failing heart even though the glycoside may have a direct positive inotropic effect in both failing or nonfailing cardiac muscle.

Therapeutic Effects The principle of hemodynamic homeostasis in the human body is to maintain blood pressure in large arteries. This is in contrast to the coronary system in which the flow rate is autoregulated. Because the systemic circulation is regulated to maintain constant blood pressure, any influence of a reduced force of cardiac contraction to lower the blood pressure triggers regulatory mechanisms. These are increases in sympathetic discharges to the heart and vascular system and activation of the renin-angiotensin-vasopressin system. The volume of the circulating blood may also increase. Attempts of the body to increase blood pressure by constricting the peripheral blood vessels and by increasing total peripheral resistance result in a decrease of perfusion of many organs except for the heart. The positive inotropic effect of cardiac glycoside reverses these changes and improves tissue perfusion. This is the primary beneficial effect of cardiac glycosides.

Cardiac glycosides do not have a direct action to improve energetic efficiency of muscle contraction. Increases in force of cardiac contraction are associated with a corresponding increase in energy utilization. In the failing heart, however, the glycoside decreases end-diastolic volume, and thereby reduces wall tension necessary to develop the required intraventricular systolic pressure. Because the hemodynamic work of blood ejection can be achieved with a smaller wall tension, the net energetic efficiency of hemodynamic work is improved by the cardiac glycosides in patients with chronic heart failure.

Cardiac glycosides do not have direct diuretic effects unless injected into the renal artery in high concentrations; however, glycosides do produce notable diuretic effects in edematous patients with congestive heart failure. This effect results from improved tissue perfusion and reversal of changes in the renin-angiotensin-vasopressin system and on reflex adjustments in patients with congestive heart failure.

The Glycosides and Na$^+$, K$^+$-ATPase Both the positive inotropic and toxic effects of the cardiac glycosides result from binding of the glycoside to the same receptor, the Na$^+$, K$^+$-ATPase of the myocardial sarcolemma. A moderate (20% to 40%) inhibition of Na$^+$, K$^+$-ATPase or the sodium pump causes the therapeutic effect, whereas a greater sodium pump inhibition elicits toxic reactions. A significant positive

inotropic effect of the glycosides requires a dose that is 50% to 60% of the toxic dose. This is the primary reason that all cardiac glycosides have a narrow margin of safety.

Catecholamines, Xanthine Derivatives, and Newer Positive Inotropic Drugs

Catecholamines such as norepinephrine, epinephrine, or isoproterenol are not useful as positive inotropic drugs in patients with either acute or chronic heart failure for several reasons. The action of these drugs is extremely short, making it impractical to maintain a positive inotropic effect, especially because these drugs cannot be given orally. The vasoconstrictive effects of high doses of norepinephrine or epinephrine are undesirable because of reduction in tissue perfusion. Moreover, these drugs cause dysrhythmias or sensitize the heart to other drugs or conditions that may cause dysrhythmias. Finally, catecholamines shorten the duration of muscle contraction and increase heart rate, and thereby markedly reduce the energetic efficiency of heart muscle.

Dopamine and dobutamine have fewer chronotropic effects compared to the catecholamines just mentioned. Partial agonists for β_1-adrenergic receptors (e.g., prenalterol or xamoterol) may have the advantage of causing limited stimulation of the β_1-receptors and simultaneously blocking the stimulatory effects of endogenous catecholamines. Some β_2-adrenergic receptor agonists have also been tested as possible positive inotropic drugs. Dopamine infusion has favorable hemodynamic effects in chronic heart failure. To circumvent the problems of a short duration of action and the need for parenteral administration, several drugs that are absorbed following oral administration and converted to dopamine in the body have been tested as possible cardiotonic drugs. These include levodopa and ibopamine. All these drugs, however, appear to cause arrhythmias. Moreover, stable long-term effects cannot be obtained with many of these drugs because of the down regulation of adrenergic receptors that occurs during chronic agonist treatments.

Classical phosphodiesterase inhibitors, e.g., caffeine and theophylline ethylenediamine, increase force of cardiac contraction by elevating tissue cAMP concentrations. The action of these drugs, however, is nonselective for the heart and not potent. In contrast, the newer phosphodiesterase inhibitors that are selective for phosphodiesterase III produce prominent hemodynamic effects. The prototype drug, amrinone, however, has been reported to have side effects such as gastrointestinal intolerance (anorexia, abdominal pain, diarrhea), headache, fever, liver function abnormalities, and thrombocytopenia. These effects are unrelated to its cardiac action. Therefore when milrinone was introduced as having enhanced inotropic potency, it was thought that it might be largely devoid of these side effects. This drug, however, has had only limited clinical use because of its low efficacy. Many phosphodiesterase III inhibitors are presently under development as possible replacements for the digitalis glycosides as positive inotropic drugs.

Controversy still exists as to whether the positive inotropic effects of these drugs are mainly mediated through phosphodiesterase inhibition or by other mechanisms and whether the improvement of hemodynamics in the patient with chronic heart failure is the result of the positive inotropic action or vasodilation. A prominent feature of most of these drugs is vasodilation, expected from their mechanism of action. Vasodilation is effective in patients with congestive heart failure.

Alternative Treatments for Congestive Heart Failure

Congestive heart failure is a condition in which the heart fails to meet body demands and results from a reduced force of contraction. Therefore the cardiac glycosides and related positive inotropic drugs have been used with some success in treating these patients. There are, however, many problems associated with the chronic use of cardiac glycosides, and alternative drugs or alternative treatments are being used.

Because the basic problem of congestive heart failure is the relative deficiency in the force of cardiac contraction with respect to the demand for blood supply to various body organs, a reduction in demand should be effective in treating the condition. This may be achieved by nonpharmacological therapies such as reducing physical activity, instituting emotional rest, and restricting salt and water intake. In addition, pharmacological reduction of cardiac workload can be achieved by reducing afterload and preload of the heart (the hemodynamic load to the heart after or before systole) by lowering systemic blood pressure, dilating blood vessels to reduce peripheral resistance,

and reducing circulating blood volume. For example, a combination of an antihypertensive drug and a diuretic is frequently successful in treating patients with congestive heart failure, especially when used in conjunction with a positive inotropic drug.

Unlike cardiac glycosides that may constrict blood vessels by their action on sympathetic nerve terminals, most newer positive inotropic drugs dilate blood vessels, increasing the force of cardiac contraction as a result of inhibiting phosphodiesterase III. Therefore these drugs have the inherent property of reducing afterload. This is apparently an additional advantage of the phosphodiesterase inhibitors, although increases in heart rate that frequently occur are a distinct disadvantage.

An argument against this treatment is that it is palliative and does not correct the underlying basic heart failure. In this regard, treatment with positive inotropic drugs is also palliative, with the true underlying mechanisms responsible for reduction in the force of cardiac contraction not addressed.

In fact, chronic therapy with digoxin or amrinone, which forces the failing heart to work harder, may increase risk factors and is suspected of accelerating the progression to myocardial failure, although this has not been substantiated. In contrast, a reduction in work load of the failing heart reduces the risk factors. An acceptable alternative therapeutic regimen appears to be vasodilator therapy alone or combined with a cardiac glycoside and a diuretic.

SIDE EFFECTS, CLINICAL PROBLEMS, AND TOXICITY

Two major problems associated with the use of cardiac glycosides are the narrow margin of safety and the inability of these drugs to retard or reverse the basic process that causes the heart to fail. The therapeutic indices of various cardiac glycosides are 1.5 to 3.0, depending on the degree of the positive inotropic effect required. If a large positive inotropic effect is necessary, the required dose of the glycoside is close to its toxic dose. Therefore the glycoside concentration in plasma should be kept within a narrow therapeutic window to maintain the drug effect without inducing toxicity.

Individual variation in glycoside sensitivity of the heart makes it difficult to achieve a correct maintenance dose for the patient, especially when drug con-

Table 15-3 Factors that Influence Digitalis Sensitivity of the Heart

	Glycoside Binding to the Sodium Pump	Reserve Capacity of the Sodium Pump	Therapeutic Index
Increased Na$^+$ influx*	Enhanced	Reduced	Reduced
Decreased plasma K$^+$	Enhanced	Reduced	Reduced
Decreased sodium pump units†		Reduced	Reduced
Hypercalcemia	No change	No change	Reduced
Magnesium depletion	No change	No change	Reduced

*Tachycardia, electrical cardioversion, ischemic border zone.
†Hypothyroidism, old age.

centrations approaching toxic are required to meet the therapeutic need. Several factors are known to affect tolerance of patients to the cardiac glycosides (Table 15-3). Old age, hypothyroidism, and hypoxemia reduce the tolerance of the heart to cardiac glycosides, probably by reducing the reserve capacity of the sodium pump. Hypokalemia, tachycardia, and electrical cardioversion also reduce the reserve capacity and, in addition, promote glycoside binding to Na$^+$, K$^+$-ATPase. Acute myocardial infarction or ischemia markedly reduces the margin of safety because tolerance to toxic reactions is reduced, whereas inotropic potency is unchanged. Under these conditions, the use of the cardiac glycosides may not be warranted because a therapeutically useful positive inotropic effect may not be obtained before the onset of toxicity. Hypercalcemia and magnesium depletion also reduce tolerance of patients to glycoside toxicity. Newer positive inotropic drugs, which are relatively unaffected by these conditions, may be useful in treating the patient when the margin of safety for the glycosides and the magnitude of obtainable positive inotropic effects are expected to be reduced.

When treatment of a patient with chronic heart failure and marked edema is initiated with a combination of glycoside and diuretic, an initially adequate dose of the glycoside will soon become toxic unless the maintenance dose is reduced as K$^+$ is lost from the body, or the plasma K$^+$ concentration is maintained by means of potassium supplementation. Because K$^+$ has a great influence on glycoside actions, it is essential to monitor the K$^+$ concentration as well as the glycoside concentration in plasma.

Hypokalemia has a profound effect on the digitalis sensitivity of the heart. A lower extracellular K$^+$ promotes glycoside binding to Na$^+$-ATPase, and inhibits turnover of the sodium pump. Under these conditions, the sensitivity of the heart to the positive inotropic effect of the glycoside is increased, resulting from enhanced glycoside binding to the sodium pump.

Because both therapeutic and toxic effects of the glycosides are mediated by increased Ca^{++} loading of the sarcoplasmic reticulum, hypercalcemia or magnesium depletion increases sensitivity of the heart to both therapeutic and toxic actions of the glycoside. Again, the margin of safety is reduced.

In patients with acute myocardial infarction, tolerance of the affected area (e.g., the margin of the ischemia area) to digitalis toxicity is markedly reduced because of an elevation in intracellular Na$^+$; however, the glycoside sensitivity of the nonischemic area, at which the positive inotropic effect can be produced, is not altered. In these patients, the glycoside may not produce an adequate positive inotropic effect before the onset of toxicity and therefore its use is not recommended.

Toxic manifestations of the glycoside overdose may be modified by the sympathetic influence to the heart. Blockade of the β-adrenergic receptors increases tolerance of the heart to the arrhythmogenic actions of the glycoside. Animal experiments, however, indicate that β-adrenergic receptor blockade or surgical removal of sympathetic influence to the heart does not alter the lethal dose. Therefore, extreme caution is needed when β-adrenergic receptor blockers are used to treat manifestations of digitalis toxicity. With or without β blockers, death most often results from ventricular fibrillation.

Extracardiac manifestations of digitalis toxicity are largely mediated by the actions of the glycoside on neuronal tissues and secretory organs. These include anorexia, nausea, vomiting, excessive salivation, headache, epigastric distress, abdominal pain and diarrhea, yellow vision, muscle twitch, fatigue, stupor, visual disturbances, and neurological pain. Psychotomimetic effects including disorientation, confusion, depression, aphasia, delirium, hallucination, and convulsions may also be caused, especially in elderly patients.

Cardiotonic drugs may have effects on other organs and tissues. The cardiac glycosides have negligible effects on skeletal muscle because (1) these cells do not have a powerful Na^{++} exchanger and (2) transmembrane Ca^{++} does not play an important role in contractile activation. The glycosides have only a minor effect on renal salt and water excretion. It requires a direct infusion of high concentrations of the cardiac glycoside into the renal artery to cause diuresis. These results suggest that the sodium pump and the Na^+/Ca^{++} exchanger do not play important roles in renal salt and water excretion or that the renal sodium pump has a large reserve capacity. Thus the effects of the cardiac glycosides are relatively selective for the heart even though these drugs act on an Na^+, K^+-ATPase that is present in most cells and has important functions.

Ca^{++} ions play an important role as a messenger in neuronal and secretory cells. High doses of cardiac glycosides therefore facilitate neuronal transmission and stimulate secretory cells. The central nervous system, however, is relatively unaffected by digoxin or digitoxin because their access to the brain is limited even though they have a high lipid solubility. The prominent effects of the glycosides on the nervous system are observed with systems that lie outside the blood-brain barrier, such as sensitization of baroreceptors, chemoreceptors, and cells within the chemoreceptor trigger zone.

The primary symptom of digitalis toxicity is dysrhythmias caused by suppression of AV conduction. Ventricular premature contractions triggered by oscillatory afterpotentials that originate in Purkinje fibers may also be superimposed. These dysrhythmias may be reversed to a normal sinus rhythm by K^+ when the plasma K^+ concentration is low or within the normal range. K^+ is sometimes effective against glycoside-induced dysrhythmias because it stimulates sodium pump activity, reduces the glycoside binding to Na^+, K^+-ATPase, and probably alters membrane conductance to cations. When the plasma K^+ concentration is high, antidysrhythmic drugs such as lidocaine, procainamide, or propranolol can be used.

Phenytoin is also useful in treating dysrhythmias; however, several instances of sudden death have been reported when phenytoin is administered to a patient with glycoside toxicity. Perhaps the most dramatic treatment for digitalis toxicity is the use of a specific antibody preparation raised against digoxin. This preparation is administered IV and acts by binding serum digoxin. The complex is excreted rapidly by the kidneys.

Quinidine should not be used to treat digoxin-induced dysrhythmias because it interacts pharmacokinetically with the glycoside. Quinidine reduces the apparent volume of distribution and renal clearance of digoxin. Therefore when quinidine is given to patients receiving digoxin, the digoxin concentration in plasma increases. The initial increase in plasma digoxin concentration that occurs when quinidine is administered to patients maintained on the glycoside is caused by a decrease in the apparent volume of digoxin distribution. Digoxin concentration, however, is maintained at a high value as long as quinidine is concomitantly administered unless the digoxin concentration is adequately reduced. This latter effect of quinidine results from a reduced renal clearance of digoxin.

The reduction in the apparent volume of digoxin distribution results from the competitive displacement of the glycoside by quinidine from mutual binding sites. Because of the competitive nature of the interaction, the degree of quinidine-induced increase in digoxin concentration is proportional to the dose of quinidine. These mutual binding sites are not the pharmacological or toxic receptors for the glycoside. Therefore the glycoside binding to the receptor site increases because the displaced glycoside combines with Na^+, K^+-ATPase and enhances the toxic effects of the glycoside. Pharmacokinetic interactions between quinidine and digitoxin are less prominent. This is because the mutual binding sites for quinidine and the glycoside account for a significant fraction of non-Na^+, K^+-ATPase binding sites for digoxin but represent a small fraction for digitoxin, which has a large apparent volume of distribution. In addition to quinidine, many drugs have been reported to have pharmacokinetic interactions with digoxin; however, significant increases in plasma digoxin concentration may be observed only with high doses of verapamil, nifedipine, amiodarone, or quinine, in contrast to quinidine, which may precipitate digoxin toxicity at relatively low doses.

CLINICAL PROBLEMS

DIGITALIS GLYCOSIDES

Overdose produces cardiac dysrhythmias

Therapeutic window is narrow and care must be taken in prescribing an appropriate dosage schedule

Greater binding of the glycosides and potential toxicity at low serum K^+ concentrations; caution needed when used with diuretics

BIPYRIDINES

Limited to short-term parenteral use

TRADENAMES

In addition to generic and fixed combination preparations, the following tradenamed materials are available in the United States.

Corotrope, milrinone
Crystodigin, digitoxin
Digibind, digoxin immune Fab (ovine)
Inocor, amrinone
Lanoxin, digoxin

Other drugs that interact with the cardiac glycoside through various mechanisms are amphotericin B, chlorthalidone, ethacrynic acid, furosemide, and thiazides, which increase the therapeutic and toxic effects of the glycoside and reduce the margin of safety by enhancing K^+ excretion. Large glucose infusions may also reduce serum K^+. Calcium preparations, reserpine, succinylcholine, and sympathomimetics may also precipitate digitalis toxicity. Propranolol may augment bradycardia caused by the cardiac glycoside. Barbiturates, phenytoin, and phenylbutazone may enhance metabolism of the glycoside and thereby reduce therapeutic and toxic effects, whereas cholestyramine combines with digitoxin in the intestine and enhances elimination of the glycoside.

The primary problems are summarized in the box above. Problems with catecholamines and xanthines are discussed in Chapters 10 and 32, respectively.

REFERENCES

Akera T: Effects of cardiac glycosides on Na^+, K^+, ATPase. In Grief K, ed: experimental pharmacology, 56/1: Cardiac Glycosides, Berlin, 1981, Springer-Verlag.

Akera T and Brody TM: The role of Na^+-K, ATPase in the inotropic action of digitalis, Pharmacol Rev 29: 187, 1977.

Colucci WS, Wright RF, and Braunwald E: New positive inotropic agents in the treatment of congestive heart failure, N Engl J Med 314: 290; 349, 1986.

Grupp G: Selective updates on mechanisms of action of positive inotropic agents, Mol Cell Biochem 76: 97, 1987.

Lee CO: 200 years of digitalis: the emerging central role of sodium ion in the control of contractile force, Am J Physiol 249: C367, 1985.

Marban E and Smith TW: Digitalis. In Fozzard HA, Haber E, Jennings RB et al., eds: The heart and cardiovascular system, Scientific Foundation, vol 2, New York, 1986, Raven Press.

Maskin CS, LeJemtel TH, and Sonnenblick EH: Inotropic drugs for the treatment of the failing heart, Cardiovasc Clin 14: 1, 1984.

Schwartz A, Lindenmayer GE, and Allen JC: The Na^+, K^+, ATPase: pharmacological, physiological and biochemical aspects, Pharmacol Rev 27: 3, 1975.

Calcium Antagonists

MAJOR DRUGS

nifedipine
verapamil
diltiazem

THERAPEUTIC OVERVIEW

It was observed in 1964 that the effects of prenylamine and verapamil on cardiac papillary muscle preparation were indistinguishable from the effects of Ca^{++} withdrawal. These drugs, like Ca^{++} withdrawal, inhibited contractile force without inhibiting the action potential and produced excitation-contraction uncoupling. These drug effects were reversed by excess Ca^{++}, β-adrenergic agonists, and cardiac glycosides. Verapamil and prenylamine, together with other drugs that inhibited the excitation-contraction coupling, were termed *calcium antagonists* to indicate that they counteract the effect of Ca^{++} on the contractile system.

The primary action of these drugs is inhibition of the inward movement of Ca^{++} through voltage-dependent Ca^{++} channels located in cell membranes. To reflect this effect, the terms *slow channel blockers, slow channel inhibitors, calcium channel blockers, calcium channel inhibitors,* and *calcium entry blockers* have also been used as alternatives to *calcium antagonists.*

Calcium antagonists, a structurally heterogenous group of drugs, are effective in the treatment of several cardiovascular disorders, particularly angina pectoris, supraventricular tachycardias, and hypertension. Several other conditions such as migraine, Raynaud's phenomenon, and posthemorrhagic cerebral vasospasm appear, in some clinical trials, to be favorably influenced by calcium antagonists. Therefore the potential therapeutic spectrum of these drugs is rapidly increasing. The therapeutic overview is summarized in the box.

Angina pectoris is the clinical syndrome of transient cardiac ischemia caused by coronary artery disease. It is characterized by severe retrosternal chest pain or pressure that in typical cases radiates to the left shoulder, left arm, and/or to the back. Exertional (stable), variant (Prinzmetal's), and unstable angina are the three clinical forms of this disease. The un-

Calcium antagonists: act by inhibiting Ca^{++} movement into cells
Disease states where effective:
Angina pectoris
Supraventricular tachycardia
Hypertension
Migrane
Raynaud's phenomenon
Posthemorrhagic cerebral vasospasm
Other names
Calcium channel blockers
Slow channel blockers
Slow channel inhibitors
Calcium channel inhibitors
Calcium entry blockers

derlying pathological condition is atherosclerosis and the related ischemia resulting from inadequate blood perfusion of an area of the myocardium. Ischemia can develop from either decreased blood supply or increased metabolic demand. Although angina pectoris is defined primarily as a "supply" defect, an increased metabolic demand is also frequently required to cause symptoms.

Exertional (exercise-induced) angina most frequently occurs in patients with atherosclerosis of the coronary blood vessels. Typically, these patients are relatively free from symptoms at rest, suggesting that the supply of oxygen and nutrients to the heart and the removal of the metabolic products by the venous blood are adequate as long as there is no excess load on the heart. Upon exercise, heart rate and blood pressure increase, which results in increased cardiac work and hence increased demand for oxygen and nutrients. The blood flow through the narrow, atherosclerotic coronaries to the myocardium becomes limited. When the increased demand exceeds supply, ischemia develops that may cause the typical array of symptoms and signs, including chest pain and depression of the ST segment. The symptoms can be alleviated by interventions that either increase the supply of oxygen and nutrients and/or decrease the demand for them. Therefore if the ischemia is removed, the anginal symptoms disappear.

Variant (Prinzmetal's) angina was originally recognized as a variant form (hence the name) in that it is the result of transient narrowing of a large epicardial coronary artery. The vasospasm frequently develops at a sclerotic narrowing but can also occur on the normal segment of the coronary artery. The symptoms occur at rest, typically at night or in the early morning, and include severe chest pain; unlike the stable form of angina, elevation of the ST segment is recorded during the episodes of pain. It has been shown that "focal vasospasm" is the hallmark of this form of angina.

The most severe form of the three types of angina is unstable angina that is diagnosed when symptomatic episodes increase in frequency, severity, or duration. Chest pain occurs at rest (day or night) and often is associated with reversible electrocardiographic changes. Advanced atherosclerosis together with coronary vasospasm may underlie this clinical syndrome.

A group of cardiac rhythmic disturbances termed supraventricular tachycardias may represent another important disease that benefits from treatment with some of the calcium antagonists. Supraventricular tachycardias include paroxysmal supraventricular tachycardia, atrial fibrillation, and atrial flutter. The pathological mechanisms involved in the development of these cardiac rhythmic disorders are described in Chapter 14. The atrioventricular (AV) node, which plays a key role in the mechanisms of these dysrhythmias, depends on the influx of Ca^{++} through drug-sensitive, voltage-dependent Ca^{++} channels. Therefore supraventricular tachycardias are sensitive to treatment with some calcium antagonists. However, of the three drugs available in the United States, only verapamil and diltiazem are useful in inhibiting conduction through the AV node.

The third major condition where calcium antagonists have significant therapeutic value is hypertension. The neurohumoral control of blood pressure, the mechanisms assumed to be involved in hypertension, and the large variety of drugs used for the treatment of hypertension are described in Chapters 12 and 13. There is no question, however, that the calcium antagonists are an exciting new modality in the treatment of some types of hypertension.

Raynaud's phenomenon is a peripheral vascular disease characterized by vasospastic attacks of digital arteries frequently precipitated by cold or emotional stress. This disease can effectively be treated by calcium antagonists, particularly dihydropyridines, because of their ability to abolish vasospasm.

MECHANISMS OF ACTION

Membrane Actions

Calcium antagonists act by inhibiting the influx of Ca^{++} into the cells through specific voltage-dependent calcium channels located in cell membranes. Calcium channels are membrane-spanning, funnel-shaped glycoproteins that function like ion selective valves (Figure 16-1). They form a water-filled pore that opens and closes to permit Ca^{++} to move in the direction of its electrochemical concentration gradient. When conformational changes in the channel macromolecule occur, the activation (A) and inactivation (I) "gates" move into and out of an occluding position. This determines opening and closing of the channel pore. Ca^{++} binding sites present in the pore ensure ion selectivity for the channels. Phosphorylation sites, as well as drug and toxin binding sites of the channel macromolecule, play important roles in the regulation of the channel. It should be emphasized that the exact macrostructure of the channel protein(s), putative gates, and other regulatory sites is unknown at this time; the structure shown in Figure 16-1 is speculative. In the case of the rabbit skeletal muscle Ca^{++} channel, the α_1 subunit polypeptide contains four sections, each of which has six membrane-spanning segments (S_1-S_6). The S_4 segment appears to be a highly preserved structure characteristic of voltage-dependent ion channels.

The primary modulator of voltage-dependent Ca^{++} channels is the membrane potential (voltage). The existence of three voltage-dependent conformations has been postulated (Figure 16-2): a resting state in which the pore is closed by the A gate; an open state in which both gates are open; and an inactivated state in which the channel is closed by the I gate. Under resting conditions, when the voltage-dependent calcium channels are closed and the membrane potential is -60 to -100 mV (intracellular with reference to extracellular), depending on the cell type, the free intracellular Ca^{++} concentration ($<10^{-7}$ M) is more than four orders of magnitude lower than the extracellular free Ca^{++} concentration (1.5×10^{-3} M). This large concentration gradient represents an enormous driving force for Ca^{++} and can be maintained only by a membrane that is largely impermeable to Ca^{++} and contains active transport systems that pump Ca^{++} out of the cytosol. The intact cell membrane fulfills these requirements. Upon excitation, a

rapid depolarization of the membrane follows. When the membrane potential reaches -40 mV, voltage-dependent Ca^{++} channels open and Ca^{++} enters the cell. This is followed by inactivation (closing) of Ca^{++} channels. Before the next depolarization occurs, Ca^{++} channels must recover from inactivation and be ready for opening from a resting closed conformation.

Besides membrane potential, other modulators, both endogenous and exogenous, also affect voltage-dependent Ca^{++} channels. These include hormones, neurotransmitters, inorganic ions, toxins, and drugs (see box). The drugs that act directly on Ca^{++} channels include both Ca^{++} agonists and Ca^{++} antagonists. Many chemical compounds are known to inhibit voltage-dependent Ca^{++} channels, but only those that have their primary effect on Ca^{++} channels are discussed here. The most selective drugs belong to one of the following three chemical groups: 1,4-dihydropyridines, phenylalkylamines, and benzothiazepines (Table 16-1). The differences in the chemical structures (Figure 16-3) show that the drugs commercially available in the United States are completely different; hence one could expect that they may bind to three distinct receptors. Therefore one should not regard the calcium antagonists as belonging to a single class of drugs but rather to three different subtypes.

Voltage-dependent calcium channels play a specific role in the excitation-contraction-relaxation cycle (Figure 16-4). Under resting conditions, when the in-

---

CALCIUM CHANNEL MODULATORS

Membrane potential (voltage)
Hormones and neurotransmitters (e.g., epinephrine) can regulate in two different ways:
  By activating protein kinases (A and/or C) that phosphorylate the channel
  Through the guanine nucleotide binding (G) proteins that directly link β-receptors to calcium channels
Inorganic ions; Co^{++}, Ni^{++}, and Cd^{++} are inhibitors.
Toxins
  Activators such as maitotoxin
  Inhibitors such as ω-conotoxin
Drugs
  Agonists
  Antagonists

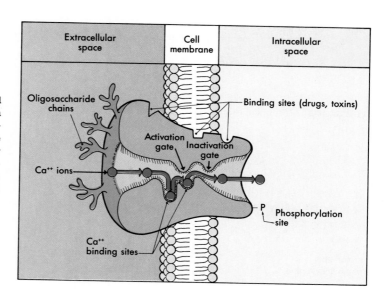

FIGURE 16-1 Schematic diagram of calcium channel glycoprotein positioned in cell membrane. The ion channel is assumed to contain activation *(A)* and inactivation *(I)* gates that are moved or altered by the potential difference across the membrane and by drugs so as to open or close the channel to the transmembrane flux of Ca^{++}. A site of phosphorylation is shown. The detailed geometry and mechanism of the channel are still speculative.

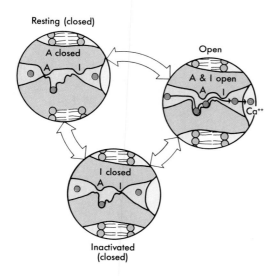

FIGURE 16-2 Three voltage-dependent conformations (states) of calcium channels. The ion channel (pore) is "open" to the transmembrane flux of Ca^{++} only when both the proposed activation *(A)* and inactivation *(I)* sites are open. In the "closed" states, either the *A* or *I* sites are not open. Top view of channel is shown on the left.

Table 16-1 Drugs Affecting Calcium Channels: Pharmacological and Structural Classifications

	1,4-dihydropyridines	phenylalkylamines	benzothiazepines
Calcium antagonists	nifedipine nimodipine nicardipine isradipine	verapamil desmethoxyverapamil D-600	diltiazem TA-3090
Calcium agonists	(−)-S-Bay K-8644 (+)-S-202-791 CGP-28392		

FIGURE 16-3   Chemical structures of calcium antagonists.

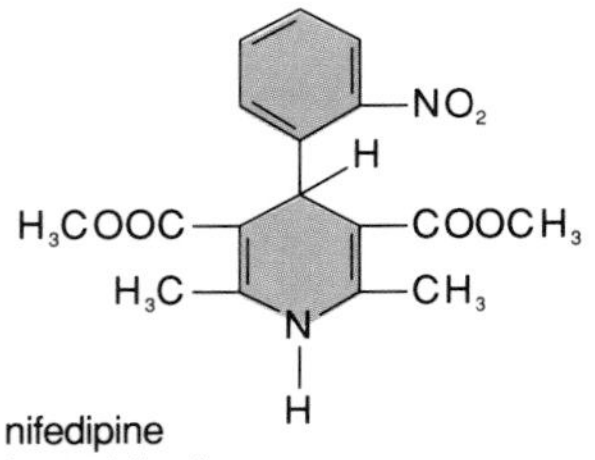

nifedipine
(dihydropyridine)

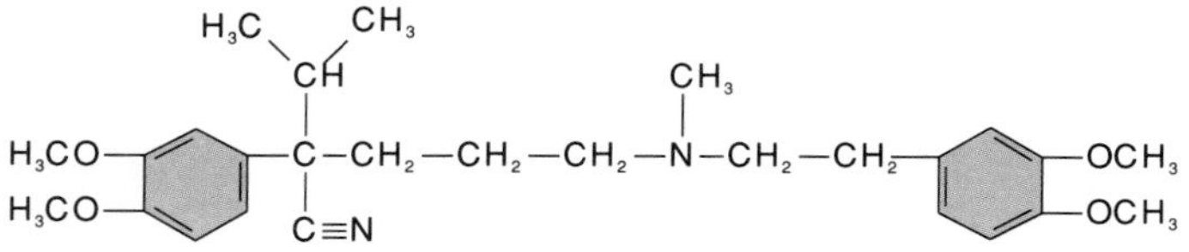

verapamil
(phenylalkylamine)

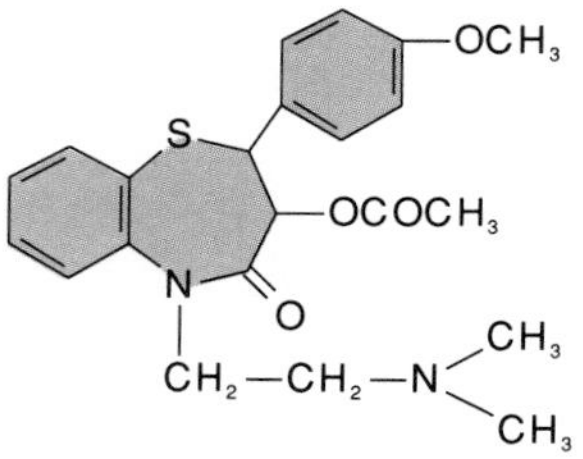

diltiazem
(benzothiazepine)

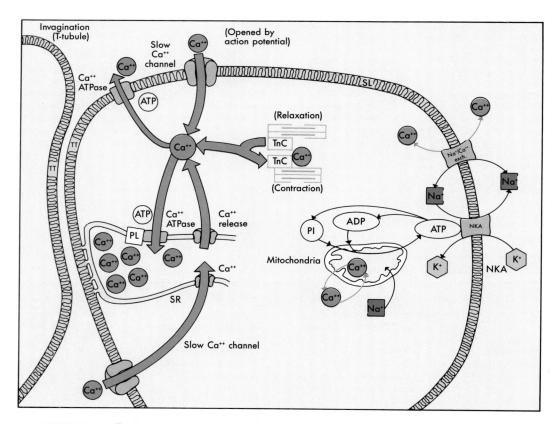

FIGURE 16-4   Excitation-contraction coupling in cardiac cells. *tt*, T-tubule; *SR*, sarcoplasmic reticulum; PL, phospholamban; *NKA*, sodium-potassium-ATPase (see text).

tracellular Ca^{++} concentration is low ($<10^{-7}$ M), the regulatory proteins (troponin I, T, and C and actomyosin) prevent interaction of actin and myosin filaments with each other; and the muscle is relaxed. When the intracellular Ca^{++} concentration increases ($>10^{-7}$ M) from the influx of Ca^{++} through Ca^{++} channels and the release of Ca^{++} from internal stores, Ca^{++} occupies specific Ca^{++} binding sites on troponin C (cardiac and skeletal muscle) and calmodulin (vascular smooth muscle). These then interact with other regulatory proteins and enzymes (e.g., troponin I) in cardiac and skeletal muscle and myosin light chain kinase in smooth muscle, facilitating cross-bridge formation between actin and myosin and activating contraction. When Ca^{++} channels close and the Ca^{++}-ATPase system pumps Ca^{++} out of the cytosol into intracellular stores and to the extracellular space, the cytosolic Ca^{++} concentration decreases to its resting level, Ca^{++} dissociates from Ca^{++} binding proteins, activation of contractile proteins is reversed, actin dissociates from myosin, and muscle relaxation occurs. Thus drugs that affect Ca^{++} channels will also affect muscle contraction. While calcium agonists produce an increase in contraction, calcium antagonists induce muscle relaxation.

Drug and Receptor Interactions

The interaction of the Ca^{++} channel modulators with Ca^{++} channels is complex. Three distinct but allosterically interacting receptors exist for the three different chemical classes of drugs (Figure 16-5): 1,4-dihydropyridines (nifedipine-like drugs), phenylalkylamines (verapamil-like drugs), and benothiazepines (diltiazem-like drugs). All these receptors are located on the same (α_1) subunit of the voltage-dependent Ca^{++} channels.

The effects of Ca^{++} antagonists are membrane potential (voltage) dependent. This phenomenon can be explained with a modulated receptor model. This model, first developed to explain voltage-dependent effects of local anesthetics on Na^+ channels, has been extended and used to explain the voltage-dependent effects of Ca^{++} channel-inhibiting drugs on Ca^{++} channels. This model postulates that channels are similar to allosteric enzymes that alter their conformations and hence affinities for substrates on binding of allosteric modulators. Specifically, the modulated receptor model assumes that the channel macromolecule alters its affinity for the drugs when its conformation ("state") is changed by the membrane poten-

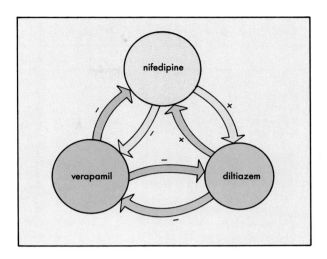

FIGURE 16-5   Allosteric interactions occur among the nifedipine (NIF), verapamil (VER), and diltiazem (DTZ) binding sites of the voltage-dependent Ca^{++} channels. All three binding sites are located on the same subunit.

tial (note open and inactivated states, Figure 16-2). It is assumed that drugs bind to the inactivated channel state with much higher affinity than to the resting and open states. This mechanism may explain why these drugs are more effective on inactivated than on open or resting channels.

The binding and effects of Ca^{++} antagonists are stereoselective. Generally, stereoisomers of the same compound produce qualitatively the same effects, with one stereoisomer being more effective than the other. In a few special situations, the stereoisomers produce opposite pharmacological effects. While the (R)-enantiomers of Bay K-8644 and 202-791 (two recently synthesized experimental 1,4-dihydropyridine derivatives) act like Ca^{++} antagonists, the (S)-enantiomers are Ca^{++} agonists. Exactly how mirror-image drugs can produce opposite effects is unknown. It has been postulated that either conformational alterations occur in the "receptor" and/or separate binding sites exist for agonists and antagonists.

 ## PHARMACOKINETICS

Dosages of different Ca^{++} channel inhibitors and the mode of administration are determined by several factors, including the nature of the disease state and the overall condition of the patient. Therefore the treatment regimen should always be individualized.

Table 16-2   Pharmacokinetic Parameters

	nifedipine	verapamil	diltiazem
Absorption	>90%	>80%	>90%
Bioavailability	45-70%	10-20%	45%
Protein binding	95%	90%	80%
Volume of distribution	1.2 L/kg	4 L/kg	5.3 L/kg
Metabolism	Liver	Liver	Liver
First-pass	30-40%	85%	50%
Active metabolite	None	norverapamil	desacetyl diltiazem
Metabolite activity (% of parent drug)	Zero	20-30%	40-50%
Renal excretion	85%	75%	85%
$t_{1/2}$, hr	4	5	4
Administered	Oral	Oral, IV	Oral
Onset of action	15 min (2-3 min, 1)*	1-2 hr	15 min
Peak effect (time after administration)	1-3 hr	3-5 hr	30 min

*Sublingual.

A low dose is recommended at the onset of treatment with subsequent increases to within the normal range until the desired therapeutic effect is reached. For a rapid effect, sublingual or IV administration of the drug may be required. When verapamil is given IV for treatment of supraventricular tachycardias, the ECG and blood pressure should be monitored; drug administration should be discontinued as soon as the desired effect is reached or signs of cardiodepression appear. The mode of administration and pharmacokinetic parameters are summarized in Table 16-2.

The gastrointestinal absorption of nifedipine is essentially complete (>90%). Due to extensive first-pass metabolism by the liver, however, only 45% to 70% of the administered drug reaches the systemic circulation. In blood, 95% of nifedipine is bound to plasma proteins. The steady state apparent volume of distribution is 1.2 L/kg body weight. Nifedipine is metabolized to three inactive metabolites in the liver, and these are excreted in the urine. The elimination half-life is about 4 hours but is longer in patients with compromised hepatic function.

Absorption of verapamil from the gastrointestinal tract is effective (>80%), but the bioavailability is very low (10% to 20%); this results from the intensive first-pass metabolism by the liver. In the systemic circulation, 90% is bound to plasma proteins. The steady state volume of distribution is 4 L/kg. Norverapamil, an active metabolite, has a potency approximately 20% to 30% that of verapamil. Metabolites are excreted in the urine with an elimination half-life of

about 5 hours; again much longer in patients with hepatic disease.

Diltiazem is almost completely absorbed from the gastrointestinal tract. Because of first-pass hepatic metabolism, the bioavailability is only 45%. Once absorbed, approximately 80% of diltiazem is bound to plasma proteins. The apparent volume of distribution is approximately 5.3 L/kg. Desacetyl diltiazem is an active metabolite with an activity of about 40% to 50% of its parent compound. Elimination half-life of diltiazem is about 4 hours but is longer in patients with hepatic diseases.

 RELATION OF MECHANISMS OF ACTION TO CLINICAL RESPONSE

In many cardiovascular diseases (i.e., Prinzmetal's angina, hypertension, and Raynaud's phenomenon), constriction of high resistance vessels occurs, possibly associated with abnormally high cytosolic free Ca^{++} concentrations. It is possible that abnormal contractile proteins, with perhaps increased affinity for calcium, are present that change endothelial cell function. Other factors may play important roles. Elevated cytosolic Ca^{++} may result from either an excessive influx of Ca^{++} or incomplete removal of Ca^{++} by Ca^{++}-ATPases and Na^+/Ca^{++} exchange processes. In any event, a rational therapeutic intervention is inhibition of Ca^{++} influx, which may induce vascular smooth muscle relaxation.

Table 16-3 Comparative Clinical Effects of Calcium Antagonists

	nifedipine	verapamil	diltiazem
Coronary dilatation	+ + +	+ +	+ + +
Peripheral vasodilation	+ + +	+ +	+
Contractility	+ *	—	0
Heart rate			
Resting	+ + *	—	0
Exercise increase	+ *	—	—
Artrioventricular conduction	0	—	—

+, Positive effect; −, negative effect; 0, no effect.
*Indirect, reflex response to peripheral vasodilation.

Endogenous and exogenous modulators that inhibit Ca^{++} channels are listed in the box. From these, only Ca^{++} channel inhibiting and activating drugs (and some toxins) act selectively on voltage-dependent Ca^{++} channels. Other drugs such as β-adrenergic agonists act on Ca^{++} channels indirectly, by activating cAMP-dependent protein kinase, which phosphorylates channel subunit(s) and thereby results in an increase in the probability of openings. β-adrenergic blocking agents act by inhibiting the binding of β agonists, thereby preventing activation of Ca^{++} channels through β receptors.

All excitable tissues contain voltage-dependent Ca^{++} channels and high affinity, reversible, and stereospecific binding sites for Ca^{++} channel-inhibiting drugs. However, calcium antagonists do not affect every tissue equally. Possible reasons for tissue-selective effects are listed in the box. In the first instance, some tissues rely primarily on exogenous Ca^{++} (atrioventricular node) and are more sensitive to these drugs than other tissues (skeletal muscle) that require little or no external Ca^{++} for function. Second, subtypes of voltage-dependent Ca^{++} channels exist that show different sensitivities for Ca^{++} channel inhibitors. The best characterized are the L-type channels (long-lasting, large channels), the T-type channels (transient, tiny channels), and the N-type channels (found in neuronal tissue and resembling neither of the other two in kinetics and inhibitor sensitivity). Of these channel subtypes, only the L-type channels are sensitive to Ca^{++} channel-inhibiting drugs. Since the distribution of the channel subtypes differs in various tissues, drug sensitivity of the tissues is also different. In addition, even the L-type Ca^{++} channels are different in various tissues with respect to their affinities for calcium antagonists. Third, these drugs bind to the receptors with higher affinity under depolarized rather than polarized conditions. Since the resting membrane potential differs in various tissues, the binding and effects of these

drugs also vary. Finally, frequency dependence indicates that the inhibition of channels by these drugs is altered by the rate of stimulation. The underlying mechanism for the frequency-dependence appears to be inhibition of the recovery of the channel from inactivation. Recovery occurs during the time available between stimuli. Only those channels that have recovered from inactivation can reopen on the next stimulus. At high frequencies, the channels affected by these drugs do not function because they have not recovered from inactivation during the short time available between stimuli. Thus drugs of this type seem to be very effective at high rates of stimulation. In contrast, at low frequencies all channels (those affected by the drug and those not affected) may completely recover from inactivation before the next stimulus arrives. Therefore drug inhibition of Ca^{++} channels is minimal or absent at low stimulation rates. Chemically different drugs show different degrees of frequency dependence. Verapamil shows much more frequency dependence than does nifedipine; diltiazem appears to be intermediate.

The effects of one calcium antagonist should not be extrapolated to another of a different subtype because drugs belonging to different subtypes have different pharmacological effects (Table 16-3).

Nifedipine

The pharmacological effects of nifedipine are related to inhibition of the L type of voltage-dependent Ca^{++} channels in vascular smooth muscle. This drug has a relatively selective effect on arterial resistance vessels. By dilating coronary blood vessels and increasing coronary blood flow, particularly through narrowed coronary arteries (e.g., by vasospasm), nifedipine increases oxygen and nutrient supply to the ischemic myocardium. By increasing coronary blood flow, nifedipine also enhances the removal of metabolic products from the ischemic area. As a result of the dilation of peripheral arterial high resistance vessels, the arterial blood pressure (afterload) decreases. Although the decrease is more significant in hypertensive patients than in normotensive individuals, any sudden decrease in blood pressure in both normotensives and hypertensives can result in a reflex increase in heart rate and contractility. If the reflex increase in contractility is stronger than the direct negative inotropic effect of nifedipine, the overall result observed may be a slight increase or no effect, rather than a decrease in contractility. Pulmonary vascular resistance and mean pulmonary arterial pressure are also decreased by nifedipine. These effects, together with the previously described effects, produce a favorable hemodynamic condition for patients suffering from angina pectoris and mild congestive heart failure simultaneously. However, there is always the potential danger that nifedipine may exacerbate incipient heart failure already present because of the direct negative inotropic action of the drug.

Nifedipine, in contrast to verapamil and diltiazem that inhibit atrioventricular conduction, has no significant effect on atrioventricular nodal conduction in vivo. Nifedipine is preferable to verapamil and diltiazem in those patients who have an underlying defective atrioventricular conduction problem (e.g., sick sinus syndrome). Nifedipine lowers esophageal sphincter pressure, may inhibit peristalsis, and, by inducing a sympathetic discharge, increases the plasma renin activity. However, not all of these effects are observed in every patient.

Stable, variant (Prinzmetal's), and unstable angina and hypertension are favorably influenced by nifedipine. Nifedipine can be used alone or in combination with nitrates or β blockers. Acute episodes of hypertension can be treated with sublingual nifedipine. In mild to moderate hypertension, nifedipine has an efficacy equivalent to β blockers or diuretics. Although it is effective alone, its use in combination with a low dose of β blockers is particularly efficacious because the reflex increases in heart rate and plasma renin activity produced by nifedipine are attenuated by the β blocker.

In addition, nifedipine is effective in the treatment of Raynaud's phenomenon. It has been successfully employed in some studies in the treatment of ischemic pain immediately after myocardial infarction and for prevention of coronary artery spasm, which frequently occurs during coronary catheterization and coronary artery bypass surgery.

Verapamil

Verapamil was the first selective Ca^{++} channel inhibitor available for treatment of cardiovascular disorders. Like nifedipine, verapamil has both coronary and peripheral vasodilator effects. Verapamil is a more potent, negative inotropic agent than nifedipine. This results from nifedipine's more potent activation of the baroreceptor reflex, secondary to the decrease in peripheral resistance. In contrast to nifedipine, verapamil also produces a potent depression of atrioventricular conduction. As a result, verapamil is the drug of choice for the treatment of supraventricular tachycardias. Verapamil is also effective for the treatment of angina pectoris and hypertension. The reflex increase in adrenergic tone due to a sudden decrease in blood pressure mitigates, but does not overcome, the strong direct negative inotropic and chronotropic effects of verapamil. Because of these prominent cardiodepressant effects, verapamil is generally contraindicated in congestive heart failure.

Diltiazem

Diltiazem has some pharmacological effects similar to those of nifedipine but resembles verapamil in its other actions. Like all Ca^{++} antagonists, diltiazem increases coronary blood flow and decreases an elevated blood pressure. Similar to verapamil, diltiazem inhibits atrioventricular conduction, although less potently than verapamil.

Diltiazem has many therapeutic uses. It is effective in all types of angina, particularly in those forms where coronary vasospasm is involved. Diltiazem has about the same efficacy as nifedipine in dilating coronaries but produces fewer side effects. It can be prescribed with sublingual glyceryl trinitrate or with isosorbate trinitrate for the treatment of angina pectoris. Diltiazem is effective in decreasing hypertension but in these same doses fails to decrease the blood pressure in normotensive individuals. It has less negative inotropic and chronotropic effects than do the β-adrenergic blocking drugs. In paroxysmal supraventricular tachycardia, diltiazem, like verapamil, slows the ventricular response to atrial tachycardia and in many cases restores a regular sinus rhythm. Orally administered diltiazem is useful in preventing the development of paroxysmal supraventricular tachycardia and decreases the ventricular response in atrial fibrillation and flutter by slowing atrioventricular conduction. Other disorders that are favorably influenced by diltiazem include Raynaud's phenomenon, migraine, and esophageal mobility disorders. Present data indicate that it may also reduce the incidence of reinfarction.

SIDE EFFECTS, CLINICAL PROBLEMS, AND TOXICITY

Problems and side effects are summarized in the box and Table 16-4. Most side effects result from excessive vasodilation or cardiodepression (i.e., negative inotropic and chronotropic effects). In most patients side effects such as dizziness, headache, and flushing decrease or disappear on decreasing the dose. In others, discontinuation of the drug may be necessary. Although true withdrawal symptoms are not observed, sudden withdrawal of a large dose of a calcium antagonist may in rare cases cause precipitation of angina. Neither tachyphylaxis nor tolerance occurs with these drugs.

With nifedipine use, side effects may occur in 17% to 20% of patients, primarily but not exclusively because of excessive vasodilation. Headache, dizziness, flushing, ankle edema, hypotension, and nasal congestion can be mitigated by reducing the dose. If unsuccessful, discontinuation of the drug may be necessary and substitution of another calcium antagonist indicated. Excessive lowering of blood pressure may exacerbate myocardial ischemia.

During verapamil treatment, side effects occur in about 8% to 10% of the patient population and may result from excessive vasodilation and from blockade of the atrioventricular node. During its oral administration, the most frequent side effects are constipation, headache, nausea, dizziness, and ankle edema. Constipation does not appear to be a problem with either nifedipine or diltiazem. It is possible that verapamil produces this side effect by acting on autonomic receptors. Rare side effects are galactorrhea and reversible hepatic damage. Adverse effects with overdoses include hypotension, atrioventricular block, bradycardia, congestive heart failure, and (rarely) ventricular asystole. Verapamil toxicity, like the effects of all calcium antagonists, may be reversed with isoproterenol alone, or in combination with IV calcium gluconate.

CLINICAL PROBLEMS

NIFEDIPINE

Problems in 17%-20% of patients
    Major: Hypotension
             Headache
             Peripheral edema

VERAPAMIL

Problems in 8%-10% patients
    Major: Cardiodepression
  Moderate: Hypotension
             Atrioventricular block
             Peripheral edema
    Minor: Headache
             Constipation

DILTIAZEM

Problems in 2%-5% of patients
    Minor: Hypotension
             Peripheral edema
             Atrioventricular block
             Cardiodepression

Table 16-4 Comparative Adverse Effects of Calcium Channel Inhibitors

	nifedipine	verapamil	diltiazem
Percentage occurrence	17%-20%	8%-10%	2%-5%
Hypotension	+ + +	+ +	+
Headache	+ + +	+	0
Peripheral edema	+ + +	+ +	±
Constipation	0	+	0
Atrioventricular block	0	+ +	+
Cardiodepression	0	+ + +	+

+ + +, Large response; + +, medium response; +, small response; ±, variable response; 0, no response.

Side effects are rare (2% to 5%) during diltiazem treatment and occur mainly at high doses. Headache, flushing, and hypotension can occur from excessive vasodilation, and atrioventricular block may result from depression of the atrioventricular node.

Before the administration of calcium antagonists to patients concurrently on digitalis preparations, two possible drug interactions must be considered. Depression of the atrioventricular conduction may occur because of the combined depressive effects of digitalis and calcium channel inhibitors on the atrioventricular node. Digitalis toxicity may also occur if the renal clearance of digoxin is reduced by calcium channel antagonists.

The combination of nifedipine with β blockers for the treatment of hypertension can be advantageous because, although both drugs decrease blood pressure, the reflex effects of nifedipine (increase in heart rate and plasma renin activity) are reduced by the β blocker. However, with this combination of drugs, decreased doses are required to prevent severe hypotension. Nifedipine, although it has no significant effect on atrioventricular conduction, produces a small negative inotropic effect in the presence of β-blockade. Therefore this combined therapy is not recommended in patients with impaired ventricular function. Combination of verapamil and β blockers may cause severe hypotension, atrioventricular block, and/or heart failure. In several studies, diltiazem and β blockers have been used safely, but again caution should be observed. From all of the studies published to date, it appears that among the calcium channel antagonists, diltiazem is preferable if monotherapy is desired.

REFERENCES

Chaffman M and Brogden RN: Diltiazem: a review of its pharmacological properties and therapeutic efficacy, Drugs 29:387, 1895.

Janis RA, Silver PJ, and Triggle DG: Drug action and cellular calcium regulation, Adv Drug Res 16:309, 1987.

Morad M, Nayler W, Kazda S et al, eds: The calcium channel: structure, function and implications, New York, 1988, Springer-Verlag.

Sorkin EM, Clissold SP, and Brogden RN: Nifedipine: a review of its pharmacodynamic and pharmacokinetic properties, and therapeutic efficacy, in ischemic heart disease, hypertension and related cardiovascular disorders, Drugs 30:182, 1985.

Triggle DJ and Janis RA: Calcium channel ligands, Ann Rev Pharmacol Toxicol 27:347 ,1987.

Vaghy PL, Williams JS, and Schwartz A: Receptor pharmacology of calcium entry blocking agents, Am J Cardiol 59:9A, 1987.

Vanhoutte PM, Paoletti R, and Govoni S, eds: Calcium antagonists: pharmacology and clinical research, Ann NY Acad Sci Vol 522, 1988.

Wray DW, Norman RI, and Hess P, eds: Calcium channels: structure and function, Ann NY Acad Sci Vol 560, 1989.

TRADENAMES

In addition to generic and fixed combination preparations, the following tradenamed materials are available in the United States.

Adalat, nifedipine
Calan, verapamil
Cardane, nicardipine
Cardizem, diltiazem
Isoptin, verapamil
Israpidine, PN200-110
Nimotop, nimodipine
Procardia, nifedipine

CHAPTER 17

Vasodilators

MAJOR DRUGS

nitroglycerin and nitrates
hydralazine
sodium nitroprusside
captopril, enalapril, and lisinopril
minoxidil
prazosin

 THERAPEUTIC OVERVIEW

Vasoconstriction, increase in tone of blood vessels, is the cause of many chronic and acute medical problems. Generally this reduction in blood vessel diameter results in blood flow reduction, causing inadequate nourishment and oxygenation of the organ or tissue and a decrement in function. Vasodilators reduce these effects by promoting relaxation of resistance and/or capacitance vessels. Among the conditions that require therapeutic intervention by vasodilator drugs are: (1) hypertension, where the goal is to reduce blood pressure; (2) congestive heart failure, where for a variety of reasons there may be a reduction in the pumping ability of the heart and the aim is to decrease myocardial work; (3) coronary insufficiency, where the goal is to promote an effective blood flow to the coronary vasculature and also to decrease myocardial work; (4) peripheral vascular disease, with a need for increased blood flow; and (5) the need for hemostasis by pharmacological means, where the goal is to reduce blood flow to the surgical field so that the surgeon may have a relatively blood-free environment (see box on p. 224).

Vasodilator drugs primarily considered here are those compounds that relax vascular smooth muscle by a direct action on that tissue, one that is independent of extrinsic autonomic innervation or hormonal effects. The use of several vasodilator agents in the treatment of essential hypertension, including those drugs that produce vasodilation indirectly, is considered in Chapter 13. A discussion of coronary insufficiency resulting in angina and the efficacy and use of calcium channel blocking agents in this condition is found in Chapter 16. However, a number of other vasodilator drugs are also used for this problem and are discussed in this chapter.

> **THERAPEUTIC OVERVIEW**
> **VASODILATOR DRUGS**

CLINICAL PROBLEM	GOAL OF DRUG INTERVENTION
Hypertension	Decrease blood pressure
Congestive heart failure	Increase cardiac output and decrease oxygen consumption
Coronary insufficiency	Increase effective flow to coronary arteries and decrease oxygen consumption
Peripheral vascular disease	Increase blood flow to the ischemic area
Hemostasis	Decrease blood flow to surgical field

Pulmonary hypertension occurs most frequently secondary to lung or cardiac diseases that enhance pulmonary blood flow and venous pressure or pulmonary vascular resistance. This increase in pulmonary artery pressure may result from genetic defects, left ventricular failure, chronic obstructive lung disease, or other causes. The primary treatment is to correct the underlying problem. However, vasodilators do have an important role as adjunctive therapy. Here the goal is to reduce pulmonary arterial pressure. Beneficial effects have been reported with nitrates, hydralazine, and calcium channel blocking agents.

Ischemic heart disease is characterized by angina pectoris, chest pain that may radiate along the inner portion of one or both arms or to the back. Vasodilators, specifically the nitrates, are mainstays in management. There are several different types of angina, depending on whether the disease is atherosclerotic in origin, or the result of coronary artery spasm, or a combination of both. Angina may also be classified according to whether the pain is exertional or occurs more frequently at rest. These differences are discussed in Chapter 16. However, irrespective of the type of angina, the purpose of pharmacological intervention is to bring about vasodilation of the coronary arteries or redistribution of blood flow in the heart and/or a reduction in the oxygen demands of the heart. Vasodilators, such as the nitrates, provide no permanent beneficial effect on the underlying pathology but merely afford temporary symptomatic relief.

Recent studies indicate that vasodilator therapy is extremely effective in the treatment of chronic congestive heart failure. In the past, drugs used more frequently for treating congestive heart failure were those that increased the force of cardiac contraction (digitalis glycosides) and minimized sodium and water retention (diuretics). Cardiac glycosides, affect only two of the several determinants of cardiac function—contractility and heart rate. Vasodilators can be useful in the treatment of congestive heart failure, reducing either *preload, afterload,* or both. Whether or not preload or afterload is affected depends on the specific action of the vasodilator on the arteriolar and venous vessels. Patients who are refractory to cardiac glycosides frequently do well if treated with vasodilators. Among the direct-acting vasodilators used to treat congestive heart failure are the nitrates, hydralazine, minoxidil, and sodium nitroprusside. Other vasodilators that are effective but act by other mechanisms are considered in Chapter 13.

Vasodilators are also used to treat peripheral vascular disorders. Direct-acting vasodilators, α-adrenergic blockers, calcium channel blocking drugs, and angiotensin converting enzyme inhibitors, are used to treat Raynaud's phenomenon. Vasodilators do not appear effective in increasing blood flow when organic obstruction is significant. In some instances, the use of vasodilator therapy may actually be harmful in that blood is shunted away from diseased areas (see below).

Vasodilator therapy is a useful adjunct to general anesthesia in reducing blood flow in certain radical surgical procedures and in situations where successful surgery depends on a relatively blood-free surgical field. Hypotension may also be desirable in procedures that ordinarily result in significant blood loss. The direct-acting smooth muscle relaxant, sodium nitroprusside, is frequently used because of its short duration of action. Vasodilators may also be used to control hypertension during surgery. Short-acting ganglionic blocking agents, because of their hypotensive action, are sometimes used to provide a suitable surgical field.

The major problem with the use of vasodilators is the so-called *steal* phenomenon. Some data suggest that the use of vasodilator drugs to promote blood flow to ischemic or diseased tissue is limited. It appears that the small blood vessels around the ischemic area are already significantly dilated. Thus the vasodilators may do little to enhance flow in the ischemic region. However, in the normal nonischemic areas where the small blood vessels are not dilated, there is an increase in blood flow with vasodilator therapy. By shunting blood to these areas, vasodilators may actually be reducing flow to the ischemic region by the *steal* mechanism.

 ## MECHANISMS OF ACTION

The commonly used vasodilators are listed in Table 17-1.

Control of Vascular Smooth Muscle Tone

Vascular smooth muscle contraction, like the contractions of other smooth muscle throughout the body, is ultimately regulated by the intracellular calcium concentration, $[Ca^{++}]_i$. There are two mechanisms by which excitation contraction coupling occurs in vascular smooth muscle. These are *electromechanical,* which results in the increase of intracellular calcium via changes in the membrane potential, and *receptor-mediated,* where the effects of the binding of an agonist to a receptor ultimately leads to an increase in $[Ca^{++}]_i$. In vascular smooth muscle the primary mechanism is receptor-mediated excitation contraction coupling, and cell depolarization is not required for contraction. The receptor-mediated excitation-contraction coupling is at least in part brought about by the hydrolysis of phosphoinositides, subsequently releasing diacylglycerol and inositol 1,4,5-trisphosphate (IP_3). How these second messengers lead to an increase in $[Ca^{++}]_i$ is described in Chapters 2 and 8.

When Ca^{++} enters the smooth muscle cell via the voltage-operated calcium channel or is released from intracellular sites by IP_3, it combines with calmodulin. The Ca^{++}-calmodulin complex activates myosin light chain kinase (MLCK), which in turn phosphorylates the myosin light chain (MLC). It is this phosphorylation of the myosin light chain that promotes the interaction of myosin ATPase and actin and cross-bridge formation, leading to the initiation of a transient increase in vascular smooth muscle contraction (Figure 17-1). The sustained maintenance of tension is provided by latchbridge formation.

Roles of cAMP and cGMP

When cAMP concentration is elevated, cAMP-dependent protein kinase is activated. This kinase phosphorylates many proteins, including MLCK, which results in a decrease of MLCK activity and ultimately in a diminution of the rate of MLC phosphorylation and relaxation (see Figure 17-1). The mechanism of the inhibition of MLCK activity apparently is related to decreased affinity of Ca^{++}-calmodulin for MLC kinase when this kinase is phosphorylated. Thus, β-adrenergic agonists, such as isoproterenol, which increase cAMP concentrations, are capable of relaxing vascular smooth muscle by the above mechanism. It is also apparent that appropriate phosphodiesterase inhibitors capable of blocking the degradation of cAMP may promote smooth muscle relaxation by increasing the cAMP concentration. It is of interest that MLCK is also a substrate for cGMP protein kinase.

Table 17-1 Mechanisms and Sites of Action of Selected Vasodilator Drugs

Drug	Mechanism	Vessels Affected
nitroglycerin and nitrates	Direct effect, conversion to nitric oxide*, increase in cGMP	Venous
hydralazine	Direct effect, partially EDRF-dependent formation of nitric oxide*, increase in cGMP	Arteriolar
sodium nitroprusside	Direct effect, conversion to nitric oxide*, increase in cGMP	Arteriolar and venous
captopril, enalapril, and lisinopril	Inhibition of angiotensin-converting enzyme	Arteriolar and venous
minoxidil	Direct effect, K⁺-channel agonist	Arteriolar
prazosin	Blockade of α-adrenergic receptor	Arteriolar and venous

EDRF, Endothelium-derived relaxing factor.
*May be nitric oxide or a chemically related unstable nitroso compound.

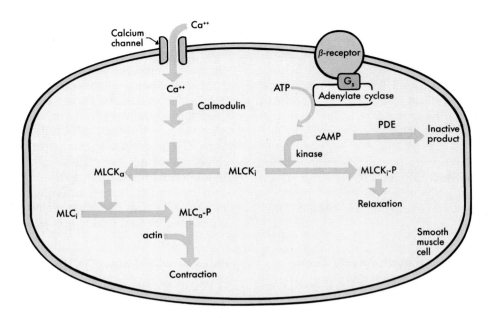

FIGURE 17-1   Possible mechanisms of contraction and relaxation in vascular smooth muscle. Contraction is initiated by the Ca^{++}-calmodulin complex, which activates myosin light chain kinase (*MLCK*). The latter phosphorylates myosin light chain (*MLC*), leading to contraction. Relaxation by β-adrenergic agonists, such as isoproterenol, that increase cAMP and cAMP kinase activity, results in phosphorylation of MLCK to give an inactive phosphorylated form. Subscripts: *(a)* active, *(i)* inactive.

Cyclic GMP plays a prominent role in the mechanisms by which the nitrovasodilators (e.g., nitroglycerin, other nitrates, and sodium nitroprusside) relax vascular smooth muscle. There is evidence that these nitro compounds are converted to nitric oxide (or to an unstable nitroso compound) and promote the accumulation of cGMP by activating a soluble guanylate cyclase within the smooth muscle cell. This increase in cGMP activates cGMP-dependent protein kinase in a manner analogous to the activation of cAMP-dependent protein kinase by cAMP. Although the mechanism by which the activated cGMP-dependent protein kinase leads to vascular smooth muscle relaxation has not been unequivocally explained, a working hypothesis is that the kinase reduces MLCK activity and/or results in the dephosphorylation of the MLC by activating myosin light chain phosphatase (MLCP) (Figure 17-2). An alternative hypothesis that also involves cGMP is that compounds that elevate cGMP concentrations in vascular smooth muscle produce their effects via a cGMP-induced inhibition of phosphoinositide hydrolysis, thereby decreasing the concentrations of second messengers that release Ca^{++}. Other possibilities

are increased sequestration of Ca^{++} into the sarcoplasmic reticulum or activation of the membrane Ca^{++} pump, leading to extrusion of free calcium.

Endothelial Cells and Smooth Muscle Relaxation

It is now recognized that the endothelium that lines vascular smooth muscle plays a regulatory role in the function of the muscle. In addition to many other important activities (e.g., fluid exchange and maintenance of a nonthrombogenic environment), the endothelial cell controls hemodynamics of the cardiovascular system by the generation and release of a number of vasoactive substances such as prostacyclin, a potent smooth muscle relaxant, and two other vasoactive substances that may function as regulatory molecules. These are called the *endothelium-derived relaxing factor* (EDRF) and the *endothelium-derived constricting factor* (EDCF) or endothelin. Because some vascular smooth muscle dilators may act via the generation and release of EDRF, this substance is discussed further.

EDRF was discovered about 10 years ago when it

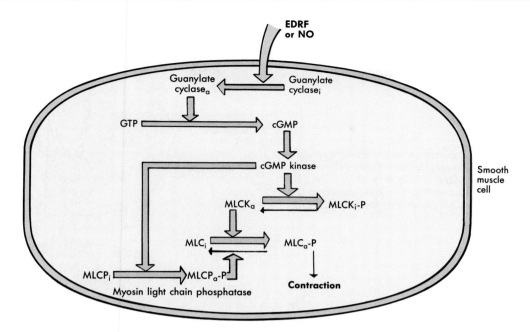

FIGURE 17-2   Possible mechanisms of vasodilation of vascular smooth muscle by endothelium-derived relaxing factor (*EDRF*) or nitric oxide (*NO*). Guanylate cyclase is activated, increasing cGMP concentration and cGMP-dependent protein kinase activity. The latter may cause a decrease in MLCK activity indirectly by phosphorylating MLCK or possibly increasing MLC phosphatase activity (MLCP), thereby reducing vascular smooth muscle contraction. Alternative mechanisms involve inhibition of phosphatidylinositol 4,5 bisphosphate hydrolysis to IP_3, sequestration of Ca^{++} into the sarcoplasmic reticulum, or activation of the membrane Ca^{++} pump, stimulating extrusion of Ca^{++}. Subscripts: *(a)* active, *(i)* inactive.

was demonstrated that the application of acetylcholine, later shown to trigger the release of EDRF, could relax isolated rabbit aorta only if the internal endothelium of that tissue was intact and undamaged. This work later led to the identification of EDRF as nitric oxide (NO) or a closely related unstable chemical entity. Subsequent evidence has shown that among the clinically important vasodilators, hydralazine may owe a part of its vasodilating action to its ability to release EDRF. Other endogenous agents such as bradykinin, histamine, ATP, ADP, substance P, acetylcholine, thrombin, and arachidonic acid are all endothelium-dependent vasorelaxants that act primarily on resistance vessels and depend on the release of EDRF for their vasodilating properties (Figure 17-3).

The source of the nitric oxide is not clear, but some evidence suggests that the nitrogen comes from L-arginine.

There is presently adequate morphological evidence that gap junctions or connecting arborizations

exist between endothelial cells and vascular smooth muscle cells. Thus, there is an opportunity for chemical signal transduction between these two cell types, and the release of EDRF from endothelium cells for relaxation of smooth muscle cells is one example. Another example is that of prostacyclin, which is synthesized by endothelial cells during prostaglandin (Chapter 18) metabolism and released locally by endogenous substances such as histamine to induce vascular dilation. Thus some agents cause vasodilation by releasing EDRF from the endothelium to the smooth muscle cell (see Figure 17-3) and others do not involve EDRF.

As indicated above, the nitrovasodilators produce their relaxant effects by increasing intracellular cGMP concentrations. It is possible that EDRF may have an important role in the regulation of basal vascular smooth muscle tone through its continual release from the endothelium to maintain high steady state concentrations of cGMP. Although some of the nitrorelaxants act via stimulation of soluble guanylate cy-

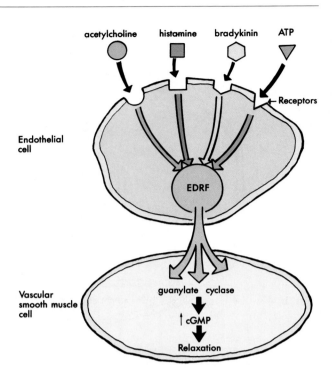

FIGURE 17-3   Endothelium-dependent relaxation produced by vasodilators. These substances act on the endothelial cell at their respective receptors to release EDRF or nitric oxide (see text). The latter diffuses into the vascular smooth muscle cell, increases guanylate cyclase activity and cGMP, and promotes relaxation.

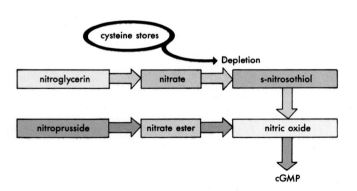

FIGURE 17-4   Intracellular conversion of nitroglycerin and nitroprusside to nitric oxide by separate pathways. Tolerance to nitroglycerin may result from a depletion of cysteine.

clase of smooth muscle cells to increase cGMP, another endogenous smooth muscle dilator, atrial natriuretic peptide (ANP), acts via stimulation of a particulate form of guanylate cyclase.

The tolerance of vascular smooth muscle to the nitrovasorelaxants such as nitroglycerin apparently results from impaired biotransformation of the parent compound to yield nitric oxide. Nitroglycerin is converted to a nitrite and then to an unstable *S*-nitrosothiol in the presence of cysteine. The *S*-nitrosothiol spontaneously decomposes to nitric oxide. Tolerance to nitroglycerin presumably results from inadequate cysteine stores. Cross-tolerance to sodium nitroprusside does not occur because nitroprusside is converted to nitric oxide by an alternative pathway not requiring cysteine (Figure 17-4).

Vasodilator Drugs

The organic nitrate vasodilator drugs include the prototype nitroglycerin plus isosorbide dinitrate, erythrityl tetranitrate, and pentaerythritol tetranitrate. The chemical structures are shown in Figure 17-5. Structures of other vasodilators (hydralazine, minoxidil, enalapril, prazosin, and captopril) are shown in Chapter 13.

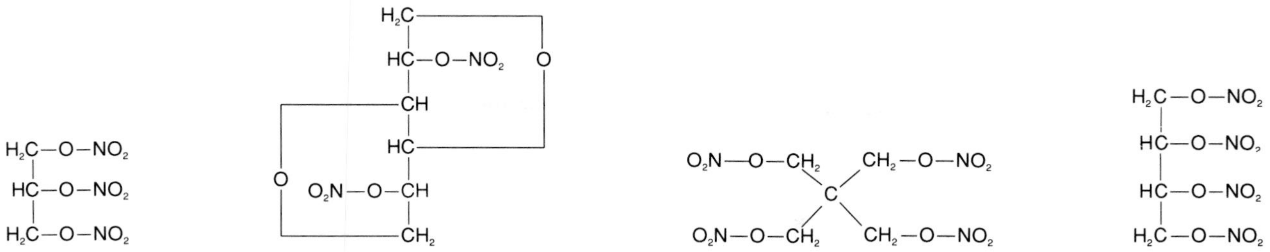

nitrogylcerin (glyceryl trinitrate) — isosorbide dinitrate — pentaerythritol tetranitrate — erythrityl tetranitrate

FIGURE 17-5 Structures of some commonly used nitrates.

Table 17-2 Pharmacokinetic Parameters

Drug	Route of Administration	Onset (min)	Duration (hr)	$t_{1/2}$ (terminal) (min)	Disposition
nitroglycerin	Sublingual	1-2	0.75-2	1-4	M
	Oral, topical	—	4-8	—	M
	IV	—	—	1-4	M
	Aerosol	2	0.5-1	1-4	M
	Transdermal	—	10-14	—	M
isosorbide dinitrate	Oral, chewable	3	4-6	240	M*
	Sublingual	3	0.75-2	60	M*
erythrityl tetranitrate	Oral, sublingual	—	6-8	—	M
pentaerythritol tetranitrate	Oral, chewable	—	6-8	—	M

M, Metabolized.
*Active metabolite, large first-pass effect.

PHARMACOKINETICS

The pharmacokinetic parameter values for nitrate vasodilators are summarized in Table 17-2.

Organic nitrates are almost completely absorbed from the GI tract and fairly completely from the buccal mucosa. After sublingual administration, peak plasma concentrations are achieved in 1 to 2 minutes. Absorption is much slower with topical ointments and transdermal patches, and plasma concentrations attained with transdermal preparations are lower and more variable than those with ointment. The nitrates are metabolized in liver by glutathione nitrate reductase (e.g., nitroglycerin is rapidly converted to inorganic nitrite and to de-nitrated metabolites). Isosorbide dinitrate is also metabolized by hepatic glutathione reductase and converted to inactive products, as well as to an active metabolite, 5-isosorbide mononitrate. This may account for the longer duration of antianginal activity of the parent compound. Isosorbide dinitrate is also used in therapy of intractable chronic congestive heart failure, frequently in combination with other vasodilators that cause relaxation of resistance vessels.

Sublingual nitroglycerin is the mainstay of therapy

in anginal attacks and is also used prophylactically. It is rapid in onset and inexpensive. Sublingual isosorbide dinitrate is also available and has a longer duration of action than does nitroglycerin. The nitroglycerin aerosol spray appears to be as effective as the sublingual tablets. The transdermal patches are not as effective as the oral, timed-release preparations, largely because of the variable absorption through the skin. As a result of tolerance development, those transdermal patches that are left in place for 24 hours are ultimately ineffective for the treatment of angina, even if the dosage is increased. However, patches that deliver 10 mg or more nitroglycerin can be effective if the patches are removed for a 10 to 12 hour period daily.

RELATION OF MECHANISMS OF ACTION TO CLINICAL RESPONSE

Vasodilators in Angina

The objectives in the treatment of angina are to reduce the oxygen requirements of the heart and to increase blood flow to the coronary vasculature. Vasodilator therapy is used to terminate an acute anginal episode or prophylactically to prevent an anginal attack or increase the exercise tolerance of the patient. This is accomplished with antianginal agents by promoting the redistribution of blood to the subendocardium of the ischemic zone. Normally, blood flow to the subepicardial and subendocardial regions is evenly distributed. During ischemia, however, subendocardial blood flow is more severely compromised. Vasodilators such as the nitrates partially correct this imbalance by selectively dilating the large epicardial vessels, thus shunting blood to the more ischemic subendocardium. The vasodilator drugs affect both arteriolar and venous vessels, with specific compounds having a greater or lesser effect on either vascular bed. These differences influence the selection of particular drugs.

The organic nitrates are the mainstays of antianginal therapy and have been effectively used for this purpose for about 100 years. The prototype drug is nitroglycerin, which acts directly to increase cGMP and produce dilation of the venous vasculature. This action decreases venous return, ventricular volume, and blood pressure. In addition to affecting preload, the organic nitrates can reduce after-load at higher drug concentrations by dilating peripheral resistance

vessels, which leads to a reduction in arterial blood pressure. In spite of the possibility that central aortic pressure may fall, the nitrates effectively increase flow to the ischemic area by the regional redistribution of blood as previously described. Although the nitrates apparently dilate both normal and diseased coronary arteries and collaterals and are effective in both classic and variant angina, the primary effect is on the peripheral circulation and not on the coronary vessels. However, it is possible to produce an effect directly on the coronary vasculature by intracoronary or IV injection of nitrates. Nitrates are available in many dosage forms, including sublingual, transdermal, and longer-acting oral preparations. The choice of nitrate preparation depends on the necessity for a rapid onset or a longer duration of action. In addition to vascular smooth muscles, nitroglycerin and other nitrates also relax bronchiolar, gastrointestinal, urethral, and uterine muscles.

Other drugs that are used in the treatment of angina are the calcium channel blocking drugs (Chapter 16) and the β-adrenergic receptor blockers, which owe their effectiveness in angina to hemodynamic properties that reduce oxygen demand on the heart by decreasing heart rate and blood pressure, particularly during exercise (Chapter 13).

Vasodilators in Chronic Congestive Heart Failure

Vasodilator therapy is now widely used for the treatment of chronic congestive heart failure, particularly when the patient has not responded adequately to drugs that increase the force of cardiac contraction or to diuretics. Increased survival of patients under a vasodilator regimen has been demonstrated. The determinants of cardiac function are preload, afterload, contractility, and heart rate (Figure 17-6). Among the major mechanisms by which vasodilators increase cardiac performance are afterload reduction, preload reduction, and the resulting increased left ventricular diastolic compliance. Afterload reduction, by use of other vasodilators and *high* concentrations of nitrates, is accomplished by dilating arterioles and thereby decreasing systemic vascular resistance. This increases cardiac output and tissue perfusion. Venodilators, including low doses of nitrates, predominantly decrease preload, reducing systemic and pulmonary venous pressures. Ventricular volume is also affected by the decreasing preload. The venodilators do not increase the force of contraction, and the heart

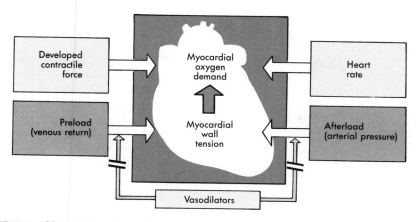

FIGURE 17-6   Mechanism of vasodilator action in the therapy of chronic congestive heart failure. The four main determinants of cardiac function act to determine the myocardial oxygen demand. Nitrates decrease preload and afterload but leave work (force and heart rate) unchanged, thereby decreasing oxygen demand.

rate is generally unchanged, so that the work of the heart remains the same. The overall effect therefore is a reduction in myocardial oxygen consumption and demand upon the heart. The vasodilator drugs may also improve left ventricular diastolic performance by shifting the diastolic pressure-volume curve to the left (i.e., to pump the same volume at a lower pressure). This shift also moves the ventricular function curve to the left, demonstrating an improvement in left ventricular performance.

Vasodilators used to treat chronic congestive heart failure will influence preload, afterload, or both. Among the agents used are the direct-acting agents (nitrates, hydralazine, and nitroprusside), the α-adrenergic receptor blocker (prazosin), and the angiotensin converting enzyme inhibitors (captopril, enalapril, and lisinopril). Long-term treatment with hydralazine alone is only minimally effective in treatment of congestive heart failure, but the combination of hydralazine with a nitrate, isosorbide dinitrate, effectively decreases mortality. Minoxidil is also generally not very effective when used alone.

Vasodilators in Peripheral Vascular Disease

Peripheral vascular diseases are either vasospastic or occlusive. In Raynaud's disease, a vasospastic disorder, blood flow to the extremities is reduced as a result of a reversible vasoconstriction. Therefore vasodilators may be helpful to these patients by dilating the blood vessels of the skin. On the other hand, vasodilators are of limited usefulness in occlusive dis-

ease with a physical obstruction, and they do not generally improve flow to either skeletal muscle or skin. A wide variety of drug classes has been used in the treatment of peripheral vascular diseases including α-adrenergic blockers, calcium channel blockers, prostaglandins, β-adrenergic agonists, and direct-acting vasodilators. Nitroglycerin ointment may be helpful as an adjunctive agent in Raynaud's phenomenon. Other nonspecific vascular smooth muscle vasodilators such as cyclandalate, papaverine, ethaverine, and nicotinyl tartrate have been used but are of questionable efficacy in the treatment of peripheral vascular disorders.

Vasodilators in Hemostasis

Vasodilators may be utilized as aids during surgical procedures. They can be used to provide a more satisfactory surgical field, to minimize large blood volume losses, and to improve cardiac performance by reducing preload or after-load. Controlled hypotension may also be utilized in hypertensive patients to provide a dry surgical field; trimethaphan, a ganglionic blocking agent, and sodium nitroprusside, a direct-acting smooth muscle vasodilator are often used. Because trimethaphan may produce undesirable autonomic and cardiac side effects and since sodium nitroprusside has a shorter duration of action, the latter is the preferred agent. Care must be used, however, in the administration of nitroprusside because it acts directly to dilate both resistance and capacitance vessels, thus presenting a potential hazard.

CLINICAL PROBLEMS

VASODILATORS

Postural hypotension
Tachycardia

NITRATE VASODILATORS

Postural hypotension
Tachycardia
Headache
Tolerance/physical dependence
Methemoglobinemia

TRADENAMES

In addition to generic and fixed combination preparations, the following tradenamed materials are available in the United States.

Cardilate, erythrityl tetranitrate
Isordil, Sorbitrate, Dilatrate; isosorbide dinitrate
Nitrostat, Nitrocine, Deponit, Nitrodisc, Nitrogard, Nitrol, Nitrolingual, Nitro-Dur, Transderm-Nitro, Nitro-Bid, Nitrong; nitroglycerin
Peritrate, pentaerythritol tetranitrate

SIDE EFFECTS, CLINICAL PROBLEMS, AND TOXICITY

As with all vasodilators, postural hypotension and tachycardia are adverse effects of nitrate therapy. Vascular headache is quite common but rapidly disappears on continued nitrate use. Tolerance to the vascular effects of nitrate does occur; however, this is not of great clinical significance, except possibly in the treatment of chronic congestive heart failure. Cross-tolerance exists between nitroglycerin and the other nitrate esters, but this and other nitrate tolerance can be reduced by only a short period of nitrate abstention. Postural hypotension can be minimized by careful adjustment of the dose and by having the patient avoid the upright position when taking the rapid-acting preparations. Physical dependence to the nitrates has been observed in munitions workers exposed continuously to very high concentrations. In these individuals, withdrawal from the industrial environment may result in angina. This phenomenon is not observed in patients normally taking therapeutic doses of nitrates, but can occur in individuals who have been taking large doses for a long time.

Nitrates can be reduced to nitrites, which in turn can oxidize the ferrous iron of hemoglobin, converting it to methemoglobin. The latter reduces oxygen delivery to tissues. Methemoglobinemia is not a problem with normal nitrate therapy but may be observed in accidental poisoning or overdose.

Problems associated with nitroprusside, prazosin, hydralazine, the angiotensin converting enzyme inhibitors, and minoxidil are discussed in Chapter 13.

The clinical problems caused by nitrate vasodilators are summarized in the box.

REFERENCES

Furchgott RF and Zawadzki JV: The obligatory role of endothelial cells in the relaxation of arterial smooth muscle by acetylcholine, Nature 288:373, 1980.

Ignarro LJ: Biological actions and properties of endothelium-derived nitric oxide formed and released from artery and vein, Circ Res 65:1, 1989.

Needleman P, Jakschik B, and Johnson EM: Sulfhydryl requirement for relaxation of vascular smooth muscle, J Pharmacol Exp Ther 187:324, 1973.

Palmer RMJ, Ferrige AG, and Moncado S: Nitric oxide release accounts for the biological activity of endothelium derived relaxing factor, Nature 327:524,1987.

Peach MJ, Loeb AL, Singer HA and et al.: Endothelium derived vascular relaxing factor, Hypertension 7:I-94, 1985.

Rapoport RM and Murad F: Agonist-induced endothelium dependent relaxation in rat thoracic aorta may be mediated through cGMP, Circ Res 52:352, 1983.

Schocken DD, and Hollaway JD: Vasodilators in the treatment of congestive heart failure, Rational Drug Ther 22:1, 1988.

Schwartz AB, and Chatterjee K: Vasodilator therapy in chronic congestive heart failure, Drugs 26:148, 1983.

Vanhoutte PM, Rubanyi GM, Miller VM et al.: Modulation of vascular smooth muscle contraction by the endothelium, Ann Rev Physiol 48:307, 1986.

Waldman SA and Murad F: Cyclic GMP synthesis and function, Pharmacol Rev 39:163, 1987.

18

Prostaglandins and Related Autacoids

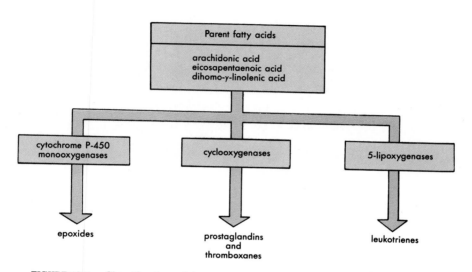

FIGURE 18-1   Classification of the major eicosanoids of pharmacological interest.

ABBREVIATIONS

ADH	antidiuretic hormone
AVP	vasopressin
EPA	eicosapentaenoic acid
K_D	dissociation constant
LTA, LTB, LTC	leukotrienes
PGD, PGE, PGF, PGG, PGH, PGI	prostaglandins
PLA$_2$	phospholipase A$_2$
PLC	phospholipase C
RNA	ribonucleic acid
TxA$_2$, TxA$_3$	thromboxanes

THERAPEUTIC OVERVIEW

Prostaglandins form one branch of a larger family of endogenous compounds known as *eicosanoids*, which constitute a diverse group of oxygenated unsaturated 20-carbon fatty acids. The eicosanoids exert profound effects on practically all cells and tissues and thus provide potential targets for pharmacological intervention in the treatments of several disease states.

The chemical classification of the major eicosanoids, including the prostaglandins, is summarized in Figure 18-1.

Most of the eicosanoid biochemical pathways of pharmacological interest originate with arachidonic acid, the parent compound, a major component of mammalian membrane phospholipids. Because of the diversity of in vivo biochemical and physiological actions attributed to the prostaglandins and other eicosanoids, numerous therapeutic applications for these agents are anticipated. Unfortunately actual clinical applications are fewer than expected, although continued research into their mechanisms of action may result in additional uses of analogs of therapeutic value.

The principal circumstances or organs where therapy with prostaglandins (and related leukotrienes) is currently available or may be possible are summarized in the box, p. 240, with chapters noted in which the clinical applications are discussed. The main thrust of this chapter is an overview of the pharmacological implications of prostaglandins.

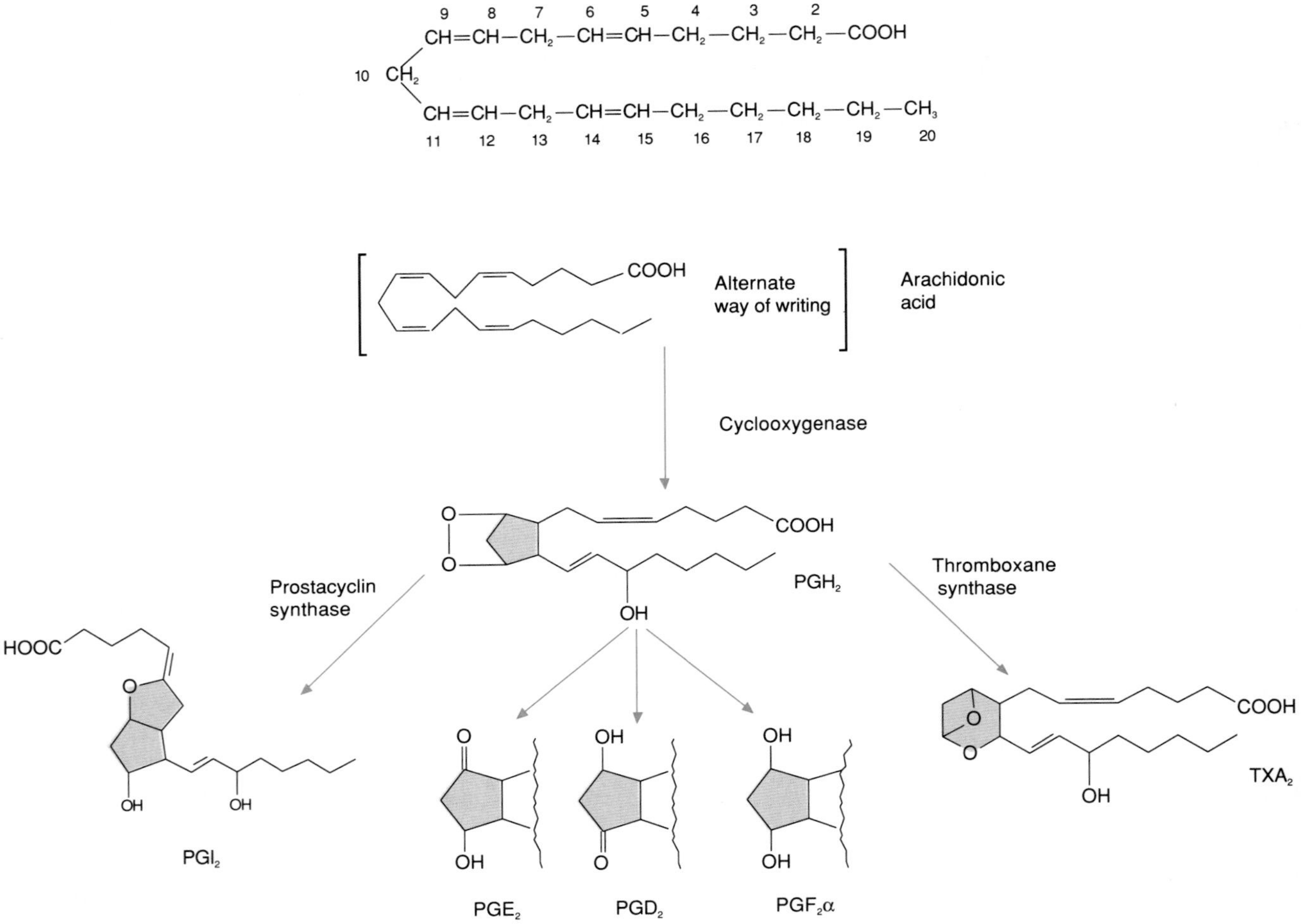

FIGURE 18-2   Chemical structures and nomenclature of principal prostaglandins. *PG*, Prostaglandin; *Tx*, thromboxane; *PGI₂*, prostacyclin. PGE₂, PGD₂, and PGF₂ₐ differ from endoperoxide PGH₂ as indicated.

RELATION OF MECHANISMS OF ACTION TO CLINICAL RESPONSE

Chemical Structures and Nomenclature

The structures and nomenclature of the prostaglandins are summarized in Figure 18-2. The primary prostaglandins, PGE_2 and $PGF_{2\alpha}$, are unsaturated fatty acid derivatives that contain 20 carbon atoms dispersed in a cyclopentane ring; they originate from common intermediates, the cyclic endoperoxides, PGG_2 and PGH_2. The nature of the substitution on the pentane ring is denoted by a capital letter (e.g., D, E, F). The endoperoxide PGH_2 is also metabolized into two unstable and highly biologically active compounds: (1) thromboxane A₂, TxA_2, distinguished by a six-membered oxane ring instead of the pentane ring, and (2) prostacyclin (PGI_2), a bicyclic ring system closed by an oxygen bridge between carbons 6 and 9. TxA_2 has a short chemical half-life, less than 1 minute at body temperature. The inactive hydrolysis products, TxB_2 and 6-keto-$PGF_{1\alpha}$ arise nonenzymatically from TxA_2 and PGI_2, respectively. All of these products (thromboxanes, prostaglandins, and prostacyclin) are derived from unsaturated 20-carbon essential fatty acids, primarily arachidonic acid, a major component of membrane phospholipids. The numbering designation of arachidonic acid, 20:4, indicates 20 carbon atoms and 4 double bonds. The compounds that retain two double bonds in their alkyl side-chains are denoted by the subscript. Examples of prostaglandins derived from all three parent compounds (see Figure 18-1) are shown in Figure 18-3. Several products generated from eicosapentaenoic acid (EPA) are less potent than corresponding products derived from arachidonic acid. The number of double bonds in the side-chains usually does not fundamentally alter the biological properties of prostaglandins; for example, prostaglandins E_1, E_2, and E_3 have similar effects on smooth muscle. However, there are exceptions; for example, PGE_1 resembles

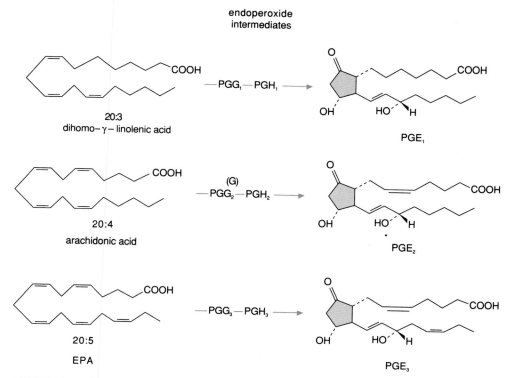

FIGURE 18-3   Nomenclature for prostaglandins originating from the parent compounds. *EPA,* Eicosapentaenoic acid. (Eicosa, containing 20 carbon atoms.)

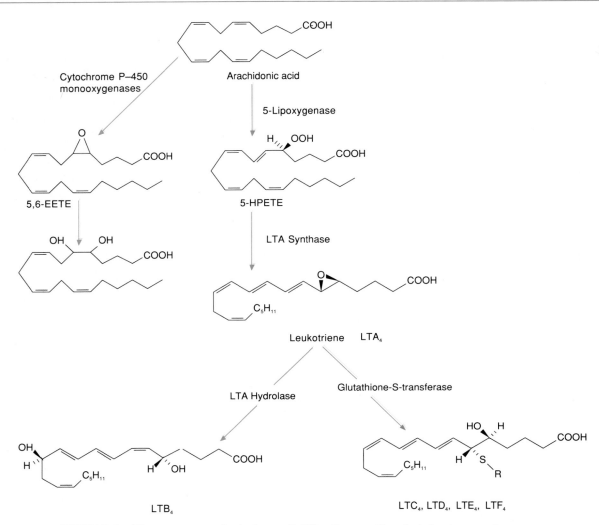

FIGURE 18-4   Lipoxygenase and cytochrome P-450 pathways. Chemical structures and nomenclature of principal leukotrienes. LTC$_4$, LTD$_4$, LTE$_4$, and LTF$_4$ differ from LTA$_4$ in the R-groups. Cytochrome P-450 monooxygenases oxidize arachidonic acid to several epoxides (EETE, epoxyeicosatetraenoic acids) and diols. 5-HPETE, unstable hydroperoxy-eicosatetraenoic acid.

PGI$_2$ in its ability to inhibit platelet aggregation, a property not shared with PGE$_2$.

Some differences in potency are noted. For example, TxA$_3$ is less potent than TxA$_2$ relative to aggregation of platelets and constriction of blood vessels. The leukotriene LTB$_5$ is relatively impotent as a chemotactic agent when compared to LTB$_4$. These differences in platelet aggregatory potency between the thromboxanes, TxA$_2$ versus TxA$_3$, and in chemotactic activity between the leukotrienes, LTB$_4$ versus LTB$_5$, constitute part of the rationale for dietary supplementation with EPA, which is found primarily in marine animals residing in cold waters. The addition of EPA to the diet, either in purified form or by consuming cold water fish, is a novel therapeutic strategy in the prevention of thrombosis (reduces formation of TxA$_2$) and of other vascular complications, as well as moderating the inflammatory response (reduces formation of LTB$_4$).

The lipoxygenase and cytochrome P-450 pathways are summarized in Figure 18-4.

Synthesis of Prostaglandins and Other Eicosanoids

Three pathways for the enzymatic conversion of arachidonic acid have been identified: cyclooxygenase, lipoxygenases, and cytochrome P-450-dependent monooxygenases. These pathways are shown schematically in Figure 18-1.

Metabolism and Concentrations of Prostaglandins

With the exception of seminal fluid, prostaglandins are not stored but are synthesized in response to diverse stimuli and enter the extracellular space. Prostaglandins and thromboxane act primarily as local hormones (autacoids), their biological activities usually restricted to the cell, tissue, or structure where they are synthesized. Concentrations of PGE_2 and $PGF_{2\alpha}$ in arterial blood are very low because of pulmonary degradation, which normally removes more than 90% of these prostaglandins from the venous blood as it passes through the lungs. Prostacyclin escapes pulmonary metabolism and therefore may act as a circulating hormone, although under basal conditions concentrations are thought to be less than 5 pg/ml, below the threshold required for biological effects. The initial and most important step in the breakdown of prostaglandins results in their rapid inactivation through oxidation of the 15-OH group catalyzed by 15-OH prostaglandin dehydrogenase, an enzyme widely distributed in the body.

The influence that adjacent or invading cells exert on arachidonic acid metabolism by a particular cell type can determine the quantity and species of prostaglandin, leukotriene, and other oxygenated arachidonic acid metabolites produced. These arachidonic acid metabolites can then affect the secretory activity and functional state of platelets, white cells, and endothelial cells. For example, the rate of formation of PGI_2 by endothelial cells greatly influences the ability of platelets to aggregate, through an effect mediated by PGI_2 on elevating platelet cAMP concentrations, resulting in diminished platelet TxA_2 formation. Platelets, in turn, may act as donors of prostaglandin endoperoxides to the metabolic machinery of the endothelium, resulting in further increases in PGI_2 formation. This cooperative interaction favoring PGI_2 formation by blood vessels is facilitated by the evolving platelet plug adherent to the vascular wall. Thrombosis and inflammation provide ideal circumstances for promoting transcellular metabolism of eicosanoids. Arachidonic acid released from activated platelets can act as a precursor for further metabolic transformation in neutrophils, events that are facilitated when platelet cyclooxygenase is blocked by aspirin-like drugs. These platelet-neutrophil interactions influence the therapeutic effects, as well as complications, of low-dose aspirin therapy thought to derive exclusively from inhibition of platelet thromboxane generation.

Another example of platelet-neutrophil interactions to consider in developing therapeutic approaches occurs with angina (Chapter 16). The elimination of one coronary vasoconstrictor agent, thromboxane, may not prevent angina because a second endogenous vasoconstrictor, LTC_4, will be unopposed by therapeutic interventions directed only against thromboxane. Thus cells may donate substrate to receiving cells either as unmodified arachidonic acid or as an arachidonate metabolite. This can result in activation, augmentation, or suppression of the activity of the receiving cell. In addition, the range of activity of the receiving cell may be increased by providing an arachidonate metabolite that is transformed to a product ordinarily not synthesized by the receiving cell.

Not all cells synthesize prostaglandins despite the claims of some investigators. For example, there are segments of the nephron that lack cyclooxygenase or show negligible capacity to transform added arachidonic acid to prostaglandin. In contrast, within the vasculature, cyclooxygenase is found in abundance, although the principal products vary longitudinally along the vasculature and cross-sectionally within the blood vessel wall (e.g., endothelium versus vascular smooth muscle). Within the coronary circulation the larger blood vessels synthesize principally PGI_2, whereas in microvessels PGE_2 predominates.

Prostaglandins are usually released in bursts into the extracellular space immediately after synthesis in response to a stimulus. Under unusual circumstances, prostaglandins may achieve relatively high concentrations in circulating blood: PGD_2 in human mastocytosis, PGE_2 in some solid tumors with metastases to bone, and PGI_2 in pregnancy. In a small group of patients having solid tumors that metastasize to bone, the associated hypercalcemia, related to elevated PGE_2 concentrations, responds to treatment with aspirin-like drugs. In late pregnancy, the gravid uterus may serve as a reservoir of prostacyclin, which is released into the systemic circulation. In addition, diseases of the lung associated with shunting of blood to the systemic circulation, thereby bypassing the lungs, can result in elevated prostaglandin concentrations in arterial blood.

Under basal conditions, PGI_2 concentrations in blood are less than 5 pg/ml ($\sim 10^{-11}$ M), well below the threshold that produces vasoactive and myotropic effects. Whether the pulmonary vascular bed can act as a reservoir for release of prostacyclin into the systemic circulation, as proposed, is not established but remains a possibility. Biological effects of prostaglandins at 10^{-11} M have been reported in erythrocytes and cardiac myocytes. For example, PGE_1 at this concentration alters the shape of red blood cells and stimulates formation of cyclic AMP (cAMP) by cardiac myocytes. However, the minimum prostaglandin concentration that elicits biological effects in most instances approaches 10^{-9} M, a valve identical to the reported dissociation constant (K_D) of prostaglandin receptors.

Mechanisms of Prostaglandin Action

Prostaglandins exert their effects by binding to specific membrane receptors. The K_D of such receptors for endogenous ligands are seldom as low as 10^{-11} M, the usually cited plasma concentration of prostaglandins. It is inefficient for the K_D to be below the basal concentration of endogenous ligand, because receptors would be permanently saturated. The K_D is the ratio of the reverse- and forward-rate constants of the association reaction of a ligand with its receptor. The forward-rate constant has an upper limit at which the reaction becomes diffusion controlled. A K_D below 10^{-11} M indicates that a low concentration of ligand is effective. A low dissociation-rate constant indicates a slow response time and a long recovery time after a stimulus. This is appropriate for the long-term response to some hormones, but is inefficient where rapid responsiveness is necessary, as is the case with prostaglandin-dependent mechanisms.

Prostaglandin synthesis and action appears to be receptor-mediated and to involve second messengers. Prostaglandins and other eicosanoids thus can influence other second messenger systems through modification of guanylate and adenylate cyclases and ultimately through mobilization of Ca^{++} from cellular stores. There is evidence that eicosanoid-dependent mechanisms act within the neuron of origin and externally at nerve endings to modulate autonomic transmission. It therefore seems likely that eicosanoids have intracellular actions in addition to the effects that register at the cell membrane.

Prostaglandins affect the cell of origin and neighboring cells by binding to specific membrane receptors linked via G proteins to adenylate cyclases, possibly guanylate cyclases, and lipases (Figure 18-5). Prostaglandins, after release, are usually denied entrance into cells, presumably because the lipid bilayer

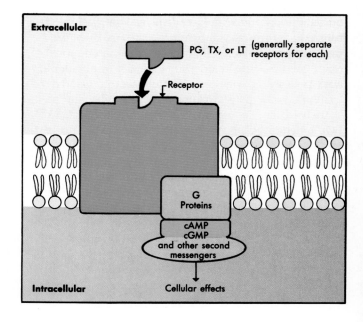

FIGURE 18-5   Eicosanoids act through specific membrane receptors, mainly G protein types with various second messenger systems. *PG*, Prostaglandins; *Tx*, thromboxanes; *LT*, leukotrienes.

is impermeable to prostaglandins. The endoperoxide, PGH_2, may be an exception because it may enter some cells to be transformed into PGI_2, although cell surface enzymes also may be chiefly responsible for metabolism of PGH_2. In the lung, renal proximal tubules, thyroid plexus, and ciliary body of the eye, an active transport system that demonstrates saturation kinetics is responsible for the rapid uptake of prostaglandins from extracellular fluids. Prostaglandins differ in their affinity for this transport system. PGE_2 and $PGF_{2\alpha}$, unlike PGI_2, have high affinity, thus accounting for removal and subsequent metabolism of PGE_2 and $PGF_{2\alpha}$ within the lung in contrast to PGI_2, which passes intact through the pulmonary circulation. It is possible to inhibit this transport system, which resembles the organic acid secretory system of the renal proximal tubules, with probenicid, the prototypical inhibitor of proximal tubular secretion. The diuretic drug, furosemide, and other organic acids also inhibit this uptake in the lung, kidney, and possibly in the brain and eye. One of the effects of this class of drugs is to increase prostaglandin concentrations in blood, urine, and perhaps spinal fluid.

Several guanine nucleotide-binding regulatory (G) proteins mediating transmembrane signaling are the basis for cell, tissue, and species specific effects of PGE_2, the prototypical prostaglandin modulator. Whether inhibition or stimulation of adenylate cyclase follows binding of PGE_2 to a specific receptor presumably depends on the nature of the G protein coupling the receptor to the catalytic unit of the adenylate cyclase system. The tissue specific functional changes induced by PGE_2 include vasodilation, bronchodilation, promotion of salt and water excretion, inhibition of lipolysis, glycogenolysis, and fatty acid oxidation.

A practical therapeutic application of suppressing the effects of PGE_2 on adenylate cyclase can be demonstrated in Bartter's syndrome, a disease characterized by excessive renal prostaglandin production associated with diuresis, kaliuresis, natriuresis, and hyperreninemia. Inhibition of cyclooxygenase activity with nonsteroidal antiinflammatory drugs results in improvement in these patients by allowing expression of salt- and water-retaining hormonal influences, chiefly those of angiotensin II and AVP. The effect of these pressor peptides is blunted by high prostaglandin concentrations intrarenally, particularly PGE_2. For example, by inhibiting the action of antidiuretic hormone (ADH) on adenylate cyclase in the collecting tubules, elevated PGE_2 concentrations prevent water retention by ADH. Further, PGE_2 promotes salt excretion (presumably via an adenylate cyclase-related mechanism) by inhibiting Na^+ and Cl^- cotransport in the thick ascending limb of the loop of Henle. Suppression of prostaglandin synthesis with a nonsteroidal antiinflammatory agent partially corrects the depletion of extracellular fluid volume in these patients.

In contrast to PGE_2-induced relaxation of vascular smooth muscle, the less frequently encountered contraction of smooth muscle produced by PGE_2 is probably linked to Ca^{++} mobilization consequent to stimulating PLC via a receptor coupled to a G_p (phospholipase) protein. This regulatory protein, as noted, is linked to PLC, which catalyzes the generation of IP_3 from PIP_2, resulting in elevation of cytosolic Ca^{++}. This mechanism is also thought to be the principal one involved in the actions of $PGF_{2\alpha}$, leading to contraction of smooth muscle.

PGI_2 produces effects by interacting with a single type of high-affinity cell surface PGI_2 receptor with wide distribution. PGI_2 binding is linked via a G_s regulatory protein to stimulation of adenylate cyclase, increased cAMP concentrations, and inhibition of platelet aggregation. The high density of PGI_2 receptors in the vasculature is reflected in the vasodilator potency of PGI_2, an effect related to elevation of cAMP concentrations in vascular smooth muscle.

TxA_2 receptors have been identified on the plasma membranes of platelets, blood vessels, bronchial smooth muscle, and mesangial cells of glomeruli. The prostaglandin endoperoxides, PGG_2 and PGH_2, also bind to thromboxane receptors. Because there is evidence of different receptor subtypes, it may be possible to design antagonists that block platelet TxA_2 receptors while sparing vascular receptors. This therapeutic discrimination can be important in eliminating unwanted side effects of antagonists (e.g., avoiding reductions of blood pressure while reducing platelet aggregation ability).

Administration of a prostaglandin or one of its analogs, if continued long enough, will result in loss of responsiveness to its biological effects. This agonist-specific desensitization is termed *homologous*, because the response to other agonists interacting with specific receptors is not lost. Desensitization of the prostacyclin receptor does not appear to relate to altered coupling of the receptor either to G_s or to the catalytic unit of adenylate cyclase. It is possible to distinguish two forms of desensitization involving thromboxane receptors, one occurring rapidly, within minutes, and resulting from impaired coupling of the G protein to the thromboxane receptor. The other form takes hours and may involve phosphorylation of occupied receptors followed by sequestration of the receptor. This "down regulation," represents a net loss of receptor sites, expressed as decreased binding of the agonist and results from sequestration/internalization of the receptor. Recovery of the sensitivity of these receptors appears to depend on de novo protein synthesis, reflecting synthesis of new receptors.

For prostaglandin-effected changes in responsiveness of a nonprostaglandin receptor such as the adenosine A_2 receptor, the term *heterologous desensitization* is used. This form of receptor unresponsiveness requires a longer exposure to the agonist and represents, in the case of receptors linked to adenylate cyclase, not only decreased responsiveness to other agonists but also to agents acting at a postreceptor step. The biochemical determinants of heterologous desensitization have not been fully defined and differ among hormones. It has been related to a change in G_s or its coupling with the catalytic unit of adenylate cyclase.

Prolonged infusion of prostacyclin or a prostacyclin analog, (e.g., iloprost) in patients with peripheral vascular disease produces decreased platelet sensitivity to these agonists (Figure 18-6). This form of desensitization derives from changes in the G_s protein linking the receptor to adenylate cyclase. The production of platelet desensitization by infusion of prostacyclin or a PGI_2 analog limits the therapeutic benefit obtained from this group of agents because, in most conditions in which PGI_2 is given, one of the purposes of therapy is to reduce vascular complications resulting from enhanced platelet aggregation. However, when the infusion is stopped, platelets demonstrate increased tendency to clump (hyperaggregatory ability), a potentially dangerous side effect in patients who are at risk because of underlying cardiovascular disease.

Prostaglandins and other eicosanoids act at or near their sites of synthesis to "coordinate net biological responses" of a tissue. As coordinators of cellular and tissue function, a major biological activity of prostaglandins is to modulate the activity of hormones and neurotransmitters. The concept that eicosanoids act locally as modulators of peptide hormones and neurotransmitters aids in understanding the multiple and overlapping spheres of biological activity and diverse

effects of prostaglandins and other arachidonic acid metabolites. For example, peptide-induced metabolism of arachidonic acid by cells within a segment of the nephron or the vasculature results in changes in the intensity and range of activities of the peptide.

THERAPEUTIC AREAS OF PROSTAGLANDIN AND OTHER EICOSANOID INTERVENTION

PROSTAGLANDINS

Platelet aggregation	Chapter 21
Uterine motility	Chapter 40
Cardiac arterial insufficiency	Chapter 15
Vasoconstriction	Chapter 13
Bronchodilation/bronchoconstriction	Chapter 57
Renal tubule stimulation	Chapter 19
Inflammation	Chapter 29
Gastric ulcers	Chapters 58, 59
Myocardial infarction prophylaxis	Chapters 20, 29

LEUKOTRIENES

Allergy response (anaphylaxis)	Chapter 60

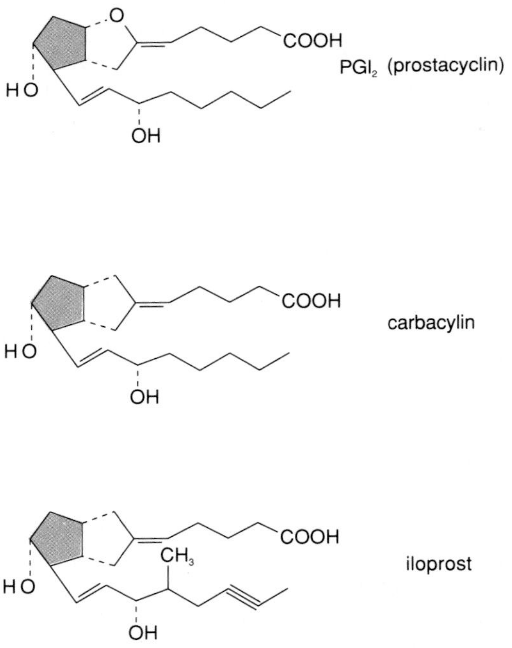

FIGURE 18-6   Two stable analogs of PGI_2.

PHARMACOKINETICS

Prostaglandins and their pharmacokinetics and side effects are discussed in the individual chapters noted in the box.

RELATION OF MOLECULAR ACTIONS TO CLINICAL RESPONSE

Therapeutic applications of the eicosanoids have failed to meet the high expectations of more than a decade when PGI_2, a natural antagonist to TxA_2, was discovered and synthesized. Attempts to use authentic PGI_2 to forestall or ameliorate myocardial infarction, cerebral ischemia, and other manifestations of arterial insufficiency are restricted by the hypotension, headache, and flushing attendant with its administration by IV infusion. Nonetheless, patients with peripheral vascular disease benefit from PGI_2 infusions of several hours into the femoral artery of the involved leg. Close arterial infusion of PGI_2 is associated with less troublesome side effects because of the selective route of administration and the consequently smaller dose of prostacyclin required to achieve therapeutic goals. However, because its use is restricted to patients under direct medical supervision, it has limited therapeutic application.

The development of prostacyclin analogs that stimulate platelet receptors (preventing aggregation) while sparing vascular prostacyclin receptors (avoiding unwanted hypotension) is a therapeutic objective. This assumes that significant differences exist between prostacyclin vascular and platelet receptors. Recent developments suggest that it is possible to discriminate between these receptors with novel synthetic analogs of PGI_2 that act as full agonists on platelets while showing only partial agonist activity on blood vessels.

Prostaglandin Analogs

PGE_1 and PGE_2 inhibit basal, as well as stimulated, gastric acid production and pepsin secretion in response to feeding, vagal stimulation, or administration of histamine or pentagastrin. These antiulcer properties of E series prostaglandins have been exploited in the development of analogs that are active orally. One analog, the methylester prodrug, misoprostol, a 15-deoxy-16 hydroxy-16-methyl PGE that resists degradation by the principal catabolizing enzyme, the 15 OH prostaglandin dehydrogenase, has proven useful for the treatment of peptic ulcers. Misoprostol must first be deesterified to the active acidic form. An unwanted side effect of PGE (and $PGF_{2\alpha}$) analogs is gastrointestinal (GI) hypermotility and associated diarrhea, consequences of the contractile effects of E series prostaglandins on GI smooth muscle. However, in appropriate dosage misoprostol is usually devoid of major side effects. The antiulcer properties of PGE analogs are related to stereospecific binding to a PGE-type receptor located on the plasma membrane of gastric parietal cells.

In addition to the treatment of peptic ulcer disease, PGE analogs can prevent gastric ulcers and promote healing of those caused by nonsteroidal antiinflammatory drugs. The propensity of aspirin-like drugs to cause GI ulcers is a consequence of eliminating the prostaglandin contribution to maintenance of mucosal integrity. That prostaglandins have protective actions on the gut mucosa distinct from their ability to inhibit secretory activity has occasioned the assignment of a "cytoprotective" action to prostaglandins and their analogs. This action of prostaglandins is manifest in their protecting the gastric mucosa from damage after topical application of injurious compounds.

There is one type of inhibitory activity of PGE analogs that must be monitored closely because it can affect the immune response; that is, suppression of cells participating in inflammation and immune responses. PGE_2, and by extension its analogs, can influence the inflammatory and immune responses by affecting activation, mobilization, and secretion of neutrophils, basophils, mast cells, and lymphocytes. For example, the inhibitory effect of PGE_2 on LTB_4 release from activated neutrophils, has been linked to stimulation of neutrophil adenylate cyclase by the prostaglandin. A similar mechanism operating through adenylate cyclase is thought to serve as the basis for PGE modulation of the activity of other cells involved in either the immune or inflammatory response.

Aspirin and Thrombosis

The dynamic interplay at the platelet-endothelium interface between proaggregatory vasoconstrictor and antiaggregatory vasodilator mediators determines the outcome of arterial insufficiency, thrombosis, and ischemia. The key components are TxA_2 and PGI_2, with those interventions that favor PGI_2 production while lowering formation of TxA_2 having the greatest benefit. Aspirin inhibits cyclooxygenase irreversibly by covalent acetylation of the cyclooxygenase. Thus therapeutic strategies strive to maximize the effect of aspirin on platelet cyclooxygenase, while sparing as much as possible, the effect of cyclooxygenase on endothelial cells. Unlike the endothelium, platelets lack nuclei and cannot synthesize new cyclooxygenase to replace that inactivated by aspirin. The effects of aspirin therefore continue for the life of the platelet, more than 10 days. Thus, deficient platelet production of thromboxane cannot be corrected until new platelets are formed, whereas vascular cyclooxygenase, after inhibition, can be replaced by new cyclooxygenase reflecting the synthetic capacity of the endothelial cell.

The resulting low dose aspirin strategy limits the opportunity for aspirin to enter the systemic circulation to inhibit vascular cyclooxygenase but still allows aspirin to act on platelet cyclooxygenase in the portal circulation (from the site of absorption of aspirin to its metabolism by the liver).

Dietary Unsaturated Fatty Acids

Additional evidence for an eicosanoid component in the development of experimental and human disease is provided by studies based on manipulating dietary fatty acids. Investigators have used the following approaches:

1. Using essential fatty-acid-deficient diets to reduce formation of arachidonate metabolites
2. Increasing dietary linoleic acid, the precursor of arachidonic acid, to increase arachidonate metabolites, particularly PGE_2 and PGI_2
3. Increasing dietary EPA to modify the activity of cyclooxygenase and lipoxygenases and, thereby, the nature and the biological activity of the eicosanoids formed by these enzymes.

The third category has received the greatest attention because it carries considerable promise for the amelioration and, possibly, prevention of diseases of the heart, blood vessels, kidneys, and lungs. The Eskimos of Greenland demonstrate a much lower incidence of myocardial infarction and lesser degrees of atherosclerosis when compared to other northern Europeans of comparable age. Their relative insusceptibility to vascular disease is attributed to the high content of EPA in their diet, derived primarily from cold-water fish and mammals. EPA is a poor substrate for cyclooxygenase but competes effectively with arachidonic acid for metabolism by oxygenases, a factor contributing to the antiplatelet activity of EPA. The result of the operation of these factors, and others, set in motion by increased intake of EPA, favors the balance of antiaggregatory vasodilator eicosanoids. Thus, EPA supplementation of the diet in humans has reportedly produced less reactive platelets and diminished vascular reactivity.

REFERENCES

Knapp HR and Fitzgerald GA: The antihypertensive effects of fish oil, N Engl J Med 320:1037, 1989.

Nicosia S and Patrono C: Eicosanoid biosynthesis and action: novel opportunities for pharmacological intervention, FASEB J 3:1941, 1989.

Smith WL: The eicosanoids and their biochemical mechanisms of action, Biochem J 259:315, 1989.

Diuretics: Drugs That Increase Excretion of Water and Electrolytes

(see p. 244)

ABBREVIATIONS	
ADH	antidiuretic hormone
BUN	blood urea nitrogen
cGMP	cyclic guanosine monophosphate
ECF	extracellular fluid
mRNA	messenger RNA
PAH	p-aminohippuric acid
pH	logarithm of the reciprocal of the H ion concentration
TALH	thick ascending loop of Henle

MAJOR DRUGS
osmotic diuretics
carbonic anhydrase inhibitors
thiazides and thiazide-related agents
Loop diuretics, types I and II
potassium sparing agents
aldosterone antagonists
pteridines
pyrazinoyl guanidines

 THERAPEUTIC OVERVIEW

Diuretics are widely used in clinical medicine; over 100 million diuretic prescriptions are written annually in the United States. The disorders for which they are used are summarized in the box on p. 244. The variety of conditions for which certain drugs in this group show efficacy is diverse, ranging from hypertension and congestive heart failure to nephrogenic diabetes insipidus, hypercalciuria, glaucoma, and certain forms of epilepsy. The major therapeutic effects sought include the following:

1. Reduction of generalized edema
2. Correction of specific ion imbalances
3. Reduction of blood pressure (see Chapter 13)
4. Reduction of rate of formation of intraocular fluid
5. Reduction of pulmonary capillary wedge pressure

Diuretics have been used for many years to mobilize and excrete the surplus salt and water that accumulate in the tissues of patients with heart failure, cirrhosis of the liver, or nephrosis. The excessive extracellular fluid (ECF) volumes in such patients result from the inability of the kidneys to excrete Na^+ at high enough rates so that sufficient water also is eliminated. Some of the earlier diuretic agents (e.g., mercurials) have been supplanted by drugs that are safer, have more desirable pharmacokinetics, or show greater ion selectivity. At present, there are five types of diuretic drugs: loop diuretics, carbonic anhydrase inhibitors, thiazides, osmotic diuretics, and potassium-sparing diuretics (see box).

Diuretics suppress the tubular reabsorption of some of the major ions filtered through renal glomeruli. As a result of the increased excretion of ions, urine flow rate, responding to the osmotic force of the additional ions, also rises. Most of the various diuretic drugs interfere with the tubular transport of Na^+ and/or Cl^-. Carbonic anhydrase inhibitors are the only exceptions to this generalization. Once the mainstays of oral diuretic therapy, the carbonic anhydrase in-

THERAPEUTIC OVERVIEW*

LOOP DIURETICS

Used in acute pulmonary edema to reduce pulmonary capillary wedge pressure and left ventricular filling pressure

Used in hypercalcemia to increase calcium excretion

Used in cirrhosis of liver, congestive heart failure (acute and chronic), nephrotic syndrome, and renal failure to increase excretion of NaCl and water

Used in hypertension to reduce blood pressure or augment action of other antihypertensives

Used in impending or incipient renal failure as a preventative (mechanism unknown)

Used in chemical intoxication to increase urine flow rate to "wash out" toxin

CARBONIC ANHYDRASE INHIBITORS

Used in cystinuria to alkalinize tubular urine

Used in epilepsy (mechanism unknown)

Used in glaucoma to reduce intraocular fluid formation

Used in cirrhosis of liver, congestive heart failure (acute or chronic), nephrotic syndrome, and renal failure to increase excretion of NaCl and water

THIAZIDES

Used in cirrhosis of the liver, congestive heart failure (acute or chronic), nephrotic syndrome, and renal failure to increase excretion of NaCl and water

THIAZIDES—cont'd

Used in hypercalciuria and renal calcium stones to decrease calcium excretion

Used in nephrogenic diabetes insipidus (see text)

Used in toxemia of pregnancy to reduce blood pressure (controversial)

Used in hypertension to reduce blood pressure or augment action of other antihypertensives

OSMOTIC DIURETICS

Used in cirrhosis of the liver, congestive heart failure (acute or chronic), nephrotic syndrome, and renal failure to increase excretion of NaCl and water

Used in impending or incipient renal failure as a preventative (mechanism unknown)

Used in hypertension to reduce blood pressure or augment actions of other antihypertensives

POTASSIUM-SPARING DIURETICS

Used in cirrhosis of the liver, congestive heart failure (acute or chronic), nephrotic syndrome, and renal failure to increase excretion of NaCl and water

Used in hypertension to reduce blood pressure or augment actions of other antihypertensives

*Osmotic diuretics are not used when natriuresis is required. Renotoxic substances (e.g., cisplatin, cyclosporine, or iodinated contrast medium), shock, or trauma during protracted surgery may induce acute renal failure. Diuretics sometimes abort or prevent failure when given in anticipation of the impending event or in the early stages of development. In rare cases, diuretics other than the loop variety are used in chemical intoxication to increase urine flow and thereby "wash out" the toxin.

hibitors act on the transport of $NaHCO_3$, not NaCl. Because Na^+ is the chief cationic constituent of extracellular fluid, its urinary excretion with accompanying anions inevitably reduces the ECF volume. Reduction of ECF helps in the treatment of the edema that often accompanies malfunction or failure of organs as structurally or functionally diverse as heart, liver, or kidney. Although the pathophysiological origins of these organic disorders differ, salt and water retention is a unifying feature, and an abnormally enlarged extracellular fluid compartment is the common thread that prompts the use of diuretics.

If a diuretic drug merely increases the flow of urine,

without increasing net sodium excretion, the therapeutic benefit derived from the resulting contraction of the ECF is short-lived; concentrations of electrolytes in ECF rise and the subject would increase water intake, replenishing the lost water. Thus to correct the salt and water imbalances of most edematous patients, there must be an increase in the excretion of sodium. There are, however, occasions when it is desirable to increase the flow of urine but not the excretion of salt. Mannitol and other drugs of the osmotic class are employed for this purpose. Mannitol increases urine flow rate but does not augment Na^+ excretion materially unless the usual clinical dosage is exceeded. Clearly, the generic term, *diuretic*, is used broadly to describe the action of osmotic drugs. The more accurate label, *water diuretic*, is preferable. Osmotic agents are not used in the treatment of generalized edema unless there is evidence of coexisting hyponatremia. Effective reduction of the ECF can be sustained only by drugs that interfere with systems directly involved in the reabsorptive transport of major ions of extracellular fluid. Drugs of this category, often called *natriuretics*, increase the net urinary excretion of sodium chloride or sodium bicarbonate.

Although it is possible to predict with reasonable assurance whether a given patient will respond adequately to a particular class of diuretic or exhibit relative refractoriness, the magnitude of the response is not predictable from one day to the next. Factors other than the usual pharmacokinetic and pharmacodynamic considerations come into play. Response to diuretics is moderated by internal homeostatic mechanisms sensitive to body fluid volumes and osmolar concentrations. Magnitude of the diuretic response depends on the preexisting physiological status and the type and severity of the disorder. For example, individuals who take a thiazide daily for even a short period of time may develop a relative refractoriness that is not a true tolerance to the drug but rather originates from activation of compensatory salt-retaining mechanisms. Similarly, cirrhotic patients with ascites often do not respond at all to a diuretic because homeostatic mechanisms for adjusting salt and water balance apparently signal the existence of depleted ECF when, in fact, the tissues are water-logged.

The purpose of diuretic intervention in the treatment of edema is to normalize the volume of the ECF compartment without distorting electrolyte concentrations. The size of the ECF compartment is largely determined by the body's total content of sodium. There are two reasons for this: (1) sodium is the predominant cation of the ECF and thus is available in quantities sufficient to influence the osmotic distribution or redistribution of large amounts of water, and (2) movements of sodium between the extracellular and intracellular compartments are controlled by active transport mechanisms that are regulated in turn by a variety of integrating mechanisms. The existence of multiple points of control ensures that blockade or failure of one mechanism evokes compensatory responses in others.

To maintain electrolyte and water balance, the uri-

nary excretion of sodium and water must equal intake minus the sum of all losses through other routes. This requirement could not be met if the periodic fluctuations in blood pressure, which occur in all humans, produced equivalent changes in blood flow to the kidneys. It is necessary therefore that wide swings in renal blood flow be dampened when blood pressure fluctuates. In addition, adjustments in the renal tubular handling of sodium and fluid should come into play as rapidly as the need arises.

To achieve the first requirement, an intrarenal autoregulatory mechanism controls arteriolar resistance and the glomerular capillary pressure, thereby preventing wide swings in renal blood flow and glomerular filtration rate. Adjustments in sodium transport rates, both short-term and long-term, are achieved through the integrated activity of renal mechanisms and extrarenal factors discussed in the next section.

To achieve the second requirement in the control of sodium, potassium, and passive water transport in nephrons, the dominant factors are aldosterone, antidiuretic hormone, and atrial natriuretic hormone. These hormones are discussed in a later section.

 ## MECHANISMS OF ACTION

Renal Transport

The names of the parts of the nephron, as used in this discussion, are based primarily on functional properties (Figure 19-1). Because diuretic agents often influence the rates of transport of sodium (Na^+), potassium (K^+), hydrogen (H^+), chloride (Cl^-), bicarbonate (HCO_3^-), and urate, the renal mechanisms of transport of these ions are reviewed before discussion of the mechanisms of action of the diuretic agents.

Tubular Reabsorption: Proximal Transport
The glomerular filtration rate of healthy human adults is usually in the range of 1.7 to 1.8 ml/min/kg. At least 99% of this filtrate must be transferred from tubular lumen back to the blood. Although paracellular (between cells) reabsorption of fluid and electrolytes takes place, the primary pathway is lumen to cell to interstitial fluid to capillary. In the process, two membranes, both permeable to water, must be traversed. The process is initiated in the proximal tubule by the active transport of sodium ions. Passage of filtered sodium into the cell generates an osmotic gradient for the nearly simultaneous movement of water. Since

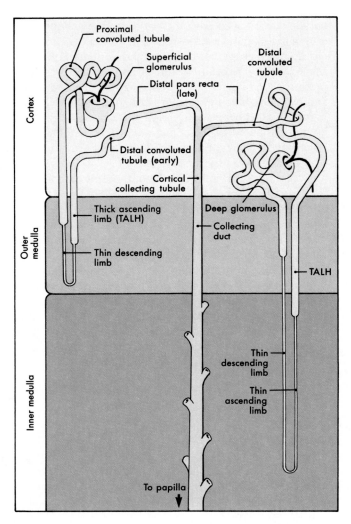

FIGURE 19-1   Renal tubular segments. Distal convoluted tubule: early distal tubule; distal pars recta late; distal tubule and cortical collecting tubule. *TALH*, thick ascending loop of Henle.

anions, chiefly but not exclusively chloride (see below), follow the same route as sodium, charge separation is minimal and electroneutrality of the reabsorbate is maintained. This efficient operation is responsible for the reabsorption of two thirds or more of the Na^+ filtered and, because it is accomplished isosmotically, the reabsorption of the same fraction of glomerular fluid. When glomerular filtration rate increases, excretion of salt and water also increases but fractional reabsorption in the proximal tubule does not change. This phenomenon is called *glomerulo-*

tubular balance. Glomerulotubular balance moderates, but does not entirely eliminate, the effects of alterations in the GFR on salt and water excretion.

The essential elements of sodium translocation are shown diagrammatically in Figure 19-2. Two steps are involved: entry across the luminal membrane and egress across the basolateral membrane. The latter process is the crucial one, for it not only involves the expenditure of metabolically-derived energy but also governs entry into the cell from the lumen. Egress is an active process (i.e., movement is "uphill" or against the prevailing electrochemical gradient), fueled by the energy released when ATP is converted to ADP by a Na-K-dependent ATPase located in the basolateral membrane. As shown in panel A of Figure 19-2, three Na^+ ions are ejected from the cell into the interstitial space; simultaneously two K^+ ions gain entry. The resultant change in the cellular concentration of Na^+ and the loss of one positive charge create a favorable electrochemical gradient for the passive entry of Na^+. The electronegative cell attracts positively charged sodium ions from the lumen (electrical gradient) and the low concentration of cellular sodium resulting from its active egress promotes continual entry (chemical or concentration gradient). The process is self-sustaining and proceeds as long as ATP and enzyme are available. It should be understood that the charge separation created when an extra Na^+ ion leaves the cell is largely dissipated by flow of other positive and negative ions in the vicinity. Healthy proximal tubular cells, however, remain slightly electro-negative with respect to the lumen.

The concentration gradient favors the passive return of the potassium ions, which were initially countertransported (see below) by the ATPase pump from interstitial fluid into the cell, back to the interstitial space. There are about 35 times as many Na^+ ions in extracellular fluid as there are K^+ ions. Obviously, the supply of potassium needed for the operation of the sodium pump would be inadequate if recycling of potassium between cell and interstitial fluid did not take place.

Because electrical and concentration gradients for passage of luminal sodium into proximal tubular cells are favorable, entry is essentially passive. It is facilitated, however, by attachment to or interaction with unidentified channel or carrier-protein receptors. Three types of entry mechanisms are presently recognized: diffusion with chloride; cotransport with un-

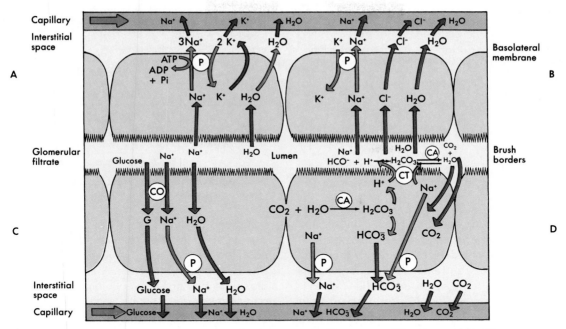

FIGURE 19-2   Transport in the proximal tubule. *P*, Sodium pump; *CO*, cotransport; *CT*, countertransport; *CA*, carbonic anhydrase, in cytoplasm and brush border, ATPase only in basolateral membrane (see text).

charged molecules or acidic anions; and countertransport with hydrogen ion.

Diffusion with chloride, quantitatively the most important, is depicted in Figure 19-2, panel B. Movement of both ions into the cell is downhill. The osmotic transfer of fluid from the lumen into the cell and thence into the interstitial space increases the concentration of chloride in the lumen, thereby accelerating both its diffusive entry across the luminal membrane against the small electrical gradient and its egress through the basolateral membrane. Chloride is also cotransported with sodium. Finally, it appears that in the inner cortical straight portion of the proximal tubule at least, chloride ions can penetrate the tight junctions between cells, traveling from lumen to interstitial space without entering the cell.

Cotransport with uncharged molecules or acidic anions is illustrated in panel C. This type of transport involves the joint, unidirectional passage of two chemical species, one "downhill" and one "uphill". In the proximal tubule, a variety of substances may be cotransported with sodium. The list includes glucose,

phosphate, amino acids, and urate.

The last mechanism, countertransport with hydrogen ion, important in acid-base regulation, is shown in Figure 19-2, panel D. It is operative not only in the proximal tubule but also in the late portion of the distal segment and is located in the luminal membrane. Sodium ions enter the cell from the lumen in exchange for hydrogen ions originating in the cell. Since the concentration of cellular H^+ is low, the reaction proceeds in the direction: $CO_2 + H_2O \rightarrow H_2CO_3 \rightarrow H^+ + HCO_3$. Thus a constant supply of hydrogen ions is furnished for countertransport with sodium. Dissociation of the carbonic acid formed by intracellular hydration of carbon dioxide provides both hydrogen ions and bicarbonate anions. The HCO_3 ions are cotransported with Na^+ across the basolateral membrane into interstitial fluid and subsequently back into the bloodstream. The cytoplasmic hydration reaction occurs spontaneously but at a rate too slow to accomplish the reabsorption of the massive load of bicarbonate filtered (normally more than 4000 mEq/24 hrs). The catalyst, carbonic anhydrase, ensures that

Table 19-1 Summary of Reabsorption in the Proximal Tubule*			
Component	Filtered	Reabsorbed	Entering Loop
	mEq/24 hr		
Na^+	25,200	17,640	7560
Cl^-	19,440	13,414	6026
K^+	810	405	405
HCO_3^-	4320	3825	648
H_2O	180 liters	126 liters	54 liters

*Representative values for a 70 kg human.

Table 19-2 Summary of Reabsorption in the Loop of Henle*			
Component	Entering Loop	Reabsorbed	Entering Distal Tubule
	mEq/24 hr		
Na^+	7560	6300	1260
Cl^-	6026	4860	1166
K^+	405	324	81
HCO_3^-	648	little	<648
H_2O	54 liters	27 liters	27 liters

*Representative values for a 70 kg human.

little or none of the filtered bicarbonate will be excreted. The result of coupling of Na-H countertransport to carbonic anhydrate-mediated hydration and rehydration of CO_2 is the preservation of body bicarbonate. Each HCO_3^- ion saved can buffer one H^+. The Na^+ ions exchanged for H^+ are removed from the cell by the sodium pump.

The final step is transfer from the interstitial fluid into peritubular capillaries. Reabsorptive transport systems of the proximal tubule deposit large amounts of fluid and solutes in the interstitial space. This deposit tends to raise pressure in the interstitium and must be removed if reabsorption is to continue. Theoretically, the sodium can reenter the sodium-depleted cell, pulling anions and water with it. When this occurs, the active transport mechanism re-extrudes it. The permeable peritubular capillary can easily carry away reabsorbed fluids and solutes. Pushed by interstitial pressure and pulled by the oncotic pressure of intracapillary proteins (higher in postglomerular than in preglomerular capillaries), filtered fluid and solutes return to the bloodstream.

In summary, the convoluted and straight portions of the proximal tubule reabsorb approximately 70% of the filtered water and sodium, 69% of the chloride, 85% of the bicarbonate, and 50% of the potassium filtered through the glomerular membranes (Table 19-2). These percentages are relatively constant, even when filtered quantities increase or decrease. As a result, minor fluctuations in glomerular filtration rate do not influence fluid and electrolyte excretion very much. The driving force for reabsorption of water and electrolytes is the sodium pump. Passive movements of the other ions and of water are initiated and sustained by the active transport of sodium across the

basolateral membranes. Osmotic equilibrium with plasma is maintained to the end of the proximal tubule. Most of the filtered bicarbonate is not actually reabsorbed from the lumen; it is converted to carbon dioxide and water in the vicinity of the brush border membranes within which large concentrations of the catalyst, carbonic anhydrase, are found. The direction of this reaction is $H_2CO_3 \rightarrow CO_2 + H_2O$ (established by the high concentration of carbonic acid in luminal fluid resulting from secretion of hydrogen ion). A carbonic anhydrase isoenzyme in the cellular cytoplasm catalyzes the formation of carbonic acid, the source of the cellular hydrogen ion exchanged for luminal sodium and of the bicarbonate ion, which exits with sodium across the basolateral membranes (see Figure 19-2, D). Thus newly formed bicarbonate replaces the bicarbonate removed from plasma through glomerular filtration.

Tubular Reabsorption: Transport in the Loop of Henle Diuretic agents exert no discernible action in the descending limb of the loop of Henle. The cells of this portion of the renal tubule are probably not equipped with specialized transporting systems. They are relatively impermeable to sodium and chloride but do permit water to diffuse easily from the lumen to the medullary interstitium where higher osmotic pressures are encountered. The following segment discusses the transporting functions of the ascending limb, an important site of action of the "loop" (also called *high-ceiling*) diuretics.

In contrast to the proximal tubule, the ascending limb of the loop of Henle transports chloride uphill, the intracellular chloride concentration exceeding that predicted by the Nernst equation. The system, present in a variety of transporting epithelia, is aptly

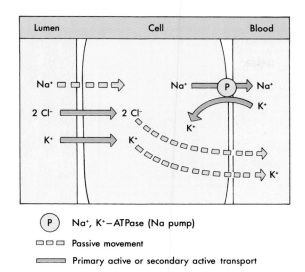

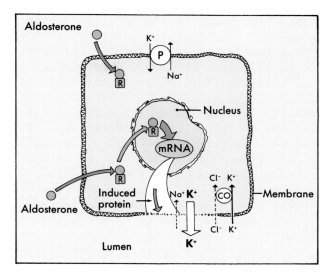

<table>
<tr><td>(P)</td><td>Na⁺, K⁺–ATPase (Na pump)</td></tr>
</table>

(P) Na$^+$, K$^+$–ATPase (Na pump)

▭▭▭ Passive movement

▬▬▬ Primary active or secondary active transport

Net result: reabsorption of Na$^+$ K$^+$ 2 Cl$^-$ ions

FIGURE 19-3   The Na$^+$, K$^+$, 2Cl$^-$ cotransport system in cells of the ascending limb of the loop of Henle.

FIGURE 19-4   Cellular action of aldosterone. *CO*, Cotransport (see text for details).

called Na$^+$, K$^+$, 2Cl$^-$ cotransport. Its activity depends on the simultaneous presence of these three ions in luminal fluid. A schematic model of the system is presented in Figure 19-3. The major source of energy required to drive it is the Na$^+$, K$^+$-ATPase of the peritubular membrane. A favorable electrochemical gradient (with the lumen positive) prompts the "downhill" entry of a sodium ion into the cell, and a transporter in the membrane facilitates the cotransport of a potassium ion and two chloride anions "uphill." The cell, now overloaded with chloride, releases the ion into the interstitium. Potassium passively reenters the lumen, shuttling back and forth. The ascending limb is highly permeable to the three cotransported ions but not to water. Accordingly, the fluid in the ascending limb remains in the lumen and is progressively diluted. The countercurrent mechanism in the renal medulla depends on the activity of this cotransport system, and drugs that block cotransport diminish the ability of the kidney to excrete urine that is either more concentrated or more dilute than plasma.

In summary, fluid is reabsorbed from the lumen of the descending limb as it pushes progressively deeper into medullary areas of higher osmotic pressure. Electrolyte concentrations increase to a maximum at the bend and then gradually decrease as the Na$^+$, K$^+$,

2Cl$^-$ cotransport mechanism and sodium pump, working in tandem, achieve the reabsorption of sodium and potassium chloride. The quantitative relationships are shown in Table 19-2. Thick ascending limb cells reabsorb about 25% of the filtered NaCl and 40% of the potassium, whereas the entire loop reabsorbs only 15% of the fluid. Loop cells do not exchange H$^+$ for luminal Na$^+$ and thus probably process only small quantities of HCO$_3^-$, if any.

Tubular Reabsorption: Distal Tubule and Collecting Duct Transport In contradistinction to the proximal tubule and loop of Henle, quantitative reabsorption of water and electrolytes in the distal tubule and collecting ducts is much less and quite variable. NaCl is reabsorbed against an electrochemical gradient. Because the early distal tubule is relatively impermeable to water, removal of NaCl amplifies an already unfavorable concentration gradient and probably limits the effectiveness of the sodium pump.

The amount of sodium and potassium present in the final urine is tightly controlled by aldosterone released from the adrenal cortex. The hormone penetrates cells of the late distal segment and attaches to a cytosolic receptor (Figure 19-4). The hormone-receptor complex then migrates to the nucleus where it induces the formation of a specific messenger RNA (mRNA). The newly formed mRNA leaves the nucleus to direct the production of a protein that enhances the permeability of the apical (luminal) membrane of the cell to Na^+ and K^+. Increased entry of substrate feeds the sodium pump and thus speeds reabsorption.

Because the pump simultaneously carries interstitial K^+ across the basolateral membrane, the cellular concentration of this ion increases. This is the first step in the secretion of potassium. But potassium is also actively transported inward, across the apical membrane, by a cotransport system. Thus it is free to move passively down its concentration gradient through either membrane. Because sodium entry from the lumen is electrogenic, the resultant electrical negativity attracts potassium (i.e., completes the final secretory step). Predominance of secretion or reabsorption generally depends on the dietary intake of potassium, the principal determinant of plasma concentration. When plasma K^+ is high, basolateral entry increases and net secretion is demonstrable; when it is low, the basolateral pump is less effective and reabsorption predominates. By indirectly rousing the activity of the sodium pump, aldosterone promotes sodium retention and potassium loss.

The final equilibratory steps take place in medullary collecting ducts. Small amounts of NaCl and potassium are reabsorbed. In the presence of antidiuretic hormone (ADH), water moves out of the lumen, following the medullary osmotic gradient established by ion transport in the ascending limb. A quantitative summary of fractional reabsorption of water and sodium of each tubular sgement is shown in Figure 19-5. The data are based on average values for a 70 kg adult in good health living in a moderate climate. Plasma sodium concentration is 140 mEq/L and glomerular filtration rate is 125 ml/min. The proximal tubule reabsorbs more sodium than water; the entire distal tubule and medullary collecting system extract less than 5% of filtered sodium.

Tubular Secretion and Bidirectional Transport of Organic Acids and Bases With the exception of two classes, osmotic agents and competitive inhibitors of aldosterone, all of the diuretics in clinical use release or accept a proton at the pH of body fluids. Thus these drugs exist in the body both as uncharged molecules and as charged organic ions. In large measure, this duality of chemical form determines transport of the drugs in the body, how quickly they undergo transport from a particular site, and what actions they exert in the kidney and other organs.

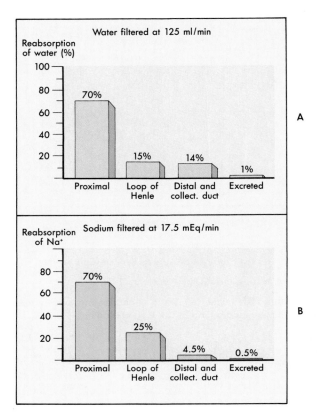

FIGURE 19-5   Summary of renal reabsorption of filtered water (**A**) and sodium (**B**) for a 70 kg human (see text).

Proximal tubular secretion of diuretic anions and cations illustrates the profound impact of electrical charge on the delivery of drugs to renal receptors and on their rapid decline in plasma. Two generic secretory systems that transport organic ions from blood to urine reside in the proximal tubule. One handles organic acids (anions as A^- form of acid HA), and the second transports organic bases (cations as BH^+ form) of base B, (see Chapter 5). The chief characteristics of these systems are:

1. At least one step in the transport process is active (uphill) and against the concentration gradient, although metabolic energy is furnished indirectly
2. The systems are saturable (fixed number of carriers)
3. The systems are susceptible to competitive inhibition by other transported organic ions bearing the charge

The lack of any specific structural requirement sup-

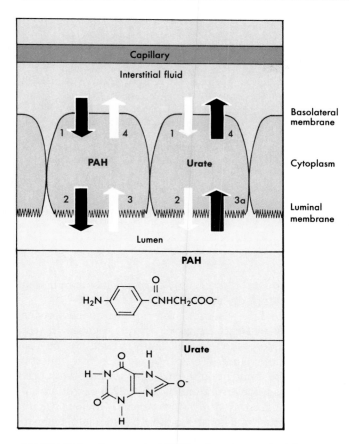

FIGURE 19-6   Transport of PAH and urate, see text for explanation. Unfilled arrows are quantitatively much less than filled arrows (see text).

ports the conjecture that these two secretory mechanisms serve primarily as "glomerular backups" for the urinary excretion of a large number of endogenous and environmental chemicals, especially but not exclusively, solutes of low molecular weight that bind to plasma proteins and thus are not freely filtered through glomerular membranes. In addition to most of the diuretics, organic acids and bases that are secreted include acetylcholine and choline, bile acids, uric acid, *p*-aminohippuric acid (PAH), epinephrine, norepinephrine, histamine, and morphine.

The tubular transport of two major acids, PAH and uric acid, is summarized in Figure 19-6. Step 1 is the same for both acids. A membrane transporter carries Na^+ downhill and PAH or urate uphill in the same direction across the basolateral membrane into the cells. Step 1 may also be accomplished by an ex-

change (countertransport) for a cellular anion. The cell, now loaded with PAH or urate, readily loses these substances to the urine as they move downhill to complete step 2 with the help of a transporter in the brush border. Step 3, movement back into the cell by exchange with a cellular anion, is either insignificant for PAH or is prevented by the large concentration gradient favoring movement of that organic anion into the urine. Although reabsorption is demonstrable in some species and can be inhibited by probenecid, a classical competitive inhibitor, the high renal extraction of PAH (usually 88% or more, equivalent to the renal plasma flow to which tubules are exposed) indicates that very little is reabsorbed.

Bidirectional transport of urate, on the other hand, is well established. Quantitatively, reabsorption exceeds secretion by a wide margin. Entry from the lumen is accomplished through two mechanisms: in step 3a by cotransport of urate with Na^+ or by cotransport of filtered lactate with Na^+ into the cell, followed by exchange between urinary urate and cellular lactate. The process is completed in step 4 by a mechanism that has not been identified but surely involves the participation of a transporter. Proximal tubular reabsorption of urate is an avid process. Less than 10% of the filtered urate is excreted, yet segments of the nephron other than the proximal tubule do not actively transport significant quantities of urate, and passive reabsorption is relatively insignificant. Depletion of sodium and contraction of the extracellular fluid volume accelerate the reabsorption of sodium. This leads, also, to increased cotransport of uric acid. Secretory transport of organic bases are discussed briefly for the potassium-sparing diuretics in a later section.

Atrial Natriuretic Hormone

In 1984 the structure of a "natriuretic factor," a salt-losing hormone long thought to be involved in the control of ECF, was identified. The hormone is a peptide found in granules in atrial myocardial cells, hence the name *atrial* natriuretic hormone or factor (also *atriopeptin*). The active peptide arises from a prohormone of 126 amino acid residues. This hormone is also detectable in other tissues, including the nervous system. Basal concentrations are present in blood and increase when ECF expands, blood pressure rises, or the dietary intake of salt is raised. The hormone increases renal blood flow and glomerular

Table 19-3   Diuretic Drugs

Type	Prototype	Primary Site of Action	Mechanism
Osmotic	mannitol	Entire tubule	Osmotic pressure
Carbonic anhydrase inhibitors	acetazolamide	Proximal and late distal	Decrease formation of H^+ in cells
thiazides	hydrochlorothiazide	Early distal	Decrease NaCl entry into cells
thiazide-related	chlorthalidone	Early distal	Decrease NaCl entry into cells
Loop I	ethacrynic acid	Ascending limb	Inhibit Na^+, K^+, $2Cl^-$ cotransport,
Loop II	furosemide	Ascending limb	Inhibit Na^+, K^+, $2Cl^-$ cotransport,
K-sparing			
aldosterone antagonists	spironolactone	Late distal	Compete for aldosterone receptors
pteridines	triamterene	Late distal	Decrease Na^+ entry into cells
pyrazinoyl guanidines	amiloride	Late distal	Decrease Na^+ entry into cells

filtration rate, though not invariably or uniformly. Atrial natriuretic hormone also increases the excretion of sodium, probably by exerting a direct action on the renal tubule. It causes vasodilation and can reduce blood pressure. Its precise mechanism of action has not been established, but its effects appear to be mediated by cGMP. It is possible that atrial natriuretic hormone acts on tubular reabsorption from locally produced hormone release. Onset of action is rapid but duration is brief. The hormone thus appears to be an ideal endogenous substance for restoring equilibrium rapidly when body fluid volume goes awry.

Diuretics

Types of Drugs The five major types and several subtypes of diuretics are listed in Table 19-3. In all cases the primary site of action is the renal tubule. The transport of Na^+, Cl^-, HCO_3^-, water, and to some extent K^+, H^+, and organic ions is affected and the concentrations of these ions undergo change.

The diverse assortment of operational transport mechanisms present in the kidney and the fact that each segment does not possess a full complement (the Na^+, K^+-ATPase, or sodium pump is the only one common to all renal transporting cells) supports the following assertions:

1. The pattern of excretion of electrolytes depends on the class of agent administered.
2. The maximal response is limited by the site of action of the agent being used.
3. The effects of two or more drugs belonging to different classes is additive, and possibly syn-

ergistic, if their sites or mechanisms of action are not the same.

In the first assertion, the pattern of electrolytes probably will vary between agents because in reasonable doses none of the diuretics acts directly on the sodium pump. Thus the selection of a diuretic should be founded on the magnitude of the response, on the particular pattern of electrolyte excretion desired, and on a case by case basis. Obviously, preconditions such as the state of electrolyte balance and severity of the disorder for which therapy is initiated are also considerations.

Osmotic Diuretics Osmotic agents are unique among the drugs classified as diuretics. They do not interact with receptors or directly block any renal transport mechanism. The pharmacological activity of this group depends entirely on the osmotic pressure exerted by the drug molecules in solution. When present in the ECF, the drugs attract cellular water, causing it to shift into the extracellular compartment; in the renal tubular lumen, osmotically active molecules oppose the movement of water into the cells. Because the relationship between magnitude of effect and concentration of drug in solution is linear, all agents used clinically are small molecules, which minimize the size of the dose.

Mannitol is the leading compound, although urea, glycerol, and isosorbide also are used. The structural formulas are shown in Figure 19-7. During the administration of mannitol, its molecules diffuse from the bloodstream into the interstitial space, where the increased osmotic pressure draws water from the cells to increase the ECF volume. Glomerular filtration of mannitol into the tubular urine then initiates the di-

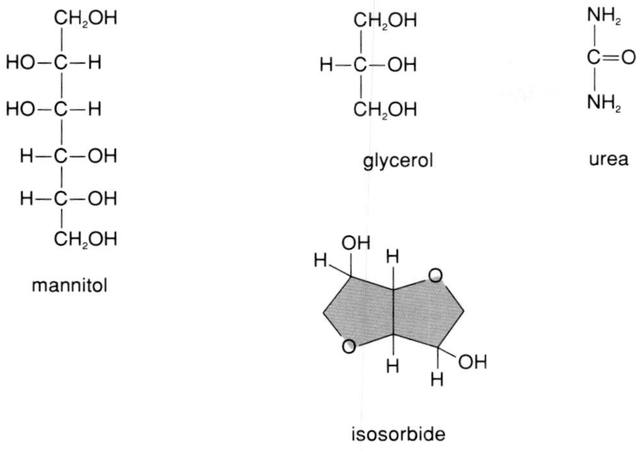

FIGURE 19-7   Osmotic diuretics.

uretic response. In the proximal tubule, molecules of mannitol retard the passive interdependent reabsorption of water that normally follows the active transport of sodium. In effect, the osmotic force of unreabsorbable solute in the lumen opposes the osmotic force of reabsorbable sodium. Isosmolality of the urine is preserved because molecules of mannitol replace the sodium ions reabsorbed. There is a reduction in the reabsorbed fraction of water and thus an increase in the amount entering the loop of Henle. Although osmotic agents do not act directly on the sodium transport mechanism, the rate of transport of sodium is affected. The luminal fluid concentration of the ion decreases when sodium is transported and water does not follow the sodium. This results in a change in the sodium concentration gradient and leads to a return flux of sodium chloride into the lumen, and ultimately to a small increase (relative to water) in the excretion of sodium. Urinary loss of sodium is dependent on dosage but is invariably less than the fractional excretion of water. The initial dilution of plasma electrolytes induced by acute expansion of the ECF volume reverses when renal excretion of water catches up. Overzealous administration of mannitol may result in hypernatremia, hyperkalemia, and volume depletion.

Under normal circumstances, reabsorption of NaCl in the thick ascending limb increases when proximal tubular reabsorption is repressed. This compensatory response fails to occur during osmotic diuresis, possibly because mannitol increases medullary blood flow, an action that washes out the countercurrent gradient. The NaCl concentration of fluid in the thick

ascending limb is much reduced, and this indirectly diminishes the efficiency of the Na^+, K^+, $2Cl^-$ cotransport system. Transport of sodium and water is decreased. Ascending limb cells are thus an important site of natriuretic action. Distal segments and medullary collecting ducts, responsible for transport of only a small fraction of filtered sodium, are unable to cope with the large salt and water loads presented during osmotic diuresis.

Carbonic Anhydrase Inhibitors   Carbonic anhydrase is a metalloenzyme that contains one zinc atom per molecule. High concentrations are present in human red blood cells, liver, and secretory epithelia of the kidney, intestine, pancreas, choroid plexus, and ciliary processes of the eye. There are five major isoenzymes in mammalian tissues. All catalyse the reversible reaction of water and carbon dioxide to form carbonic acid. The prevailing direction of this reaction is established by the pH of the medium. A rise of pH increases the rate of hydration and a fall increases dehydration. For example, the activity of cytoplasmic isoenzyme II in the proximal tubule accelerates the formation of carbonic acid, the primary source of the cellular hydrogen ion that is secreted into the lumen by the Na^+, H^+ cotransport mechanism and of the cellular bicarbonate that replaces the filtered ion. Isoenzyme IV in contiguous brush border membranes dehydrates the luminal carbonic acid formed from secreted hydrogen ion and filtered bicarbonate. Secretion of H^+ thus mediates the preservation of plasma bicarbonate, and the brush border enzyme lowers the gradient against which H^+ is transported. Sulfanilamide-type compounds such as acetazolamide, methazolamide, and dichlorphenamide reversibly inhibit carbonic anhydrase, resulting in increased urine flow and sodium excretion. The chemical structures of these drugs are shown in Figure 19-8.

Thiazide Diuretics   This type of diuretic drug was discovered from attempts to find compounds that increase the excretion of NaCl rather than $NaHCO_3$. The basic structure (Figure 19-9) comprises a heterocyclic (benzothiadiazide) ring and an unsubstituted sulfamyl ($-SO_2NH_2$) group. Thiazide-related diuretics are formed by altering the ring structure. Hydrochlorothiazide is formed by addition of hydrogen at positions 3 and 4. This minor change improves oral absorption, increases diuretic potency, and substantially reduces carbonic anhydrase activity.

The major site of action of thiazides is the early distal tubule. Suppression of sodium and chloride

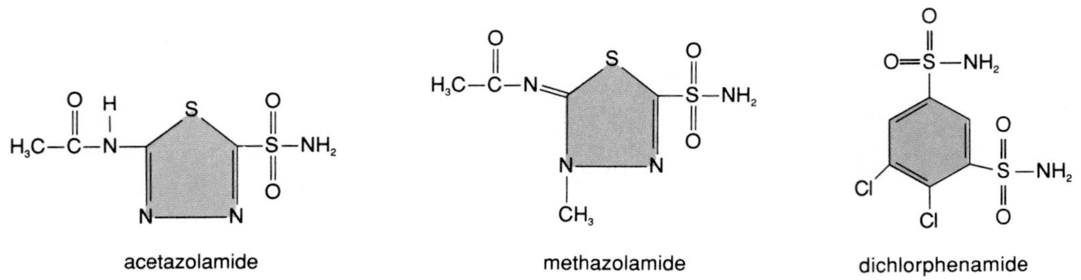

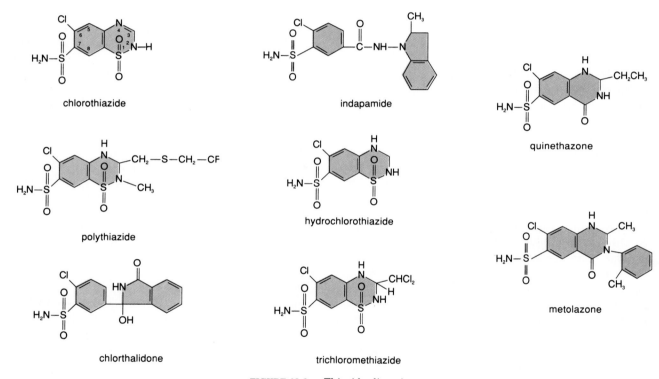

FIGURE 19-8   Carbonic anhydrase inhibitors.

FIGURE 19-9   Thiazide diuretics.

transport at this locus increases the delivery of these two ions, along with fluid attracted osmotically, to the later portions of the nephron. There, a small fraction of the sodium ion in excess is reabsorbed and replaced with potassium. Because only 15% or less of the glomerular filtrate reaches the early distal segment, the magnitude of the diuretic effect is more limited than that induced by agents that act earlier (e.g., in the loop of Henle). Thiazides interfere with the electroneutral passage of NaCl from lumen to cells.

Chlorothiazide in recommended doses may inhibit bicarbonate transport in the proximal tubule, but most of the thiazides and thiazide-related drugs are weaker inhibitors of carbonic anhydrase, and do not affect bicarbonate at usual therapeutic doses.

Loop Diuretics   Loop diuretics satisfy the need for agents capable of generating larger responses than those produced by thiazides. Acting on the ascending

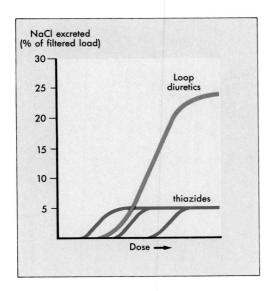

FIGURE 19-10   Schematic dose-response curves comparing thiazides to loop diuretics.

furosemide

ethacrynic acid

bumetanide

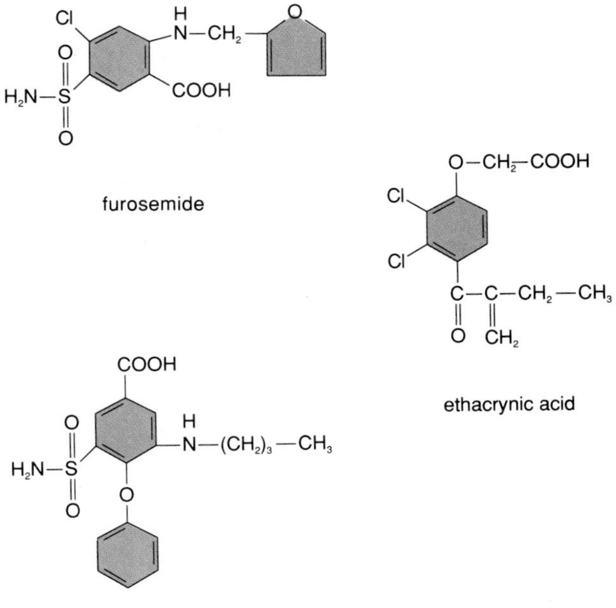

FIGURE 19-11   Loop diuretics.

limb, loop diuretics can inhibit the reabsorption of as much as 25% of the glomerular filtrate (Figure 19-10) and are often effective when thiazides do not suffice. Greater efficacy confers greater ability to distort fluid and electrolyte balance. Overdoses of thiazides are usually tolerated, but overdoses of loop agents may evoke serious consequences. Nevertheless, loop diuretics are remarkably safe when used properly.

Three loop diuretics are available in the United States (Figure 19-11). Ethacrynic acid and furosemide are prototypes of loop I and II drugs, respectively. Bumetanide, of the same class as furosemide, is considerably more potent and differs pharmacokinetically, but otherwise is similar to the older drug. Ethacrynic acid attaches to sulfhydryl groups in vivo, a reaction formerly considered the antecedent of diuresis. This opinion no longer prevails because several natriuretic compounds with related structures do not react chemically with sulfhydryl groups in vitro. Loop diuretics suppress reabsorption of NaCl in the ascending limb. Recent evidence suggests that furosemide competes with chloride for a binding site on the Na^+, $K+$, $2Cl^-$ cotransporting system. Although ethacrynic acid also inhibits this transport mechanism, efforts to identify the molecular mechanism have been unsuccessful. The drug can inhibit Na^+, K^+-ATPase, but only at concentrations that greatly exceed those achieved with therapeutic doses.

Both drugs reach their site of action by first entering the urine upstream and then passing with luminal flow into the loop and thence into cell membranes. Proximal tubular secretion is thus an important component of the delivery mechanism. Drugs that block tubular secretion (e.g., probenecid) influence the temporal response to loop diuretics but do not abolish their effects. Evidence that ancillary sites of action are present in segments of the nephron other than the ascending limb is largely discounted on the assumption that a proximal tubular action would be annulled downstream and a distal action, in any event, would be trivial. This overlooks the fact that loop diuretics interfere with reabsorptive transport in the loop. Thus full compensation may not be possible.

Potassium-Sparing Diuretics The potassium-sparing diuretics comprise three pharmacologically distinct groups: steroidal aldosterone antagonists, pteridines, and pyrazinoylguanidines. One drug from each group is available in the United States. Locus of action for all is the late distal segment in which they interfere with sodium reabsorption and potassium secretion, though each operates through a different molecular mechanism. Diuretic activity is weak because fractional sodium reabsorption in the late

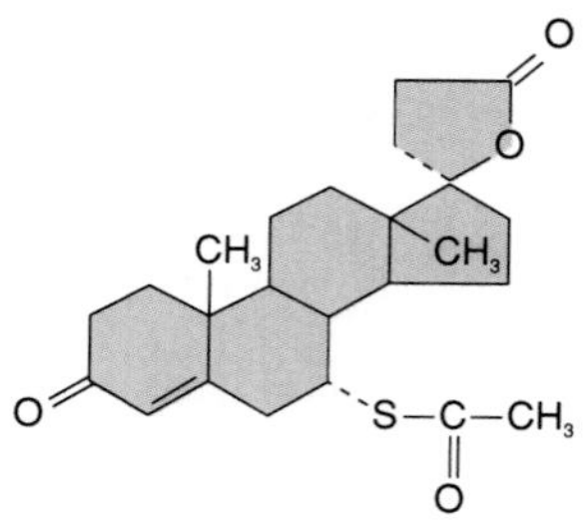

spironolactone

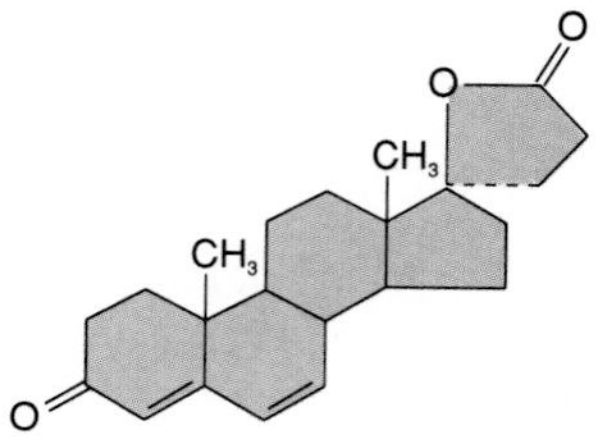

canrenone

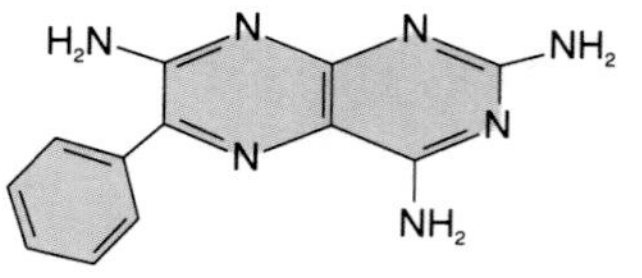

triamterene

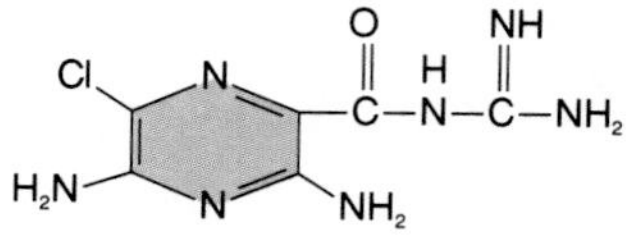

amiloride

FIGURE 19-12   K$^+$-sparing diuretics.

distal segment usually does not exceed 3% of the filtered load. For this reason, potassium-sparing drugs are ordinarily used in combination with thiazides or loop diuretics, often in a single preparation, to restrict potassium losses and sometimes to augment diuretic action. Use as single agents is infrequent.

Spironolactone (Figure 19-12) is an analog of aldosterone. Spironolactone and its major metabolite, canrenone, attach to aldosterone receptors in the kidney and elsewhere and act as competitive inhibitors of the endogenous hormone.

Triamterene and amiloride (see Figure 19-12) are structurally diverse but use the same primary site of action. The molecular mechanisms of action probably differ somewhat but the results are virtually identical. Triamterene is an aminopteridine chemically related to folic acid. Amiloride is a pyrazinoylguanidine. Both are organic bases secreted in the proximal tubule. Prevailing evidence indicates that basolateral movement into the cell is downhill and egress through the luminal membrane is uphill, with transporters involved in both cases. Triamterene and amiloride prevent entry of luminal sodium into cells of the late distal tubule. The molecular mechanism of this action is unknown. It may involve closure of sodium channels, which produces a selective reduction in permeability

of the membranes to sodium. Because sodium transport at this site is electrogenic, failure of entry dispels the electrical gradient between cell and lumen, and thus cancels a critical force that draws intracellular potassium into the urine. Although the drugs are weak diuretics and natriuretics, potassium is conserved and chloride is excreted with sodium. These two agents may also increase bicarbonate excretion and interfere with urinary acidification. Amiloride can reduce sodium-hydrogen exchange in the proximal tubule and possibly also downstream. Some investigators believe that a portion of the natriuretic response to triamterene is related to inhibition of Na$^+$, K$^+$-ATPase. Amiloride also depresses the renal clearance of calcium, an action that is coupled with the inhibition of sodium reabsorption in the late distal segment. In contrast to spironolactone, triamterene and amiloride are active in the presence or in the absence of circulating aldosterone.

PHARMACOKINETICS

The pharmacokinetic parameters for diuretic agents are summarized in Table 19-4.

Since mannitol is not readily absorbed from the

Table 19-4 Pharmacokinetic Parameters

Drug	Administration	Absorbed	Plasma Protein Binding (%)	Onset (hour)	$t_{1/2}$ (hour)	Disposition*
mannitol	IV	Poor	—	—	0.25-0.33	R (~100%)
acetazolamide	Oral/IV	Good	90	1	5	R (~100%)
methazolamide	Oral	Fair	—	—	14	R
chlorothiazide	Oral	Poor	—	—	—	R (main), B
hydrochlorothiazide	Oral	Good	—	1	8-10	R (main), B
chlorthalidone	Oral	Poor	—	3	—	R (main), B
metolazone	Oral	Good	—	1	—	R (main), B
furosemide	Oral/IV	Good	>95	—	1	R (40%), M
bumetanide	Oral/IV	Good	—	1	—	M*
ethacrynic acid	Oral/IV	Good	—	0.5	—	R (main), M*
spironolactone	Oral	Fair	>90	2-4	—	M*, R, B (15%)
triamterene	Oral	Good	60	—	2	R, M, B
amiloride	Oral	Good	—	—	6	R (50%), B (40%)

R, Renal (parent drug); *M*, metabolized; *B*, biliary.
*Active metabolite.

intestine and large doses are required to produce a significant effect, it is administered IV as a bolus or by drip over an extended period of time. It distributes in extracellular fluid. Excretion is almost entirely by glomerular filtration, with about 90% appearing in the urine within 24 hours. Less than 10% is reabsorbed in the renal tubule and a similar quantity is metabolized, probably in the liver. The plasma half-life is approximately 15 to 20 minutes.

Isosorbide and glycerol are administered orally to reduce intraocular pressure before opthalmological surgery. Urea is rarely given by mouth because it induces nausea and emesis. It is administered IV as an aqueous solution containing dextrose or invert sugar. Urea, glycerol, and isosorbide are metabolized extensively.

Acetazolamide is well absorbed from the gastrointestinal (GI) tract. More than 90% of the drug is plasma protein bound. Because it is relatively insoluble in lipid, it does not readily penetrate cellular membranes or cross the blood-brain barrier. The highest concentrations are found in tissues that contain large amounts of carbonic anhydrase (e.g., renal cortex, red blood cells). Renal effects are noticeable within 30 minutes and are usually maximal at 2 hours. Acetazolamide is not metabolized but is excreted rapidly by glomerular filtration and proximal tubular secretion. The half-life is about 5 hours and renal excretion is essentially complete in 24 hours. In com-

parison, methazolamide is absorbed more slowly from the GI tract, and its duration of action is long, with a half-life of about 14 hours. Heretofore, topical preparations of carbonic anhydrase inhibitors were ineffective. However, newer sulfonamides can penetrate the cornea in amounts sufficient to inhibit carbonic anhydrase as well as oral acetazolamide. The first of these compounds, MK 927, is in clinical trial and appears to be effective and devoid of the particularly troublesome side effects (e.g., depression, malaise) associated with oral administration to patients with glaucoma.

Individually, the thiazides differ considerably with respect to pharmacokinetic properties. Plasma protein binding varies from 10% to 95% but extensive binding does not prevent access to the site of action. Free drug enters the lumen by filtration and by organic acid secretion and subsequently diffuses or is transported to its site of action.

Each thiazide and thiazide-related drug possesses singular attributes with respect to potency, onset, and duration of action. For example, the diuretic action of chlorthalidone, a thiazide-related drug, is slow in onset but remains for 24 hours or more; cyclopenthiazide is 100 times as potent as hydrochlorothiazide. Time-course of action and potency are manifestations of solubility in lipid, highly soluble members of the thiazide family possessing larger apparent volumes of distribution and lower renal clearances. All of the agents, however, appear to share the same mechanism of action. Dose-response curves are parallel, and maximal responses (efficacy) are similar. Hydrochlorothiazide is not metabolized. The major route of disappearance is renal, with elimination by glomerular filtration and proximal tubular secretion. Biliary excretion is a second less prominent route.

Although chlorothiazide has adequate bioavailability when given orally, it is not extensively absorbed from the GI tract. Absorption is dose-dependent in the therapeutic range; about 20% of a 250 mg dose enters the systemic circulation but only 10% of a 500 mg dose is absorbed. Either the absorptive site is easily saturated or poor water solubility interferes. Hydrochlorothiazide is approximately 70% bioavailable and its fractional absorption is not dose-dependent. This drug has a large apparent volume of distribution, and the plasma concentration provides a rapid (1 hour) onset of action. The half-life is 8 to 10 hours.

The loop diuretic, ethacrynic acid, is well absorbed. Onset of action of an oral dose is extremely rapid, with the peak effect occurring in 1 to 2 hours and diuresis continuing for 6 to 8 hours. Ethacrynic acid is conjugated with glutathione, which subsequently forms an ethacrynic acid-cysteine adduct that is more potent than the parent drug. Because ethacrynic acid is poorly soluble in lipid, the apparent volume of distribution is small. Plasma protein binding is extensive and the compound and its metabolites are excreted in the urine by filtration and proximal tubular secretion. Elimination via the intestine is augmented through biliary transport and accounts for about one third of the administered dose.

Furosemide is practically insoluble in lipid and almost totally bound to plasma protein (>95%). Well absorbed from the GI tract, its onset and duration of action match those of ethacrynic acid, and it is excreted via the same routes. The average therapeutic dose excreted unchanged is 30% to 50%, and the elimination half-life is approximately 1 hour. Half-life increases in patients with renal insufficiency or cirrhosis. The liver forms an inactive glucuronide.

Spironolactone is poorly soluble in aqueous fluids. Bioavailability of an oral dose is approximately 90% in some but not all commercial preparations. The drug is rapidly metabolized in the liver. Canrenone, the predominant metabolite, is responsible for roughly 80% of the potassium-sparing effect. Canrenone binds extensively to plasma protein (98%). Its half-life varies

from 10 to 35 hours, and it is excreted in urine and bile along with smaller quantities of additional metabolites. Tubular secretion of canrenone has been reported but unmetabolized drug is not detectable in urine. The onset of action is extremely slow, with peak response sometimes occurring 48 hours or more after the first dose; effects gradually wane over a period of 48 to 72 hours.

Oral absorption of triamterene in humans is rapid and almost complete in healthy subjects. Half-life is about 2 hours. Approximately 60% of the parent drug and 90% of the major metabolite, a sulfate conjugate, are bound to plasma proteins. Up to 70% is excreted in the urine, but only a small fraction is unchanged. A considerable quantity is metabolized in the liver, and biliary excretion is significant. Most patients respond during the first day of treatment but the maximum is not reached for several days.

When amiloride is administered orally, about 50% of the dose is recovered in the urine and 40% in the feces. The half-life is 6 hours, with action usually beginning in 2 hours and lasting about 24 hours. Amiloride is not metabolized.

 ## RELATION OF MECHANISMS OF ACTION TO CLINICAL RESPONSE

Osmotic Diuretics

Mannitol is usually the drug of choice because its properties best satisfy the requirements for an efficient osmotic diuretic. It is inherently nontoxic, freely filtered through glomeruli, essentially nonreabsorbable from tubular fluid, and not readily metabolized. Urea, glycerol, and isosorbide are less efficient as osmotic agents because they penetrate cellular membranes. As drug molecules are reabsorbed, luminal concentration falls and the tendency to retain filtered fluid diminishes. Patients treated with mannitol may develop mild hyperkalemia acutely. Although the origin of this action is not firmly established, it is likely that bulk flow of potassium accompanies the osmotic-induced discharge of water from cells into the interstitium. Mannitol increases the excretion of a number of important ions. The list includes potassium, bicarbonate, phosphate, calcium, and magnesium. Losses are usually modest and clinically unimportant. Nevertheless, it is prudent to be aware of the potential imbalances that may be induced in patients receiving prolonged therapy or in those in whom concentrations of these electrolytes are already distorted.

It is a common clinical impression that mannitol improves renal hemodynamics in a variety of situations of impending or incipient renal failure. There is supporting evidence in some clinical studies but dissenting reports abound and the topic is controversial. Mannitol does not increase glomerular filtration rate or renal blood flow in humans, as it clearly does in some laboratory species.

Because they penetrate into the aqueous compartment in trace amounts only, osmotic drugs reduce the volume and pressure of the aqueous humor by extracting fluid from it. Hence, they may be used for the short-term treatment of acute glaucoma. Similarly, infusions of mannitol are used to lower the elevated intracranial pressure of cerebral edema associated with tumors, neurosurgical procedures, or other conditions. Osmotic agents cause the redistribution of body fluid, increase urine flow rate, and accelerate the renal elimination of filtered solutes. These effects are often sought in the treatment of many clinical disorders.

These drugs are also administered prophylactically to prevent the development of renal failure associated with severe traumatic injury, cardiovascular and other complicated surgical procedures, or therapy with cisplatin and other renotoxic drugs. Efficacy and mechanism of action in such instances are not well established. Based on studies in experimental animal models, many investigators claim that mannitol dilates renal blood vessels that are in the constricted state and, by causing the rate of urine flow to increase, prevents obstruction of the renal tubules and further reduction in glomerular filtration.

Mannitol is occasionally used to promote renal extraction of bromides, barbiturates, salicylates, or other drugs in overdosed individuals.

Carbonic Anhydrase Inhibitors

The popularity of carbonic anhydrase inhibitors as diuretics has waned because of (1) rapid tolerance development, (2) increased urinary excretion of bicarbonate with inevitable acidotic manifestations when these drugs are given daily, and, most importantly, (3) because of the advent of more suitable agents. Nevertheless, acetazolamide can be administered for short-term therapy, especially in combi-

nation with other diuretics to patients who are resistant or who do not respond adequately to other agents. The rationale for using a combination is based on summation of sites of action. It is occasionally used in the treatment of chronic open-angle glaucoma.

Acetazolamide is also used effectively in the prevention and treatment of acute mountain sickness and to alkalinize the urine. All three of the carbonic anhydrase inhibitors (see Figure 19-8) are used to treat epilepsy.

Thiazide Diuretics

The development of chlorothiazide offered the opportunity, for the first time, to treat edematous patients with a diuretic agent that was orally effective, well tolerated, and relatively safe. Also, it was discovered that chlorothiazide potentiates the antihypertensive response to ganglionic blocking agents and is mildly antihypertensive when used alone. This drug, however, has largely been supplanted by hydrochlorothiazide, a much weaker carbonic anhydrase inhibitor but a more potent chloruretic agent, and by other newer compounds. All of the thiazides act in the same way, with the differences among them due largely to pharmacokinetic characteristics and inherent carbonic anhydrase inhibitory activity.

The renal effects of thiazides are dependent in large measure on (1) the physiological state of water and electrolyte balance at the time they are administered and (2) the functional status of the kidneys, cardiovascular system, and liver. A large dose may be ineffective in a patient with severe renal hepatic disease whereas a standard dose can produce a tremendous diuretic response in a severely edematous patient whose renal and hepatic functions are relatively normal.

Effects on Potassium and Magnesium When the natriuretic action of a diuretic is exerted proximal to the late portion of the distal segment (i.e., in advance of the site where aldosterone action is prominent) the agent increases the excretion of potassium. Such is the case for thiazides and for loop diuretics (discussed later). There are three cogent reasons for this increase: (1) more sodium and water delivered to the aldosterone exchange site, where reabsorption of larger amounts of sodium and dilution of luminal fluid enhance the secretion of potassium; (2) contraction of the ECF, causing an increase in secretion of aldosterone; and (3) hypochloremic alkalosis induced by diuretics promoting potassium excretion. The fraction of patients who develop hypokalemia or display evidence of potassium depletion while on long-term thiazide dosing is quite variable. Young people with hypertension treated with thiazides may have no effects or become only slightly hypokalemic. Others develop clear signs of deficiency. That hypokalemia generated by thiazides results in increased ventricular ectopy has been questioned by some investigators. The Medical Research Council trial found no difference in mortality and cardiac events between hypertensive patients who take thiazides and those who are undergoing β-blocker therapy. Nevertheless, even mild hypokalemia should be avoided, especially in cirrhotic patients, those taking cardiac glycosides, patients with diabetes, and the elderly. Disturbances in insulin and glucose metabolism can often be prevented if potassium depletion is avoided. Measures for preventing or correcting potassium deficiency are discussed below.

Although reabsorption of magnesium takes place primarily in the proximal tubule, thiazides and loop diuretics can accelerate its excretion. Magnesium depletion in patients on chronic diuretic therapy is occasionally reported and is considered by some clinicians to be a risk factor in the development of ventricular dysrhythmias. The addition of potassium-sparing diuretics reportedly prevents magnesium loss.

Effects on Calcium Under most conditions, a parallel relationship exists between sodium and calcium excretion in the urine. Measures that alter the elimination of one of these ions alter the second similarly. This association does not exist when thiazides are used. Paradoxically, sodium reabsorption is reduced while calcium reabsorption is increased. The underlying mechanism involves contraction of the ECF volume. Acutely, thiazides do not enhance calcium reabsorption. When administered repeatedly, however, they display a hypocalciuric action. This action can be overcome merely by restoring salt and water losses. Thus dissociation between sodium and calcium transport begins only when volume contraction opposes the natriuretic response.

Thiazides are now widely used to prevent the formation of recurrent calcium stones. The serum calcium concentration often increases, but the rise is modest and rarely causes a problem.

Effects on Uric Acid Thiazides increase the serum concentration of urate. Two mechanisms are involved: increased proximal tubular reabsorption and reduced tubular secretion of urate. The former, like calcium reabsorption, depends on contraction of the ECF volume. Volume reduction enhances fractional sodium reabsorption, and sodium carries urate with it (cotransport). Depletion of ECF volume alone elevates serum urate concentration. Replacement of thiazide-induced salt and water loss lessens the effect of thiazides on serum urate. The extent to which suppression of urate secretion contributes to urate retention is not defined.

More than 50% of patients on long-term thiazide therapy develop hyperuricemia. In the majority, elevation of urate is modest and does not precipitate gout unless the patient is afflicted with the primary disease or possesses a gouty diathesis. Currently, there is no reason to believe that the risk of hyperuricemia outweighs the benefits of thiazide therapy in patients who do not have a history of gout.

Other Effects Carbohydrate intolerance may develop in nondiabetics and usually worsens in diabetic patients on chronic thiazide therapy. The cause is not established but has variously been attributed to such factors as suppression of insulin secretion, resistance to insulin action, or increased glycogen breakdown. In most instances, carbohydrate tolerance returns to the predrug levels within a year after the thiazide is withdrawn. Another disturbance associated with chronic thiazide therapy is a small rise in serum lipids and lipoproteins. Low-density lipoprotein-cholesterol and triglyceride concentrations may increase during short-term therapy but total cholesterol and triglyceride concentrations usually return to baseline values in studies of more than 1 year in duration. It has been suggested that this action on lipids is linked to glucose intolerance, and that both of these metabolic disturbances are, in part, consequences of potassium depletion.

Clinical Indications and Uses The primary indications for thiazides are listed in the box on p. 244. In general, these agents are employed for the treatment of congestive heart failure, other conditions in which edema is a common feature, adventitiously in nonedematous patients when reduction of ECF volume is beneficial, and in hypertension. Reduction of blood pressure in patients with hypertension results, in part, from contraction of ECF volume (see Chapter 13). This occurs acutely, leading to a decrease in cardiac output with compensatory elevation of peripheral resistance. Vasoconstriction then subsides, enabling cardiac output to return to normal values. Augmented synthesis of vasodilator prostaglandins is reported and may be a crucial factor for long-term maintenance of a lower pressure even though ECF volume tends to return toward normal (see Chapter 18).

Thiazides also are employed in the treatment of vasopressin-resistant diabetes insipidus. In these patients, urine is copious and dilute, while plasma is hyperosmotic. Chronic administration of thiazides increases the osmolarity and reduces urine flow in this condition. The mechanism hinges on the removal of sodium from the ECF, an action that inevitably contracts ECF volume. The proximal tubule then overreabsorbs sodium. Urine flow rate diminishes and urine osmolality rises when sodium transport in the early distal segment is inhibited by the diuretic. Drug therapy in this instance is most effective in combination with dietary salt restriction.

Loop Diuretics

Response to loop agents is extremely sensitive to dose. At the low end of the dosage spectrum, NaCl losses are equivalent to those obtained with thiazides; at high doses, massive amounts of salt are excreted. Two decisive factors adjust the magnitude of the response: (1) the existing status of the salt and water balances and (2) the delivery of drug to the site of action. Contraction of ECF volume is an example of the first factor. Salt and water depletion invariably lessens the diuretic response by enhancing proximal and distal tubular reabsorption of sodium. Renal insufficiency is an example of the second. Less drug reaches critical receptors when some of the pathways (glomeruli or proximal tubules) are destroyed. Loop diuretics also increase the excretion of potassium, calcium, magnesium, and protons, and all of the electrolyte depletion phenomena associated with thiazides may occur. Similarly, carbohydrate intolerance and hyperlipidemia have been reported.

Loop diuretics initially produce a slight rise in the excretion of urate. On continued administration, however, this effect is reversed and retention of urate becomes evident. The second event undoubtedly depends on contraction of the ECF volume (discussed under thiazides). Furosemide and ethacrynic acid may increase renal blood flow for brief intervals during which urinary excretion of prostaglandin E is elevated. IV injections of furosemide reduce pulmonary

arterial pressure and peripheral venous compliance. Indomethacin, an inhibitor of prostaglandin synthesis, interferes with all of these actions. Vascular phenomena of this sort occurring in the kidney and elsewhere precede the onset of diuresis. The therapeutic value of loop diuretics in pulmonary edema may be attributable in part to stimulation of prostaglandin synthesis in the lung.

Common clinical indications for loop diuretics are listed in the box on p. 244. In most cases, their employment overlaps that of thiazides, but there are some major differences. The greater efficacy of loop agents often enables their successful use in evoking diuresis in edematous patients with disturbances of cardiovascular, renal, or hepatic origin. For example, an oliguric patient whose glomerular filtration rate is only 10% of normal derives no benefit from a thiazide but may respond well to a large dose of a loop diuretic. In addition, furosemide is an important adjunct in the treatment of acute pulmonary edema. The drug increases pulmonary and peripheral venous compliance, thereby affording rapid relief, and then maintains these beneficial effects by reducing the plasma volume. The initial vascular effects are not linked to actions on the renal tubule (venodilation occurs in anephric patients).

Many investigators report that thiazides or related drugs, especially longer-acting members of each group, are more effective than loop agents for reducing blood pressure. Others, citing evidence of lesser effects on carbohydrate metabolism and plasma lipids, prefer furosemide. The 1988 Report of the Joint National Committee on Detection, Evaluation, and Treatment of High Blood Pressure does not address this question. Loop diuretics are used to lower serum calcium concentrations of patients with hypercalcemia. Isotonic saline is often coadministered to maintain the glomerular filtration rate.

Potassium-Sparing Diuretics

Depletion of body potassium with or without significant lowering of serum K^+ concentration (only 2% of total body potassium is present in ECF) is probably the most common side effect of diuretic therapy. Hypokalemia of sufficient magnitude creates many problems and may be life-threatening. These problems may include impairment of neuromuscular function, cardiac dysrhythmia, intestinal disturbances, and partial loss of the ability to concentrate urine. Predisposition of diuretics to potassium-wasting is especially worrisome during the treatment of congestive heart failure. In patients on digitalis preparations and a diuretic, diuretic-induced hypokalemia can ensue and sensitize the heart to the toxic effects of the cardiac glycoside.

Measures to elude the hazards of potassium deficit or to correct an established deficit are plentiful, but success is not guaranteed. The first steps are precautionary: dietary intake of large amounts of potassium, avoidance of excessive NaCl intake, and monitoring of serum K^+ concentrations. If serum potassium concentrations do not stabilize at an acceptable value, supplements of KCl may be prescribed; however, compliance may be a problem. The most effective therapeutic measure is to add a potassium-sparing diuretic to the therapeutic regimen, but KCl supplements should be *discontinued* if a K^+ sparing agent is used.

Spironolactone Uses Spironolactone is most effective in patients with primary or secondary hyperaldosteronism and is ineffective in patients with nonfunctional adrenal glands. The drug prevents the attachment of aldosterone to a cytosolic receptor in the late distal segment of the nephron (see Figure 19-4). Consequently, the hormonal stimulus to formation of new protein ceases. In the absence or reduction in amount of this protein, the permeability of the luminal membrane to sodium and potassium decreases, with the result that sodium excretion is enhanced and potassium secretion is diminished. Entry of potassium across the basolateral membrane also abates. Additional actions in both the proximal and distal tubule have been reported. These involve the transport of protons and bicarbonate anions and appear to depend on the hormonal status of the recipient. They may be related to intrinsic glucocorticoid activity or to one of the implicit steroidal effects of spironolactone.

Spironolactone is used for correction of hypokalemia. The drug is also administered alone, with thiazides, or a loop diuretic, to reduce the ECF volume without causing potassium depletion or hypokalemia. The drug is especially appropriate for the treatment of cirrhosis with ascites, a condition invariably associated with secondary hyperaldosteronism. It is also employed to boost natriuresis when the response to agents acting on the ascending limb or early distal tubule is inadequate. Although its natriuretic action is weak, spironolactone lowers blood pressure in patients with mild or moderate hypertension and is frequently prescribed for this purpose.

Triamterene and Amiloride Use Triamterene and amiloride are generally used in combination with potassium-wasting diuretics, especially when maintenance of normal serum potassium concentrations is clinically important (e.g., patients with dysrhythmias, receiving a cardiac glycoside, or with low serum potassium concentrations). Fixed combination preparations are generally not appropriate for initial therapy but may be more expedient when the dosage schedule is demonstrated to be correct. Since these drugs possess a different site and mechanism of action from those of thiazides or loop agents, they are sometimes administered together to increase the response in patients who are refractory to a single agent. There are few circumstances that mandate use of either drug alone.

SIDE EFFECTS, CLINICAL PROBLEMS, AND TOXICITY

Effective diuretic therapy alters the volume and composition of the extracellular fluid compartment—the reason for using the drugs. However, it is difficult to achieve the desired objectives entirely, and the volume and composition changes are often not attained or are exceeded. Moreover, it is not possible to restrict the effects of these drugs only to those desired for the therapeutic purposes. Accordingly, the repeated use of diuretics is frequently associated with shifts in acid-base balance and changes in serum electrolyte concentrations. Two shifts frequently encountered when diuretics are administered continuously include potassium depletion and hyperuricemia. Since these changes are manifestations of the molecular mechanism of action of the drugs, they are difficult to avoid in most patients unless counteractive measures are taken. It is best to anticipate the occurrence of such side effects. Patients at risk include the elderly, those with severe disease of any kind, individuals taking cardiac glycosides, and the malnourished. Supplemental intake of potassium (dietary or oral KCl) or the concomitant use of potassium-sparing diuretics with thiazides or loop diuretics is often successful. Elevation of urate rarely, if ever, precipitates an attack of gout in patients who are not disposed to the disease.

Paradoxical diuretic-induced edema may be observed in patients with hypertension when abrupt withdrawal of diuretics is initiated after a period of chronic use. Similarly, "idiopathic edema" appears to

CLINICAL PROBLEMS

OSMOTIC DIURETICS

Acute increase in ECF volume and serum potassium concentration, nausea and vomiting, headache

CARBONIC ANHYDRASE INHIBITORS

Metabolic acidosis, tolerance, drowsiness, fatigue, CNS depression, paresthesias, hypersensitivity thiazides and thiazide-related agents (see Table 19-5)

LOOP DIURETICS

Hypokalemia, hyperuricemia; metabolic alkalosis; hyponatremia; hearing deficits (usually associated with concurrent use of ototoxic antibiotics) in patients receiving large IV doses; watery diarrhea with ethacrynic acid

POTASSIUM-SPARING DIURETICS

aldosterone inhibitors: hyperkalemia, gynecomastia, hirsutism, menstrual irregularities
triamterene: hyperkalemia, megaloblastic anemia in patients with cirrhosis
amiloride: hyperkalemia, increase in blood urea nitrogen, glucose intolerance in diabetes mellitus

Table 19-5 Adverse Reactions to Thiazides and Related Drugs

Reaction	Examples
Depletion phenomena	Hypokalemia, dilutional hyponatremia, hypochloremic alkalosis, hypomagnesemia
Retention phenomena	Hyperuricemia, hypercalcemia
Metabolic changes	Hyperglycemia, hyperlipidemia, hypersecretion of renin and aldosterone
Hypersensitivity	Fever, rash, purpura, anaphylaxis
Other	Azotemia (in patients with poor renal function); cholecystitis; pancreatitis, withdrawal edema

be associated with irregular use or abuse of diuretics among women who are concerned with their weight and appearance. It is probable that the edema in these instances is also caused by sudden withdrawal after a period of use. The designation "idiopathic" is incorrect, because the subjects lose all traces of edema when they are weaned from salt-losing drugs. These findings are not surprising. Chronic use of diuretics results in a persistent elevation of plasma renin activity and the development of secondary aldosteronism. When it is necessary to discontinue diuretic therapy, stepwise reduction over a period of a few weeks combined with reduction of sodium intake is recommended. The main problems are summarized in the box.

Osmotic Diuretics

Acute expansion of the ECF engendered by osmotic diuretics increases the work load of the heart. Patients already in cardiac failure are especially susceptible and may develop pulmonary edema. They should not be treated with these drugs. Underlying heart disease in the absence of frank congestive failure, although not an absolute contraindication, is a serious risk factor. Rapid expansion of the plasma volume can precipitate congestive failure and pulmonary congestion. Mannitol is sometimes given to restore urine flow in oliguric or anuric states when the cause is due to extrarenal factors (e.g., hypovolemia, hypotension). In these cases, the response to a test dose should be evaluated before therapeutic quantities are administered.

Severe volume depletion and hypernatremia may result from the prolonged administration of mannitol unless sodium and water losses are replaced. Mild hyperkalemia is often observed, but intolerable elevations of potassium are not apt to occur except in patients with diabetes, patients with adrenal insufficiency, or those whose renal function is severely impaired.

Carbonic Anhydrase Inhibitors

Among the side effects of carbonic anhydrase inhibitors are metabolic acidosis, drowsiness, fatigue, CNS depression, and parathesias. Hypersensitivity reactions are rare.

Thiazides

Because most complications of thiazide therapy are direct manifestations of their pharmacological effects, adverse events are usually predictable. The list in Table 19-5 includes adventitious hazards that have no apparent relationship to the descriptive pharmacology of the drugs. Although relatively uncommon, the latter are usually more serious. Thiazides should be used cautiously in patients with renal insufficiency. Alterations in fluid and electrolyte balance may precipitate hepatic coma in such patients. Thiazides reduce the clearance of lithium and, as a rule, should not be administered concomitantly. Though not an absolute contraindication, the drugs are not recommended during pregnancy unless the anticipated benefit justifies the risk. Thiazides cross the placenta and appear in breast milk. Anuria and precedent hypersensitivity to sulfonamides are absolute contraindications.

Loop Diuretics

The depletion phenomena and metabolic derangements listed in Table 19-5 occur also with loop diuretics; azotemia may be noted in conjunction with disturbances in electrolyte balance. Normal serum calcium concentrations are usually maintained even though urinary excretion of the ion increases initially; losses of calcium are not sustained during long-term therapy probably because the ECF volume undergoes contraction. Nevertheless, hypocalcemia and rare cases of tetany are documented. Hypersensitivity reactions of the sulfonamide variety may be seen with furosemide.

Vertigo and deafness sometimes develop in individuals receiving large IV doses of loop diuretics, but coadministration of an aminoglycoside antibiotic (known to be ototoxic) and impaired renal function may also need to be present for this toxic reaction to occur. It is prudent to avoid concurrent use of ototoxic antibiotics and loop agents. Additional drug interactions occur with indomethacin (decreased activity of the loop diuretic), warfarin (displacement of the anticoagulant from plasma protein), and lithium (decreased clearance and increased risk of lithium toxicity).

All diuretics are contraindicated in anuric patients.

Potassium-Sparing Diuretics

The most serious adverse reaction encountered during therapy with spironolactone is hyperkalemia. Serum potassium should be monitored periodically even when the drug is administered with a potas-

---

TRADENAMES

In addition to generic and fixed combination preparations, the following tradenamed materials are available in the United States.

Aldactone, spironolactone
Anhydron, cyclothiazide
Aquatag, benzthiazide
Bumex, bumetanide
Diamox, acetazolamide
Diucardin, hydroflumethiazide
Diulo, metolazone
Diuril, chlorothiazide
Dyrenium, triamterene
Edecrin, ethacrynic acid
Enduron, methyclothiazide
Esidrix, hydrochlorothiazide
Exna, benzthiazide
Hydrodiuril, hydrochlorothiazide
Hydromox, quinethazone
Hygroton, chlorthalidone
Lasix, furosemide
Lozol, indapamide
Metahydrin, trichlormethiazide
Midamor, amiloride hydrochloride
Naqua, trichlormethiazide
Naturetin, bendroflumethiazide
Neptazane, methazolamide
Proaqua, benzthiazide
Renese, polythiazide
Saluron, hydroflumethiazide
Zaroxolyn, metolazone

---

sium-wasting diuretic. Patients at highest risk are those with low glomerular filtration rates and any individuals who take potassium supplements concurrently. Simultaneous use of supplements and a potassium-sparing agent is contraindicated.

Gynecomastia may occur in men, possibly as a consequence of binding of canrenone to androgen receptors; decreased libido and impotence have also been reported. These actions are dose-related. Women may develop menstrual irregularities, hirsutism, or swelling and tenderness of the breast. Triamterene and amiloride may cause hyperkalemia, even when a potassium-wasting diuretic is part of the therapeutic program. This risk is highest in patients with limited renal function (e.g., renal insufficiency, diabetes, and elderly patients). Additional complications include elevated serum blood urea nitrogen (BUN) and uric acid, glucose intolerance, and GI disturbances. Triamterene may contribute to or initiate formation of renal stones, and hypersensitivity reactions may occur but are rare. The drugs are contraindicated in patients with hyperkalemia, individuals taking potassium supplements in any form, or in severe renal failure with progressive oliguria. Anuria is always a contraindication for diuretics.

REFERENCES

Brater DC: Resistance to loop diuretics, Drugs 30:427, 1985.

Cafruny EJ: Diuretics: Encyclopedia of human biology, vol. 3, San Diego, 1991, Academic press (in press).

Cragoe EJ Jr, ed: Diuretics: chemistry, pharmacology, and medicine, New York, 1983, John Wiley & Sons, Inc.

Lant A: Clinical pharmacology and therapeutic use, Drugs 29; Part I, 57; Part II, 162, 1985.

Shackleton R, Wong NLM, and Sutton RAL: Distal (potassium-sparing) diuretics. In Dirks JH and Sutton RAL, eds: Diuretics: physiology, pharmacology, and clinical use, Philadelphia, 1986, WB Saunders Co.

Weiner IM: General pharmacologic aspects of diuretics. In Dirks JH and Sutton RAL, eds: Diuretics: physiology, pharmacology, and clinical use, Philadelphia, 1986, WB Saunders Co.

20

Lipid-Lowering Drugs and Atherosclerosis

ABBREVIATIONS	
ACAT	acyl-CoA:cholesterol acyl trans-ferase
acetyl-CoA	acetylcoenzyme A
Apo A	apoprotein A
Apo E	apoprotein E
HDL	high density lipoprotein
HMG-CoA	hydroxy-3-methyl-glutaryl coen-zyme A
IDL	intermediate density lipoprotein
LDL	low density lipoprotein
PDGF	platelet derived growth factor
VLDL	very low density lipoprotein
EGF	epidermal growth factor

MAJOR DRUGS
bile acid ion-exchange resins
cholesterol synthesis inhibitors
fibric acid derivatives
probucol
nicotinic acid
other agents: neomycin and sitosterol

THERAPEUTIC OVERVIEW

Diseases of the heart and blood vessels are the principal causes of death in industrialized countries of the world. In the United States, more people die of such diseases than from cancer or any other illness. Of the deaths resulting from cardiovascular disease, over three fourths can be attributed to atherosclerosis and its complications. Atherosclerosis is a generalized disease of the arterial tree that usually develops in a symptom-free manner over many years. The most common manifestation of atherosclerosis is coronary heart disease, followed by stroke and peripheral vascular disease. Because it is a slowly developing disorder, treatment must be directed at causative factors and at its prevention rather than its reversal. In pri-

mates, studies demonstrate actual reversal of lipid deposits in the arterial wall and a regression of the attendant fibrous tissue. Therefore there is hope for clinical reversal in humans. Coronary artery studies in humans show increases in lumen size with a decrease in blood cholesterol concentration.

Elevated cholesterol concentrations are one of the major contributing factors in the development of atherosclerosis. Cholesterol enters the circulation from two major sources, absorption from food (exogenous pathway) and synthesis by the liver (endogenous pathway). It leaves the circulation when it is taken up by the liver to form bile acids, or taken up by other cells to form steroid hormones or inserted into membranes. When present in excess, it is taken up by fibroblasts and scavenger cells in regenerating tissues, as well as fat cells. Transport of cholesterol within the plasma is by way of lipoprotein particles.

Currently, smoking cessation and lowering plasma concentrations of cholesterol and its associated lipids are the only proven approaches to the prevention of atherosclerosis-related disorders. A variety of clinical

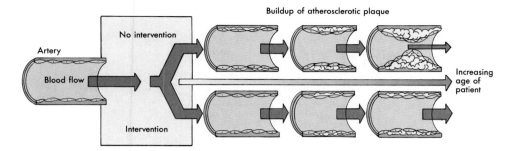

FIGURE 20-1   Atherosclerosis prevention. Intervention (treatment) involves (1) diet to decrease cholesterol and lipids, (2) cessation of smoking, (3) drugs to reduce plasma cholesterol, (4) control of blood pressure, and (5) control of diabetes (see text).

studies demonstrate the feasibility of lowering cholesterol with diet and drugs such as niacin, clofibrate, bile-acid binding resins, gemfibrozil and lovastatin (Figure 20-1). Two classical clinical trials show a reduction in total cholesterol and low density lipoprotein and elevation in high density lipoprotein fractions to be clearly associated with a reduced incidence of coronary artery event rates (angina, myocardial infarction, coronary bypass surgery needs, or positive treadmill testing.). In general, for every percentage point that the cholesterol concentration is lowered, a 2% lowering of the risk of coronary heart disease occurs.

The metabolism of cholesterol and fatty acids and their associated lipid transport particles (the lipoproteins), occurs in the gut, liver, and the peripheral tissues. Drugs that alter cholesterol concentrations act, for the most part, by altering the kinetics of one or more parts of the metabolic cycle. Production and secretion of bile formed from cholesterol by liver cells or hepatocytes is necessary for the emulsification of dietary fat and cholesterol before absorption. The majority of the secreted bile is reabsorbed during the digestive process and recycled, but approximately one third is lost in the stool. Interruption of this cycle by bile-acid binding resins such as cholestyramine, colestipol, and the antibiotic neomycin, results in reduced gastrointestinal (GI) absorption of cholesterol and dietary fats. The prevention of the reabsorption of bile acids has the secondary effect of causing the hepatocyte to synthesize increased amounts of bile. Because cholesterol is the necessary precursor for bile formation, the increased cholesterol utilization reduces the total body pool of cholesterol by promoting

---

THERAPEUTIC OVERVIEW

ANTILIPID DRUGS

Goal: prevention of myocardial infarction and other atherosclerotic disorders such as stroke and peripheral vascular disease

Approach: prophylactic use to reduce formation of atherosclerotic plaque and subsequent narrowing of lumen in cardiac arteries

Primary risk factors:
  High blood cholesterol and certain lipids
  High blood pressure
  Smoking
  Overweight
  Sedentary lifestyle

---

an increase in certain receptors and subsequent removal of the fraction that binds to these receptors.

Therapeutic uses of lipid-lowering drugs are summarized in the box.

Cholesterol Balance

The dynamics of cholesterol ingestion, synthesis, metabolism, and elimination are summarized in Figure 20-2. Dietary intake can vary from 0 to 1000 mg per day; of that, between 30% and 75% is absorbed. Normal endogenous synthesis is between 600 and 1000 mg/day. About 750 to 1250 mg will be secreted in the bile each day. Of that secreted in bile, about one half will be reabsorbed and the remainder ex-

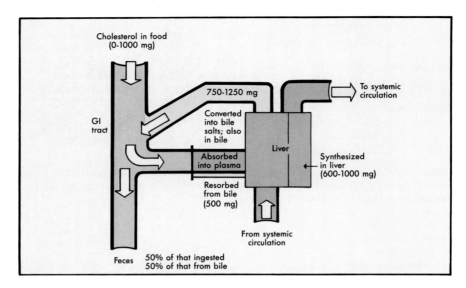

FIGURE 20-2   Total body balance of cholesterol, showing input by ingestion and liver synthesis, output by nonabsorption into feces, conversion into bile salts, delivery in bile salts to small intestine, partial reabsorption from bile, and delivery as lipoproteins into systemic circulation. Quantities shown are approximate daily amounts.

creted in the stool. The total body pool of cholesterol is estimated to be in excess of 125 gm, of which at least 90% is in cell membranes.

De novo synthesis of cholesterol is the second and generally the major source of cholesterol. Although cholesterol can be synthesized in most cells of the body, the most active cells are in the adrenal glands and the liver. Because liver mass is so much greater, synthesis in the liver is critical to the total body burden of cholesterol. The synthesis of cholesterol originates with acetylcoenzyme (acetyl-CoA), a key intermediate linking glycolysis; the citric acid cycle; and fatty acid degradation. The in vivo synthesis of cholesterol from acetyl-CoA involves 21 distinct steps, and is summarized in Figure 20-3. The first step, the irreversible conversion of 3-hydroxy-3-methyl-glutaryl coenzyme A (HMG-CoA) to mevalonic acid, is rate-limiting. The rate of synthesis is influenced by several factors, including the following:

1. Time of day
2. Inhibition by fasting
3. Enhancement by excessive food intake or obesity
4. Composition of diet

Diets rich in saturated fats result in a rise in serum cholesterol, whereas the substitution of either unsaturated fats or carbohydrates generally is accompanied by decreases in serum cholesterol.

In addition to the effects of diet, a variety of factors at the cellular level affect the rate of cholesterol synthesis. Cellular concentrations of cholesterol are in dynamic equilibrium with the concentrations of certain lipoproteins, discussed later.

The liver is the primary organ for cholesterol uptake and degradation. Most of the cholesterol is converted to bile acids, which in turn are secreted into the intestine to emulsify ingested fats. The bile acids are then reabsorbed and recycled. The total bile pool mass is estimated at 2 to 3 gm and is recycled about six times per day. About 50% of the cholesterol secreted in the bile is reabsorbed as part of a chylomicron and the remainder excreted in the feces. The rapid recycling normally limits the need for high levels of synthesis of bile acids. Cholesterol is also secreted in the bile as free cholesterol. Because it is fairly insoluble, large amounts of bile are required for solubilization. The enhanced synthesis and increased excretion of cholesterol in the bile is the probable cause

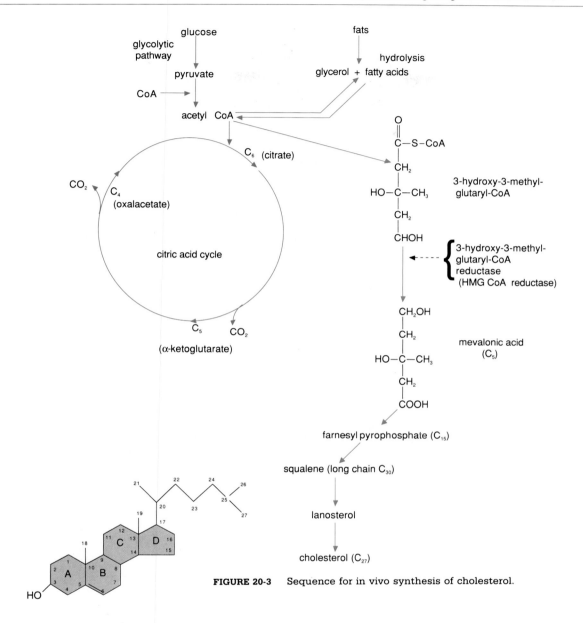

FIGURE 20-3   Sequence for in vivo synthesis of cholesterol.

of development of cholesterol-containing gall stones in obesity, just as the increased ratio of cholesterol to bile in patients on clofibrate therapy apparently makes them more likely to develop gallbladder disease.

Transport of cholesterol and other lipids in plasma and other body fluids is accomplished by encasing the lipid in protein coats to form lipoprotein particles. The nomenclature and characteristics of the lipoprotein particles are summarized in Figure 20-4. Larger lipoprotein particles undergo size reduction through the action of lipases. Delivery of smaller particles to specific cells for the use of the cholesterol or triglycerides occurs through the binding of lipoprotein particle components to receptors on the cell wall.

The largest of the lipoprotein particles is the chylomicron, composed of approximately 85% to 95% triglyceride and 3% to 6% cholesterol. The shell is composed of phospholipid, cholesterol, and several apoproteins (A, B48, CI, CII, CIII, and E). The chylomicron

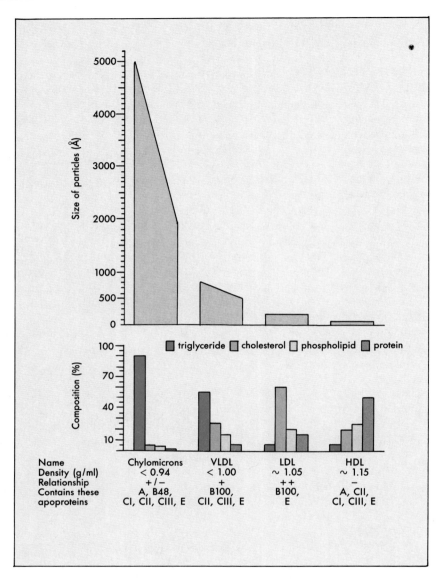

FIGURE 20-4   Summary of nomenclature, approximate composition, size, and relative athero-genic potential of lipoprotein particles, which serve as transport vehicles for cholesterol and triglycerides *VLDL*, Very low density lipoproteins; *LDL*, low density proteins; *HDL*, high density lipoproteins; +, definite relationship; −, no relationship (+ and − refer to relationship of concentration to atherogenic potential).

is formed in the gut wall, and ranges in size from 2000 to 5000 Å. Its principal role is the transport of absorbed fats to adipose tissue. As the chylomicron leaves the gut, it acquires the apoprotein CII whose presence triggers the enzyme lipoprotein lipase in the capillary wall. The triglyceride is released from the chylomicron and cleaved into free fatty acids and glycerol. The chylomicron remnants, containing apoprotein A (Apo A), apoprotein B (Apo B), and apoprotein E (Apo E) but having lost Apo CII and Apo CIII, return to the venous blood and are eventually removed by specific receptors on hepatic cells. This route is the principal method of transport of dietary fat and is often referred to as the *exogenous pathway*.

Endogenous transport of triglycerides is by very low density lipoprotein (VLDL). Synthesized principally by liver and to a lesser extent by the gut, these particles are approximately $\frac{1}{100}$ of the volume (500 to 800 Å diameter) of chylomicrons. In contrast to the chylomicrons, the source of triglyceride in the VLDL is from fatty acids synthesized by the liver or released by adipose tissue. In addition to cholesterol and phospholipid, the wall of VLDL particles contains apoproteins B 100, CII, CIII, and E. The internal composition is about 50% to 60% triglyceride and 20% to 30% cholesterol. The presence of the Apo CII in the VLDL particle again activates lipoprotein lipase; the presence of Apo E allows the VLDL fragments after lipolysis to be bound by the same hepatic receptors that bind chylomicron fragments.

As the VLDL particles are reduced by lipoprotein lipase cleavage, a substantial percentage of the particles are transformed to a size and density classified as *intermediate density lipoprotein* (IDL) and are about 6% of the volume of the VLDL particles. IDL particles suffer two fates. Significant amounts are bound to receptors on hepatocytes, which recognize the Apo E, and the remainder lose the Apo E as they lose further triglyceride. Such contracted particles are known as *low density lipoprotein* (LDL) and have a size that is about 2% of the VLDL particle or $\frac{1}{5000}$ the volume of a chylomicron. LDL particles contain about 50% to 60% cholesterol, less than 10% triglyceride, and have one molecule of Apo B 100 on the surface.

Apo B 100 is recognized by the LDL receptors in pits located on the cell walls of hepatocytes and peripheral cells. When the LDL particle binds to the receptor, the LDL particle and the associated receptor are transported into the cytoplasm by a process known as *receptor-mediated endocytosis*. The LDL particle is then incorporated into lysosomes and separated from the receptor, which is recycled. The coating of the particle is removed, and the esterified cholesterol is hydrolyzed and released as free cholesterol.

The released cholesterol has the following three major effects on cholesterol metabolism:

1. The intracellular concentration of cholesterol affects the cellular content of hydroxy-3-methyl-glutaryl-coenzyme A (HMG-CoA) reductase. Thus as cholesterol concentrations rise, the internal synthesis of cholesterol falls.
2. Rising concentrations of cholesterol stimulate the activation of the enzyme acyl-CoA:cholesterol acyl transferase (ACAT).
3. Rising concentrations of cholesterol inhibit the transcription of LDL receptor into messenger RNA while falling concentrations increase transcription.

This third effect enables cells to adjust their cholesterol concentrations according to need. For example, dividing fibroblasts, which need new membranes, have up to 40,000 receptors per cell whereas quiescent fibroblasts appear to have only one tenth as many receptors. Decrease in the number of LDL receptors is the basis for familial hypercholesterolemia. The heterozygous form appears in about 1 in 500 individuals whereas the homozygous form is rare (1 in 1,000,000). Actually, various genetic defects impair LDL receptor genesis but the end result is much the same. Heterozygotes have serum cholesterol concentrations about two times normal and account for about one twentieth of those who have heart attacks before age 60. Homozygotes have cholesterol concentrations six times normal and may show evidence of coronary artery disease at a very early age. Many homozygotes die before age 10 to 12 and almost all have had a myocardial infarction by age 20. The elevated blood cholesterol concentrations can be directly related to a reduction in the number of LDL receptors. Roughly 25% of the cholesterol is removed by the scavenger pathway.

The remaining type of lipoprotein particle is the high density lipoprotein (HDL). It is relatively small, approximately 80 Å in diameter, and thus has a volume of about 0.12% of the VLDL particle. HDL contains Apo A and Apo CII; however, smaller amounts of Apo CI, Apo CIII, and Apo E are also present. It is formed from nascent HDL synthesized in the liver or as a "spin off" fragment as the lipolysis of chylomicron or VLDL fragments progresses. HDL is the major vehicle for the transport of cholesterol from the peripheral tissues to the liver for utilization or excretion.

Drug Mechanisms

Bile Acid Sequestrants If the predominant source of excess cholesterol is dietary, in contrast to receptor defects, then alteration of the digestion and absorption of cholesterol-rich fatty foods is an approach to decreasing cholesterol concentrations and lipoprotein metabolism. As previously noted, bile acids and cholesterol are secreted into the gut and bile acids play a critical role in the emulsifying of

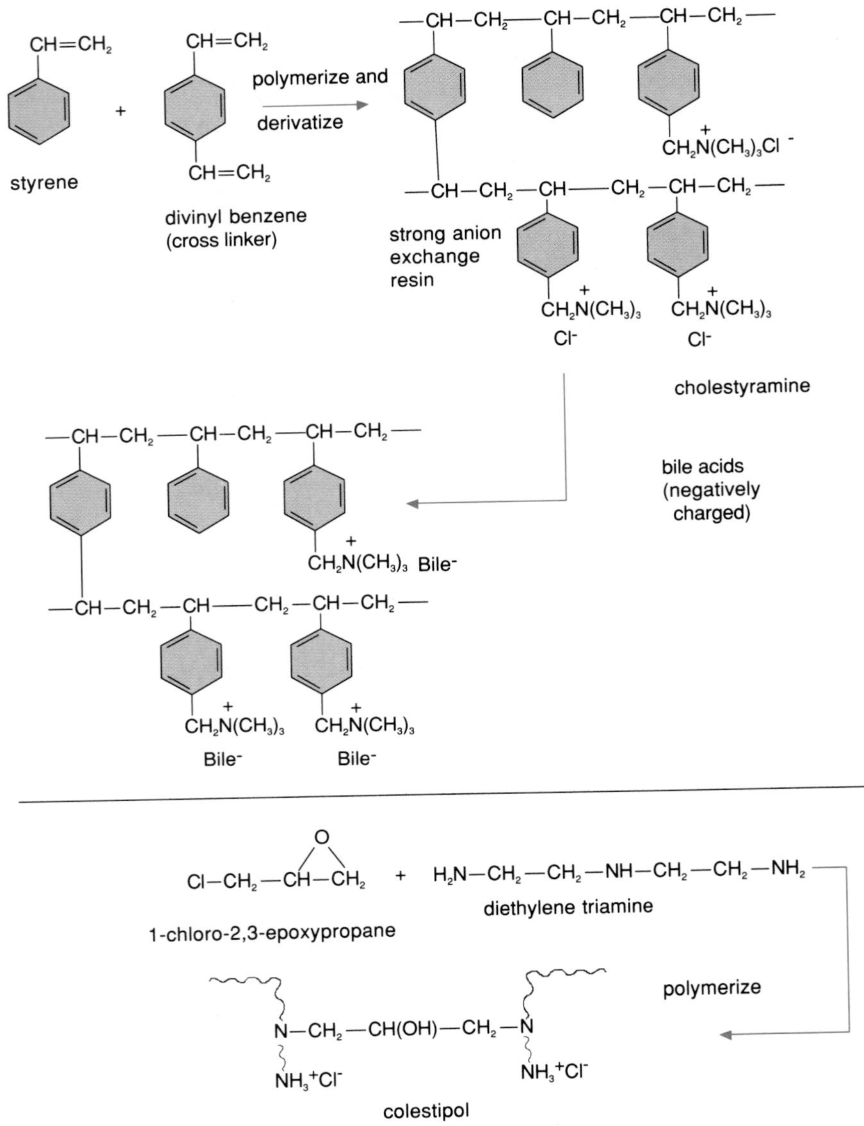

FIGURE 20-5   Anion exchange resins for ingestion to remove bile acids. Resins act by exchanging Cl^- for negatively charged bile salt anion and passing out the gut with the stool.

ingested fats. Several bile acid ion-exchange resins are available for clinical use.

Cholestyramine and colestipol are the two resins approved for use in the treatment of hypercholesteremic states. Cholestyramine is a large copolymer of styrene and divinyl benzene with fixed cationic sites provided by trimethylbenzylammonium groups. It is administered as the chloride salt, with anion exchange of bile acids for chloride occurring in the gut

(Figure 20-5). Colestipol is another copolymer formed from dimethylenetriamine and chlorepoxypropane, having fixed cation sites available for exchange of chloride and ionized bile acids. Both resins are insoluble and are administered as suspensions that are indigestible and pass unaltered in the stool. The bound bile acids are thus excreted. As previously noted, the usual bile acid pool is 2 to 3 gm but is recycled up to six times per day. When bile acids are

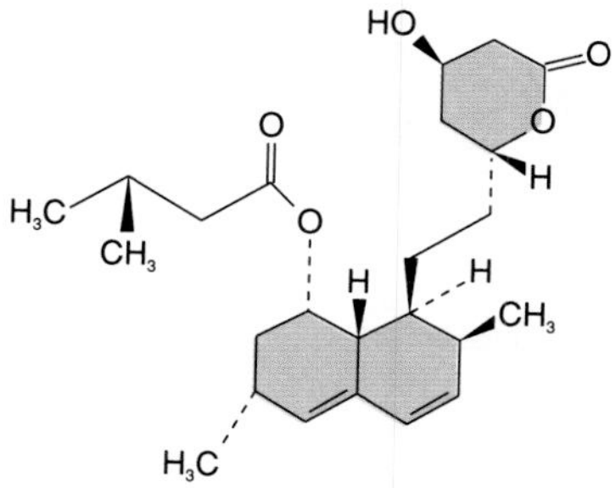

FIGURE 20-6   Structure of lovastatin.

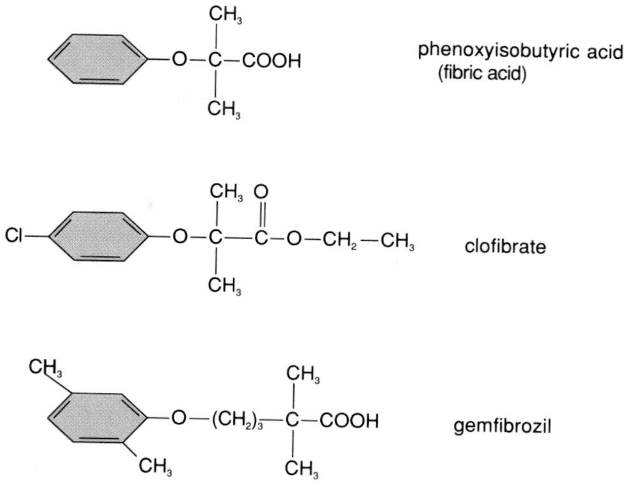

FIGURE 20-7   Fibric acid-based compounds that lower plasma cholesterol and triglycerides.

removed from the enterohepatic recirculation, there is a stimulus to synthesize increased bile acids. The resultant increase in cholesterol synthesis by hepatic cells results in an increase in LDL receptors and greater hepatic uptake of LDL. Circulating concentrations of LDL fall between 20% to 35% with maximum doses of bile acid sequestrants; at the same time VLDL and plasma triglyceride concentrations may rise as much as 20%. Usually this latter effect disappears within 2 to 3 months but the changes are not predictable. In some subjects in whom triglyceride elevation is a major finding, resins are contraindicated. There is no consistent effect on HDL concentrations with resin administration, but they often rise slightly.

Inhibitors of Cholesterol Synthesis Lovastatin and a series of similar compounds under development inhibit the enzyme HMG-CoA reductase, which is the initial rate-limiting step in cholesterol synthesis (Figure 20-3). The inhibition of cholesterol synthesis, particularly in the hepatocyte, results in an increased need for exogenous (extracellular) cholesterol. This need is met by increased uptake of LDL particles, which are rich in cholesterol. As increased catabolism of LDL occurs, plasma concentrations of LDL fall and less LDL is available to react with cellular elements in the blood and blood vessel walls.

The structure of lovastatin is shown in Figure 20-6. It appears to act as a competitive inhibitor for the active site on the enzyme with a much higher affinity than HMG-CoA.

Fibric Acid Derivatives Phenoxyisobutyric acid, also known as *fibric acid,* is the base compound for several drugs that lower plasma cholesterol and triglyceride concentrations. Clofibrate and gemifibrozol are the two currently available drugs of this class.

Their structures are shown in Figure 20-7. These drugs have multiple sites of action. Clofibrate and gemfibrozil increase the amount of cholesterol secreted into the bile and thereby increase the amount lost in the feces. Peripheral lipoprotein lipase activity is also increased, accelerating the peripheral mobilization of fats and thereby facilitating their return to the liver. These agents alter the rate of synthesis of several apoprotein components that form the receptor recognition site of the surface of lipoprotein particles, thus allowing the uptake of these particles by the liver.

Clofibrate is the original fibric acid derivative tested for the treatment of dysbetalipoproteinemias, first reported in 1962. Early metabolic balance studies indicated a significant increase of neutral sterols, but a decrease in acid sterols in the feces of patients on clofibrate. These findings suggest increased fecal excretion of cholesterol and a decline in bile acid excretion. Such a hypothesis is confirmed by increased cholesterol in the bile.

More recent work demonstrates that clofibrate uniformly increases extrahepatic lipoprotein lipase activity but not hepatic lipase activity. Thus the triglyceride lowering effect of clofibrate may be due to increased efficiency of removal of VLDL, as well as reduced VLDL secretion by the liver.

Clofibrate was used in several clinical trials in which long-term changes in cholesterol and triglycerides were noted. Significant side effects, including an increase in cholelithiasis (gall stones), cardiac arrhythmias, and seeming increase in malignancies in subjects on active drug versus placebo, have caused the drug to fall out of favor.

Gemfibrozil is a newer fibric acid derivative. Although the full range of activity and its underlying mechanism of action are not known, several factors are recognized: (1) alteration of the rates of synthesis of apoproteins CII and CIII, with increases in CII in comparison to CIII result in activation of extrahepatic lipoprotein lipase and (2) increased rate of synthesis of Apo AI and AII and thus increased formation of HDL particles. However, these mechanisms do not explain the increased cholesterol content in the bile and the decreased resorption of cholesterol from the small intestine.

Gemfibrozil, in several clinical trials, lowered serum concentrations of triglycerides and cholesterol. It is currently approved for treatment of persons with very high concentrations of serum triglycerides (>750 mg/dl). Such concentrations pose a risk not in terms of atherogenesis but in the occurrence of episodes of abdominal pain and pancreatitis. In a recent Finnish study, 4081 asymptomatic men (ages 40 to 55 years) with primary dyslipidemia (non-HDL cholesterol greater than 200 mg/dl and triglyceride concentrations up to 700 mg/dl) received 600 mg of gemfibrozil or placebos. The group (2051) who received gemfibrozil showed a 10% increase in HDL, a decline of non-HDL cholesterol by 14% and of triglycerides by 43% in the first 2 years of the study. In the final 3 years of the study, there was a 2% decline in HDL and a slight rise in triglycerides (12%) and in non-HDL cholesterol (0.4%). The dropout rate was 29.9%. The total number of cardiac end points in the gemfibrozil group was 56 (27.3/1000) compared to 84 in the placebo group (41.4/1000). This overall reduction difference of 34% is statistically significant by several tests. It should be noted that although there was a significant decrease in both mortal and nonmortal cardiovascular events, the rate of death from carcinoma was the same in the two groups. The all-cause mortality in the two groups remained the same. Similar discrepancies in mortality rate change have been reported in other trials of lipid-lowering agents as well.

Other fibric acid derivatives such as finofibrate and bezafibrate are currently under investigation. Although their overall mechanisms of action appear similar, there are some differences in their effect on various lipoprotein fractions.

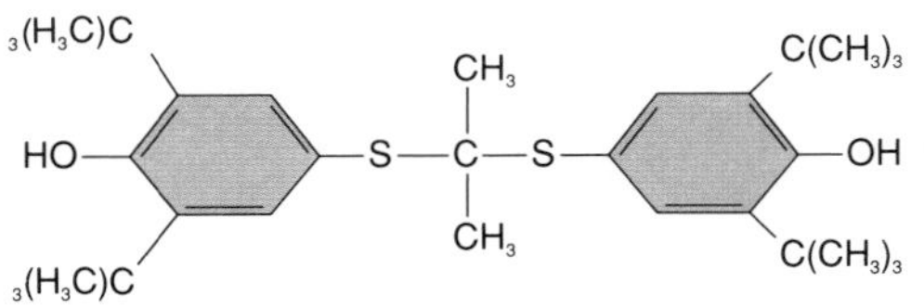

FIGURE 20-8   Probucol.

Probucol Probucol is a unique antilipemic compound that is not related in structure to any other lipid-lowering drug (Figure 20-8). Based on animal and clinical studies, two separate mechanisms of action are suggested. Its effect on atherosclerotic lesions is independent of its effect on cholesterol lowering. Decreases in peripheral accumulations of cholesterol occur independent of changes in total serum cholesterol concentrations. Its full spectrum of activity is not understood (similar to many of the drugs used in lowering cholesterol), but enhanced synthesis of apo E messenger RNA in peripheral tissues appears to be significant. Apo E appears to play a critical role in the peripheral mobilization of cholesterol, its movement to the liver, the increased catabolism in the liver, and its increased elimination in the bile. More recent work suggests that probucol is incorporated in LDL particles and that it functions as an antioxidant. Its presence inhibits the formation of pathogenic cholesterol esters and the conversion of tissue macrophages to foam cells when they incorporate the LDL particles. In most studies, probucol lowers plasma cholesterol by 10% to 25%. Therapy appears to be effective for up to 10 years.

Nicotinic Acid Niacin or nicotinic acid was found, in the mid-1950s, to lower triglycerides and serum cholesterol. It was successfully used as one treatment arm of a coronary drug trial to reduce the rate of myocardial reinfarction.

Hepatic uptake of the released free fatty acids and the synthesis of VLDL is reduced by nicotinic acid. In addition, the clearance of chylomicrons and VLDL from the plasma is enhanced. The mechanism for this phenomena in humans is not clear. In rats, lipoprotein lipase activity is increased but such increases in activity have not been demonstrated in humans. The increased catabolism of VLDL results in a decrease in LDL and an increase in the HDL particles containing apoprotein A (Apo A). Central to the action of niacin is its inhibition of the release of free fatty acids from tissue fat stores. The effect of niacin on cholesterol lowering can be enhanced by taking it with resins. A full dose of niacin reduces LDL concentrations by 10% to 15%; when taken in conjunction with resins, a 60% to 70% reduction is often reported. However, side effects, including intense flushing and pruritis, limit the acceptance and usefulness of this drug as a cholesterol-lowering agent.

Other Agents Two other agents, neomycin and sitosterol, have been used to lower plasma cholesterol by effects on the GI tract. Neomycin, an aminoglycoside antibiotic, which is poorly absorbed, lowers plasma cholesterol by an average of 22% in clinical studies. The mechanism is unclear. Binding of exogenous and bile-secreted cholesterol; precipitation of fatty acids, cholesterol, and bile acids; and alteration of GI bacterial flora all are proposed as mechanisms of action.

It is claimed that side effects of 0.5 to 1.0 gm doses of neomycin per day clear within several weeks of therapy. However, 14% of patients stop taking neomycin because of troublesome diarrhea. Larger doses of neomycin (>20 gm/day) are associated with steatorrhea, deafness, and impairment of renal function. Pretreatment auditory testing and use only in patients without renal functional compromise is indicated.

Because doses of neomycin greater than 1.0 gm/day have been associated with interference with digoxin absorption, it is necessary to monitor plasma concentrations of digoxin when taken concurrently with neomycin.

PHARMACOKINETICS

As a class, the pharmacokinetics of these drugs have not been well studied.

Lovastatin is administered as the inactive lactone. Of the administered dose about 30% is absorbed and all but about 5% of the absorbed dose is taken up by the liver in the first passage. On uptake by the hepatocytes it is hydrolyzed to the β-hydroxy acid, which is the active form and the principal metabolite. The major route of excretion is fecal (83%), whereas only 10% appears in the urine. In plasma, lovastatin is highly bound to plasma proteins and crosses the blood-brain and placental barriers. Absorption is enhanced by administration with a meal. Concentrations peak within 4 hours of the time of dosing.

Probucol is hydrophobic; as a result, about 10% of

Table 20-1   Pharmacokinetic Parameters

lovastatin	Administered orally, 30% absorbed, given as prodrug, metabolized to active form Disposition: 85% to feces, 10% to urine first pass effect >95% bound to plasma proteins
gemfibrozil	Administered orally Disposition: 90% metabolized, $t_{1/2}$ 1.5 hr
probucol	Administered orally, 10% absorbed, remains in fatty tissue for months
cholestyramine	Administered orally, not absorbed
colestipol	Administered orally, not absorbed
niacin	Administered orally Disposition: metabolized
neomycin	See Chapter 47

the administered dose is absorbed and significant amounts of the drug persist in fatty tissues after cessation of therapy. Absorption can be enhanced by administering the drug with meals. The full magnitude of decline in blood lipid concentrations is not seen immediately. About 60% of the decline is seen within 6 weeks, and it is often 6 to 12 months before the full effect is appreciated. The average decline in concentration of serum cholesterol with probucol is 10% to 25%.

The half-life of niacin in plasma is approximately 1 hour. It is rapidly converted to nicotinamide, which has no effect on lipid metabolism. When given by mouth, peak concentrations are achieved within 1 hour.

Pharmacokinetic parameters are summarized in Table 20-1.

RELATION OF MECHANISMS OF ACTION TO CLINICAL RESPONSE

Pathophysiology of Lipid Metabolism and Development of Atherosclerosis

To rationally use drugs that potentially alter the development and course of atherosclerosis, an understanding of the current concepts of atherogenesis is necessary. Current theory states that atheromatous plaques develop in arteries as a "response to injury." The exact nature of the injury may be obscure but certain locations in arteries such as branching sites,

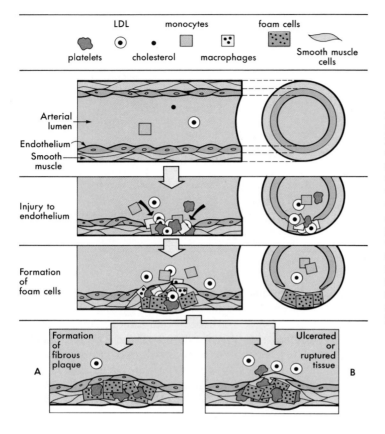

FIGURE 20-9   Development of an atheromatous plaque. An injury to the endothelial lining allows LDL particles, monocytes, and platelets to enter the smooth muscle tissue. Inflammation at the injury site triggers the conversion of monocytes to macrophages, which scavenge the LDL particles and cholesterol to form enlarged foam cells (xanthoma cells). Smooth muscle cells, foam cells, platelets, and LDL particles form fibrous plaques. The plaques form in two ways: **A,** at the interface between the endothelium and the smooth muscle tissue, leaving an elevation in the repaired endothelium, or **B,** as an ulcerated or ruptured lesion in the endothelium that protrudes into the lumen. Both types of plaque result in narrowing of the lumen and restricted blood flow.

which are subject to turbulent rather than laminar flow, appear more susceptible to plaque development than other sites. Factors contributing to the development of atherosclerotic lesion include elevated blood pressure, elevated cholesterol concentrations, elevated plasma transport lipid concentrations, and cigarette smoking. The discussion that follows focuses on cholesterol and the plasma lipids.

The response to injury hypothesis proposes that the initial event is some form of injury or disruption of the endothelial lining of arteries. High concentrations of the plasma lipid, particularly LDL cholesterol, are thought to be toxic to the vascular endothelium, but other factors such as oxidation of LDL particles and formation of antibodies also may be involved. Fatty streaks are the first manifestation of intimal injury. They can often be seen at autopsy in the arteries of children and young adults who have died suddenly. With time, the fatty streak progresses and becomes converted to a fibrous plaque. The fibrous plaque consists of a fibrous matrix of intimal smooth muscle cells

surrounded by large amounts of both intra- and extracellular lipids. Coronary and other vascular disease occurs when the plaque becomes large enough to compromise the flow of blood through the vessel. Plaque formation is summarized in Figure 20-9.

In monkeys, pigs, dogs, rabbits, and pigeons fed a lipid-rich diet, lesions similar to those seen in humans develop. Because it is not possible to determine the progression of atherosclerotic lesions in humans with any exactitude, most of our current knowledge of plaque formation is based on animal models.

In monkeys fed a high-fat, high cholesterol diet, the following sequence occurs:

1. After 2 weeks, clusters of leukocytes (principally monocytes) can be seen attached to the arterial endothelium or lining cells of the arteries, especially at or near branching points of the vessels.
2. On tissue cross-section an inward migration of the monocytes from the lumen to the smooth muscle layers is observed.

3. Large amounts of lipid have accumulated and taken on the appearance of foam cells.

4. Over the following weeks to months, there is continuing attachment of monocytes and continued migration into the vessel wall.

5. The fatty streak enlarges as a result of continued inward migration and accumulation of smooth muscle cells, which migrate and grow from their origin in the muscularis layer of the vessel (see Figure 20-9).

As this heterogeneous group of cells of various origins increases in number, the previously intact junctions between the endothelial lining cells begin to separate and retract. As a result, the early plaque is exposed to the circulating blood and its contents. These exposed cells represent a disruption of normal vessel endothelium and thus provide an opportunify for platelet adherence, aggregation, and development of mural thrombi. Increased lipid concentrations also enhance platelet adhesiveness.

In animals, it is established that the rate of formation and growth of atherosclerotic lesions depends on the rate of rise of the cholesterol concentration in plasma, the total circulating cholesterol level, and the duration of the elevation. The invasion of smooth muscle cells and their conversion into other cell types appear to be the key steps that determine the rate of growth and the extent of the fatty streak and subsequently the development of the fibrous plaque. Thus the intensity of the smooth muscle cell response ultimately determines whether clinical sequelae will develop. These cells will form the fibrous matrix of the plaque, as well as assume the appearance of foam cells with an intracellular collection of cholesterol and lipid.

The smooth muscle response is determined by a number of factors. What is known is that smooth muscle cells respond to a number of chemotactic and mitogenic factors (i.e., stimuli to move and reproduce). Among the sources of these factors are the vascular endothelium and circulating platelets. The role of platelet aggregation and the release of the granular contents of platelets as a major component of the response to endothelial injury is recognized, and modifiers of platelet response such as aspirin are being evaluated as a component in the treatment of atherosclerotic disease.

When the endothelium is intact, it prevents adherence of platelets to the vessel by the formation and release of antithrombogenic substances such as heparin and prostacyclin. Disruption of endothelial continuity or endothelial injury alters the formation and release of these substances, and in their absence the attachment of platelets with resultant aggregation or clumping may occur. Among the materials released when platelets clump are epidermal growth factor (EGF) and platelet derived growth factor (PDGF). PDGF may be the most critical in plaque formation because it is mitogenic and chemotactic to smooth muscle cells, thus causing their replication and luminal migration.

The third significant cell type that contributes to the development of the atherosclerotic plaque is the circulating monocyte. These cells are the source of histiocytes and macrophages in tissue. Indeed, subendothelial migration of monocytes is the initial step in fatty streak formation. Monocytes and their transformation product, macrophages, have multiple receptors on their cellular surfaces. Most important for the present discussion, they have receptors for LDL that are rich in cholesterol (vide supra). Macrophages accumulate LDL and cholesterol. They also secrete superoxide anions, lysosomal hydroxylases, and fibroblast growth factors and convert the cholesterol to esterified forms.

The cellular factors critical to the development of the atherosclerotic plaque have been described. Although these factors are present in animals and in humans, the development of fatty streaks and atheromatous plaques is not a universal finding. Other unknown factors determine that some animals and some humans will develop atherosclerosis and others will not.

Chronically elevated concentrations of plasma lipoprotein, particularly LDL and VLDL, have long been associated with an increased incidence of atherosclerosis. It is by the development of elevated concentrations of these lipoproteins that atherosclerosis can be induced in experimental animals. Under normal conditions the incorporation of these lipoproteins into cells is controlled by the number of cellular receptors. At higher concentrations, other modes of entrance of lipids into the cell occur. Receptor number is controlled by the need of the cell for cholesterol and certain genetic factors. The critical mechanisms that link excess cholesterol, LDL, and VLDL and the development of atherosclerosis are not well established, but various factors are known. First, it has been proposed that alterations in the ratio of cholesterol to phospholipid in the cell membrane will alter membrane viscosity. Thus endothelial malleability may be distorted, particularly at sites of intravascular stress or turbulence. If correct, this is a partial explanation for the early attachment of lymphocytes and platelets at these sites, as well as the cause for retraction of the endothelium over fatty streaks. Second, the presence of excess lipoprotein in macrophages may result in oxidation products toxic to the endothelium. Furthermore, the recruitment of antibodies to the oxidation products may be another factor. In conclusion, although atherosclerosis is described as a response to injury, the exact nature of the injury, or in fact if any injury is necessary, is still unclear.

The strongest positive correlations between lipoproteins and atherosclerosis exist for LDL. Impressive evidence derives from studies from lipid research clinics that performed an integrated series of epidemiologic community-based studies, as well as primary prevention trials. When total and LDL cholesterol concentrations are compared, there is a consistent rise in those concentrations during adulthood. Total cholesterol and LDL concentrations gradually increase in women until age 70. In men, concentrations increase until age 50 with a subsequent plateau until age 70, and then a decline. The pattern, however, is not one of a simple constant increase, and thus the ratios between various fractions continuously change. Because HDL and LDL cholesterol concentrations are independent of each other, the information derived from the measurement of each has additive value in the prediction of future coronary heart disease. The strongest quantitative clinical data provide the relationship between serum cholesterol and coronary heart disease mortality rate, shown in Figure 20-10. These studies also demonstrate that the major determinants of lipoprotein concentrations are dietary and genetic. The major factors affecting lipoprotein concentrations are shown in the box.

FACTORS AFFECTING LIPOPROTEIN CONCENTRATIONS

Dietary*
  Total calories
  Calories from fat
  Cholesterol intake
Anthropometric*
  Weight to height ratio (obesity)
Behavioral*
  Smoking
  Exercise
  Alcohol intake
Race
Genetic
Sex
  Estrogen concentrations (endogenous and exogenous)*
Other diseases, including diabetes*

* Modifiable factors.

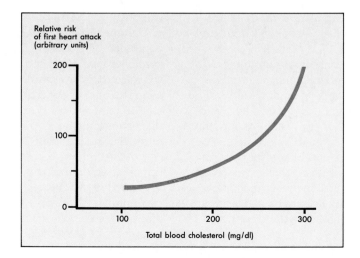

FIGURE 20-10   Summary of relationship between blood cholesterol concentrations and relative risk of initial heart attack.

In contrast to the positive correlation between LDL concentrations and the development of atherosclerotic disease, epidemiologic studies demonstrate an inverse relationship between HDL concentrations and the risk of atherosclerotic disease. However, although several studies show that lowering LDL concentrations reduces the incidence of atherosclerotic disease, it has not been demonstrated that raising HDL concentrations alone will reduce the risk of future disease. Many of the dietary changes such as reducing the total fat in the diet, making a greater percentage of the fats consumed polyunsaturated, and increasing the fraction of total calories obtained from carbohydrates, which are recommended to reduce LDL concentrations, enhance HDL turnover.

Drug and Dietary Interventions

A number of drugs that enhance HDL concentrations have other adverse effects that preclude their use. Estrogens cause increases in HDL concentrations, but when estrogens are used in men after a first myocardial infarction, there is an increased incidence of recurrent infarction. Drugs such as barbiturates induce hepatic microsomal enzyme activity and also enhance HDL concentrations; but their other effects preclude their usefulness in this disease.

The administration of probucol, which seemingly enhances reverse cholesterol transport, results in decreased concentrations of HDL-cholesterol. Nicotinic acid and the fibric acid derivatives clofibrate, gemfibrozil, and bezafibrate result in increased HDL concentrations. Cholestyramine, colestipol, and lovastatin appear to have little or no effect on HDL-cholesterol concentrations.

There are several forms of HDL and the confusion generated by these divergent findings may be related to the type of HDL present and the relative content of various apoproteins. As knowledge of lipoprotein transport and metabolism increases, it is clear that many of the apparent defects in the system, as well as the mechanism of action of several of the drugs mentioned, depend on the rate of synthesis and catabolism of several apoproteins. Measurement of various apoprotein concentrations may be superior in predicting atherosclerotic disease and drug action but techniques for measuring apoproteins are still too complex for routine use and the critical epidemiological studies have not been completed at this time.

The best treatment of atherosclerosis appears to be that directed at altering the major risk factors associated with its development. Lowering lipid concentrations should be accompanied by weight control, smoking cessation, and blood pressure control.

Because most individuals with elevated cholesterol concentrations acquired those increases on the basis of diet, the basic recommendations for reduction of cholesterol are decreasing calories and lowering the

Table 20-2   Summary of Dietary Recommendations

Phase	Typical American Diet	Phase I Modification of AHA	Phase II Modification of AHA
Fat (% calories)	40	30	25
Saturated fats (% calories)	17	10	7
Protein (% of calories)	15	15	15
Carbohydrates (% of calories)	45	55	60
Cholesterol (mg)	500	300	200
U/S (ratio of unsaturated to saturated)	1.5:1	2:1	2.5:1
CLASSIFICATION OF CHOLESTEROL CONCENTRATIONS			
Total blood cholesterol:	<200 mg/dl	Desirable	
	200-239 mg/dl	Borderline	
	≥240 mg/dl	High	
LDL-cholesterol (blood):	<130 mg/dl	Desirable	
	130-159 mg/dl	Borderline	
	≥160 mg/dl	High risk	
HDL-cholesterol (blood):	>35 mg/dl	Desirable	

proportion of the diet composed of saturated fat. Current recommendations of the American Heart Association and the National Heart, Lung, and Blood Institute are summarized in Table 20-2.

The effect of dietary intervention varies widely in the population. However, dietary intervention enhances the effectiveness of concurrent drug therapy. If dietary intervention is attempted first and does not lower cholesterol to acceptable concentrations, various pharmacologic agents are available. The argument for dietary change as the initial step is based on the following four considerations:

1. It is the most physiologic approach
2. The change should be life long
3. None of the drugs is without known or potential side effects
4. Drug therapy is relatively expensive, costing 1 to 2 dollars per day

SIDE EFFECTS, CLINICAL PROBLEMS, AND TOXICITY

Clinical problems are summarized in the box.

Resin Therapy

Resin therapy is not without difficulty. Resins are insoluble and have the consistency of fine sand. They must be mixed with fluids to be ingested. They tend to cause GI bloating, excess flatus, and constipation with associated nausea and indigestion. A diet high in fluids and fiber is necessary to minimize these effects and prevent impaction.

Because of the exchange of chloride ion for bile acids, excess chloride absorption may result in a hyperchloremic metabolic acidosis. Transient rises in alkaline phosphatase and transaminase also have been reported.

Because of the binding of bile acids and the removal of their emulsifying action, excess fat may appear in the stool, causing steatorrhea. Although the potential for interfering with fat-soluble vitamins exists, experts disagree as to whether or not supplementation of fat soluble vitamins is indicated. The binding properties of the resins may interfere with the absorption of thiazide diuretics, phenobarbital, thyroxine, warfarin, and digitalis preparations that undergo enterohepatic circulation. It is advisable to separate the administration of these resins and other therapeutic agents by several hours. The use of resins

---

CLINICAL PROBLEMS

LOVASTATIN

Increases serum transaminase; produces some increase in creatine phosphokinase and GI distress

RESINS

Lead to bloating and constipation; produce unwanted removal of chloride ions, dietary components, and drugs

PROBUCOL

Causes GI distress; prolongs Q-T interval

CLOFIBRATE

Produces cholelithiasis; possibly carries a carcinoma risk

GEMFIBROZIL

Possibly produces same problems as clofibrate; interacts with oral anticoagulants

NIACIN

May exacerbate cardiac dysrhythmias, gout, gallbladder disease, and liver disease; causes GI distress and intense flushing and pruritis

NEOMYCIN

Shows poor absorption, produces diarrhea, impairs renal function, interferes with digoxin absorption

---

in persons with elevated concentrations of cholesterol and particularly LDL has demonstrated the ability to lower the risk of coronary heart disease.

Lovastatin

Myalgias and transient elevations of creatine phosphokinase have been reported in patients on lovastatin therapy. In cardiac transplant patients receiving immunosuppressive drugs such as cyclosporin, almost 30% develop myositis within 1 year of starting lovastatin. In a few of these patients, myositis progressed to severe rhabdomyolysis and acute renal failure. About 5% of patients taking gemfibrozil and immunosuppressives have a similar reaction. In early studies about 11% of patients had increased creatine phosphokinase concentrations that were twice normal. In comparative trials, 9% of patients on cholestyramine and 2% of patients on probucol showed similar increases. Marked and persistent increases in serum transaminase occur in nearly 2% of adult patients who receive lovastatin for longer than 12 months. Changes in transaminase concentrations are common reasons for drug cessation. Enzyme changes usually appear at some time between 3 and 12 months of therapy. With cessation of therapy the elevations of transaminase gradually return to normal. It is recommended that patients have their transaminase concentrations measured every 3 months for the first 15 months of therapy.

Discontinuing the drug is recommended in any patient who develops a risk factor that would dispose to renal failure secondary to rhabdomyolysis (i.e., severe infection, hypotension, major surgery, trauma, or uncontrolled seizures).

Up to 10% of patients have GI symptoms, including diarrhea, constipation, dyspepsia, excess flatus, abdominal pain/cramps, and nausea. In double blind trials, headache was a complaint twice as frequent in patients receiving lovastatin as those given a placebo.

Since lovastatin inhibits the synthesis of cholesterol, the potential for inhibition of the synthesis of adrenal and gonadal steroid hormones, as well as bile acids, exists; however, substantial evidence indicates that such inhibition does not occur. None of the other end products of mevalonic metabolism such as dolichol, required for glycoprotein synthesis, or ubiquinone, used for mitochondrial electron transport, appear to be significantly affected by such inhibition. Because lovastatin reduces serum cholesterol by increasing receptor-mediated uptake of LDL, it is of little use in patients with homozygous familial hypercholesterolemia because these patients lack such receptors. Other than the adverse reactions and laboratory test changes described above, there appear to be few interactions of lovastatin with other drugs.

Fibric Acid Derivatives

Clofibrate use has diminished because of the occurrence of significant side effects such as an increased incidence of cholelithiasis and the possible increased incidence of carcinoma. In a study by the World Health Organization there was a significantly higher all cause mortality in patients on clofibrate compared to those taking placebo (36% difference). In the Coronary Drug Project study, there was no difference in mortality between those taking a placebo and those taking clofibrate. These studies suggest that there was an increased incidence of thrombosis and the development of claudication in patients taking clofibrate. Studies of gemfibrizol in Finland do not indicate the same associations.

Both agents tend to enhance the anticoagulant effect of warfarin and associated compounds. Thus doses of warfarin often must be reduced by as much as 50% when a fibric acid derivative is added to the patient's treatment. Other side effects with these drugs are principally GI and consist of abdominal pain, and, less frequently, nausea, vomiting, and diarrhea.

Probucol

Side effects of probucol include dyspepsia, abdominal pain, nausea, vomiting, flatulence, and diarrhea. The latter are probably due to increased bile flow. Prolongation of the Q-T interval on the electrocardiogram is seen in a significant number of patients. In monkeys fed atherogenic high cholesterol diets and probucol, an increased incidence of sudden death was reported. In dogs given high doses of probucol, sensitization of the myocardium to epinephrine and resultant ventricular fibrillation have been reported. These effects appear to be species specific and have not been reported in humans or in other animal species.

Drug interactions appear to be minimal. There is little advantage in using this agent in conjunction with clofibrate because further lowering of serum cholesterol does not occur.

Niacin

Side effects are generally noted within 30 minutes of niacin ingestion. Intense flushing and pruritus of the trunk, face, and arms generally occurs. This probably is due to prostaglandin E_1 release and can be partially inhibited by taking 325 mg of aspirin 60 minutes before taking the niacin. In addition, there are various other GI side effects including vomiting, diarrhea, and dyspepsia. Elevations of transaminases, as well as creatine phosphokinase concentrations, are common. Serum uric acid rises and there is an increased incidence of gouty arthritis in patients treated with nicotinic acid. Based on several studies there appears to be an increased incidence of cardiac dysrhythmias, including (but not limited to) atrial fibrillation. Side effects limit the usefulness of niacin as a cholesterol-lowering drug.

REFERENCES

Brown MS and Goldstein JL: How LDL receptors influence cholesterol and atherosclerosis, Sci Am 251(5):58, Nov 1984.

Goldstein JL and Brown MS: Hyperlipidemia in coronary heart disease: a biochemical genetic approach, J Lab Clin Med 85:15, 1975.

Green MS, Heiss G, Rifkind MB et al.: The ratio of plasma high-density lipoprotein cholesterol: age-related changes and race and sex differences in selected North American populations, Circulation 72(1):93, 1985.

Grundy SM: HMG-CoA reductase inhibitors for treatment of hypercholesterolemia, N Engl J Med 319(1):24, 1988.

Johnson WJ, Bamberger MJ, Latta RA et al.: The bidirectional flux of cholesterol between cells and lipoproteins, J Bio Chem 26(13):5766, 1986.

Manninen V, Elo MO, Frick HM et al.: Lipid alterations and decline in the incidence of coronary heart disease in the Helsinki heart study, JAMA 260(5):641, 1988.

Oster G and Epstein AM: Cost-effectiveness of antihyperlipemic therapy in the prevention of coronary heart disease, JAMA 258(17):2381, 1987.

Report of the national cholesterol education program expert panel on detection, evaluation, and treatment of high blood cholesterol in adults, Arch Intern Med 148:36, 1988.

Strandberg TE, Van Hanen H, and Miettinen TA: Probucol in long-term treatment-of-hypercholesterolemia, Gen Pharmacol 19(3):317, 1988.

Zilversmit DB: Atherogenesis: a postprandial phenomenon, Circulation 60(3):473, 1979.

Drugs Affecting Coagulation, Fibrinolysis, and Platelet Aggregation

ABBREVIATIONS

APTT	activated partial thromboplastin test
AT-III	antithrombin III
a_2PI	a_2-antiplasmin or a_2-plasmin inhibitor
cAMP	cyclic adenosine monophosphate
PGI_2	prostaglandin I_2
PT	prothrombin time
rt-PA	recombinant DNA-derived tissue plasminogen activator
$t_{1/2}$	half-life
TXA_2	thromboxane A_2
μ-PA	urokinase plasminogen activator
V_a	apparent volume of distribution
vWF	von Willebrand factor

MAJOR DRUGS

anticoagulants
fibrinolytics
platelet aggregation agents

 THERAPEUTIC OVERVIEW

Pathways that lead to blood clot formation and clot lysis are activated and inhibited by a complex variety of endogenous blood and tissue components and by numerous exogenous materials. The full range of activators and inhibitors and how they interact to stim-ulate or modify coagulation, fibrinolysis, or platelet aggregation in a variety of disease states is only partially understood. In the majority of patients, the clot formation and clot lysis systems function so that neither excessive bleeding nor the formation of unwanted thrombi are a problem. However, in a significant number of cases, particularly involving cardiovascular disease states, coagulation fibrinolytic-platelet systems are important in the development of improved therapeutic approaches. An important recent consideration is vascular endothelium cells and how they modulate the activation, inhibition, and storage of coagulation-fibrinolytic-platelet constituents. This accents the importance of in vivo rather than in vitro data in gaining a better understanding of the clot forming-dissolution systems.

The reasons for therapeutic intervention into the coagulation-fibrinolytic-platelet systems are (1) to partially inhibit the coagulation of platelet systems or (2) to stimulate the lysis of an already formed but unwanted thrombus. Certain surgical procedures such as hip-joint replacement or artificial heart valve insertion, in which whole blood comes in contact with foreign materials, result in situations that show a propensity for activation of thrombus formation. Here, the prophylactic administration of anticoagulants, usually heparin or coumarin, is effective in diminishing unwanted thrombus formation. In such as deep vein thrombosis, acute myocardial infarction or pulmonary embolism where a thrombus already has formed, rapid activation of the fibrinolytic system to obtain lysis of the thrombus plus initiation of anticoagulation to minimize further clot formation are ef-

ANTICOAGULATION (HEPARIN, COUMARINS)

Arterial thrombus
Atrial fibrillation
Cardiomyopathy
Cerebral emboli
Hip surgery
Open heart surgery
Vascular prosthetic devices
Valvular heart disease
Vascular prosthetic devices
Venous thromboembolism

FIBRINOLYSIS (UROKINASE, STREPTOKINASE, TISSUE PLASMINOGEN ACTIVATOR)

Acute myocardial infarction
Deep vein thrombosis
Pulmonary embolism

ANTIPLATELET AGGREGATION (ASPIRIN, DIPYRIDAMOLE, SULFINPYRAZONE)

Cerebral vascular accident
Coronary artery by-pass surgery and postoperation period
Postmyocardial infarction
Transient ischemic attack
Unstable angina pectoris

FACTOR REPLACEMENT (FACTORS VIII AND IX)

Hemophilia

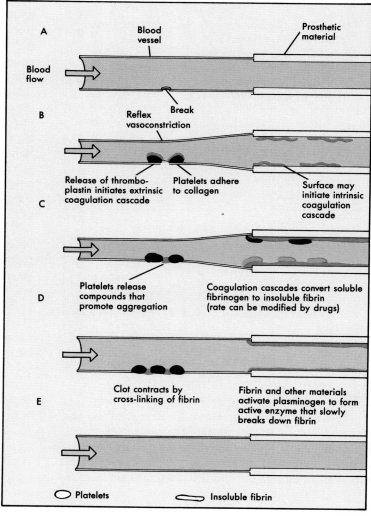

FIGURE 21-1 Main interactions of coagulation, platelet, and fibrinolytic systems. **A,** Presence of a prosthetic material in contact with blood or of a break in vessel wall causes rapid initiation of coagulation system and of platelet adhesion in **B.** This leads to plugging of break or coating of foreign surface. **C,** Retraction of clot now occurs over longer time period. **D,** Activation of fibrinolytic system takes place for slow degradation of fibrin clot to produce a more normal environment, **E,** after the new membrane cells repair the break.

fective. The use of drugs to minimize platelet aggregation is receiving major study for the prophylactic treatment of a wide range of cardiovascular diseases. Clinical trials have evaluated the efficacy of antiplatelet aggregation drugs as long-term prophylactic agents following myocardial infarction. The results, although controversial, appear promising.

Therapeutic use of anticoagulant, fibrinolytic and antiplatelet drugs are summarized in the box.

 ## MECHANISMS OF ACTION

The interactions of the coagulation, fibrinolytic, and platelet systems are summarized in Figure 21-1.

Coagulation

Activation of the coagulation system can be accomplished through contact of blood proteins with foreign surfaces or with damaged tissue. In either case, activation is propagated by sequential conversion of a series of inactive proteins into catalytically active protease enzymes (Figure 21-2). Each protein is designated by a clotting factor number, for example, factor X (inactive form) or X_a (active form). Factors V_a and VIII_a have no inherent activity but serve as cofactors. Several factors require the formation of a factor-Ca^{++}-phospholipid complex for the factor to exert its catalytic action.

The two major types of clinically used anticoagulants, heparin and coumarins, act by blocking the coagulation sequence to give the same result (i.e., a reduction in fibrin deposition). However, the mechanisms of blockade between the two types of anticoagulants differ markedly.

Commercial heparin is a linear anionic polymer made up of partially sulfated 2.6-disulfoglucosamine, 2-sulfoiduronate, and β-glucuronate residues in the ratio of roughly 3:2:1, with Na^+ or Ca^{++} as the cation (Figure 21-3). Commercial heparin is obtained by extracting hog intestinal mucosa or beef lung to give a mixture of polymer chains of approximately 5,000 to 30,000 daltons (average about 16,000 daltons) molecular weight.

Heparin acts by binding to an endogenous 58,000 dalton glycoprotein, antithrombin III (AT-III), which serves as the major inhibitor of the serine protease clotting enzymes, especially for factors X_a and II_a. AT-III inhibits these serine enzymes by formation of a stable 1:1 molar complex between the enzyme active site and position Arg385 or Ser386 of AT-III, but the specific bonds are not known. Heparin binds to a different site on AT-III. The heparin binding is thought to produce a marked conformational change in AT-III, leading to an enhanced rate of inhibition, particularly of X_a and II_a, but also of IX_a, XI_a, and XII_a (Figure 21-4). Commercial heparin can be separated into two fractions based on its in vitro affinity for AT-III. It is not clear whether the low (major fraction) and high (minor fraction) binding affinity is needed for significant in vitro inhibition of factors X_a or II_a. Recent clinical interest is on the use of heparin fragments, originally thought to be of too low a molecular weight to be effective but which in vivo produce a clinically useful anticoagulant effect. This low molecular weight heparin (4500 to 5000 daltons), which is produced by enzymatic or chemical hydrolysis of longer chains of natural heparin, appears to exert its anticoagulant action with fewer side effects. Whether the low molecular weight and natural heparins act by the same mechanism is not known.

The sites of action of heparin are plasma and probably also the surface of vascular endothelial cells. Heparin anions are rapidly taken up by the endothelium, with the intracellular heparin concentration 100 times that in circulating blood.

Coumarins, typified by warfarin (Figure 21-5), make up the second major type of clinically used anticoagulants. The major chemical component is the 4-hydroxy-substituted coumarin ring system. Coumarins act by blocking vitamin K regeneration during enzymatic modification of several endogenous clotting proteins. These vitamin K-dependent proteins include clotting factors II (prothrombin), VII, IX, and X and proteins C and S. These six proteins have several glutamic acid residues, which normally undergo liver microsomal enzyme carboxylation to form dianionic residues (carboxylated factor II in Figure 21-6) that function as binding sites for Ca^{++} ions. Thus carboxylation provides the template for clotting factor−cofactor-Ca^{++}-phospholipid positioning that places clotting factors in their correct spatial positions and catalytically active conformations. Coumarins inhibit the enzymes that catalyze the reduction of vitamin K epoxide to regenerate the active hydroquinone form of the vitamin (see Figure 21-6). Coumarins thereby inhibit the synthesis of functional clotting factors II, VII, IX, and X but have no direct effect on already synthesized factors. Therefore, there is a sig-

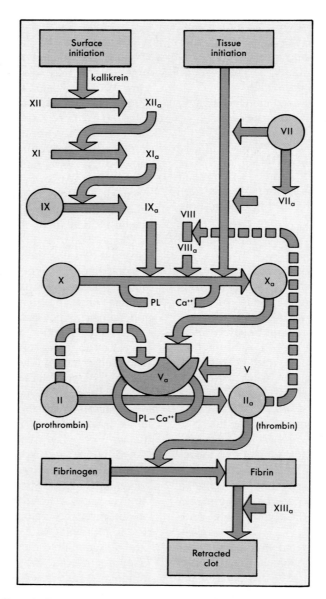

FIGURE 21-2   Coagulation sequence. In activated forms *(subscript a)*, Factors XII, XI, X, IX, VII, and II function as serine protease enzymes. They propagate activation cascade by cleaving a small peptide from the next protein in sequence. Factors, II, VII, IX, and X require vitamin K for completion of synthesis. Factors V_a and VIII_a are cofactors that enhance rates of activation of II and X, respectively. Calcium ions and phospholipd *(PL)* are required to hold factors and cofactors in correct spatial relationships. Factor XIII_a is a transglutaminase that catalyzes formation of crosslinks between fibrin strands. Initiation of extrinsic (tissue) route occurs when tissue thromboplastin contacts Factor VII or VII_a. Initiation of intrinsic (surface) route occurs through activation of factor XII by contact with negatively charged nonendothelium surfaces and is aided by presence of kallikrein and high molecular weight kininogen.

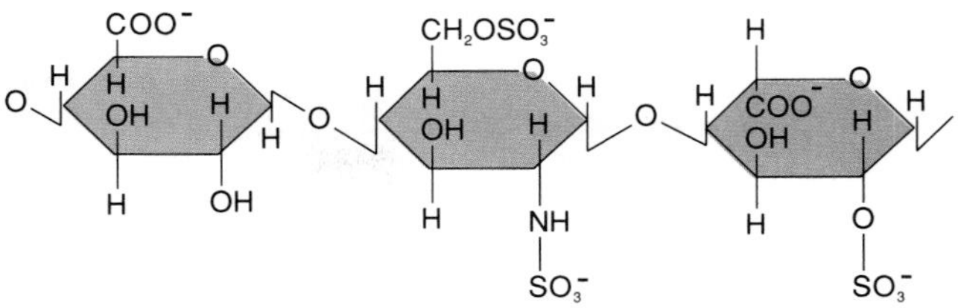

FIGURE 21-3   Heparin. β-D-glucuronic acid *(left)*; sulfated D-glucosamine *(center)*; sulfated *L*-iduronic acid *(right)*. The sequence of these three groups varies.

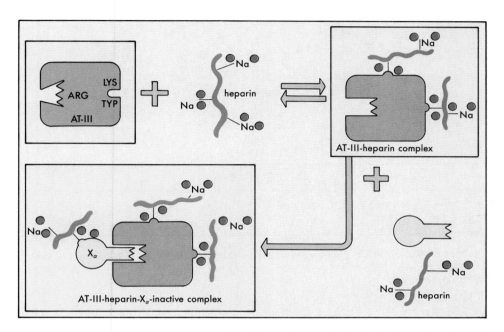

FIGURE 21-4   Mechanism of AT-III *(red)* inhibition of factor X_a *(yellow)* with sodium heparin *(blue-green)*. AT-III is an endogenous protease inhibitor to which heparin and serine protease clotting enzymes, particularly factors X_a or II_a, bind. Heparin is binding to two different sites on AT-III. The most prevalent theory suggests that heparin inhibits factor X_a by enhancing the rate of formation of the AT-III-X_a complex. However, a possible role for additional binding of heparin to X_a, either through the same or different heparin molecules that bind to AT-III, is not ruled out.

FIGURE 21-5   Warfarin. Structure of coumarin anticoagulant showing asymmetric center of carbon atom in active metabolite.

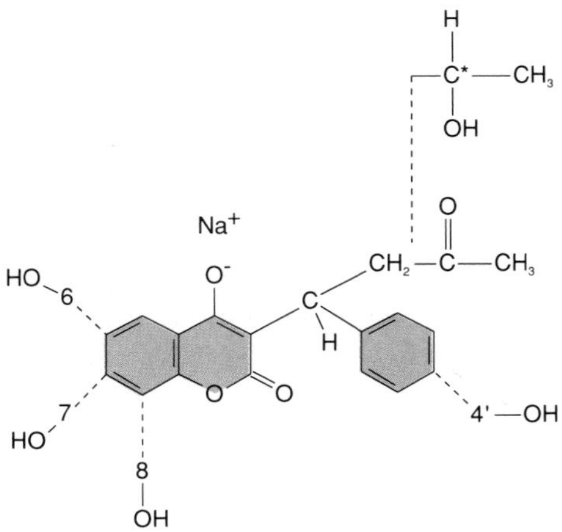

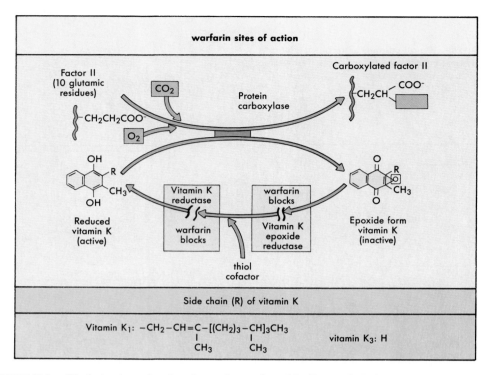

FIGURE 21-6   Warfarin sites of action shown for prothrombin (factor II). *R,* Side-chain of vitamin K.

nificant time delay before the anticoagulant effect is observed clinically.

Protein C, a serine protease, is another natural anticoagulant. When circulating thrombin binds to thrombomodulin found on the surface of vascular endothelium cells, the product becomes a strong activator of protein C and generates the anticoagulant action through inhibition of clotting factors V_a and VIII_a. Protein S is a cofactor required for the factor V_a and VIII_a inactivation. Because the natural anticoagulant action of protein C is reduced by coumarins, the concentration of protein C may be a consideration in patients in which warfarin therapy proves difficult to control clinically.

Protein C has a relatively short half-life (10 hours) compared to other serine proteases affected by coumarins. There is a period during early anticoagulation with warfarin when the concentration of functional protein C is very low while that for other proteins is normal. An exception is factor VII, which also has a short half-life. During this time, usually the first 3 days of coumarin therapy, the patient is susceptable to clot formation. Therefore heparin must be continued until all of the other affected proteins are at low concentra-

tions (approximately 3 days). This overlap should occur despite a prolonged prothrombin time (the test used to monitor warfarin action) because the prothrombin time will increase early because it is most sensitive to low concentrations of factor VII. If in switching from heparin to warfarin the heparin is terminated too early, re-thrombosis may occur.

Fibrinolysis

The in vivo lysis of fibrin clots requires the conversion of endogenous plasminogen into active protease plasmin. In normal circulating whole blood most of the plasmin is inactive, complexed with endogenous plasmin inhibitor, α_2-antiplasmin or α_2-plasmin inhibitor (α_2PI). If a fibrin clot is present, a high concentration of fibrin is found on the clot surface (Figure 21-7). Plasminogen is a single-chain protein of 92,000 to 94,000 daltons molecular weight. The activation of plasminogen involves enzymatic cleavage to form a two-chain protein, linked through disulfide bridges, which is catalytically active plasmin. The major types of commercially available plasminogen activators are (1) protease enzymes, urokinase (μ-PA) and strepto-

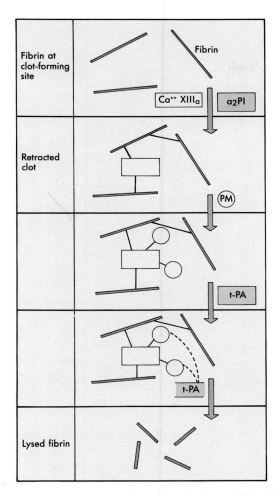

FIGURE 21-7   Clot retraction catalyzed by factor XIII_a to form crosslinks between fibrin strands or through α_2 PI (plasmin inhibitor). Plasminogen *(PM)* binds to α_2 PI. For lysis, t-PA binds first to fibrin and then acts on circulating or bound plasminogens to produce plasmin, which at high enough local concentration hydrolyzes the fibrin strands.

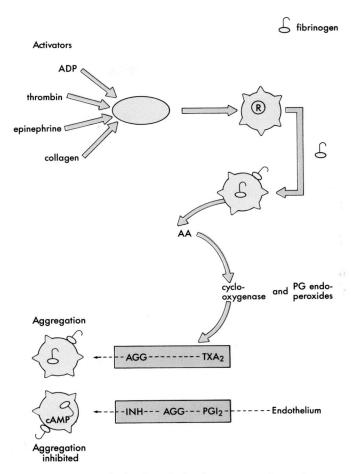

FIGURE 21-8   Activation of platelets causes shape change that exposes fibrinogen receptors *(R)* on platelet surface and allows fibrinogen to bind. This stimulates platelet binding to von Willebrand factor (which is bound to injury site) and arachidonic acid *(AA)* release. AA leads to synthesis of TXA_2, a strong stimulant of platelet aggregation. PGI_2 from vascular endothelium raises intraplatelet cAMP, which reorients platelet membrane to block fibrinogen binding and inhibit platelet aggregation. *AGG*, aggregation; *INH*, aggregation inhibited.

kinase and (2) recombinant DNA-derived tissue plasminogen activator (rt-PA) released by endothelial cells. Urokinase, which originates in human kidney cells, and streptokinase, which is of bacterial origin, exert their major fibrinolytic action throughout the plasma. A major advantage of t-PA is that it must first bind to fibrin before it can activate plasminogen (see Figure 21-7). The major portion of the lysis action with t-PA is thus localized at the clot and not distributed throughout the circulatory system. However, hemorrhagic events still can be a major problem with t-PA. The human-derived rt-PA is produced in ge-

netically engineered cell lines. Some nonfibrinolytic clot lysis may occur due to release of proteolytic enzymes by leukocytes.

Platelet Aggregation

Activation and subsequent aggregation of platelets is a key feature that can lead to thromboembolic complications of cardiovascular disease states. Several pathways are available for initiation of platelet aggregation; the sequence shown in Figure 21-8 is best understood. Platelet activation produces a shape change, exposing receptors that can bind to fibrinogen tightly. Fibrinogen and another protein, von Willebrand factor (vWF), act as adhesives, with vWF providing mainly injury-site-to-platelet and fibrinogen mainly platelet-to-platelet adhesion. Exposure of platelet fibrinogen receptors can be reversed by elevated intraplatelet concentrations of cAMP, so that compounds that lead to increased platelet cAMP produce inhibition of platelet adhesion and aggregation. Platelet activation leads to the formation of the potent aggregation promotor, thromboxane A_2 (TXA_2) within platelets. Prostacyclin (PGI_2) released by vascular endothelial cells, increases intraplatelet cAMP and blockade of platelet aggregation. Several therapeutic approaches are available for reducing platelet aggregation. Low dose aspirin, dipyridamole, and sulfinpyrazone are the principal agents (Figure 21-9). Ticlopidine, dazoxiben, and suloctidil are newer agents undergoing clinical trials. A 1989 comparison of aspirin with ticlopidine (both administered daily) demonstrates a reduction of stroke but a greater increase of side effects. Aspirin irreversibly inhibits cyclooxygenase via acetylation of a threonine at the active site of the enzyme, and thereby blocks the synthesis of the powerful platelet aggregation inducer TXA_2. Aspirin also blocks the synthesis of the endogenous antiaggregation compound PGI_2 but the duration of the synthesis blockade is much longer for TXA_2 than for PGI_2. Aspirin may also produce additional platelet aggregation effects, but the mechanism is not known. In addition, the detailed mechanism by which TXA_2 causes platelets to aggregate is not clear (see Chapter 18). Epinephrine causes platelet aggregation by binding to platelet α-receptors to produce decreased intraplatelet concentrations of cAMP and therefore reduced availability of fibrinogen receptors.

In 1989 the results of a study of 22,000 U.S. participants extending over 5 years showed a 44% reduction in risk of myocardial infarction for those age 50 or older receiving aspirin as compared to placebo. The relative risk of ulcer was 22% greater in the aspirin group; the relative risk of the aspirin group for stroke and cardiovascular death remained inconclusive.

Dipyridamole (see Figure 21-9) is a phosphodiesterase enzyme inhibitor, and thus might be expected to produce its antiaggregation effect by inhibiting the breakdown of intraplatelet cAMP. An explanation that better fits the data is that dipyridamole inhibits

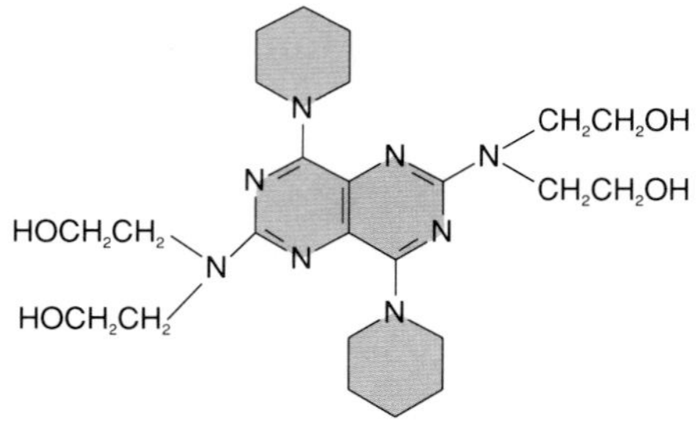

dipyridamole

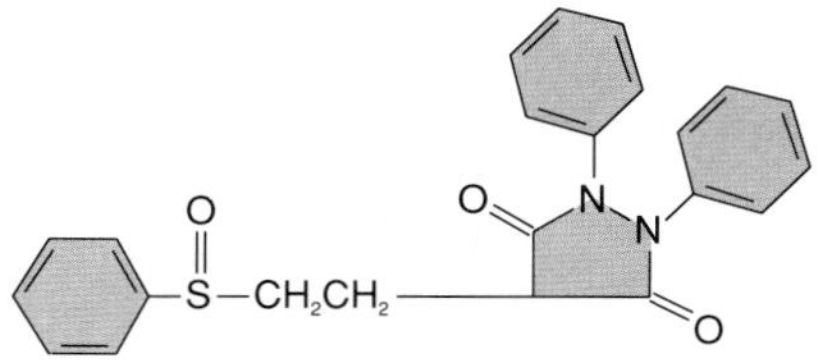

sulfinpyrazone

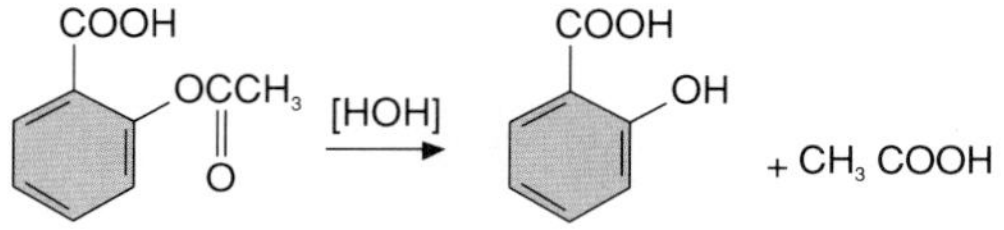

aspirin   salicyclic acid

FIGURE 21-9   Antiplatelet aggregation drugs.

adenosine transport into erythrocytes, thus elevating plasma concentration of adenosine. Adenosine in turn stimulates adenylate cyclase to elevate cAMP; therefore the platelet antiaggregation effect of dipyridamole appears to be linked to elevated intraplatelet concentrations of cAMP.

Sulfinpyrazone (see Figure 21-9) exerts its platelet antiaggregation effect by competitive inhibition of platelet cyclooxygenase, thereby blocking the synthesis of TXA_2. Sulfinpyrazone is metabolized to the sulfoxide reduction product, which is 100 times more active than the parent drug.

PHARMACOKINETICS

The principal pharmacokinetic parameters of the anticoagulants, fibrinolytic activators, and antiplatelet aggregation drugs are given in Table 21-1. Warfarin is typical of the oral anticoagulants. Because of

Table 21-1   Pharmacokinetic Parameters

Drug	Administered	Absorption	$t_{1/2}$ (hour)	Disposition	Plasma Protein Binding (%)
heparin*	IV, SC	No	1.5 (IV)	†	Trace
16,000 MW			3.0 (SC)		
5,000 MW	IV, SC	No	2.2 (IV)	R	Trace
			3.8 (SC)		
warfarin	Oral	good	40 ± 12	M (main), R	97
dipyridamole	Oral	fair	11.6	M (main)	91-99
sulfinpyrazone	Oral	—	3	M	98-99
salicylic acid	IV	good	2-3	M, R	50-70
streptokinase*	IV, intracoronary	No	0.35 after activated	M (?)	—
urokinase*	IV, intracoronary	No	0.3	M (liver)	—
t-PA*	IV	No	0.2	M (?)	—

R, Renal; *M*, metabolism.
*Activity in units.
†Taken up by vascular endothelium and RES (reticuloendothelial system).

the different mechanisms of action, the maximum heparin anticoagulant effect after a single dose is immediate, whereas that of warfarin takes 36 to 48 hours in humans. Warfarin is metabolized in the liver. The only warfarin metabolite that has anticoagulant activity is the alcohol (see Figure 21-5), but the concentration of this metabolite is low, the activity is greatly reduced, and it is usually of little clinical importance. Warfarin is strongly bound to plasma albumin, whereas heparin shows little binding to albumin or to other nonclotting-related plasma proteins. The half-life and bioavailability of low molecular weight heparin differs significantly from that of the longer chain drug. Aspirin hydrolysis to salicylic acid occurs rapidly, with a $t_{1/2}$ of 15 to 20 minutes and salicylic acid is metabolized by four different routes; the products are eliminated in the urine.

RELATION OF MECHANISMS OF ACTION TO CLINICAL RESPONSE

Unwanted thrombus can be treated with fibrinolytic activators. However, observing the progress of thrombus dissolution may be difficult. When clinically warranted, invasive radionuclide or contrast angiography, impedance plethysmography, or Doppler ultrasound can be used to confirm and follow a clot. In some cases external monitoring of the changes in radiation level is used to assess the disappearance of the thrombus.

The common use of anticoagulants and antiplatelet aggregation compounds is to prevent a thromboembolic disease state from occurring. In these cases nonspecific clotting tests usually are used to establish the degree of deviation from normal clot forming activity. For heparin, the activated partial thromboplastin test (APTT) is normally used to monitor the degree of anticoagulation; with warfarin, the one stage prothrombin time (PT) is the standard laboratory test. These procedures consist of mixing patient plasma (citrated to remove calcium) with commercial tissue extracts that restore calcium and certain clotting factors and measuring the time in seconds for a clot to form. The presence of anticoagulant will prolong the time necessary to form a clot. The clinical guidelines vary depending on the specific APTT or PT reagents and the disease being treated.

Anticoagulant effect of coumarins can be expressed as the fractional inhibition of the prothrombin synthesis rate, compared to the synthesis rate in the absence of drug. Although this method of measuring the anticoagulant effect is too complex for routine clinical use, the approach provides a useful method for defining the mechanisms of warfarin drug interactions. Warfarin is used clinically as a racemic mixture, with the (−) S isomer producing about 1.5 times the anticoagulant effect of the (+) R isomer.

The anticoagulant effect of heparin can be reversed

rapidly with protamine sulfate; the effect of warfarin is reversible with vitamin K$_1$ but rapid reversal can be achieved by transfusing fresh or frozen plasma that contain the clotting factors. Vitamin K$_1$ has no effect on warfarin absorption, metabolism, or protein binding.

Platelet aggregation tendencies are monitored using standard aggregrometer tests. Platelet function is assessed by measuring the bleeding time, a standard coagulation test.

SIDE EFFECTS, CLINICAL PROBLEMS, AND TOXICITY

The major problem with all of these agents is bleeding, even when used in therapeutic doses. Thrombocytopenia (heparin), drug interactions (warfarin), and platelet aggregation by other drugs also pose significant problems (see box).

Roughly 1% to 10% of heparinized patients develop thrombocytopenia. When associated with arterial thrombosis, this side effect can be extremely serious and even fatal. Platelet counts may drop well below 100,000 platelets/mm^3, with the drop most evident 6 to 12 days after the start of heparin administration. The mechanism appears to involve an immune reaction similar to that of other drug-induced thrombocytopenias. Heparin binds to the platelet membrane and stimulates the formation of platelet membrane antibodies, which activate complement C$_3$ and lead to platelet aggregation. The usual treatment is to stop the use of heparin. So far, no guidelines are available to predict which patients are most likely to have this complication.

CLINICAL PROBLEMS

HEPARIN

Produces hemorrhage, thrombocytopenia, hypersensitivity; when use is discontinued, hypercoagulability

WARFARIN

Produces hemorrhage, drug interactions, drug metabolism enzyme induction; some resistant subjects

STREPTOKINASE

Produces bleeding disorders (activator not localized to clots) and antibodies; lowers fibrinogen concentrations

UROKINASE

Produces bleeding, although less than streptokinase; lowers fibrinogen concentrations; expensive

t-PA and rt-PA

Degrades circulating fibrinogen; requires tighter binding to fibrin; expensive

ASPIRIN

Blocks TXA$_2$ synthesis in nonplatelets; acetylates AT-III and may affect coagulation; does not inhibit thrombin-induced platelet aggregation

---

Table 21-2 Drug Interactions with Warfarin and Other Drugs Given Concurrently

Other Drug	Interaction Mechanism
allopurinol	↓ metabolism (?)
aminoglutethimide	↑ metabolism (enzyme induction)
anabolic steroids	↓ clotting factor synthesis (?)
	↑ clotting factor degradation (?)
barbiturates	↑ metabolism (enzyme induction)
carbamazepine	↑ metabolism (enzyme induction)
chloral hydrate	displace from albunim
chloramphenicol	↓ dicumarol metabolism
cholestyramine	reduced absorption from gut
cimetidine	↓ metabolism
clofibrate	several possibilities
disulfiram	↓ metabolism (?)
erythromycin	↓ metabolism
glucagon	↓ clotting factor synthesis (?)
glutethimide	↑ metabolism (enzyme induction)
griseofulvin	↑ metabolism (enzyme induction)
heparin	direct action on clotting factors, interferes with prothrombin time
mefanamic acid	displace from albumin
metronidazole	↓ metabolism
nalidixic acid	displace from albumin
phenylbutazone	↓ metabolism and displace from albumin
rifampin	↑ metabolism (enzyme induction)
salicylates	↓ clotting factor synthesis, reduced platelet adhesion and release reactions
sulfinpyrazone	↓ metabolism
sulfonamides	displace from albumin, also ↓ metabolism
thyroid stimulants	↑ clotting factor degradation
tolbutamide	accumulation from hepatic enzyme induction by dicumarol
vitamin K (large doses)	↑ clotting factor synthesis

Drugs Affecting Coagulation, Fibrinolysis, and Platelet Aggregation   **293**

Because chronic warfarin administration often extends over many months or years, the likelihood of a patient on warfarin receiving other drugs concurrently is very high. There is a major possibility for drug interactions with warfarin because of its high degree of binding to plasma albumin and its metabolic mode of elimination (Table 21-2).

Several drugs normally used therapeutically for the treatment of other disease states also influence the anticoagulant, fibrinolytic, or platelet systems. Long-term use of the oral hypoglycemic, chlorpropamide, decreases concentrations of t-PA, but changing to a second generation drug such as glipizide (see chapter 39) will eliminate this problem. Benzodiazepines inhibit platelet aggregation by decreasing the release of arachidonic acid. The calcium channel blocker, verapamil, also causes a decrease in platelet aggregation, probably via reduced TXA_2 generation. The opposite effect, namely enhanced platelet aggregation, has been associated with cimetidine use in the treatment of peptic ulcer.

TRADENAMES

In addition to generic and fixed combination preparations, the following tradenamed materials are available in the United States.

ANTICOAGULATION

Aquamephyton, vitamin K_1
Calciparine, heparin calcium
Coumadin, warfarin sodium
Hemofil-T, factor VIII
Koate-HT, factor VIII
Konyne-HT, factor IX
Profilate, factor VIII
Profilnine, factor IX
Proplex, factor IX (also with II, VII, and X)
Prothar, factor IX

FIBRINOLYSIS

Abbokinase, urokinase
Activase, restriction tissue
    plasminogen activator (rt-PA)
Kabikinase, streptokinase
Streptase, streptokinase

PLATELET ANTIAGGREGATION

Anturane, sulfinpyrazone
Bayer, aspirin
Persantine, dipyridamole
SK-Dipyridamole, dipyridamole

REFERENCES

Collins R, Serimgeour A, Yusuf S et al.: Reduction in fatal pulmonary embolism and venous thrombosis by preoperative administration of subcutaneous heparin, N. Engl J Med 318:1162, 1988.

Esmon CT: The regulation of natural anticoagulant pathways. Science 235:1348, 1987.

Fasco MJ, Hildebrandt EF, and Suttie JW: Evidence that warfarin anticoagulant action involves two distinct reductase activities, J Biol Chem 257:11210, 1982.

Loscalzo J and Braunwald E: Tissue plasminogen activator, N Engl J Med 319:925, 1988.

Schröder R, Neuhaus KL, Leizorovicz A et al.: A prospective trial of intravenous streptokinase in acute myocardial infarction (ISAM), N Engl J Med 314:1465, 1986.

Steering Committee Physicians' Health Study Research Group: Final report on the aspirin content of the ongoing physicians' health study, N Engl J Med 321:129, 1989.

TIMI Study Group: Comparison of invasive and conservative strategies after treatment with intravenous tissue plasminogen activator in acute myocardial infarction, N Engl J Med 320:618, 1989.

Vesterqvist O: Rapid recovery of in vivo prostacyclin formation after inhibition of aspirin, Eur J Clin Pharmacol 30:69, 1986.

CNS: DRUGS AFFECTING BEHAVIOR, PSYCHOTIC STATE, PAIN SENSATION, MUSCLE CONTROL, AND SLEEP

Drugs affecting the central nervous system (CNS) play an increasingly important role in the modern world. Mankind has experienced the effects of mind-altering drugs throughout recorded history, and a large number of compounds with specific and therapeutically useful effects on brain and behavior have been discovered and characterized over the last half century (Table IV-1). Drugs acting on the CNS are now among the most widely used of all drugs. These drugs have dramatically improved the quality of life for many people with diverse medical problems. Discovery of the general anesthetics was an absolute prerequisite for the development of surgery, and continued advances in the development of anesthetics, sedatives, narcotics, and muscle relaxants have made possible the complex microsurgical procedures in common use today. Discovery of antipsychotic drugs in the 1950s revolutionized the treatment of schizophrenia and other psychiatric disorders. Although possessing many potentially serious side effects, the well-regulated use of antipsychotic drugs allows many people to lead happy and productive lives in society instead of being confined to mental institutions. Other drugs act on the CNS to reduce pain or fever, relieve seizures and movement disorders associated with neurological diseases, or control mood and motivational states such as depression, mania, anxiety, arousal, or appetite. Proper use of such compounds results in marked increases in the quality of health care.

The increasing therapeutic utility of drugs affecting the CNS and the nonmedical use of these compounds have increased dramatically. Historically, alcohol, caffeine, and nicotine have been used to alter mood and behavior and are still widely used. However, increasing awareness of the addictive and potential toxic effects of alcohol and nicotine has led to legal restrictions on their marketing and use. Many stimulants, depressants, and antianxiety agents intended for medical use are obtained illicitly and used for their mood-altering effects. Although the short-term effects of these drugs may be useful, exciting, or pleasurable, excessive use often leads to physical dependence and/or toxic effects that result in long-term problems. Illicit "recreational drugs" such as heroin and cocaine are major problems in society. The

Table IV-1   Drugs That Act on the CNS and Are Commonly Used in Medical Practice, Arranged by Their Approximate Period of Introduction

Period of Drug Introduction	Indication for Use
BEFORE 1900	
morphine	Pain
caffeine	Drowsiness
nitrous oxide	Surgery
aspirin	Pain, fever, inflammation
1900 TO 1950	
barbiturates	Epilepsy
phenytoin	Epilepsy
meperidine and analogs	Pain
antihistamines	Wakefulness
SINCE 1950	
halothane and related fluoro-carbons	Surgery
lithium carbonate	Bipolar affective disorders
chlorpromazine and related phenothiazines	Psychoses
chlorprothixene and related thioxanthines	Psychoses
haloperidol and related buty-rophenones	Psychoses
monoamine oxidase inhibitors	Depression
tricyclic antidepressants	Depression
mixed agonist/antagonist opioids	Pain
methadone	Opiate dependence
opioid antagonists	Opiate overdoses
clonidine and related imidazolines	Hypertension
diazepam and related benzodiazepines	Anxiety
primidone, ethosuximide, carbamazepine and valproic acid	Epilepsy
most nonsteroidal anti-inflammatory agents	Pain, inflammation
L-DOPA	Parkinson's disease
amantadine	Parkinson's disease
"Second generation" antidepressants	Depression
bromocriptine and other dopamine agonists	Parkinson's disease
baclofen and related drugs	Spasticity

extremely high abuse liability of these drugs often results in physiological and/or psychological addiction, with their severe attendant social problems.

The increasing use and abuse of centrally acting drugs results in intense interest in the mechanisms by which these drugs act. It is useful to understand the specific molecular targets on which these drugs act, the physiological processes affected by the interactions of these drugs with their target molecules, and the relationship of such physiological changes to the complex mood and behavioral effects caused by these drugs. Such information is valuable in maximizing the therapeutic efficacy of centrally acting drugs, while minimizing their toxic effects, addiction liability, and abuse potential.

The complexity of the CNS makes this a formidable task. The brain is composed of many billions of neurons and glial cells, with most neurons having many processes and hundreds or thousands of interconnections with other neurons. The CNS functions directly or indirectly as sensor, integrator, and regulator of all bodily processes. Because it is also the center of consciousness and thought, it is not surprising that this area of biology is one in which the functional and organizational principles are still not well understood. The spectacular advances in cell and molecular biology that have occurred over the past decade have begun to yield new techniques, approaches, and tools for studying the brain.

Because of the complexity of the brain, the molecular targets through which various drugs alter function are often poorly understood. Much of what is known about the mechanisms by which drugs affect the CNS relates observed actions on specific molecular processes to known mood-altering or behavioral actions of drugs. Studies on the mechanism of actions of these drugs often follow the pattern outlined in Figure IV-1. Drugs with demonstrated behavioral actions are examined to determine if they have specific cellular or biochemical actions. When a biochemical effect is identified, other drugs with similar behavioral profiles are also studied. If they cause similar biochemical actions with potencies similar to their behavioral potencies, this action is postulated to be involved in the behavioral actions of the drug. This hypothesis is then tested with other compounds and experimental approaches. Clearly, this type of approach results in only correlative information and

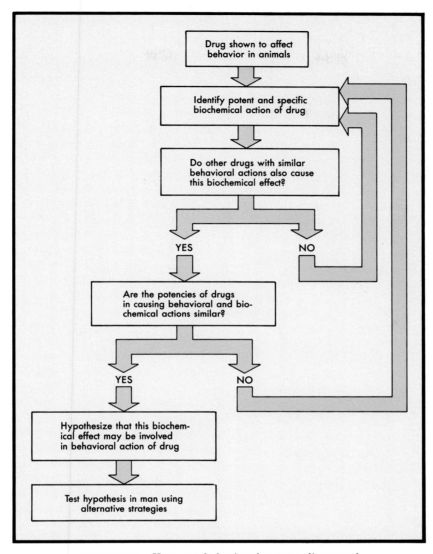

FIGURE IV-I   How mood-altering drugs are discovered.

cannot prove that a drug acts by a particular mechanism. In many cases, this is the best approach currently available for studying the mechanisms of action of centrally acting drugs.

Chapters in this section describe drugs used for the therapeutic modification of behavior (psychoses, Chapter 23; mood, Chapter 24; and anxiety, Chapter 25), control of epilepsy (Chapter 26) and movement disorders (Chapter 27), diminish pain sensations (Chapters 28 to 30), control inflammation (Chapter 29), and provide relief for sleep disorders (Chapter 33). The nontherapeutic role of alcohol (Chapter 31) and mind-changing, often addictive abused drugs (Chapter 32) are also described.

22

Pharmacological Organization of the CNS

ABBREVIATIONS	
ACTH	adrenocorticotropic hormone
ATP	adenosine triphosphate
cAMP	cyclic adenosine monophosphate
DOPA	dihydroxyphenylalanine
GABA	γ-aminobutyric acid
MAO	monoamine oxidase

To understand the effects of drugs on the central nervous system (CNS), it is important to have a basic understanding of the cellular physiology and biochemistry of the brain. A review of the basic biology of the CNS is provided in this chapter, with an emphasis on the molecular processes thought to be specific targets for drug actions. Although drugs act at many sites in the brain, many of the most selective and useful drugs appear to act specifically at chemical synapses. Because this is the predominant site of information transfer and integration, it is also an ideal target for affecting specific brain functions. For this reason, the chemistry and physiology of synaptic transmission is heavily emphasized.

CELLULAR BUILDING BLOCKS

Cell Types

The two major classes of cells in the CNS are neurons and glia. Each has many morphologically and functionally diverse subclasses (Figure 22-1). Neurons

exhibit many different shapes, some quite complex and elaborate. They share many characteristics with other epithelial cells in the body but also have unique properties well suited for the transfer and integration of information.

There are four general morphological regions in neurons: the cell body, dendrites, axon, and axon terminals. The cell body (or *soma*) is the region surrounding the nucleus, where the main organelles of the cytoplasm are grouped to perform the basic processes necessary to maintain the cell. Arising from the cell body are elaborate branching processes, *dendrites,* the parts of the neuron where incoming messages from other neurons are usually received. The cell body also gives rise to an elongated tube called an *axon,* a cablelike process that can be very long (up to 1 meter). Near its termination, the axon has characteristic structural features, often dividing into many fine branches, each of which terminates in a specialized ending called an *axon terminal* or *synaptic bouton.* Other types of axons exhibit multiple dilated regions *(varicosities)* near the termination point. These presynaptic structures are the sites where electrical signals passing down axons are converted into chemical messages for transmission to nearby cells.

Although most neurons have these four characteristic features, their relative prominence varies dramatically in different cells (see Figure 22-1). A feature of neurons is that they branch in widely different patterns (much like trees). Some neurons have only a single major process extending from the cell body (which may, however, branch) and are thus called *unipolar neurons.* Others have two (bipolar) or more (multipolar) major processes arising from the cell

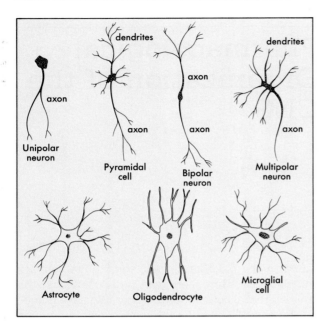

FIGURE 22-1   Types of cells in the CNS: selected examples.

body. Although most neurons have one axon, a few have more than one and some function without any axon. The largest variability occurs in the length of the axon and the number and branching of the dendrites. Classification by shape, number of processes, arborization, or similar anatomical criteria can give only limited insight into neuronal function. Therefore neurons are usually classified by their localization and functional properties and the types of neurotransmitters that they synthesize and to which they respond.

Although glial cells outnumber neurons in the CNS, their precise functions are poorly understood. It is thought that glial cells provide various passive support services for the neurons, the major components involved in information transfer and integration. This is analogous to the role played by connective tissue in other parts of the body. Recent evidence suggests that glial cells contain many types of neurotransmitter receptors and ion channels, and the possibility that glial cells are also actively involved in information transfer and integration is increasingly likely.

The glial cells in the CNS are the astrocytes, oligodendrocytes, and microglia (see Figure 22-1). There are at least two main types of astrocytes, distinguished by morphology and surface antigens. The main functions of astrocytes appear to be (1) the phys-

ical separation of different nerves and nerve pathways from each other, (2) assistance in repairing nerve injury, and (3) modulation of the metabolic and ionic microenvironment of nerve cells. Oligodendrocytes generally have fewer and thinner branches than astrocytes and are responsible for formation of the myelin sheath around axons in the CNS. Microglia are small cells scattered throughout the nervous system that proliferate after injury or degeneration. These cells move to the site of injury and transform into large macrophages (phagocytes), which remove the debris.

It is tempting to think simplistically of a network of information-processing neurons embedded in a matrix of inert glial cells, much as patterns of semiconductor material are etched on a background of inert substrate in the manufacture of integrated circuits. The more that is learned about glial cells, however, the more obvious it becomes that such a view is incorrect. Glial cells help control the environment of neurons and may play an essential role in many of their functions.

Functional Compartmentalization of Neurons

The complex structures of neurons (and to a lesser extent glial cells) suggest that there must be substantial compartmentalization of function. Not surprisingly, this functional compartmentalization is also reflected in a compartmentalization of intracellular organelles (Figure 22-2). The organelles necessary for synthesis of macromolecules and general cell maintenance are mainly in the cell body, although they can also be in dendrites. These include the nucleus containing the genetic information; the ribosomes, Nissl substance, and endoplasmic reticulum for synthesis of proteins; and the Golgi complex for storing, processing, and concentrating secretory proteins. Mitochondria, for energy production through glycolysis or the citric acid cycle, are also present in the cell body. The axon contains a large number of neurofilaments and microtubules, which also extend into dendrites and cell bodies. These play a major role in transporting substances between the different parts of nerve cells. Dendrites also contain mitochondria for energy production, as well as some neurotransmitter-containing vesicles. The nerve terminals and varicosities are specialized for neurotransmitter release and mainly contain mitochondria and large numbers of neurotransmitter-containing synaptic vesicles.

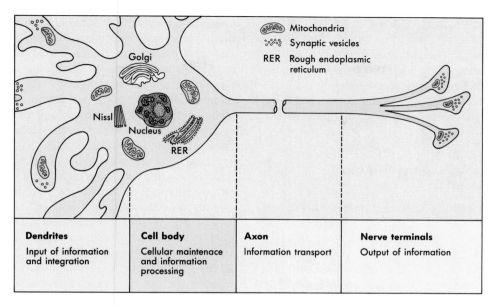

| Mitochondria |
| Synaptic vesicles |
| RER   Rough endoplasmic reticulum |

| **Dendrites** | **Cell body** | **Axon** | **Nerve terminals** |
| Input of information and integration | Cellular maintenace and information processing | Information transport | Output of information |

FIGURE 22-2   Structural components of nerve cells.

Such anatomical compartmentation has major implications for nerve cell function. The most obvious is the need for transport of macromolecules from their sites of synthesis in the cell body to the specific parts of neurons in which they perform their functions. For example, proteins essential for the function of synaptic vesicles must be synthesized in the ribosomes of the cell body and transported to axon terminals. This is accomplished by the microtubules and neurofilaments extending throughout the neuron in a process called *axonal* or *axoplasmic* transport. Axonal transport can be "slow" (1 mm/day) or "fast" (>100 mm/day). Fast and slow are used in a relative sense here; fast axonal transport could take many days to transport a substance from the cell body to the end of a long axon. Similar types of transport processes also occur in highly branched dendrites.

Neurons must fire rapidly and repetitively to transmit information, and it is important that supplies of neurotransmitter at the axon terminals be readily replenished. Fast axonal transport is an inefficient way to ensure a constant supply of transmitter in the terminals of a rapidly firing neuron. Neurons circumvent this problem by synthesizing most neurotransmitters locally in the nerve terminals. The major exception to this generalization are peptide neurotransmitters, which require ribosomes for synthesis. The peptides

are synthesized as larger precursor molecules in the cell body and must be transported to the axon terminals. This is only one of the fundamental differences between peptide and other neurotransmitters, which are discussed further below.

Another consequence of the complicated morphology of neurons is in their response to incoming signals. Integration of these messages occurs mainly at the axon hillock. This is the area where the axon arises from the cell body and where action potentials that will traverse down the axon are generated. Small changes in membrane potential occurring in the distal parts of highly arborized dendrites will have a smaller effect on the membrane potential of the axon hillock than will similar changes occurring more proximally. The extensive branching of the dendrites confers a spatial aspect to all incoming signals, which, in addition to the temporal and quantitative aspects of the signal, forms part of the message received by the neuron.

Clearly, neurons are extremely complex cells that have evolved highly specialized subcellular regions for performing specific tasks. The complicated morphology of neurons is an important aspect of their role in the input, processing, and output of information. A neuron by any other shape would probably not function nearly as well.

ELECTRICAL PROPERTIES OF NEURONS

Most information transfer and processing in the CNS is accomplished by alterations in electrical currents flowing across neuronal membranes. It is therefore important to have a firm understanding of how charge differences across nerve cell membranes are controlled.

Pumps, Channels, and the Resting Membrane Potential

Similar to other biological membranes, the membranes of nerve cells are composed of lipid bilayers stabilized by hydrophobic interactions. As such, they present physical barriers to free diffusion of water-soluble molecules between the intracellular and extracellular compartments. The electrical properties of nerve cells are generated by the ability of their surface membranes to control the movement of charged molecules (ions) and to selectively concentrate them on only one side of the membrane. The resulting ion gradients result in a charge difference (voltage) across the membrane, referred to as a *potential difference* or *membrane potential.* The membrane potential is one of the major mechanisms by which information is stored and processed in the CNS.

There are two classes of protein molecules spanning the cell membrane whose primary functions are to control ion movement. "Pumps" actively move charged ions from one side of the membrane to the other, selectively concentrating them against their concentration gradient in an energy requiring manner. "Channels," as described in Chapter 2, are molecular pores in the membrane that allow specific species of ions to pass. Channels can exist in two states—open or closed—although some investigators suggest the existence of a third state in which the channel cannot be activated. Ions generally traverse a channel from high to low concentration. In addition to pumps and channels, there is a constant relatively small permeability of the cell membrane to ions, referred to as the *leak current.*

The relative distribution of three ions, sodium, potassium, and chloride, is the primary determinant of the membrane potential of nerve cells. Although the total concentrations of these three ions are similar, their distribution across the membrane is different. Sodium and chloride are found in high concentration outside the cell, whereas potassium is in high concentration inside the cell. These concentration gradients constantly encourage sodium to leak into the cell, and potassium to leak out. The gradients are supported by continuous exchange of sodium and potassium by the sodium-potassium ATPase. This membrane-spanning enzyme pump exchanges three sodium ions from the intracellular fluid for two potassium ions from the extracellular fluid using energy obtained from hydrolysis of ATP. Because the ions exchanged by this enzyme are positively charged, the activity of this pump generates a small unequal charge distribution across the membrane and sets the stage for the resting membrane potential.

The presence of ion channels selectively permeable to sodium or potassium causes an unequal distribution of charge across the membrane (Figure 22-3). Chloride ions are distributed passively across most nerve cell membranes and make little contribution to resting membrane potential, although they can be important in determining electrical responses to incoming signals. At rest, the nerve cell membrane is most permeable to potassium, because most sodium channels are closed but many potassium channels are open. Positively charged potassium ions flow down their concentration gradient out of the cell, leaving behind a relative negative charge as a result of the large nonpermeant anionic proteins inside the cell. As the inside of the cell becomes increasingly negative, it is more difficult for a positive charge to leave the cell, and potassium outflow slows. Eventually the concentration gradient and the electrical potential difference cancel and there is no further net ionic movement.

Because potassium is selectively allowed to flow out, the inside of the neuron is negative with respect to the outside. Although this "resting membrane potential" is due mainly to selective permeability to potassium, some sodium channels are also open at rest. This allows some sodium to enter and reduce the magnitude of the resting membrane potential. In practice, the resting membrane potential of different cells ranges between -90 and -40 mV, depending on the relative activity of various pumps and channels.

Action Potentials

Nerve cells can carry electrical signals over long distances without any loss of signal strength. This is accomplished by the action potential—a regenera-

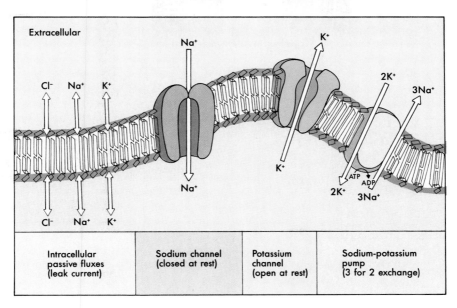

FIGURE 22-3   Primary determinants of resting membrane potential in nerve cells.

tive, all-or-none phenomenon that actively propagates electrical impulses rapidly down axons to their nerve terminals. The ionic basis of action potentials was discovered about 40 years ago and the molecular basis for this phenomenon has recently been elucidated.

Inputs to nerve cells consist of graded changes in membrane potential caused by the actions of neurotransmitters and modulators. Such "synaptic potentials" are spatially and temporally summated in the cell body. When the strength of these inputs is sufficient to cause a substantial reduction in membrane potential at the base of the axon *(axon hillock),* an action potential is generated. This is caused by a complex sequence of events initiated by the change in membrane voltage, which is summarized in Figure 22-4.

The primary components in the generation and form of an action potential are ion channels in the cell membrane whose permeability changes when the transmembrane electrical potential is altered. Such channels are called *voltage-dependent* or *voltage-gated,* as described in Chapter 2, since the change in transmembrane voltage can be thought of as opening or closing a "gate" over the pore.

Initiation of the action potential is caused by opening of voltage-dependent sodium channels at the axon hillock. These channels are usually closed at the nor-

mal resting membrane potential, preventing the high concentration of sodium in the extracellular fluid from entering the cell. When the membrane is depolarized, these channels open and allow sodium to flow into the cell down its concentration gradient. This influx of positive charge depolarizes the cell further, opening more voltage-dependent sodium channels. This is the self-regenerating part of an action potential, because opening sodium channels causes further depolarization, resulting in opening of more sodium channels. These channels are the site of action of local anesthetics that, by blocking sodium influx, prevent regenerative action potentials and conduction of nerve impulses.

If sodium influx continues, the cell becomes completely depolarized. However, sustained depolarization causes an automatic inactivation of the voltage-dependent sodium channels, shutting off sodium influx. The channels not only close, but also become refractory to reopening. There is also a concurrent but independent opening of voltage-dependent potassium channels, allowing an increased outflow of potassium ions to counterbalance the inflow of sodium ions. Potassium channels inactivate very slowly and often remain open as long as the membrane is depolarized. Potassium efflux causes the membrane potential to return to its normal resting value when the sodium channels are inactivated.

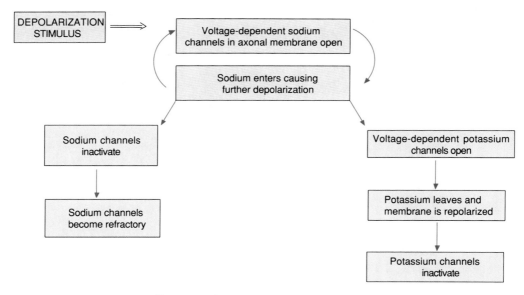

FIGURE 22-4   Sequence of events occurring during an action potential.

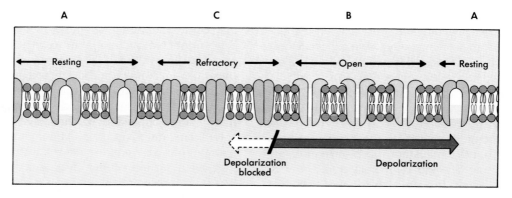

FIGURE 22-5   Unidirectional nature of axonal impulse conduction. Sodium channels are depicted as being in the resting **(A)**, open **(B)**, or refractory **(C)** state. The refractory channels prevent the depolarization from proceeding in more than one direction.

The inactivation of voltage-dependent sodium channels results in impulse conduction that is unidirectional (Figure 22-5). When the newly opened channels inactivate and become refractory, they form an effective block to further depolarization. Therefore, depolarization can proceed only in a forward direction, toward resting channels that have not recently been opened. The inactivated refractory channels are eventually returned to their normal resting state and can participate in subsequent action potentials.

The voltage-dependent sodium and potassium channels involved in the action potential are proteins whose structures have recently been determined by gene cloning and sequencing techniques. The voltage-dependent sodium channel, consisting of four internally homologous repeating regions joined together by regions extending in the cytoplasm, is described in Chapter 2.

Speed of Axonal Conduction

In many situations messages must be sent quickly along long axons. The speed of conduction of the action potential is controlled by the passive spread of

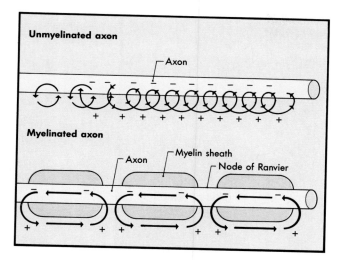

FIGURE 22-6 Spread of current in unmyelinated and myelinated axons.

depolarization into adjacent regions of the axon, causing the opening of more voltage-gated sodium channels. This spread of depolarization is not instantaneous and is the rate-limiting factor in action potential propagation.

One way to increase the speed of conduction of action potentials is to increase the diameter of the axon. Since internal resistance to current flow decreases as the axon diameter increases, axons with a larger diameter will conduct impulses more rapidly than those with a smaller diameter. Increasing the axon diameter also causes an increase in the membrane capacitance (ability to separate and store charge), thus further facilitating the spread of depolarization down the axon.

There are practical limitations to axon size, and myelination also increases the speed of action potential propagation. This is the process of wrapping a surface membrane of oligodendrocytes (or Schwann cells in peripheral nerves) around nerve axons in tight concentric layers. The number of layers can be very high (20 to 300) and provides a dramatic increase in membrane resistance to current flow. The myelination is interrupted every 1 to 2 mm by bare stretches of axon, called *nodes of Ranvier*. These nodes contain very high densities of voltage-dependent sodium channels (up to 12,000 per square micron), whereas the axon under the myelin contains few, if any, of these channels. The myelin provides a very effective insulator with a high resistance and low capacitance,

and current can only flow at the myelin-free nodes of Ranvier. Current, therefore, tends to flow along the fiber to the next node rather than leak back across the membrane. Each node responds with an active regenerative depolarization to the spread of depolarization from the preceding node. The impulse essentially jumps from node to node (Figure 22-6), rapidly speeding up impulse conduction. Such conduction is very efficient; since less active membrane is required, fibers can be smaller, and less energy is required to restore the ionic gradients. It is common in higher organisms, where it plays an important role in facilitating high speed conduction.

The presence and characteristics of voltage-dependent ion channels make the axon uniquely suited for long-distance transmission of information. The next step to be considered is the transmission of information between neurons and their target cells.

SYNAPTIC TRANSMISSION

Effective transfer and integration of information in the CNS require that neurons pass information encoded by action potential frequency to adjacent neurons or other target cells. Because the axon terminal is usually separated from adjacent cells by an intercellular gap of 20 nm or more, there must be some way for the signal to cross this gap. This is usually accomplished by specialized areas of communication around axon terminals, referred to as *synapses*.

Synapses

As the axon approaches its point of termination it exhibits a variety of subcellular specializations, previously discussed. Most prominent are the appearance of varicosities and synaptic boutons filled with mitochondria and large numbers of synaptic vesicles. These are referred to as *synaptic terminals* because they form the transmitting portion of the synapse. The synaptic terminals usually form a specialized contact zone with the adjacent cell, referred to as the *postsynaptic* cell, since it forms the receiving portion of the synapse. This contact zone is usually identified by thickening of the postsynaptic membrane. Sometimes a similar thickening is observed in the presynaptic membrane, although this is more variable. It is across this junction, a synaptic terminal filled with vesicles to a postsynaptic specialization on the adjacent cell, that information must be transmitted.

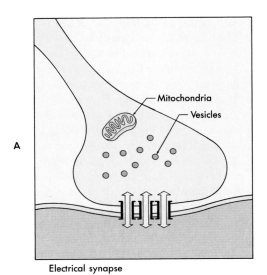
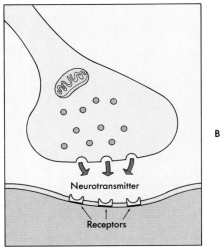

Electrical synapse   Chemical synapse

FIGURE 22-7   Electrical and chemical synapses. **A,** Electrical synapses have channels bridging the gap between presynaptic and postsynaptic neurons. These "gap junctions" allow free, bidirectional passage of ions and small molecules. **B,** Chemical synapses do not have gap junctions and rely on chemical mediators to transfer information.

It was originally thought that the depolarization of the axon terminal might, through passive electrical influences, directly affect the membrane potential of the postsynaptic cell. It rapidly became clear, however, that nerves could also release chemical messengers conveying messages to postsynaptic cells. It is now known that there are two different and apparently unrelated types of synapses: electrical and chemical. Electrical synapses are common in invertebrates and lower vertebrates, and chemical synapses predominate in higher organisms.

A comparison of electrical and chemical synapses is shown in Figure 22-7. In electrical synapses, large protein channels physically bridge the gap between the presynaptic and postsynaptic membrane, thereby connecting the cytosol of the two cells. These channels are similar to the gap junctions often found connecting epithelial cells in the body. They allow free passage of ions and other small molecules from the interior of one cell to the interior of another cell, in either a forward or a reverse direction. When an action potential invades an electrical synapse, the resulting influx of positive charge in the presynaptic terminal can flow directly into the postsynaptic cell and cause a local depolarization in the postsynaptic cell.

The geometry of most synapses in the mammalian CNS indicates that the electrical communication is not of prime importance. A very small presynaptic terminal with a high resistance could not deliver enough current to depolarize a large postsynaptic cell, even with essentially no resistance at the synaptic junction. In fact, most synapses in the human brain use chemical messengers to transfer messages across the synaptic junction (see Chapter 2). An action potential arriving at a chemical synapse has no direct electrical connection with the postsynaptic cell. Rather, the depolarization of the presynaptic terminal causes the release of a chemical mediator (neurotransmitter) into the extracellular fluid between the presynaptic and postsynaptic cells (the *synaptic cleft*). The neurotransmitter then diffuses across the synaptic cleft to act on the postsynaptic cell membrane to deliver its message. The postsynaptic cell must then respond in some appropriate fashion to the received message.

Chemical synapses require a greater degree of specialization than electrical synapses. The presynaptic terminal must have specialized mechanisms for storing neurotransmitters and releasing them in response to a depolarization stimulus. The postsynaptic cell must have specialized receptors for detecting the presence and identity of different neurotransmitters and initiating appropriate changes in cell physiology or metabolism. Finally, there must be efficient mech-

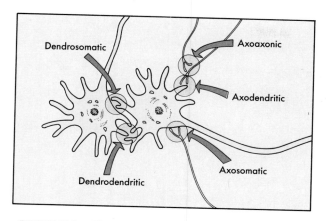

FIGURE 22-8   Types of synaptic connections in the CNS.

anisms for formation, degradation, and reutilization of neurotransmitters to ensure rapid onset and offset of arriving messages. To a large extent, it is these specializations of chemical synapses that are the sites of action for many centrally acting drugs.

All synapses show some degree of morphological specialization, although the extent of specialization varies dramatically. Classification of synapses based on morphological criteria is often as difficult and unrewarding as classification of neurons on the basis of shape, discussed previously. Examination of the extremes of synaptic specialization can, however, illustrate some general factors important to synaptic communication.

A synapse is the juxtaposition between the transmitting element of one neuron and the receiving element of another neuron. It is clear, however, that information does not pass only from axon terminals to dendrites. The classical concept of input at dendrites, processing in the cell body, transmission over the axon, and output at the presynaptic terminals (see Figure 22-2) is too simplistic. In fact, most parts of the neuron may contain both sending and receiving roles. Dendrites can also store neurotransmitters and release them in response to changes in membrane potential, and therefore function as a "presynaptic" element. Targets for released neurotransmitters include not only dendrites, but also the cell soma, the initial segment of the axon, and the axon terminals. Examples of possible types of synaptic connections between neurons are illustrated in Figure 22-8. Communication from an axon to a dendrite is referred to as an *axodendritic* synapse, from a dendrite to an axon as *dendroaxonic*, and between two axons as

axoaxonic. Note that in some "reciprocal" synapses there can be impulse traffic in both directions when appropriate synaptic specializations are present.

Other criteria by which synapses can be classified include the distance between the presynaptic terminal and the postsynaptic target (i.e., the distance the released neurotransmitter must diffuse to its site of action). If the terminal is closely apposed to the postsynaptic membrane, the transmitter will be released at its site of action, have little opportunity to diffuse, and thus act on only a small target area. Conversely, if the terminal is farther away, the transmitter will have to diffuse farther and will have access to a wider target area. Such synapses are referred to as *directed* and *nondirected*, respectively (Figure 22-9).

The peripheral nervous system contains extreme examples of each of these types of synapses (see Chapters 8 to 11). A directed synapse is exemplified by the neuromuscular junction between somatic motor nerves and skeletal muscles (see Chapter 11). Here, the presynaptic terminals terminate very close (20 to 30 nm) to the postsynaptic membrane, which sends out extensively invaginated ramifications that almost surround the terminal and greatly restrict the diffusion of the released neurotransmitter, acetylcholine. A nondirected synapse is exemplified by the junction between postganglionic sympathetic nerves and their target organs in the autonomic nervous system (see Chapter 10). Here, the neurotransmitter (norepinephrine) is released from varicosities relatively distant (up to 400 nm) from the nearest cell. Few, if any, postsynaptic specializations are observed and the released neurotransmitter appears to act on a relatively large target area.

Most synapses in the CNS lie somewhere between these two extremes. Synaptic clefts are usually relatively narrow (20 to 30 nm), but there is a large heterogeneity in the postjunctional area and the postsynaptic specializations on the target cells. These can be subdivided as "simple" or "specialized" based on whether or not there are clear anatomical subspecializations. Synaptic terminals also have been subclassified on the basis of the types of synaptic vesicles they contain. There are various types of synaptic vesicles in neurons, ranging from 30 to 400 nm diameter, with different shapes and electron densities. Although these different types of vesicles probably contain different types of transmitters, it is not yet possible to determine the neurotransmitter based on the

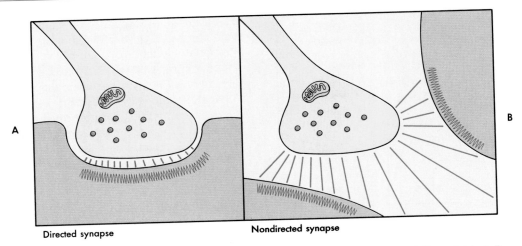

A, Directed synapse

B, Nondirected synapse

FIGURE 22-9   A, In directed synapses, the site of transmitter action is spatially restricted. **B,** In nondirected synapses, the transmitter can diffuse over a much wider target area.

type of vesicles contained in neurons.

Clearly, synapses are heterogeneous; however, the functional implications of the heterogeneity have not been determined. Similar to the classification of neurons discussed previously, morphological classification of synapses suggests some general principles about how neurons communicate, but has not provided specific insight into the function of particular synapses.

Neurotransmitters

Neurotransmitters are the substances nerve cells use to communicate with each other. Although this is a simple definition, it is remarkable how much disagreement there is over which substances function as neurotransmitters in the CNS. Part of the controversy is caused by the methodological difficulties involved in isolating and identifying neurotransmitter substances. However, there is also substantial discussion about the directedness and specificity of synaptic communication and the types of messages encoded by specific intercellular mediators.

The chemical messengers that are released by cells to send signals to other cells vary between two extremes. One extreme includes hormones, which are secreted into the blood, diffuse throughout the body, and act on many different target cells. The other extreme includes neurotransmitters at "directed" synapses, which are secreted into the extracellular space,

act solely on the patch of postsynaptic membrane surrounding the nerve terminal, and are inactivated before they can diffuse further. In such cases, the distinction between hormones and neurotransmitters is obvious.

However, some substances are not easily classified. Antigen-stimulated histamine release from mast cells can be highly localized to the area immediately adjacent to the immune insult. Prostaglandins released locally from platelets may have short-lived effects on nearby vascular smooth muscle contractility before being rapidly inactivated. Similarly, some neurotransmitters have larger or more diverse target areas, such as in the "nondirected" synapses discussed previously. These examples do not fall clearly into hormone or neurotransmitter categories.

The dilemma has no obvious solution. Classification of intercellular messengers is based primarily on the type of cell from which they are released. Neurons secrete neurotransmitters; other cells secrete hormones. Further subclassification might be based on the relative speed, duration, specificity of action, or distance traveled by the released messenger. Neurotransmitters may have highly localized action, neuromodulators slightly large target areas, and neurohormones diffuse to still more distant sites. However, the net result is that the terms *neurotransmitter, neuromodulator,* and *neurohormone* are used interchangeably. For simplicity, the term *neurotransmitters* is used here to indicate any messenger substance released from neurons, regardless of its specificity or localization of action.

Identification of Neurotransmitters The following common sense criteria are necessary to establish whether a particular substance is responsible for conduction of an impulse across an identified synapse:

1. The suspected neurotransmitter substance must be present in the nerve terminals and the cell must be capable of making or accumulating the substance and inactivating it
2. The substance must be released on nerve stimulation and exogenous application of the substance must mimic nerve stimulation
3. Drugs with known effects on enzymes and receptors for the proposed transmitter must affect the nerve stimulated response in a predicted manner

Although these criteria should be met for a substance to be considered a neurotransmitter at a particular synapse, it is impossible to fulfill all of these criteria for most synapses. Particularly in the CNS, where various heterogeneous cells are closely apposed and intermingled, such specific information is often unavailable. In practice, the relative importance of these different lines of evidence is a matter of controversy.

Because of these complicating factors, there is little direct information about the identities of the neurotransmitters at the large majority of synapses in the mammalian brain. A few compounds have been unequivocally identified, particularly in the peripheral nervous system. There is also substantial evidence for a large number of other compounds that are thought to play a neurotransmitter role in the brain.

Classes of Neurotransmitters Substances thought to be neurotransmitters at various synapses in the mammalian brain are an extremely heterogeneous group of compounds. They range from the small two-carbon amino acid, glycine, to large peptides composed of 30 to 40 covalently bonded amino acids (see box), with subclassification on the basis of chemical structure. Examples of structures from each class are shown in Figure 22-10.

Interestingly, neurotransmitters can also be subdivided on the basis of their functional roles in other cells. First, there are the substances that have no other known function in mammalian physiology. These include three of the biogenic amines (acetylcholine, norepinephrine, and dopamine), one amino

SUBSTANCES THOUGHT TO PLAY A NEUROTRANSMITTER ROLE IN MAMMALIAN BRAIN	
BIOGENIC AMINES	**PEPTIDES**
acetylcholine	carnosine
dopamine	thyrotropin releasing hormone
norepinephrine	enkephalins
epinephrine	angiotensin II
histamine	cholecystokinin
serotonin	oxytocin
	vasopressin
AMINO ACIDS	bradykinin
GABA	dynorphin
glutamate	luteinizing hormone releasing
glycine	hormone
aspartate	substance P
	substance K
NUCLEOTIDES AND NUCLEOSIDES	neurotensin
	α-melanocyte stimulating hormone
adenosine	bombesin
ATP	somatostatin
	secretin
	vasoactive intestinal peptide
	β-endorphin
	glucagon
	calcitonin-gene-related peptide
	neuropeptide Y
	ACTH
	corticotropin releasing factor
	insulin

acid (γ-aminobutyric acid [GABA]), and a few of the peptides (e.g., neuropeptide Y, calcitonin-gene related peptide, and substance P). There is a large second class of substances that function as hormones in other tissues but also serve as neurotransmitters. These include three other biogenic amines (epinephrine, histamine, serotonin) and all of the remaining peptides. The third class includes the three remaining amino acids, which are important building blocks in the formation of peptides and proteins (glutamate, glycine, aspartate). Finally, there are the nucleotides (adenosine and ATP), which serve prominent roles in energy metabolism. Clearly, neurons co-opt a variety

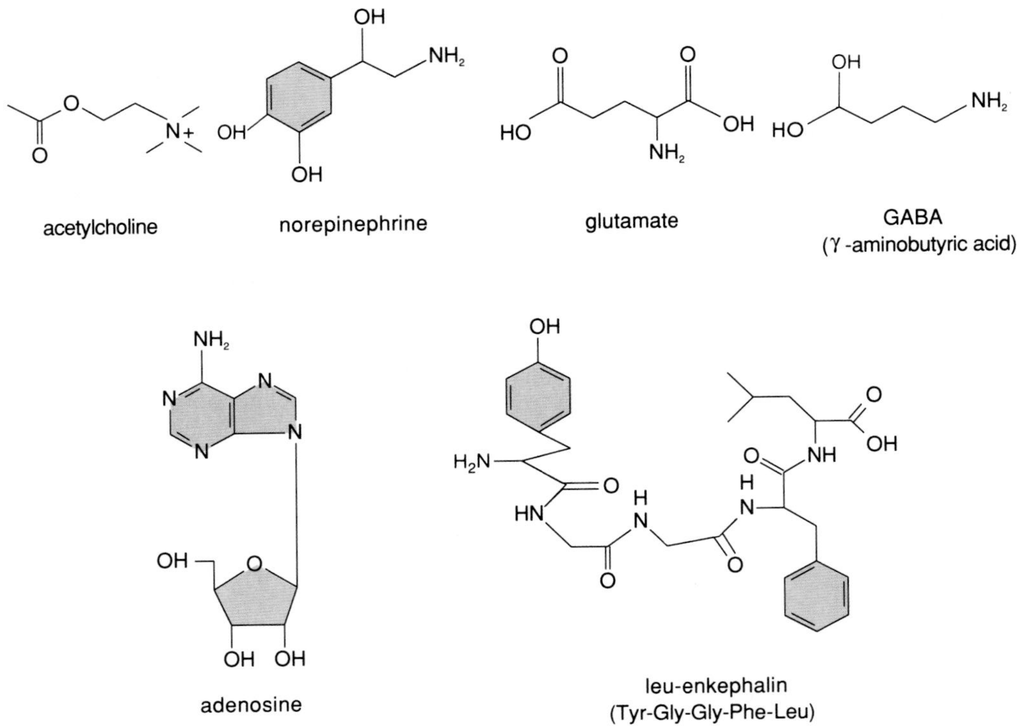

acetylcholine   norepinephrine   glutamate   GABA
                                                                  (γ-aminobutyric acid)

adenosine   leu-enkephalin
                                       (Tyr-Gly-Gly-Phe-Leu)

FIGURE 22-10   Structures of selected neurotransmitter candidates.

of compounds to serve as intercellular messengers, involving some unique structures but making use of many compounds with other important functional roles.

It is believed that a single neuron will release the same neurotransmitter from all of its synapses. This concept assumes that during development some process of differentiation determines the type of neurotransmitter that a given neuron will synthesize, store, and release. We now know that this process can be influenced by the external environment of the neuron. By manipulations of growth conditions, sympathetic neurons that would normally synthesize and release norepinephrine can be made to synthesize and release acetylcholine. However, after such differentiation occurs it is usually permanent, and the neuron cannot be reversed to a norepinephrine-releasing phenotype. This implies that if the identity of a neurotransmitter can be ascertained at one synapse, one can assume that the same neurotransmitter is released at all of the potentially thousands of synapses that neuron might form with different target cells.

Cotransmitters It was assumed for many years that a single neuron would synthesize and release only *one* neurotransmitter. We now know that this is not true. Advances in neurotransmitter localization by immunocytochemical techniques and microchemical analysis of released substances indicates that some neurons can synthesize, store, and release more than one neurotransmitter. Although this phenomenon was first identified in developing neurons, it is also observed in an increasing variety of mature, fully-differentiated neurons. Two or more proposed neurotransmitter substances are often localized to the same presynaptic terminal, and up to four neuropeptides have been localized to a single neuron.

Two transmitter substances co-localized in a single neuron are shown, in some instances, to be co-released in response to depolarization of the neuron. In some cases, both substances cause identifiable physiological effects when applied to the postsynaptic cell, although this is difficult to demonstrate. These observations necessitate major revisions in the classical concept of chemical synaptic transmission. Instead of thinking about a single chemical signal

Stimulation
frequency

Separate
storage
vesicles

Co-stored
in same
vesicles

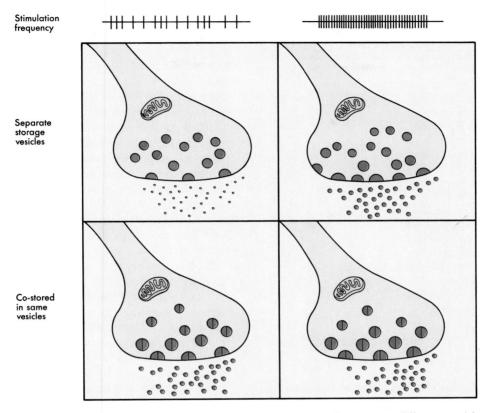

FIGURE 22-11   Release patterns for cotransmitters stored in the same or different vesicles. Note that the frequency of release will be the same if the two substances are stored in the same vesicles but can be different if they are stored in different vesicles.

being responsible for transmitting a single message from the presynaptic nerve terminal to the postsynaptic cell, the possibility of multiple signals carrying independent, complementary, or mutually reinforcing messages must be considered. These multiple signals are referred to as *cotransmitters*.

Several intriguing ramifications to the concept of cotransmitters have implications for pharmacology. First, would the cotransmitters be stored in the same, or different, vesicles? If they are stored in the same vesicles, a constant ratio of the two substances should be released regardless of the depolarization stimulus. However, if they are stored in different vesicles, one transmitter could be released preferentially in response to low frequency nerve impulses while the other could require a higher frequency to cause release (Figure 22-11). The two substances might then convey different messages to the postsynaptic cell about the frequency of impulse traffic in the presynaptic terminal. In fact, supposed cotransmitters are sometimes found stored in separate vesicles, and sometimes in the same vesicles, suggesting that both types of situations may exist in the brain.

There are similar questions about the targets of the cotransmitters. In a directed synapse, one might expect that both substances would be directed to the same restricted postsynaptic target area. However, in a less-directed synapse, one could envision a situation in which each substance has an anatomically distinct target. One substance might transfer messages to adjacent neurons, while the other controls local metabolic processes and activities of nearby glial cells. There is little evidence as to whether cotransmitters might be targeted to anatomically distinct structures in higher organisms, although such evidence is obtained in invertebrates.

Analysis of the presence of cotransmitters in a wide variety of individual neurons reveals a definite

---

COEXISTENCE OF NEUROTRANSMITTERS (FOUND EXPERIMENTALLY)

acetylcholine/vasoactive intestinal peptide
acetylcholine/substance P
norepinephrine/somatostatin
norepinephrine/enkephalins
norepinephrine/neurotensin
norepinephrine/neuropeptide Y
norepinephrine/ATP
dopamine/cholecystokinin
dopamine/neurotensin
epinephrine/neuropeptide Y
epinephrine/enkephalin
epinephrine/neurotensin
serotonin/substance P
serotonin/thyrotropin releasing hormone
serotonin/enkephalin
vasopressin/cholecystokinin
vasopressin/dynorphin
oxytocin/enkephalin

---

pattern (see box). With few exceptions, one member of each pair of cotransmitters appears to be a peptide. This fact and several unique features of neuropeptides suggest the possibility that the large variety of peptides in nerve terminals may not be neurotransmitters in the classical sense, that is, transmitting messages to the postsynaptic cell based on the frequency of action potentials arriving from the cell body. Rather, they may play some more subtle, long-term role in such information transfer, possibly enhancing the message of another "primary" transmitter.

Several features of peptides seem to make them unsuitable for rapid and reversible information transfer known to occur between neurons. First, and most obvious, peptides cannot be synthesized locally in the region in which they are released, because (as previously discussed) there are no ribosomes in nerve terminals. This prevents rapid replenishment of peptide transmitters, and would seem to be an inefficient mechanism for providing transmitter to the nerve terminals. Second, peptides are usually at least 1000 times more potent in causing effects on postsynaptic cells than are other transmitters. This raises the question whether the effects of such potent compounds could be rapidly reversed. In fact, the effects of peptides are usually much longer-lasting and much more

difficult to reverse than are the effects of other transmitter substances. So far, it is difficult to identify specific and rapid mechanisms for terminating the actions of peptides after synaptic release, and it appears that simple diffusion from the site of action plays a major role (see below). This also does not indicate a role in rapid synaptic communication.

All of these considerations raise the question as to whether peptides are really neurotransmitters. Many of the established criteria for neurotransmitters are met by some peptides, but no peptide has met them all for a given synapse. Conversely, several other transmitters (including acetylcholine, norepinephrine, GABA, and glutamate) fulfill all of the criteria necessary to be regarded as neurotransmitters at particular synapses.

In considering the possibility of cotransmitters, however, the criteria for identification of neurotransmitters must be revised. Obviously, if a neuron is releasing more than one neurotransmitter, the application of a single substance cannot be expected to mimic the postsynaptic effects of nerve stimulation. Rather it is necessary to isolate and apply all of the substances released by the neuron at the same time. Similarly, pharmacological modification of the effects of a single substance might not have the same effect on the response to nerve stimulation, because other substances might also be released that would cancel out the pharmacological intervention.

Synthesis, Storage, and Inactivation of Neurotransmitters A number of centrally acting drugs exert their effects by altering the synthesis, storage, or inactivation of specific neurotransmitters. Although the mechanisms involved are almost as varied as the diverse types of molecules that function as neurotransmitters, a few important generalizations can be made about these processes.

The nerve terminal must be able to rapidly replenish its supplies of neurotransmitter to enable continuous transfer of incoming information across the synaptic cleft, even after high frequency stimulation. The enzymes necessary for synthesizing neurotransmitters must be made on the ribosomes in the cell body, and are then transported and concentrated in nerve terminals. The precursor molecules from which neurotransmitters are made are usually common molecules such as amino acids, sugars, and nucleotides, which are widely distributed throughout the body. These substances are readily available to nerve terminals and are often actively concentrated there to facilitate transmitter synthesis. Finally, the neurotransmitter itself or one of its major breakdown products is often effectively recaptured after release, thus allowing efficient reutilization of the available raw material. The major exception to these generalizations are the peptides, as discussed previously.

To ensure accurate transfer of information across the synapse, neurons have complex mechanisms for regulating the synthesis and concentrations of neurotransmitter within the nerve terminal. Synthesis of neurotransmitters is controlled by the amount and activity of enzymes of synthesis, the availability of substrates, and the presence of catalytic cofactors necessary for optimal enzyme activity. One of these three factors is usually responsible for controlling the synthesis of a single type of transmitter. Synthesis of acetylcholine is regulated mainly by the availability of the substrate choline. Conversely, synthesis of norepinephrine is regulated mainly by the activity of the first (of four) enzymes in the synthetic pathway, tyrosine hydroxylase (see Chapters 8 and 10). The activity of this enzyme is regulated by the concentration of one of its cofactors, tetrahydrobiopterin, and through a negative feedback mechanism by the concentrations of its products, dopamine and norepinephrine.

Most neurotransmitters are stored in the synaptic vesicles, which are prominent features of nerve terminals. Concentration into vesicles appears to be responsible for maintaining a ready supply of transmitter in a convenient ready-to-use packet and for protecting transmitters from breakdown by intracellular enzymes. These vesicular packets are then available for exocytotic release. Recent discussion includes the possibility of nonvesicular release of some neurotransmitters (see Chapter 9) (possibly by opening of channels in the terminal membrane). However, there is good evidence that vesicles are actively involved in storage and release of most transmitters, and the vesicle hypothesis is still generally accepted.

After release, the transmitter acts on its target to cause a response. To ensure reversibility of action and allow for further information transfer across the synapse, the transmitter must be rapidly inactivated. The two highly effective ways of terminating the actions of neurotransmitters are (1) rapid enzymatic breakdown by extracellular degradative enzymes in the synaptic cleft and (2) rapid reuptake into the nerve terminal by specific, high affinity pumps in the plasma membrane. Both mechanisms provide rapid and efficient termination of transmitter action. An effective, but much slower, way of terminating the action of transmitter is by simple diffusion from the site of action. Diffusion is more effective in nondirected synapses than in highly directed synapses, because diffusion in directed synapses is greatly reduced by morphological barriers. Transmitter can also be removed by nonspecific absorption into tissues (i.e., partitioning into neuronal or glial structures caused by the chemical properties of the transmitter—without involvement of specific energy-requiring uptake pumps). This process, although effective, can be slow. If a released transmitter persists in the synapse for a long time, a new signal cannot get through. Therefore, the slow processes of diffusion and nonspecific uptake are thought to be generally less important methods of transmitter inactivation than are the more rapid processes of degradation and active reuptake.

Released neurotransmitters are usually reutilized in some form. This helps replenish transmitter concentrations and prevents local depletion of substrates and/or cofactors in nerve terminals. The most efficient mechanism is the rapid reuptake of the neurotransmitter itself, and subsequent reuptake into synaptic vesicles. Norepinephrine and dopamine appear to be directly reutilized in this efficient manner, removing the necessity for further synthesis and reducing the amount of energy required. Other transmitters are degraded by enzymes in the synaptic cleft and the breakdown products are subsequently reutilized for further transmitter synthesis. For example, acetylcholine is hydrolyzed down into choline and acetate in the synaptic cleft, and the choline is actively reconcentrated into the cell.

Information on the synthesis, storage, and degradation of many of the heterogeneous group of compounds serving as neurotransmitters in the brain (see box) is presented in the chapters in this section and in Chapter 8 for acetylcholine and norepinephrine. However, some differences in neurotransmitter life cycles are illustrated schematically in Figure 22-12 using acetylcholine, norepinephrine, GABA, and a peptide transmitter as representative examples. The major differences include the following:

1. Synthesis in the cell soma (peptide), nerve terminal cytosol (acetylcholine, GABA) or vesicle (norepinephrine)
2. Uptake of transmitter (acetylcholine, GABA, peptide) or precursor (norepinephrine) into vesicles

3. Inactivation by enzymatic hydrolysis (acetylcholine), active reuptake (norepinephrine), nonspecific uptake (GABA), or diffusion (peptide)

4. Reutilization of transmitter (norepinephrine, GABA) or hydrolysis product (acetylcholine), or neither (peptide) for further transmitter synthesis

5. Control of synthesis by substrate availability (acetylcholine) or enzyme activity (norepinephrine, GABA, peptide)

Release of Neurotransmitters The arrival of an action potential at a nerve terminal causes a depolarization of the terminal membrane, resulting in exocytotic release of neurotransmitter from synaptic vesicles. Although the physiological characteristics of such "excitation-secretion coupling" are well established, the molecular events linking depolarization of the terminal to release of neurotransmitter are only now beginning to be understood.

Calcium provides the essential link between depolarization and transmitter release. If calcium is removed from the extracellular fluid, there is no release of neurotransmitter in response to depolarization of nerve terminals. Calcium must, therefore, be added to the list of ions (sodium, potassium, and chloride) that are critical to the function of neurons. However, calcium often plays a fundamentally different role than the other three ions. Sodium, potassium, and chloride function mainly as charge carriers, important in maintaining the electrical properties of neurons. Although calcium can also function as an important charge carrier (i.e., in cardiac action potentials), it plays a more important role in regulating metabolic activity. This is because the total concentration of calcium in the CNS (1 to 2 mM), is much lower than that of either sodium, potassium, or chloride (100 to 150 mM)), which are therefore more likely to contribute significantly to total charge distribution.

Similar to sodium, the concentration of calcium is much higher in the extracellular fluid surrounding neurons than in the cytoplasm. This gradient is maintained by continuous active extrusion of calcium by energy-requiring pumps in the plasma membrane and also by active sequestration of calcium by intracellular

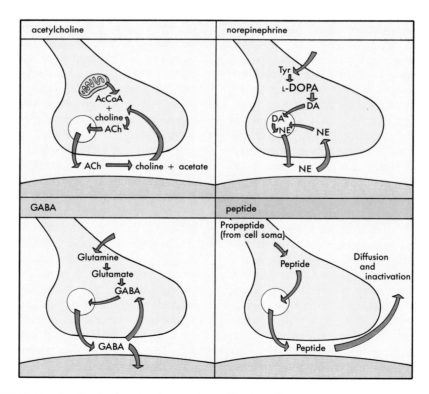

FIGURE 22-12   Synthesis, inactivation, and reutilization of selected neurotransmitters. *ACh*, Aceytlcholine; *NE*, norepinephrine; *GABA*, γ-aminobutyric acid.

organelles, particularly the mitochondria. The net result is a calcium concentration gradient substantially larger than that of sodium and potassium, a concentration about 10,000 times higher in the extracellular than in the intracellular fluid.

When the resting membrane of the nerve terminal is depolarized by arrival of an action potential, there is a large influx of free calcium. This is caused by the opening of voltage-dependent calcium channels concentrated in the membrane of the nerve terminal. These channels are much like the voltage-dependent sodium channels discussed previously. At the normal resting potential, the channels are mainly closed and impermeable to calcium; however, depolarization causes them to open (probably by some rearrangement of charge in the channel protein, as with sodium channels). When open, they selectively permit passage of calcium down its concentration gradient into the cell.

The influx of calcium into the nerve terminal initiates processes that result in endocytosis of synaptic vesicles and release of neurotransmitters. However, the molecular mechanisms by which calcium influx promotes exocytosis of synaptic vesicles is poorly understood. The increase in intraterminal calcium probably alters the conformation of certain enzymes or structural proteins in the synaptic vesicle and/or the plasma membrane, which eventually causes fusion of

these two structures, although the specific events have yet to be elucidated.

The exocytotic release of neurotransmitters by synaptic vesicles appears to be responsible for neurotransmitter release in packets of discrete size, known as *quanta*. Postsynaptic changes in membrane potential caused by low presynaptic nerve activity are always an integer multiple of some basic unitary size. This implies that the amount of transmitter released in response to varying degrees of depolarization is not continuously variable, but is due to release of greater or fewer numbers of preformed packets. The correlation with synaptic vesicles is obvious, and it is tempting to speculate that one vesicle contains one quantum of transmitter. However, in some cases, a physiological quantum may sometimes represent the simultaneous release of several vesicles. The extent of depolarization therefore will determine the number of vesicles that undergo exocytosis, the number of quanta released, and the size of the postsynaptic response.

After exocytosis, the terminal must decrease the high concentration of calcium to prevent continued release of neurotransmitter and allow incoming signals to initiate additional transmitter release. This is accomplished by inactivation of the voltage-dependent calcium channels in response to continued depolarization. After the channels close, the active

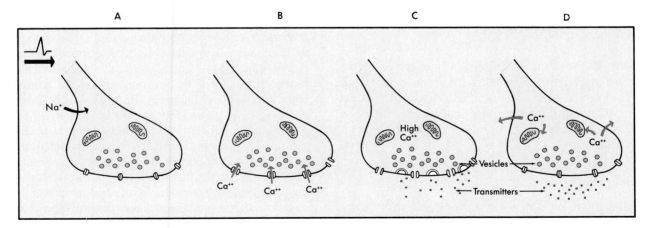

FIGURE 22-13   Sequence of events linking depolarization of a nerve terminal to release of neurotransmitter. **A,** Action potential arrives at nerve terminal and depolarizes resting membrane potential. **B,** Voltage-gated calcium channels open, allowing influx of calcium down its concentration gradient. **C,** The increased intracellular calcium promotes fusion of transmitter-containing synaptic vesicles with plasma membrane, resulting in exocytosis of vesicular contents. **D,** Calcium channels rapidly inactivate and the intracellular calcium is returned to normal by sequestration into mitochondria and active extrusion from the cell.

processes normally responsible for keeping calcium concentrations low within the cell again come into play. These include active extrusion of calcium by membrane pumps and active sequestration by the mitochondria and other intracellular organelles. The net result is a return to normal resting concentrations of intracellular calcium until the next action potential reopens the voltage-dependent channels.

The steps linking arrival of an action potential to neurotransmitter release from nerve terminals are summarized in Figure 22-13. It is important to note that voltage-dependent calcium channels in nerve terminals are different from those in other tissues. The calcium channel antagonists are an important class of drugs whose primary mechanism of action is a use-dependent blockade of voltage-dependent calcium channels in cardiac and smooth muscle (see Chapter 26). However, there are distinct subtypes of these channels that can be distinguished by their electrical and pharmacological properties. The calcium channel antagonists that effectively block the channels most often found in cardiac and smooth muscle (L-type) have no effect on most of the voltage-dependent calcium channels found in nerve terminals (N-type). This is fortunate because if calcium channel antagonists also blocked neurotransmitter release, their toxicity would undoubtedly prevent them from being therapeutically useful.

POSTSYNAPTIC ACTIONS OF NEUROTRANSMITTERS

When released, neurotransmitters are effective only if they interact with receptors on their target cells. The specificity of neuronal interactions is based on the type of transmitter released and on the types of receptors that are present for the transmitter to activate.

Receptors

Receptors are the sensors by which cells detect incoming messages. They are responsible for detecting the presence, identity, and concentration of transmitters released into the extracellular space. They must also initiate the sequence of molecular events that will alter postsynaptic cell physiology in a manner appropriate to the incoming message. Progress has been made in the identification and characterization of neurotransmitter receptors over the past two decades, the amino acid sequences are known for many neurotransmitter receptors, and some specific ideas on the structures of several receptors are available. These are discussed in detail in Chapters 2 and 32 and are not repeated here. Instead, emphasis is placed on the functional actions and interactions of receptors that are of special interest to the CNS.

Receptors have highly specialized recognition sites with rigid structural requirements for binding transmitter. They usually bind only one type of transmitter, although other natural and synthetic drugs also may bind to the receptor with high affinity. Because they are recognition molecules, receptors are named by the type of neurotransmitter that activates them. Although most receptors recognize only a single transmitter, each transmitter can activate more than one subtype of receptor. As more specific and selective drugs are developed, it becomes clear that each transmitter probably acts on a (sometimes large) family of different receptor subtypes.

The rank order of potencies of a series of structurally diverse compounds for activating a receptor (agonists) or inhibiting the response to receptor activation (antagonists) is considered to be diagnostic of the receptor subtype. If a receptor in another cell or tissue shows a similar order of potencies, it is probably of the same subtype. However, if the order of potencies is different, the subtypes must be different. As more and more closely related subtypes are distinguished, the differences between their binding properties sometimes become very subtle and difficult to distinguish. There is no uniform nomenclature for receptor subtypes. Each of the subtypes can often be further subdivided. For example, there are at least eight subtypes of cholinergic and seven subtypes of adrenergic receptors identified so far (Figure 22-14).

Determination of receptor structures by gene cloning and sequencing has had a major impact in this area. Cross-hybridization studies reveal many different gene products that code for closely related receptor subtypes. For example, up to eight genes that code for different cholinergic receptor subtypes have been identified (see Figure 22-14). Some of these different gene products have no detectable differences in binding properties (determined with currently available drugs) and thus do not fit the classical criteria for receptor subtypes. This raises the possibility that receptors might be classified by primary structure (amino acid sequence), rather than by their li-

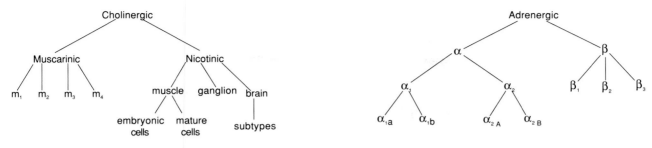

FIGURE 22-14   Families of cholinergic and adrenergic receptors.

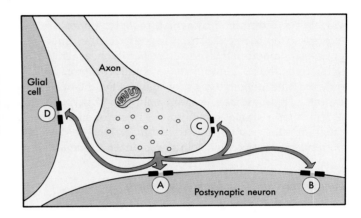

FIGURE 22-15   Potential targets for transmitter released from nerve terminal. Transmitter can activate receptors on a postsynaptic cell adjacent to the release site *(A)* or at some distance away *(B)*, on its on its own presynaptic nerve terminal *(C)*, or on adjacent neurons or glial cells *(D)*.

gand binding properties (see Chapter 2). In most cases, changes in receptor structure are associated with changes in ligand binding properties. Although differences in ligand binding properties will always be diagnostic of potentially useful differences between receptor subtypes, structural differences may or may not. Thus, the traditional pharmacological approach to receptor classification may still have advantages to classification based on primary structure.

Localization and Coexistence of Receptor Subtypes

The presence or absence of appropriate receptors determines whether a particular cell or area of cell membrane responds to transmitter. As discussed in Chapters 2 and 32, hormone receptors can be located in the plasma membrane, responding to external signals, or intracellularly, requiring incoming chemical messengers to penetrate the cell. Neurotransmitter receptors are almost always located in the external plasma membrane, ensuring rapid onset of incoming

messages, as well as rapid removal of transmitter. This allows rapid and repetitive information transfer.

In some directed synapses such as the neuromuscular junction, receptors are highly clustered in the areas of postsynaptic membrane surrounding the nerve terminal. This is relatively unusual, however, and receptors are usually less highly localized. In neurons, receptors are often diffusely spread over the dendrites, cell soma, and axon terminals. Functional receptors on axons have not been demonstrated. although receptor molecules undergoing transport to nerve terminals can be identified in axons. Receptors are also commonly found on glial cells, suggesting that these cells also respond to released neurotransmitters.

Thus transmitter released from a nerve terminal can have several targets (Figure 22-15). It can obviously act on the immediately adjacent postsynaptic membrane. However, depending on its rate of inactivation it can also diffuse relatively far from the synapse and act on an "extrasynaptic" area of the postsynaptic cell, or of adjacent neurons or glial cells. In addition, many transmitters also activate receptors on the nerve terminals from which they are released. These are called *autoreceptors* because they respond to the transmitter released from the cell on which they are located. Activation of autoreceptors provides feedback relating to the quantity of transmitter in the synaptic cleft and regulates further synthesis and release of transmitter.

Many different types of receptors can coexist on a single cell. This includes multiple receptors for different transmitters, as well as multiple subtypes of receptors for a single transmitter. The types of receptors on particular neurons or glial cells will obviously be determined by which receptor genes are expressed by that cell. This is another of the differentiated characteristics of brain cells, which, as usual, is highly variable. Neurons may contain receptors for only a single transmitter or for many different transmitters. Neurons may contain only one subtype of receptor for a single transmitter or many or all of the different subtypes for that transmitter. This has important implications for neurotransmitter actions.

Responses to Receptor Activation

The response of a particular neuron to released neurotransmitter depends as much on the type of receptors available as on the type of transmitter released. It is important to realize that *a given neurotransmitter does not always cause the same postsynaptic effect.* An example of this is found in the peripheral nervous system, where neuronally released acetylcholine causes relaxation of cardiac muscle and contraction of skeletal muscle through different receptor subtypes. Similarly, release of a given transmitter in the CNS can cause different postsynaptic effects, depending on the type of receptors available for it to activate.

Receptors initiate signals in neuronal and glial cells by the types of signal transduction mechanisms outlined in Chapters 2 and 32. In the CNS, however, the most important signal transduction mechanisms are those occurring in the external cell membrane. Thus the primary effect of receptor activation is usually a direct influence on an ion channel or activation of one of the large family of G-proteins (see Chapter 2). Ion channels controlled directly by transmitters are usually referred to as *chemically gated channels,* because the channel permeability is altered by direct binding of the transmitter to the channel protein. Activation

of different G-proteins may activate specific ion channels or, more generally, alter the activity of a membrane-bound enzyme that synthesizes or releases a second messenger inside the cell (cyclic AMP, inositol trisphosphate, diacylglycerol, and arachidonic acid). These second messengers produce metabolic effects on the cell, prominent among which are activation of protein phosphorylation via protein kinase activation and release of intracellular calcium.

Because much information in the nervous system is encoded electrically, released transmitters usually alter the membrane potential of their postsynaptic targets. These local alterations in membrane potential are called *synaptic potentials.* Although it is obvious how activation of chemically gated channels, where the channel is an integral part of the receptor protein, can produce synaptic potentials, the mechanisms by which activation of receptors linked to G-proteins can occur are less intuitively evident because channels that are not part of the receptor protein may be involved. The effects of G-protein–linked receptors appear to be mediated by alterations in ion channels, although these are generally more roundabout than those caused by chemically gated channels, but are equally effective. The general mechanisms by which receptor activation can result in synaptic potentials are diagrammed schematically in Figure 22-16. Regardless of the intermediary steps, receptor activation eventually alters charge distribution across the membrane by altering ion channel permeability.

Comparison of the direct and relatively circuitous routes by which receptor activation can alter permeability of ion channels in the nervous system (Figure 22-16) raises another interesting aspect of transmitter action. This is the speed with which the signal is initiated and terminated. Opening of channels in response to direct binding of transmitters on the channel molecule is clearly much faster than the cascade of events including G-protein activation, enzyme activation, formation of a second messenger, protein kinase activation, and phosphorylation of a channel. It is consequently suggested that receptors mediating synaptic responses can be divided into two general classes based on the time latency of their synaptic potentials. Chemically gated channels would be responsible for "fast" information transfer whereas receptors stimulating second messenger formation would take longer to initiate signals. Termination of the signals is also different. Chemically gated channels rapidly close when transmitter is removed,

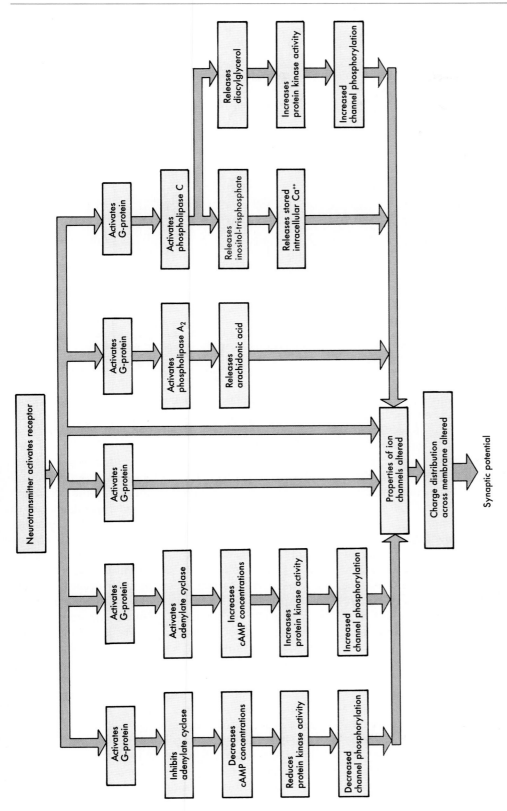

FIGURE 22-16 Mechanisms by which transmitter-receptor interactions can result in synaptic potentials. Ion channels may be of two types: (1) those that are part of the receptor protein and activated by chemical gating and possibly by some G-proteins and (2) those that are located elsewhere and activated through G-proteins. Properties of ion channels include their voltage dependency.

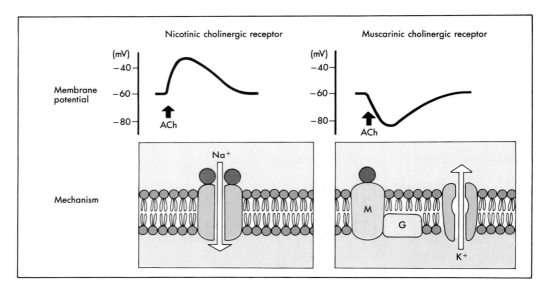

FIGURE 22-17   Activation of different receptors by acetylcholine can cause opposite effects on resting membrane potential. Activation of the nicotinic subtype *(left)* opens a chemically gated channel to allow sodium to enter and depolarize the cell. Activation of the muscarinic subtype *(right)* activates a G-protein, which in turn opens a potassium channel, leading to potassium efflux and hyperpolarization of the cell.

whereas the biochemical events caused by activation of G-protein–linked receptors might persist for substantially longer periods of time after removal of transmitter. Figure 22-16 also shows that the number of intermediate reactions linking G-protein activation to channel permeability alterations vary greatly with different transduction mechanisms, suggesting that responses should not be classified as simply fast or slow, but with various gradations of latency.

As previously mentioned, the availability of specific receptors determines the type and magnitude of response caused by release of a given transmitter. Because each transmitter can activate a family of different receptors associated with distinct signal transduction mechanisms, a single transmitter may cause completely different effects on different cells. Figure 22-17 illustrates one example. Acetylcholine causes depolarization of the resting membrane potential in one cell through activation of nicotinic receptors gating sodium influx. In a separate cell, acetylcholine causes hyperpolarization through activation of muscarinic receptors gating a potassium channel through an intermediary G-protein. Such transmitter-induced depolarization and hyperpolarization are called *excitatory* and *inhibitory* postsynaptic potentials, respectively (see Chapter 2). Thus a

synaptic connection cannot be classified as excitatory or inhibitory based solely on the identity of the released transmitter but must include the type of receptor that it activates.

The situation is complicated further by the fact that multiple receptor subtypes for one transmitter can coexist on a single cell. This raises the possibility that one transmitter can deliver multiple messages to the same cell. These messages may be opposing, complementary, or completely independent. For example, in Figure 22-18 various combinations of adrenergic receptors can be present on the same cell. The β_1 subtype activates adenylate cyclase through a G-protein (G_s). Because the α_2 subtype inhibits adenylate cyclase through a different G-protein (G_i), the presence of both subtypes will result in mutually antagonistic signals caused by the neurotransmitter norepinephrine. In a like manner, additive signals can be generated by the copresence of the β_2 subtype, which also activates adenylate cyclase through G_s, or independent signals can be generated by the copresence of the α_1 subtype that activates phospholipase C (see Figure 22-18). Obviously, the response of a cell to a single transmitter will depend on the types and relative proportions of receptor subtypes present in the target membrane.

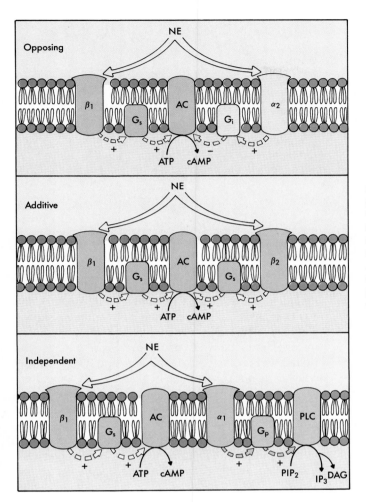

FIGURE 22-18   Activation of multiple receptors by a single transmitter: effects on signal transduction. Coactivation of more than one receptor subtype for norepinephrine can result in second messenger responses, which are opposing, additive, or independent. G-proteins shown for stimulatory (G_s), inhibitory (G_i), and phospholipase (G_p). *NE*, Norepinephrine; *AC*, adenylate cyclase; *ATP*, adenosine triphosphate; *cAMP*, cyclic adenosine monophosphate; *PLC*, phospholipase C; *PIP_2*, phosphatidylinositol 4, 5-bisphosphate; *IP_3*, inositol 1,4,5-trisphosphate; *DAG*, 1,2-diacylglycerol.

Similar situations can arise when different types of transmitters act on specific receptors in the same cell. Incoming messages may be opposing, complementary and/or independent, and each released transmitter can cause excitatory or inhibitory potentials, or both, depending on the receptors present. The function of the neuron is to integrate all of these multiple messages, from a single transmitter or from multiple transmitters, to control the impulse activity of its own axon.

ALTERATIONS IN SYNAPTIC EFFICIENCY

The information output of a neuron is encoded in the rate at which it initiates action potentials at the axon hillock. Because action potentials are an all-or-none phenomenon, their quantitative and temporal characteristics usually do not vary. Degree of depolarization and length of time necessary for repolarization are similar for all action potentials in a particular axon. Therefore a uniform depolarization may cause a uniform release of neurotransmitter quanta, and activation of a given terminal may always result in the same postsynaptic response. In this case, a particular synapse could be thought of as a simple on/off circuit, like a switch. The terminal could be either active or inactive, but when active it would always send the same message to the postsynaptic cell.

However, this is not the case. The strength of a synaptic connection is not uniform and can be altered by a variety of mechanisms. Although an action potential always causes an invariant depolarization of a nerve terminal, the net effect on the postsynaptic cell

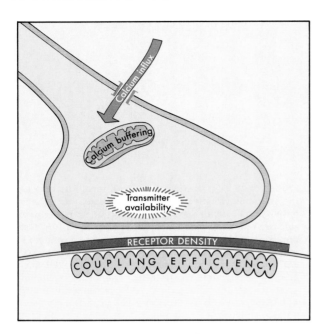

FIGURE 22-19 Major factors controlling efficiency of synaptic transmission (see discussion in text).

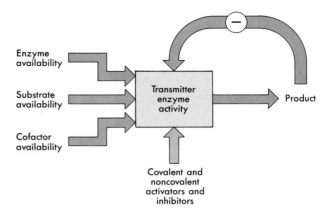

FIGURE 22-20 Factors controlling transmitter synthesis (see discussion in text).

can vary substantially depending on the recent and long-term history of the terminal. In fact, a nerve terminal might be more accurately compared to a rheostat than a simple on/off switch because its output is continuously variable between certain upper and lower limits. Such alterations in synaptic efficiency can occur in either the synaptic terminal, the postsynaptic cell, or both, by a variety of mechanisms. The most important of these are illustrated schematically in Figure 22-19. In the synaptic terminal, alterations in depolarization-evoked calcium influx, intracellular buffering of calcium, or transmitter synthesis and availability can result in changes in the amount of neurotransmitter released by nerve terminal depolarization. On the postsynaptic side, changes in receptor density and/or coupling efficiency can alter the response to a given concentration of released transmitter. These modifications may form the cellular basis of learning and memory, and also play an important role in the tolerance and dependence that are observed on chronic administration of many centrally acting drugs.

Alterations in Transmitter Release

Depolarization-evoked release of neurotransmitters is caused by opening of voltage-dependent calcium

channels. As discussed previously, the resulting influx of calcium causes exocytosis of neurotransmitter-containing vesicles. The quantity of transmitter released in response to depolarization is mainly controlled by two factors: (1) the concentration of intracellular calcium and (2) the availability of transmitter. Each of these is carefully regulated by the neuron and can be increased or decreased as the situation warrants.

Transmitter synthesis must be carefully controlled to ensure that a constant supply of messenger molecules is available to transport information across the synaptic cleft. Synthesis must be increased when nerve activity is high, and decreased when it is low. In addition, one way in which a neuron might change the amount of transmitter released in response to a single depolarization stimulus is by modifying its rate of synthesis. Increasing or decreasing the concentration of transmitter will alter the amount released in response to depolarization and consequently alter the postsynaptic response.

The factors controlling transmitter synthesis are diagrammed in Figure 22-20 and are subject to the following three major types of regulatory control:

1. The amount of synthetic enzyme can be increased by *induction*. This is a slow process, requiring new enzyme protein synthesis in the cell soma, which must then be transported to the terminal. Therefore its major role is probably in long-term regulation of transmitter release.
2. Activity of already existing enzymes can be *regulated* by several mechanisms, including activation or inhibition by covalent modifications

such as phosphorylation, or allosteric "feedback" inhibition by increased concentrations of product (transmitter). Regulation is rapid (and rapidly reversible) and is probably important in acute regulation of transmitter concentrations.

3. *Substrate availability* regulates the synthesis of several transmitters, and the availability of precursors may influence the concentration of neurotransmitter released in response to depolarization. This type of regulation is also rapid in onset, although the rate of reversal depends on the rapidity with which substrate concentrations can be normalized.

Although a nerve terminal is usually depolarized to a constant potential by an incoming impulse, the magnitude of the resulting increase in cytosolic calcium can vary. Several factors control depolarization-evoked increases in cytosolic calcium. These include the resting membrane potential, the density and state of calcium channels, and the ability of the cell to sequester or extrude the incoming calcium. Because exocytotic release of transmitter is directly proportional to the concentration of free calcium in the nerve terminal, such variations in calcium concentrations will be directly reflected in variations of amount of transmitter released.

One way of altering depolarization-evoked transmitter release from a nerve terminal is through axoaxonic synapses (see Figure 22-8). Release of transmitter from one nerve terminal can act on receptors on another nerve terminal to increase or decrease the amount of transmitter released in response to an action potential. Axoaxonic synapses that increase transmitter release are called *sensitizing* and those that decrease transmitter release *inhibitory*. There are various mechanisms by which activation of receptors on the nerve terminal can alter transmitter release. A common mechanism is through alterations in resting membrane potential in the nerve terminal, which affects the concentration of calcium attained in response to an action potential. When the membrane is slightly depolarized, resting calcium influx is increased and normal cytosolic concentrations are higher. Action potentials will then result in a higher cytosolic calcium concentration and greater transmitter release. Opposite effects are observed with hyperpolarization, in which the resulting calcium concentrations in response to action potentials are lower, and less transmitter is released.

Another mechanism by which activation of receptors on presynaptic terminals can alter transmitter

release is by altering the properties of the voltage-dependent channels in the terminal membrane. Second messenger induced alterations in phosphorylation of calcium and potassium channels have shown to alter their gating characteristics. If the number of functional voltage-dependent calcium channels is reduced, depolarization opens fewer channels and causes a smaller increase in calcium and less transmitter release. If the number of functional voltage-dependent potassium channels is reduced, it is harder to repolarize the membrane and depolarization causes a greater increase in calcium and more transmitter release.

Axoaxonic synapses translate incoming information from other neurons into changes in transmitter release. However, alterations in the strength of a synaptic connection can also occur based solely on the recent history of the cell, in the absence of external synaptic input. One of the best studied of such alterations is the process called *habituation*, in which repetitive stimulations of a single synaptic connection cause progressively smaller postsynaptic potentials. This is the classic dilemma in which an initial stimulus results in a large behavioral response, but repetitive stimulations cause increasingly smaller responses. In neurons, such habituation appears to be due to a progressive inactivation of the voltage-dependent calcium channels of the nerve terminals caused by the persistent activation. This results in a decrease in calcium influx and a decreased release of transmitter.

The other mechanism by which transmitter release is often controlled is the rate at which calcium is removed from the cell or sequestered into intracellular sinks, particularly the mitochondria. In situations of intense nerve stimulation, so much calcium flows into the cell that the mechanisms for extruding and sequestering calcium become overloaded. The sinks become "full" and the cell is less able to reduce cytosolic calcium to its normal resting concentration. The resting calcium concentration increases markedly, causing an increase in basal and depolarization-evoked transmitter release. This phenomena is referred to as *facilitation* and is often observed after a train of high frequency impulses. A similar phenomenon occurs in skeletal muscle, where it is referred to as *post-tetanic potentiation*. The same mechanism is involved (i.e., a transient saturation of the normal calcium-buffering system) resulting in a residual build-up of calcium and increased transmitter release. Facilitation can also be caused by other mechanisms such as slow inactivation of potassium channels, leading to slower repolarization and increased transmitter release.

Alterations in Postsynaptic Sensitivity

Alterations in transmitter availability and calcium homeostasis occur in the presynaptic terminal to change the amount of transmitter released in response to depolarization. Other modifications can occur in the target cell to alter the postsynaptic response to a given concentration of transmitter. The clearest example is when multiple inputs converge on a single postsynaptic target and initiate competing signals. Transmitter released from one terminal may cause an inhibitory postsynaptic potential, whereas transmitter released from an adjacent terminal may cause an excitatory postsynaptic potential. The effect of activation of one input will reduce or cancel out the effect of activation of the other input. Such synaptically induced hyperpolarizations that reduce the magnitude of excitatory postsynaptic potentials are referred to as *postsynaptic inhibition.*

The postsynaptic response to a single input can also be varied independently by adaptational responses of the postsynaptic cell. The cell can increase or decrease its response to transmitter in response to changes in synaptic input, much like increasing or decreasing the gain on an amplifier. If an incoming nerve fires more rapidly than normal the postsynaptic cell receives more transmitter and often decreases its responsiveness to further input. This phenomenon is called *desensitization* or *subsensitivity* and protects the cell from excessive stimulation. Conversely, reductions in the normal impulse traffic tends to increase cellular responsiveness; a phenomenon called *supersensitivity.* This magnifies the effect of incoming signals and is useful for amplifying available information when signal traffic is reduced.

Desensitization and supersensitivity can be caused by changes in the density of receptors for transmitter in the postsynaptic membrane or the efficiency with which these receptors are coupled to changes in cell physiology. Chronic activation of a synaptic connection can decrease the density of receptors in the postsynaptic cell membrane, whereas chronic decreases in synaptic activation can result in increases in receptor density. Similar effects can be observed when the postsynaptic receptors are continuously activated or inhibited by chronic agonist or antagonist treatment (Figure 22-21). Such changes in

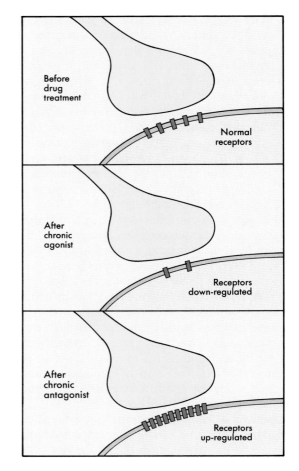

FIGURE 22-21 Chronic treatment with agonists or antagonists can alter postsynaptic receptor density and/or responsiveness ("up" and "down" regulation of receptors).

receptor density are usually relatively slow in onset and only slowly reversible. For example, increasing receptor density requires importing new receptor protein from the cell body, and reversing such an increase would necessitate degrading these newly acquired receptors. Thus changing receptor density is usually a long-term (days to weeks) adaptive response to changes in synaptic input.

Probably of more importance, the postsynaptic cell can regulate the efficiency with which receptor activation is coupled to changes in cell physiology. These changes usually occur at the level of the coupling of the receptor to channel opening or second messenger production, and can be extremely rapid in onset and termination of activation. This makes

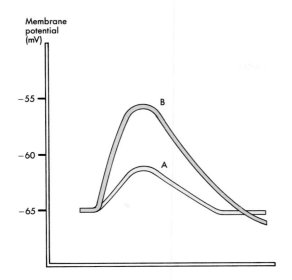

FIGURE 22-22   Excitatory postsynaptic potentials to low frequency nerve stimulation before *(A)* and after *(B)* high frequency stimulation of hippocampal CA1 neurons. The increased response after high frequency stimulation is called *long-term potentiation,* because it can persist for weeks.

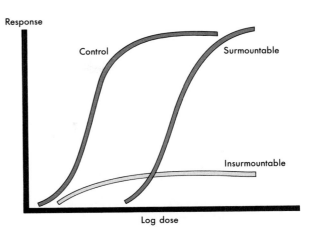

FIGURE 22-23   Types of tolerance. Insurmountable tolerance is often caused by presynaptic depletion of transmitter. Surmountable tolerance is often caused by a decrease in postsynaptic receptor density or coupling efficiency.

them ideal for rapid control of the efficiency of synaptic transmission. Often these changes in coupling efficiency are due to increases or decreases in covalent modifications of the receptors, G-proteins, channels, or enzymes responsible for second messenger synthesis. Some of these are discussed in Chapter 32.

An alteration of postsynaptic responsiveness that has received recent attention is the phenomenon of "long-term potentiation," observed after high frequency stimulation of synaptic inputs to hippocampal pyramidal cells. After a train of high frequency impulses, activation of a synaptic input causes a membrane depolarization about twice as large as that observed before the intense stimulation (Figure 22-22). This appears to be due to an increased release of the transmitter glutamate and modifications in the response of the postsynaptic cell to glutamate. These modifications are very interesting because they occur within minutes but can persist for weeks. Thus this may be a biochemical version of (relatively) long-term memory. Although the precise mechanisms involved in long-term potentiation have not been identified, they may involve long-term changes in phosphorylation of certain proteins such as the excitatory amino acid receptor channels (see Chapter 2).

As mentioned previously, alterations in synaptic efficiency are probably responsible for many types of learning and memory, and are also responsible for the adaptive responses to chronic drug administration. The characteristics of presynaptic and postsynaptic alterations suggest that they might result in different patterns of adaptive responses. For example, depletion of a transmitter from the presynaptic terminal reduces the effect of a drug whose actions require release of that transmitter. This effect could not be overcome no matter how intense the stimulus. Conversely, postsynaptic reductions in receptor coupling efficiency might cause a reduced responsiveness to that drug, although a high enough concentration of drug might still be able to initiate a full response. Such "insurmountable" and "surmountable" types of tolerance to drug action are illustrated in Figure 22-23. Understanding the mechanisms by which synaptic efficiency is altered can be useful in predicting the types of adaptive responses that might occur.

ORGANIZATION OF THE NERVOUS SYSTEM

The individual cells in the CNS are organized into circuits of varying sizes and complexities. These circuits control the processes necessary for survival of the organism and coordination of function. Such circuits range from simple two-neuron rapid reflex arcs

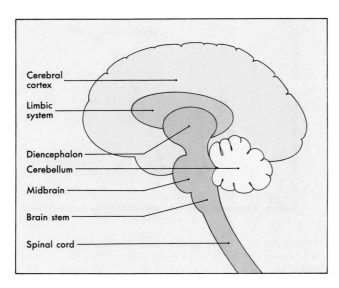

FIGURE 22-24   Major brain regions.

to enormous networks of cells controlling complex functions such as sensation, motor activity, mood, and motivation. Although the relationship between individual cells and the complex functions mediated by large neural systems are not well understood, some general principles of organization have been identified and are useful when thinking about the mechanisms by which drugs affect the CNS.

Major Subdivisions

Specialized areas of the brain have evolved to perform particular functions in higher vertebrates. This localization of function can be appreciated by a quick review of the major subdivisions of the CNS (Figure 22-24). The cerebral cortex is the largest region of the brain where most sensory, motor, and associational information is processed, and where integration of many somatic and vegetative functions occurs. The limbic system consists of a variety of structures lying beneath the neocortex that integrate emotional state with motor and visceral activities. The cerebellum, which resides behind the cerebral hemispheres, provides complex sensorimotor coordination. The midbrain and brain stem relay information from the cerebral hemispheres and limbic system to the spinal cord, and provide central integration of essential reflexive acts. The spinal cord extends caudally from the brain stem and receives, sends, and integrates sensory and motor information.

Each of these regions is heterogeneous and can be subdivided into many smaller regions and groups of cells with diverse functions, many of which were extensively studied. Although obviously interesting and important, the gross anatomy of the brain does not shed much light on the mechanisms by which drugs affect the brain. The effects of drugs are determined more by the phenotype and activity of the individual cells in which their molecular targets are located, and the types of neural relays in which those cells participate, than in the particular brain region in which the cells are located.

Types of Circuits

Neuronal systems are usually subdivided into two major types, *hierarchical* and *diffuse*. Hierarchical systems transmit information in a sequential manner from one neuron to the next, providing a highly directed and precise flow of information. Diffuse systems, as the name implies, are less directed and extend many divergent connections to a variety of target cells. Activation of diffuse systems affects large areas of the CNS simultaneously, often in a relatively uniform manner. Conceptually, hierarchical and diffuse systems can be thought of as multicellular analogs of directed and nondirected synapses (see Figure 22-9). Hierarchical systems provide a highly specific and directed flow of information, whereas diffuse systems blanket a much wider target area; much like serial and parallel information processing (Figure 22-25). These represent two extremes and many neuronal systems combine aspects of both types of information processing.

Many of the pathways involved in sensory perception and motor control involve hierarchical and diffuse processing. In hierarchical pathways, information is detected in sensory cells, transmitted to relay cells, and finally to sensory fields in the cerebral cortex. Motor information is output from the motor cortex through intermediate relays to the spinal motor neurons controlling muscles. The neurotransmitters involved have not been clearly identified; however, excitatory amino acids, acetylcholine, and certain peptides have been implicated at specific synapses. The sequential nature of these connections results in highly orderly information transfer, although interrup-

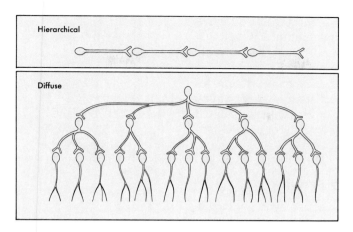

FIGURE 22-25   Hierarchical and diffuse systems of neural networks provide for serial and parallel information processing.

tion at any point in the sequential pathway will cause complete interruption of the system.

As might be expected, diffuse systems have less well-defined and specific functions. They appear to have major importance in many integrated functions of the brain, such as mood, arousal, emotion, and motivational states. Certain of the biogenic amines (norepinephrine, serotonin, and dopamine) and some peptides are implicated as neurotransmitters in diffuse systems. These neurons extend multiple branching axons to many target cells and can affect many brain regions in a simultaneous and relatively uniform manner. Interference with diffuse systems does not result in the dramatic loss of information transfer observed when hierarchical systems are interrupted. Interruption of diffuse systems results in more subtle changes in brain activity, consistent with modulatory roles in more global aspects of CNS function.

Drugs can interact with hierarchical and diffuse systems in specific ways. Actions on hierarchical systems usually result in highly specific and defined effects. For example, anticonvulsants specifically block the hyperactivity of motor and sensory systems, analgesics specifically block transduction of sensory pain information, and antiemetics block vomiting reflexes. The actions of each of these classes of drugs are caused by interruption of highly directed and specialized information flow. Drugs acting on diffuse systems cause effects that, although specific, are more difficult to define. These include drugs for treatment of depression, psychoses, anxiety, and sleep disorders. Although the actions of these drugs are specific,

they are not due simply to interruption of information flow. They appear to be caused by subtle modifications occurring throughout the entire system, rather than blockade of transmission at particular synapses.

Tonic Activity

Another important characteristic of neuronal systems is their level of tonic activity. In the absence of synaptic input, neurons can exist in either of two states. They can be totally quiescent by maintaining a constant and uniform polarization of their cell membrane, or they can initiate action potentials at uniform intervals by spontaneous graded depolarizations. Neurons that automatically generate action potentials are called *pacemaker* cells (such as those in the sinoatrial node of the heart) and their spontaneous activity is often due to a constant inward leakage of sodium greater than that extruded by the sodium-potassium pump. The ability of neurons to generate their own rhythmic impulse activity is another area that functionally distinguishes them from electrical circuits, which always require external input for activity. Thus neurons can require external drivers or they can generate their own patterns of impulse activity.

In a similar manner, systems of neurons can require external stimuli for activity or demonstrate spontaneous activity, depending on the pacemaker activity of their individual components. Clearly, a system with an intrinsic spontaneous activity will have different characteristics from a quiescent system. Although both can be activated, only a spontaneously active system can be inhibited. Drugs that inhibit neuronal function (e.g., anesthetics and other CNS depressants) may have quite different effects depending on the pattern of activity of the neuronal system involved. Any system with a constant level of activity (either intrinsic or externally driven) will be inhibited by such drugs, whereas the activity of a quiescent system will be unaffected.

Excitatory and Inhibitory Systems

The net effect of activation of one neuronal system generally will be to increase or decrease information outflow from the CNS or increase or decrease the activity of another neuronal system in the brain. Whether activation of a particular neural system is excitatory or inhibitory depends primarily on the neurotransmitters released at the output synapse(s) and the types of receptors on the target cells (discussed previously). This has important consequences for drug action.

As discussed, any tonically active neural network can have its activity increased or decreased by excitatory or inhibitory control systems, respectively. This type of bidirectional regulation means that the effect of a drug cannot necessarily be predicted based solely on its effect on isolated neurons. A drug that reduces neuronal firing can activate a neural system by reducing a tonically active inhibitory input. Conversely, a drug that increases neuronal firing can inhibit by activating an inhibitory input (Figure 22-26). Thus a "depressant" drug may in some circumstances cause excitation, and a "stimulant" drug may in some cases cause sedation. A well-known example of this is the stimulant phase that is frequently observed after ingestion of ethyl alcohol. Ethanol is a general neuronal depressant and the initial stimulation is due to depression of an inhibitory control system. This effect occurs only at low concentrations of ethanol; higher concentrations cause a uniform depression of nerve activity. A similar "stage of excitement" can sometimes be observed during induction of general anesthesia, which is also due to the removal of tonically active inhibitory control systems.

Normal physiological variations in this activity of neuronal systems can also alter the effects of centrally acting drugs. Anesthetics are generally less effective in hyperexcitable patients and stimulants are less effective in more sedate patients. This is probably due

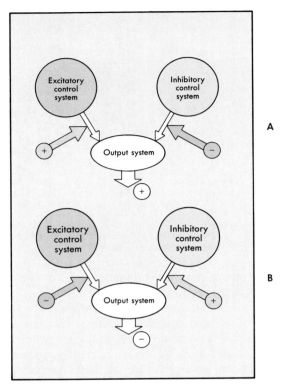

FIGURE 22-26   **A,** Neuronal output can be increased by increasing a tonic excitatory control or decreasing a tonic inhibitory control. **B,** Output can be reduced by decreasing tonic excitatory control or increasing tonic inhibitory control.

to the presence of varying levels of excitatory and inhibitory control systems, which alter sensitivity to drug-induced manipulation. The effects of other stimulant and depressant drugs administered concurrently will also alter responses to centrally acting drugs. Depressants are generally additive with depressants, and stimulants are additive with stimulants. For example, ingestion of ethanol potentiates the depression caused by barbiturates and can be fatal. However, the interactions between stimulant and depressant drugs are more variable. Stimulant drugs usually physiologically antagonize the effects of depressant drugs, and vice versa. Because such antagonism is due to activation or inhibition of competing control systems and not to neutralization of the effect of the drugs on their target molecules, concurrently administered stimulants and depressants usually do not completely cancel the effects of the other drug.

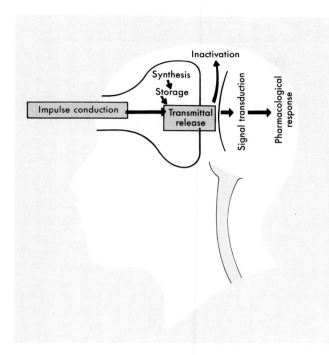

FIGURE 22-27   A pharmacologist's view of the brain.

Table 22-1 Targets for Selected Centrally Acting Drugs

Cellular Target	Class of Drugs
Membrane lipid	general anesthetic drugs
cyclooxygenase	nonsteroidal antiinflammatory drugs
Voltage-dependent sodium channels	local anesthetics
L-type voltage-dependent calcium channels	calcium channel blockers
opioid receptors	opioid analgesics
opioid receptors	opioid antagonists
GABA receptors	benzodiazepines
GABA receptors	barbiturates
adrenergic receptors	clonidine
histamine receptors	antihistamines
dopamine receptors	antipsychotic drugs
adenosine receptors	caffeine
monoamine oxidase	MAO inhibitors
dopamine synthesis	L-DOPA
norepinephrine reuptake	tricyclic antidepressants
serotonin reuptake	tricyclic antidepressants
dopamine reuptake	amantidine
phosphatidylinositol breakdown	lithium
cAMP breakdown	caffeine (?)

SITES OF DRUG ACTION

Almost all drugs with primary actions on the CNS cause their effects by modifying some aspect of chemical synaptic transmission. Thus, a "pharmacologist's view of the brain" is much like the famous "New Yorker's view of the United States," in which New York and surrounding boroughs dominate the landscape, with the rest of the country squeezed into a small area as an unimportant afterthought. Similarly, pharmacologists magnify the importance of chemical synapses and relegate the remainder of the brain to supporting status (Figure 22-27).

Target Molecules

Drugs act on specific molecular targets to alter cell function. The distribution of these targets determines which cells are affected by a particular drug and is the primary determinant of the specificity of drug action.

Drugs acting on the CNS can be divided into several major classes, based on the distribution of their specific target molecules (Table 22-1). Drugs that act on molecules expressed by all types of cells (DNA, lipids, and structural proteins) are said to have "general" actions. Other drugs act on molecules that are expressed in essentially all neurons, but not in other cell types. These drugs are called *neuron-specific*, and usually interact with the pumps and channels that maintain the electrical properties of neurons. Some drugs interact specifically with the macromolecules involved in synthesis, storage, release, actions, and inactivation processes associated with particular neurotransmitters. The targets for these transmitter-specific drugs will be expressed only by neurons synthesizing or responding to certain neurotransmitters; consequently these drugs will have more discrete and limited actions. The various targets for transmitter-specific drugs can be any of the large variety of macromolecules involved in the life cycle of different transmitter molecules (see Figure 22-27). Finally, some drugs mimic or interfere with specific signal transduction systems shared by a variety of different receptors. Such signal-specific drugs will affect responses to activation of various different receptors that utilize the same pathway for initiating signals in their target cells.

Although examples of these four drug categories are found in clinical practice, the transmitter-specific drugs are clearly the largest class. Some of the known and suspected target molecules for centrally acting drugs are listed in Table 22-1. The transmitter-specific drugs are most common, probably because their specific target molecules have a more limited distribution than those of the general neuron-specific, or even the signal-specific, classes. The more limited distribution of target molecules for transmitter-specific drugs often results in a greater specificity of drug action, and is reflected clinically by a lower incidence of unwanted side effects.

Specificity

Although drugs exert their primary actions by interacting with the specific target molecules previously discussed, they also have other actions. No drug causes only a single specific effect, because few if any drugs bind to only a single molecular target. At higher concentrations, most drugs can interact with a wide variety of biological molecules, often resulting in functional alterations to the cell.

To be therapeutically useful, drugs must specifically interact with their target molecules without disrupting normal cellular activity. There is usually a range of concentrations in which a drug will affect its specific target molecule without affecting other cellular processes. However, higher drug concentrations will always have other effects, and the size of the "window of selectivity" is variable with different drugs (see Therapeutic Ratio, Chapter 2). Sometimes it can be fairly large (e.g., benzodiazepines), and other times it will be quite small (e.g., barbiturates). Such selectivity is always relative, however, and it is important to remember that all drugs will also have other "nonspecific" actions, particularly at higher concentrations.

Some drugs have potent actions on so many different processes in the CNS that it is difficult to identify their primary molecular targets. Some of these drugs may cause their therapeutic effects by combinations of specific effects on multiple cellular processes. Others may exert their primary actions

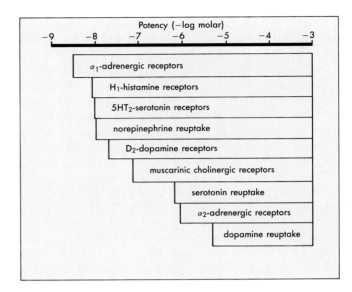

FIGURE 22-28   Potency of chlorpromazine in inhibiting various receptors and reuptake pumps. Note that this drug has multiple actions at low concentrations.

through interaction with a single cellular target, and the simultaneous interaction with other targets does not influence the primary effect of the drug. For such drugs, the window of selectivity is very small, and use of these compounds is often associated with a wide spectrum of unwanted side effects. For example, the antipsychotic drug chlorpromazine is thought to exert its beneficial effects on schizophrenia by blocking D_2 dopamine receptors. However, chlorpromazine blocks many different monoamine receptors and uptake pumps with various potencies (Figure 22-28). Some of the molecular effects of chlorpromazine occur in concentrations lower than those required to block D_2 dopamine receptors, whereas some occur at higher concentrations. Figure 22-28 clearly illustrates that the window of selectivity of chlorpromazine is essentially nonexistent. This is one of the reasons why the use of chlorpromazine (similar to many other antipsychotic drugs) is associated with a wide range of unwanted side effects, including drowsiness (histamine receptor blockade), dry mouth and blurred vision (muscarinic cholinergic receptor blockade), and orthostatic hypotension (α-adrenergic receptor blockade). Also, the fact that any administered dose of chlorpromazine will affect multiple molecular targets makes it difficult to separate out which effects are important for its therapeutic actions.

This example demonstrates some of the difficulties involved in determining the mechanisms by which drugs affect CNS function. As discussed early in this chapter, it is challenging enough to attempt to relate specific biochemical actions of drugs to observed changes in mood or behavior. To this challenge must be added an appreciation for the cellular and molecular complexity of neurons and their transmitters, a recognition of the plasticity of synaptic connections, and the likelihood of multiple targets for drug action within the brain. Clearly, how psychoactive drugs exert their effects on a molecular level are only beginning to be understood.

Despite these obstacles, important discoveries about how centrally acting drugs work continue. Manipulating brain biochemisty and physiology with specific drugs and observing the effects on integrated behavioral parameters is one of the few approaches currently available for relating the function of brain cells with complex integrated behaviors. Increased understanding results in an increasingly sophisticated appreciation of the relationship between the cellular components of the brain and its global functions. Such information will be useful in the future for rational design of drugs for various diseases of the CNS. Another result will be the intrinsic satisfaction of understanding more about the genesis and control of human thought and emotion. Although understanding the actions of drugs on the CNS poses a great challenge, it also promises great rewards.

REFERENCES

Cooper JR, Bloom FE, and Roth RH: The biochemical basis of neuropharmacology, ed 5, New York, 1986, Oxford University Press.

Kandel ER and Schwartz JH: Principles of neural science, New York, 1981, Elsevier Science Publishing, Inc.

Shepherd GM: Neurobiology, New York, 1983, Oxford University Press.

23 Antipsychotic Agents

CHAPTER 23

ABBREVIATIONS

cAMP	cyclic adenosine monophosphate
GABA	γ-aminobutyric acid
IM	intramuscular, intramuscularly
IV	intravenous, intravenously
$t_{1/2}$	half-life

MAJOR DRUGS

phenothiazines
thioxanthenes
butyrophenones

THERAPEUTIC OVERVIEW

Psychosis is a severe disturbance of brain function in which normal perceptions of the environment are disrupted. Manifestations of this disorder include auditory and/or visual hallucinations, intense suspicion, feelings of persecution or control by external forces (paranoia), depersonalization, and attachment of excessive personal significance to daily events, called *ideas of reference.*

For therapy, it is important to distinguish psychosis from delirium, in which a patient has hallucinations and impaired cerebral functions. Delirium almost always has a definable etiology, is transient, and occurs in the course of drug intoxication or withdrawal, whereas psychosis is usually of unknown etiology, possibly of longer duration, and often not associated with drugs.

Many causes of psychoses are acute, self-limiting situations not requiring pharmacological intervention and include infections, inflammatory brain diseases, metabolic disturbances, or exposure to drugs or toxins. Of greater concern are the causes of chronic psychosis, since these longer-term disorders account for the majority of antipsychotic drug usage. A significant proportion of patients with dementias, most having Alzheimer's type of pathology, develop psychoses of varying intensity during their illness. As the population ages and the number of elderly with dementing illnesses increases, this group of patients will constitute a greater percentage of individuals using antipsychotic drugs. Older patients also have special concerns regarding drug side effects, which may be more pronounced.

The majority of antipsychotic drugs are used to treat schizophrenia and related diseases, including psychosis associated with depression and manic-depressive illness. These conditions are usually life-long and disabling. The following conditions appear to be associated with schizophrenia:

1. A set of core clinical symptoms, genetic risk factors, and natural disease progression
2. Neuropathological, radiological, and functional brain imaging abnormalities
3. The fact that antipsychotic drugs are efficacious in alleviating certain symptoms

Schizophrenia is the most prevalent and disabling of the adult psychotic disorders. It afflicts about 1%

of the population worldwide and before "deinstitutionalization" of the mentally ill, accounted for over half of all hospitalized patients. Many of the nation's homeless are chronic schizophrenic patients. This disorder is considered lifelong, with the initial episode occurring typically during young adulthood, although indications may appear in young children. The disorder first presents as positive symptoms (i.e., hallucinations, delusions, paranoia, ideas of reference) that appear in isolation or combination. Frequently, the symptoms develop rapidly (over days to weeks) and are extensive. This initial "psychotic incident" is commonly resolved with drug therapy but rarely spontaneously and is usually followed by recurrent acute psychotic breaks. Recurrence occurs frequently with medication noncompliance. For about half of patients with schizophrenia, the onset of positive symptoms is followed within a few years by the appearance of negative symptoms, which must occur in the absence of signs of depression, and are characterized by apathy, social withdrawal, anhedonia, and extreme inattentiveness to or lack of motivation to interact with the environment. Unfortunately, these negative symptoms are usually progressive, not responsive to currently available medication, and represent the major source of disability for many patients.

Psychotic symptoms also occur in affective disorders (see Chapter 24). These psychoses are characterized by positive symptoms, although severely depressed patients with hallucinations and delusions exhibit negative symptoms from the depression. The psychotic symptoms respond to antipsychotic drugs equally as well as in schizophrenia, suggesting that a common underlying mechanism for producing psychoses exists.

Certain drugs also can produce altered states that appear similar to endogenous psychoses but do not reproduce the true characteristics of psychoses as experienced by patients with psychiatric illness. These drugs include the hallucinogens such as natural and man-made amphetamines (mescaline), substituted indoles (dimethyltryptamine), and lysergic acid derivatives (LSD). These drugs produce intense visual hallucinations, depersonalization, and altered perception of the environment. The production of psychoses with prominent paranoid features also results from long-term use of amphetamine or cocaine. Because both of these drugs are believed to act by enhancing dopamine concentrations at dopaminergic synapses, results support the "dopamine hypothesis

---

THERAPEUTIC OVERVIEW

PSYCHOSES IN WHICH DRUGS ARE USED EFFECTIVELY
Schizophrenia
Affective disorders
Acute idiopathic psychoses
Certain drug-induced psychoses

THERAPY APPROACHES
Symptomatic treatment
Positive symptoms (schizophrenia, affective disorders) respond to medication
Negative symptoms often do not respond to medication

---

of schizophrenia" as the etiology of positive psychotic symptoms.

The therapeutic approaches and major considerations in the treatment of psychoses are summarized in the box.

 ## MECHANISMS OF ACTION

The first antipsychotic drug that relieved symptoms of psychoses rather than merely provided sedation was chlorpromazine. This led to the development of other phenothiazines, also known as neuroleptics (*leptos,* seize). The structures of some of the clinically used phenothiazines are shown in Figure 23-1. The structures of additional nonphenothiazine antipsychotic drugs used clinically are shown in Figure 23-2. Of the nonphenothiazine drugs, pimozide is a potent and long-lasting member, molindone is of intermediate potency, and haloperidol is one of the most potent and widely used antipsychotic drugs in the world.

Multiple lines of investigation suggest that the unifying principle of antipsychotic action of these drugs is the reduction of dopamine synaptic activity in the limbic forebrain. The efficacy of neuroleptics in relieving positive schizophrenic symptoms, psychotic symptoms in other neuropsychiatric diseases, and psychosis associated with amphetamine and cocaine toxicity appears to reside in this mechanism. The multiplicity of the drug side effects, however, apparently results from interference with synaptic trans-

phenothiazine nucleus

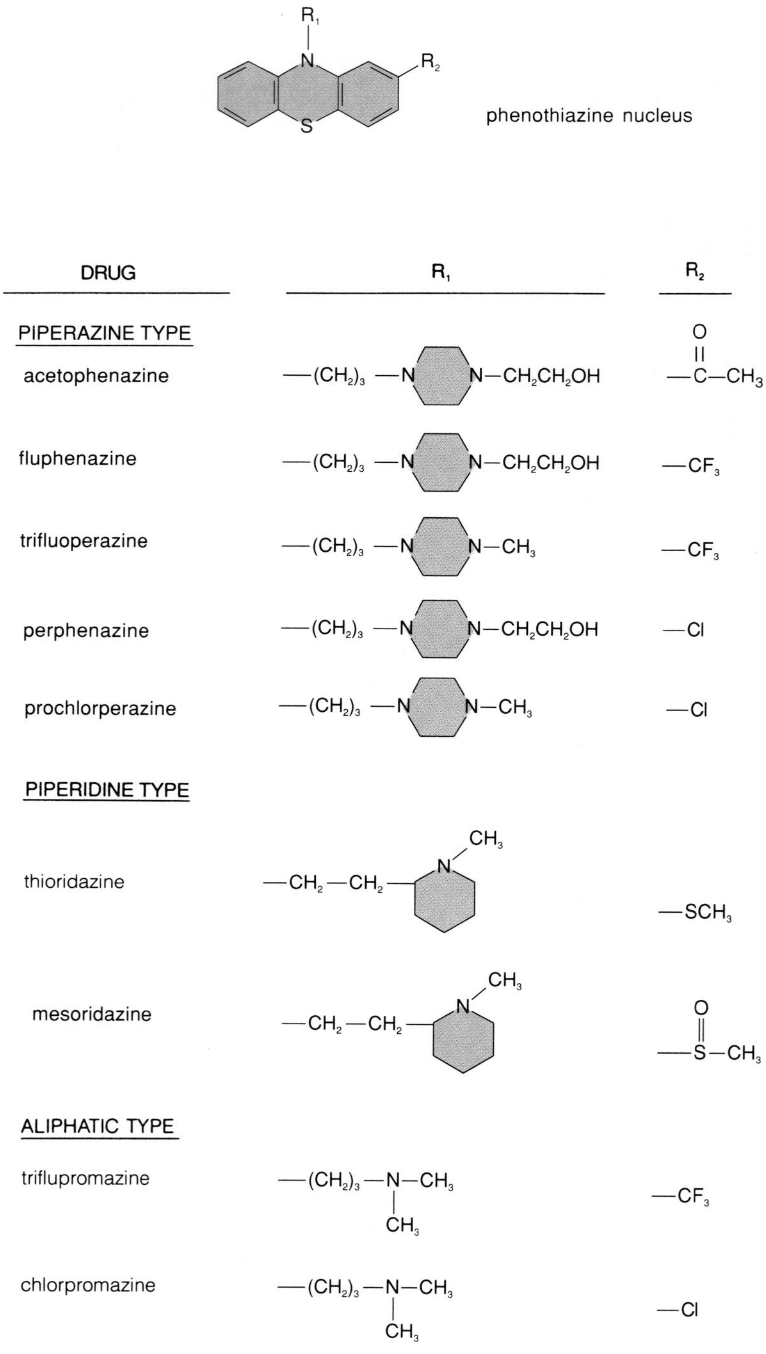

DRUG	R_1	R_2
PIPERAZINE TYPE		
acetophenazine	$-(CH_2)_3-N\!\!\bigcirc\!\!N-CH_2CH_2OH$	$-\overset{\overset{\displaystyle O}{\|}}{C}-CH_3$
fluphenazine	$-(CH_2)_3-N\!\!\bigcirc\!\!N-CH_2CH_2OH$	$-CF_3$
trifluoperazine	$-(CH_2)_3-N\!\!\bigcirc\!\!N-CH_3$	$-CF_3$
perphenazine	$-(CH_2)_3-N\!\!\bigcirc\!\!N-CH_2CH_2OH$	$-Cl$
prochlorperazine	$-(CH_2)_3-N\!\!\bigcirc\!\!N-CH_3$	$-Cl$
PIPERIDINE TYPE		
thioridazine	$-CH_2-CH_2-\bigcirc\!\!\!N-CH_3$	$-SCH_3$
mesoridazine	$-CH_2-CH_2-\bigcirc\!\!\!N-CH_3$	$-\overset{\overset{\displaystyle O}{\|}}{S}-CH_3$
ALIPHATIC TYPE		
triflupromazine	$-(CH_2)_3-N(CH_3)-CH_3$	$-CF_3$
chlorpromazine	$-(CH_2)_3-N(CH_3)-CH_3$	$-Cl$

FIGURE 23-1   Structures of phenothiazine antipsychotic agents.

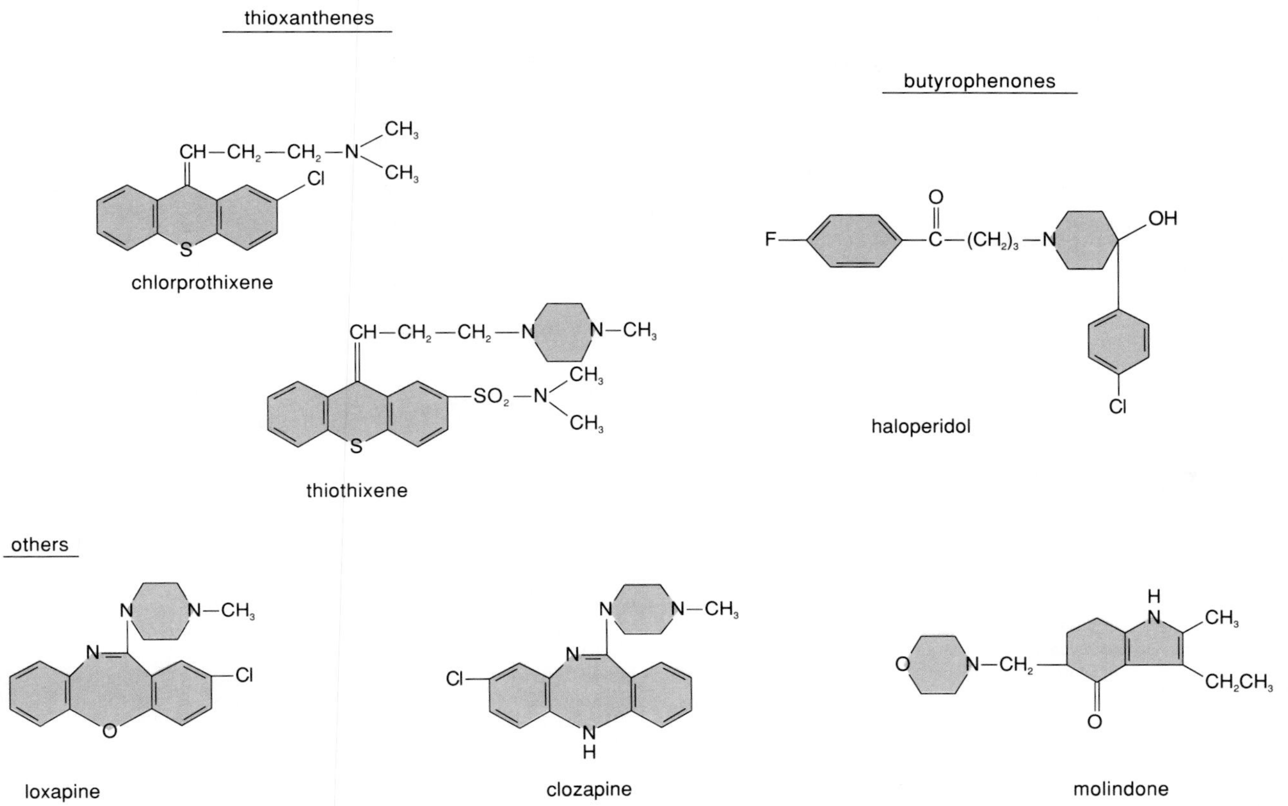

FIGURE 23-2   Structures of nonphenothiazine antipsychotic agents.

mission at other (nondopamine) neurotransmitter systems.

Anatomy and Physiology of Dopamine Pathways

There are four major dopamine pathways in the mammalian forebrain (Figure 23-3). Nerve cell bodies of origin are clustered in nuclei in the rostral midbrain of three of these pathways, with the borders between the nuclei not always well defined. These nuclei have been shown to contain dopamine neurons. Anatomically, the most distinctive nuclei are the paired *substantia nigra neurons,* whose axons ascend rostrally in the nigrostriatal pathway to provide dopaminergic innervation of the corpus striatum (caudate and putamen). The substantia nigra neurons selectively degenerate in Parkinson's disease (Chapter 15). A closely paired nucleus, the ventral tegmental area,

lies medial and dorsal to the substantia nigra and its dopamine neurons provide two ascending pathways: (1) the mesolimbic, which provides dopamine innervation of forebrain limbic structures, especially the nucleus accumbens in the ventral striatum, and (2) the mesocortical, which provides dopamine innervation of the frontal and cingulate cortex. The fourth dopamine nucleus, the *arcuate,* is in the hypothalamus, projects to the median eminence, and releases dopamine directly into the hypophyseal portal circulation. Dopamine is then carried to the anterior lobe of the pituitary where it can inhibit prolactin release.

Midbrain dopamine neurons have similarities and differences in their firing properties and regulation of transmitter synthesis and release. Many neurons have the same type of slow regular discharge, but others fire in bursts of higher frequency. In particular, mesocortical neurons fire faster and with greater bursting than most mesolimbic neurons. In addition, the reg-

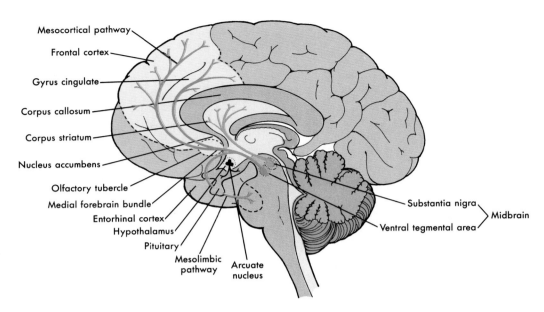

FIGURE 23-3   Anatomy relevant to dopamine neurons thought to be involved in actions of antipsychotic agents. Dopamine neurons in substantia nigra and ventral tegmental area lead to ascending nigrostriatal and mesolimbic/mesocortical pathways, respectively, which ascend in medial forebrain bundle to their forebrain targets. The nigrostriatal pathway terminates in the corpus striatum (caudate/putamen). Major mesolimbic targets are the nucleus accumbens, olfactory tubercle, and entorhinal cortex. Mesocortical innervation is primarily to the medial frontal cortex and cingulate gyrus. Tuberoinfundibular dopamine neurons in the arcuate nucleus project to the median eminence (pituitary stalk).

ulation and effects of neuroleptics on the firing rates of these midbrain dopamine cells differ. Acute, behaviorally active doses of all classes of neuroleptics increase the firing rates of some neurons but not certain neurons that make up the mesocortical pathway. The latter neurons normally fire at elevated rates at baseline compared to the former group but are relatively insensitive to neuroleptics. These and additional results demonstrate the presence of somatic autoreceptors for dopamine, activation of which decreases cell firing, and acute blockade of these autoreceptors by neuroleptics that increases firing.

Firing of dopamine nerve cells leads to depolarization of dopamine nerve terminals in the forebrain and coupled release of dopamine into the synaptic cleft. Dopamine is also manufactured in nerve terminals from the dietary amino acid tyrosine, first by hydroxylation in the 3 position to L-DOPA followed rapidly by decarboxylation to dopamine (see Chapter 10, Figure 10-1). Many in vitro and in vivo studies demonstrate the presence of additional dopamine autoreceptors on forebrain dopamine nerve terminals.

These presynaptic receptors control the release of dopamine after nerve terminal depolarization and synthesis of dopamine on a minute-to-minute basis.

Thus mesolimbic dopamine neurons and associated nerve endings possess impulse-, release-, and synthesis-modulating presynaptic dopamine receptors, which provide an intrinsic mechanism for regulation of dopamine synaptic transmission. The neuron and endings are capable of monitoring synaptic dopamine concentrations and fine-tuning firing rates, depolarization-release, coupling, and synthesis of dopamine to meet demands.

Pharmacology of Dopamine Receptors

Postsynaptic receptors for dopamine are of two major classes, D_1 and D_2, defined functionally by degree of coupling to second messenger systems and pharmacologically by interaction with selective agonists and antagonists. D_1-dopamine receptors are characterized by positive coupling through a stimulatory guanine nucleotide protein, Gs, to activation of adenylate cyclase and intracellular production of cAMP. D_2 receptors in certain tissues are coupled through an inhibitory guanine nucleotide protein G_i and/or G_o to adenylate cyclase; activation of D_2 receptors in some cases inhibits D_1-induced increase in cAMP synthesis. Recently D_2 receptors have been shown to reduce turnover of inositol phosphates, suggesting that they might also influence the inositol trisphosphate-diacylglycerol second messenger systems (see Chapter 2).

Dopamine, the naturally occurring agonist, interacts with D_1 and D_2 receptors, and both receptors are found in high density in striatum and accumbens. Most striatal neurons have D_1 responses and most accumbens neurons have D_2 responses.

Dopamine postsynaptic responses can be mediated by either D_1 or D_2 receptors, whereas presynaptic receptors appear to be exclusively the D_2 subtype. In addition, D_2 receptors on midbrain dopamine neurons (i.e., presynaptic receptors) and on striatal neurons (i.e., postsynaptic receptors) open a potassium channel and would be expected to hyperpolarize neurons and slow firing rates. Ionic responses to activation of D_1 receptors are not yet known.

A remarkable property of all "classical" neuroleptic drugs (phenothiazines, thioxanthines, butyrophenones) is that their binding affinity to brain D_2 receptors correlates closely with their clinical potency as antipsychotics. Although all of these drugs also bind to D_1 receptors, there is no demonstrable association between D_1-receptor binding and clinical potencies.

The dopamine synapse mechanism is supported by clinical results that demonstrate the ability of neuroleptics to block behavioral actions of dopamine agonists and to increase the turnover (i.e., rate of synthesis and degradation) of dopamine. In addition, systemic administration of neuroleptic drugs blocks the electrophysiological effects of dopamine on postsynaptic neurons.

 ## PHARMACOKINETICS

Most neuroleptic drugs are highly lipophilic, bind avidly to proteins, and tend to accumulate in highly perfused tissues. Oral absorption is often incomplete and erratic, whereas intramuscular (IM) injection is more reliable. With repeated administration, variable accumulation occurs in body fat and possibly in brain myelin. Half-lives are generally long, so that a single daily dose is effective. An esterified derivative of fluphenazine requires dosing only once every few weeks. After long-term treatment and drug administration is stopped, therapeutic effects may outlast significant blood concentrations by days or weeks. This may result from tight binding of parent drug and/or active metabolites in the brain.

Metabolism of antipsychotic drugs usually starts with oxidation by hepatic microsomal enzymes, followed by glucuronidation and excretion in the urine. After long-term use, the rate of conversion of the parent drug increases slightly, causing a mild metabolic

Drug	Administration	$t_{1/2}$ (hr)	Disposition	Active Metabolite
acetophenazine				
fluphenazine HC1	Oral, IM	20	M	
trifluoperazine HC1				
perphenazine HC1	Oral, IM			
prochlorperazine	Oral, IM, IV			
thioridazine HC1	Oral			
mesoridazine				
triflupromazine				
chlorpromazine	Oral, IM, IV	30	M	+
chlorprothixene				
thiothixene	Oral, IM			
haloperidol	Oral, IM	18 (decanoate 3 wks)	M	
loxapine	Oral		R	
molindone HC1	Oral		M (95%)	
clozapine	Oral	24	M	

Table 23-1 Pharmacokinetic Parameters

M, Metabolized; *R*, renal.

tolerance; however, monitoring the blood concentration of drug is generally not useful in preventing this problem. In individual patients, very wide variations in blood concentrations of antipsychotic agent can still achieve control of symptoms. Thioridazine, because of its prominent anticholinergic activity in the gastrointestinal (GI) tract, may display erratic absorption after oral administration. Even with regular dosing, especially in older patients, periods of inadequate or excessive blood concentrations of drug may result. The pharmacokinetic parameter values for the antipsychotic agents are listed in Table 23-1.

RELATION OF MECHANISMS OF ACTION TO CLINICAL RESPONSE

All Types of Psychoses

Acute neuroleptic treatment can block all assayable dopamine receptors within hours and induce a state of immobility without sedation (cataplexy), but also without immediate control of psychotic symptoms. It is thus unlikely that blockade of postsynaptic dopamine receptors alone explains the antipsychotic action of neuroleptic drugs.

Typically, antipsychotic effects with neuroleptics require several weeks or longer to appear, in spite of adequate dosages and serum drug concentrations. An explanation for this delay in clinical effect is that the acute neuroleptic action at release-modulating presynaptic receptors increases synaptic dopamine concentrations and overrides receptor blockade. As tolerance develops to this presynaptic receptor phenomenon, postsynaptic blockade becomes more effective. Also, onset of clinical effect may depend on suppression of midbrain dopamine neuron firing, as observed in animal tests.

It is likely that both of the above explanations are operative. Evidence for presynaptic receptor compensation of dopamine receptor blockade can be concluded from the observation that few Parkinsonian-like side effects appear acutely in normal or psychotic individuals given neuroleptics. This is in spite of the demonstration that virtually all available dopamine receptors in striatum are occupied by drug. In contrast, individuals with Parkinson's disease and little dopamine synaptic reserve can be sensitive to low doses of neuroleptic and develop a severe exacer-

bation of their Parkinson's symptoms rapidly (over hours). Evidence for the delayed loss of spontaneous midbrain neuronal firing involves delay in clinical antipsychotic effects and the delayed appearance of Parkinsonism in nonParkinsonian patients.

The proven antipsychotic efficacy of atypical neuroleptic drugs, exemplified by clozapine, requires careful scrutiny of the mechanism of relief of psychosis. Whereas classical neuroleptic drugs tend to interact more selectively with D_2 compared to D_1 receptors, atypical drugs possess little D_2/D_1 selectivity, at least in receptor studies. These two neuroleptic classes are further distinguished by the very low incidence of the Parkinsonian side effects of clozapine and its virtual inability to cause tardive dyskinesia (discussed under side effects).

Evidence suggests that atypical neuroleptic drugs alter dopamine synaptic function selectively in the mesolimbic system, in terms of acute increases in dopamine turnover and chronic suppression of neuronal firing. It is likely that elucidation of the mechanism(s) underlying this dopamine pathway selectivity will provide additional information regarding antipsychotic efficacy.

Modern antipsychotic drugs allow many schizophrenics to lead productive lives outside hospitals or less restrictive lives within hospitals. Unfortunately, for about half of patients with schizophrenia, classical neuroleptics are not effective in controlling positive symptoms. The progression of negative symptoms also leads to progressive deterioration.

Many proposals for empiric drug therapy of schizophrenia have evolved over the years. For severely disturbed and highly agitated psychotic patients, rapid administration of a neuroleptic (every 1 to 2 hours) is used in preference to more gradual dosing. This protocol likely induces cataplexy more rapidly, because it commonly involves administration of the potent drug haloperidol, but does not provide any more rapid relief of positive psychotic symptoms.

All antipsychotic drugs are equally efficacious but differ dramatically in potency and side effects. Treatment choices are empiric and there is no scientific rationale for having a patient take more than one neuroleptic at a time, except during drug changeover.

The common cause of relapse of psychotic symptoms is noncompliance with medication, and there is the suggestion that the ultimate outcome in schizophrenia varies inversely with the number of psychotic breaks. Maintaining drug compliance, which is one of the most important aspects of physician-patient relationships in this disease, may determine lifelong disease severity. Finally, more is involved in the care of these unfortunate individuals than judicious drug prescribing. Lifelong psychological and social support contributes greatly to quality of life and may influence the frequency and/or severity of psychotic episodes.

Nonschizophrenic Psychoses

Psychosis associated with depression may require concomitant treatment with an antidepressant (see Chapter 24) and a neuroleptic. Such combinations are usually safe and well tolerated but some combinations should be avoided. Inhibitors of monoamine oxidase (MAO) in current use in the United States are nonselective and tend to lower blood pressure. Such drugs should probably not be used with neuroleptics possessing α-adrenergic antagonist activity such as chlorpromazine, which also can lower blood pressure and frequently cause orthostatic hypotension. Many tricyclic antidepressants possess significant anticholinergic activity and should be given carefully with neuroleptics that are also strong anticholinergics (i.e., thioridazine).

Psychosis associated with manic-depressive illness, also known as *bipolar affective disease,* is usually treated with combinations of lithium and a neuroleptic. For most bipolar patients the neuroleptic can be cautiously reduced and stopped once the psychotic symptoms are under good control, and maintenance prophylactic therapy is continued with lithium.

Psychosis associated with dementias occurs frequently in elderly patients, usually an individual with early Alzheimer's-type dementia who functions reasonably well during daylight hours, but encounters greater confusion, delusions, and hallucinations in the early evening. For many dementia patients, psychotic thinking or greater preponderance of symptoms occurs during daylight hours. These individuals frequently respond well to low doses of a nonsedating neuroleptic such as haloperidol. In these patients, neuroleptics with significant anticholinergic activity should be avoided because of increased risk of worsening defective memories and inducing toxic delirium.

SIDE EFFECTS, CLINICAL PROBLEMS, AND TOXICITY

Neuroleptic drugs are replete with side effects. Many side effects occur early during treatment and result from neuroleptic blockade of additional receptors in the central and peripheral nervous systems; others appear later in the course of treatment.

Most neuroleptics have some effect at muscarinic cholinergic receptors, ranging from little (haloperidol) to marked (thioridazine). Treatment is associated with dry mouth and less frequently with dry eyes, urinary hesitation (in males with prostate problems), blurred vision, decreased sweating, and constipation. The anticholinergic activity of thioridazine probably underlies its reduced tendency to cause Parkinson's disease but may also lead to anticholinergic-induced memory impairment or delirium in the elderly.

Actions at peripheral α-adrenergic receptors and at H_1 histamine receptors by chlorpromazine can cause orthostatic hypotention and sedation, respectively. Phenothiazines appear to lower seizure thresholds with seizure disorders, with a much smaller influence by butyrophenones.

Blockade of D_2 receptors on pituitary lactotroph cells leads to increased serum prolactin concentrations in both males and females, with the increase in females sufficient to produce breast engorgement and galactorrhea.

Chronic neuroleptic treatment commonly leads after several weeks to mild clinical symptoms of Parkinson's disease, manifested by combinations of masked facies, bradykinesia, limb rigidity, and rest tremor. In individuals with reduced synaptic dopamine reserve, such as those with preclinical Parkinson's disease, the result may be life-threatening. For individuals with mild symptoms of Parkinson's disease, symptomatic treatment with muscarinic antagonists (trihexyphenidyl, benztropine) or amantadine is usually effective and no interruption in neuroleptic treatment is necessary. For those with more severe symptoms of Parkinson's disease, either the neuroleptic must be stopped or dopamine replacement therapy must be started.

Akathisia is a common neuroleptic side effect and frequently occurs without objective alterations in movement. It is an intensely uncomfortable sensation, with patients often appearing hyperactive, but is treatable with anticholinergic agents.

Acute dystonic reactions frequently take the form of sudden spasms of the neck and ocular muscles and can be neuroleptic induced. These typically occur early in the course of neuroleptic therapy in younger patients and are rapidly reversed with parenteral anticholinergic drugs (benztropine or diphenhydramine).

After months to years of neuroleptic treatment, about 10% to 30% of patients develop tardive, or late-appearing movement disorders, *tardive dyskinesia*. This commonly appears in older patients or individuals with some form of additional brain insult (prior head injury, mental retardation). The dyskinesias can be clinically indistinguishable from those of patients with Huntington's disease or patients with Parkinson's disease experiencing dyskinesias with dopamine-mimetic therapy. Most tardive dyskinesia is little more than a cosmetic inconvenience or social embarrassment, but occasionally dyskinesias can interfere with chewing and swallowing food, breathing, or walking. All classical neuroleptic drugs can produce tardive dyskinesia, with the frequency for each drug depending on use. Experience suggests that clozapine has an extremely low frequency of producing tardive dyskinesia.

The known ability of classical neuroleptic drugs to induce dopamine receptor supersensitivity, coupled with the observation of similar movement disorders in patients with Parkinson's disease receiving dopamine-mimetic therapy, led to an initial hypothesis that tardive dyskinesia arises from neuroleptic-induced production of supersensitive dopamine receptors. The major argument against this hypothesis is that receptor supersensitivity can be produced with several days of neuroleptic treatment, but tardive dyskinesia in humans requires months to years to appear. Subsequent research showed that tardive dyskinesia appears to result from decreased γ-aminobutyric acid (GABA) transmission in certain basal ganglia outflow pathways, but required an intact dopaminergic nigrostriatal pathway for its clinical expression.

Treatment of tardive dyskinesia involves withdrawal from neuroleptic therapy, if possible. In such patients, about half experience marked reduction or loss of adventitious movements within 18 months of stopping the neuroleptic. For the remainder, the movements may be permanent. If dyskinetic movements are severe, treatments with increasing doses of reserpine are frequently helpful but carry a significant risk of depression. Limited experience with the

---

CLINICAL PROBLEMS WITH ANTIPSYCHOTIC DRUGS

Failure to control negative effects
Significant toxicity
   Parkinsonian-like syndrome
   Akathisia
   Tardive dyskinesia
   Autonomic, endocrine, and cardiac effects
   Neuroleptic malignant syndrome (NMS)
Poor concentration or dose-effect relationship
Drug treatment choices are empiric

TRADENAMES

In addition to generic and fixed combination preparations, the following tradenamed materials are available in the United States.

PHENOTHIAZINES

Compazine, prochlorperazine
Mellaril, thioridazine
Permitil, fluphenazine
Serentil, mesoridazine
Stelazine, trifluoperazine
Thorazine, chlorpromazine
Tindal, acetophenazine
Trilafon, perphenazine
Vesprin, triflupromazine

OTHERS

Haldol, haloperidol
Leponex, clozapine
Loxitane, loxapine
Moban, molindone
Navane, thiothixene
Taractan, chlorprothixene

GABA-mimetic drug progabide is encouraging, but further studies are needed. Clozapine also appears, in limited clinical experience, to have an antidyskinetic effect in some patients with tardive dyskinesia.

Neuroleptic-malignant syndrome is a rare but serious side effect of neuroleptic therapy that can be lethal. It can arise at any time in the course of neuroleptic treatment and shows no definite predilection for age, duration of treatment, neuroleptic, or dose.

The diagnosis is based on the rapid development over hours to days of fever, autonomic instability, altered sensorium to include delirium or coma, muscular rigidity, leukocytosis, and elevated serum creatine phosphokinase activity. Treatment includes immediate cessation of neuroleptic, induction of muscular weakness with dantrolene or paralytic agents, treatment with a dopamine agonist, and supportive measures. Neuroleptic-malignant syndrome appears to be an idiosyncratic reaction to dopamine receptor blockade, possibly in hypothalamic areas. The clinical problems are summarized in the box.

REFERENCES

Hollister LE: Drug treatment of schizophrenia, Psychiat Clin North Amer 7:435, 1984.

Meltzer H, ed.: Psychopharmacology: the third generation of progress, New York, 1987, Raven Press.

Seiden LS an Balster RL, eds.: Behavioral pharmacology: the current status, New York, 1985, Alan R Liss, Inc.

Trimble MR and Zarifian E, eds.: Psychopharmacology of the limbic system, New York, 1985, Oxford University Press.

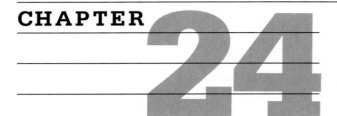

CHAPTER 24

Drugs For Affective (Mood) Disorders

<table>
<tr><td colspan="2" align="center">ABBREVIATIONS</td></tr>
<tr><td>ACh</td><td>acetylcholine</td></tr>
<tr><td>5-HT</td><td>5-hydroxytryptamine</td></tr>
<tr><td>MAO</td><td>monoamine oxidase</td></tr>
<tr><td>GABA</td><td>γ-aminobutyric acid</td></tr>
</table>

<table>
<tr><td align="center">MAJOR DRUGS</td></tr>
<tr><td>tricyclic antidepressants
monoamine oxidase inhibitors
fluoxetine
trazodone</td></tr>
</table>

 ## THERAPEUTIC OVERVIEW

Affective disorders are characterized by severe disturbances of mood and range from depression (unipolar affective disorder) to manic-depressive illness (bipolar affective disorder). These disorders are accompanied by multiple derangements of normal biological processes, including neuroendocrine circadian rhythms. In severe forms, patients develop positive psychotic symptoms (see Chapter 23) and become separated from reality, producing psychotic depression or manic-depressive psychosis.

All persons experience periods of despondency and despair, as well as feelings of extreme well-being. One view is that depression and manic-depressive disorders represent extreme expressions of otherwise normal emotional swings. Although this has conceptual appeal, the biology of affective disorders suggests that these illnesses represent major alterations in normal brain function.

Depression is one of the most underdiagnosed and undertreated of the medical illnesses. About 10% of the adult population can expect to experience a period of depression serious enough to require medical

intervention during a lifetime. Many depressions occur as a result of definable life stresses, whereas other depressions occur without identifiable stresses and are considered *endogenous.*

Typical symptoms of depression include continuous sadness, anhedonia (loss of interest and pleasure in activities), crying spells, emotional lability, and feelings of guilt, worthlessness, and hopelessness. Some individuals exhibit symptoms characterized by anxiety and agitation, particularly the elderly. Depression requiring medical treatment is usually accompanied by biological abnormalities, termed *vegetative signs,* which include decreased appetite, weight loss, gastrointestinal (GI) disturbances (frequently constipation), fatigue, difficulty concentrating, and loss of libido. Depression also causes disturbances of sleep, characterized by early morning awakening. Many depressed persons have alterations in the activity of the hypothalamic-pituitary-adrenal axis. Depression can impair the immune system and may lead to increased susceptibility to infection and risk of cancer.

Manic symptoms are truly the opposite of depression. Whereas depressed patients are at risk of death by suicide from a feeling of hopelessness, manic patients are at risk of physiological exhaustion from lack

---

THERAPEUTIC OVERVIEW

AFFECTIVE DISORDERS

Unipolar

Depression or mania (not both)

Bipolar

Recurring depression and mania (both)

THERAPY

Act on biogenic amines to inhibit amine transport
   and density of amine receptors
Several mechanisms involved
Successful therapy requires several months
Produce significant side effects

---

of sleep and endless activity. Patients with mania invariably experience depression at least once and, more frequently, cycle between the two states with an individually consistent cycle length, usually measured in months. Rare individuals have cycle lengths measured in days or even hours and are called *rapid cyclers* if their cycle length is less than 3 months.

Drugs can be used to treat depression, control manic symptoms, and prevent relapse into mania or depression. However, chronic use of certain drugs such as opiates, sedative-hynotics, and agents that interfere with the synthesis or storage of bioamines can lead to depression. The main therapeutic considerations for treatment of depression and manic symptoms are summarized in the box.

MECHANISMS OF ACTION

Biogenic Amine Systems

Although the primary biochemical abnormalities responsible for depression and manic-depressive illnesses remain unknown, most drugs used in treating these illnesses appear to act through the brain biogenic amine systems. Both norepinephrine and 5-hydroxy tryptamine (5-HT) (also called *serotonin*) neuronal cell bodies are present in the brainstem. In the floor of the fourth ventricle, paired locus ceruleus nuclei contain norepinephrine cell bodies whose axons ascend in dorsal and ventral bundles to provide nor-

adrenergic innervation of the entire forebrain (Figure 24-1). 5-HT containing neurons in the dorsal and median raphe nuclei provide 5-HT innervation of the forebrain (Figure 24-1). The organization and physiology of the dopamine nuclei and pathways are similar to those discussed in Chapter 23. The various biogenic amine neuronal systems share physiological similarities. The nerve cells fire slowly and regularly, although their circadian patterns of firing and responses to stress may differ. Most cell bodies and nerve terminals possess neurotransmitter receptors, at least of the impulse-modulating and release-modulating varieties, which provide regulation of neuronal firing rates and the degree of depolarization-neurotransmitter release coupling. There are also interconnections between different types of biogenic amine systems, for instance, communication from the locus ceruleus through γ-aminobutyric acid (GABA) interneurons to raphe neurons. Thus firing of locus ceruleus cells disinhibits raphe cells.

Antidepressant Drugs

Three classes of drugs are used clinically in the treatment of depression: (1) tricyclic antidepressants, (2) monoamine oxidase (MAO) inhibitors, and (3) atypical antidepressants.

The tricyclics are the most widely prescribed antidepressant group. Several active metabolites of parent antidepressants are also available for separate clinical use as active drugs (see pharmacokinetics). The structures of some of the clinically used tricyclic antidepressants are shown in Figure 24-2. Structures of several atypical antidepressants are shown in Figure 24-3.

The tricyclic antidepressants act primarily by inhibiting cellular reuptake of amines, although other actions also occur. All biogenic amine transmitters are conserved and their synaptic actions terminated by substrate-selective nerve terminal reuptake systems as discussed in Chapter 10. These active transport, energy-driven systems appear to be common sites of action of tricyclic antidepressants with varying degrees of selectivity towards inhibiting norepinephrine and dopamine compared to 5-HT carriers (Figure 24-4).

The atypical antidepressant fluoxetine appears to be a very specific inhibitor of nerve terminal 5-HT transport. This is important because other atypical antidepressants, exemplified by trazodone, have

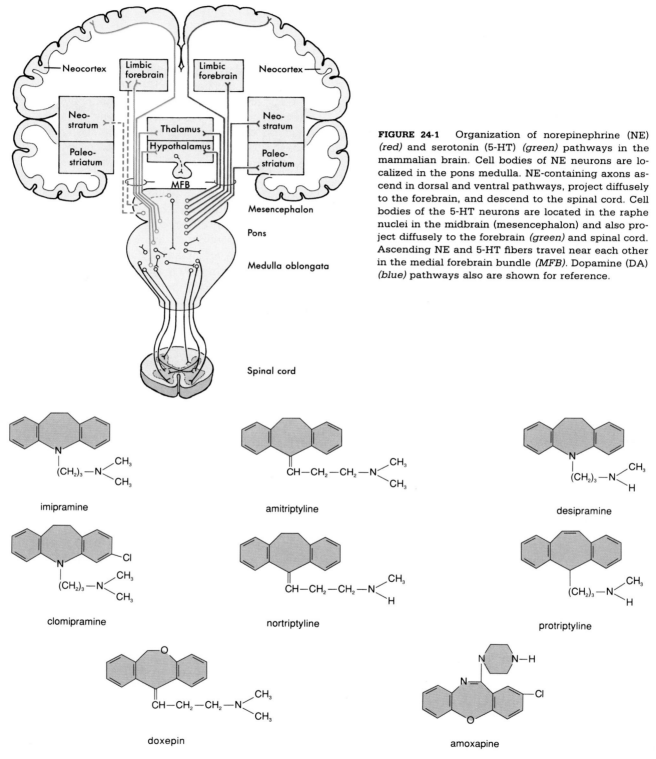

FIGURE 24-1 Organization of norepinephrine (NE) *(red)* and serotonin (5-HT) *(green)* pathways in the mammalian brain. Cell bodies of NE neurons are localized in the pons medulla. NE-containing axons ascend in dorsal and ventral pathways, project diffusely to the forebrain, and descend to the spinal cord. Cell bodies of the 5-HT neurons are located in the raphe nuclei in the midbrain (mesencephalon) and also project diffusely to the forebrain *(green)* and spinal cord. Ascending NE and 5-HT fibers travel near each other in the medial forebrain bundle *(MFB)*. Dopamine (DA) *(blue)* pathways also are shown for reference.

FIGURE 24-2 Chemical structures of major types of clinically used tricyclic antidepressants.

MAO inhibitors

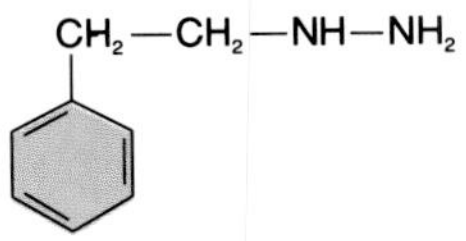

CH_2—CH_2—NH—NH_2

phenelzine

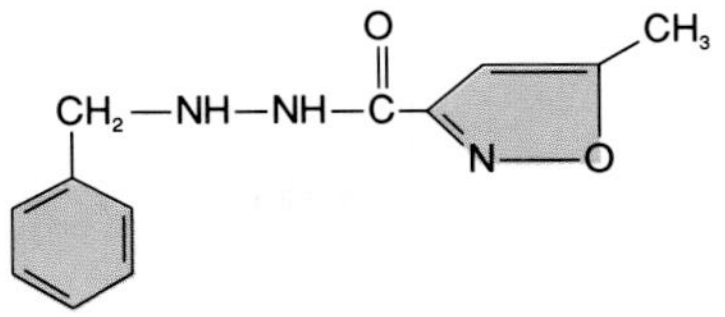

CH_2—NH—NH—$\overset{\overset{\displaystyle O}{\|}}{C}$—$\underset{isoxazole}{}$ CH_3

isocarboxazid

$\underset{\displaystyle CH}{\overset{\displaystyle CH_2}{\diagup\diagdown}}$CH—CH—$NH_2$

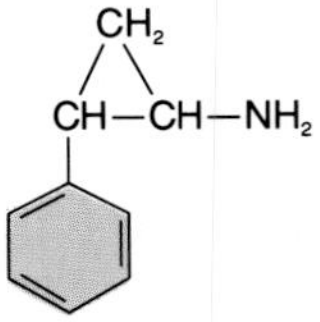

tranylcypromine

tetracyclic

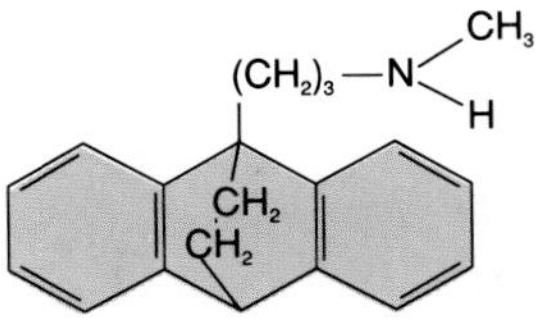

$(CH_2)_3$—$N\overset{\displaystyle CH_3}{\underset{\displaystyle H}{}}$

maprotiline

atypical

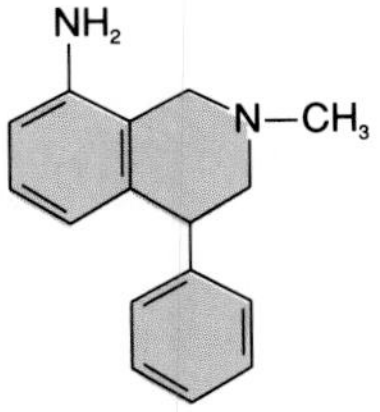

NH_2

N—CH_3

nomifensine

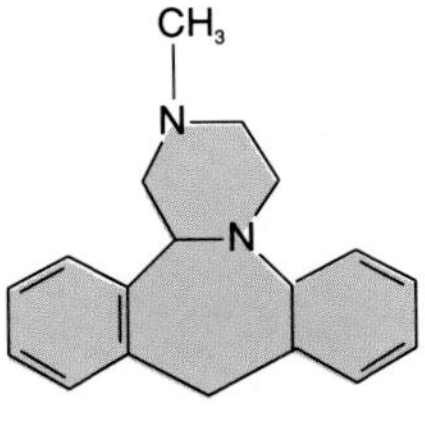

CH_3

N

N

mianserin

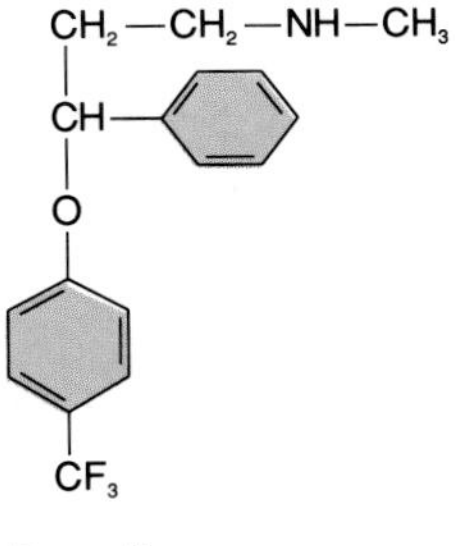

CH_2—CH_2—NH—CH_3

CH

O

CF_3

fluoxetine

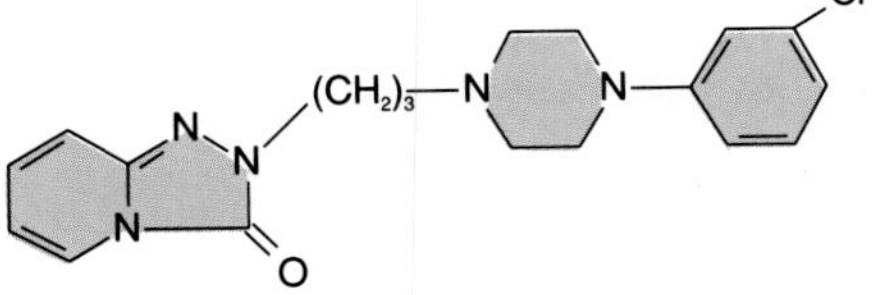

$(CH_2)_3$—N N

Cl

N
N

N

O

trazodone

$\overset{\overset{\displaystyle O}{\|}}{C}$—$CH$—$CH_3$

NH—$C(CH_3)_3$

Cl

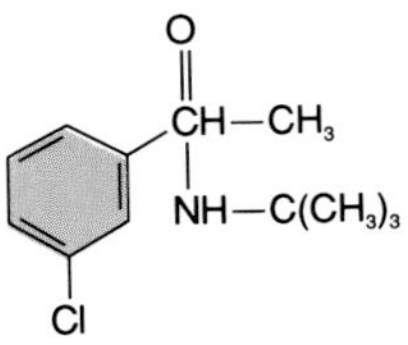

bupropion

FIGURE 24-3 Chemical structures of MAO inhibitors and atypical non-tricyclic antidepressants used in the United States.

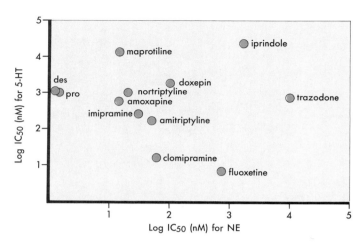

FIGURE 24-4   Relative abilities of antidepressants to inhibit norepinephrine (NE) and serotonin (5-HT) uptake into nerve terminals. An IC_{50} value is the concentration of drug that blocks 50% of the high-affinity uptake of NE or 5-HT into nerve terminals measured in vitro. A smaller IC_{50} means the drug is more potent in inhibition of uptake. *des*, desipramine; *pro*, protriptyline.

much weaker effects on nerve terminal amine transport (see Figure 24-4). In this figure, the binding affinities of the antidepressant drugs for 5-HT and NE receptors are shown in a single plot. Iprindole and trazodone are the least selective drugs shown. Fluoxetine is the most selective for 5-HT receptors, and desipramine (des) and protriptyline (pro) are most selective for NE receptors.

The structures of the MAO inhibitors used clinically in the United States are also shown in Figure 24-3. MAO catalyzes the metabolism of the biogenic amines. Two MAO inhibitors, phenelzine and isocarboxazid, are "suicide substrates" for MAO, in that these drugs become irreversibly bound to and inactivate the active site of the enzyme. The third available agent, tranylcypromine, is also irreversible. Because MAO is a mitochondrial enzyme and is synthesized slowly, virtually complete and continuous inhibition is possible. MAO activity appears important for regulation of intraneuronal stores of amine transmitters, particularly in nerve endings.

There are two major isoenzymes of MAO: types A and B. A is selectively inhibited by clorgyline (not used clinically in the United States) and primarily degrades 5-HT. B is selectively inhibited by deprenyl (used in the United States for treatment of Parkinson's disease, see Chapter 15) and primarily degrades phenylethylamine and dopamine. Currently available MAO inhibitors used for treating depression are relatively nonselective for the A or B isoenzymes. Clin-

ical studies indicate that selective inhibition of type B MAO does not improve depression. Thus antidepressant activity appears to reside primarily in inhibition of the A isoenzyme.

The time-course of antidepressant clinical effects and binding to various neuroreceptors differ widely. The effects of antidepressant drugs to inhibit biogenic amine transport and MAO degradation of biogenic amines can be demonstrated within hours after administration to animals. But the clinical effects of long-term administration of these drugs on biogenic amine receptor systems require several weeks of treatment to develop. The recognized effects of long-term antidepressant treatment on potency of amine receptor binding in experimental animals is summarized in Table 24-1. Although consistent reduction in β-adrenergic receptor density can be understood as a result of (1) tricyclic inhibition of norepinephrine uptake, (2) increase in synaptic norepinephrine concentrations, and (3) resulting receptor desensitization, the mechanism behind the tricyclic-induced increase in α_1-adrenergic receptor binding is less obvious. Tricyclic effects on 5-HT function include reductions or increases in receptor binding for $5\text{-}HT_1$ and $5\text{-}HT_2$ subtypes but increased physiological responsiveness to activation of 5-HT pathways or to the direct application of 5-HT to neurons (see p. 347). Chronic treatment with MAO inhibitors lowers biogenic amine receptor binding and responsiveness for all subtypes (see Table 24-2).

Table 24-1   Relative Binding Affinities of Antidepressants on Amine Receptors

| Drug | ACh | Relative Binding of Drug to Receptor* (%) | | |
		α_1-Adrenergic	α_2-Adrenergic	H_1
amitriptyline	100	92	100	30
protriptyline	49	12	11	.06
doxepin	25	100	77	100
imipramine	18	32	24	.2
clomipramine	13	52	24	—
nortriptyline	6	36	36	.2
maprotiline	6	27	8	—
amoxapine	3	48	29	—
desipramine	3	18	11	.01
iprindole	.6	.4	9	.03
fluoxetine	.4	.3	6	—
trazodone	.01	34	77	.006

ACh, Muscarinic cholinergic receptor; H_1, histamine receptor.
*Binding to receptor is determined in vitro with transmitter and then IC_{50} concentration of drug is determined at each receptor type. The relative affinities are calculated as IC_{50} of most potent drug/IC_{50} of related, less potent drug and the result multiplied by 100. Thus, for ACh, amitriptyline IC_{50} = 1 nM and doxepin IC_{50} = 4nM.

Table 24-2   Effects of Long-Term Antidepressant Treatment on 5-HT Neurotransmission*

| Drug Class | Site | | | |
	Somatodendritic Presynaptic Receptor	Nerve Terminal Presynaptic Receptor	Postsynaptic Receptor	Net Effect
tricyclic antidepressant	0	0	increase	increase
MAO inhibitor	decrease	0	0/decrease	increase
5-HT uptake blocker	decrease	decrease	0	increase

0, No effect.
*Studies in animals with antidepressant drugs administered daily for 2 to 3 weeks; drug effects on presynaptic and postsynaptic receptors determined electrophysiologically by direct application of 5-HT or 5-HT agonists to 5-HT neurons (presynaptic receptors) or cortical neurons (postsynaptic receptors); net effect on 5-HT transmission determined by direct stimulation of 5-HT pathways.

Obviously, no single biochemical effect can explain the mechanism of action of antidepressant drugs. It is unlikely that inhibition of biogenic amine uptake or degradation, in isolation, can correct the fundamental chemical abnormalities of depression. However, the available data suggest that manipulation of biogenic amine synaptic transmission is involved in antidepressant action.

One hypothesis is that antidepressants increase the efficiency of transmission through 5-HT pathways but by different molecular mechanisms. The evidence on relative binding affinities for various amine recep-

tors in experimental animals is summarized in Table 24-1. In these studies and those of Table 24-2, long-term administration of drugs shows that: (1) typical tricyclic drugs increase physiological sensitivity of postsynaptic 5-HT receptors; (2) MAO inhibitors (type A only) decrease presynaptic receptor sensitivity on 5-HT neurons and nerve endings; (3) 5-HT uptake blockers, exemplified by fluoxetine, also decrease presynaptic receptor sensitivity without altering sensitivity of postsynaptic 5-HT receptors. The net effect of each of these alterations is to increase 5-HT synaptic transmission if the firing rates of 5-HT neurons are normal. Although these effects of antidepressant drugs are found after 14 to 21 days of treatment, acute drug administration produces effects frequently opposite and predictable based on their mechanisms of action in vitro.

Antimanic Drugs

Lithium salts and carbamazepine are the primary drugs used in the treatment of manic disorders. The structure of carbamazepine is shown in Chapter 14 because this drug also is used in the treatment of epilepsy.

Acute (48 hour) lithium treatment enhances 5-HT neurotransmission but does not affect 5-HT postsynaptic receptor sensitivity or 5-HT neuron firing rates. Longer-term lithium administration to animals does not produce any consistent alteration in biogenic amine receptor density or function but does inhibit production of receptor supersensitivity, whether the supersensitivity is the result of denervation or long-term antagonist blockade of receptor sites. Lithium also interferes with biogenic amine second messenger systems through inhibition of catecholamine-stimulated adenylate cyclase and inositol trisphosphate/diacylglycerol production at therapeutically relevant concentrations.

Although structurally similar to tricyclics, carbamazepine does not efficiently block norepinephrine uptake or decrease the number of β-adrenergic receptors. Carbamazepine inhibits release of norepinephrine, possibly by acting as a mixed agonist-antagonist at adenosine receptors. Inhibition of norepinephrine release may account for the ability of carbamazepine to increase firing of locus ceruleus neurons.

Table 24-3 Pharmacokinetic Parameter Values

Drug*	$t_{1/2}$*	Disposition	Bioavailability (%)	Active Metabolites
TRICYCLICS				
amitriptyline	10-30	M	30-60	nortriptyline
amoxapine	8	M	—	7,8-OH
clomipramine	20-40	M	—	desmethyl
desipramine	15-60	M	60-70	—
doxepin	8-25	M	15-45	desmethyl
imipramine	10-25	M	30-75	desipramine
nortriptyline	15-55	M	50-80	10-OH
protriptyline	55-124	M	75-95	—
TETRACYCLIC				
maprotiline	25-60	M	40-75	desmethyl
ANTIMANIC				
carbamazepine	10-20	—	70	—
lithium salts	8-40	R (95%)	100	none
ATYPICAL				
bupropion	8-16	M	—	yes
fluoxetine	24-72	M	—	norfluoxetine
mianserin	10-27	—	30-75	—
nomifensine	2-4	—	—	—
trazodone	6-11	M	—	m-chlorophenyl-piperazine
MAO INHIBITORS				
phenelzine	—	M	—	—
tranylcypromine	—	M	—	—
isocarboxazid	—	M	—	—

M, Metabolized; *R*, renal.
* Oral administration.

PHARMACOKINETICS

Pharmacokinetic parameters for drugs used in the treatment of affective disorders are listed in Table 24-3.

Antidepressants

Tricyclics are lipophilic and well absorbed after oral administration; they distribute widely in tissues of the body. The oral bioavailability of most antidepressants is reduced because of first-pass metabolism by the liver. Drug disposition is predominately by metabolism. Some tricyclic tertiary amines undergo demethylation to form active secondary amines. The degree of demethylation varies widely among patients, tends to stabilize for a given patient, and necessitates assay of serum concentrations of both parent drug and active metabolites. The anticholinergic activity of many of these drugs can interfere with the rate of absorption of the tricyclic and other concomitantly administered drugs.

Tricyclics have long half-lives, frequently more than 24 hours, which allows once a day dosing. This feature can improve compliance, which is a major factor in achieving therapeutic success. The atypical antidepressant fluoxetine is notable for having a half-life of 2 to 3 days for the parent drug and 7 to 9 days for the biologically active metabolite, norfluoxetine.

MAO inhibitors are well absorbed after oral administration. Those that produce irreversible inhibition have very long half-lives as a result of slow turnover of the enzyme. Drug abstinence for 2 to 3 weeks is necessary for MAO activity to return to near normal and such an abstinence is necessary before introduction of other drugs, in particular tricyclic antidepressants. Some of the MAO inhibitors are inactivated by hepatic acetylation, the rate of which is under genetic control. Adequacy of dosing can be assayed by measuring platelet MAO activity, with greater than 65% inhibition associated with improved therapeutic response.

Antimanic Drugs

Lithium salts are rapidly and completely absorbed from the intestinal tract and distribute within a few hours into extracellular water and finally into total body water. Lithium concentrations in brain extracellular space at steady-state are about half serum concentrations. Lithium is filtered by the glomerulus and extensively reabsorbed (about 80%) in the tubules, where it competes with sodium ion for reabsorption. Lithium excretion is enhanced by sodium loading and inhibited by sodium depletion. Conditions such as congestive heart failure, ascites, or cirrhosis, which lead to sodium and fluid retention, can increase lithium reabsorption and lead to toxic concentrations. Diuretics that inhibit distal sodium reabsorption can increase lithium reabsorption and produce toxicity. In general, marked changes in sodium intake or excretion should be avoided in patients on lithium.

Serum lithium concentrations peak within a few hours of each dose and then decline in a biphasic elimination pattern. Individual pharmacokinetics vary among patients but tend to be constant for a given person.

RELATION OF MECHANISMS OF ACTION TO CLINICAL RESPONSE

Patients with affective disorders, in particular unipolar depression, have altered physiological activity and receptor responsiveness of neuroendocrine systems and sleep-wake cycles, which are influenced strongly by brain biogenic amine pathways. Antidepressant drug therapy can normalize amine receptor responses but the critical receptor system(s) necessary for therapeutic activity are unclear. Evidence in experimental animals suggests that increased synaptic transmission through the 5-HT system may represent a necessary and possibly sufficient mechanism of action of antidepressant drugs.

The therapeutic efficacy of atypical antidepressant drugs, some of which do not significantly block amine transport or inhibit MAO, suggests that neither of these biochemical actions is ultimately responsible for antidepressant efficacy. Although depression encompasses a reproducible core of clinical symptoms, individual patients may be biochemically or "synaptically" heterogenous and more responsive to particular antidepressants. In large clinical studies, however, no single antidepressant has demonstrated superior efficacy.

It is unclear which, if any, of the known biochemical actions of lithium is responsible for its antimanic and mood-stabilizing properties. Based on available data, a reasonable hypothesis is that unipolar affective disease derives at least in part from a deficiency of forebrain 5-HT neurotransmission, and bipolar affective disease arises from abnormalities in postsynaptic actions of biogenic amine transmitters, either at receptor sites or postreceptor transduction machinery.

Therapy of psychotic depression and depression with significant suicide risk typically involves a tricyclic agent combined with a neuroleptic if severe agitation or positive symptoms are present. The choice of initial agent is somewhat empirical, but drugs with strong anticholinergic activity should be avoided or used cautiously in elderly patients and avoided in patients with dementia, prostatism, or narrow-angle glaucoma.

Because of the cardiac toxicity and anticholinergic side effects of typical tricyclic antidepressants, atypical antidepressants are used increasingly as first-line drugs for unipolar illness. As a result, fluoxetine is the most commonly prescribed antidepressant in the United States.

The major cause of treatment failure is inadequate dosing for too short a period of time. Serum drug concentrations are useful as guidelines for adequacy of dosing. Response times for improvement of affect vary among individuals but usually are in the range of 3 to 6 weeks. Failure of drug therapy can be followed by electroconvulsive therapy. In fact, electroconvulsive therapy consistently produces the fastest improvement in affect in the greatest percentage of patients and is now the treatment of first choice for many depressed elderly.

Patients with mania (bipolar) are at risk of physiological exhaustion and require hospitalization to initiate drug therapy and attend to nutrition, hydration, and rest. Treatment is initiated with lithium carbonate in divided daily doses and a neuroleptic or a sedative-hypnotic (usually benzodiazepine), depending on the presence of psychosis or severity of agitation. Lithium exerts an antimanic effect, but the delay in onset of this effect necessitates initiating therapy to provide rapid sedation and rest.

Patients with documented bipolar disease usually require maintenance therapy with lithium to prevent relapse into mania or depression. Patients refractory to lithium often respond to carbamazepine, with the latter begun at low doses and increased slowly to maintenance. Frequent monitoring of serum concentrations ensures adequate dosing and prevention of toxic side effects.

SIDE EFFECTS, CLINICAL PROBLEMS, AND TOXICITY

Clinical problems are summarized in the box.

Tricyclic Antidepressants

Most of the side effects of tricyclic antidepressants result from their interactions at various central and peripheral nervous system receptor sites. The common side effects arise from antagonism at muscarinic cholinergic receptors (especially with amitriptyline) and include dry mouth, blurred vision, constipation, delayed bladder emptying, and confusion. Sedation reflects activity mainly at histamine H_1 receptors (especially with doxepin) and orthostatic hypotension arises from antagonism at peripheral α-adrenergic receptors (see Table 24-2). Side effects with widely used fluoxetine include arousal, insomnia, and changes in appetite.

An important side effect not related to specific receptor antagonism is cardiac toxicity. Tricyclics

---

CLINICAL PROBLEMS

TRICYCLIC ANTIDEPRESSANTS
Autonomic and Cardiovascular Side Effects

Hypotension
Tremors
Blurred vision
Cardiac dysrhythmias

Toxic Overdoses: Problem With Long-Term Therapy

Loss of consciousness
Acidosis
Hypotension
Cardiac dysrhythmias

MAO INHIBITORS

Hypotension
Side effects similar to those of tricyclics

LITHIUM

Small therapeutic index
Toxicity serious
Interacts with thiazide diuretics

should be used cautiously if at all in patients with cardiac conduction defects, particularly those in acute myocardial infarction. Cardiac toxicity is the most serious side effect of tricyclic drugs. This toxicity results in part from the quinidine-like actions of tricyclic drugs on cardiac muscle.

Patients with known seizure disorders may have seizure recurrence with addition of tricyclics. This may occur from lowering of the seizure threshold and alteration of metabolism of anticonvulsant drugs by tricyclics.

Overdosage with tricyclics can be life-threatening, mainly as a result of cardiac toxicity and/or seizures deriving from anticholinergic toxicity. Relative to antipsychotic drugs, tricyclics have lower therapeutic indices, and serious overdosage can occur with a 1 week supply of drug. Tricyclic drugs potentiate the sedative actions of other central nervous system (CNS) depressants such as alcohol, barbiturates, and benzodiazepines. Finally, tricyclic drug administration to a patient with bipolar illness, usually presenting as depression without a history of mania, can precipitate acute mania or rapid cycling.

Monoamine Oxidase Inhibitors

Therapy with MAO inhibitors usually proceeds without significant side effects. However, this is a deceptive situation because the catabolic capacity of the body to deaminate drugs and natural products is severely impaired. The diminished catabolic capacity is dramatically demonstrated by the appearance of a hypertensive crisis. This occurs after ingestion of foods containing tyramine, a naturally occurring amine that potently releases norepinephrine from sympathetic nerve endings and normally is degraded by intestinal MAO type A. Tyramine is commonly found in pickled fish, aged cheeses, and red wines. The hypertensive crisis can be severe and lead to intracranial bleeding or other severe organ damage. Selective inhibitors of MAO type B appear to be free of this tyramine problem, but have questionable efficacy as antidepressants.

MAO inhibitors should not be coadministered with tricyclic antidepressant drugs because of the possibility of producing central hyperexcitation syndrome. The mechanism of production of high fever, delirium, and hypertension in this drug interaction is obscure. Other reported adverse drug interactions occur between MAO inhibitors and opiates, anesthetics, sedatives, and sympathomimetic amines. These potentially severe side effects limit the use of MAO inhibitors in the United States.

Lithium

Lithium use is complicated by its low therapeutic index and is best monitored by frequent checking of serum lithium concentrations. Many patients receiving lithium develop a fine intention or postural tremor similar to that seen in essential tremor. If troubling, this tremor frequently responds to β-adrenergic antagonists.

The problems associated with lithium use are GI-related (nausea, vomiting, diarrhea). As many as one third of the patients receiving lithium develop benign, diffuse, nontoxic goiter and become clinically euthyroid, in spite of increased circulating thyroid stimulating hormone. True hypothyroidism is rare, but thyroid status should be followed regularly in patients on lithium. Some patients experience disturbing polyuria, and many of these have increased urinary concentrations of antidiuretic hormone. Rare cases of nephrogenic diabetes insipidus have been attributed to lithium. Delayed impairment of renal function not due to altered free water metabolism has also been described, but its relation to lithium concentrations is not clear. Toxic doses of lithium cause permanent renal damage in animals; some patients on long-term lithium have abnormal renal biopsies, particularly those with polyuria.

Thyroid and renal complications may result from the ability of lithium to inhibit adenylate cyclase stimulation by a variety of hormones, including thyroxine and antidiuretic hormone. Serious lithium toxicity is usually related to increased serum concentrations and primarily affects the CNS. Varying signs and severity of toxic encephalopathy, including coma, are observed. Finally, lithium has potential fetal toxicity and its use in pregnancy must be questioned and closely regulated.

Most carbamazepine toxicity is related to elevated serum concentrations that affect the CNS, commonly with confusion, sedation, or progressive ataxia. Carbamazepine toxicity is easily treated by a reduction in dose. Serious toxic reactions are rare and cause bone marrow agranulocytosis or liver allergic hepatitis.

TRADENAMES

In addition to generic and fixed combination preparations, the following tradenamed materials are available in the United States.

TRICYCLIC ANTIDEPRESSANTS

Anafranil, clomipramine
Asendin, amoxapine
Aventyl, nortriptyline
Elavil, amitriptyline
Norpramin, desipramine
Sinequan, doxepin
Tofranil, imipramine
Vivactil, protriptyline

MAO INHIBITORS

Marplan, isocarboxazid
Nardil, phenelzine sulfate
Parnate, tranylcypromine sulfate

OTHERS

Desyrel, trazodone
Ludiomil, maprotiline
Prozac, fluoxetine

REFERENCES

Baldessarini RJ: Chemotherapy in psychiatry: principles and practice, Cambridge, Mass, 1985, Harvard University Press.

Cooper JR, Blim FE, and Roth RH: The biochemical basis of neuropharmacology, ed. 5, New York, 1986, Oxford University Press.

Gold PW, Goodwin FK, and Chrousos GP: Clinical and biochemical manifestations of depression, N Engl J Med 319:348, and 413, 1988.

Iversen SD, ed.: Psychopharmacology: recent advances and future prospects, New York, 1985, Oxford University Press.

Meltzer H, ed.: Psychopharmacology: the third generation of progress, New York, 1987, Raven Press.

Rech RH and Gudelsky GA, eds.: 5-HT agonists as psychoactive drugs, Ann Arbor, Mich, 1988, NPP Books.

Seiden LS and Balster RL, eds.: Behavioral pharmacology: the current status, New York, 1985, Alan R Liss, Inc.

CHAPTER

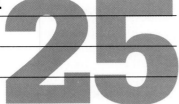

Drugs to Treat Anxiety and Related Disorders

THERAPEUTIC OVERVIEW

ANXIETY
Normal
Pathologic

DRUGS
Anxiolytics or minor tranquilizers
benzodiazepines
    Enhance chloride ion channel current through
    GABA system
    5-HT system may be involved

MAJOR DRUGS

benzodiazepines
buspirone

THERAPEUTIC OVERVIEW

Anxiety is the most prevalent symptom in mental illnesses, but it also occurs normally and may have adaptive value. Normal anxieties are of short duration and are generally marked by dissatisfaction, unhappiness, or apprehension. Normal anxiety is usually event-related and not under the subject's control. Under severe stress, normal individuals may experience periods of increased muscle tension, exaggeration of the discomfort of minor aches and pains, irritability, or sadness. These generally reflect an extension of normal anxiety. However, research suggests that pathological anxiety is not an exaggeration of normal anxiety but may stem from inheritable traits. This leads to attempts to classify anxiety based on symp-toms, but such classification is far from satisfactory, because of considerable overlap in the symptoms of anxiety disorders and depressive states. Generally the treatments of *normal* anxiety and *pathological* anxiety involve the same drugs.

Previously, anxiety was treated with alcohol, opiates, or barbiturates. Meprobamate was introduced in the 1950s as a more selective antianxiety drug, but subsequently was found to have barbiturate-like actions. Benzodiazepines, introduced in the late 1960s, were the first drugs to relieve anxiety without producing sedative effects. Buspirone, a more recent drug, may effectively treat anxiety with fewer side effects. The antianxiety drugs are known as *anxiolytics* and *minor tranquilizers*.

Therapeutic approaches to the treatment of anxiety disorders are summarized in the box (above).

MECHANISMS OF ACTION

The benzodiazepines are primary agents for the treatment of anxiety. Chlordiazepoxide, diazepam, oxazepam, lorazepam, chlorazepate, halazepam, prazepam, and alprazolam are in clinical use in the United States. These agents have virtually replaced the barbiturates, meprobamate, and other sedative-hypnotic drugs previously used in the treatment of anxiety. Buspirone is another type of antianxiety drug that is more effective than benzodiazepines in some patients. The chemical structures of the benzodiazepines and buspirone are shown in Figure 25-1.

Benzodiazepines bind to γ-aminobutyric acid (GABA) type A receptors to impart an allosteric effect on GABA-controlled opening of the chloride channel associated with this receptor complex. The GABA neurotransmitter-receptor system in the central nervous system (CNS) is the major inhibitory biochemical pathway in the mammalian brain, especially in the amygdala region and spinal cord. Peripheral GABA receptors and pathways exist but appear to have little relevancy to anxiolytic actions of benzodiazepines.

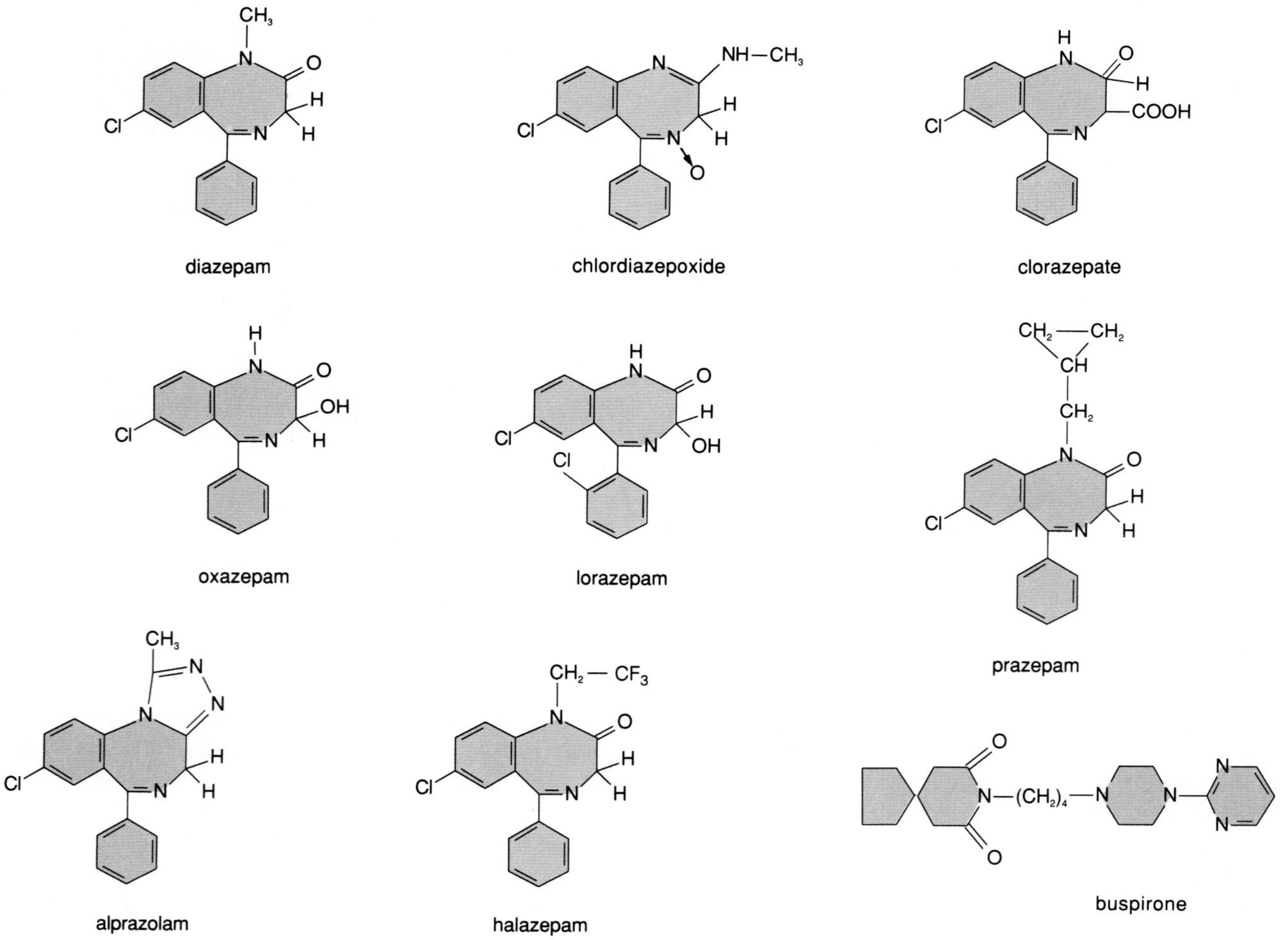

diazepam

chlordiazepoxide

clorazepate

oxazepam

lorazepam

prazepam

alprazolam

halazepam

buspirone

FIGURE 25-1   Chemical structures of anxiolytic benzodiazepines and buspirone.

Barbiturates also bind to the same receptor and exert an allosteric effect on GABA-controlled opening of the same chloride channels, but the binding sites for barbiturates and benzodiazepines are thought to be different. The type A GABA-benzodiazepine-chloride channel complex is described further in Chapter 2 and in Figure 25-2 (shown as the postsynaptic GABA receptor, but presynaptic GABA systems also exist).

Binding of benzodiazepines or barbiturates to GABA type A receptors results in increased chloride channel ion current. Both types of compounds produce allosteric modulation of the GABA effects and agree with the experimental observations that GABA must be present at sufficiently high concentrations before the channels can open. Binding of benzodiazepines increases the frequency of chloride channel openings, whereas binding of a barbiturate such as pentobarbital prolongs the duration of the chloride channel open time. It appears that a large fraction of the brain benzodiazepine sites implicated in sedative,

muscle relaxant, and anticonvulsant activities are coupled to GABA type A receptors and chloride ion channels. However, quantitative differences must exist among different drug-receptor complexes in terms of the efficacy of various benzodiazepine drugs, because (1) some members of this class act as sedatives, (2) others are anticonvulsants, and (3) still others have greater muscle relaxant activity.

The role of the GABA receptor in the mechanism of antianxiety action of the benzodiazepines is more controversial. Not all data support the coupling of benzodiazepine and GABA type A receptors to influence anxiety states, and acute (compared to long-term) administration of benzodiazepines may modulate other neurotransmission systems besides GABA. Modified transmitter turnover rates after long-term administration of certain benzodiazepines have been observed with glycine, muscarinic acetylcholine, dopamine, 5-hydroxytryptamine (5-HT), norepinephrine, and GABA. In addition, there is evidence that an endogenous benzodiazepine binding site ligand may exist, but efforts to isolate and purify such a material are incomplete. Another factor is the lack of correlation among benzodiazepines between efficacy of anxiolytic effects and the sedation, muscle relaxation, or anticonvulsant properties attributed to some of these drugs.

Furthermore, the latter effects show tolerance fairly rapidly on repeated drug treatment, whereas relief of anxiety does not show tolerance. Thus it is suggested that a Type I benzodiazepine receptor may be responsible for the anxiolytic actions of these drugs and a Type II benzodiazepine receptor may account for the other central actions. Dopaminergic and serotonergic (5-HT) innervations to the amygdala have been examined for changes after benzodiazepine treatment. Both show acute reduced activity, but the decreased dopamine turnover shows rapid tolerance development. Therefore, 5-HT activity in the amygdala may be anxiety-promoting, and its interruption by a benzodiazepine drug could explain the antianxiety effect. The development of buspirone and other second-generation antianxiety agents that affect brain 5-HT mechanisms gives further impetus to theories of a 5-HT causation for anxiety. It is conceivable that GABA- and 5-HT-modulating brain systems are involved, each having greater or lesser control according to the type of anxiety that predominates in a particular patient.

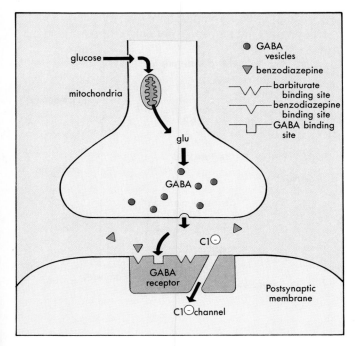

FIGURE 25-2   GABA-benzodiazepine postsynaptic system. Presynaptic system not shown. *Glu,* Glutamic; *GABA,* γ-aminobutyric acid.

A seemingly novel class of antianxiety drugs was introduced with buspirone, which has a chemical structure reminiscent of butyrophenones (haloperidol, see Chapter 24). This agent appears to be a partial agonist at dopamine and $5-HT_{1A}$ receptors and causes minimal sedation and muscle relaxation when used to treat anxiety.

PHARMACOKINETICS

The pharmacokinetic parameter values for the benzodiazepines and buspirone are summarized in Table 25-1.

The benzodiazepines differ in their lipid solubility, rate of metabolism to active metabolites and/or inactive products, relative potencies, and plasma half-lives of parent drug versus active metabolites. Several of the drugs are metabolized to more active species as summarized in Figure 25-3. When given orally, there is a latent period that is largely reflective of the distribution phase. The maintenance dosage is a function of the elimination phases of the parent and/or active metabolites. Many of the benzodiazepines and their metabolites bind tightly to plasma proteins. For example, the free fraction of alprazolam in plasma represents about 30% of the total drug, whereas less than 2% of diazepam remains unbound in plasma.

The parent benzodiazepines are slowly absorbed when administered orally, with the exception of diazepam and clorazepate. Diazepam enters the brain rapidly after absorption into the blood stream. It also redistributes rapidly from brain to peripheral tissues after a single dose. After a single IV administration,

the effective concentration of diazepam in the brain is maintained for less than 2 hours because concentrations during much of the elimination period are below the threshold value for pharmacological activity. This contrasts with lorazepam (a compound with a lower lipid solubility), which after a single IV dose may continue to have pharmacological effects for 6 to 8 hours, despite the elimination half-life of lorazepam being less than that of diazepam. When administered repeatedly, diazepam and its active metabolites accumulate, with the active metabolites often exceeding the concentration of the parent compound. Sudden termination of long-term treatment can result in slowly developing withdrawal as a result of the long elimination half-lives of diazepam and metabolites. Lorazepam, administered repeatedly, is less likely to accumulate because of its shorter elimination half-life and because its metabolites are inactive. As tolerance develops, there may be a "breakthrough" of rebound anxiety. In addition, when lorazepam and other benzodiazepines with short elimination half-lives are stopped abruptly after long-term treatment, more rapid and intense withdrawal signs may be expected. For this reason, it is advisable to reduce the use of lorazepam, oxazepam, or alprazolam gradually after chronic administration. Clorazepate, halazepam, and prazepam act only as prodrugs; their

Table 25-1 Pharmacokinetic Parameter Values for Anxiolytic Benzodiazepines

Drug	$t_{1/2}$ (hour)	Disposition
chlordiazepoxide	5-30	M*
clorazepate	30-200	M*
lorazepam	10-20	M
oxazepam	5-15	M
diazepam	20-70	M*
alprazolam	8-20	M*

M, Metabolized.
* Active metabolite.

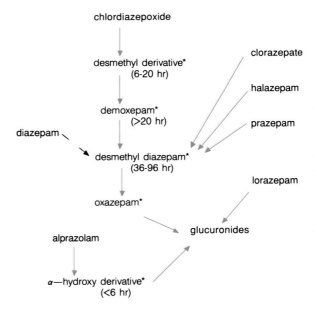

FIGURE 25-3   Metabolism pathways for anxiolytic benzodiazepines. Numbers in ( ) are disposition half-lives. *Active metabolites.

anxiolytic activity is mediated by the formation of their active metabolites.

Hepatic metabolism of benzodiazepine occurs by oxidation, with aliphatic hydroxylation of *N*-dealkylation, or by glucuronide conjugation. Oxidative processes yield active metabolites; glucuronidation yields only inactive products. Oxidative processes, but not conjugating mechanisms, are often greatly reduced in rate in elderly patients and slowed by liver disease and certain drugs (cimetidine, estrogens). Thus under these conditions, the use of oxazepam or lorazepam may be advisable because these benzodiazepines are metabolized directly to the glucuronide rather than requiring intermediate oxidative steps. In subjects using chronic barbiturates, one may anticipate a more rapid elimination of diazepam and chlordiazepoxide on the basis of the induction of hepatic oxidative enzymes by the barbiturates.

RELATION OF MECHANISMS OF ACTION TO CLINICAL RESPONSE

A difficulty in defining a therapy for the treatment of anxiety arises from the heterogeneity of the symptoms. Anxiety states include the following:
1. Panic disorders with or without agoraphobia
2. Simple phobias
3. Social phobias
4. Obsessive-compulsive disorders
5. Generalized (less dramatic and/or less specific) anxiety disorders

Although drug therapy of anxiety disorders has improved, psychotherapy and behavioral interventions continue to be the most effective long-term treatments, with a combination of pharmacological and behavioral approaches more effective than either one alone.

Anxiety symptoms that are secondary to other major mental disorders (medical illness, psychosis, depression) are best addressed by controlling the primary illness. Benzodiazepines are effective in controlling nonpsychotic anxiety of a general nature. Their best application appears to involve intermittent use or limited terms (4 to 8 weeks) of treatment for acute or intermittent anxiety reactions. There is the danger with long-term treatment of developing psychic and/or physical dependence, as well as disturbances in intellectual functioning and motor dexterity. The use of buspirone offers an attractive alter-

native when long-term treatment is required because this nonbenzodiazepine antianxiety drug overcomes most of the disadvantages of the benzodiazepines.

If panic attacks are present, tricyclic antidepressants or monoamine oxidase (MAO) inhibitors appear to be the most effective drug therapy (see Chapter 24). Benzodiazepines are generally not effective but can alleviate symptoms of generalized anxiety associated with panic reactions. Alprazolam appears to be unique among the benzodiazepines in having a selective antipanic efficacy, making it a drug of choice in this disorder. Benzodiazepines are usually not effective when depression is associated with anxiety, but alprazolam may again represent an exception because it also appears to exert some antidepressant activity.

Benzodiazepines are used for anxiolytic and sedation effects before surgery and general anesthesia (see Chapter 30), during alcohol withdrawal (see Chapter 31), and for treatment of epilepsies and seizures (see Chapter 26) in addition to treatment of anxiety states. GABA mechanisms are implicated in inhibitory modulation relating to sleep, skeletal muscle tone and coordination, and tonic control of forebrain excitability for cognitive and emotional functions. Therefore as diazepam enhances GABA activity relating to many basic CNS functions, it is not surprising that the drug also causes sedation or hypnosis, muscle relaxation, ataxia, and anticonvulsant effects.

Recent advances in antianxiety therapy have resulted from the introduction of buspirone and related drugs that appear to act at 5-HT$_{1A}$ receptors. Buspirone does not act directly with benzodiazepine or GABA receptors, does not potentiate the depression of alcohol, and apparently has little addiction liability. Nevertheless, it appears to be as effective in controlling symptoms of generalized anxiety as the benzodiazepines. It may be somewhat slower in onset than benzodiazepines. Moreover, buspirone is not as active as diazepam against nervous states identified with increased muscle tension but may be more active in controlling frustration and hostility. Another potential advantage is that abrupt withdrawal after prolonged treatment with buspirone does not result in rebound anxiety as observed with benzodiazepines. Because elderly patients are susceptible to the general depressant effects of benzodiazepines, buspirone could be the agent of choice for these patients. Buspirone may exert some antidepressant activity similar to other drugs that bind to 5-HT receptors. The benzodiazepines, when used intermittently, are most effective in situation-dependent anxieties, whereas buspirone is more effective in chronic anxieties with symptoms of irritability and hostility. The tricyclic antidepressants (which also act via 5-HT) are superior to the benzodiazepines in the treatment of panic and phobic disorders (see Chapter 24).

SIDE EFFECTS, CLINICAL PROBLEMS, AND TOXICITY

Clinical problems are summarized in the box.

Benzodiazepines are widely prescribed for treatment of anxiety problems. When associated with heart problems, benzodiazepines reduce psychological-based and somatic tone-based anxiety. These drugs appear relatively safe for short-term use (less than a few months). However, long-term use (more than 6 months) is controversial because of the documented prevalence of withdrawal problems and dependence. In addition, 25% of hospitalizations for drug toxicity and overdoses appear due to benzodiazepines, including those self-inflicted, with some fatalities resulting. In long-term users, rebound anxiety often occurs if the drug is stopped abruptly. Withdrawal symptoms (anxiety, insomnia, fatigue, sweating, tremors, nausea, and increased sensory perception) also occur in some patients when the drug dose is gradually diminished.

The CNS effects of these agents and their active metabolites increase inhibitory functions, mainly through GABA. Even after large doses, these agents have only moderate effects on processes subserving vital functions. Sedation, with dulling of attention, spinal reflexes, and sensory acuity, is observed, and

memory disturbed. When sleep is induced by benzodiazepines (see Chapter 33) there is minimal suppression of rapid eye movement (REM) (in contrast to the barbiturates), although stage 4 slow-wave sleep may be suppressed to a greater extent.

The benzodiazepines spare respiratory and cardiovascular functions, perhaps because the medullary brain centers utilize few inhibitory synapses using benzodiazepine-GABA$_{1A}$ coupled chloride channels. Skeletal muscle relaxation occurs, at least in part, from effects on brainstem motor systems. Occasionally, an alcohol-like intoxication marked by paradoxical excitement, aggressiveness or hostility, and even increased anxiety is induced in a particular patient. Tolerance and physical dependence that sometimes occurs with long-term treatment arises more slowly and to a lesser degree than with barbiturates and other sedative-hypnotics. Psychological dependence develops less readily than with other classes of CNS depressant drugs. However, patients who achieve significant relief of anxiety after long-term use of a benzodiazepine may be reluctant to discontinue the drug. Many of these agents have active metabolites with long half-lives, which further complicates drug withdrawal. Newer agents with short half-lives (e.g., alprazolam) and without active metabolites may show rebound anxiety effects and a greater tendency for withdrawal seizures. Cross-tolerance between benzodiazepine and other sedative-hypnotics or alcohol is the basis for treatment of withdrawal from barbiturate, meprobamate, or alcohol dependence using diazepam, chlordiazepoxide, or clonazepam. Other

---

CLINICAL PROBLEMS

Nonanxiolytic CNS effects of benzodiazepines
  Sedation
  Muscle relaxation
  Anticonvulsant effects
  Tolerance may develop
  Withdrawal seizures may occur

TRADENAMES

In addition to generic and fixed combination preparations, the following tradenamed materials are available in the United States.

Ativan, lorazepam
BuSpar, buspirone
Centrax, prazepam
Librium, chlordiazepoxide
Paxipam, halazepam
Serax, oxazepam
Tranxene, clorazepate
Valium, diazepam
Xanax, alprazolam

side effects are minimal with the benzodiazepine compounds.

Some older drugs are occasionally employed as anxiolytics. Among these are the antihistamines, hydroxyzine, and diphenhydramine, which are sedative and have anticholinergic properties. They do not induce cross-tolerance with benzodiazepines, barbiturates, meprobamate, or alcohol, nor do they produce physical or psychological dependence.

REFERENCES

Biggio G, and Costa E, eds.: Chloride channels and their modulation by neurotransmitters and drugs, New York, 1988, Raven Press.

Busto V, Sellers EM, Naranjo CA et al.: Withdrawal reactions after long-term therapeutic use of benzodiazepines, N Engl J Med 315:854, 1986.

Costa E, ed.: The benzodiazepines, New York, 1983, Raven Press.

CHAPTER 26

Drugs for Seizure Disorders (Epilepsies)

ABBREVIATIONS

GA	generalized absence seizures
GABA	γ-aminobutyric acid
GTC	generalized tonic-clonic seizures
NMDA	*N*-methyl-*D*-aspartate

MAJOR ANTIEPILEPTIC DRUGS

carbamazepine
phenytoin
valproate
ethosuximide
phenobarbital
primidone
clonazepam

 THERAPEUTIC OVERVIEW

Epilepsy is a chronic disorder characterized by recurrent self-limited seizures with excessive discharges throughout localized or generalized groups of neurons in the brain. About 0.5% of the population suffers from epilepsy. Seventy-five percent of these individuals have their first seizure before the age of 18. Recurrent seizures, if frequent, interfere with the patient's ability to perform day-to-day activities; how-

ever, judicious use of antiepileptic medications allows about 75% of epileptic patients to be seizure-free.

Identification of seizure type is important because antiepileptic medication is selected accordingly. The current classification of seizure types is listed in Table 26-1. Partial seizures arise at specific foci in the forebrain and have identifiable symptoms, ranging from disorders of sensation or thought to convulsive movements of parts of the body. Partial seizures are termed *simple* if no alteration of consciousness occurs and *complex* if consciousness is impaired or lost. In partial complex seizures, motor activity often appears as nonreflex actions that can be complicated and seemingly purposeful. Partial seizures can become secondarily generalized to involve the entire brain. General seizures involve large areas of the brain, are bilateral in their initial manifestations, and are associated with impairment of consciousness from the outset. They may range from absence seizures with only impaired consciousness to generalized tonic-clonic seizures in which widespread convulsive activity takes place.

Often an epileptic syndrome can be identified that consists of an etiology of the seizures; a natural history, including certain clinical findings; a family history; and a prognosis. Recognition of a syndrome will help determine whether or not medication is necessary and, if so, how long it should be continued. In addition, identification of the syndrome has genetic implications. Juvenile myoclonic epilepsy (Janz syndrome) is an example of an epileptic syndrome that is marked by generalized tonic-clonic seizures, usually occurring on awakening, that first develop in ad-

Table 26-1 Classification of Seizures, Frequency, and Clinical Manifestations

	Frequency (%)	Clinical Manifestations
PARTIAL (FOCAL) SEIZURES		
Simple partial	10	No impairment of consciousness; focal motor, sensory, or speech disturbance
Complex partial	35	Impaired consciousness; dreamy dysaffective state, with or without automatisms
Partial seizures, secondarily generalized	10	
GENERAL SEIZURES		
Tonic-clonic	30	Loss of consciousness, falling Rigid extension of trunk and limbs (tonic phase) Rhythmic contraction of arms and legs (clonic phase)
Absence	10	Impaired consciousness with staring spells, with or without eye blinks
Myoclonic, atonic (atypical)	4	Myoclonic jerks (shock-like contractions), loss of muscle tone, falling, "drop attacks"
UNCLASSIFIED EPILEPTIC SEIZURES	1-8	Includes all other seizures

olescence. The patient often has early morning myoclonus as well. Considering only the type of seizure could lead to selection of a specific drug; however, identification of the syndrome indicates the use of a different drug. Seizures are easily controlled by drugs, usually administered for life.

All individuals can experience seizures. Brain insults associated with fever, sedative or opioid drug withdrawal, hypoglycemia, hyponatremia, extreme acidosis, or alkalosis can result in seizure, but if the condition is corrected the seizure does not recur. The causes of isolated seizures and epilepsy (recurrent seizures) are summarized in the box (see p. 362).

The occurrence of a single seizure requires a decision as to whether or not to treat the patient. Factors associated with a higher risk of seizure recurrence include neurological deficits, an abnormal electroencephalogram (EEG), abnormal neuroimaging studies, or a family history positive for epilepsy. If any predisposing factors are present, treatment with antiepileptic drugs should be considered. Otherwise it may be appropriate to wait until a second seizure occurs.

An example of a single seizure occurrence is the febrile convulsion, which occurs in up to 5% of children, constitutes a relatively benign disorder of early childhood, and is characterized by general convulsive seizures occurring during an acute febrile illness. The majority of febrile convulsions are brief and uncom-

plicated with the overall risk of developing epilepsy less than 4%; the majority of children do not require drug treatment. However, if there are neurological abnormalities, the febrile seizure is longer than 15 minutes, or there is a history of nonfebrile convulsions in parents or siblings, then limited treatment with antiepileptic drugs may be warranted.

The goal of antiepileptic drug therapy (see box, p. 362) is to prevent seizures while minimizing side effects with the simplest drug regimen. After initiation of therapy, if seizures continue and further increases in dosage are inadvisable because of dose-related side effects, at least one and sometimes more alternative drugs should be tried as monodrug therapy before considering the use of two drugs simultaneously. Discontinuation of antiepileptic medication after several seizure-free years depends on the diagnosis (type of seizure and epileptic syndrome), etiology, and response to therapy. With certain epileptic syndromes, antiepileptic drugs may be stopped, but in others, such as recurrent seizures secondary to a structural lesion, antiepileptic medication should be continued for life.

When seizures recur so close together that baseline consciousness is not regained between seizures, *status epilepticus* exists. The patient is considered to be in status epilepticus when seizures last at least 30 minutes. Status epilepticus is a medical emergency with a mortality rate of 15% or less.

CAUSES AND THERAPY OF SEIZURES

CAUSES

Birth and perinatal injuries
Vascular insults
Head trauma
Congenital malformations
Metabolic disturbances (e.g., serum sodium, glucose, calcium, urea)
Drugs or alcohol, including withdrawals from barbiturates and other CNS depressants
Neoplasia
Infection
Genetic
Idiopathic
Hyperthermia in children

THERAPY

Monodrug therapy is preferable to polydrug therapy because of:
Lower incidence of adverse effects
Avoidance of drug interactions
Improved patient compliance
Lower medication costs
Success with monodrug therapy depends on:
Correct seizure classification and diagnosis
Appropriate drug choice for seizure type
Optimal drug administration and serum monitoring

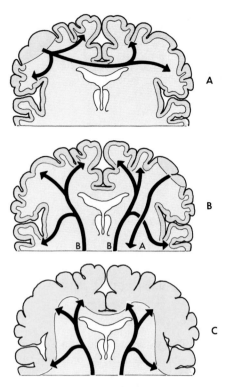

FIGURE 26-1   Schematic representation of seizure spread. **A,** Focal seizure with spread to adjacent and contralateral cortical regions. **B,** Focal seizure with secondary generalization. Seizure discharge activates subcortical centers *(A)*, which then activate entire cortex *(B)*. **C,** Primary generalized absence seizure in which thalamocortical relays are thought to act on a diffusely hyperexcitable cortex.

MECHANISMS OF ACTION

Seizure Mechanisms

The pathophysiology of epilepsy is not fully understood for any of the seizure types previously described. However, it is known that multiple mechanisms are involved. Some mechanisms operate in one seizure type and do not operate in others, but no seizure type is explained by a single mechanism. Currently, the pathophysiology of focal seizures is better understood than for general type seizures. A focal seizure (Figure 26-1, *A*) arises when pathological alterations in a restricted region of the brain initiate a seizure. Additional features serve to synchronize neurons into epileptic discharges and to propagate the discharges to areas surrounding the focus (Figure 26-1, *B* and *C*).

Available Drugs

The structures of the mainline antiepilepsy drugs available in the United States are shown in Figure 26-2. The drugs include carbamazepine, phenytoin, valproate, ethosuximide, phenobarbital, primidone, and clonazepam. Additional drugs used secondarily in the treatment of epileptic seizures, but not discussed further, include clorazepate dipotassium, diazepam, ethotoin, methsuximide, phensuximide, phenacemide, paramethodione, mephenytoin, and trimethadione.

Drug Mechanisms

There are several points in the initiation and growth of a seizure at which antiepileptic drugs may act (Figure 26-3). The first is to block abnormal epi-

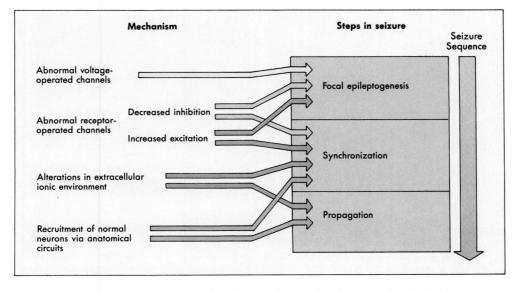

carbamazepine

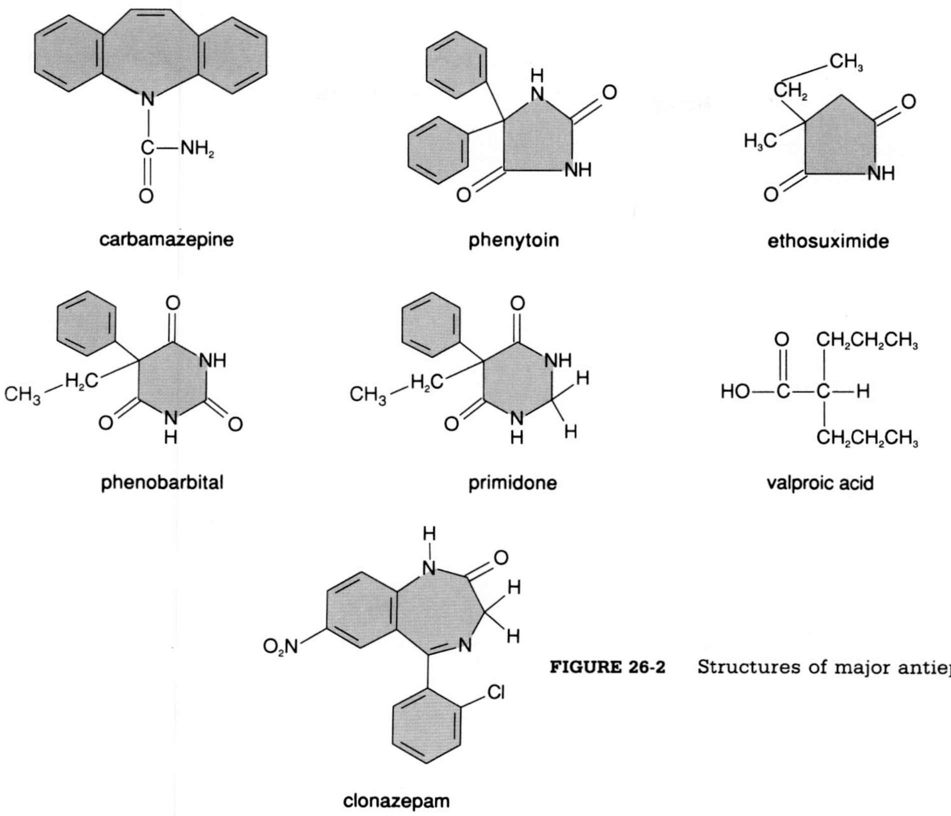

phenytoin

ethosuximide

phenobarbital

primidone

valproic acid

clonazepam

FIGURE 26-2   Structures of major antiepileptic drugs.

FIGURE 26-3   Cellular mechanisms of epileptic seizures. A seizure can be divided into three phases: (1) focal epileptogenesis *(initiation)*, (2) *synchronization* of the surrounding neurons, and (3) *propagation* of the seizure discharge to other areas of the brain. Arrows indicate steps in seizure sequences where drugs may act.

leptic events within single neurons. The second is to block or slow the synchronization of epileptic discharges among neurons involved in the seizure. A third point is to block the propagation of seizure activity. A drug may act via multiple mechanisms and have actions at one or more points.

At least four different mechanisms are involved in the genesis and spread of epileptic discharges, and all are amenable to disruption by drugs. The first includes alterations in neuronal membrane function such as changes in voltage-regulated ion channels in neuronal membranes. These changes lead to excessive depolarization (paroxysmal depolarization shift)

or excess action potential firing (loss of inactivation). Examples are carbamazepine and phenytoin, which reduce repetitive firing of neurons by producing a use-dependent blockade of sodium channels (Figure 26-4). By prolonging the inactivated state of the sodium channel and thus the relative refractory period, phenytoin and carbamazepine do not alter the first action potential but reduce the likelihood of repetitive action potentials. The neurons retain their ability to generate action potentials at the low frequencies operational in physiological states. In this way these drugs do not alter normal brain activity but can suppress epileptic discharges.

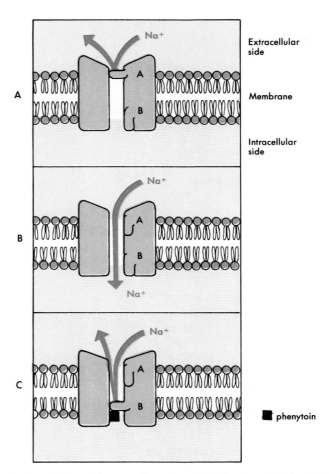

FIGURE 26-4   Action of phenytoin on sodium channel. **A,** Resting state in which sodium channel activation gate *(A)* is closed. Arrival of an action potential in **B** causes depolarization and opening of activation gate *(A)* and Na$^+$ ions flow into the cell. When depolarization continues **(C),** an inactivation gate *(B)* moves into the channel. Phenytoin prolongs the inactivated state of the sodium channel presumably by preventing reopening of the inactivation gate *(B).*

The second broad mechanism of drug-modifiable genesis and spread of epileptic discharge is decreased inhibition, which allows excessive neuronal firing to occur. γ-Aminobutyric acid (GABA) is the major inhibitory neurotransmitter in the forebrain. GABA opens receptor-operated chloride channels that lead to hyperpolarization and make epileptic firing less likely to occur. In experimental animals, increased GABAergic inhibition has antiepileptic activity, whereas administration of agents that diminish GABAergic inhibition causes seizures. The GABA receptor/channel complex contains the receptor site for the transmitter GABA (this is a prime target for antiepileptic drug action) and also includes benzodiazepine and barbiturate recognition sites (see Chapter 13). Binding of a benzodiazepine (diazepam, chlorazepam, lorazepam) modulates the effectiveness of inhibition by increasing the frequency of chloride channel opening when GABA combines with its receptor. Barbiturates interact with the GABA receptor at a binding site adjacent to the chloride channel but separate from the benzodiazepine site. Some barbiturates have GABA-mimetic (direct action on chloride channels) and GABA-potentiating effects (prolonging the opening of chloride channels achieved by a given amount of GABA). Barbiturates that are effective antiepileptic compounds (suppressing seizures with minimal sedation) have strong GABA-potentiation but no GABA-mimetic actions. Some barbiturates suppress seizures but are not useful clinically as antiepileptics because of the resultant strong sedative effects through GABA-mimetic action. Valproic acid may enhance the GABA inhibitory system, but this is controversial and an exact mechanism has not been elucidated. A new drug undergoing clinical trials (γ-vinyl-GABA) is an irreversible inhibitor of GABA transaminase, the enzyme that metabolizes GABA. γ-Vinyl-GABA increases GABA concentrations, augments inhibition, and functions as an antiepileptic agent. The effectiveness of γ-vinyl-GABA against partial seizures has been shown in clinical trials in Europe.

Adenosine, which decreases neurotransmitter release from terminals (presynaptic effect) and binds to adenosine receptors that activate second messengers (postsynaptic effect), is an effective antiepileptic agent in experimental animals. Carbamazepine interacts with the adenosine system causing enhanced inhibition and reduced epileptogenesis, including focal development of epileptic discharges, synchronization of discharges, and seizure propagation throughout the brain.

A third mechanism by which drugs interrupt the genesis and spread of epileptic discharges is by reducing excitation. Excitatory neurotransmission is mediated predominantly through glutamate or related compounds. One type of glutamate receptor, the N-methyl-D-aspartate (NMDA) receptor, may have a role in epileptogenesis. The NMDA receptor is predominantly involved in high frequency discharges, such as occur with seizures, and is activated only minimally in physiological neuronal activity of the brain. Antagonists of the NMDA receptor are anticonvulsants in animal and in vitro models of epilepsy. A drug that effectively reduces abnormal excitatory transmission by blocking the NMDA receptor could reduce focal epileptogenesis, slow synchronization of the discharge, and slow or block spread of the seizure.

A fourth mechanism involved in drug-interrupted genesis and spread of epileptic discharges is an alteration in the extracellular concentrations of potassium and calcium. During seizures, the extracellular concentrations of potassium increase and calcium decreases. Both changes cause greater excitability of neurons and may promote seizure initiation and spread. Phenytoin acts by suppressing epileptic discharges in an altered ionic environment. The ability of phenytoin to produce frequency dependent blockade of action potentials is augmented when extracellular potassium is elevated to concentrations characteristic of seizure activity. This makes phenytoin more effective in epileptic tissue than in normally functioning brain areas.

Absence seizures are characterized by the sudden appearance of spike-wave discharges synchronized throughout the brain, as noted by modified electroencephalographic patterns compared to that of generalized tonic-clonic seizures or partial seizures (Figure 26-5). Thalamic neurons may play a role in the generation of thalamocortical rhythms, including the paroxysmal discharges of absence seizures. The thalamic neurons generate depolarizations based on calcium currents that may be a crucial cellular mechanism in the generation of normal and abnormal thalamocortical rhythms. Recent results suggest that certain antiepileptic drugs block absence seizures by reducing calcium currents in these thalamic neurons.

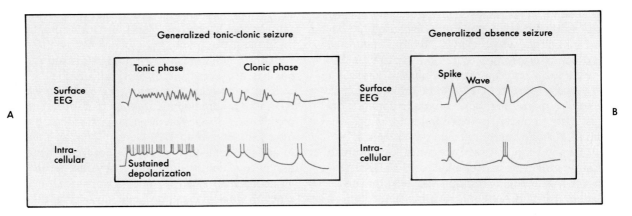

FIGURE 26-5   Neuronal correlates of paroxysmal discharges. **A,** A tonic-clonic seizure begins with a tonic phase of rhythmic high-frequency discharges (recorded by surface EEG) with cortical neurons undergoing sustained depolarization with generation of protracted trains of action potentials (recorded intracellularly). Subsequently, the seizure converts to a clonic phase characterized by groups of spikes on the EEG and periodic neuronal depolarizations with clusters of action potentials. **B,** Absence seizures are distinguished by the spike and wave discharge that is recorded on the surface EEG. During the spike phase, neurons generate short duration depolarization and a burst of action potentials, but unlike in **A,** do not show sustained depolarization nor produce sustained repetitive firing of action potentials. This difference may explain why drugs that are effective against sustained firing in vitro are effective against tonic-clonic seizures in humans, but not absence seizures.

 PHARMACOKINETICS

Pharmacokinetic parameter values are summarized in Table 26-2 for antiepileptic drugs.

Valproic acid is a liquid at room temperature, but formulations are available to allow valproic acid to be given in capsule form. A new formulation containing equal proportions of valproic acid and sodium valproate is enteric-coated to reduce GI side effects.

Because antiepileptic drugs are used to treat a chronic medical condition they must be absorbed orally and cross the blood-brain barrier. All of the antiepileptic drugs are metabolized to a significant extent and all bind to plasma proteins, many to a high degree. This is important clinically because the usual determinations of blood concentrations indicate total drug (bound plus free) in the serum. Concentrations of the free fraction of antiepileptic drugs can be measured but the tests are expensive and time-consuming to carry out. In addition, there is less experience with what constitutes a therapeutic range for free drug concentrations than for total drug concentration. Therefore the determination of free drug concentrations is reserved for special circumstances.

The metabolism of phenytoin is characterized by saturation kinetics (see Chapter 5) that arise because the liver enzymes that catalyze phenytoin metabolism become saturated and operate at maximum velocity when serum concentrations rise above a certain value. This phenomenon at lower doses results in an essentially linear relationship between the dose of phenytoin and serum concentration of the drug. At higher doses a much greater rise in serum concentration develops for a given increase in dose. The dose at which this transition occurs varies from patient to patient but is usually in the range of 400 to 600 mg/day. As a result, doses of phenytoin must be individualized to avoid the toxicity associated with excessive concentrations or the lack of seizure control associated with too low a serum concentration of drug.

Phenobarbital is also metabolized in the liver and causes induction of liver microsomal enzyme systems. Thus phenobarbital typically accelerates its own metabolism and that of other drugs taken concurrently. Phenobarbital has a long half-life and takes several weeks of dosing to reach steady state unless a loading dose is used. Primidone is metabolized in the liver to phenobarbital with all its actions and side

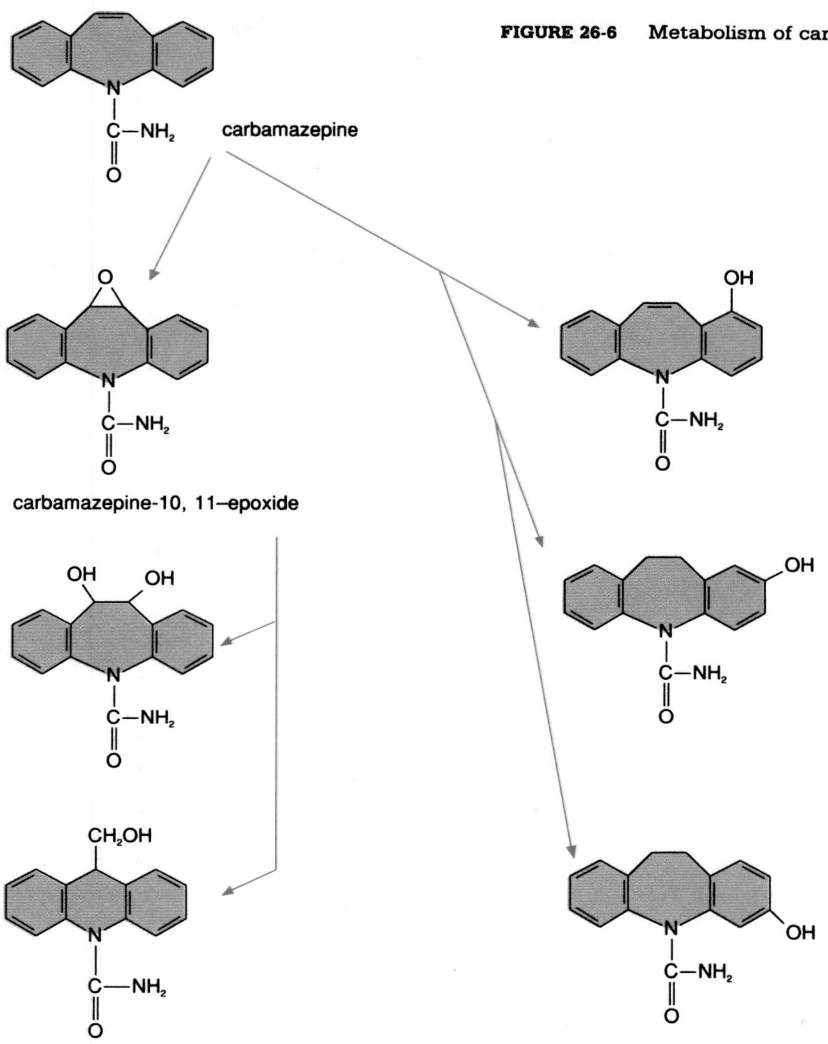

FIGURE 26-6   Metabolism of carbamazepine.

carbamazepine

carbamazepine-10, 11–epoxide

Table 26-2   Pharmacokinetic Parameter Values

Drug	Administered	$t_{1/2}$ (hour)*	Disposition	Bound to Plasma Proteins (%)
carbamazepine	Oral	10-15	M (60%),† R (40%)	75
phenytoin	Oral	12-36	M (95%), R (5%)	90
phenobarbital	Oral	48-144	M (75%), R (25%)	50
primidone	Oral	6-15	M (60%),† R (40%)	10
ethosuximide	Oral	24-60	M (80%), R (20%)	10
valproic acid	Oral	6-15	M (>95%)	90
clonazepam	Oral	24-36	M (>95%)	>50

M, metabolized (in liver); *R*, eliminated unchanged by renal mechanisms.

* Age dependent.

† Produces an active (antiepileptic) metabolite.

effects and to phenethylmalonamide, which also has some antiepileptic action.

Carbamazepine is metabolized in the liver to produce a 10,11 epoxide, which is relatively stable and accumulates in the blood (Figure 26-6). This metabolite has antiepileptic properties, and some believe that the epoxide is a contributor to the neurotoxicity that often develops in patients taking carbamazepine. Carbamazepine also induces its own metabolism, with the rate of metabolism of carbamazepine increasing during the first 4 to 6 weeks so that larger doses become necessary to maintain constant serum concentrations.

Ethosuximide is hydroxylated in the liver and has a long half-life that allows for once-a-day dosing. However, the GI side effects are frequently intolerable with once-a-day dosing and are reduced with divided dosing. The half-life of ethosuximide and the other antiepileptic agents varies with the age of the patient and exposure to other drugs.

Many antiepileptic drugs are available as brand name and generic products, but differences in formulation result in a wide range of bioavailability among the several preparations of a given drug. This can lead to problems in seizure control when formulations are changed and should be considered in prescribing antiepileptic drugs.

RELATION OF MECHANISMS OF ACTION TO CLINICAL RESPONSE

Treatment of Epilepsies

The first line and alternative drugs for epilepsy types of seizure are listed in Table 26-3 with serum-concentration ranges usually thought to be therapeutic. However, these therapeutic ranges are determined empirically from general clinical experience in diverse and heterogeneous populations of epileptic patients and should not be taken as absolute recommendations for individual patients.

Antiepileptic Drugs During Pregnancy

Because antiepileptic agents are taken for many years or for a lifetime, the issue of taking these drugs during pregnancy must be addressed. During pregnancy, seizures increase in 25% of epileptic women, do not change in frequency in 50%, and decrease in frequency in 25%. The possibility of seizures, or even status epilepticus, with hypoxia and other metabolic changes places the epileptic mother and her child at risk. However, the teratogenic properties of antiepileptic drugs is also a concern. The epileptic mother is at heightened risk for obstetrical complications and her child at increased risk for perinatal difficulties. Children of mothers who have epilepsy have an increased risk of malformations even if antiepileptic drugs are not used during pregnancy. No antiepileptic drug has been shown unequivocally to cause birth defects, but none has proven absolutely safe either. Thus, the issues involved with the use of antiepileptic drugs in pregnancy are complex.

In some patients it may be possible to discontinue antiepileptics. If not, monodrug therapy and the smallest possible dose of the antiepileptic agent should be used. Studies show that the highest incidence of birth defects occurs with multiple drug use. A number of drugs, including phenytoin and carbamazepine, are linked to particular fetal cardiac defects, cleft lip and palate, and craniofacial anomalies, but not all clinicians agree that these are specific effects rather than examples of a more general syndrome. There is evidence that trimethadione is teratogenic and this drug should be avoided. Valproic acid is cited as causing neural tube defects in 1% to 2% of offspring of mothers with epilepsy.

Profound changes in the distribution and metabolism of antiepileptic drugs occur in pregnant women, resulting in a decrease of serum total drug concentrations, and monitoring of serum drug concentrations at regular intervals before, during, and after pregnancy is advised. However, a change in serum concentration does not necessarily mandate a change in daily drug dosage.

The newborn of mothers who have received phenobarbital, primidone, or phenytoin during pregnancy may develop a deficiency of vitamin K dependent clotting factors that can result in serious hemorrhage during the first 24 hours of life. This can be prevented by administration of vitamin K to the newborn shortly after birth.

Treatment of Status Epilepticus

The general strategy for treating *status epilepticus* involves support of cardiovascular and respiratory systems and treatment of seizure activity (Table 26-4). Initially a rapidly acting antiepileptic such as IV

Table 26-3 Treatment of Epilepsies

Seizure Disorder	Drug Therapy	Therapeutic Serum Concentrations (µg/ml)
Primary generalized tonic-clonic (grand mal)		
Drugs of choice	carbamazepine	6-12
	phenytoin	10-20
	valproate†	50-100
Alternatives	phenobarbital	15-35
	primidone	6-12
Partial, including secondarily generalized		
Drugs of choice	carbamazepine	6-12
	phenytoin	10-20
Alternatives	phenobarbital	15-35
	primidone	6-12
General absence (petit mal)		
Drugs of choice	ethosuximide	40-100
	valproate*	50-100
Alternative	clonazepam	.013-.072
Atypical absence		
Myoclonic, atonic		
Drug of choice	valproate†	50-100
Alternative	clonazepam	.013-.072

*First choice if primary generalized tonic-clonic also present.
†Not approved unless absence involved.

Table 26-4 Treatment of Status Epilepticus in Adults

	Drugs of Choice	Initial Dose	Rate (mg/min)	Repeat Doses
INITIAL	Diazepam, IV	5-10 mg	1-2	5-10 mg every 20-30 min
	Lorazepam, IV	2-6 mg	1	2-6 mg every 20-30 min
FOLLOW-UP	Phenytoin, IV	15-20 mg/kg	30-50	100-150 mg every 30 min
	Phenobarbital, IV	10-20 mg/kg	25-50	120-240 mg every 20 min

diazepam or lorazepam (longer duration) is given to stop the seizures. Because the effect wears off rapidly, long-term antiepileptic therapy with IV phenytoin or phenobarbital is also instituted. Phenobarbital is more sedating and, when the effects are added to the CNS depression produced by the benzodiazepine, can lead to respiratory compromise. Therefore IV phenytoin is more frequently used as the second drug. It, however, has the potential side effects of hypotension and/or cardiac arrhythmias if administered too rapidly. If status epilepticus develops during withdrawal of a particular drug (e.g., phenobarbital or the benzodiazepines) then consideration should be given to reinstating that compound.

SIDE EFFECTS, CLINICAL PROBLEMS, AND TOXICITY

Clinical problems for antiepileptic drugs are summarized in the box.

Side Effects and Toxicity

Antiepileptic drugs cross the blood-brain barrier and thus have potential for systemic and neurologic toxicity (see box). These side effects may be dose-related or idiosyncratic. Dose-related side effects are common at higher serum concentrations and can be reduced by lowering the drug dose. Idiosyncratic reactions are unique to a particular patient and drug combination and may pose a serious risk to the patient that often necessitates stopping the drug.

In several studies, side effects of antiepileptic drugs are reported in 30% to 50% of patients. However, these are frequently tolerable and require only physician interaction with the patient and monitoring. In other cases, the side effects can be reduced or eliminated by changing the dose or administration schedule. In 5% to 15% of patients another antiepileptic drug must be prescribed because of toxicity. With some of the antiepileptic agents, it is common to experience side effects when drug administration is initiated, but patient counseling and incremental dose increase can result in the tolerance to side effects and not hinder the chronic use of the drug.

Patients often initially experience nausea and visual disturbances with carbamazepine. This can be minimized by slow incremental increases in total daily dosage until the desired dose is reached. In addition, hematological effects may be encountered, particularly leukopenia or thrombocytopenia. These may disappear with continued use or may persist as a dose-dependent side effect. The most problematic hematologic effect is depression of granulocytes in the blood. If good seizure control is achieved and other serious side effects are absent, an absolute granulocyte count of ≥1000 is acceptable. An aplastic anemia syndrome is associated with carbamazepine, but it is very infrequent (<1/50,000) and appears to be idiosyncratic. Other idiosyncratic reactions with carbamazepine include rash in 5% of cases and rare hepatitis. Dose-related side effects for carbamazepine include nausea, dizziness, visual symptoms, and, infrequently, inappropriate antidiuretic hormone secretion. Four percent of children receiving carba-

CLINICAL PROBLEMS
carbamazepine
Autoinduction of metabolism
Nausea and visual disturbances (dose-related)
Granulocyte suppression
Aplastic anemia (idiosyncratic)
phenytoin
Ataxia and nystagmus (dose-related)
Cognitive impairment
Hirsutism, coarsening of facial features, gingival hyperplasia
Saturation metabolism kinetics
phenobarbital
Sedation, cognitive impairment
Behavioral changes
Induction of liver enzymes
primidone
See phenobarbital
valproic acid
Tremor
Nausea and vomiting
Elevated liver enzymes
Weight gain
ethosuximide
Stomach aches and vomiting
Hiccups
clonazepam
Sedation and lethargy
Ataxia
Tolerance to antiepileptic effects

mazepine show agitation or violent behavior that necessitates discontinuation of the drug. Use of serum concentrations of carbamazepine to assess toxicity can be problematic because the 10,11 epoxide (see Figure 26-6) may also cause toxicity.

The common idiosyncratic reaction with phenytoin is a rash (5% of cases); less common reactions are hepatitis, a lupus-like connective tissue disease, lymphadenopathy, and pseudolymphoma. Dose-related side effects are more common and include ataxia and nystagmus, commonly detected with total serum concentrations >20 μg/ml; profound encephalopathy in a few cases; and the more common slight dulling of cognitive performance, especially at high doses. Children may develop choreiform movements with phenytoin that may abate with lowering of the dose. Other side effects with chronic phenytoin therapy are hirsutism, coarsening of facial features, and gingival hyperplasia. These should be considered when prescribing phenytoin for children.

Side effects likely to appear early with valproic acid include nausea, vomiting, and lethargy. The availability of enteric coated tablets of valproic acid has significantly decreased the GI side effects. Allergic reactions such as rashes are rare, but elevation of liver enzymes and blood ammonia in patients receiving valproic acid is common. This is important because fatal hepatitis may occur in patients taking valproic acid; overall the risk is small (approximately 1 per 40,000 but heightened considerably for patients <2 years of age treated with multiple antiepileptic drugs). Some experimental studies indicate that other antiepileptic drugs such as phenobarbital may promote the formation of toxic metabolites of valproic acid. Thus valproic acid should be avoided in the high risk patient. In other patients, liver function tests are usually monitored and mild elevations of liver enzymes are tolerated. Valproic acid is also reported to cause pancreatitis. Two uncommon dose-related side effects of valproic acid are thrombocytopenia and changes in coagulation parameters, secondary to depletion of fibrinogen. These changes usually are not serious clinically, although they may be associated with bruising, and can often be reduced by lowering the drug dosage. Other side effects of valproic acid are weight gain, alopecia, and tremor.

A frequent side effect of phenobarbital is depression of CNS function, resulting in drowsiness. This may occur during initiation of phenobarbital therapy or as a dose-dependent phenomenon later in the treatment. Idiosyncratic reactions with phenobarbital are rare but include rash (3%) and bone marrow suppression. Common side effects in children include motor hyperactivity, irritability, decreased attention, or mental slowing. The side effects of primidone are similar to those for phenobarbital.

Skin rashes occur during treatment with ethosuximide and are idiosyncratic. Dose-related side effects include GI problems (stomach aches and vomiting) and hiccups. Tolerance to these effects may develop. Ethosuximide may also lead to bone marrow suppression. The side effects of clonazepam relate to its depressive action on the CNS, causing sedation and lethargy, or ataxia.

Drug Interactions

Antiepileptic drugs may interact with each other in two ways (Table 26-5): (1) one compound alters the

Table 26-5   Antiepileptic Drug Interactions

Drug	Interaction Mechanism
ANTIEPILEPTIC DRUGS	
carbamazepine, with:	
phenobarbital	Increased metabolism to epoxide
phenytoin	Decreased carbamazepine effect (increased metabolism)
phenytoin, with:	
primidone	Increased conversion of primidone to phenobarbital
valproic acid, with:	
clonazepam	May precipitate nonconvulsive status epilepticus
phenobarbital	Increased phenobarbital toxicity (decreased metabolism)
phenytoin	Increased phenytoin toxicity (displacement from binding)
OTHER DRUGS	
Antibiotics	Elevates serum concentrations of phenytoin, phenobarbital, or carbamazepine
Anticoagulants	Some antiepileptic drugs (particularly phenytoin and phenobarbital) augment metabolism of coumadin anticoagulants
cimetidine	Displaces benzodiazepines (and possibly phenytoin and valproic acid) from plasma proteins
isoniazid	Increased toxicity of phenytoin (inhibits metabolism)
oral contraceptives	Antiepileptics increase metabolism
salicylates	Compete for plasma protein binding sites, especially with phenytoin and valproic acid
theophylline	Carbamazepine and phenytoin may decrease effects of theophylline

metabolism of another by inducing hepatic enzymes or by competing for reactive sites on those enzymes, or (2) one drug changes the binding of another to plasma proteins. For example, valproic acid may increase the toxicity of phenobarbital or phenytoin by decreasing the hepatic metabolism of phenobarbital or displacing phenytoin from plasma binding sites.

Antiepileptic drugs can also interact with nonantiepileptic drugs, for example, the propensity of antibiotics (isoniazid, chloramphenicol, erythromycin) to elevate serum concentrations of phenytoin, phenobarbital, or carbamazepine. Cimetidine frequently

---

TRADENAMES

In addition to generic and fixed combination preparations, the following tradenamed materials are available in the United States.

PRIMARY ANTIEPILEPTIC DRUGS

Klonopin, clonazepam
Depakene, Depakote; valproic acid
Dilantin, phenytoin
Luminal and others, phenobarbital
Mysoline, primidone
Tegreto, carbamazepine
Zarontin, ethosuximide

SECONDARY ANTIEPILEPTIC DRUGS, INCLUDING ADJUNCTS

Celontin, methsuximide
Diamox, acetazolamide
Mebaral, mephobarbital
Mesantoin, mephenytoin
Milontin, phensuximide
Paradione, paramethadione
Peganone, ethotoin
Phenurone, phenacemide
Tranxene, clorazepate
Tridione, trimethadione

DRUGS FOR THE TREATMENT OF STATUS EPILEPTICUS

Ativan, lorazepam
Valium, diazepam

---

displaces benzodiazepines from plasma proteins and may do the same with phenytoin and valproic acid. Salicylates also compete for plasma protein binding sites, especially with phenytoin. Some antiepileptic drugs decrease the concentration of coumadin anticoagulants by augmenting coumadin metabolism. Antiepileptics also hasten the metabolism of oral contraceptives, resulting in a contraceptive failure rate threefold above the normal.

A few specific interactions needing emphasis include the combination of valproic acid and benzodiazepines, which may precipitate absence status epilepticus in some unusual cases, and the exacerbation of absence seizures by carbamazepine, phenytoin, and phenobarbital.

REFERENCES

Consensus Statement on Febrile Seizures, In Nelson KB and Ellenberg JH, eds.: Febrile seizures, New York 1981, Raven Press.

Drugs for Epilepsy, Med Lett Drugs Ther 31:1, 1989.

Dreifuss FE: Classification of epileptic seizures and the epilepsies, Pediatr Clin North Am 36:265, 1989.

Levy RH, Mattson RH, Meldrum BS, et al.: Antiepileptic drugs, ed. 3, New York, 1989, Raven Press.

MacDonald RL and McLean MJ: Anticonvulsant drugs: mechanisms of action. In Delgado-Escueta AV, Ward AA, Woodbury DM et al.: Basic mechanisms of the epilepsies, molecular and cellular approaches, Adv in Neurology, New York, 1986, Raven Press.

CHAPTER 27

Drugs for the Treatment of Movement Disorders and Spasticity

ABBREVIATIONS	
COMT	catechol-O-methyl transferase
DAG	diacylglycerol
DOPAC	dihydroxyphenylacetic acid
GABA	γ-aminobutyric acid
5-HTP	5-hydroxytryptophan
IP$_3$	inositol trisphosphate
L-DOPA	L-dihydroxyphenylalanine
MAO-B	monoamine oxidase type B
MPP$^+$	N-methyl pyridinium ion
N-MPTP	N-methyl-4-phenyl tetrahydro-pyridine
PI	phosphatidyl inositol

MAJOR DRUGS
L-DOPA
dopamine agonists
deprenyl
anticholinergic drugs
benzodiazepines
baclofen

THERAPEUTIC OVERVIEW

Movement disorders involve abnormalities of voluntary and involuntary movement but generally do not include those that arise because of stroke or seizures. Although there are many possible schemes to categorize movement disorders, a useful initial classification is to divide them into hypokinetic-rigid disorders and hyperkinetic-choreic disorders.

The hypokinetic-rigid syndromes consist of (1) Parkinson's disease, (2) additional systems that degenerate coupled with Parkinson's disease, and (3) drug-induced Parkinsonism. The distinction between Parkinson's disease and look-alike system degenerations is sometimes difficult to detect at the early stages, but is ultimately of great therapeutic importance. Parkinson's disease responds well to pharmacological in-

tervention, whereas the others do not. Examples of systems degenerations include progressive supranuclear palsy (parkinsonism + abnormalities of ocular gaze), olivopontocerebellar atrophy (parkinsonism + ataxia), and Shy-Drager syndrome (parkinsonism + autonomic failure).

Parkinson's disease is a progressive disorder of voluntary movement that affects 1% to 2% of the population over 60 years of age and has an average onset age in the 50s and 60s. Clinical symptoms of Parkinson's disease expressed by most patients include four primary manifestations: (1) resting tremor, typically 4 to 6 Hz and beginning in one limb, (2) rigidity, or increased resistance to passive stretching of muscles, (3) bradykinesia, or slowness in initiating and carrying out voluntary movements, and (4) impaired postural reflexes, with a resulting tendency to fall backwards or forwards easily. Several drugs are useful in the treatment of Parkinson's disease symptoms.

Systems that undergo degenerations coupled with parkinsonism are much more difficult to treat. Drug therapy of these conditions is empirical and generally unsatisfactory. Patients with occasional progressive supranuclear palsy have improved ocular gaze when treated with tricyclic antidepressant drugs. Patients with parkinsonism symptoms have been helped with high doses of dopamine agonists. Ataxia in olivopontocerebellar atrophy may improve with L-5-hydroxytryptophan, the amino acid precursor of serotonin. Orthostatic blood pressure decreases associated with Shy-Drager syndrome usually respond to liberalization of salt intake, mineralocorticoid supplementation, or to direct α-adrenergic receptor agonist (ephedrine) treatment.

Drug-induced parkinsonism generally results from treatment with neuroleptic drugs or with metoclopramide, a potent and selective dopamine D_2 receptor antagonist. In patients receiving neuroleptic drugs for treatment of psychiatric disorders (Chapter 23), concomitant administration of anticholinergic drugs and/or amantadine usually controls the "extrapyramidal" side effects. Neuroleptics must be administered with caution to patients with known Parkinson's disease, even at an early stage, because such patients may experience life-threatening worsening of their Parkinson's disease symptoms.

The hyperkinetic syndromes consist of a group of disorders known as tics, myoclonus, tremors, dystonia, dyskinesia-chorea (including tardive dyskinesia), and Wilson's disease.

Spasticity is a less well-defined disorder that has elements of hypokinetic and hyperkinetic signs and symptoms and is controlled by pharmacological intervention.

These different disease states and the drugs used to treat each are summarized in the box.

 ## MECHANISMS OF ACTION

L-DOPA Therapy

Parkinson's disease is the result of diminished concentrations of the neurotransmitter dopamine within the CNS. The mechanisms by which Parkinson's disease can be treated include replacement of the lost dopamine. Replacement may be by administration of the amino acid precursor L-dihydroxyphenylalanine (L-DOPA). L-DOPA is rapidly decarboxylated before entering the brain, but inhibitors (e.g., carbidopa) (see Chapter 10) of peripheral decarboxylase activity are available for better control of CNS dopamine concentrations. The synthesis and degradation pathways for dopamine and L-DOPA are shown in Figure 27-1.

THERAPEUTIC OVERVIEW FOR MOVEMENT DISORDERS

HYPOKINETIC MOVEMENT DISORDERS

Idiopathic Parkinson's disease
    Primary agents—carbidopa/L-DOPA; bromocriptine; pergolide
    Secondary agents—trihexyphenidyl; benztropine; amantidine
    Protective agent—deprenyl
Olivopontocerebellar atrophy
    carbidopa/5-HTP* (latter for ataxia)
Progressive supranuclear palsy
    bromocriptine; pergolide (for parkinsonism); amitriptyline (for ocular gaze)
Shy-Drager syndrome
    mineralocorticoid; ephedrine

HYPERKINETIC MOVEMENT DISORDERS

Tics
    neuroleptics
Myoclonus
    carbidopa/5-HTP* (for anoxic myoclonus); benzodiazepines; baclofen
Essential tremor
    propranolol; primidone; clonidine
Parkinsonian tremor
    anticholinergics
Dystonias
    anticholinergics; *C. botulinum* toxin

CHOREA

Huntington's disease
    neuroleptic drugs
Tardive dyskinesia
    reserpine; L-DOPA; clonidine

SPASTICITY

benzodiazepine; baclofen

*5-HTP, 5-hydroxytryptophan.

In dopamine agonist therapy, L-DOPA exerts a therapeutic benefit by entering the brain and being converted to dopamine, the endogenous agonist. Subsequent to the introduction of L-DOPA, additional agents have been developed that exert direct agonist effects at dopamine receptors. Apomorphine is the oldest of the known agonists, but it is used only in experimental situations and is not considered here.

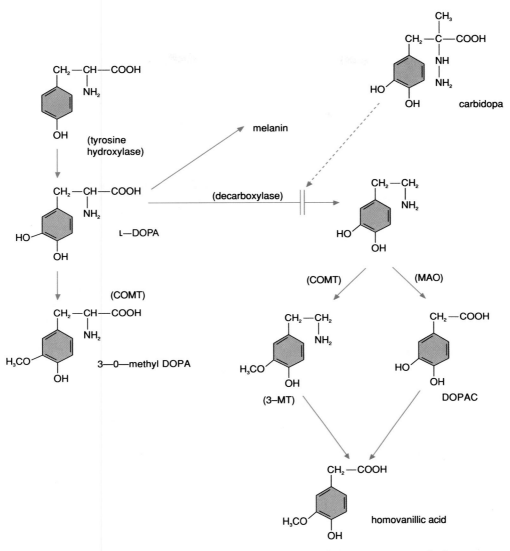

FIGURE 27-1   Pathways of synthesis and catabolism of L-DOPA, structures of relevant compounds. L-DOPA is normally synthesized in dopamine neurons from dietary L-tyrosine. Exogenous L-DOPA is methylated to 3-0 methyl-DOPA by catechol-0-methyl transferase (COMT). The majority of L-DOPA given to Parkinson's disease patients can be lost by decarboxylation if carbidopa is not given concomitantly. In the brain, dopamine formed from L-DOPA is ultimately catabolized to homovanillic acid.

Two direct dopamine agonists, bromocriptine and pergolide, are available for use, and additional dopamine agonists are in various stages of development and may be introduced in the near future. The chemical structures of bromocriptine and pergolide are shown in Figure 27-2.

Dopamine agonists bind to dopamine receptors, of which at least two major classes (D_1 and D_2) are known. D_1-receptors operate through a secondary messenger system that couples ligand-receptor binding to a stimulatory guanine nucleotide, binding G_s-protein to adenylate cyclase to produce increased cAMP production. D_2-receptors are also coupled to adenylate cyclase but through an inhibitory G_i-protein

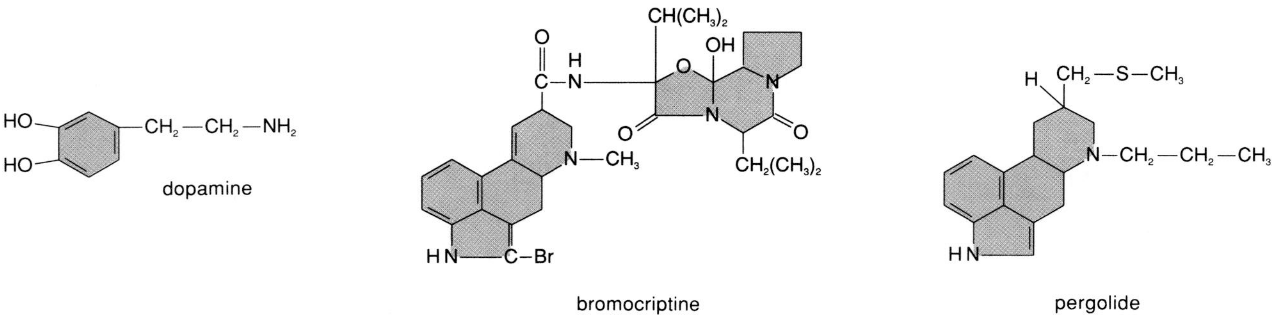

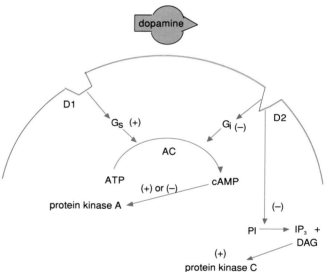

FIGURE 27-2   Structures of the dopamine agonists bromocriptine and pergolide. Note that both of these agonists contain the basic structure of dopamine.

FIGURE 27-3   Second messengers involved in the mechanisms of action at D_1- and D_2-dopamine receptors. D_1-receptors couple to adenylate cyclase (AC) through a stimulatory guanine nucleotide binding protein (G_a) to increase the intracellular production of cAMP from ATP. cAMP stimulates phosphorylation of a variety of cellular proteins by protein kinase A. D_2-receptors couple to AC through an inhibitory G-protein (G_i) to decrease cAMP production. D_2-receptors also reduce the rate of conversion of phosphatidyl inositol (PI) to inositol trisphosphate (IP_3) and diacylglycerol (DAG). DAG stimulates protein phosphorylation by protein kinase C.

that decreases cAMP production. Brain D_2-receptors also decrease the turnover rate of diacylglycerol (DAG)(Figure 27-3).

Detailed information on the structures and functions of D_1- and D_2-receptors is available, but it is still unclear whether the altered cAMP or DAG production observed in vitro with these receptors is responsible for the therapeutic effects of dopamine agonists observed in vivo. However, it is known that both receptor subtypes are present in high densities in those brain regions that receive dopamine terminals, and that simultaneous activation of both receptor subtypes in experimental parkinsonism in animals is necessary for maximum physiological and behavioral responses. D_2-receptors are also present on dopamine nerve cell bodies and endings (autoreceptors), where they control firing rates and modulate dopamine synthesis and release. Because Parkinson's disease is associated with pronounced and progressive loss of dopamine neurons, effects of dopamine-agonist drugs on presynaptic autoreceptors in Parkinson's disease patients is probably of little functional significance.

Our present knowledge of dopamine D_2-receptors is much greater than that of D_1-receptors. Activation of D_2-receptors hyperpolarizes neurons by increasing potassium conductance of both brainstem dopamine neurons and neurons that receive dopamine terminals. The D_2-receptor has been cloned and shown to consist of seven hydrophobic transmembrane segments connecting cytoplasmic and extracellular loops, thus sharing structural features similar to those of other biogenic amine receptors that couple to G-proteins. It is of interest that blockade of D_2-receptors by neuroleptic drugs is associated with their ability to produce parkinsonism in patients taking such drugs.

Anticholinergic Drugs

The mainstay of Parkinson's disease therapy is attempted replacement of lost dopamine synaptic function with L-DOPA-carbidopa and/or direct-acting dopamine agonists. Before the introduction of these drugs, muscarinic anticholinergic drugs had been used for decades as the only known medical treatment for Parkinson's disease. Several anticholinergic drugs are still used for treating early Parkinson's symptoms and are particularly effective in ameliorating tremor, with generally much less efficacy in treating rigidity and bradykinesia. They differ only in potency and have the same spectrum of side effects from blockade of central (memory loss, confusion) and peripheral (dry mouth, decreased sweating, constipation, impaired bladder function) muscarinic receptors.

Another drug used in early treatment of Parkinson's disease is amantadine (see box, p. 374). Amantadine appears to increase dopamine release from preserved dopamine terminals and is thus effective mainly in early Parkinson's patients.

Protective Therapies

A major advance in Parkinson's disease treatment stems from a consideration of the possible etiologies for dopamine cell death, which causes the disease. The appearance in the early 1980s of rapidly progressive, severe parkinsonism in young heroin addicts led to the identification of N-methyl-4-phenyl tetrahydropyridine (N-MPTP, Figure 27-4) as the contaminant in a synthetic opiate preparation used by the addicts. MPTP was subsequently shown to be a "pro-toxin," which is oxidized by brain monoamine oxidase type B (MAO-B) to N-methylpyridinium ion (MPP⁺, Figure 27-4). MPP⁺ is then selectively trans-

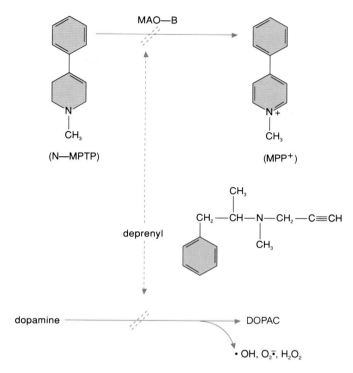

FIGURE 27-4 Potential mechanisms of protective action of deprenyl in Parkinson's disease. Deprenyl blocks the oxidation by MAO-B of the dopamine neuron protoxin H-methyl-4-phenyltetrahydropyridine (N-MPTP) to the toxic derivative N-methylpyridinium ion (MPP⁺). Deprenyl also blocks the normal intraneuronal oxidation of dopamine to dihydroxyphenylacetate (DOPAC), during which free radicals (hydroxyl, OH; superoxide, O_2^-; and peroxide H_2O_2) can be formed.

ported into and concentrated in dopamine nerve endings, where it inhibits mitochondrial respiration, resulting in death of dopamine neurons. When given to older monkeys, MPTP produces an excellent pathological and biochemical model of human Parkinson's disease. The discovery of MPTP-induced parkinsonism revolutionized thinking about possible etiologies of Parkinson's disease and, more importantly, lead to appropriate testing of the hypotheses.

In addition to possible MPTP-like neurotoxicity from substituted pyridines in the environment, dopamine neurons are considered to be susceptible to damage from free radicals formed during oxidative deamination of dopamine by MAO-B (Figure 27-4). Both the "free radical" and "neurotoxin" hypotheses of Parkinson's disease etiology are undergoing testing in a nationwide trial by a MAO-B inhibitor, deprenyl, with or without large doses of vitamin E (α-tocopherol) in patients with Parkinson's disease with early disease symptoms. Preliminary results from both the large trial and a smaller pilot study show that MAO-B inhibition with deprenyl slows the progression of Parkinson's disease symptoms independently of improving the symptoms. It is still not known if vitamin E therapy will be an effective protective agent.

Spasticity

Several drugs that act by binding to GABA receptors are useful in treatment of spasticity. Benzodiazepine drugs potentiate the ability of GABA to open chloride ion channels when GABA binds to GABA type A postsynaptic receptors. The benzodiazepines are discussed further in Chapter 25.

Baclofen is an agonist at GABA type B receptors. This is primarily a presynaptic receptor in the brainstem and spinal cord that is localized to terminals of dorsal root afferent fibers. Activation of GABA type B receptors inhibits neurotransmitter release, probably by inhibition of inward calcium current. The structure of baclofen is shown in Figure 27-5 (see Chapter 25 for structures of benzodiazepines).

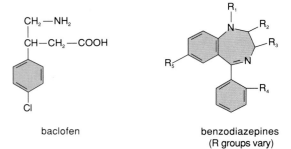

FIGURE 27-5   Structure of baclofen (β-*p*-chlorophenyl-GABA) and benzodiazepines.

 PHARMACOKINETICS

The serum half-life of L-DOPA is short, usually in the range of 1 to 2 hours. A major route of L-DOPA catabolism in the periphery is by 3-O-methylation to 3-O-methyl DOPA (Figure 27-1). The enzyme responsible for this process, catechol 3-O-methyltransferase, has high activities in liver and erythrocytes. With daily use of L-DOPA, particularly in higher doses, 3-O-methyl DOPA serum concentrations increase, mainly as a result of its long serum half-life (around 100 to 150 hours). Elevated 3-O-methyl DOPA blood concentrations have been shown to interfere with the therapeutic action of L-DOPA by competing with L-DOPA for passage across the blood-brain barrier.

Most patients with Parkinson's disease with moderately advanced symptoms improve substantially by taking carbidopa/L-DOPA 3 or 4 times per day, in spite of the short serum half-life of L-DOPA. The longevity of L-DOPA action in these patients probably derives from the ability of surviving dopamine neurons to store dopamine formed from L-DOPA. The pharmacokinetic parameters are summarized in Table 27-1.

RELATION OF MECHANISMS OF ACTION TO CLINICAL RESPONSE

L-DOPA in Parkinson's Disease

A major improvement in L-DOPA therapy occurred with the recognition that 95% of orally administered L-DOPA is lost by decarboxylation before entering the brain unless coadministration of a protective agent is included. Sites of decarboxylation include the intestinal wall, liver, and brain capillaries. Coadministration of peripheral decarboxylase inhibitors (e.g., car-

Table 27-1   Pharmacokinetic Parameters

Drug	Administered	$t_{1/2}$ (hr)	Disposition
L-DOPA	oral	1-2	M (main)
baclofen	oral	—	R (main)
	intrathecal	4-5 in CSF	
bromocriptine	oral	4-6	M (main)
pergolide	oral	—*	M (about 100%)

M, Metabolism; *R*, renal.

*No parent drug detected in plasma after oral administration.

bidopa) with L-DOPA reduced by several-fold the daily DOPA requirements and eliminated peripheral side effects for most patients.

Relief by L-DOPA of Parkinson's disease symptoms in humans and behavioral deficits of experimental parkinsonism in animals depend on access of L-DOPA to brain tissue and decarboxylation to dopamine. A member of the large neutral class of amino acids, L-DOPA is transported by sodium-dependent, carrier-mediated diffusion across tissue barriers. These transport systems in the various tissues are similar if not identical in substrate requirements, and facilitate L-DOPA passage across the intestinal mucosa, blood-brain barrier, and neuronal membrane. At each of these sites, L-DOPA must compete for transport with other large neutral amino acids, and it has been shown that L-DOPA entry into brain can be blocked by raising serum concentrations of competing amino acids. Thus some patients with Parkinson's disease can improve their response to L-DOPA by staggering the doses between meals or by minimizing protein intake during the day.

Dopamine Agonists

Both bromocriptine and pergolide bind to D_1- and D_2-receptors. In in vitro experiments, bromocriptine acts as a D_2 agonist and a D_1-receptor mixed agonist-antagonist. Pergolide is approximately 10-fold more potent than bromocriptine as a dopamine-receptor agonist and has less D_1-antagonist action, at least in vitro. Clinically, both drugs effectively treat Parkinson's disease symptoms in both early and late phases of the disease. Both drugs have been shown to function well as supplements to L-DOPA when Parkinson's disease patients develop irregular responses to L-DOPA and can stabilize clinical symptoms. It is likely that their potent D_2-agonist properties, when combined with the D_1-properties of L-DOPA (after conversion to dopamine), exert maximum clinical effects in a similar fashion to treatment of experimental parkinsonism in animals.

Deprenyl Therapy

In contrast to dopamine agonists, anticholinergics and amantadine, which are symptomatic therapies of Parkinson's disease, daily therapy with deprenyl constitutes protective therapy, that is, protects the surviving dopamine neurons and lessens the rate of progression of symptoms. Whether deprenyl therapy will prolong the time of good response to L-DOPA/carbidopa remains to be demonstrated, although theoretically this should also occur. Deprenyl has also been approved for concomitant administration with L-DOPA in more advanced Parkinson's disease patients experiencing fluctuations in response to L-DOPA. It appears to be moderately effective for some patients and presumably acts by inhibiting the degradation of dopamine by MAO-B. Deprenyl is free of typical MAO inhibitor side effects when taken in low MAO-B selective doses. Thus very few side effects are produced by deprenyl in the dose used for Parkinson protective or supplemental therapy.

Therapy of Hyperkinetic Disorders

Hyperkinetic movement disorders encompass a broad spectrum of abnormal signs and symptoms. The descriptive classification of hyperkinetic syndromes does not provide clues as to etiology. For the vast majority of these disorders no underlying consistent pathophysiology is known, but there may be known causes. In general, pharmacotherapy is empirical.

Tics The tic disorder most commonly treated with drugs is Tourette's syndrome, which begins in childhood and is associated with vocalizations, abnormal gestures, and frequently with obsessive-compulsive personality. Neuroleptic drugs are helpful in controlling both the simple and complex tics in Tourette's syndrome. As with any prolonged neuroleptic treatment, there is a risk of producing tardive dyskinesia (see Chapter 24).

Myoclonus Myoclonus is frequently a symptom of metabolic encephalopathy (i.e., renal failure) or drug toxicity, and treatment must be directed at the underlying cause(s). It is important to establish if the myoclonic movements are accompanied by EEG changes, so-called cortical myoclonus, in which case anticonvulsant drugs may be helpful. Another secondary cause of myoclonus is hypoxic-ischemic brain injury. Such individuals recover from their coma only to develop disabling myoclonic jerks when attempting to use their limbs. Their "action myoclonus" is frequently responsive to 5-hydroxytryptophan when given with carbidopa to block peripheral decarboxylation.

Idiopathic myoclonic disorders are difficult to treat. Those which respond at all to drugs tend to respond to benzodiazepines or baclofen. Sedation is frequently the limiting side effect.

Tremors Other than Parkinson's disease tremor discussed previously, the most commonly seen tremor disorder and that most responsive to medication is benign essential tremor, also known as adrenergic, or familial tremor. In contrast to the rest tremor of Parkinson's disease, essential tremor is not apparent at rest and is evoked by use of the affected limb(s) or body part (voice), or postural use of associated muscles (i.e., head-neck). Essential tremor is generally faster (8 to 12 Hz) than parkinsonian tremor, exacerbated by caffeine, and suppressed by small quantities of ethanol. About 75% of essential tremor patients respond to nonselective β-adrenergic antagonist drugs, usually in small doses relative to those used to treat hypertension or angina. Those not responsive to β-adrenergic blockers may respond to the anticonvulsant, mysoline, or the presynaptic α-adrenergic agonist, clonidine.

Dystonia Dystonia may begin and remain focal, affecting only one area of the body, but can also begin focally and evolve into generalized dystonia. Some generalized dystonia is inherited in an autosomal dominant fashion, particularly the type found among Ashkenazi Jews.

Two very common forms of focal dystonia involve forced eyelid closure (blepharospasm) or twisting of the neck to one side (torticollis), frequently in combination with pulling of the neck backwards (retrocollis). Although occasionally patients with such focal dystonias improve with benzodiazepines or baclofen, improvement is often partial, transient, and complicated by side effects. A recent addition to the armamentarium for treating dystonia is injection of *Clostridium botulinum* toxin into dystonic muscles. Botulinum toxin injection inhibits presynaptically the release of acetylcholine from motor nerve endings and produces an effective, long-lasting denervation of involved muscles.

The only consistently effective medical therapy for generalized dystonia is high-dose anticholinergic drugs. After a slow upward titration of dose, such drugs as trihexyphenidyl are tolerated in surprisingly high doses by generalized dystonia patients, sometimes with substantial improvement.

Dyskinesia-Chorea Although these two terms describe the same clinical phenomena, *dyskinesias* generally refer to "choreic" drug side effects, whereas *choreas* occur in the course of natural diseases. The most commonly encountered dyskinesia is that arising in the natural history of Parkinson's disease

treated with L-DOPA. This dopa-dyskinesia can also be seen with direct dopamine agonists, and it is presently unknown whether these patients treated exclusively with dopamine agonists (i.e., no L-DOPA) have a lower incidence of dyskinesia later in their disease. Optimal management of DOPA-dyskinesias is presently unclear.

Tardive Dyskinesia Tardive dyskinesia is a choreic movement disorder arising late in the course of neuroleptic treatment. Recent data from tardive dyskinesia produced experimentally in animals and analysis of brains obtained from tardive dyskinesia patients suggest that a deficiency of GABA in certain basal ganglia nuclei is consistently present. This GABA deficiency hypothesis is also supported by the ability of GABA antagonists injected into the same basal ganglia areas to produce chorea in primates, and the efficacy of experimental GABA agonist to relieve tardive dyskinesia movements.

No such specific therapy is available for tardive dyskinesia. Disabling cases, which can be dramatic, but also are rare, frequently respond to carefully titrated high doses of reserpine. The major side effects of this treatment are orthostatic blood pressure drops and mental depression. Less severe tardive dyskinesia may respond paradoxically to carbidopa/L-DOPA or to clonidine treatment. The appearance of tardive dyskinesia must always yield evaluation of need for continued neuroleptic treatment and, if still indicated, minimum effective neuroleptic dose (Chapter 24).

Chorea naturally occurs in the course of Huntington's disease, an autosomal dominantly inherited neurodegenerative disorder. The marked loss of GABA neurons in the brains of Huntington's disease patients suggests similarities to tardive dyskinesia. However, limited trials of GABA-mimetic therapies have not been successful. Agents that block dopamine receptors (neuroleptic drugs) or deplete dopamine stores (reserpine, tetrabenazine) are occasionally helpful in this otherwise dismal disease.

Wilson's Disease Hepatolenticular degeneration must always be considered in the differential diagnosis of hyperkinetic movement disorders, particularly in young adults. Wilson's disease arises from an autosomal recessively inherited defect in the synthesis of ceruloplasmin, a copper-transporting serum protein. Over time, copper accumulates in all tissues, particularly in brain and liver. Progressive neurological (with or without hepatic) dysfunction develops, which is partially reversible with dietary copper re- striction and daily use of a copper-chelating agent (penicillamine) to accelerate copper excretion.

Spasticity Spasticity is a constellation of clinical signs that develops when lower motor neurons (an- terior horn cells and gamma motor neurons) are chron- ically disconnected from their upper motor neuron innervation. Signs of spasticity include increased re- sistance to sudden muscle stretch, increased speed and amplitude of muscle stretch reflexes, weakness and appearance of primitive limb reflexes, such as Babinski's sign. The symptom of spasticity that most frequently leads to treatment is muscle spasms, which can occur either spontaneously or from sensory stimulation.

Drugs useful in the treatment of spasticity include benzodiazepines and baclofen. They are equally ef- fective in both treating spasticity and producing un- wanted CNS side effects, mainly sedation.

Recently, baclofen administered intrathecally (into the spinal subarachnoid space) resulted in good con- trol of spasticity symptoms with minimal side effects. As the technology improves for chronic intrathecal drug delivery, control of spasticity symptoms with minimal side effects may become a common reality.

SIDE EFFECTS, CLINICAL PROBLEMS, AND TOXICITY

For most Parkinson's disease patients, after 3 to 5 years of smooth response to L-DOPA, fluctuations in response appear and become more troublesome over time. These fluctuations initially appear as "wearing off," which is the reappearance of Parkinson's symp- toms at the end of each dosing interval. This problem is usually responsive to both increases in the L-DOPA dose and decreases in dosing interval. Later in the course of the disease, "peak dose dyskinesias" be- come apparent. These are involuntary choreic move- ments of face and/or limbs that typically occur within 30 to 60 minutes after taking L-DOPA, fade as the patient becomes nearly normal for a period of time, and then are followed by "wearing off." Later in the course of the disease many patients develop the most troublesome problem of "random on-off" swings. These are sudden changes in parkinsonian disability, frequently manifested as freezing spells of variable duration that occur randomly and independently of L- DOPA dose.

CLINICAL PROBLEMS

L-DOPA (PARKINSON'S)

Fluctuations in response; confusion and hallucina- tions; problems with L-DOPA uptake (by food)

BACLOFEN (SPASTICITY)

Major side effect is sedation

DEPRENYL

Protective doses have very few side effects

TRADENAMES

In addition to generic and fixed combination prepa- rations, the following tradenamed materials are available in the United States.

Artane, trihexyphenidyl
Cogentin, benztropine
Lioresal, baclofen
Mysoline, primidone
Parlodel, bromocriptine
Permax, pergolide
Sinemet, carbidopa/L-DOPA
Symmetrel, amantadine

The above fluctuations in response to L-DOPA can be eliminated by administering L-DOPA IV at a con- tinuous rate. Pharmacokinetic studies in Parkinson's disease patients show that peripheral metabolism of L-DOPA is no different between normal individuals and Parkinson patients in the early stages without fluctuations. The sudden fluctuations in clinical re- sponse thus appear to arise from abnormal drug ac- tion dynamics of L-DOPA, most likely from decreased capacity of brain tissue both to store dopamine formed from L-DOPA and to buffer synaptic dopamine concentrations as L-DOPA enters the brain.

Both direct dopamine agonists and carbidopa/L- DOPA have similar CNS side effects. Of these, the most troubling and frequently dose-limiting is con- fusion and hallucinations. Fortunately, most Parkin- son's disease patients do not suffer this side effect, and it seems to occur in Parkinson's patients who suffer from concomitant dementia. Both direct do-pamine agonists and L-DOPA can exacerbate psy-chosis in prone individuals and must be used very cautiously in that population. Lastly, a severe aki-netic-rigid condition mimicking neuroleptic malig-nant syndrome can occur if dopamine agonist therapy is rapidly withdrawn from Parkinson's patients with more advanced symptoms. The clinical problems are summarized in the box, p. 381.

REFERENCES

Parkinson Study Group: Effect of deprenyl on the progres-sion of disability in early Parkinson's disease, N Engl J Med 321:1364, 1989.

Weiner WJ and Lang AE: Movement disorders, Mount Kisco, NY, 1989, Futura Publishers.

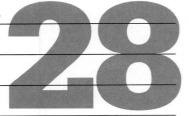
Pain Control with Narcotic Analgesics

MAJOR DRUGS

opioid analgesics

opioid antagonists

 THERAPEUTIC OVERVIEW

Pain sensation is complex and variable. Experiences considered painful by one individual may not be equally painful to another person and may vary in the same individual depending on the circumstance. One aspect of pain is that there are both physiological (discriminative) and psychological (affective) components. Subjective experiences (e.g., "phantom limb" pain) make it clear that there is a strong psychological component to pain.

Several groups of compounds are used to relieve pain, depending on the severity and duration and on the nature of the painful stimulus. These drugs are classified in several ways.

Drugs used to relieve pain without causing unconsciousness are called *analgesics* and are subdivided into three groups according to their ability to relieve mild, moderate, or severe pain. Mild analgesics are termed *non-narcotic* and include such agents as aspirin (Chapter 29). This chapter primarily covers the narcotic (opioid) analgesics used to control moderate to severe pain, of which morphine is the prototype. Included in this chapter is a discussion of opioid antagonists, partial agonists, and mixed agonists/antagonists.

The Sensation of Pain

The specific anatomical pathways that transmit pain impulses within the CNS are summarized in Figure 28-1. Two different types of nociceptive (noxious) stimuli are intense enough to be perceived as pain and can be alleviated by opioid drugs. One type, sometimes called somatic pain, consists of an intense, localized sharp or stinging sensation. This is mediated by fast-conducting lightly myelinated A-delta fibers that have a high threshold (i.e., require a strong mechanical stimulus) and enter into the spinal cord through the dorsal horn where they terminate mostly in lamina I of the cord.

The second type of pain, sometimes called visceral pain, is characterized as a diffuse, dull, aching, or burning sensation. This type is mediated by largely unmyelinated, slower-conducting C fibers that are polymodal (i.e., mediate mechanical, thermal, and chemical stimuli). These C fibers also enter the spinal cord through the dorsal horn, where they terminate mostly in the outer layer of lamina II. The ascending tracts are the paleospinalthalamic and the neospinalthalamic.

Endogenous pain control systems descend the spinal cord through the dorsolateral funiculus to the spi-

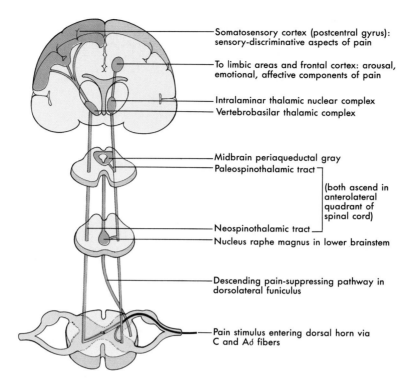

Somatosensory cortex (postcentral gyrus): sensory-discriminative aspects of pain

To limbic areas and frontal cortex: arousal, emotional, affective components of pain

Intralaminar thalamic nuclear complex
Vertebrobasilar thalamic complex

Midbrain periaqueductal gray
Paleospinothalamic tract ⎤
                            ⎥ (both ascend in
                            ⎥ anterolateral
                            ⎥ quadrant of
                            ⎥ spinal cord)
Neospinothalamic tract ⎦
Nucleus raphe magnus in lower brainstem

Descending pain-suppressing pathway in dorsolateral funiculus

Pain stimulus entering dorsal horn via C and Aδ fibers

FIGURE 28-1   Schematic diagram of the paleospinothalamic (red) and neospinothalamic (purple) pain-transmission pathways and the descending pain-suppression pathway (blue).

nal dorsal horn where they inhibit neurons that are activated by nociceptive stimuli. The higher centers connected to these descending systems include the periaqueductal gray region and various subregions of the medulla (e.g., the *nuclei raphe magnus, nuclei reticularis magnocellularis,* and *nuclei reticularis paragigantocellularis lateralis*). These regions contain opioid receptors, and the ability of morphine to inhibit the perception of nociceptive stimuli may involve the activation of these descending pathways.

Although much remains to be learned about the neurotransmitters involved in both the afferent nociceptive and descending antinociceptive pathways, prime candidates for the afferent pathways include peptidergic neurotransmitters (e.g., substance P, somatostatin, vasoactive intestinal polypeptide, cholecystokinin, and calcitonin gene-related peptide). The descending antinociceptive pathways appear to involve norepinephrine and serotonin as neurotransmitters, as well as endogenous opioid peptides. The spinal cord also contains opioid receptors, which are mainly localized within laminae I to III of the dorsal horn and within the tract of Lissauer. The highest

---

SUMMARY OF THERAPEUTIC ASPECTS OF NARCOTIC ANALGESICS

DESIRED EFFECT IS TO RETAIN CONSCIOUSNESS
Mild to moderate analgesics (see Chapter 29)
Narcotic analgesics
      Morphine and related opioid receptor agonists
      Opioid receptor antagonists
Antidiarrheal action

---

density of opioid receptors is localized in the inner segment of lamina II.

Since pain is both a sensation (objective feeling) and an emotion (subjective feeling), it is not surprising that opioid drugs affect one of these components more than the other. A continuous, dull pain is more effectively relieved by opioid drugs than is a sharp, intermittent pain. At usual therapeutic doses, opioid drugs can markedly increase the ability to tolerate pain, while the capacity to perceive it may be little affected. Higher doses, however, also have the ability to interfere with pain perception.

The therapeutic aspects of narcotic analgesics are summarized in the box.

 ## MECHANISMS OF ACTION

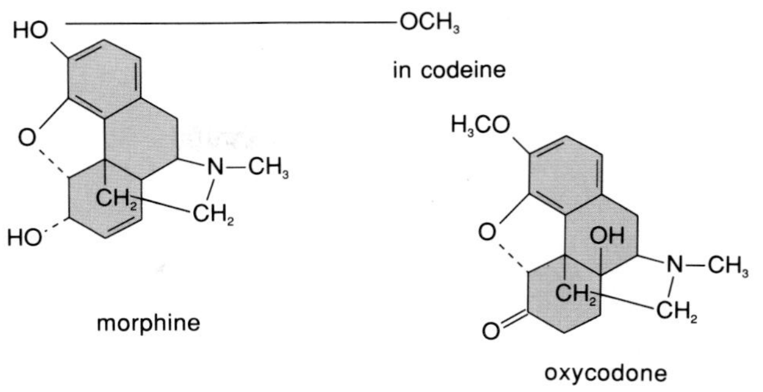

Morphine is the prototype opioid. The structure of morphine and related compounds are shown in Figure 28-2. Although sap from the unripe seed pods of the opium poppy plant, which contains morphine, was being used medicinally as early as 400 to 300 BC, not until the early 1800s was morphine isolated; in the 1900s its chemical structure was determined. By the mid-1900s, it was known that only a small fraction of a dose of morphine crosses the blood-brain barrier into the CNS to produce analgesia. In addition, the presence of binding sites in CNS membranes was used to show that the analgesic levo-isomer of an opioid could bind with high affinity, but the inactive dextro-isomer could not. In addition, drugs known to be specific opioid antagonists were also shown to bind to these sites with high affinity, which provided a mechanism to explain why antagonists can block the analgesic, as well as other agonist effects of morphine and related opioid agonists.

Opioid Receptors and Endogenous Opioid Peptides

It is now established that there are multiple types of opioid receptors in the CNS designated as μ, κ, σ, and δ, with evidence that additional classes of subclasses may exist. μ Receptor activation in the brain is presumed to be responsible for the analgesic effect of morphine-like drugs. *K* receptors, which exist in the brain and spinal cord, also appear capable of producing analgesia, particularly at the spinal level. The majority of the psychotomimetic effects of opioid drugs (e.g., dysphoria and hallucinations) are apparently mediated by *σ* receptors; however, it is doubtful that *σ* receptors are strictly "opioid" in character, as they appear also to be activated by such nonopioid compounds as phencyclidine. The fourth type of opioid receptor, the δ, has a different distribution in the brain and is thought to be the primary receptor for endogenous opioid pentapeptides known as enkephalins. These receptors are found not only in the

brain and spinal cord, but also in some peripheral tissues.

The synthetic, semi-synthetic, and naturally occurring opioid analgesics have pharmacological effects similar to those of the endogenous opioid peptides. The first endogenous opioid peptides to be identified, methionine-enkephalin and leucine-enkephalin, eventually led to the identification of three different classes of endogenous opioid peptides. Each of these is derived from a different genome. One gene encodes for the precursor peptide pro-opiomelanocortin, which is cleaved to produce an opioid peptide called β-endorphin. The second gene encodes for pro-enkephalin A, which gives rise to methionine-enkephalin, and the third encodes for pro-dynorphin, which gives rise to the dynorphin family of opioid peptides. Both pro-enkephalin A and pro-dynorphin also contain the pentapeptide sequence of leucine-enkephalin. The structures of these three types of endogenous peptides and the pathways for their production are shown in Figures 28-3, 28-4, and 28-5.

The pharmacological profiles of the several families of opioid peptides are described on p. 387. Dynorphin A action has agonist activity at κ receptors. β-endorphin binds to both μ and δ receptors and in addition to a new type of opioid receptor, the ε receptor. Progress in purification and characterization of opioid receptors should further our understanding.

β-endorphin and dynorphin are located predominantly in the pituitary gland, but also exist in the CNS proper. The three types of peptides have a distinct distribution throughout the CNS, indicating separate enkephalinergic (δ receptors) neurons, endorphi-

FIGURE 28-2   Chemical structures of morphine and related compounds. Codeine results when the OH of morphine is replaced by OCH_3.

Primary Gene Product:

H₂N— | SIGNAL / —— / γ MSH / —— / ACTH / —— / ß–MSH / ß–endorphin | —COOH

ß-endorphin: Tyr—Gly—Gly—Phe—Met—Thr—Ser—Glu—Lys—Ser—Gln—Thr—Pro—Leu—Val—
Thr—Leu—Phe—Lys—Asn—Ala—Ile—Ile—Lys—Asn—Ala—Tyr—Lys—Lys—Gly—Leu

FIGURE 28-3   Order of compounds encoded by the pro-opiomelanocortin peptide gene and amino acid sequence of β-endorphin. The same gene also encodes for adrenocorticotrophic hormone (ACTH) and a family of melanocyte stimulating hormones (MSH), as well as for other peptides.

Primary Gene Product:

H₂N— | SIGNAL / — / ME / ME / — / MERGL / — / Peptide E / — / MERP | —COOH

Peptide—E: Try—Gly—Gly—Phe—Met—Arg—Arg—Val—Gly—Arg—Pro—Trp—Trp—Met—
Asp—Tyr—Gln—Lys—Arg—Tyr—Gly—Gly—Phe—Leu

ME: Tyr—Gly—Gly—Phe—Met   (δ>μ>κ)

LE: Tyr- -Gly—Gly—Phe—Leu   (δ>μ>κ)

MERP: Tyr—Gly—Gly—Phe—Met—Arg—Phe   (δ>μ>κ)

MERGL: Tyr—Gly—Gly—Phe—Met—Arg—Gly—Leu   (δ>μ>κ)

FIGURE 28-4   Order of opioid peptide sequence encoded by the pro-enkephalin A gene and the amino acid sequences. The order of preference in binding to brain membrane receptor types is shown in parentheses (either δ, μ, or κ). Note that ME differs from LE by the substitution of leucine for methionine at the C-terminus. MERP is met-enkephalin enlarged by arginine (R) and phenylalanine (P) at the C-terminus. MERGL is met-enkaphalin enlarged by arginine R, glycine (G), and leucine (L) at the C-terminus. E begins with the met-enkephalin *(ME)* sequence and ends with the leu-enkephalin *(LE)* sequence.

Primary Gene Product:

| SIGNAL /—— /α –Neoendorphin / —— / Dynorphin-A / Dynorphin–B / | —COOH

dynorphin—A: Tyr—Gly—Gly—Phe—Leu—Arg—Arg—Ileu—Arg—Pro—Lys—Leu—Lys—Trp—Asp—
Asn—Gln   (κ>μ>δ)

dynorphin—B: Tyr—Gly—Gly—Phe—Leu—Arg—Arg—Gln—Phe—Lys—Val—Val—Thr   (κ>μ>δ)

α—neo—endorphin: Try—Gly—Gly—Phe—Leu—Arg—Lys—Tyr—Pro—Lys   (κ>δ>μ)

leu—enkephalin: Tyr—Gly—Gly—Phe—Leu   (δ>μ>κ)

FIGURE 28-5   Order of opioid peptide sequence encoded by pro-dynorphin gene and the amino acid sequences. The order of preference in binding to brain membrane receptor types is shown in parentheses (either δ, μ, or κ). Note that all of the opioid products of this gene begin with the leu-enkephalin sequence.

nergic (μ and δ receptors) neurons, and dynorphinergic (κ receptors) neurons. Small amounts of the peptides released appear in human cerebrospinal fluid (CSF). CSF also contains appreciable amounts of incompletely processed opioid peptides with the leuenkephalin-Arg[6]-and met-enkephalin-Lys[6]-amino acid sequences. The endogenous opioid peptides are involved with the modulation of pain sensory mechanisms and may be important in other body processes as well. It is possible that the endogenous opioid peptides are involved in the regulation of respiration, the disturbance of which is a very significant side effect of the opioid analgesic drugs. Finally, it has been shown that some endogenous opioid peptides exist in tissues and organs other than the brain. Some are present in the GI tract, one of the sites of action of opioid drugs. The roles of endogenous opioid peptides in regulating normal respiratory function and normal intestinal function have not been well characterized.

Many details of the molecular action of morphine are still not known. The opioid receptors are located on the membranes of neurons, and the interaction of agonists with these receptors generally leads to decreased firing rates or reduced excitability. Agonists of μ receptors increase the outward flux of potassium ions, which makes the neuron less excitable and thus less calcium enters the neuron when stimulated. Agonists of κ receptors more directly inhibit the entry of calcium into neurons by decreasing influx through voltage-dependent calcium channels. These findings support the idea that increasing calcium concentrations attenuate the effects of morphine, and conversely, decreasing calcium concentrations increase the potency of morphine. Agonists of μ and δ receptors also decrease neuronal cAMP synthesis. The effect of morphine on pain perception is different from the effect of a local anesthetic. Local anesthetics (Chapter 30) interfere with pain perception by decreasing conduction along the axon. Opioids have very limited activity on neuronal conduction. Often after receiving an effective dose of an opioid drug, patients relay to their physician, "It hurts, but who cares?" Such drugs are useful in treating the psychological or emotional component of pain. Unlike aspirin and the nonnarcotic analgesics, opioid drugs do not have antiinflammatory activity. Because of the ability of many opioid drugs to release histamine, their intracutaneous injection can lead to a mild inflammatory reaction.

OPIOIDS ACTING ON μ RECEPTORS

morphine	diphenoxylate
codeine	loperamide
hydromorphins	fentanyl
oxymorphine	alfentanil
levorphanol	sufentanil
oxycodone	methadone
meperidine	1-α-acetylmethadol
alphaprodine	propoxyphene

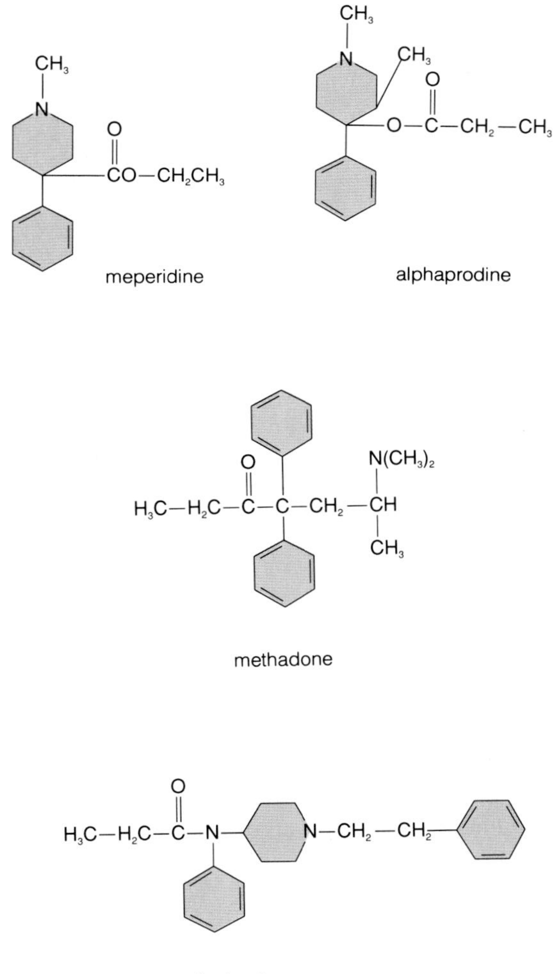

FIGURE 28-6   Chemical structures of additional opioid analgesics that act as agonists at μ receptors (in addition to those in Figure 28-2).

Partial μ agonist

buprenorphine

κ Receptor agonist

nalorphine dinicotinate

Agonist-antagonist

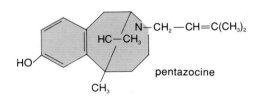

pentazocine

Antagonist

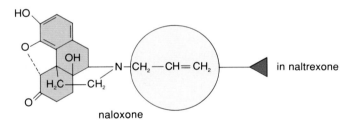

in naltrexone

naloxone

FIGURE 28-7   Several partial μ or κ receptor agonists and antagonists.

Opioid Drug Types

Opioid analgesic drugs can be grouped into four categories according to the opioid receptor subtype and whether the compounds act as agonists or antagonists.

The drugs that act primarily at μ receptors as agonists are listed in the box.

The chemical structures of some of these drugs are shown in Figure 28-6.

Additional drugs that act as partial agonists at μ receptors, including buprenorphine, are shown in Figure 28-7. Structures of the antagonists naloxone and naltrexone also are shown in Figure 28-7.

PHARMACOKINETICS

The pharmacokinetic parameter values for the opioid analgesic drugs are summarized in Table 28-1.

Morphine is usually administered IM and varied bioavailability limits oral administration to low-dose preparations of opium (e.g., paregoric) used for treating diarrhea. Oral preparations are also used in some terminally ill cancer patients to limit the discomfort of frequent injections. The bitter taste of morphine limits sublingual use.

Levorphanol, fentanyl, and methadone, with longer half-lives than durations of action, may accumulate

Table 28-1 Pharmacokinetic Parameters

Drug	Administration	Elimination t $_{1/2}$ (hr)	Disposition	Analgesia Duration (hr)
morphine	IM, IV, SC	2.9	M* (main)	4-5
hydromorphone	oral, SC	2.6	M	4-5
oxymorphone	IM, IV, SC	(?)	M (main)	4-5
oxycodone	Oral	(?)	M	4-5
levorphanol	SC, Oral	11	M	4-5
buprenorphine	IM, IV, SC	5	—	5-9
meptazinol		1.6	M	1-2
methadone	Oral, SC	25	M	3-5
propoxyphene	Oral	3.3	M† (main)	1-3
meperidine	IM, Oral	3.2	M† (main)	2-4
alphaprodine	IV, SC	2.2	—	1-2
fentanyl		3.7	—	0.5
alfentanil		1.6	—	<0.5
sufentanil		2.6	—	0.5
pentazocine	Oral, IM	2.9	—	3-4
butorphanol	IM, IV	2.7	—	3-4
nalbuphine	IM, SC, IV	5.1	—	4-5
naloxone	Oral	1.2	M* (main)	1-4 ‡
naltrexone		9.7	M†	10-24‡
codeine	Oral, SC	—	M† (main) (converted to morphine)	—

M, Metabolized.
*Large first pass effect.
†Active metabolite.
‡Duration of antagonistic action.

in plasma and tissue. Duration of the action of methadone can increase up to 12 hours with repeated dosing, making it difficult to titrate individual patients. After IV administration of a single dose, fentanyl, alfentanil, and sufentanil have rapid onsets of action. Their short durations of action relative to their plasma half-lives is because of redistribution from the brain to peripheral tissues. Fentanyl is 80% to 85% bound to plasma protein, whereas alfentanil and sufentanil are 90% to 95% bound. In comparison, morphine is only about 30% bound to plasma proteins. Many opioid analgesics undergo extensive "first pass" metabolism after oral administration. For example, studies of the oral use of morphine in cancer patients have indicated a variable bioavailability ranging from 15% to 49%. The decreased bioavailability of morphine orally, when compared to morphine given parenterally, is largely due to first pass metabolism of morphine via glucuronide formation. The major urinary metabolite of morphine is morphine-3-glucuronide. This 3-position is substituted with a methyl group in oxycodone and codeine, which have greater bioavailability (50% to 65%). The major urinary metabolite of codeine is codeine-6-glucuronide. Methadone and levorphanol also have reasonably good oral bioavailability (approximately 50%).

Some opioid drugs also have active metabolites. For example, meperidine is metabolized in part to normeperidine, which has about one half the analgesic potency of meperidine, but with greater excitatory effects than meperidine. Administration of meperidine in frequent high dose intervals, particularly in patients with decreased renal function, can lead to an accumulation of normeperidine and result in excitatory symptoms, including seizures. Repeated dosing with propoxyphene leads to its accumulation as well as the accumulation of an active metabolite, norpropoxyphene. These accumulations are accompanied by an increased half-life of propoxyphene (3.3 to 11.8 hours) and norpropoxyphene (6.1 to 39.2 hours). The major unconjugated metabolite of naltrexone, 6-β-naltrexol, can achieve higher plasma concentrations than naltrexone itself and has a half-life of approximately 11 hours. Although 6-β-naltrexol possesses opioid antagonist activity, it is considerably less potent than naltrexone.

RELATION OF MECHANISMS OF ACTION TO CLINICAL RESPONSE

Major Effects of Opioid Analgesics

Clinical use of opioid analgesics consists primarily of balancing the analgesia produced against adverse side effects. Morphine and most other opioid analgesics elicit a mixture of stimulatory and inhibitory effects, with the major sites of activity for these drugs being the brain and GI tract. Areas of the brain receiving input from the ascending spinal pain-transmitting pathways are rich in opioid receptors, with a major effect of opioid analgesics being a depression of neuronal activity. This increases the pain threshold

---

SUMMARY OF DEPRESSANT AND STIMULANT EFFECTS OF MORPHINE

DEPRESSANT EFFECTS

Suppression of pain, analgesia
Drowsiness and decreased mental alertness, sedation
Decreased respiration, increased intracranial pressure
Decreased myocardial oxygen demand
Suppression of cough, antitussive
Decreased peristalsis
Inhibition of fluid and electrolyte accumulation in intestinal lumen
Decreased gastric acid secretion
Inhibition of emetic center
Slight decrease in body temperature
Decreased release of gonadotropin leuteinizing hormone (LH) and follicle stimulating hormone (FSH)

STIMULANT EFFECTS

Euphoria
Constriction of pupils, miosis
Stimulation of chemoreceptor trigger zone
Increased tone of intestinal smooth muscle
Increased tone of sphincter of Oddi, increased biliary pressure
Increased tone of detrusor muscle
Increased tone of vesical sphincter
Increased release of prolactin and antidiuretic hormone
Proconvulsant in overdose

---

and sedation, and is often accompanied by euphoria. Although morphine and other opioids produce drowsiness and promote sleep, this clearly is not the cause of the analgesia. The depressant and stimulant effects of morphine are summarized in the box.

An important specific effect of opioid drugs on the CNS is their ability to depress the cough reflex (antitussive). Commonly used opioids, except meperidine, possess antitussive activity. The prototype antitussive drug is codeine. Only *l*-isomers of opioids are analgesic. However, both *d* and *l* isomers possess anti-tussive activity. This has led to the development of a number of compounds (e.g., dextromethorphan) for use as antitussives. The advantage of dextro-isomers, e.g., dextromethorphan, which is active orally, is that they do not produce physical dependence. The dependence liability of opioid drugs, like analgesia resides in the levo-isomer. Care should be observed in using levo-isomers as antitussives in patients who show a high propensity for dependence liability or a pattern of drug abuse. *d*-Isomers are often used as antitussives and are found in a variety of nonprescription cough remedies.

Opioid analgesics depress respiratory function with the same doses that produce analgesia. This effect is due to depression of respiratory centers in the brain stem and to depression of respiratory reflexes. This leads to respiratory failure from overdose and is also one of the most limiting side effects of these drugs.

Although CNS depression is usually the overriding effect of the opioid drugs, certain excitatory effects are sometimes observed. These include restlessness, delirium, mania, and strychnine-like stimulation of the spinal cord. They do not occur in all individuals and are more prevalent with specific opioids.

A stimulatory effect observed with most opioids is constriction of the pupils (miosis). The increased activity of neurons in the Edinger-Westphal nucleus of the oculomotor (third cranial) nerve leads to increased parasympathetic tone. The pupillary constriction aids in the clinical identification of heroin addicts. Ophthalmic application of parasympatholytic agents (e.g., scopolamine) blocks opioid-induced miosis.

Opioid drugs sometimes cause nausea and vomiting, especially in ambulatory patients, while at other times they block these effects. Nausea and vomiting are induced by stimulation of the chemoreceptor trigger zone in the area postrema of the medulla. This stimulatory action is tempered by an inhibitory effect of opioid drugs on the vomiting (emetic) center in the lateral reticular formation of the medulla.

A second major site of action of opioid drugs is the GI tract. Actions on the GI tract can be either therapeutically useful or produce marked side effects, especially in patients requiring opioids for prolonged periods of time. Since opioid drugs produce constipation, they are used effectively in treating diarrhea. Clinically significant tolerance does not develop to this effect.

The mechanisms by which opioids produce constipation involve (1) prolongation of stomach emptying time, (2) decreased propulsive contractions of the small intestine and increased tone of the large intestine to slow transit, and (3) increased tone of the anal sphincter and inattention to normal sensory stimuli for defecation. In addition, the antidiarrheal actions of opioids may also involve blockage of ion and water flow into the intestinal lumen caused by certain bacterial toxins (e.g., cholera toxin).

Other effects of morphine-like opioids on smooth muscle include increased bile duct pressure and increased sphincter tone, leading to difficulty in micturition. Morphine therefore is contraindicated in treatment of biliary colic. Atropine is used to decrease this effect of morphine without interfering with analgesia. Agonist-antagonist drugs, discussed later, usually cause little, if any, increase in biliary pressure. The morphine-induced increase in the tone of the vesical sphincter may be tempered by a reduced volume of urine production. Conversely, agonists of κ receptors can produce a water diuresis.

Morphine and other opioid drugs have limited effects on the cardiovascular system at therapeutic doses, especially in supine patients. However, depressant effects may be observed at higher doses. Occasionally, orthostatic hypotension may occur. Morphine is useful to treat pain and apprehension in myocardial infarction. It is also useful in treating acute pulmonary edema left ventricular failure because it reduces the left ventricular work by peripheral pooling of blood. In contrast, some agonist-antagonist opioids (e.g., pentazocine and butorphanol) increase ventricular afterload and myocardial oxygen requirement. These deleterious hemodynamic effects can result in extension of an infarct. Pentazocine and butorphanol are not recommended for use in patients with acute myocardial infarction.

A major therapeutic use of opioids is as preanesthetic agents before surgery to produce analgesia, sedation, reduced anxiety, and decreased needs for general anesthetic agents. Some opioids (e.g., morphine or fentanyl) may be used as the major agent in balanced anesthesia, especially for cardiac surgery. Nonopioid benzodiazepines (e.g., diazepam) are also often used as preanesthetic agents; however, they do not produce analgesia.

Opioid Analgesics that Interact Primarily with μ Receptors

Morphine Morphine, widely used to relieve severe pain, does not affect other sensory modalities, including touch, taste, smell, or hearing. The IV and spinal uses of morphine are limited to patients whose respiratory function is carefully monitored for potential respiratory depression. Respiratory depression from morphine administered intrathecally is avoided by elevating the upper body to prevent the rostral flow of morphine in cerebrospinal fluid. Spinal administration of morphine has the advantages of increased potency and duration, reduced incidence of side effects, and temporary relief from tolerance that develops in patients who require long-term analgesia, such as patients with terminal cancer. However, severe itching, not relieved by antihistamines, or urinary retention, especially in elderly men, may prevent spinal use. In general, the therapeutic ratio (see Chapter 1) of morphine is quite good.

Heroin Heroin, diacetyl morphine (Figure 28-2), is used orally for pain relief in European countries and has been tested in the United States. Because of its great propensity for intravenous abuse, it has no legal medical use in the United States. Heroin is two or three times as potent as morphine, but is not more effective than morphine in treating acute pain. Its use in chronic pain is controversial and some have proposed that heroin should be legalized in treating patients with terminal cancer.

Heroin must be converted in the body to 6-acetylmorphine and morphine to produce analgesia. The 3-acetyl group is removed at least in part by plasma and tissue esterases. The 6-acetylmorphine produced, as well as heroin itself, penetrates the blood-brain barrier much more readily than morphine. Heroin and 6-acetylmorphine transported into the brain can undergo enzymatic deacetylation to produce morphine. Since heroin does not have a high affinity for opioid receptors, the analgesic effects of heroin are likely mediated by morphine and 6-acetylmorphine. The increased potency of heroin over morphine thus involves the greater penetrability into the brain of the acetylated forms of morphine. Therefore, heroin has the same spectrum of pharmacological effects as morphine.

Codeine Codeine, the most commonly used opioid analgesic, is often used with acetaminophen. Codeine is less efficacious than morphine, but it is nevertheless a useful agent in the relief of mild to moderate pain. Codeine has more predictable bioavailability than morphine after oral administration. Codeine is the prototype antitussive agent and is less addicting at therapeutic doses than is morphine. Codeine does not have a high affinity for opioid receptors, but since it is partially metabolized to morphine, a part of its analgesic activity is morphine-related.

Other Morphine Congeners Other morphine-like analgesics available include hydromorphone, oxymorphone, levorphanol, and oxycodone (see Figure 28-2). Compared with an analgesic dose of morphine, hydromorphone is about 8 times as potent, oxymorphone 10 times, levorphanol 5 times, and oxycodone is equipotent. They are as effective as morphine for moderate to severe pain and have similar durations of action. Except for hydromorphone, these have greater bioavailability than morphine orally, retaining about half of their analgesic potencies compared to their effect when administered parenterally. All have addiction potentials similar to morphine.

Meperidine and Other Phenylpiperidine Derivatives Meperidine is widely used to treat moderate to severe pain. It does not have a morphine-like chemical structure but is a piperidine derivative. Meperidine has a faster onset of action than morphine, with analgesic effects 10 minutes after SC or IM injection and 15 minutes after oral administration. However, it has a shorter duration than morphine because of its more rapid metabolism. Its effects last from 2 to 4 hours compared to 4 to 5 hours for morphine. The shorter duration may account, at least in part, for the decreased constipation and decreased biliary spasm. Its slightly lower addiction potential is still considerable, as indicated by its history of extensive abuse, particularly by physicians and paraprofessionals. Meperidine and other phenylpiperidine derivatives do not have useful antitussive activity.

Another phenylpiperidine agent, alphaprodine, is more potent but with a shorter duration of action (1 to 2 hours) than meperidine. It is useful in obstetrical, urological, and orthopedic procedures where rapid analgesia of short duration is needed.

Diphenoxylate and loperamide are used only as antidiarrheal agents and use is limited to oral administration. Although doses of diphenoxylate higher than those required for antidiarrheal activity can produce morphine-like euphoria, analgesia, and physical dependence, chronic abuse potential is limited by the addition of atropine to preparations of diphenoxylate. Atropine causes undesirable parasympatholytic side effects when taken in high doses. The relative insolubility of diphenoxylate in aqueous solutions also prevents intravenous abuse. Loperamide, which also has low aqueous solubility, binds to intestinal tissue, and most of what is absorbed undergoes efficient enterohepatic circulation, leading to low systemic blood concentrations and poor distribution to the brain. Both antidiarrheal agents are considered to have low abuse potential, with that of loperamide being less than that of diphenoxylate. Loperamide has recently been made available in a nonprescription antidiarrheal preparation. Opioid antidiarrheal agents are contraindicated in diarrheal diseases accompanied by high fever or blood in the stools.

Fentanyl and Derivatives Fentanyl, alfentanil, and sufentanil are extremely potent opioid drugs of the piperidine series. Fentanyl is about 80 times as potent as morphine, with a much shorter duration of action following a single IV injection (about 30 minutes), a result of redistribution from brain to peripheral tissues. Alfentanil is about one fourth as potent as fentanyl, and sufentanil is 5 to 10 times as potent as fentanyl. Both have shorter durations of action than fentanyl. Given IV, these opioids are used primarily as a component of balanced anesthesia for certain surgical procedures, and their use generally requires mechanical ventilation. The muscle rigidity that high doses of these agents sometimes produce can interfere with artificial ventilation. Administration of a muscle relaxant may also be necessary.

Fentanyl and related compounds must be used cautiously in balanced anesthesia, as a number of cases of a delayed respiratory depression have been reported.

Lofentanil is 6000 times as potent as morphine and has a significantly longer duration of action. It binds so tightly to opioid receptors that its effects cannot be antagonized by narcotic antagonists. These characteristics increase the possibility of death from overdose of fentanyl derivatives. Also, a number of deaths among heroin addicts have occurred from illicit production and use of 3-methylfentanyl (China White), which has nearly 1000 times the potency of heroin.

Methadone and Its Congeners Methadone is a synthetic opioid analgesic not structurally related to morphine. Its potency is equal to or slightly greater than that of morphine, with a similar duration of action after a single dose. Methadone has greater bioavailability than morphine by oral administration. These properties, in addition to its longer half-life, have led to its widespread use as a heroin substitute in treatment programs for opioid addiction.

A methadone congener, l-α-acetylmethadol, has been tested as an alternative to methadone in treatment of addicts because of its ability to suppress appearance of withdrawal signs in an addict (i.e., maintain physical dependence) as long as 72 hours after a single oral dose. The long duration of action is probably related to the formation of long-acting metabolites.

Propoxyphene is chemically similar to methadone but is much less potent and less effective. Its use is limited to oral administration and, when compared to oral codeine, is about one half to two thirds as potent. Propoxyphene is not effective for treating severe pain. Against mild to moderate pain it is about as effective as aspirin. Although propoxyphene has less abuse liability than codeine, its use has declined recently following reports of poisoning and death from overdose, particularly when taken in combination with alcohol, tranquilizers, or other CNS depressants. Many deaths occurred from deliberate overuse, abuse, or suicide attempts. Toxicity of propoxyphene is characterized by respiratory and CNS depression. However, seizures, cardiotoxic effects, and pulmonary edema can also occur. Some effects are antagonized by naloxone.

Opioid Analgesics That Are Partial μ Receptor Agonists

Buprenorphine is an opioid agonist of μ receptors displaying some properties not typical of most morphine-like drugs. In the therapeutic range, doses of buprenorphine that are equianalgesic with morphine also depress respiration to a similar extent, but the onset of this depression is delayed. Once developed, the respiratory depression caused by buprenorphine is only partially reversible by the narcotic antagonist, naloxone. Buprenorphine can antagonize the greater respiratory depressant effects of the higher doses of morphine or fentanyl that are sometimes used during cardiac surgery and still provide postoperative analgesia in such cases. Buprenorphine causes less euphoria than morphine, and physically dependent subjects on buprenorphine experience a milder but prolonged morphine-like abstinence syndrome that cannot be precipitated by naloxone. These features are characteristic of a compound that is only a partial agonist of μ receptors and that dissociates from these receptors very slowly. It also appears to be a κ receptor antagonist. Buprenorphine has somewhat less abuse liability than morphine.

Meptazinol is an investigational drug in the United States that is used in the United Kingdom. Unlike other opioid analgesics, meptazinol does not produce as much respiratory depression in therapeutic doses as does morphine. It also produces less miosis, and does not have antidiarrheal properties. However, it may produce a higher incidence of nausea and vomiting than morphine. It has poor oral bioavailability (<10%) and a shorter duration of action (2 hours) than morphine. Although not recognized as an opioid by experienced addicts and although no physical dependence has been noted with chronic administration, meptazinol possesses antagonist activity and thus can precipitate withdrawal symptoms in subjects dependent on other opioid drugs. Its analgesic effects can be blocked by naloxone. Meptazinol may be a selective agonist of a postulated subtype of μ receptor, denoted as the μ_1 opioid receptor.

Opioid Analgesics That Are Agonists of κ Receptors

Nalorphine, Levallorphan and Cyclazocine Analgesic properties of nalorphine are equivalent to morphine, but it produces dysphoria rather than the euphoria observed with morphine. Nalophine has significantly less addiction liability than morphine. Other synthetic opioids, levallorphan and cyclazocine, have similar properties to those of nalorphine. Unfortunately, a high incidence of dysphoric side effects at analgesic doses has discouraged the development of these drugs for use as opioid analgesics. Nalorphine and levallorphan enjoyed wide use as opioid antagonists to treat opioid overdose until the development of drugs with more specific antagonist activity such as naloxone.

Pentazocine Pentazocine was the first compound in the series of agonist-antagonist analgesics to be used clinically. Pentazocine is less potent than morphine, and appears to be less efficacious, particularly when an anxiolytic effect is desired. It requires 3 to 4 times as much pentazocine to be equianalgesic to morphine when given IM. Pentazocine is also active when given orally in somewhat higher doses. Unlike morphine, as the doses of pentazocine are increased above the therapeutic range, the respiratory depression caused by pentazocine does not increase to the point of causing death. Thus, there appears to be a ceiling effect to the respiratory depressant effect of pentazocine and other related opioid antagonist-analgesics. In overdose cases there is less risk of death from respiratory depression than with morphine-like analgesics. However, increasing the dose of pentazocine above the therapeutic range also results in progressively higher incidence of psychotomimetic side effects, including the inability to suppress unpleasant thoughts, dysphoria, and hallucinations.

Butorphanol Unlike pentazocine, butorphanol is only given parenterally because of its low bioavailability (about 17%) after oral administration. A comparison of butorphanol with other drugs given IM for the relief of postoperative pain indicates that butorphanol has up to 7 times the potency of morphine, 40 times that of meperidine, and 20 times that of pentazocine. Butorphanol has antitussive activity, but is not used for this purpose. The incidence of psychotomimetic side effects is less than that with pentazocine.

Nalbuphine Nalbuphine also is only given parenterally. Its analgesic potency is approximately the same as that of morphine and 3 to 4 times that of pentazocine. It may have a slightly longer duration of action than pentazocine, but its peak analgesic effect is less, and the incidence of psychotomimetic side effects is less than with pentazocine.

The possibility that pentazocine, butorphanol, and nalbuphine can produce analgesia, at least in part, by acting as partial agonists on μ receptors has not been ruled out. Like the partial μ-receptor agonist buprenorphine, these agonist-antagonist drugs can precipitate a withdrawal syndrome in persons who are highly physically dependent upon morphine-like drugs. Nalbuphine has greater antagonistic activity

at analgesic doses than do the other agonist-antagonist analgesics. Pentazocine, nalbuphine, and butorphanol generally have much less excitatory effect than morphine on smooth muscles, so constipation and exacerbation of biliary colic are rarely encountered. The most common side effect of these agonist-antagonist opioids is sedation. Diuretic effects of these drugs have not been reported in humans, although butorphanol has a limited diuretic effect in animal studies, which has led to the postulate that it may be a partial agonist of κ receptors.

Opioids Used Solely as Antagonists

Naloxone Naloxone was the first drug with relatively pure antagonist activity to become available for treating opioid overdose and has now largely replaced nalorphine and levallorphan for this use. A major caution with this use of naloxone is that the patient must be carefully monitored for possible recurrence of respiratory depression because the duration of action of naloxone is short relative to the duration of the depressant effects of most opioid agonists. This short duration is circumvented by using multiple injections of naloxone until the patient is out of danger. The great utility of naloxone, which is administered IV, is that a physically dependent patient can be titrated very carefully to reverse the respiratory depression without precipitating a severe withdrawal syndrome. Naloxone has a higher affinity for μ receptors than for κ receptors. This might explain why a higher dose of naloxone is required to reverse the respiratory depression caused by pentazocine-like drugs than that caused by morphine-like drugs. The observation that naloxone produces a significant increase in blood pressure in various forms of shock (e.g., from acute spinal cord injury or septicemia) suggests the possible use of this drug to counteract the deleterious hemodynamic effects of endogenous opioids that are apparently released during shock.

Naltrexone Naltrexone is another opioid antagonist that, unlike naloxone, has a relatively good bioavailability after oral administration. It also is about three times more potent than naloxone and has a much longer duration of action. These advantages over naloxone have led to the experimental use of naltrexone as an "extinction" therapy in the treatment of opioid addiction. The chronic oral use of naltrexone has been associated with a low but significantly increased incidence of headache and other manifes-

Table 28-2 Summary of Clinical Responses Produced by Opioid Analgesics

Drug	Analgesia	Antitussive	Constipation	Respiratory Depression	Abuse Liability
morphine	+ + +	+ +	+ + +	+ + +	+ + +
heroin	+ + +	+ +	+ + +	+ + +	+ + + +
codeine	+	+ +	+ +	+	±
hydromorphone	+ + +	+ +	+ +	+ + +	+ + +
oxymorphone	+ + +	+	+ +	+ + +	+ + +
oxycodone	+ +	+ +	+ +	+ +	+ + +
levorphanol	+ + +	+ +	+ +	+ + +	+ + +
buprenorphine	+ + / + + +	±	+	+ + / + + +	±
meperidine	+ + / + + +	—	±	+ + +	+ +
alphaprodine	+ + / + + +	—	±	+ +	+
methadone	+ + +	+ +	+ +	+ + +	+ +
propoxyphene	+	—	±	+	+
pentazocine	+ + / + + +	—	±	+ + / + + +	+
butorphanol	+ + / + + +	+	±	+ + / + + +	+
nalbuphine	+ + / + + +	—	±	+ + / + + +	±

+ + + +, Strongest effect; +, weak effect; ±, weakest effect.

tations of pain, and an elevation of serum transaminase concentration that then returns to normal upon discontinuation of the drug.

Very recently, naltrexone has been used experimentally to treat apneic disorders that appear to be associated with elevated concentrations of β-endorphin-like immunoreactivity in the CSF. These include the infant apnea syndrome, which may be involved in some cases of sudden infant death syndrome (SIDS); Rett syndrome, only observed in girls and involving a number of neurological problems in addition to respiratory disturbances; and several disorders in which naltrexone blocks apnea and enhances seizure control by antiepileptic drugs. Naltrexone does not appear to be useful for the treatment of apnea in premature infants; theophylline is the drug treatment of choice.

Summary of Clinical Responses

The major effects of the opioid analgesics are summarized in Table 28-2.

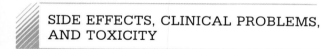

SIDE EFFECTS, CLINICAL PROBLEMS, AND TOXICITY

Respiratory depression, constipation, opioid abuse and addiction, development of tolerance, and devel-

opment of physical dependence are the most troublesome side effects and problems associated with the use of opioid analgesics.

Respiratory Depression

Except for the investigational drug meptazinol, all of the strong analgesics produce a comparable degree of respiratory depression at equianalgesic doses, regardless of whether they act predominantly at μ or κ opioid receptors. Although the respiratory depression produced by therapeutic doses of these agents is generally not deleterious to patients with normal respiratory and cardiovascular function, great caution should be exercised when administering these agents to patients with compromised respiratory function (e.g., those with sleep apnea, asthma, or emphysema). Opioid drugs are contraindicated during an asthmatic attack and in patients with head injury that may have caused brain trauma. The respiratory depression produced by therapeutic doses increases the pCO_2, which in turn causes cerebral vasodilation and increased intracranial pressure that can worsen brain trauma. Mechanical ventilation to prevent increase in pCO_2 can be used to prevent increased intracranial pressure.

Since respiratory depression occurs at therapeutic doses, it often is a limiting factor in the use of opioid analgesics in obstetrics. If an opioid analgesic is administered to the mother, it can cross the placenta and cause respiratory depression in the newborn. Obviously women who abuse opioids also place their offspring in jeopardy.

Tolerance and Physical Dependence

Tolerance, best described as the need for an increased dose of drug to produce the same pharmacological effect, is associated with continuous use of opioid analgesics. Rate and degree of tolerance development are related to the frequency, dose, and length of time the drug is used. Although the molecular mechanism for opioid tolerance is unknown, several studies with animals and cultured neurons have indicated that tolerance may involve multiple types of adaptation by neuronal cells that possess cell membrane opioid receptors. Mechanisms include decreased affinity for agonists or decreased number of cell membrane opioid receptors and decreased efficiency of coupling between agonist-occupied receptor and cellular response. Alternate hypotheses for tolerance include a compensatory increase (or decrease) in excitability of target neurons or tissues innervated by neurons that possess the opioid receptors and recruitment of a redundant pathway to bypass the inhibited functional pathway.

Whatever the mechanism(s), tolerance does not develop uniformly to all actions of the opioid drugs. For example, with chronic morphine administration, less tolerance develops to the constipating and miotic effects than to the analgesic effect, so that as the dose of morphine is increased to achieve the desired level of analgesia, it is always accompanied by these side effects.

Another related characteristic of tolerance involves cross-tolerance. Although generally accepted that tolerance to one opioid confers cross-tolerance to other opioids, recent animal studies indicate that the degree of cross-tolerance may not be equal. Theoretically, two mechanisms could account for unequal cross-tolerance at the receptor level. First, if two different types of opioid receptors (e.g., μ and κ) mediate the same type of response (e.g., analgesia), development of tolerance to drugs that interact primarily with κ receptors, for example, should leave the response mediated by μ-receptor agonists relatively intact. Second, different agonists of the same type of receptor may differ in their ability to produce a given degree of response. Thus one drug may produce a

response by occupying only 10% of the receptors that mediate that response, whereas the elicitation of the same response by another drug may require the 50% occupation of those receptors. This difference in coupling efficiency is sometimes referred to as a difference in intrinsic activity. As tolerance develops, the intrinsic activity of drugs that require occupancy of a large fraction of receptors in the nontolerant state may fall off faster than the activity of drugs that require occupancy of a smaller fraction of receptors. Therefore it may be possible to at least partially circumvent or delay the tolerance problem by appropriate switching of drug therapies. However, this possibility has not been exploited clinically. It is important to remember that switching from chronic administration of a μ receptor agonist to a κ or partial μ agonist could result in the precipitation of a withdrawal syndrome, unless there is an opioid-free period between the administration of the two drugs. For patients requiring chronic opioid administration to relieve pain, addition of a nonnarcotic analgesic to the therapeutic regimen often provides beneficial additive effects.

Another major adverse effect of opioid analgesics is their propensity for producing both psychic and physical dependence (see also Chapter 21). Psychic dependence is best characterized by the continued desire or craving for a substance. Individuals can be psychically dependent on many things, in addition to many drugs. Physical dependence is observed when the cessation of administration of a substance (abstinence) causes physical signs of withdrawal. The distinction between psychic and physical dependence becomes less clear when one considers that both emotional and vegetative body functions are modulated by neurotransmitters and hormones acting on receptors and that many drugs alter such systems. Opioid drugs clearly produce both psychic and physical dependence.

Although physical dependence can develop with relatively low doses of morphine-like drugs, seldom does a patient become dependent with short term therapy. Opioid physical dependence is probably closely related to the development of tolerance, as the physical signs of withdrawal generally represent physiological actions opposite to acute actions of opioid drugs. For example, if an acute opioid effect is constipation, the corresponding physical withdrawal sign is diarrhea. The typical features and time course of withdrawal from morphine-like drugs are

Table 28-3 Symptoms and Their Time Course Following Withdrawal of Morphine and Morphine-like Drugs

Time After Withdrawal	Symptoms
6-12 hr	Drug-seeking (purposive) behavior; nonpurposive signs, such as restlessness, lacrimation, rhinorrhea, sweating, yawning.
12-24 hr	Restless sleep for several hours (yen) and feeling more miserable than before after awakening; irritability, tremor, dilated pupils, anorexia, gooseflesh.
24-72 hr	Increased intensity of above signs plus weakness, depression, nausea, vomiting, intestinal cramps, diarrhea, alternate chills and flushes, various aches and pains, increased heart rate and blood pressure, involuntary movements of arms and legs, dehydration and possible electrolyte imbalances.
Later	Above symptoms of autonomic hyperactivity alternate with brief periods of restless sleep and gradually decrease in intensity until addict feels better in 7 to 10 days, but may still exhibit strong craving for the drug. In addition, some mild signs may be detectable for up to 6 months. Delayed growth and development of infants born to addicted mothers may be detected for up to 1 year.

summarized in Table 28-3. The intensity of a given abstinence sign is not always proportional to the degree of physical dependence. This is because physical dependence and tolerance are dynamic phenomena that undergo constant adjustments according to the concentration of agonist present at the receptors. If an agonist has a long half-life (e.g., methadone), agonist withdrawal results in a milder, though more prolonged, withdrawal than that which occurs if agonist activity is suddenly blocked by the injection of the antagonist, naloxone. Generally the overall intensity of naloxone-precipitated withdrawal is directly related to the degree of physical dependence. The intensity of abstinence withdrawal, however, may be modified by environmental factors. For example, some soldiers who used large doses of heroin in Vietnam returned home and did not go through severe withdrawal when they stopped using heroin. Such observations indicate that the phenomenon of physical dependence is much more complicated than previously believed. The extent to which endogenous opioid peptides may function to modify the withdrawal syndrome is unknown. Single-dose physical dependence in ex-addicts has been demonstrated in both clinical and animal studies, indicating that one cycle of physical dependence and withdrawal apparently causes long-lasting changes that increase the liability for initiating another cycle of dependence (recidivism). The relative contributions of psychic dependence and protracted physical dependence to recidivism, as well as the extent to which endogenous

opioid peptides may play a role in this problem, are also unknown.

Abuse Liability

The capacity of an opioid drug to produce physical dependence requiring continued drug use to suppress unpleasant withdrawal symptoms is only one of the factors that contribute to the abuse liability of an opioid (see also Chapter 21). Other factors include the drug's ability to produce euphoria, the occurrence of toxic side effects when the dose is increased beyond the usual therapeutic range, and the ability to suppress abstinence symptoms caused by withdrawal of other agents in this class. Of these factors, the degree to which a drug induces euphoria or positively-reinforcing effects is a major one in determining abuse liability and drug-seeking behavior. The intensity of the euphoric effect depends to some extent upon the physical characteristics of the drug. A high degree of lipid solubility that allows the drug to rapidly penetrate the blood-brain barrier after IV administration leads to a shorter latency and more intense euphoria. On the other hand, the drug must be sufficiently soluble in water so that it can be injected IV. Heroin has both of these characteristics.

It is generally thought that analgesics acting through κ receptors (e.g., pentazocine) produce less euphoria and have less overall abuse liability than do the morphine-like drugs. In 1977, however, some addicts discovered that the combination of the antihistamine tripelennamine with pentazocine was just as euphoric as heroin and the IV abuse of this mixture became widespread. This led to more control over the distribution of pentazocine, and since 1983 one oral form of this drug has included a small amount of naloxone hydrochloride to discourage IV abuse by dependent individuals. Because of extensive first-pass metabolism by the liver when administered orally, this amount of naloxone does not antagonize the analgesic effect of pentazocine, but if administered IV, naloxone blocks the euphoric effect of pentazocine.

Pharmacological Treatment of Opioid Addiction

The most widely used treatment of addiction is the substitution method in which methadone is administered in place of the opioid drug being abused. As with cross-tolerance to morphine-like drugs, there is also cross-dependence among the members of this class, which allows the orally active methadone to substitute for the opioid drug. The methadone, supplied free by specially licensed clinics, hopefully reduces the engagement of addicts in criminal activities to meet costs. That methadone is active orally also removes the possibility of infection from the sharing of needles and syringes. This is particularly important because of the increased incidence of acquired immunodeficiency syndrome (AIDS) among intravenous drug abusers (Chapters 21 and 51).

The original theory of methadone treatment of addiction is based on first maintaining a high degree of tolerance, so that no euphoric "high" is experienced with heroin, and then gradually decreasing the methadone. The rationale for this theory is that the addicts will not undergo as severe a withdrawal as they do with the abrupt withdrawal characteristics of opioid drugs that have a shorter half-life than methadone. One of the problems has been that withdrawal from methadone, at least in some patients, has been equal to or worse than withdrawal from the injected opioid drugs, particularly with withdrawal duration. However, methadone maintenance is effective, and is widely used to treat opioid addiction.

A second method for treating opioid addiction involves the oral use of an opioid antagonist such as naltrexone. Although this treatment has not been widely used clinically, it is being tested in patients

---

CLINICAL PROBLEMS

RESPIRATORY DEPRESSION
With essentially all strong analgesics

CONSTIPATION
Beneficial effects in diarrhea, undesirable effects with nondiarrheal conditions

TOLERANCE
Degree varies with action, may get cross-tolerance between different opioids

PHYSICAL AND PSYCHIC DEPENDENCE PRODUCED
Withdrawal problems and abuse liability

---

who appear particularly motivated to become drug free. The patient is taken off all opioid drugs and goes through withdrawal, and then is treated with a long-acting antagonist. The theory behind opioid antagonist therapy is that if subsequent injections of an opioid are received, the antagonist will block the euphoric effect of the drug, thereby discouraging further opioid use. During the withdrawal phase, some clinics use the α_2-adrenergic agonist clonidine to suppress withdrawal signs that appear to result from excessive activity of the autonomic nervous system. Clonidine does not alleviate the dysphoria or drug craving that occurs during withdrawal.

The major difference between these two types of treatment is that in one methadone is substituted for another opioid drug and the patient does not go into withdrawal, while in the other (antagonist) approach the patient must go through complete withdrawal and be completely devoid of opioid drugs before treatment with an opioid antagonist begins. Otherwise, the antagonist could precipitate an immediate and severe withdrawal syndrome.

One major problem with both of these types of treatment is the high frequency of drug administration. Methadone or naltrexone must be taken at least once a day by the patient coming to the clinic, but thus far the longer acting l-α-acetylmethadol has not gained clinical acceptance. However, the shorter-acting drugs necessitate more frequent appearance of the addict or post-addict at the treatment center,

TRADENAMES

In addition to generic and fixed combination preparations, the following tradenamed materials are available in the United States.

Alfenta, alfentanil HCl

Astramorph, MS Contin, MSIR, Roxanol, morphine sulfate

Buprenex, buprenorphine

Darvon, propoxyphene HCl

Demerol, meperidine HCl

Dilaudid, hydromorphone HCl

Dolophine, methadone HCl

Levo-Dromoran, levorphanol tartrate

Narcan, naloxone HCl

Nubain, nalbuphine HCl

Numorphan, oxymorphone HCl

Pantopon, opium alkaloids HCl

Roxicodone, oxycodone HCl

Stadol, butorphanol tartrate

Sublimaze, fentanyl citrate

Synalgos-DC, dihydrocodeine

Talwin, pentazocine HCl

Trexan, naltrexone HCl

thus providing opportunity for important psychological support, and removal of this psychological support may be detrimental to the value of the therapy with the longer duration drugs.

The clinical problems with the opioid analgesics are summarized in the box.

REFERENCES

Basbaum AI and Fields HL: Endogenous pain control systems: brainstem spinal pathways and endorphin circuitry, Ann Rev Neurosci 7:309, 1984.

Bobill JG, Sebel PS, and Stanley TH: Opioid analgesics in anesthesia: with special reference to their use in cardiovascular anesthesia, Anesthesiology 61:731, 1984.

Foley KM and Inturrisi CE: Analgesic drug therapy in cancer pain: principles and practice, Med Clin North Am 71(2): 207, 1987.

Millan MJ: Multiple opioid systems and pain, Pain 27: 303, 1986.

Yaksh TL: Opioid receptor systems and the endorphins: a review of their spinal organization, J Neurosurg 67: 157, 1987.

CHAPTER 29

Pain and
Inflammation
Control with
Nonnarcotic
Analgesics

ABBREVIATIONS	
HGPRT	hypoxanthine guanine phospho-ribosyltransferase
PPi	pyrophosphate
PRPP	5-phosphoribosyl-l-pyrophosphate

 THERAPEUTIC OVERVIEW

Nonnarcotic analgesics are used to treat (1) mild pain and/or elevated body temperature, (2) arthritis and other inflammatory disorders, and (3) gout and hyperuricemia. These disorders may be acute or chronic and affect large segments of the population. Although symptoms may be extremely undesirable and often disabling, these disorders generally are not life threatening. The mild to moderate pain of headache, myalgia, neuralgia, and arthralgia that generally arises from integumental structures, and certain kinds of postoperative pain and dysmenorrhea can usually be treated with analgesics such as aspirin and acetaminophen or with several nonsteroidal antiinflammatory compounds. These drugs also are antipyretic agents, and aspirin, because of its ability to inhibit platelet aggregation, is also useful in the prophylaxis of myocardial infarction.

The arthritic disorders include rheumatoid arthritis, juvenile arthritis, ankylosing spondylitis, psoriatic arthritis, Reiter's syndrome, and osteoarthritis. They are characterized by inflammation and subsequent tissue damage. Although immunological factors play an important role in the etiologies of these diseases,

the precise pathogenesis is largely unknown. Thus many different chemical classes of drugs are being used on an empirical basis to treat these conditions.

Gout, a disorder characterized by the deposition of uric acid crystals in joints, is accompanied by hyperuricemia. Hyperuricemia may also be present secondary to diseases or can result from other drug treatment. Therapies for acute or chronic arthritides conditions and underlying hyperuricemia can be successfully carried out with the drugs described in this chapter.

The therapeutic control of mild pain, inflammation, and gout is summarized in the box.

 MECHANISMS OF ACTION

Nonnarcotic Drugs Used to Treat Pain and Fever

Drugs used to reduce mild to moderate pain and fever include acetylsalicylic acid (aspirin), diflunisal, salsalate, acetaminophen, ibuprofen, naproxen, and fenoprofen.

The mechanism by which these drugs act to reduce mild to moderate pain is based on the relationship between drugs such as aspirin and prostaglandin synthesis. Studies in humans have shown that IV administration of certain prostaglandins elicits headache and pain and produces hyperalgesia, sensitizing the individual to stimuli that normally would not produce pain. Aspirin and related compounds inhibit the enzyme cyclooxygenase and prevent the formation of

TREATABLE WITH NONNARCOTIC ANALGESICS

Mild to moderate pain—headache
　　　　　　　　　myalgia
　　　　　　　　　neuralgia
　　　　　　　　　postoperational pain
　　　　　　　　　dysmenorrhea

TREATABLE WITH ANTIPYRETICS

Elevated temperature

TREATABLE WITH A WIDE RANGE OF DRUG TYPES

Arthritis—rheumatoid
　　　　　juvenile
　　　　　ankylosing spondylitis
　　　　　osteoarthritis
　　　　　immunological factors

TREATABLE WITH SEVERAL DRUG CLASSES

Gout/hyperuricemia

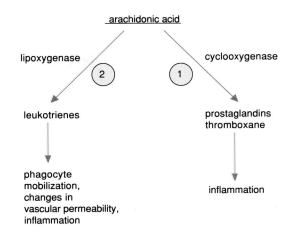

FIGURE 29-1　Proposed mechanisms of action of nonnarcotic analgesics. Most nonnarcotic analgesics act at *(1)* to block prostaglandin and thromboxane formation, and several antiinflammatory agents may also act at *(2)* to block leukotriene formation. (See Chapter 18 for more details.)

prostaglandin endoperoxides, PGG and PGH, which are normally formed from arachidonic acid (Figure 29-1). The details are described in Chapter 18. The production of all prostaglandins derived from these endoperoxides therefore is blocked. Prostaglandins are not stored within cells so their release depends on their de novo biosynthesis. Practically all mammalian cells synthesize prostaglandins; however, the efficacy of inhibitory drugs varies with the tissue. Thus drug selection is based on pain location. In contrast to the effects of the opioids, cyclooxygenase inhibitors act locally to block pain rather than to influence its recognition in the brain.

The chemical structures of some of the analgesic and antipyretic compounds are shown in Figure 29-2. Acetaminophen and related structures are shown in Figure 29-3.

The ability of aspirin-like drugs to reduce fever depends on their inhibition of prostaglandin E_2 biosynthesis within the preoptic hypothalamic region, which regulates body temperature. Fever usually is caused by viral or bacterial infections. Certain cell wall products of pyrogenic microorganisms stimulate the synthesis and release of a pyrogen that enters the central nervous system and promotes prostaglandin release in the hypothalamus. The cyclooxygenase inhibitors lower elevated body temperature by blocking prostaglandin synthesis.

Antiinflammatory Drugs

The inflammatory response is mediated by a host of endogenous compounds, including immunological and chemotactic factors, proteins of the complement system, histamine, serotonin, bradykinin, leukotrienes, and prostaglandins. Both leukotrienes and prostaglandins are major contributors to the symptoms of inflammation. Prostaglandins E_2 and I_2 promote edema and leukocyte infiltration and enhance the pain-producing properties of bradykinin. The leukotrienes increase vascular permeability and further increase the mobilization of endogenous mediators of inflammation. As already noted, by blocking cyclooxygenase activity, the salicylates and related nonsteroidal antiinflammatory drugs prevent the formation of endoperoxides and subsequent prostaglandin metabolites. The lipoxygenase pathway, which converts arachidonic acid to leukotrienes (Figure 29-1 and Chapter 18), is inhibited by some antiarthritic agents but not by salicylates. Several antiinflammatory drugs block prostaglandin biosynthesis and leukotriene generation, while others weakly inhibit cyclooxygenase but have primary actions on lipoxygenases. Some antiinflammatory drugs also inhibit superoxide anion

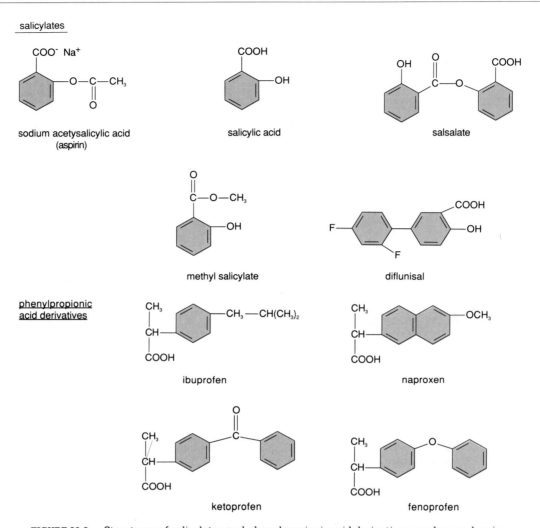

FIGURE 29-2   Structures of salicylates and phenylpropionic acid derivatives used as analgesics, antipyretics (some), or antiinflammatory drugs.

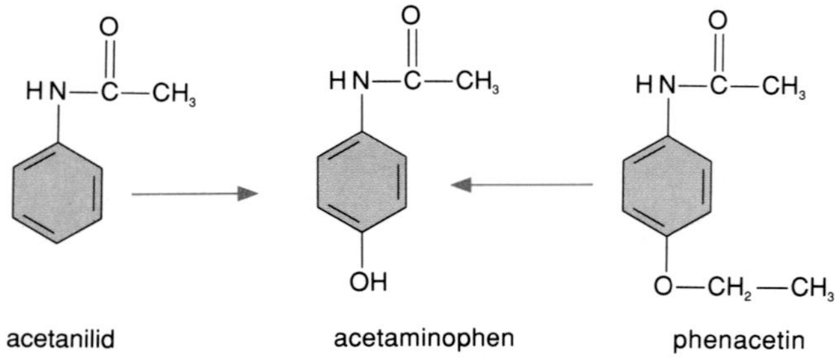

FIGURE 29-3   Structures of *p*-aminophenol derivatives, including acetaminophen.

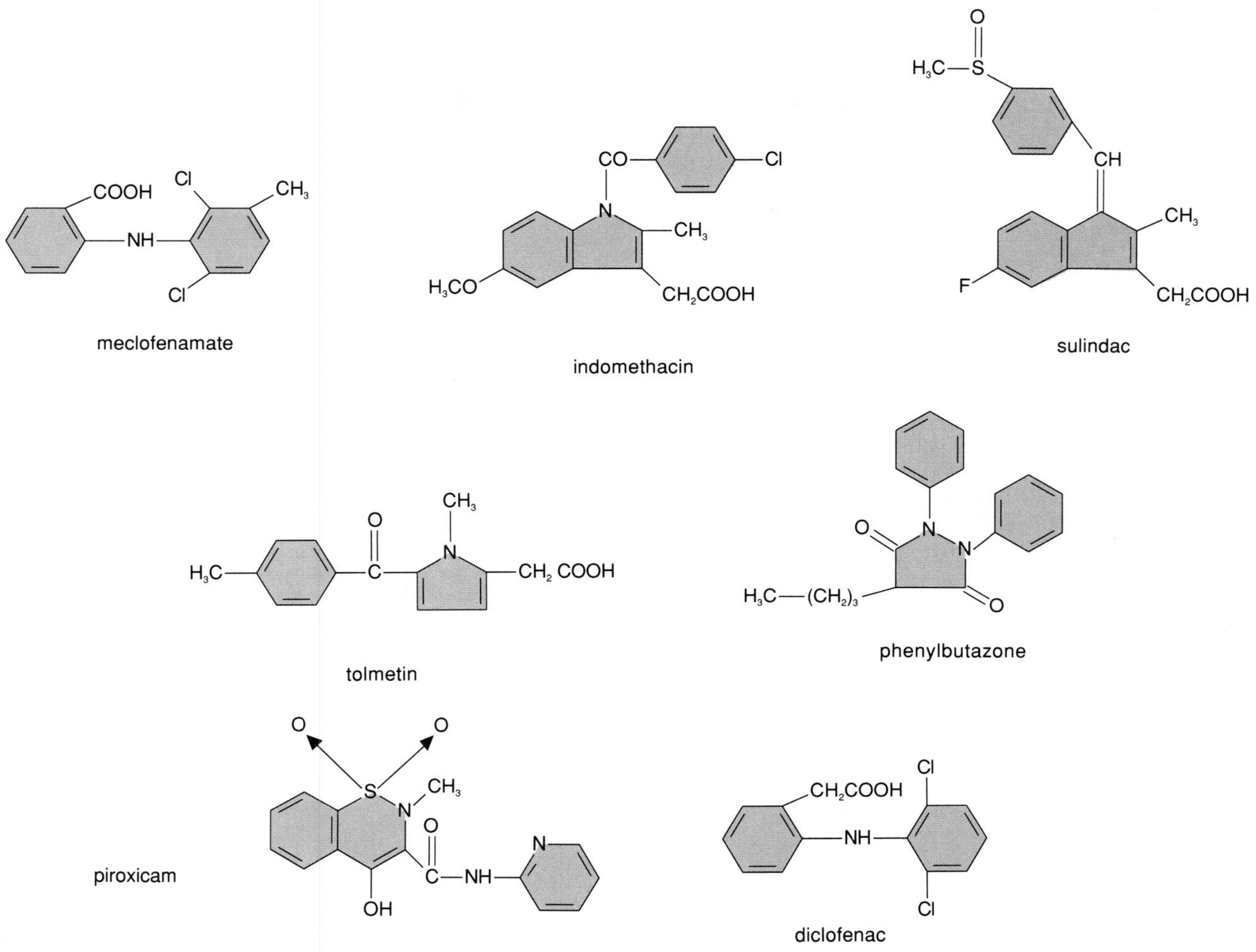

FIGURE 29-4   Structures of drugs used in treatment of arthritis and other inflammatory disorders (see also Figure 29-2).

generation, leukocyte aggregation, phagocytosis, and lysosomal enzyme release.

Drugs used to treat arthritic and other inflammatory disorders are listed here (see also Figures 29-2 and 29-4):

salicylates: aspirin, salsalate, sodium salicylate, diflunisal

phenylpropionic acids: ibuprofen, naproxen, fenoprofen, ketoprofen

pyrrole acetic acid derivatives: indomethacin, sulindac, tolmetin

anthranilic acid derivatives: meclofenamate, diclofenac

a pyrazolon: phenylbutazone

an oxicam: piroxicam

antimalarial compounds: chloroquine, hydroxychloroquine (Chapter 54)

gold compounds: aurothioglucose, gold sodium thiomalate, auranofin

others: penicillamine (Chapter 45), azathioprine (Chapter 43), prednisone (Chapter 35), prednisolone (Chapter 35)

When rheumatoid arthritis does not respond to conventional drug therapy, remission-inducing drugs are sometimes added to the treatment regimen. These include the gold salts, antimalarials, penicillamine, corticosteroids, and immunosuppressants. These agents are sometimes palliative but relatively toxic; they act by mechanisms that are not well understood.

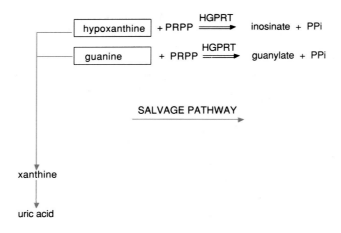

PRPP = 5-phosphoribosyl-1-pyrophosphate

HGPRT = hypoxanthine-guanine phosphoribosyltransferase

FIGURE 29-5   Salvage pathway for recycling of purine bases to form nucleotides, inosinate, and guanylate. A decrease in the salvage pathway activity can lead to an increase in uric acid formation.

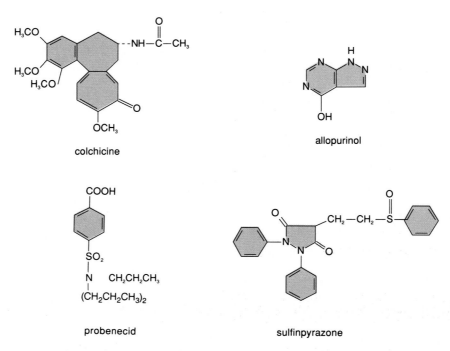

FIGURE 29-6   Some of the drugs used to treat gout.

Drugs Used to Treat Gout and Hyperuricemia

The reasons for overproduction of uric acid and decreased uric acid secretion in primary hyperuricemia are unknown. This condition usually is classified as an inborn error of metabolism. Overproduction can be caused by a deficiency of hypoxanthine-guanine phosphoribosyltransferase activity or to increased phosphoribosyl pyrophosphate synthetase. Both enzymes can produce increased concentrations of 5-phosphoribosyl-l-pyrophosphate (PRPP), a key intermediate in the salvage pathway for purines and uric acid formation (Figure 29-5). The reduced capacity to excrete uric acid results from decreased renal tubular secretion and/or increased tubular reabsorption.

Drugs frequently used to treat acute gouty arthritis are colchicine and indomethacin. Adrenal steroids are also sometimes used, and phenylbutazone, although extremely toxic, can be effective in refractory patients. Several newer antiinflammatory nonsteroidal agents (sulindac, ibuprofen, naproxen, fenoprofen) are also clinically effective in acute gout. Probenecid, sulfinpyrazone, and allopurinol are effective in chronic gout and other conditions where it is essential to decrease plasma uric acid concentrations. (See Figure 29-6 for chemical structures.)

In gout, body fluids become supersaturated with urate and needlelike crystals of urate precipitate in tissues. This deposition causes pain and inflammation. Phagocytosis of crystals by polymorphonuclear leukocytes takes place. Leukocytes migrate to the inflamed area, break open as a result of lysosomal enzymes acting on the leukocyte plasma membrane, and empty into the joint. Colchicine acts by binding to a cellular microtubular protein, tubulin, causing microtubules to disaggregate. The intact microtubules help maintain cell structure, influence movement of intracellular organelles, and participate in exocytotic release of cell substances. By affecting microtubule disaggregation, colchicine prevents the movement of leukocytes and reduces the release of urate crystals.

Allopurinol, used to reduce the blood concentration of urate in chronic gout, is an analog of hypoxanthine. Allopurinol is a better substrate for xanthine oxidase than is hypoxanthine and, when oxidized, forms oxypurinol (alloxanthine). The latter compound is an irreversible, i.e., "suicide," inhibitor that binds very tightly to the catalytic site of xanthine oxidase. Inhibition of xanthine oxidase results in decreased blood urate concentrations and increased excretion rates of the more water-soluble xanthine and hypoxanthine (Figure 29-7).

In some patients reduced excretion of uric acid results from decreased renal tubular secretion and/or increased tubular reabsorption. Thus, agents that promote the excretion of urate are also useful in the treatment of hyperuricemia and related conditions. Such uricosuric agents include probenecid and sulfinpyrazone, which increase urate excretion by competing for the renal tubular acid transporter so that less urate is reabsorbed (Figure 29-8). Normally, about 90% of filtered urate is reabsorbed, with only 10% excreted.

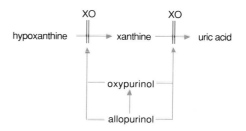

FIGURE 29-7   Blockade of uric acid synthesis by allopurinol and its oxidation agent, oxypurinal. *XO,* xanthine oxidase.

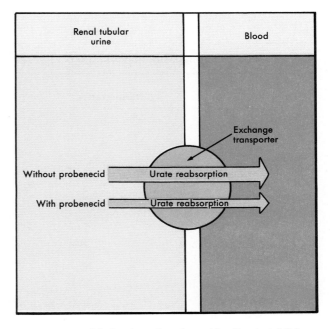

FIGURE 29-8   Mechanism of probenecid action to inhibit urate reabsorption.

Uricosuric agents promote excretion via the renal tubular organic acid transporter. Urate from the tubular fluid is taken up by the transporter and exchanged for an organic or inorganic ion, countertransported in the opposite direction. Thus the transporter acts as an ion exchanger. Uricosuric drugs in the tubular lumen compete with urate for the transporter, thus inhibiting the reabsorption of urate (see Chapter 19).

PHARMACOKINETICS

Pharmacokinetic parameters are summarized in Table 29-1.

Salicylates

Oral absorption of salicylates occurs rapidly from the stomach but to an even greater extent from the lower gastrointestinal tract via passive diffusion. The pH of the stomach favors absorption because salicylates are weak acids and have a low pK_a. These drugs are found in plasma within 30 minutes, and peak plasma concentrations are achieved 1 to 2 hours after oral administration.

Highly buffered effervescent solutions of aspirin are less irritating to the stomach and are more rapidly absorbed. Enteric-coated preparations are also available, but the absorption rate varies among different products. Rectal suppositories are of limited use because of the variable absorption.

Salicylates are distributed across membranes primarily by passive diffusion and can be detected in most body tissues and fluids. However, because plasma salicylate is largely ionized, only a small amount of salicylate crosses the blood-brain barrier. Aspirin and salicylic acid are bound to plasma proteins (50% to 80%).

Aspirin has a plasma half-life of 15 minutes, undergoing rapid hydrolysis to salicylate, although both acetylsalicylate (aspirin) and salicylate readily enter body tissues and fluids, as already stated. The half-life of salicylate varies from 2 to 3 hours for analgesic doses, up to 12 hours for antiinflammatory doses, and up to 20 hours at toxic doses. The primary metabolites of aspirin and salicylate are shown in Figure 29-9 (see also Chapter 5). The conjugates are inactive pharmacologically and are excreted. The percent of each metabolite (Chapter 5) depends on the metabolic pool of glucuronic acid or glycine. While salicylate is secreted by the proximal tubule, the extent of renal excretion as salicylate also can vary, since salicylate can undergo passive back-diffusion. Thus the net re-

Table 29-1 Pharmacokinetic Parameters

Drug	Administration	$t_{1/2}$ (hr)	Disposition	Plasma Protein Binding (%)
acetylsalicylate	Oral	0.25	M (100%)	50-80
		2-12*	M* (main), R*	50-80*
diflunisal	Oral	8-12	M (main), R	—
naproxen	Oral	12	M (main)	99
ibuprofen	Oral	2-4	M (main)	99
acetaminophen	Oral	1-3	M (main)	20-50
fenoprofen	Oral	2-3	M (main)	High
ketoprofen	Oral	3-5	M (main)	99
flurbiprofen	Oral	2-4	M (main)	High
meclofenamate	Oral	2-3	M, R	99
diclofenac	Oral	3-4	M (main)	High
indomethacin	Oral	5-10	M, R	90
sulindac	Oral	15	M†, R (small)	High
tolmetin	Oral	1	M, R (50%)	99
piroxicam	Oral	45	M, R (small)	99

M, Metabolized; *R*, renal elimination as unchanged drug.
*Refers to salicylic acid, active metabolite of acetylsalicylate, $t_{1/2}$ dose dependent.
† Active metabolite.

nal elimination of salicylate depends on urine pH in the tubular lumen. At alkaline pH, more free salicylate is cleared from the body. Discussed in Chapter 5, alkalinization of the urine by administration of sodium bicarbonate is used to lower toxic concentrations of salicylate. Since the conjugation of salicylate is enzyme catalyzed, the reactions can become saturated (zero order) (see Chapter 5). The limited availability of glycine and glucuronide for conjugation of salicylic acid also can cause the elimination of salicylate to follow first-order kinetics at lower doses and zero-order kinetics at higher doses. This is reflected in the plasma half-lives, which increase with dose.

The pharmacokinetics of diflunisal are similar to those of aspirin. Diflunisal is rapidly absorbed with peak plasma concentrations achieved in 2 to 3 hours. The drug is extensively conjugated to water-soluble glucuronides and excreted in the urine. Like salicylate, diflunisal exhibits zero-order elimination kinetics at high doses.

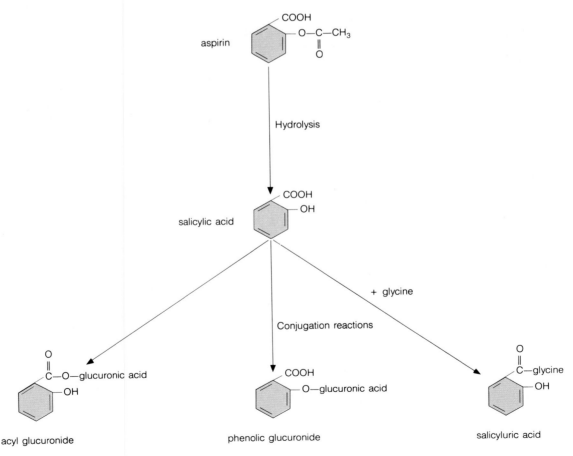

FIGURE 29-9   Metabolism of aspirin.

Acetaminophen, a very weak acid with a pK_a of 9.5, is rapidly absorbed from the gastrointestinal tract. Peak plasma concentrations are achieved within 1 hour. Distribution is relatively uniform throughout all body tissues. The parent compound is almost completely biotransformed to inactive metabolites by the liver, forming conjugates with glucuronic acid, sulfate, and cysteine, which are excreted in the urine. Overdose with acetaminophen results in the formation of a reactive intermediate, which combines with glutathione. When glutathione concentrations are depressed in the liver, toxic intermediates form adducts with hepatic proteins resulting in necrosis and resultant hepatitis.

Nonsalicylates

These drugs are all generally well absorbed after oral administration, with peak plasma concentrations occurring in 0.5 hr to several hours. Antirheumatic effects are observed after 1 to 2 weeks of treatment, and with few exceptions show a correlation between plasma concentrations and drug effectiveness. Most are avidly bound to plasma proteins, thereby increasing the potential for drug interactions. These drugs are metabolized by the liver and products are excreted by the kidney.

RELATION OF MECHANISMS OF ACTION TO CLINICAL RESPONSE

Drugs commonly used to treat mild pain, arthritis/inflammatory disorders, and gout are listed in the boxes.

Salicylates

Aspirin remains one of the most commonly used and effective agents for analgesia and antipyresis. Salicylates are used to treat headache and joint, muscle, and nerve pain of mild to moderate intensity. However, they are not effective in treatment of deep visceral pain, where the opioids are used.

Several analogs of aspirin also are used clinically, including sodium salicylate, diflunisal, salsalate, salicylic acid, and methyl salicylate. The latter two compounds are only used externally. Salicylic acid is applied topically as a keratolytic agent and methyl salicylate is used as a counter-irritant.

COMMONLY USED DRUGS USED IN THE TREATMENT OF MILD TO MODERATE PAIN

acetylsalicylic acid (aspirin)
diflunisal
salsalate
acetaminophen
ibuprofen
naproxen
fenoprofen

Several of these are also appropriately combined with narcotic analgesics for this purpose and include: aspirin (650 mg) plus codeine (32 or 65 mg), acetaminophen (650 mg) plus codeine (32 or 65 mg).

COMMONLY USED DRUGS FOR THE TREATMENT OF ARTHRITIC DISORDERS

SALICYLATES	FENAMATES
aspirin	meclofenamate
diflunisal	diclofenac
salsalate	
choline magnesium trisalicylate	**INDOLES**
	indomethacin
PROPIONIC ACID DERIVATIVES	sulindac
ibuprofen	tolmetin
naproxen	
fenoprofen	**PYRAZOLONES**
ketoprofen	phenylbutazone
flurbiprofen	oxyphenbutazone
	OXICAMS
	piroxicam

COMMONLY USED DRUGS FOR THE TREATMENT OF GOUT

colchicine
indomethacin
allopurinol
probenecid
sulfinpyrazone

Several of the drugs used to treat mild to moderate pain are also used (see text and box on p. 401).

Aspirin shows no tolerance development to its analgesic effects, no psychological or physical dependency, or addiction liability as seen with the opioids. Nor do salicylates produce CNS depression. While aspirin is extremely effective in reducing elevated body temperature, its use for this purpose has diminished because of epidemiological data that indicate a relationship between aspirin use (especially in the treatment of chickenpox or influenza infections) and the occurrence of Reye's syndrome. Since the nature of the relationship is still unclear, alternative therapy is advised, generally acetaminophen. There is a dose-dependent distinction between the analgesic and antiinflammatory actions of the salicylates. At low concentrations, the analgesic effect is devoid of antiinflammatory action, whereas at much larger concentrations and over extended time periods the antirheumatic effect is obtained. For relief of mild to moderate pain, 650 mg of aspirin is as effective as 50 mg of pentazocine, 65 mg of propoxyphene, or 650 mg of acetaminophen.

Aspirin has a long and successful history in treating rheumatic disorders. Because of side effects, this agent is sometimes not well tolerated and patient compliance is frequently a problem in long-term use. As a result several nonacetylated derivatives of aspirin are now available, but for patients who experience no side effects, aspirin is still the drug of choice.

Buffered aspirin is of some use in reducing gastrointestinal effects, although the antacid content of these preparations is quite small. A disadvantage of the buffered preparations is the large amount of sodium present, which may be undesirable for some patients. Enteric-coated tablets are also available to minimize gastric distress.

Among the nonacetylated derivatives, diflunisal is an effective cyclooxygenase inhibitor used for analgesic and antiinflammatory activities but has only weak antipyretic action. Sodium salicylate, choline salicylate, magnesium salicylate, choline magnesium trisalicylate, and salicylsalicylic acid (salsalate) are other nonacetylated compounds with similar pharmacologic effects. These agents are as effective as aspirin in treating inflammatory disorders such as osteoarthritis and rheumatoid arthritis.

Acetylsalicylate is more effective than sodium salicylate as an analgesic, antipyretic, or antiinflammatory agent. While the reason for this difference is not clear, it may result from the ability of aspirin to acetylate an active site on cyclooxygenase. Although sodium salicylate has no acetylating capacity, it does reduce prostaglandin biosynthesis in vivo. Since acetylsalicylate is metabolized to salicylate, it appears that both compounds possess similar but not equivalent pharmacological activities. Some, but not all, of the salicylates are effective inhibitors of platelet aggregation, which is related to aspirin's ability to acetylate cyclooxygenase (see Chapter 21). Because of this activity, aspirin is effective for prophylaxis of myocardial infarction, and also has been used in certain thromboembolic diseases. Diflunisal is a weak, reversible inhibitor of platelet aggregation.

Acetaminophen

Because of its lower incidence of side effects, lower potential for toxicity in the event of overdose, and better tolerance by many patients, acetaminophen is an effective alternative to aspirin for the treatment of headache, mild to moderate pain, and antipyresis. It has essentially no antiinflammatory activity. Other members of this group, such as phenacetin and acetanilid (Figure 29-3), are no longer used in the United States because of their toxic effects. Acetaminophen is a major metabolite of both of these agents (Figure 29-3). The lack of antiinflammatory action of these agents is not well understood. Acetaminophen is a weak inhibitor of prostaglandin biosynthesis, yet an effective analgesic/antipyretic. This may result from greater inhibition of cyclooxygenase in the CNS compared to peripheral tissues. No association is known between acetaminophen and Reye's syndrome and acetaminophen produces no methemoglobinemia, like acetanilid or phenacetin. Acetaminophen does not inhibit platelet aggregation (like aspirin) nor does it cause CNS depression or produce tolerance or dependence.

Phenylpropionic Acids

Among the nonsteroidal antiinflammatory drugs, several of the phenylpropionic acid derivatives are used to treat of mild to moderate pain. These include ibuprofen, naproxen, and fenoprofen. All have a lower potential for adverse side effects than aspirin and also are effective antipyretic and antiinflammatory agents. All of these agents are potent inhibitors of cyclooxygenase and have similar spectra of pharmacological activity. Clinically, 200 mg of ibuprofen or fenoprofen are equivalent in analgesic effectiveness to 650 mg of aspirin or acetaminophen. Ibuprofen is somewhat more effective than aspirin in the treatment of dysmenorrhea.

Naproxen is analgesic, antipyretic, and antiinflammatory. It is used to treat most rheumatoid disorders and acute gout. Its pharmacological properties, toxicity, and therapeutic indications are similar to those for the other nonsteroidal antiinflammatory drugs.

Fenoprofen is similar in its action to ibuprofen. It is analgesic, antipyretic, antiinflammatory, and equipotent with ibuprofen. It is an effective alternative to aspirin in the treatment of rheumatoid arthritis and osteoarthritis.

Ketoprofen also has good analgesic/antipyretic and antiinflammatory activity and is used to treat rheumatoid arthritis and osteoarthritis. It inhibits both cyclooxygenase and lipoxygenase and stabilizes lysosomal membranes. Flurbiprofen, another similar derivative, is used to treat rheumatoid arthritis, osteoarthritis, and ankylosing spondylitis.

Indole Derivatives

This group includes indomethacin, sulindac, and tolmetin. Indomethacin, introduced in the 1960s as an antiinflammatory drug, has limited clinical use as an analgesic/antipyretic because of toxicity. It is still widely used to treat acute gouty arthritis, ankylosing spondylitis, osteoarthritis in Reiter's syndrome, and psoriatic arthritis. One of the most potent inhibitors of prostaglandin biosynthesis, like colchicine, it also interferes with the migration of leukocytes, contributing to its utility in the treatment of gout. Neonates who suffer from cardiac failure as a result of incomplete closure of the *ductus arteriosus* may be helped by treatment with indomethacin. Closure of the ductus is accomplished in 70% of patients.

Sulindac is a prodrug that undergoes hepatic conversion to the sulfide to produce analgesic, antipyretic, and antiinflammatory actions. It is used in adults with rheumatoid arthritis, osteoarthritis, and ankylosing spondylitis.

Tolmetin is a suitable substitute in indomethacin intolerant patients, and is one of the few drugs suitable for treatment of juvenile arthritis, rheumatoid arthritis, osteoarthritis, and ankylosing spondylitis.

Pyrazolone Derivatives

Phenylbutazone is an effective analgesic, antipyretic, and antiinflammatory agent, but its use is limited by serious blood dyscrasias, which can occur, including leukopenia, agranulocytosis, and aplastic anemia. It should be used only after all other therapeutic regimens have failed and the risk-benefit ratio carefully evaluated. It is also an effective alternative to colchicine for treatment of acute gout and acute episodes of rheumatoid arthritis, but long-term therapy is not recommended. Oxyphenbutazone is an active metabolite of phenylbutazone with a spectrum of pharmacological activity and toxicity similar to those of the parent drug.

A new pyrazolone derivative, apazone, is a prostaglandin synthesis inhibitor related to phenylbutazone but has a lower incidence of blood dycrasias. It is used to treat rheumatoid arthritis, osteoarthritis, psoriatic arthritis, and gout and also serves as an effective uricosuric agent.

Other Antiarthritis Drugs

Meclofenamate, mefenamic acid, and diclofenac have analgesic/antipyretic and antiinflammatory action, with the antiinflammatory action of mefenamic acid weaker than the others and more toxic. Piroxicam has similar analgesic/antipyretic and antiinflammatory actions. It inhibits cyclooxygenase and is reported to inhibit neutrophil aggregation and lysosomal enzyme release. It is used to treat rheumatoid arthritis, osteoarthritis, ankylosing spondylitis, and gout.

Elemental gold compounds such as aurothioglucose, gold sodium thiomalate, and auranofin are used to suppress immune responsiveness and thereby arrest the progress of active adult and juvenile arthritis. Penicillamine has immunosuppressive actions similar to gold, but the high incidence of adverse reactions with this agent limits its use.

Several other immunosuppressive agents used to treat rheumatic disorders include highly toxic azathioprine, methotrexate, and cyclophosphamide (Chapter 43). Bone marrow depression and other toxicities limit their use to life-threatening situations where all other therapies have failed.

The pharmacology of the corticoids is considered in Chapter 35. Prednisone and prednisolone are effective when given orally, and long-acting corticoids (e.g., triamcinolone) are also available for intraarticular administration. The effects of these drugs may last from weeks to months. The corticoids are not regarded as remission-inducing drugs.

Some of the antimalarials such as chloroquine and

hydroxychloroquine also produce remission in arthritic disorders, including juvenile arthritis and systemic lupus erythematosus. They also may produce functional improvement rather than remission.

Drugs for the Treatment of Gout

Colchicine is effective in the treatment of acute gouty arthritis and appears to be relatively specific for this disease. It relieves both pain and inflammation and is frequently the first-line drug for an initial attack. These effects of colchicine are secondary to its action in blocking the mobilization of leukocytes and macrophage release of inflammatory mediators into the joint. Indomethacin and phenylbutazone are also used to treat acute urate crystal-induced gout, apparently through inhibition of urate crystal phagocytosis. The new antiinflammatory drugs fenoprofen, ibuprofen, naproxen, and sulindac also are effective in high doses and serve as alternatives to colchine for prophylactic therapy. Adrenal glucocorticoids may be effective in severe attacks that do not respond favorably to other antiinflammatory agents. The intraarticular injection of a corticosteroid can relieve pain if a single joint is involved.

Allopurinol is recommended for the therapy of chronic tophaceous gout and other hyperuricemias. Plasma and urine concentrations of uric acid are reduced because of the ability of allopurinol to inhibit xanthine oxidase and de novo purine biosynthesis. Excretion of urates is reduced, lowering the potential incidence of renal injury. Reduction in symptoms and in serum urate concentrations usually occurs in several days to 2 weeks.

In chronic gout, probenecid and sulfinpyrazone reduce plasma uric acid concentrations and prevent or reduce joint inflammation in chronic gout in patients with adequate renal function. Because acute attacks may occur, early treatment with these uricosuric agents, colchicine, or other antiinflammatory agents may be given concurrently. Other acids (e.g., salicylate) should not be given concomitantly since they compete with uric acid for the same renal transport system.

SIDE EFFECTS, CLINICAL PROBLEMS, AND TOXICITY

The most frequent problem with the salicylates is their propensity to cause gastrointestinal distress.

With larger doses used to treat rheumatoid diseases, gastrointestinal problems occur in about 20% of patients. Occult bleeding is quite common although blood loss is minimal. The nonacetylated derivatives (other than salicyclic acid) cause fewer gastrointestinal problems. Special preparations, such as buffered or enteric-coated aspirin tablets, afford some further protection. Long-term use of salicylates is believed to contribute to the incidence of peptic ulcers, and salicylates should be avoided, if possible, in patients with active ulcers. Gastritis can be reduced by taking aspirin with meals and with an adequate amount of water to ensure tablet dissolution.

With large doses of salicylate, CNS effects are prominent. So-called *salicylism* is characterized by tinnitus, hearing loss, and vertigo, reversible on reducing drug intake. These are not reliable signs of a maximally tolerated dose in elderly patients or in children, whose early signs of toxicity may vary. Slightly larger doses may stimulate the respiratory center and cause respiratory alkalosis. At moderate toxicity, a metabolic acidosis is observed, which is the consequence of impaired carbohydrate and lipid metabolism from salicylate's effect to uncouple oxidative phosphorylation.

A small number of patients are hypersensitive to aspirin and may develop a rash or an anaphylactoid reaction. They frequently have nasal polyps. Such individuals may also be sensitive to other nonsteroidal antiinflammatory drugs that inhibit prostaglandin biosynthesis. Because aspirin inhibits platelet aggregation, it should be avoided in patients who are taking coumarin or other anticoagulants. Very large doses of aspirin can produce liver injury, and this drug is not recommended in patients with chronic liver disease. There is no indication of a potential hazard in pregnant women taking occasional moderate doses of aspirin.

Acute intoxication from accidental overdose of aspirin is common in children and may have a fatal outcome. Metabolic acidosis, nausea, vomiting, stupor, and coma may develop. Hyperthermia is frequently observed. Extent of intoxication can be estimated from blood salicylate concentrations, with 50 mg/dl considered mildly toxic and 100 to 150 mg/dl potentially lethal. Treatment depends on the severity of the intoxication. Gastric lavage, activated charcoal, and alkalinization of the urine are used to reduce the body burden of salicylate. Dehydration, acidosis, and hypoglycemia, if they occur, should be corrected.

CLINICAL PROBLEMS

Gastrointestinal disturbances
Renal dysfunction
Bleeding disorders
Hypersensitivity
    dermatologic
Hematologic reaction (rare)

TRADENAMES

In addition to generic and fixed combination preparations the following tradenamed materials are available in the United States.

Ansaid, flurbiprofen
Anturane, sulfinpyrazone
Benemid, probenecid
Butazolid, phenylbutazone
Clinoril, sulindac
Cuprimine, penicillamine
Disalcid, salicylsalicylate
Dolobid, diflunisal
Feldene, piroxicam
Indocin, indomethacin
Meclomen, meclofenamate
Motrin, Advil, Nuprin, Rufen, ibuprofen
Myochrysine, gold sodium thiomalate
Nalfon, fenoprofen
Naprosyn, naproxen
Orudis, ketoprofen
Plaquentil, hydroxycloroquine
Ridaura, auranofin
Solgangal, aurothioglucose
Tanderil, oxyphenbutazone
Tolectin, tolmetin
Trisilate, choline magnesium trisalicylate
Voltraren, diclofenac
Zyloprim, allopurinol

At usual therapeutic doses, acetaminophen is remarkably safe. However, normally a small quantity of the parent compound is converted by the cytochrome P-450 mixed function oxidase system to a highly reactive toxic intermediate, which is detoxified by conjugation with glutathione. When an overdose of acetaminophen occurs, the conjugation process is overwhelmed and the toxic intermediate becomes covalently bound to hepatic macromolecules, resulting in hepatic necrosis and hepatitis, which can be fatal. Factors that decrease glutathione concentrations enhance toxicity. Treatment of the toxicity involves reducing the body burden of acetaminophen and the administration of N-acetylcysteine as a specific antidote.

Other nonsteroidal antiinflammatory drugs produce a broad spectrum of adverse effects. When large doses are used in antirheumatic therapy, the incidence of toxicity is enhanced. Most frequent and most severe reactions are gastrointestinal, dermatologic, renal, hepatic, hematologic, and immunologic in nature. CNS effects may also occur.

The main clinical problems are summarized in the box.

REFERENCES

Bloomfield SS: Analgesic management of mild to moderate pain, Ration Drug Ther 19:1, 1985.

Hart FD and Huskisson EC: Non-steroidal anti-inflammatory drugs: current status and rational therapeutic use, Drugs 27:232, 1988.

Hess EV and Tangnijkul Y: A rational approach to NSAID therapy, Ration Drug Ther 20:1, 1986.

O'Brien WM: Pharmacology of non-steroidal anti-inflammatory drugs: practical view for clinicians, Am J Med 75:32, 1983.

Rumack BH: Mechanisms of acetaminophen toxicity. In Haddad LM and Winchester J, eds: Clinical management of poisoning and drug overdose, Philadelphia, 1983, WB Saunders Co.

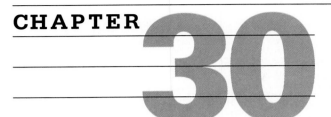

Pain Control with General and Local Anesthetics

This chapter is divided into two sections. The first considers general anesthetic agents, administered either by inhalation or IV injection. The second describes local anesthetic agents, which produce their effects at discrete anatomical sites.

General Anesthetics

 ### THERAPEUTIC OVERVIEW

Modern surgical procedures would not be possible without anesthetic agents to block the traumatic pain that would otherwise be experienced by the patient. Such agents have been available since the 1840s, when diethyl ether was first used successfully to provide anesthesia during surgical procedures on humans.

General anesthetic agents are reversible depressants of the CNS that produce a loss of sensation and consciousness. Many of the general anesthetic agents are administered by inhalation and differ in potency, speed of onset of effect, and side effects. None of the agents currently available are free of problems, although in the vast majority of surgical situations, the anesthetic agents produce the desired effects with tolerable side reactions. A second group of general anesthetic agents are administered by IV injection. The IV agents are used either alone or are administered in conjunction with inhalational anesthetics.

Several of the available general anesthetic agents

ABBREVIATIONS	
C_m	minimum anesthetic concentration
CNS	central nervous system
DNA	deoxyribonucleic acid
GABA	gamma-aminobutyric acid
IM	intramuscular, intramuscularly
IV	intravenous, intravenously
MAC	minimum alveolar concentration
pH	logarithm of the reciprocal of the hydrogen ion concentration
PN	perineural (around the nerve)
RNA	ribonucleic acid

provide highly desirable rapid induction, thus blunting the usual responses to the trauma of surgery. Most of these agents provide the desired analgesia and amnesia; not all are capable of producing the desired degree of skeletal muscle relaxation or of maintaining physiological homeostasis without depression of ventilatory drive and cardiovascular function during or

THERAPEUTIC CONSIDERATIONS FOR GENERAL ANESTHETIC AGENTS

INHALATIONAL

- Speed of onset (or time to reach unconsciousness)
- Ability to produce analgesia and amnesia
- Muscle relaxant properties
- Ease for providing moment-to-moment control
- Side effects, especially cardiovascular and respiratory depression
- Toxicity to liver
- Emergence safety and speed

INTRAVENOUS

- Speed of onset
- Pain at injection site
- Produce analgesia, amnesia, muscle relaxation
- Side effects
- Emergence safety and speed
- Rate of metabolism or redistribution

after the trauma of surgery.

The safe and effective use of general anesthetic agents is a dynamic process that must be individualized for each patient and surgical situation. The needs of both the surgical team and the patient change during the course of a surgical procedure and may alter the anesthetic requirements. For example, at different times there may be needs to (1) blunt the tachycardia and hypertension that result from an intense sympathetic nervous system stimulus, (2) produce greater relaxation of skeletal muscle, or (3) provide additional analgesia. All anesthetic interventions must be reversible, and tissue hypoxia must be prevented.

The primary therapeutic considerations in the use of general anesthetic agents are summarized in the box.

MECHANISMS OF ACTION

Inhalational Anesthetics

Inhalational anesthetics can generally induce unconsciousness within a few minutes after inhalation of the agent. Therefore, the physical or biochemical

N_2O	nitrous oxide
$CF_3—CHBrCl$	halothane
$CF_3—CHCl—O—CHF_2$	isoflurane
$CHFCl—CF_2—O—CH_2$	enflurane
$CHCl_2—CF_2—O—CH_3$	methoxyflurane
$CH_3—CH_2—O—CH_2—CH_3$	diethyl ether

FIGURE 30-1 Structures of principal inhalational general anesthetic agents.

events that produce narcosis also must occur within the same time frame. The chemical structural simplicity of the inhalational anesthetics (Figure 30-1) suggests that they do not act directly by binding to specific receptor sites. Such specific binding action would be difficult to rationalize for the anesthetic effects of elemental xenon (used successfully to anesthetize humans) or for nitrogen gas. Although the mechanism of action of inhalational anesthetics has not been established, several hypotheses are currently being examined.

One hypothesis, with which many investigators agree, is that the anesthetic produces a change in the function of an ion channel protein, brought about by a conformational modification of the protein. But whether the anesthetic acts directly on the channel protein or indirectly through surrounding neuronal cell membrane components is controversial. Experimental evidence has shown that inhalational anesthetic agents can dissolve in the lipid portion of membranes adjacent to ion channels and thereby disrupt the action of the channel (Figure 30-2). Preliminary data also have shown the process of saturable halothane binding sites, with these sites about 50% occupied at clinically relevant anesthetic concentrations. These binding sites have not been identified nor has it been established whether they are on proteins or lipids.

Neuronal cells can still generate action potentials in anesthetized subjects, although the threshold for cell depolarization is increased and the rate of rise of the action potential is reduced. The latter effect results from interference with sodium influx. One hypothesis suggests that anesthetic agents dissolve in

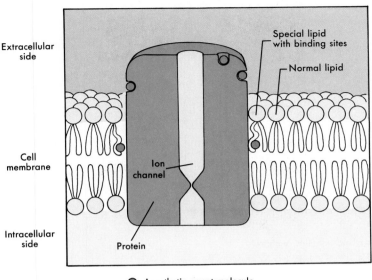

Extracellular side

Special lipid with binding sites

Normal lipid

Cell membrane

Ion channel

Intracellular side

Protein

⬤ Anesthetic agent molecule

FIGURE 30-2   Possible sites for saturable binding of halothane or other inhalational anesthetic agents to protein or lipid portions of cell membrane components.

the lipid matrix of the cell membrane and distort the channels involved in sodium conductance. Another hypothesis suggests that these changes in cellular depolarization result from differences in K^+ conductance of the cell membrane, with the channels in question being Ca^{++} dependent. Other data indicate that anesthetic agents such as halothane or diethyl ether can increase intracellular concentrations of Ca^{++} in resting cells, possibly by displacing absorbed ions, and further that halothane can induce anesthetic-activated K^+ currents, which is in keeping with the above hypothesis. Other experimental evidence also shows that isoflurane causes acetylcholine channels to oscillate between the open and closed states and suggests that the anesthetic agent may act by an allosteric mechanism. Other investigators suggest that the γ-aminobutyric acid (GABA) receptor may be the ion channel protein that is affected by inhalational anesthetic agents. Clearly, additional research is needed to resolve these many hypotheses and interesting experimental results.

The suggestion that the inhalational anesthetics act directly on lipids finds considerable support in the empirically derived correlation between anesthetic agent lipid solubility (oil/gas partition coefficient) and potency (MAC, defined later) of the agent. This re-

lationship holds over about a 100,000-fold range of anesthetizing concentrations (Figure 30-3). The implication is that the environment in which inhalational anesthetics produce their effects is hydrophobic and possibly that anesthesia occurs when a specific number of anesthetic molecules occupy a critical hydrophobic region in certain cell membranes. An earlier theory utilized the evidence that inhalational anesthetic molecules in cell membranes may expand the volume of a hydrophobic region beyond a critical size and that such expansion might alter the function of ion channels or the electrical properties of the membrane. The observation that all inhalational anesthetics can undergo reversal of anesthetic effect by increasing the atmospheric pressure supports this hypothesis.

Synaptic communication between neurons is the basis for nervous system function. Anesthetizing concentrations of inhaled agents depress synaptic transmission but have little effect on axonal transmission. It might be assumed that polysynaptic neuronal pathways would be more susceptible to the effects of inhalational anesthetics than monosynaptic pathways. However, this is not true of all neural systems that have been tested. It is likely that synapses vary in their sensitivity to anesthetic-induced depression of

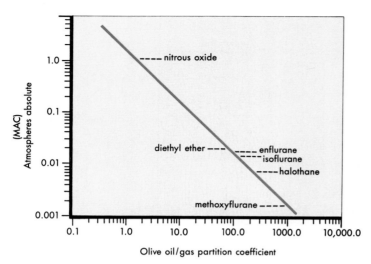

FIGURE 30-3   Relationship between potency (MAC defined in text) and lipid solubility of inhalational anesthetic agents, oil/gas partition coefficient.

transmission, and that the overall effect of an anesthetic is a result of drug-induced depression of both excitatory and inhibitory pathways.

Not all parts of the central nervous system are affected equally by all anesthetics. Cells of the substantia gelatinosa in the dorsal horn of the spinal cord, for example, are very sensitive to low concentrations of inhaled anesthetics. A decrease in function of this area interrupts sensory transmission in the spinothalamic tract, including that mediating nociceptive input. Progressive depression of ascending pathways in the reticular activating system occurs during surgical anesthesia, and depression of spinal reflex activity contributes to the skeletal muscle relaxation induced by general anesthetics.

Intravenous Anesthetics

The IV anesthetic agents frequently used clinically are the barbiturates, benzodiazepines, ketamine, etomidate, and propofol. The structures are shown in Figure 30-4. The IV agents also can induce unconsciousness very rapidly. In general, the lipid solubility of these drugs correlates with anesthetic potency. Barbiturates penetrate membranes rapidly and may alter the physical state of the membrane lipids, although the barbiturate lipophilicity may merely enable the agents to reach the site of action before metabolism occurs. Some barbiturates are convulsant rather than anesthetic, but it has not been determined if this difference is due to alternate actions on membrane lipids or to another mechanism.

Both barbiturates and benzodiazepines bind to the

GABA Type A receptor. This is a cell membrane protein receptor that has separate binding sites for GABA and agonists, benzodiazepines, barbiturates, and chloride channel blocking toxins (see Chapter 2). The benzodiazepine and barbiturate binding sites are allosteric, in that binding only of GABA or agonists can open the chloride channel, while binding of barbiturates or benzodiazepines enhances the frequency or duration of channel opening. GABA and the associated GABA type A receptor constitutes the major inhibitory neurotransmitter-receptor system in the human CNS. As such, the administration of agents that prolong GABA receptor channel open times leads to larger chloride currents and greater inhibition of CNS activity. Barbiturates enhance GABA activity and produce larger chloride currents. The mean channel open time is prolonged and the chloride currents occur in bursts that also are prolonged. The net result is barbiturate enhancement of GABA-induced CNS inhibition. The benzodiazepines also bind to allosteric sites on the GABA type A receptor and enhance GABA-induced chloride channel activity by generating larger chloride currents for the same concentration of GABA.

Etomidate, a carboxylated imidazole, also produces CNS depression through GABA mimetic action. Likewise, the effects of etomidate can be antagonized by GABA antagonists, as can those of benzodiazepines. The effects of barbiturates are not as easily reversed.

Ketamine also produces receptor mediated effects. There appears to be a receptor, with no known en-

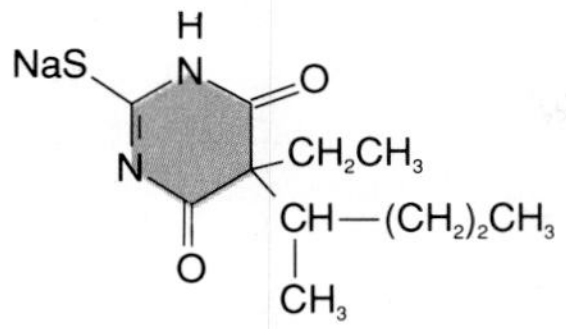

FIGURE 30-4   Structures of intravenous general anesthetics.

thiopental sodium

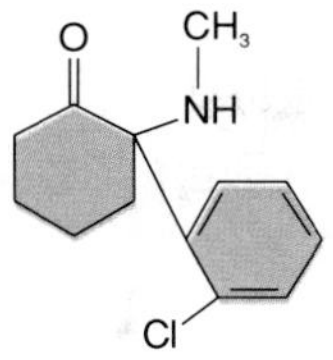

ketamine

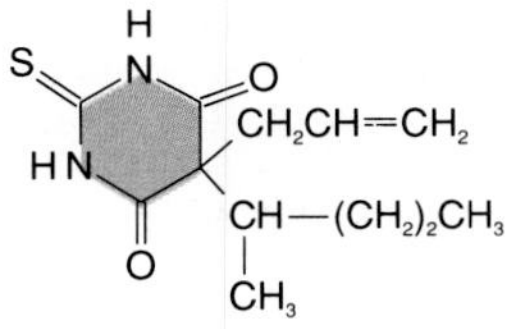

thiamylal

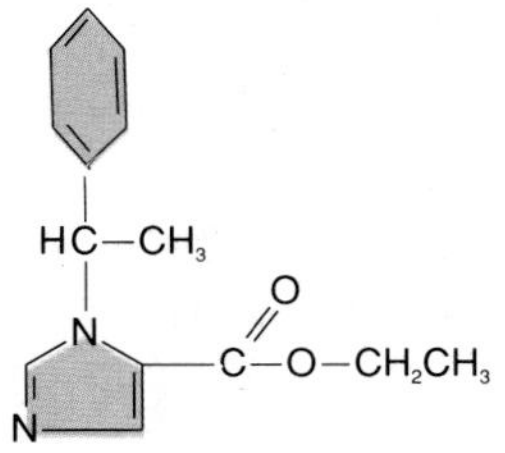

etomidate

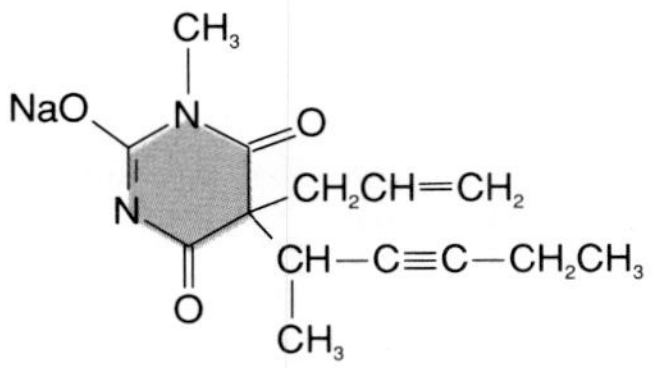

methohexital
sodium

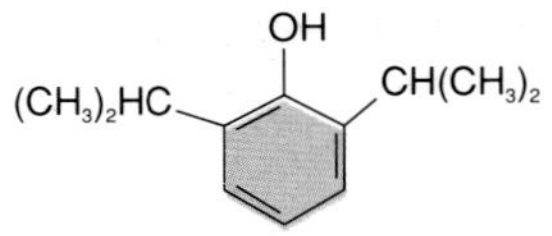

propofol

benzodiazepines

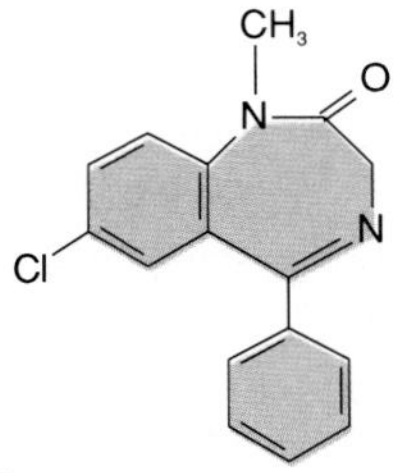

diazepam

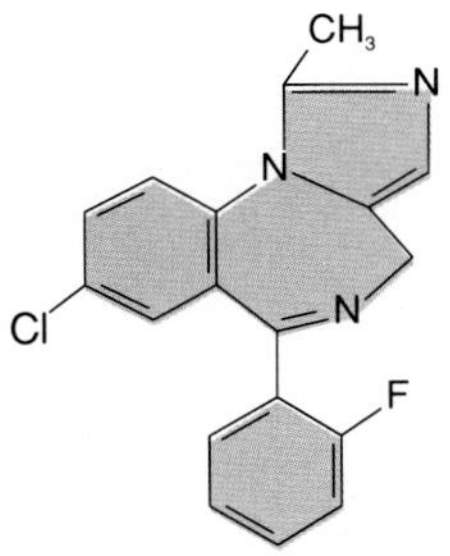

midazolam

dogenous ligand, with which ketamine interacts. Ketamine has a much weaker stimulatory interaction with sigma opioid receptors.

Little information is currently available on the mechanism of action of propofol.

PHARMACOKINETICS

The pharmacokinetic parameter values for the anesthetic agents are summarized in Table 30-1.

Table 30-1   Pharmacokinetic Parameters

Drugs	Adminis-tration	Elimination ($t_{1/2}$, hr)	Onset Time
nitrous oxide	Inhalation	—	—
halothane	Inhalation	—	—
isoflurane	Inhalation	—	—
enflurane	Inhalation	—	—
methoxyflurane	Inhalation	—	—
thiopental	IV	10-12	30-40 sec
thiamylal	IV	—	40-50 sec
methohexital	IV, rectal	3-5	—
propofol	IV	5-10	40-50 sec
ketamine	IV, IM	2-4	—
etomidate	IV	2-5	—
diazepam	IV	20-40	—
midazolam	IV, IM	1.2-12	3-5 min

* Active metabolite.

Inhalational Anesthetics

To understand (1) which variables control the rate of delivery of anesthetic gases to blood and tissues, (2) when equilibrium is achieved, and (3) how these gaseous agents are eliminated, it is essential to have some knowledge of the behavior of gases in body fluids and tissues. Nitrous oxide is the only commonly used inhalational anesthetic that is a gas at ambient temperatures and pressures. All of the other inhalational anesthetics are liquids at room temperature and pressure and require vaporization before use. The rate of onset of loss of consciousness, the rapidity and ease by which muscle relaxation can be achieved in the surgical field, and the rate and routes of disposition of the agents are the principal pharmacokinetic variables of interest with the inhalational agents.

The administration of the inhalational agents is accomplished by vaporization of the agent followed by mixing with oxygen or air and passage of the mixture through the upper airway passages into the alveolar space. The composition of the gaseous mixture is described in terms of the partial pressures of each of the components. The partial pressure of the anesthetic agent, for example, is defined as the pressure exerted by the anesthetic gas if these were the only molecules that occupied the gas space. Partial pressures are additive, with the total pressure being the sum of the partial pressures. During the administration of inhalational anesthetic agents, the total pressure of one atmosphere is made up of the partial

Table 30-2   Equivalent Molar Concentrations of Halothane in Alveoli, Blood, and Brain Tissue at Total Body Equilibrium

INSPIRED GAS/ALVEOLI

halothane administered at 1.3 times MAC
MAC = 0.75% of 1.0 atmosphere (see Table 30-3)
1.3 MAC = (0.0075)(1.3)(760 torr/atm) = 7.4 torr, partial pressure of halothane in alveoli
equivalent molar concentration of halothane in alveoli can be calculated using natural gas law: $PV = nRT$
P = 7.4 torr, partial pressure of halothane in gas phase
T = 37°C + 273 = 310°K, absolute temperature in degrees Kelvin
N = moles of halothane
V = volume, arbitrarily taken as 1.0 liter
R = gas constant, 62.3 in these units
concentration = n/V = P/RT = 7.4/(62.3)(310) = 0.00038 molar or 0.38 mM in alveoli

BLOOD CONCENTRATION OF HALOTHANE AT EQUILIBRIUM

blood/gas partition coefficient = 2.3 (see Table 30-3)
concentration = 2.3 (0.38 mM) = 0.87 mM in blood

BRAIN TISSUE CONCENTRATION OF HALOTHANE AT EQUILIBRIUM

brain white matter/gas partition coefficient = 8.2 (see Table 30-3)
concentration = 8.2 (0.38 mM) = 3.1 mM in brain white matter

SUMMARY

at equilibrium

Alveolar Gas	Blood	Brain
0.38 mM	0.87 mM	3.1 mM
7.4 torr	7.4 torr	7.4 torr

pressures of one or more anesthetic agents, oxygen, water vapor, carbon dioxide, and nitrogen. An illustration for halothane is shown in Table 30-2.

When a fluid such as blood or a tissue is exposed to a gas, some of the gas dissolves in the fluid or tissue, and equilibrium ultimately is achieved between the components in the two phases. For example, the halothane in the alveolar gaseous space rapidly dissolves in the pulmonary membranes and achieves equilibrium between the halothane concentrations in the gas and membrane phases. Halothane diffuses from the pulmonary membrane and dissolves in pulmonary blood to establish another halothane equilibrium. In like manner, equilibria are established

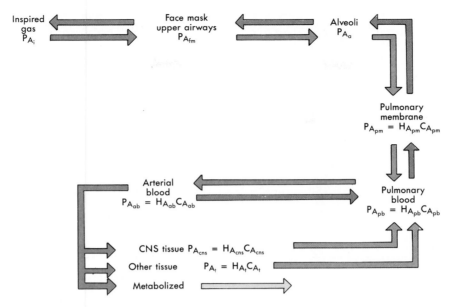

FIGURE 30-5 Pathways for uptake, distribution, and elimination of inhalational anesthetic agents. p_A, Partial pressure of agent A; H, proportionality constant; C, molar concentration of A. Other subscripts refer to anatomical regions.

between halothane in blood and brain tissue and between halothane in blood and other tissues. Anesthesia occurs only when an adequate partial pressure of halothane accumulates in brain tissue. The sequence of steps in the delivery of inhalational anesthetic agents to brain tissue is shown schematically in Figure 30-5.

The relationship between the concentration of a gas (i.e., compound A) dissolved in a fluid or tissue phase and the equilibrium partial pressure of the same compound that would exist if there was a gas phase in contact with the fluid or tissue is described by the simple equation

$$p_A = H_A (C_A)$$

where p_A is the equilibrium partial pressure of compound A in the gas phase, H_A is a proportionality constant for compound A, and C_A is the molar concentration of compound A in the fluid or tissue phase. This equation is shown in Figure 30-5 for calculating the equivalent equilibrium partial pressure of anesthetic agent for each of the fluids and tissues indicated.

It is the difference in partial pressures of anesthetic agent, not the difference in molar concentrations of dissolved agent, that determines the rate of net trans-

fer of inhalational agent between any two phases (e.g., blood and brain tissue, blood and muscle tissue, or alveolar gas and blood) (see Table 30-2).

When a difference in the partial pressure of anesthetic agent between two phases is present, such as initially when starting the administration or when a change in the surgical requirements necessitates adjustment in the concentration of agent in the inspired gas, the rate of onset of anesthesia or modification in anesthetic effects is highly dependent on the solubility of the agent in blood and tissues. This can be illustrated by comparing nitrous oxide and halothane. From Table 30-3 the blood/gas partition coefficient for nitrous oxide is 0.47 and for halothane 2.3. The partial pressure of the agent in blood increases rapidly and becomes equal with the partial pressure in the inspired gas much more rapidly for the less soluble nitrous oxide than for the more soluble halothane (Figure 30-6). With a more highly soluble agent such as diethyl ether the time to reach equivalent partial pressures is longer than for nitrous oxide or halothane.

With low solubility nitrous oxide, equilibrium is reached rapidly between the inspired air and pulmonary capillary blood. Because of its low solubility in blood, only a small fraction of the agent leaves the

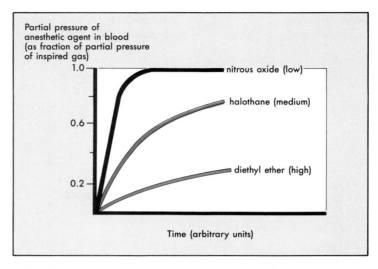

FIGURE 30-6   Uptake of inhalational anesthetic agents, showing how uptake rate varies with blood solubility of agents. *Low, medium,* and *high* refer to solubility of agents in blood. Onset of anesthesia requires the partial pressure of the agent in brain tissue to be sufficiently high.

Table 30-3 MAC and Solubility Values for Clinically Used Inhalational Anesthetic Agents in Young Adults

Anesthetic	MAC* (% of one atm)	Brain (White Matter)/Gas Partition Coefficient	Blood/Gas Partition Coefficient
nitrous oxide†	101.0	0.5	0.47
diethyl ether‡	1.92	13.5	12.0
halothane	0.75	8.2	2.3
enflurane	1.7	3.2	1.9
isoflurane	1.3	4.7	1.48
methoxyflurane	0.16	31.0	10.2

*Expressed as partial pressure of agent (in alveolar space) divided by standard total atmospheric pressure × 100.

†A MAC < 100% means a partial pressure greater than 760 mm Hg is needed, a situation that can be achieved experimentally by carrying out the measurements in a hyperbaric chamber.

‡Included mainly for comparison, not used much in the United States.

alveolus with each breath, and the blood partial pressure of nitrous oxide builds up rapidly. Because of the relatively low solubility of nitrous oxide in tissues, the tissues take up a relatively small fraction of the agent from the blood. This means that when venous blood returns to the lungs after circulating through the body, it still contains nitrous oxide, and not much more needs to be transported across the pulmonary membrane to re-equilibriate between blood and alveolar gas. Thus with a poorly soluble agent there is always a large partial pressure of agent in the alveolar

region and gas can be moved rapidly from the alveolus to blood. The resulting time for equilibration is short, and the onset of anesthesia is very rapid. With such low solubility agents, total body equilibrium in which the partial pressure of agent reaches the same value in all body fluids and tissues is achieved. It is also apparent that respiration rate has little or no influence on the onset of anesthesia with nitrous oxide, since the concentration of this agent in the alveoli is not altered significantly with each respiration.

With anesthetic agents of higher blood/gas solubility than nitrous oxide, (e.g., halothane) a larger fraction of the anesthetic agent is transferred from the alveoli to pulmonary blood during each breath, so that less agent remains in the alveoli at the end of a breath. The partial pressure difference between the alveoli and blood, and thus the driving force, is reduced, and the transport from alveolus to blood is slow. These same agents also are more soluble in tissues, and thus it takes much longer to achieve sufficiently high brain tissue partial pressure for the onset of anesthesia. With these agents, the onset time can be shortened by increasing the depth and/or rate of respiration by delivering more anesthetic to the alveoli. With the high solubility agents, total body equilibrium again is defined as attainment of the same partial pressure of agent in all body fluids and tissues, but in practice many surgical procedures are too short (1 to 6 hours) for total body equilibrium to be attained with halothane and other relatively soluble anesthetic agents.

From the standpoint of the anesthesiologist, the most desirable situation is to have a small change in the partial pressure in the inspired gas be reflected in an almost immediate equivalent change in the partial pressure of agent in the brain and therefore in the effects of the anesthesia. With highly soluble agents such rapid response is difficult to obtain and only near-equilibrium can be achieved. The low solubility nitrous oxide provides the desired rapid response but lacks the potency to achieve the deep surgical anesthetic effects by itself.

Most inhalational anesthetics are removed from the body by the same route as they enter, (i.e., via the lungs). The rates of removal by the lungs are similar to the rates of onset in that agents of low solubility are rapidly removed via the lungs and the anesthesia terminated. Agents with higher solubility are much less rapidly removed, and recovery from anesthesia is longer. Recovery can be considered to be the mirror image of onset. Partitioning of the anesthetic agents into certain tissues (e.g., body fat) may also influence recovery time. Obese individuals are not only generally more difficult to anesthetize with the more soluble anesthetics than those with a lean body mass, but termination of anesthesia is also slower.

When induction of anesthesia is slow, the gradual depression of CNS function results in obtundation of some reflexes and simultaneous hyperactivity of other neurologic functions. During an inhalation induction, which takes several minutes to complete, the patient may experience hyperacusis (more acute sense of hearing), increased airway reactivity (laryngospasm), and even sufficient motor activity to cause personal injury. This is an "excitement stage," and rapid induction by whatever means minimizes this dangerous period. Potentially dangerous hyperactivity may also occur during awakening.

Although ventilation is the major route of elimination of inhalation anesthetics, almost all such agents undergo significant metabolism. If the inhalation anesthetic was administered for several hours, there will be a significant amount of anesthetic remaining in the patient's tissues when consciousness is regained. The hepatic metabolism of such drugs as halothane is inhibited by anesthetic concentrations of halothane, but metabolic degradation by hepatic microsomal enzymes is significant when lower concentrations of drug are present. It has been estimated that as much as 9% of administered enflurane, 46% of halothane, and 75% of methoxyflurane is metabolized following a 2-hour exposure to subanesthetic concentrations of drug. Under these circumstances metabolism of isoflurane is minimal. Some of the metabolites of anesthetic agents may have toxic effects, as discussed in a later section.

Intravenous Anesthetics

IV administration of anesthetic agents produces a more rapid induction of anesthesia in the adult than does exposure to inhalation anesthetics. Because IV anesthetics are administered directly into the bloodstream, the factors that affect movement of the drug molecules from blood to brain are most important in determining the time to onset of action. Brain blood flow is the principal variable, so a patient with extremely low cardiac output and hence relatively low brain blood flow may have a delayed onset of effect. Most of the IV anesthetics have high lipid solubility and cross the blood-brain barrier rapidly. The most rapid induction of anesthesia, 30 to 50 seconds from injection to loss of lash reflex, is produced by the short-acting barbiturates and propofol. A similar degree of obtundation may require several minutes to develop following administration of benzodiazepine.

The duration of effect of IV anesthetic is determined by redistribution and/or metabolism. With only the administration of one induction dose of barbiturate, redistribution of the drug from brain into less well-perfused areas of the body (e.g., abdominal viscera, skeletal muscle, and fat) is the predominant mechanism responsible for termination of effect. This mechanism can be so efficient that within minutes of induction of anesthesia, reflex activity and then consciousness begin to return to the patient. Propofol is the most rapidly redistributed and eliminated IV anesthetic and therefore has the shortest duration of action. Full recovery of consciousness occurs later after induction of anesthesia with barbiturate or benzodiazepine than after induction with propofol. Ketamine, although it has a relatively short half-life in blood (see Table 30-1), produces prolonged sedation following an IV dose.

Problems can develop with some of the IV anesthetic agents if improper modes of injection are used. For example, the alkaline pH of sodium pentothal can cause significant local tissue irritation if injected outside a vein, and high concentrations of thiopental (5%) or methohexital (2%) when injected IV often cause venous thrombosis. Intraarterial injection of thiopental produces severe vascular injury, and barbiturates may precipitate when injected simultaneously with neuromuscular blockers into an IV tubing.

Diazepam is insoluble in water, and so is provided in a viscid solution that often produces pain when injected IV, and venous thrombosis may ensue. In contrast, midazolam is water soluble, produces little pain with IV administration, and is easily absorbed following IM injection. Ketamine may be administered IV with little risk to tissues, and IM with rapid uptake. However, etomidate may also cause pain followed by thrombophlebitis on intravascular injection. Propofol, which is insoluble in water, is available in an aqueous emulsion.

Thiopental is metabolized in the liver by oxidation, desulfurization, and hydrolysis. Significant depression of metabolism occurs during hepatic disease. Because redistribution rather than metabolism terminates the effect of a single dose of barbiturate, duration of effect of a small induction dose of barbiturate may be normal in patients with hepatic disease, but the effects of repeated doses will be prolonged. Similarly, diazepam undergoes demethylation in the liver and its plasma half-life is prolonged in patients with cirrhosis. Desmethyldiazepam, a major metabolite of diazepam, is almost as potent a sedative as diazepam and can contribute significantly to drowsiness in the first 24 hours after administration of diazepam. Midazolam is metabolized, but the metabolites are inactive.

Ketamine is demethylated by the liver to produce a weak anesthetic compound, which is then hydroxylated and/or dehydrated; alternatively the cyclohexylamine ring of ketamine may be hydroxylated. Etomidate also is metabolized, with hydrolysis by the liver of 90% of the drug. Variations in plasma albumin concentration can have a marked effect on the free fraction of etomidate. Propofol is also metabolized rapidly in the liver, and perhaps in other sites, to produce water-soluble glucuronide and sulfate conjugates.

 ## RELATION OF MECHANISMS OF ACTION TO CLINICAL RESPONSE

Inhalational Anesthetics

The potency of inhalational anesthetic agents is expressed in terms of the minimum concentration of agent in the alveolar space of a normal patient needed to prevent a response to a standard stimulus, generally a skin incision. The alveolar concentration depends on both the rates of anesthetic disappearance from the patient's pulmonary circulation and input from the vaporizer that supplies the gaseous form of the agent. Potency is not determined clinically, but a typical measurement would involve administration of the inhalational agent long enough to establish equilibrium in the anesthetic partial pressure between the gas present in the alveolus, that dissolved in the blood, and that dissolved in CNS tissues. Then the standardized painful stimulus is applied to the subject and the characteristic all-or-none withdrawal response is observed. The minimum alveolar anesthetic concentration (MAC) is defined as that concentration of anesthetic in alveolar or end-expired gas that is present when 50% of the subjects do not respond when exposed to the skin incision (MAC = 1.0). The MAC values for several clinically used agents are listed in Table 30-3.

Although MAC is a useful concept, the administration of anesthesia is usually titrated to an effect rather than to a specific dose or multiple of the MAC value. The dose-response relationship for inhalational anesthetics is steep. Over 95% of patients fail to respond to a painful stimulus at 1.3 MAC, and 50% (by definition) fail to respond at 1.0 MAC. Frequently, inhalation anesthetics are administered to produce 1.3 MAC end-tidal anesthetic concentration because few patients respond to a skin incision under those conditions. A much lower anesthetic concentration is expected to produce amnesia. However, inhalational anesthetics vary in the degree of muscle relaxation they produce during anesthetic administration and in the degree of analgesia the patient experiences during emergence from anesthesia. Inhalational anesthetics often are coadministered with nitrous oxide or IV anesthetics to assist in achieving a rapid onset of action. During surgery the intensity of the traumatic surgical stimuli may vary, requiring continual adjustments of the alveolar concentration of anesthetic agent. After administration of the anesthetic is terminated, 50% of patients will respond to a verbal command when the alveolar anesthetic partial pressure has fallen to 0.4 MAC.

It is useful in comparing agents to examine the side effects of different inhalational anesthetics at similar MAC values. Thus one might compare the depression in respiratory drive or cardiovascular function of two inhalational anesthetics at equal multiples of the MAC for each agent (i.e., at equipotent doses of anesthetic).

MAC values for a given inhalational agent change with patient age. The general trend is shown in Figure 30-7 for isoflurane. Note that the value of 1.3% from Table 30-1 corresponds to age 25 years in Figure 30-7.

Previous drug exposure can alter the amount of inhalational anesthetic required in a subject. In general, drugs that decrease the amount of anesthetic required have inhibitory effects at one or more sites in the CNS. This applies to the narcotic analgesics, benzodiazepines, and barbiturates. α_2-Adrenergic agonists, such as clonidine, stimulate the locus coeruleus, which then produces inhibitory effects regarding awareness, baroreceptor control of cardiovascular reflexes, and pain perception. Following clonidine or opioid administration, inhalational anesthetic requirements are decreased as measured by assessment of MAC and analysis of EEG spectra, respectively. Repeated administration of certain drugs may lead to changes in function and produce the opposite effect in terms of the requirements for anesthetics. For example, MAC is increased in patients tolerant to benzodiazepines, barbiturates, or ethyl alcohol. Drugs that increase activity of catecholaminergic neurons in the CNS, such as *d*-amphetamine, iproniazide, cocaine, or ephedrine, also increase MAC. Benzodiazepine antagonists and narcotic antagonists also increase MAC.

MAC, or potency, is actually of little consequence in the selection of general anesthetic agents since the more potent clinically used agents utilize only 1% to 3% of an atmosphere (Table 30-3) for frequently used initial gas mixtures that correspond to 1.3 MAC plus about 25 volume % oxygen. Thus in clinical practice only 190 to 200 torr of 760 torr available is utilized for

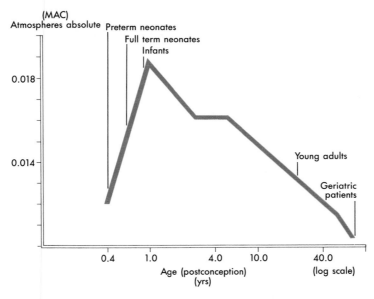

FIGURE 30-7   Trends in MAC with patient age for isoflurane.

the inhalational anesthetic and oxygen, leaving considerable leeway for the use of lower potency agents. Nitrous oxide is an exception since 1.0 MAC for this agent can be approximated only under hypoxic conditions (zero oxygen partial pressure) at a total pressure of 1 atmosphere (760 torr) (see Table 30-3). The low potency of nitrous oxide limits its use in general surgical procedures to anesthesia induction and other conditions where nitrous oxide is mixed with other anesthetic agents to minimize the amounts of the more potent agents that must be used.

Intravenous Anesthetics

The onset of anesthesia with IV anesthetic agents can be observed by administering a single dose and noting the loss of reflex activity, for example, by noting the lack of blink following touch of the eyelashes. The factors that alter the required amount of IV anesthetics are similar to those that alter the needs for inhalation. These factors that alter the volume of distribution of the anesthetic agent, including protein binding, can produce a change in the amount of agent that is needed to obtain specific reflex depression.

IV induction of anesthesia may be complicated by transient excitation of reflexes. The phenomena commonly observed vary from one drug to another. Methohexital may produce hiccups and twitching of the extremities. Etomidate and propofol may also produce myoclonic twitching or tremors. The incidence of these complications is somewhat lower following thiopental administration. Small doses of an opioid may ameliorate these excitatory effects.

When a barbiturate is used for induction or maintenance of anesthesia it may be necessary to administer an opioid or other analgesic drug. Low concentrations of barbiturate may exacerbate the patient's response to pain (hyperalgesia). Little skeletal muscle relaxation is produced by barbiturates. Etomidate and propofol also lack analgesic properties.

The state of consciousness induced by ketamine has been described as dissociative anesthesia. It differs from the narcosis induced by barbiturates and other drugs in that patients appear cataleptic with minimal sedation but experience intense analgesia and amnesia. The quality of reflex suppression by ketamine differs from that of other IV anesthetics.

SIDE EFFECTS, CLINICAL PROBLEMS, AND TOXICITY

The clinical problems with general anesthetic agents are summarized in the box.

Inhalational Anesthetics

Some of the clinically encountered side effects of the inhalational anesthetic agents are dose related, and although the needs of the surgical procedure may necessitate the accommodation of some side effects, the intensity of these unwanted effects usually can be minimal. Some of these dose related side effects include depression of respiratory drive, depression of myocardial contractility, and modified tone of vascular smooth muscles or of striated muscles. An example is shown in Figure 30-8 for the effects of several agents on mean arterial pressure under conditions of controlled ventilation and normal CO_2 concentration. With halothane, additional cardiovascular side effects may include hypotension, decreased myocardial contractile force (possibly through actions on calcium channels), lower baroreceptor response to reduced blood pressure, reduced energy needs of the heart, and increased ventricular arrhythmic action of catecholamines. These effects may differ in degree and even in direction from one inhalational anesthetic agent to another. Some effects vary with the chemical structure of the agents. For example, muscle relaxa-

---

CLINICAL PROBLEMS

INHALATIONAL AGENTS

Depression of respiratory drive
Lower response to CO_2 or hypoxia
Depressed myocardial contractility
Modified muscle tone
Gaseous space enlargement by nitrous oxide
N_2O inactivation of vitamin B_{12}
Fluoride ion toxicity from methoxyflurane
Malignant hyperthermia

INTRAVENOUS AGENTS

Depressed respiratory drive
Depressed cardiovascular function
Ketamine hallucinations and emergence delirium
Etomidate steroidogenesis inhibition

tion is provided by the halogenated ethers such as enflurane and isoflurane but not much by the halogenated hydrocarbons such as halothane. The halogenated hydrocarbons sensitize the heart to catecholamines, an effect generally not seen with the ethers.

The depression of respiratory drive includes dampened response of minute ventilation (expressed as liters/minute) to elevated CO_2 concentrations and to hypoxia. A higher concentration of CO_2 is tolerated with inhalational anesthetics than without. With anesthetics present, hypoxic conditions result in a significantly lower minute ventilation.

Because nitrous oxide is administered in relatively large quantities and is only slightly soluble in blood (blood/gas partition coefficient of 0.47), nitrous oxide may readily accumulate in any gas containing volume and present a special problem. Such volumes are normally filled with air nitrogen. A nitrogen bubble will enlarge since nitrous oxide from the blood supply enters the bubble faster than nitrogen can leave. Either the volume or pressure in the space will increase depending on the compliance of the walls of the space. Clinically important consequences as diverse as tension pneumothorax, serous otitis, increased intracranial pressure, and distended bowel may result.

Nitrous oxide inactivates vitamin B_{12} methionine synthetase and related vitamin B_{12} enzymes that are important for the synthesis of methionine and other amino acids needed for protein synthesis and for synthesis of purines and pyrimidines for DNA/RNA synthesis. Nitrous oxide undergoes reduction with simultaneous oxidation of the cobalt atom in vitamin B_{12} to inactivate this co-factor for a wide range of enzymes. Clinically, the extreme case of megaloblastic anemia, characteristic of vitamin B_{12} deficiency, may occur. Although inhibition of methionine synthetase activity may occur during nitrous oxide anesthesia, this appears to cause no harm to the routine surgical patient. The same exposure to nitrous oxide may be dangerous for the fetus, for the severely infected patient, or the patient with impaired hematopoiesis. Sedating patients with 50% nitrous oxide for 5 to 6 days has been associated with neutropenia and thrombocytopenia, and intermittent exposure to 50% nitrous oxide for 15 minutes 3 times a day for 24 days has produced megaloblastic anemia. Although high doses of folinic acid may provide protection from some effects of nitrous oxide, the clinical efficacy of this preventive strategy has not been established.

The same mechanism may be responsible for peripheral neuropathies that appear after chronic low dose exposure to nitrous oxide. The clinical presentations of numbness, tingling, poor balance, weakness, reduced reflexes, and impaired sensation of vibration, is similar to subacute combined degeneration of the spinal cord due to vitamin B_{12} deficiency. Recovery may be slow after elimination of the source of

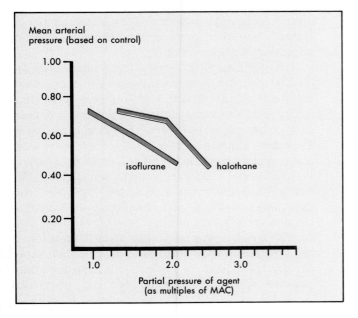

FIGURE 30-8   Cardiac-dose–related side effects of isoflurane and halothane.

nitrous oxide and supplementary administration of vitamin B_{12} may be of little therapeutic benefit.

These are some of the reasons why waste anesthetic gases must be scavenged rather than allowed to pollute the atmosphere of the surgical operating room or dental operatory.

Nephrogenic diabetes insipidus has been seen following prolonged exposure to methoxyflurane. The causative agent is the fluoride ion produced during metabolism of methoxyflurane. Serum concentrations of fluoride greater than 50 μM are likely to produce renal injury in otherwise normal humans. Patients with impaired renal function preoperatively may be more sensitive. However, 2 MAC-hours of methoxyflurane exposure (2 hours at 0.16% end-expired methoxyflurane or 4 hours at 0.08% of 1 atmosphere) are probably not likely to cause fluoride toxicity in a healthy adult. Enflurane metabolism also produces fluoride ions, but even in patients with enhanced hepatic microsomal enzyme activity (through drug-stimulated enzyme induction) the fluoride concentrations are not likely to reach nephrotoxic concentrations.

Halothane metabolism produces bromide, but this ion has no known toxic effect in the range of plasma concentrations (2.4 to 4.2 mEq/L) observed in healthy volunteers after prolonged halothane anesthesia. Sedation from bromide alone occurs at somewhat higher serum concentrations, 6 mEq/L. Bromide concentrations peak 2 days after anesthesia with halothane, making predictions of potential drug interactions difficult.

Hepatic necrosis has been noted after repeated exposure to halothane, but hepatotoxicity associated with halothane is rare, approximately 1 in 35,000. Pretreatment with barbiturate, concurrent hypoxia, and previous halothane exposure are potential causative factors in the production of hepatocyte injury, and autoimmune or hormonal mechanisms may also be involved. The mechanism may involve anesthetic induced disruption of intracellular calcium homeostasis.

All potent anesthetics studied to date are capable of inducing the potentially fatal syndrome of malignant hyperthermia. This syndrome can occur only in genetically susceptible individuals exposed to extreme environmental stress or pharmacologic triggers such as skeletal muscle depolarizers and inhalation anesthetics. The primary defect appears to involve the intracellular regulation of calcium flux in skeletal muscle. The incidence of this anesthetic complication ranges from 1 in 5000 to 1 in 250,000. The 1 in 250,000 estimate is for all anesthetics. The 1 in 5000 estimate is for potent inhalational anesthetics and succinylcholine co-administered. Dantrolene, a skeletal muscle relaxant, is the drug of choice in the prevention and treatment of malignant hyperthermia (see Chapter 11).

Intravenous Anesthetics

In general, the side effects are dose related depressions of respiratory drive and cardiovascular function. For many intravenous anesthetics, there is a very narrow margin of safety between the dose of drug that produces sufficient depression of consciousness to permit surgery and that which produces apnea. These general anesthetics may also have adverse excitatory effects on the CNS. Although it does induce anesthesia, methohexital has such excitatory effects that it lowers the seizure threshold. This may be of clinical significance in patients with a history of seizures or those receiving other drugs that may induce seizures, such as local anesthetics or subarachnoid radiographic contrast agents.

Ketamine has minimal depressant respiratory but significant dysphoric effects. Patients may recall vivid hallucinations, undergo delirium during the recovery phase of anesthesia, and experience flashbacks of these experiences at a later date, but emergence delirium can be greatly minimized by administration of a small dose of benzodiazepine before induction of anesthesia with ketamine.

The cardiovascular effects of the IV anesthetics are diverse. Depression of blood pressure may be due to histamine release as with barbiturates or more commonly to direct effects of the drug producing depression of myocardial contractility and vascular tone. Etomidate appears to have the least effect on heart rate and blood pressure, with benzodiazepines having less depressant activity than barbiturates. Ketamine, on the other hand, can significantly increase heart rate, blood pressure, and alter regional blood flow through its sympathomimetic effects.

With few significant exceptions, the IV anesthetics are relatively free of toxic effects other than those already mentioned. In patients with the metabolic disorder acute intermittent porphyria (incidence about 1 in 10,000), the administration of barbiturates or benzodiazepines for induction of anesthesia may precipitate life-threatening neurologic complications. This syndrome is characterized by colicky abdominal pain, tachycardia, hypertension, bulbar and/or pe-

ripheral neuropathy, and often psychotic behavior. In addition, etomidate may inhibit steroidogenesis, by blocking 11β-hydroxylase and cholesterol side-chain cleaving mitochondrial cytochrome P-450 dependent enzymes.

Local Anesthetics

 ## THERAPEUTIC OVERVIEW

Local anesthetics cause a reversible blockade of action potential conduction in neurons. They have many uses in medicine to make a specific section of the body impervious to the perception of painful stimuli. These uses range from dentistry, obstetrics, and procedures as simple as local infiltration for removal of a superficial skin lesion to regional anesthetics used entirely for a hip replacement, including management of postoperative pain. Therapeutic considerations are indicated in the box.

 ## MECHANISMS OF ACTION

Local anesthetics act directly on nerve cells to block their ability to transmit impulses down their axons. By blocking action potential propagation in sensory neurons, they eliminate sensations of pain. Local anesthetics are not specific to any nerve cell type and act on all sensory, motor, and autonomic neurons and all neurons in the CNS. However, by local administration the actions of these compounds can be restricted. Also, certain practical pharmacokinetic considerations make them particularly useful in blocking sensory transmission of pain impulses. The great-

est advantage of local anesthetics is their reversibility. When the drug is eliminated by metabolism or excretion, its action is terminated and the nerve resumes completely normal function. There are generally no long-term consequences of local anesthetic use. Thus these drugs are highly effective in providing regional, localized, and reversible pain relief.

The molecular targets for local anesthetic action are the voltage-dependent sodium channels that occur in all neurons. As reviewed in Chapter 22, these channels are responsible for the regenerative action potentials that occur along neuronal axons to carry messages from cell bodies to nerve terminals. Voltage-dependent sodium channels are usually closed at normal resting membrane potentials, preventing the high concentration of sodium in the extracellular fluid from entering the cell. When membranes are depolarized, these channels open and allow sodium to flow into the cell down its concentration gradient. This influx of positive charge depolarizes the cell further, opening more channels and causes a self-regenerating action potential as discussed in Chapter 22. Sustained depolarization causes an automatic inactivation of the voltage-dependent sodium channels, shutting off sodium influx, and a concurrent opening of voltage-dependent potassium channels. The resultant potassium efflux returns the membrane potential to its normal resting value.

The mechanism by which local anesthetics block conduction of nerve impulses is well understood. These drugs bind selectively to the intracellular surface of sodium channels and block the entry of sodium into the cell (Figure 30-9). By blocking sodium influx, these drugs eliminate the depolarization necessary for action potential propagation and, at sufficient concentrations, block impulse conduction. Since the binding of local anesthetics to sodium channels is

---

THERAPEUTIC CONSIDERATIONS OF LOCAL ANESTHETICS
Speed of onset
Side effects
seizures
cardiovascular depression

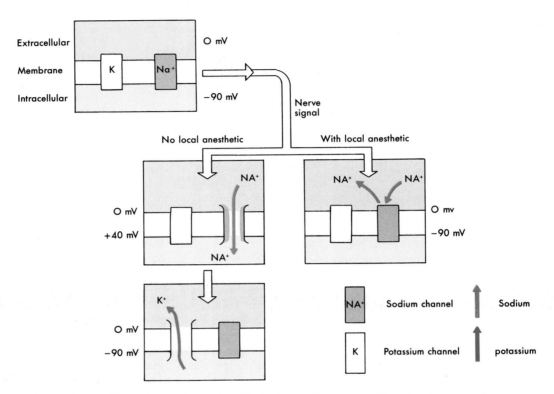

FIGURE 30-9   Transmission of nerve impulse in absence (normal conditions) and presence (nerve block) of local anesthetic agent.

completely reversible, when drug administration is stopped drug diffuses away and is metabolized and nerve function is completely restored. The ability of local anesthetic drugs to block sodium channels is highly dependent on the conformation (or state) of the channel. As discussed in Chapter 22, sodium channels exist in three major states. In ths resting state, the channels do not allow sodium influx and are highly sensitive to depolarization-induced opening, in the open state they allow sodium influx, and in the refractory state they do not allow sodium influx and are not opened by depolarization (see Figure 22-5).

Local anesthetics have different potencies in binding to the several states of sodium channels. Local anesthetics are much more likely to block sodium channels that are open or refractory and bind to resting channels with a much lower potency. This phenomenon is called *state-dependence* and has great

practical importance. Because local anesthetics will preferentialy block nerves in which sodium channels are open or refractory, they are more potent in rapidly firing nerves than in nerves in which action potentials are less frequent. Since sensory neurons often fire at substantially greater frequencies than motor fibers, sensory neurons are often preferentially blocked by a given concentration of local anesthetic.

The structures of local anesthetic drugs have a number of interesting aspects that have a direct bearing on their therapeutic actions (Figure 30-10). These drugs all contain a hydrophobic group (almost always an aromatic moiety) linked through an alkyl chain of intermediate length to a hydrophilic group (usually a tertiary amine). The presence of both hydrophilic and hydrophobic groups reflects the dual requirements for local anesthetic drug action. The drug must be partially water-soluble to be able to diffuse to the nerves

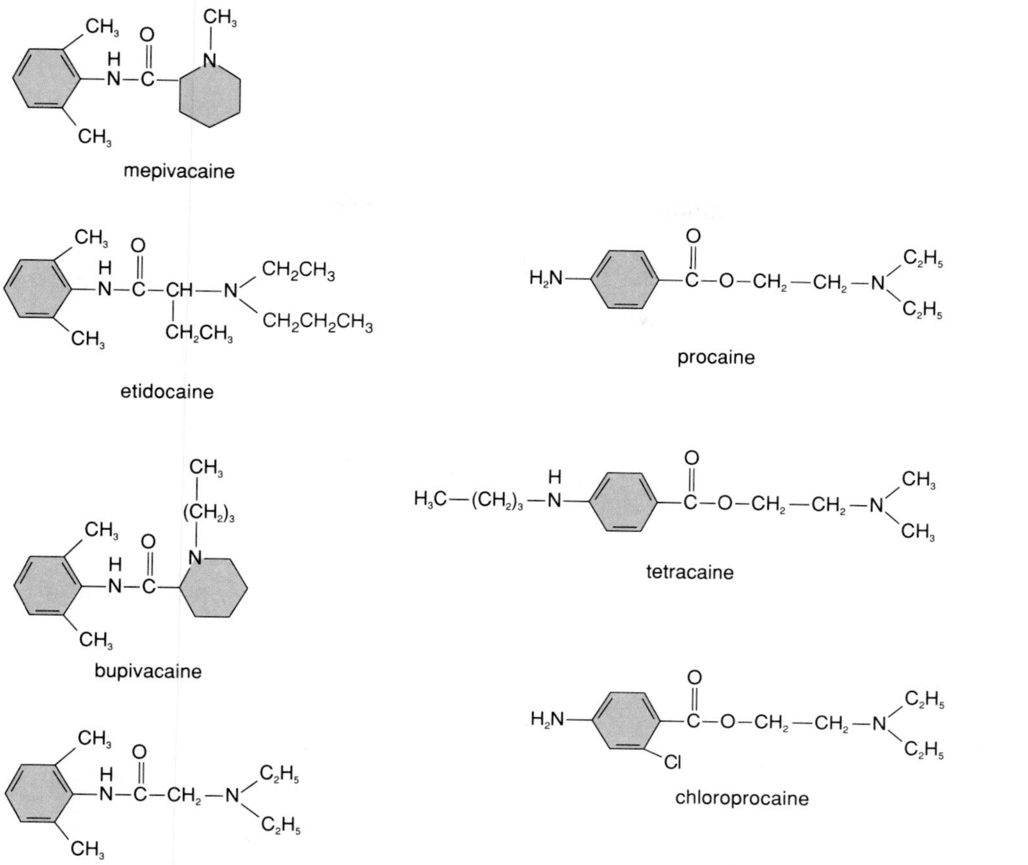

mepivacaine

etidocaine

bupivacaine

lidocaine

procaine

tetracaine

chloroprocaine

FIGURE 30-10 Structures of local anesthetic agents shown as free base forms.

to be blocked after local infection; however, it must also be sufficiently lipid-soluble to be able to penetrate the cell membrane and reach its binding site on the inner surface of the voltage-dependent sodium channels. Thus the hydrophilic tertiary amine facilitates diffusion to the cells of interest, while the hydrophobic aromatic group allows the drug to enter the cell and reach its actual site of action.

Another relevant aspect of the chemistry of these drugs is the effect of pH. Local anesthetic drugs are weak bases, with pK_a values usually in the range of 8 to 9. This means that most of the drugs will be in the charged cationic form at normal body pH. This is fortunate, since most evidence suggests that it is the cationic form of the drug that binds to and blocks the sodium channel. On the other hand, the cationic-charged form of the drug is much less likely to penetrate the cell membrane (despite the presence of the hydrophilic aromatic group) and thus is less able to reach its site of action. The constant equilibrium between cationic and unprotonated drug explains this dichotomy. As a weak base, although most drug will be protonated at physiologic pH, a certain proportion (1% to 10%) will be nonprotonated. This minor nonprotonated fraction of the drug is probably the primary species that permeates the cell membranes and accumulates in the cytoplasm. Once across the membrane, equilibrium is reestablished and most of the drug will again be protonated, facilitating sodium channel blockade.

The type of bond linking the aromatic and amine groups in local anesthetic drugs has major implications for the duration of action and toxicity of these compounds. Two types of linkages are found in the alkyl chains connecting the hydrophobic and hydrophilic regions of local anesthetic molecules. An ester linkage, as found in procaine, allows the drug to be inactivated by esterases that are widely distributed throughout the body. Because hydrolysis of the ester bond eliminates the biological activity of the drug, the presence of an ester bond usually, although not always, results in a drug with a relatively short du-

Table 30-4 Pharmacokinetic Parameter Values for Local Anesthetics

Drugs	Administration	Elimination ($t_{1/2}$, hr)	Disposition	Plasma Protein Bound (%)	Onset Time
mepivacaine	PN	1.9-3/2 (adults) 2.7-9/0 (neonates)	R, B, M, (main) —	75 —	3-20 min —
bupivacaine	PN	2.7 (adults) 8.1 (neonates)	— M	— 95	2-10 min
lidocaine	PN, IV	1.5-2	M* (95%), R	70	—
procaine	PN, IV	<60 sec	M	—	3-5 min
etidocaine	PN	2.5	M, R	95	

R, Renal; *B*, biliary; *M*, metabolism.
PN, Perineural (around the nerve).
* Large first pass effect.

ration of action. In contrast, an amide linkage, as is found in lidocaine, cannot by hydrolyzed by esterases and usually results in drugs that are longer acting. Finally, since hydrolysis of ester-type local anesthetic drugs results in metabolites that resemble para-aminobenzoic acid derivatives, ester-type local anesthetic drugs are more likely to provoke hypersensitivity reactions than amide-type local anesthetic drugs (although these actually are relatively infrequent with either drug class). This is discussed in more detail in the next section.

PHARMACOKINETICS

Local anesthetics are generally administered by injection close to the nerves to be blocked. Since the point where local anesthetics act is the inner surface of nerve membrane, agents must diffuse through tissues from the injection site to reach the appropriate nerve fibers. A number of factors influence rate of onset of anesthesia. Because local anesthetics are weak bases (forming salts by combining with acids) and have pK_a values between 8 and 9, they exist as the nonprotonated form in an alkaline or less acidic environment. The nonprotonated form more readily traverses tissue membranes to reach the site of action than does the charged or protonated form. Inside the nerve membrane, it is the latter species that interacts with sodium channel proteins and is responsible for the pharmacological effect.

Other determinants of rate of onset of local anesthesia include drug concentration and potency, drug binding to plasma protein, rate of metabolic biotransformation, and vascularity at the site of drug injection.

The latter is of primary importance in that any diffusion into blood vessels will reduce the regional drug concentration at the nerve fibers to be blocked. Vasoconstrictors, such as epinephrine, are frequently employed to prevent diffusion and reduce systemic absorption. While vasoconstrictor drugs tend to extend the duration of the less lipid-soluble agents (lidocaine, chloroprocaine, and mepivacaine) than those of the more lipid-soluble etidocaine and bupivacaine. A number of local anesthetics are marketed in combination with fixed concentrations of vasoconstrictor drugs.

Local anesthetics vary considerably in the rates at which they are converted to inactive metabolites by body tissues. Since all local anesthetics diffuse into the systemic circulation to some extent, metabolic fate becomes a prominent factor in the potential of these agents to produce undesirable side effects or overt toxicity. In addition to drug biotransformation, plasma protein binding to α_1-acid glycoprotein will also reduce the concentration of free drug in the systemic circulation.

Several local anesthetics (procaine, chloroprocaine, and tetracaine) are esters (see Figure 30-10) and are rapidly metabolically transformed to inactive products via hydrolysis by plasma cholinesterase and liver esterases. These agents generally have a relatively short half-life in the body (Table 30-4). In the absence of esterase activity, such as in spinal fluid, the duration of spinal anesthesia with the esters is considerably extended. Amide-type local anesthetics are metabolized by microsomes of the liver endoplasmic reticulum. This involves an initial *N*-dealkylation followed by hydrolysis. Relative rates of biotransformation of amide-linked local anesthetics are

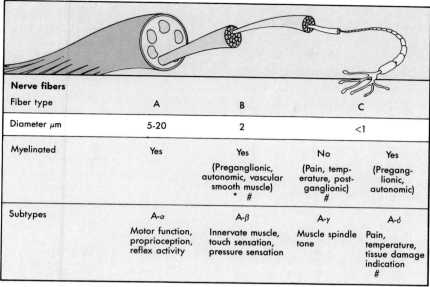

Nerve fibers				
Fiber type	A	B	C	
Diameter μm	5-20	2	<1	
Myelinated	Yes	Yes (Preganglionic, autonomic, vascular smooth muscle) * #	No (Pain, temperature, postganglionic) #	Yes (Preganglionic, autonomic)
Subtypes	A-α Motor function, proprioception, reflex activity	A-β Innervate muscle, touch sensation, pressure sensation	A-γ Muscle spindle tone	A-δ Pain, temperature, tissue damage indication #

* Spinal and peridural anesthesia
# Pain transmission fibers

FIGURE 30-11   Summary of anatomical types of nerve fibers, including those over which pain signals are conducted.

lidocaine (fastest) followed by mepivacaine and bupivacaine (slowest) (see Table 30-4). Some products of lidocaine metabolism possess local anesthetic activity.

The amides are also extensively bound to plasma proteins, and nonspecific tissue binding also occurs near the injection site. Preexisting liver disease is more likely to result in toxicity with these agents as a result of both reduced drug biotransformation and a lower plasma protein concentration, since these latter proteins are synthesized in liver.

RELATION OF MECHANISMS OF ACTION TO CLINICAL RESPONSE

Anatomical, physiological, and chemical factors all play an important role in determining the susceptibility of nerve fibers to block by local anesthetics. The rate of onset, intensity, and duration of nerve block are dramatically affected by the size, myelination, firing rate, and anatomical location of the nerves. Chemical considerations, such as pH, also have improtatn practical effects on the clinical response to these drugs. Because the same types of sodium channels are present in most types of neurons, local anesthetics block impulse conduction in all types of nerve cells, including sensory, motor, autonomic, and CNS neurons. Sodium channels also play an important role in electrically excitable muscle cells, and local anesthetics can also have prominent actions on muscle. Actions on cardiac sodium channels is the basis for some of their therapeutic uses in treating cardiac dysrhythmias (see Chapter 14), and actions on smooth and cardiac muscle explain some of their toxicity. However, local anesthetics are not equally potent and effective in all cells in which sodium channels are found. In fact, these drugs show marked selectivity between different types of neurons and muscle cells. This selectivity is based primarily on pharmacokinetic considerations of penetration, physiological aspects concerning firing rate, and anatomical considerations of nerve size and degree of myelination.

Neurons differ from each other substantially based on diameter, frequency of firing, and degree of myelination. Most pain impulses in humans are carried on two types of primary afferent fibers, Aδ and C (Figure 30-11). Aδ fibers are distributed primarily in skin and mucous membranes, are small and finely myelinated, and are associated with sensations of sharp pricking pain. C fibers are widely distributed, small and unmyelinated, and are associated with long-lasting, burning pain. Some pain impulses are also carried by myelinated B fibers.

Because the binding of local anesthetics to sodium channels is state-dependent, rapidly firing neurons, such as those carrying pain impulses as are generally blocked at lower concentrations than are more slowly firing neurons (as discussed). It is also clear that small nerve fibers are generally more sensitive than are large nerve fibers, and myelinated nerves are more sensitive than unmyelinated nerves. Size (diameter of the axon) is important because it relates to the critical length along the axon that must be affected to block transmission. Small fibers generally have shorter critical lengths than do large fibers. Myelination is important because of the different types of current spread in unmyelinated and myelinated axons (see Figure 22-6). Spread of current along myelinated fibers is generally discontinuous, involving only the small unmyelinated areas at the nodes of Ranvier. Since this involves much less surface membrane to be blocked, local anesthetics usually block myelinated fibers more effectively than unmyelinated fiber of the same size.

The situation is complicated further by considering the anatomical localization of the different nerve types. Nerve cells in the outer portion of nerve trunks will generally be exposed to higher drug concentrations than nerve cells located in the center of nerve trunks, where diffusion of drug will be restricted. Although these general principles can explain the differential sensitivity of nerve fibers to blockade by local anesthetics, it is clearly difficult to predict precisely what will happen in a given situation. There is, however, a general order in which sensory modalities are usually lost: pain first, then cold, warmth, touch, and deep pressure. Motor functions are often more resistant to local anesthetics, probably due to considerations of size, firing rate, and anatomical localization, as discussed.

Local anesthetic drugs are generally found to be less effective in infected tissues than in normal tissues. This is because infection usually results in a local metabolic acidosis, lowering the pH. As discussed, the ability of local anesthetic drugs to penetrate cell membranes depends on the acid-base equilibrium, since the small proportion of the nonprotonated form is better able to permeate cell membranes. Infection-induced acidosis upsets this equilibrium, greatly reducing the proportion of the drug in the nonprotonated form. Consequently, the ability of the

---

CLINICAL PROBLEMS WITH LOCAL ANESTHETICS

CNS seizures and convulsions at high agent concentrations

Cardiac sodium channel blockade (also used therapeutically for antiarrhythmic effects) (see Chapter 14)

---

drug to cross the cell membrane to its site of action is markedly reduced. Since local anesthetics are often used to treat pain associated with inflammation or infection, this reduced efficacy has substantial clinical relevance.

Local anesthetic drugs are widely used to provide temporary pain relief localized regions of the body. By varying the drug, its concentration, the dose of the drug, and the method by which it is administered, one can obtain a wide range of effects. A localized intensely numb area of skin can be achieved for a short time by infiltrating the area with a short-acting drug. Conversely, a mostly sensory block can be achieved by administering a dilute solution of a long-acting local anesthetic drug via an indwelling catheter to the epidural space, providing complete anesthesia while preserving motor function and a mother's ability to deliver an infant. Anesthetics can be used to provide analgesia (relief of pain) and muscle relaxation at the same time, by administering a potent compound to the central neuraxis (spinal or epidural) or a major peripheral nerve complex (for example, the brachial plexus). Dilute solutions of local anesthetics mixed with narcotics are increasingly used in postoperative pain to provide excellent analgesia with a lower total narcotic drug dose than would be required with conventional therapies. Finally, local anesthetics are used in the management of more complicated acute and chronic pain states as both diagnostic and therapeutic tools. Many different drugs are available that differ primarily in their duration of action, side effects, and toxicity.

SIDE EFFECTS, CLINICAL PROBLEMS, AND TOXICITY

Because the termination of local anesthetic action ultimately depends on movement of drug into the

be only minimally affected by local anesthetics.

Local anesthetics do have potential deleterious actions on pacemaker activity, electrical excitability, conduction times, and contractile force of the heart. Arrhythmias are also possible; however, cardiac toxicity is infrequently observed, apparently only when high blood concentrations of the anesthetic agent are attained. Cardiovascular failure has also been reported to occur, however, from small doses used in infiltration anesthesia.

Lidocaine is also used therapeutically to depress abnormal pacemaker activity in certain arrhythmogenic states (see Chapter 14). Cocaine, a potent local anesthetic, which had wide clinical use several decades ago, also has prominent side effects on the heart and the CNS (see Chapter 32). Among the local anesthetics in current use, bupivacaine is considered to be more cardiotoxic than other agents.

Local hypersensitivity reactions can result from the use of some ester-type local anesthetics, particularly procaine and related compounds. These can be ameliorated by the systemic administration of antihistaminics.

REFERENCES

Davis PJ and Cook DR, eds: Clinical pharmacokinetics of the newer intravenous anaesthetic agents, Clin Pharm 11:18, 1986.

Domino EF, ed: PCP (phencyclidine): historical and current perspectives, Ann Arbor, Mich, 1981, NPP Books.

Eger EI, ed: Anesthetic uptake and action, Baltimore, 1974, Williams & Wilkins Co.

Eger EI, ed: Nitrous oxide, New York, 1985, Elsevier.

Katz R, editor: Propofol: clinical update and implications in seminars in anesthesia, vol III, no 1, suppl 1, New York, 1988, Grune & Stratton.

Miller RD, ed: Anesthesia, New York, 1981, Churchill Livingstone.

Olsen RW, ed: Drug interactions at the GABA receptor-ionophore, Ann Rev Pharmacol Toxicol 22:245, 1982.

Roth SH and Miller KW, eds: Molecular and cellular mechanisms of anesthetics, New York, 1986, Plenum Press.

systemic circulation, side effects and toxicity can result from blockade of impulse propagation in excitable organs and tissues perfused by blood. The central, peripheral, and autonomic nervous systems and all muscle are potential targets.

CNS effects may be manifest as depression or stimulation, or both, depending on the nervous pathways affects by the local anesthetic. Depression of cortical inhibitory neurons, without the balancing depression of excitatory nerves, may result in tremor and restlessness and culminate in overt clonic convulsions, coma, and respiratory failure (see box). However, a variety of symptoms, including general depression and drowsiness, are common clinical consequences. Seizures can be treated or prevented by injecting diazepam intravenously; oxygen can protect against hypoxemia in the convulsing patient. Overdose of local anesthetics results in reduced transmission of impulses at the neuromuscular junction and at ganglionic synapses, producing weakness or muscle paralysis. Support of respiration is an important component of treatment. Smooth muscle appears to

CHAPTER 31

Alcohol

31

Ethanol is a prime example of an agent that is widely used for nonmedical purposes, is misused and abused, causes psychological and physical dependence, can be life-threatening, and causes serious social, medical, and economic problems in those cultures where its use is accepted. In this country, its use causes almost insurmountable problems. It is estimated that 65% to 70% of Americans use alcohol (i.e., ethanol) and that more than 10 million are alcohol dependent. An additional 10 million are subject to negative consequences of alcohol abuse such as arrests, automobile accidents, violence, occupational injuries, and deleterious effects upon job performance and health. About 50% of all traffic deaths are estimated to be alcohol-related. The annual cost of alcohol-related problems in the United States is over 100 billion dollars. Since individuals who abuse alcohol probably overuse the health care system, alcoholics constitute a substantial fraction of many medical practices, and a medical history designed to elicit information on alcohol use is an essential feature of a modern medical work-up. Clearly, alcohol use and abuse are significant public health problems. This chapter covers these behavioral and toxicological problems associated with the use of ethanol as a recreational drug or drug of abuse and reviews the deleterious effects of other alcohols.

USES OF ETHANOL

Ethanol is used primarily as a social drug, with only limited application as a therapeutic agent (see the box). Ethanol is used externally as a rub to lower elevated body temperature by promoting evaporation, as a rub to prevent bedsores in bedridden patients, and sometimes by injection to produce irreversible nerve block or tumor destruction. It is also effective in the treatment of methanol and ethylene glycol poisonings, where it acts competitively to prevent the conversion of these alcohols to toxic intermediates until the unmetabolized parent compounds are removed from the body (see below for details). Ethanol is sometimes prescribed for its antianxiety and sed-

Table 31-1 Some Ion Channels That Are Functionally Altered by Ethanol

Channel	Effect	Ethanol Concentration
Sodium (voltage-gated)	Inhibited	100 mM and higher
Potassium (voltage-gated)	Facilitated	50-100 mM
Calcium (voltage-gated)	Inhibited	50 mM and higher
Calcium (glutamate-activated)	Inhibited	20-50 mM
Chloride (GABA-gated)	Facilitated	10-50 mM

THERAPEUTIC OVERVIEW

Ethanol is used:

Topically to reduce body temperature and as an antiseptic

By injection to produce irreversible nerve block

By inhalation to reduce foaming in pulmonary edema

Orally for sedative effect

Orally to increase appetite

In treatment of methanol and ethylene glycol poisoning

ative properties and as an appetite stimulant. Ethanol mist is also used to reduce the frothing in acute pulmonary edema resulting from left ventricular failure.

MOLECULAR MECHANISM OF CENTRAL NERVOUS SYSTEM EFFECTS

For many years alcohol and the general anesthetic agents were assumed to share a common mechanism of action in that both (1) require millimolar concentrations to produce their effects and (2) show excellent correlation between the oil/water partition coefficients (see Chapter 30) of these agents and their ability to depress the CNS. Before the advent of ether, ethanol was used as the "anesthetic" agent before surgical intervention.

Pharmacological and genetic evidence now indicate that ethanol, like general anesthetics, "fluidizes" or "disorders" the physical structure of cell membranes, particularly those low in cholesterol. In studies with animals previously exposed to ethanol or that exhibit pharmacological tolerance to ethanol intoxication or in species genetically resistant to the effects of ethanol, the neuronal cell membrane is not readily disordered by ethanol. Also, cell membranes from animals selectively bred for sensitivity to ethanol are more easily fluidized than those obtained from animals genetically resistant to alcohol.

At the molecular level ethanol may interfere with the packing of molecules in the phospholipid bilayer of the cell membrane, thus increasing membrane fluidity. However, this fluidizing effect of ethanol is small and may not be responsible for ethanol's CNS depressant effects. However, this fluidizing effect may be relegating to lipid structures in discrete areas of the brain, such as those surrounding important neurotransmitter receptors or ion channels, and thereby generating greater CNS disruption. Current experimental techniques do not permit ethanol measurements in small enough areas of the cell membrane to explore this theory; however, at some concentrations, ethanol affects most channels and receptors. Table 31-1 lists some of the ion channels influenced by ethanol. While the significance of these findings has not been established, ethanol appears to have both inhibitory and facilitatory effects, depending on the channel. In each case, ethanol depresses the CNS. Because both barbiturates and benzodiazepines exhibit cross tolerance to ethanol, all three agents may share a common mechanism, perhaps through the GABA-benzodiazepine-chloride channel complex (see Chapter 25).

Recent studies in animals demonstrate a selective effect of low concentrations of ethanol on guanine nucleotide binding proteins. Ethanol apparently promotes the activation of G_s (see Chapter 2), thus enhancing adenylate cyclase activity. Whether this event plays an important role in the mechanism of action of ethanol in humans is not determined. It has been suggested that the adenylate cyclase system may provide a biochemical marker of genetic predisposition to alcoholism.

OBSERVED EFFECTS OF ETHANOL ON THE CENTRAL NERVOUS SYSTEM

Like the general anesthetic agents, ethanol depresses all areas and functions of the brain. As with most CNS depressants, an excitement stage is observed initially as depression of higher inhibitory centers releases the normal control mechanisms responsible for social and behavioral restraints. Thus, ethanol is described as a disinhibitor or euphoriant. The higher integrative areas of the brain are affected first, with thought processes, fine discrimination, judgment, and motor function sequentially impaired. These effects may be observed with blood ethanol concentrations of 0.05% (50 mg/dl) or lower. Specific behavioral changes are difficult to predict and depend to a large extent upon the environment and the personality of the individual. As blood ethanol concentration increases to 0.1%, errors in judgment are frequent, motor systems are impaired, and responses to complex auditory and visual stimuli are altered. Patterns of involuntary motor action are affected. Ataxia is noticeable, with walking becoming difficult, and staggering common as the blood alcohol concentration approaches 0.15% to 0.2%. Reaction times are increased and the individual may become extremely loud, incoherent, and emotionally unstable. Violent behavior may occur at these concentrations. These effects are the result of depression of the excitatory areas throughout the brain. At blood ethanol concentrations from 0.2% to 0.3%, intoxicated individuals frequently experience periods of amnesia or "blackout," with failure to recall events occurring at that time.

With increased blood ethanol concentrations to 0.25% to 0.30%, anesthesia ensues. Ethanol, although sharing many properties with the general anesthetics, is less safe as an anesthetic because of its low margin of safety (ratio of anesthetic to lethal concentration). It is also a poor analgesic. Coma in humans occurs with blood alcohol concentrations above 0.3%. The lethal range for ethanol, in the absence of other CNS depressants, is between 0.4% and 0.5%, although individuals with much higher blood concentrations have survived. Death from acute ethanol overdose is relatively rare compared to death resulting from the combination of alcohol with other CNS depressants such as barbiturates and benzodiazepines. Death occurs as a result of a depressant effect on the medulla, resulting in respiratory failure.

Tolerance and Dependence

Both acute and chronic tolerance occurs with ethanol use. The mechanism of tolerance to ethanol is not well understood but involves both metabolic tolerance and cell or tissue tolerance, with the latter sometimes called pharmacodynamic tolerance. Acute tolerance can occur within a matter of hours and can rapidly dissipate. If alcohol is ingested daily for periods of weeks to months, chronic tolerance ensues with high chronic tolerances developing in some individuals. For a given effect, approximately a doubling of blood alcohol concentrations is seen in tolerant compared to nontolerant individuals. This is much less, however, than is observed with opiate drugs where a tolerance of 10- to 30-fold can be seen. With alcohol, tolerance development has greater implications than does tolerance with other agents, because other organ systems are now exposed to much higher concentrations with deleterious consequences, particularly to the liver. While tolerance develops to some of the CNS effects with ethanol, there is only a very minor increase in the concentration of drug that produces death. The greatest degree of tolerance is attributable to cell tolerance. Apparently metabolic tolerance accounts for only about 25% of the total effect.

Both psychological and physical dependence are characteristics of chronic alcohol use. The clinical manifestations of ethanol withdrawal are divided into early and late effects. The early symptoms occur between a few hours and up to 48 hours following cessation of drinking, with peak effects around 24 to 36 hours. Tremor, agitation, anxiety, anorexia, and insomnia are some of the usual symptoms. Seizures can also occur during the early phase of withdrawal. Late withdrawal symptoms or delirium tremens are relatively rare but can be life-threatening. They consist of confusion, disorientation, auditory or visual hallucinations, disturbed sensory perception, and hyperthermia. Coma and death can occur if these are untreated. Complicating factors in alcohol withdrawal are trauma from falls or accidents, bacterial infections, and problems associated with other organ systems, such as liver and heart. The withdrawal syndrome following ethanol consumption is much more severe than that with opioids and depends largely on the blood alcohol concentration before withdrawal and the duration of the consumption. Management is aimed at preventing severe complications that may lead to a fatal outcome and includes prevention or treatment of seizures, delirium, and cardiac arrhythmias. Intravenous benzodiazepines, particularly those not converted to active metabolites, are the drugs of choice. Phenobarbital can also be used. Other barbiturates and phenothiazines should be avoided. Phenytoin should not be used unless there is a preexisting CNS disorder.

 PHARMACOKINETICS

Absorption and Distribution

The pharmacokinetic parameters for ethanol are summarized in Table 31-2. Alcohol taken orally is absorbed throughout the gastrointestinal tract. Absorption depends on passive diffusion and is governed by the concentration gradient and the area available for absorption. Several factors influence absorption, the most important being the presence of food in the stomach. This tends to dilute the alcohol, delay emptying time, and retard absorption from the small intestine (where absorption is favored because of the large surface area). Higher ethanol concentrations in the GI tract cause a greater concentration gradient and therefore hasten the rate of absorption. The absorption process continues until the alcohol concentration in the blood and that in the GI tract are at equilibrium. Since ethanol is rapidly metabolized and removed from the blood, eventually all the alcohol is absorbed from the GI tract. Ethanol vapor is also rapidly absorbed from the lung.

Once ethanol reaches the blood it is immediately distributed to other body compartments at a rate proportional to the blood flow to that area and is eventually distributed equally to total body water. Because the brain receives a high blood flow, high brain concentrations are achieved rapidly.

Metabolism and Elimination

The major pathway for the disappearance of ethanol from the body is metabolism by the liver and to a minor extent by other organs (however, see below), with metabolism accounting for about 90% of the total eliminated. Expired air contains ethanol in proportion to the vapor pressure of ethanol at body temperature. The ratio of ethanol concentrations between exhaled air and blood alcohol, 1/2100, forms the basis for the "breathalyzer" test, in which blood alcohol concentration is determined by extrapolation from analysis of the alcohol content of the expired air.

Blood alcohol determination varies with hematocrit; people living at higher altitudes have a higher hematocrit and therefore a lower water content in blood. Urine is also available for determining ethanol concentration, and spinal or ocular fluid is generally used in postmortem analyses.

Blood concentrations of ethanol can be estimated from the weight of the individual and the amount of ethanol consumed orally. These estimates are somewhat higher than actual blood concentrations unless the ethanol is given IV, because there is rapid first-pass metabolism following oral administration. After consuming comparable amounts of ethanol, women have higher blood ethanol concentrations than men, even after correcting for differences in weight. Women also are more susceptible to alcoholic liver disease. Much of the first-pass metabolism of ethanol occurs in gastric tissue. The first-pass metabolism of ethanol is about 50% less in women than in men because of lower alcohol dehydrogenase activity in

Table 31-2	Pharmacokinetic Parameters of Ethanol
Administered	Topically, orally, sometimes by inhalation, by injection into nerve trunks
Absorption	Slight topically, complete from stomach and intestine by passive diffusion, rapid via lungs
Elimination	>90% metabolized to CO_2 and H_2O by liver and other tissues, excreted in air, urine, milk, sweat
Rate of metabolism	Normally about 100 mg/kg/hr of total body burden, or 0.015%/hr; higher or lower in liver enzyme induction or in liver disease; zero order kinetics
Distribution	Total body water; Widmark factors for volume of distribution are 68% of body weight in men and 55% in women; varies widely

the female gastric mucosa. This occurs in nonalcoholic and alcoholic women and explains the increased vulnerability of women to the effects of acute and chronic alcoholism. It had been assumed earlier that the higher ethanol concentrations in women were entirely dependent on a difference in the apparent volumes of distribution between men and women. Body water content is 55% of body weight for women and 68% for men (Widmark factors). Recent studies have shown that differences do exist in the volumes of distribution of ethanol between men and women, but these differences do not account entirely for the higher ethanol concentrations in women.

Calculation of Blood Alcohol Concentration from the Amount Ingested

Physicians are frequently called on as expert witnesses in cases involving alcohol intoxication. Moreover, in the course of taking a medical history it is valuable to be able to estimate the blood alcohol concentration and the subsequent effects of the alcohol from the amount ingested. In calculating the amount of ethanol ingested, the percent of alcohol in the beverage (usually indicated on a volume/volume percentage, with 100 proof equivalent to 50% ethanol by volume) and the density of 0.8 gm for each ml of ethanol must be known. Blood alcohol concentrations (BAC) are calculated as mg of alcohol/L of blood. The legal limit for operating a motor vehicle in most states is 1000 mg/L, 100 mg/dl, or 0.1%. An example of a typical calculation for a 70 kg person ingesting 1.5 oz or 45 ml of 80 proof distilled spirits is as follows:

$$\left(\frac{80 \text{ proof}}{2} = 40\% \right) (45 \text{ ml}) = \frac{18 \text{ ml } 100\% \text{ EtOH}}{(\text{by volume})}$$

$$(18 \text{ ml}) (0.8 \text{ g/ml}) = 14.4 \text{ g EtOH (by weight)}$$

If absorbed immediately and distributed in total body water:

$$\text{BAC (male)} = \frac{14.4 \text{ g}}{(70 \text{ kg}) (0.68)} = 0.3 \text{ g/L, 30 mg/dl, 0.03\%}$$

$$\text{BAC (female)} = \frac{14.4 \text{ g}}{(70 \text{ kg}) (0.55)} = 0.37 \text{ mg/L, 37 g/dl, 0.037\%}$$

An average rate for metabolism of ethanol by nonpreconditioned individuals is 100 mg/kg body weight/hr or 7 g/hr in a 70 kg individual. Chronic

alcoholics metabolize ethanol at a higher rate, because of stimulation of the MEOS or cytochrome P-450 system (see below). In the example below, left, the man with a body burden of 14.4 g of ethanol would totally metabolize the alcohol in 2 hours.

Figure 31-1 provides an approximation of the blood alcohol concentrations in men ingesting 1 to 5 drinks in 1 hour for different body weight individuals, assuming rapid absorption. This figure emphasizes how little consumption can produce impaired motor skills and inability to drive an automobile safely, as indicated by the legal limit of 0.10% ethanol in most states and 0.08% in some states.

Enzyme Systems that Metabolize Ethanol

Most of the metabolism of ethanol takes place in the liver parenchyma catalyzed by alcohol dehydrogenase (ADH). The metabolic sequence is shown in Figure 31-2. Ethanol is metabolized to acetaldehyde by ADH, which in turn is oxidized to acetate by aldehyde dehydrogenases (ALDH). Acetate is then oxidized to CO_2 and H_2O, primarily in peripheral tissues. Both ADH and ALDH are NAD^+-dependent enzymes, with the oxidation of one mole of ethanol to acetate producing two moles of NADH. Thus, for continuation of ethanol oxidation, mechanisms must exist both for acetaldehyde removal and for recycling of NAD^+ from NADH. Liver mitochondria contain a particularly efficient form of ALDH with a very low K_m that removes the acetaldehyde. The NADH is reoxidized to NAD^+ by several mechanisms including the mitochondrial electron transport system (ETS) and the conversion of pyruvate to lactate by lactate dehydrogenase. During ethanol oxidation the concentration of NADH rises substantially, and NADH product inhibition can become rate-limiting. Another rate-limiting factor can be the amount of enzyme in liver. During fasting, ethanol metabolism decreases, an effect that can be accounted for by the decrease in liver ADH. Because of these factors, the metabolism of ethanol is limited and exhibits zero order kinetics (Figure 31-3).

The other system for metabolizing ethanol in the liver is that catalyzed by cytochrome P-450. This system has also been called the microsomal ethanol metabolizing system (MEOS) and converts ethanol to acetaldehyde. The K_m for the system is relatively high (~30mM) and normally would not be responsible for a significant fraction of ethanol metabolism. This enzyme system, however, is induced by prolonged eth-

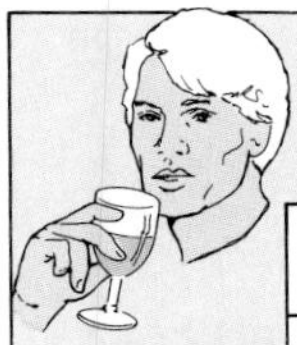

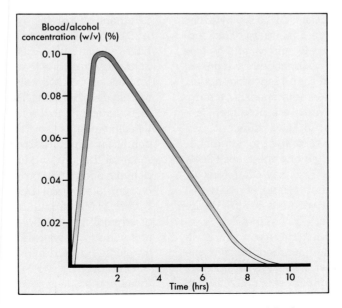

	Drinks in 1 hr				
Body weight (pounds)	1	2	3	4	5
100	.03	.06	.10	.13	.16
120	.03	.05	.08	.11	.13
140	.02	.05	.07	.09	.11
160	.02	.04	.06	.08	.10
180	.02	.03	.05	.07	.09
200	.02	.03	.05	.06	.08

Blood alcohol concentration (BAC) %

FIGURE 31-1   Approximate percentages of ethanol in blood (BAC) in male subjects of different body weights, calculated as percent, weight/volume (w/v), after indicated number of drinks. One drink is 12 oz of beer, 5 oz of wine, or 1 oz of 80 proof distilled spirits. Individuals with BAC of 0.10% or higher are considered legally intoxicated in most states; those with BAC of 0.05% to 0.09% are considered impaired. (Pink area, impaired; red area, legally intoxicated.) BAC can be 20% to 30% higher in female subjects. Note the small number of drinks that can result in a state of intoxication.

FIGURE 31-2   Metabolism of ethanol by alcohol and aldehyde dehydrogenases (see text).

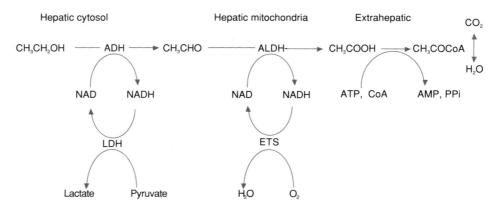

FIGURE 31-3   Disappearance of ethanol after oral ingestion follows zero order kinetics.

anol exposure and can be important in chronic alcoholism. During the oxidation of ethanol with this system, one molecule of NADPH is utilized for every molecule of ethanol oxidized to acetaldehyde. Therefore the $NADH/NAD^+$ ratio does not increase. Since this enzyme system also metabolizes other exogenous compounds, when ethanol is present, their metabolism may be inhibited in chronic alcoholics, or stimulated if the cytochrome P-450 system is induced (see Chapter 5).

Genetics of Ethanol Drug Metabolizing Enzymes

Human alcohol dehydrogenase (ADH) is a cytosolic zinc-containing dimeric enzyme made up of six separate subunits, α, β_1, β_2, and β_3 and γ_1 and γ_2 (see Table 31-3). These subunits are encoded by 3 genes, ADH_1, ADH_2, and ADH_3, and their respective alleles. Because homodimers and heterodimers exist, a number of combinations of isozymes are possible. Caucasians, Orientals, and blacks have different percentages of isozymes, which contribute to differences in the metabolism of ethanol among the races (Table 31-4). The several isozymes also have different K_m values. Most of these isozymes are saturated between 20 to 30 mM ethanol, which accounts for the disappearance curves following zero order kinetics.

The second enzyme in the ADH pathway is aldehyde dehydrogenase. This mitochondrial enzyme has a K_m of about 1 μM, so that the very large amounts of aldehyde generated are handled efficiently. This is fortunate because acetaldehyde is very reactive and potentially toxic. With this enzyme there are significant genetic differences that influence the responses

Table 31-3 ADH Genetic Model*		
Gene	**Allele**	**Subunit**
ADH_1	ADH_1	α
ADH_2	$ADH_2{}^1$	β_1
	$ADH_2{}^2$	β_2
	$ADH_2{}^3$	β_3
ADH_3	$ADH_3{}^1$	γ_1
	$ADH_3{}^2$	γ_2

* From Schuckit MA: Genetic aspects of alcoholism, Ann Emerg Med 15:991, 1986.

to ethanol. Orientals have a different mitochondrial ALDH than do Caucasians. Fifty percent of Orientals have an inactive ALDH, caused by a single base change in the gene that encodes for the enzyme. This renders some Orientals incapable of oxidizing acetaldehyde efficiently. High concentrations of acetaldehyde bring about a flushing reaction and other unpleasant effects, so that orientals with this genetic condition rarely become alcoholic. Advantage is made of the strongly undesirable response to acetaldehyde accumulation in the aversive treatment of chronic alcoholism by the use of disulfiram (Antabuse). Disulfuram inhibits ALDH and in the presence of ethanol brings about flushing, headache, nausea and vomiting, sweating, and hypotension, shortly after alcohol ingestion.

Other agents such as metronidazole, the sulfonylureas, griseofulvin, some cephalosporins, and chloramphenicol may also provoke the acetaldehyde effect. Disulfiram also inhibits dopamine β hydroxylase.

Table 31-4 Frequency of ADH$_2$ and ADH$_3$ Alleles in Racial Populations

	ADH$_2$^{1}	ADH$_2$^{2}	ADH$_2$^{3}	ADH$_3$^{1}	ADH$_3$^{2}
White-Americans	>95%	<5%	<5%	50%	50%
White-Europeans	85	15	<5	60	40
Orientals	15	85	<5	95	5
African-American	85	<5	15	85	15

OTHER TISSUES AND ORGANS AFFECTED BY ETHANOL

The effects of ethanol on other organs and tissues are also important in assessing the hazards of ethanol ingestion.

Gastrointestinal Tract

It has been known for many years that tissues other than the liver have the capacity to metabolize ethanol. The metabolism of alcohol by the stomach and small intestine contributes to first-pass metabolism (discussed previously) and the greater susceptibility of women to ethanol. The oral mucosa, esophagus, stomach, and small intestine are also exposed to higher concentrations of ethanol than other tissues of the body. Thus they are susceptible to direct toxicity from ethanol. The alcohol dehydrogenase in the GI tract is different from that in the liver and has a particularly high K_m. These tissues are also capable of metabolizing ethanol by the cytochrome P-450 system.

Acute gastritis resulting in nausea and vomiting is a result of ethanol abuse. Bleeding, ulcers, and cancer of the upper GI tract are possible consequences.

Liver

The consequences of ethanol metabolism by the liver can be devastating and contribute significantly to the pathology seen in this organ. The metabolism of ethanol causes a large increase in the NADH/NAD ratio, which produces serious biochemical disruption in liver metabolism. The cell attempts to maintain NAD concentrations in the cytosol by reducing pyruvate to lactate, leading to increased lactic acid in the liver and blood. Lactate is excreted by the kidney and competes with urate for elimination, which can increase blood urate. The excretion of lactate also apparently leads to a deficiency of zinc and magnesium. A more direct effect of increased NADH concentrations in the liver is increased fatty acid synthesis since NADPH is a necessary cofactor. Since NADH participates in the citric acid cycle, the oxidation of lipids is depressed, further contributing to fat accumulation in liver cells.

Acetaldehyde may also play a prominent role in liver damage. If there is an initial insult to the liver, the concentration of ALDH decreases and acetaldehyde is not removed efficiently, and can react with a number of cell constituents. Possible consequences to the liver of chronic alcoholism and other deleterious effects of ethanol are listed in the boxes, p. 442.

Pancreas

Ethanol is a known cause of acute pancreatitis. Repeated use can lead to pancreatic insufficiency with decreased pancreatic enzyme secretion and diabetes mellitus as possible consequences.

Endocrine System

Large amounts of ethanol decrease testosterone concentrations in men and cause loss of secondary sex characteristics and feminization. Premenopausal women who abuse alcohol may have a disruption of ovarian function seen as oligomenorrhea, hypomenorrhea, or amenorrhea. Ethanol also stimulates the release of adrenocortical hormones by increasing the secretion of ACTH.

Heart

Alcoholic cardiac myopathy is also a consequence of ethanol consumption. Other cardiovascular effects include mild increases in blood pressure and heart rate and cardiac arrhythmias.

EFFECTS OF ETHANOL ON THE LIVER

Increased NADH/NAD ratio
Increased acetaldehyde concentration
Increased lipid content
Increased protein accumulation
Decreased protein export
Increased water content
Increased oxygen uptake
Centrilobular hypoxia
Proliferation of endoplasmic reticulum
Increased cytochrome P_{450} content
Increased or decreased drug metabolism
Increased production of free radicals and lipoperoxidation products
Decreased production of coagulation factors
Increased collagen deposition
Hepatitis
Scarring
Cirrhosis
Cell death

OTHER CONSEQUENCES OF ETHANOL

Gastritis
Increased incidence of peptic ulcer
Pancreatitis
Cardiomyopathy
Portal hypertension
Cardiac dysrhythmias
Feminization in males
Cancers of upper GI tract, liver
Fetal alcohol syndrome
Wernicke-Korsakoff's syndrome

Kidney

As is well known, ethanol has a diuretic effect unrelated to fluid intake. This is caused by inhibition of secretion of antidiuretic hormone, which decreases the renal reabsorption of water.

Brain

There are several well-documented conditions resulting from excessive ethanol intake; these include Wernicke-Korsakoff's syndrome, which can result in damage of brain structures. Cerebellar atrophy, central pontine myelinosis and demyelinization of the corpus callosum are other effects of ethanol upon the brain.

Fetal Alcohol Syndrome

Although this condition has been recognized from early times, it was rediscovered in the 1970s and the general public is well aware of the hazards of drinking by pregnant women on the health of the fetus. Consequences of maternal ingestion of alcohol can include miscarriage, stillbirth, low birth weight, slow postnatal growth, microcephaly, mental retardation, and many other organic and structural abnormalities.

The incidence of fetal alcohol syndrome in some parts of the United States is estimated to be as high as 1 in 300 births.

Other Effects

Alcoholics are frequently immunologically compromised, are subject to infectious diseases, and have excess mortality to cancers of the upper GI tract as well as the liver. While the mechanism of this latter effect is not known, alcohol consumption is a risk factor for the development of cancer.

Ethanol relaxes blood vessels and in severe intoxication, hypothermia resulting from heat loss from vasodilation may occur. Several types of anemias have been described in alcoholic patients.

DIAGNOSIS OF CHRONIC ALCOHOLISM: GENETIC FACTORS

The diagnosis of chronic alcoholism in a patient is a difficult problem for the practicing physician. Success depends on a reliable history from the patient or from a member of the patients' family. If a diagnosis can be made, it is frequently difficult to manage the problem because treatment is initiated when the disorder is well-advanced.

Over the past 10 to 15 years the role of genetic factors in the development of chronic alcoholism has been identified with the hope that early intervention may be more successful. Studies involving family members and twins support a predisposition and an increased risk of alcoholism among close relatives. This conclusion that primary alcoholism is genetically influenced is based upon a number of interesting findings.

Studies among families indicate a threefold to four-fold higher risk for alcoholism in sons and daughters of alcoholic parents. Comparisons of the risk of alcoholism in identical twins versus fraternal twins should indicate if alcoholism is related to the childhood environment. Since both types of twins have similar childhood backgrounds, if alcoholism is related to the childhood environment, both identical and fraternal twins should have the same rates of development of the alcoholic disorder. Most results show that in identical twins, which share 100% of their genes, there is a twofold higher concordance for alcoholism compared to fraternal twins. In another study, alcoholic risk was assessed in children of alcoholics who were raised by adoptive parents (other than their biological parents) who were nonalcoholics. In these children there was a threefold to fourfold higher risk for alcoholism. No difference in susceptibility was detected between sons or daughters of alcoholics.

Other studies have categorized alcoholics into several subgroups. One is the alcoholism most frequently seen in men and associated with criminality, and the second is a subtype equally observed in both sexes and influenced by the environment. Genetic predisposition, however, is merely one of several factors leading to the development of alcoholism. Studies in progress are attempting to seek out possible biological markers with which to identify potential alcoholics (e.g., specific differences in blood proteins, enzymes involved in ethanol degradation, and enzymes concerned with brain neurotransmitters and signaling system components, including G-proteins) to encourage such individuals to seek assistance sooner.

TREATMENT OF ALCOHOLISM

Acute Intoxication

Emergency treatment of acute alcohol intoxication includes the maintenance of an adequate airway and support of respiration and blood pressure. In addition to its depressant actions on the CNS, other organs including the heart may be affected. It is also important to assess the level of consciousness relative to blood alcohol concentration, since other drugs may influence the apparent degree of intoxication. As a precaution a short-acting narcotic antagonist is generally administered. Hypoglycemia, ketoacidosis, and dehydration may require the administration of glucose. The loss of body fluids may also necessitate IV fluids containing potassium, magnesium, and phosphate. Thiamine and other vitamins such as folic acid and pyridoxine are administered usually with IV glucose to prevent the neurologic deficits that may occur.

Chronic Alcoholism

The effective management of chronic alcoholism includes the social and environmental, as well as the medical aspects, and also involves the family of the individual undergoing treatment. Several types of treatment are available, including group psychotherapy (e.g., Alcoholics Anonymous), and private and public clinics outside of a hospital setting. Hypnotherapy, psychoanalysis, and aversive therapy with disulfiram also have been used. Management regimens have had variable success rates, with many being no more effective over the long term than 10% to 15% of the participants.

OTHER ALCOHOLS

Methanol Intoxication

Alcoholics may accidentally or intentionally ingest methanol, which has a toxicological profile quite different from that of ethanol. The two major characteristics of methanol intoxication are optic nerve damage, which can lead to blindness, and severe acidosis. Methanol is metabolized by alcohol dehydrogenase and aldehyde dehydrogenase systems in a manner similar to ethanol, but at a much slower rate. The products of methanol metabolism are formaldehyde and formic acid, which are apparently responsible for visual damage and acidosis. Management requires maintenancee of an airway and respiration as with any intoxication, attempts to remove residual methanol, the treatment of the acidosis, and the administration of IV ethanol to retard the formation of the toxic metabolic products. Ethanol is effective since it can compete successfully with methanol for alcohol dehydrogenase and essentially saturate the enzyme (Figure 31-4). This reduces the likelihood of subsequent effects of methanol metabolites and provides the time necessary for removal of methanol from the body by dialysis if necessary.

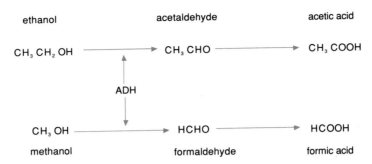

FIGURE 31-4   Ethanol has a greater affinity for alcohol dehydrogenase than does methanol, thereby reducing the conversion of methanol to its metabolic products.

Figure 31-4
Wingard CG
7-31-90

Ethylene Glycol Intoxication

This dihydric alcohol is found in antifreeze products and may also be ingested accidentally and cause severe CNS depression and renal damage. Ethylene glycol is also metabolized by alcohol dehydrogenase to glycolic and oxalic acids. Glycolic acid can cause metabolic acidosis, as with methanol intoxication, while oxalate appears to be responsible for the renal toxicity. Management is similar to that for methanol intoxication.

Isopropanol Intoxication

Isopropyl alcohol, or rubbing alcohol, is sometimes accidentally ingested and may be used by chronic alcoholics at times when ethanol may be unavailable. It is a CNS depressant and more toxic to the CNS than ethanol. Signs and symptoms of intoxication are also similar to ethanol. Toxicity is limited, however, because isopropanol produces severe gastritis with accompanying pain, nausea, and vomiting. Isopropanol is metabolized by alcohol dehydrogenase but at a much slower rate than ethanol. In severe intoxication, hemodialysis is used to remove isopropanol from the body.

REFERENCES

Abel EL: Fetal alcohol syndrome and fetal alcohol effects, New York, 1984, Plenum Press.

Deitrich RA, Dunwiddie TV, Harris RA et al.: Mechanism of action of ethanol: initial central nervous system actions, Pharmacol Rev 41:489, 1990.

Frezza M, Di Padova C, Pozzato G et al.: High blood alcohol levels in women, N Engl J Med, 322:95, 1990.

Goldstein DB: Pharmacology of alcohol, Oxford Press, 1983, Oxford Press.

Hoffman PL and Tabakoff B: Ethanol and guanine nucleotide binding proteins: selective interaction, FASEB J 4:2612, 1990.

Schuckit MA: Genetic aspects of alcoholism, Ann Emerg Med 15:991, 1986.

32

Drug Abuse

ABBREVIATION

AIDS	acquired immunodeficiency syndrome
AMP	adenosine monophosphate
cAMP	cyclic adenosine monophosphate
EEG	electroencephalogram
HIV	human immunodeficiency virus
IV	intravenous, intravenously
LSD	D-lysergic acid diethylamide
PCP	phencyclidine
pH	logarithm of the reciprocal of the hydrogen ion concentration
THC	tetrahydrocannabinol
MDMA and XTC	methylenedioxymethamphetamine

THERAPEUTIC OVERVIEW

Medical problems related to drug abuse have become an important concern of practicing physicians. These problems include (1) the treatment of acute drug overdoses, (2) the management of drug withdrawal following repeated nontherapeutic administration of drugs primarily for effects on consciousness, and (3) the long-term rehabilitation of the drug-taking behavior of these subjects.

The main types of abused substances are listed in the box, p. 446. Abused substances are defined as drugs or other materials administered repeatedly in a pattern and amount that interferes with the health or normal social/occupational functioning of the sub-

ject. This definition does not require the development of tolerance or dependence, although these often accompany substance abuse. Tolerance (Chapter 3) is characterized by a reduced drug effect with repeated use and the requirement of higher doses to produce the same effect. Since tolerance does not occur to the same extent for all effects, drug abusers who take increasing amounts of drugs risk exposure to increasing toxic effects.

Dependence (Chapter 3) is characterized by physiological and/or behavioral changes following discontinuation of drug, and these withdrawal effects can be reversed by resumption of drug administration. Physical (or physiological) dependence is characterized by typical signs and symptoms during withdrawal. The time course varies according to the rate of elimination of individual drugs or their active metabolites. Withdrawal from long-acting drugs has a delayed onset, is relatively mild, and may occur over many days or weeks (Figure 32-1, *A*), while that from more rapidly metabolized/eliminated drugs is more intense but of shorter duration (Figure 32-1, *B*). If an antagonist is administered, withdrawal signs are even more intense and of shorter duration (Figure 32-1, *C*). Physical dependence usually occurs only when substances are used over extended times with relatively continuous blood and brain concentrations achieved for days, weeks, or months. Occasional drug use does not result in physical dependence; rather, extended use produces a continuum of symptoms of increased severity, with users slipping gradually into dependence, often without fully realizing it.

Withdrawal can occur spontaneously or can be precipitated by antagonists (Figure 32-1). Spontaneous

---

SUBSTANCES OF ABUSE

OPIATES

natural opium-based compounds, morphine, codeine, heroin

OPIOIDS

other derivatives of morphine

SYMPATHOMIMETIC STIMULANTS

cocaine, amphetamines, phenmetrazine, methylphenidate

DEPRESSANTS

barbiturates, methaqualone, glutethimide, ethanol (Chapters 31 and 33)

HALLUCINOGENS

mescaline, LSD

OTHERS

phencyclidine (PCP), marihuana, inhalants, nicotine, caffeine

---

withdrawal occurs without an antagonist when drug use is discontinued. For example, when opioid-dependent individuals are given the antagonists naloxone or naltrexone, the individuals experience an immediate, intense withdrawal syndrome. Similarly, precipitated abstinence from benzodiazepines can be produced by benzodiazepine antagonists, such as flumazenil, a drug currently under development. The duration of the precipitated withdrawal syndrome is determined by the duration of action of the antagonist.

Sometimes different drugs within a pharmacological class can support physical dependence produced by other drugs in the same class. Such cross-dependence (e.g., during heroin withdrawal) can be blocked by other opioids. This is the rationale for using methadone in the pharmacotherapy of opiate dependence. Alcohol, barbiturates, and benzodiazepines also show cross-dependence to each other in that individuals tolerant to one drug in a class are usually tolerant to others in the same class.

Behavioral (or psychological) dependence usually means intense craving and drug-seeking behavior. This has not been a very useful concept because it is defined differently by different individuals.

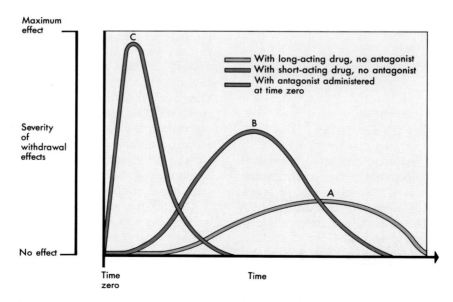

FIGURE 32-1   Schematic showing time course of severity of drug abuse withdrawal effects for drugs with long *(A)*, short *(B)* durations of action or with antagonist administered *(C)*. No antagonist present in *A* or *B*.

The property of a drug that leads to self-administration is termed *reinforcing efficacy* or *euphorigenic tendency*. Many drugs of abuse, especially the psychomotor stimulants, produce strong euphoria and feelings of well-being.

Various terms are used to describe pharmaco-therapeutic strategies for treatment of drug abuse. Maintenance therapy utilizes a drug such as methadone to maintain opioid dependence while psychological, social, and vocational therapies are used to support the user during abstinence. Detoxification is the process of treating physical dependence and can be performed abruptly or gradually by slowly reducing the drug dosage.

 ## MECHANISMS OF ACTION

Opiates

Opium is the concentrated resinous material obtained from the opium poppy. Illegal opium generally is in the form of small bricks or cakes, which are transported to areas where processing occurs. Small pieces of opium are smoked, or taken orally as an alcoholic solution, although this latter this form of opiate abuse is not common in the United States. The two principal opiates present in opium are morphine and codeine. Although total synthesis of these compounds is possible, it is difficult and expensive. All illicit morphine comes from the plant product.

The most commonly abused opioid is heroin, or diacetyl morphine, synthesized clandestinely from natural morphine. The effects of heroin and morphine are similar, but heroin is about three times more potent and therefore contains three times as many "doses" as a corresponding amount of morphine. Under experimental conditions, experienced abusers have difficulty distinguishing between equipotent doses of morphine and heroin. Other opioid agonists, including hydromorphone, meperidine, and dextropropoxyphene, produce similar effects and have similar abuse potential.

The opiates act through binding to opioid receptors, as discussed in Chapter 28. The structures of codeine and morphine are given in Chapter 28. The structure of heroin is shown in Figure 32-2.

The biological basis of opiate dependence is poorly understood. Changes may occur in opiate receptor regulation with repeated opioid exposure, but studies in animals have not found consistent evidence for changes in μ opiate receptor number or affinity, nor have consistent changes been found in the concentration or effects of endogenous opioids. A biochemical marker has yet to be found for opiate dependence. The most consistent change is increased sensitivity to opiate antagonists. Recent research has demonstrated that this sensitivity may begin with the first opiate dose, since high concentrations of antagonists can precipitate a withdrawal syndrome within a few hours after a single dose of morphine or methadone.

Sympathomimetic Stimulants

The most widely known members of this class of abused drugs are cocaine and amphetamines, but various nonamphetamine stimulants such as phenmetrazine and methylphenidate, and several weight control medications also have abuse potential. These drugs all are centrally acting sympathetic CNS stimulants that act through enhancement of catecholaminergic neurotransmission, discussed in Chapter 10.

The structure of the natural alkaloid cocaine is shown in Figure 32-2. Some similarity in structure exists between cocaine and atropine (Chapter 9). Cocaine is the principal psychoactive alkaloid present in the coca bush, cultivated principally in South America, where the chewing of coca leaves is a common practice. Cocaine is extracted from the plant and used as either the free-base or as the water-soluble hydrochloride.

The amphetamines include the dextroamphetamine salts and the *N*-methyl analog, methamphetamine. The amphetamines are synthetic compounds related structurally to the catecholamine (Figure 32-2) neurotransmitters and to substituted phenethylamine hallucinogens.

Nonamphetamine sympathomimetic stimulants such as methylphenidate and phenmetrazine are also abused. Other weight-control medications have varying degrees of sympathomimetic action and propensity for abuse. The anorectics with potent serotonergic actions, such as mazindol and fenfluramine, may produce adverse effects at higher doses, which limits their abuse potential. In prescribing weight-control medications, physicians should assess the possibility of excessive use and abuse.

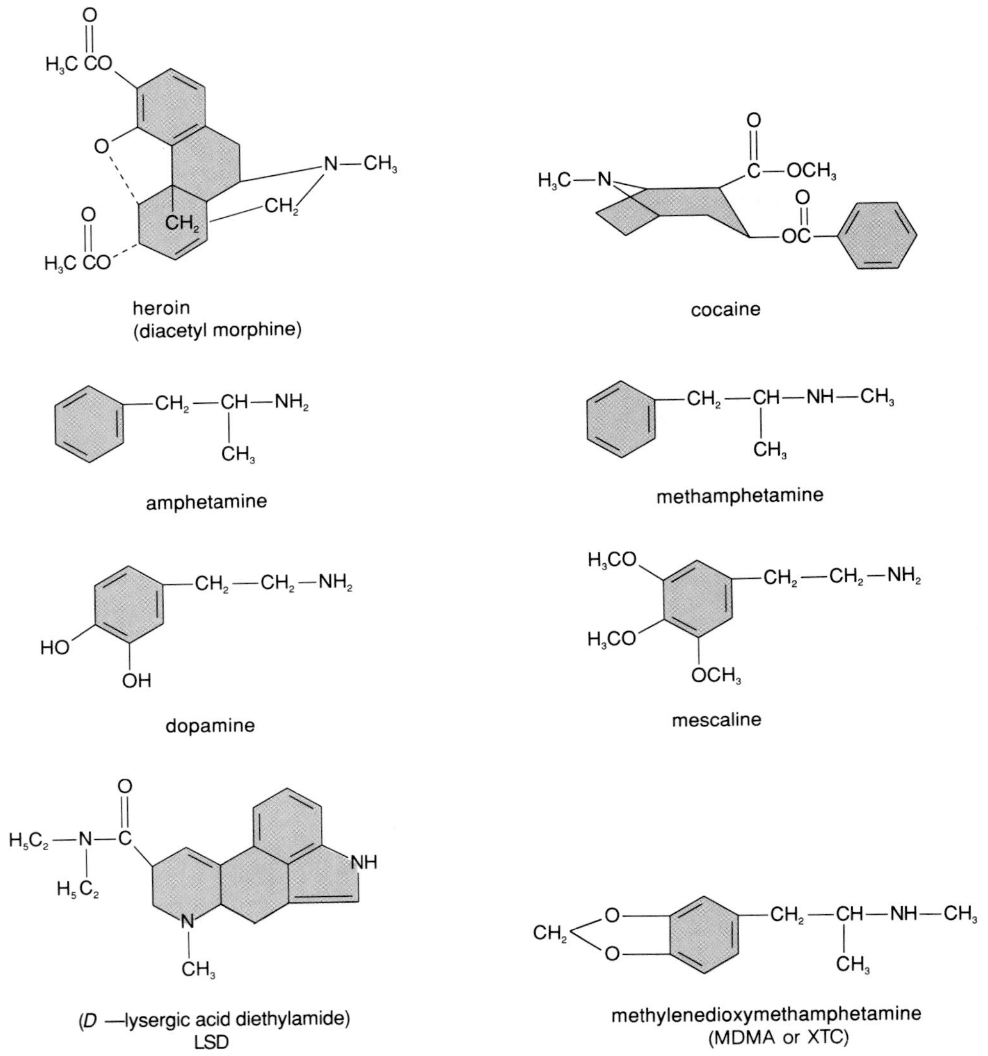

FIGURE 32-2 Structures of heroin, sympathomimetic stimulants (with dopamine included for reference), and hallucinogens.

The central effects of cocaine and amphetamines arise from enhanced catecholamine neurotransmission for dopamine synapses in the ascending mesolimbic pathways (Figure 32-3). Cocaine blocks the reuptake of dopamine into presynaptic terminal areas such as the nucleus accumbens and other parts of the median forebrain, thus enhancing dopamine action. Amphetamines also have dopaminergic actions in these regions by enhanced neurotransmitter release, inhibition of enzymatic destruction by monoamine oxidase, reuptake blockade, and/or direct postsynaptic receptor activation. Dopaminergic pathways activated by stimulant drugs are those that may have an important role in reinforcement processes in general.

CNS Depressants

Structures and mechanisms of action of barbiturates and benzodiazepines, the two major therapeutic CNS depressants that are abused, as well as ethanol (see Chapter 25) are described in Chapter 31.

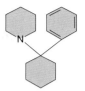

Phenylcylclohexyl piperidine
(PCP; phencyclidine)

FIGURE 32-4   Structure of phencyclidine.

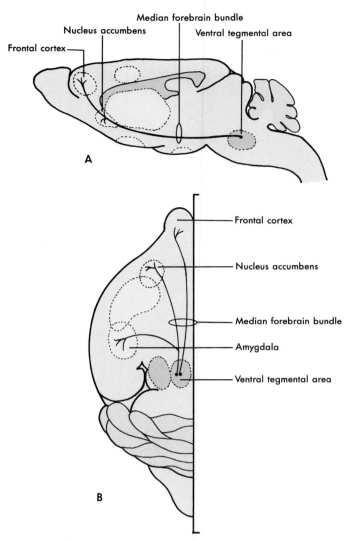

FIGURE 32-3   Schematic of ascending dopaminergic brain pathways believed to mediate the reinforcing effects of cocaine. **A,** Sagittal or sideview. **B,** Coronal or top view.

Hallucinogens

Abused hallucinogenic compounds fall into two chemical classes, the substituted phenethylamines and the indolamines. Mescaline is the prototypic substituted phenethylamine hallucinogen (see Figure 32-2). Ring-substituted amphetamines are also commonly abused, and include such compounds as methylenedioxymethamphetamine (MDMA), a compound recently referred to as *ecstacy* or *XTC* (see Figure 32-

2). LSD is the prototypic indolamine hallucinogen. Others include dimethyltryptamine and psilocybin (from mushrooms). Most of the hallucinogens have no recognized medical use. Because of the large number of chemical modifications that can be made in the substituted phenethylamine series that result in compounds that retain psychoactivity, so-called designer drugs have appeared. These are illicitly synthesized abusable compounds not subject to drug abuse control provisions. Examples of designer drugs in other classes are the potent heroin-like fentanyl derivatives (e.g., China White) and various phencyclidine analogs.

The mechanisms of hallucinogenic compounds are based on sympathomimetic actions, with recent evidence suggesting that activation of the dopaminergic 5-HT$_2$ receptor is involved (see Chapters 22 and 24 for further discussion).

Others

Phencyclidine Phencyclidine, often referred to as PCP, was originally developed as an injectable anesthetic (Figure 32-4). Ketamine, a close structural analog of PCP, is currently used clinically as an anesthetic (Chapter 30). PCP was removed from human testing because of its toxic effects. Ketamine also has this toxic potential, although the emergence of toxicity is more rapid and easier to manage. Until recently, PCP was used as a veterinary anesthetic and to capture wild animals. The type of dissociative anesthesia produced by PCP and ketamine is very dissimilar from inhalation and barbiturate anesthesia and is discussed in Chapter 30.

A unique binding site for PCP has been discovered, but the endogenous neurotransmitter acting on this binding site receptor is not known, nor is the phys-

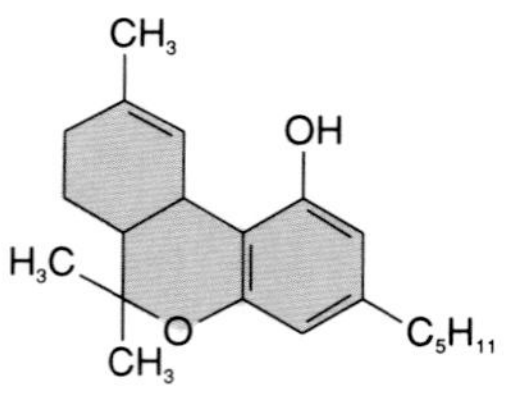

Δ^9 tetrahydrocannabinol
(THC)

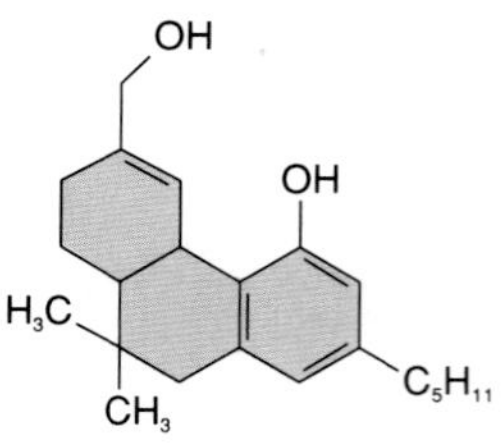

11-OH- Δ^9-THC

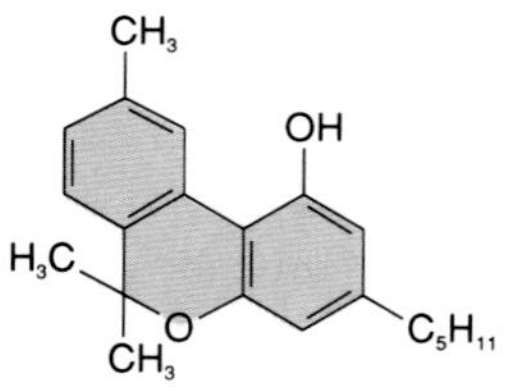

cannabinol

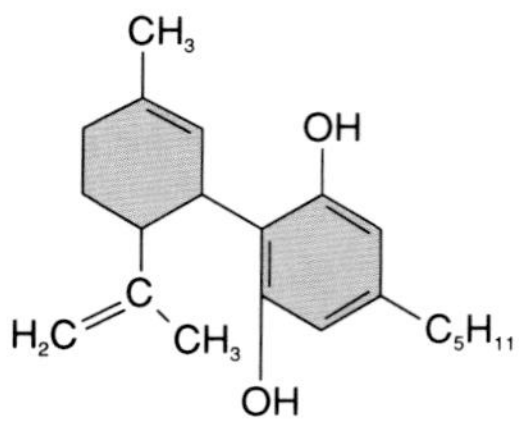

cannabidiol

FIGURE 32-5   Structures of selected cannabinoids.

iological role of PCP receptor activation understood. PCP receptors may comprise part of an ion channel regulated by the excitatory amino acid transmitter glutamate, since PCP antagonizes glutamate and offers some protection against excitotoxicity resulting from overstimulation of the *N*-methyl-D-aspartate subtype of glutamate receptors (see Chapter 2). However, it is unclear whether glutamine antagonism is the basis for the effects of PCP relevant to its abuse. Interest is developing in studying certain PCP-like drugs as possible neuroprotective agents in ischemic or concussive brain injury where glutamate may play a role.

Cannabis Cannabis sativa is the common hemp plant; however, plant varieties suitable for making rope often have little psychoactivity. The leaves and resin from *Cannabis sativa* cultivated for smoking contain chemicals referred to as cannabinoids; (-)-Δ^9-tetrahydrocannabinol (or THC) (Figure 32-5) is the major cannabinoid with psychoactivity. The plant psychoactivity resides primarily in its THC content. THC is metabolically converted to another active compound, 11-OH Δ^9-THC. Other plant cannabinoids

include cannabinol, which has weak biological activity, and cannabidiol, which is inactive. Marihuana is the dried leaf material and generally contains 1% to 3% THC. Hashish is the dried resinous material exuded by mature plants and generally contains about 10 times greater concentrations of THC than the corresponding leaf material.

PHARMACOKINETICS

Since the therapeutic uses of abused drugs are discussed in other chapters, no table of pharmacokinetic parameter values is included here.

Morphine and codeine pharmacokinetic parameters are discussed in Chapter 28. Since heroin and morphine have poor oral availability, abusers of these drugs usually resort to administration by injection or smoking. An epidemic of heroin smoking in Southeast Asia involving dusting heroin onto various smoking materials resulted in numerous cases of dependence.

For cocaine administered by smoking, absorption into the blood is rapid, leading to quick onset of action

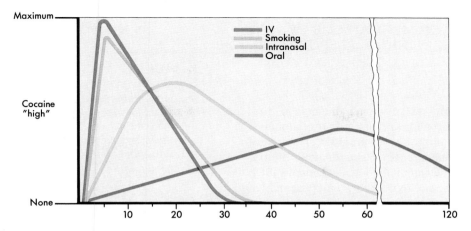

FIGURE 32-6   The intensity and time course of cocaine intoxication at equivalent doses by different routes of administration (see text).

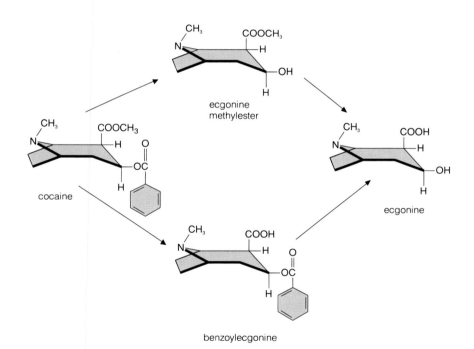

FIGURE 32-7   Deesterification pathways for cocaine metabolism by serum and liver esterases.

similar to that for IV administration (Figure 32-6). Intranasal and oral administration are slower in onset.

Cocaine is rapidly metabolized by blood and liver esterases (Figure 32-7) to a common final product with metabolites found in urine for some time. *N*-demethylation in the liver to norcocaine is a minor metabolic pathway, with corresponding deesterified norcocaine metabolites also found in the urine. Assay for cocaine metabolites in urine is the basis for establishing cocaine use. Cocaine intoxication after IV administration or inhalation generally lasts only about 30 minutes. Redosing frequently occurs in an attempt to maintain the high.

RELATION OF MECHANISMS OF ACTION TO CLINICAL RESPONSE

Opiates

Administration Most heroin abusers in the United States eventually administer the compound by IV injection. This route of administration leads to a sequence of medical problems (see the box). Heroin abusers often begin by smoking or subcutaneous (SC) injections (skin popping) of the drug, and progress to IV use (mainlining). Because heroin is relatively expensive, the most efficient use is IV because of increased response associated with this route. A particularly dangerous practice is the sharing of injection paraphernalia, since the incidence of blood-borne infection in opiate abusers is extraordinarily high. Transmission by contaminated needles has been a major vector for HIV (see Chapter 53) and other infectious diseases.

By 1988, IV drug abuse was estimated to be the mode of transmission in 28% of AIDS cases (up to 54% among females), with a disproportionate number of individuals from minority groups, particularly those residing in large industrial cities. For example, of this latter group, surveys have indicated that 34% of men with AIDS have reported IV drug abuse as the only risk factor; 80% of the women in this group with AIDS have indicated either IV drug abuse or being the sex partner of an IV drug abuser as their only risk factor. About 21% of the total IV drug abuser population in the United States are believed to be HIV carriers. Socioeconomic factors, however, may also play a contributory role.

Most heroin abusers prefer "syringes" made from eye-droppers over commercial syringes because the eyedropper allows for repeated injections. When the bulb is released, blood flows into the syringe, mixing with drug. After a short time, the mixture is reinjected. This is repeated until the drug is gone, the needle clots, or the vein is lost. If this blood-mixed drug is shared with another user, the danger of this practice can be readily appreciated.

Initial Effects The "rush" that accompanies an IV injection is quite intense. When the abuser is in withdrawal, which is not uncommon, the positive reinforcing effects of the rush are amplified by the negative reinforcing effects of instant alleviation of withdrawal sickness. The allure of this combination

MEDICAL SEQUELAE OF OPIATE ABUSE

Overdosage
Abscesses at site of injection, thrombophlebitis
Pregnancy complications and babies born dependent
Possibilities for subsequent infections:
    HIV and AIDS (see Chapter 51)
    Bacterial endocarditis
    Hepatitis and hepatic dysfunction
    Pneumonia
    Septic pulmonary embolism
    Tetanus

can hardly be overestimated. Sadly for many physically-dependent abusers who have developed tolerance to the positive reinforcing effects, all they can achieve is relief from abstinence. However, this too can motivate considerable drug-seeking behavior.

After a few minutes duration, the rush subsides, and the effects resemble those after oral dosing. The user feels relaxed and carefree, somewhat dreamy, but able to carry on many normal activities including normal conversations. Unlike someone intoxicated with alcohol or CNS depressants, the opiate abuser is difficult to diagnose on the basis of observable drug effects. Indeed, health professionals abusing opioids cannot be readily detected, and patients stabilized on methadone are able to function quite normally.

The effects of injected heroin last about 4 to 6 hours, depending on the dose. Users who are not physically dependent recover readily from the effects. Most heroin abusers do not immediately develop a dependence-producing pattern of use, but may take opiates only occasionally for many years and with insufficient frequency to become physically dependent. It is important to diagnose physically dependent from nondependent opiate abusers, since treatment strategies differ considerably. Unfortunately, most drug abuse treatments are for hard-core dependent abusers. Strategies for preventing escalation from occasional use would be highly desirable, but during this phase of the abuse cycle, users often do not come to the attention of health professionals.

Overdosage leads to unconsciousness, respiratory depression, and extreme miosis, although the latter cannot always be attributed to opiate overdose, since hypoxia can cause dilation of the pupils. An opiate antagonist such as naloxone or naltrexone can immediately reverse these effects. Before administering naloxone, one should be prepared for a rapid recovery. Since the duration of action of naloxone is shorter than that of opioid agonists, one should also be cautious that severe intoxication does not reemerge. Although naltrexone has a longer duration of action than naloxone, it is presently not available in the United States in an injectable form. It is also important not to administer too large a dose, since severe abstinence signs can be precipitated in a physically dependent patient.

Dependence The progression to physical dependence occurs gradually for most opiate abusers. The users generally feel confident that they can control their use of opiates and initially are only dimly aware that they have come to be dependent. An individual taking multiple daily recreational doses of heroin or other opioids will probably develop clinically significant dependence in a few weeks. Opiate withdrawal rarely constitutes a medical emergency, and is considerably less dangerous than unmedicated withdrawal from alcohol and barbiturates (see box).

The significance of physical dependence to the abuser is the inexorable appearance of the abstinence syndrome about 6 or more hours after the last heroin injection. Many of the signs and symptoms of withdrawal (see box) are opposite to the effects of acute opiate administration. Abdominal cramps and muscle aches, sometimes accompanied by muscle spasms and other signs of hyperexcitability, can occur in severely dependent individuals or during precipitated abstinence. Unmedicated, the syndrome reaches peak severity in about 48 hours and is over in 7 to 10 days. Unmedicated withdrawal has been termed *cold turkey* because of the gooseflesh appearance accompanying piloerection. Unmedicated opiate withdrawal is not a medical emergency and is rarely dangerous in a healthy individual. Opioids cross the placental barrier, and if the mother is opioid dependent, the newborn will undergo a withdrawal syndrome beginning 6 to 12 hours after birth. This is generally treated with paregoric or methadone. Although the long-term consequences of prenatal opioid dependence are poorly understood, it may be better to maintain the mother on methadone and treat the dependent infant than to withdraw the mother, since she may leave treatment, resume street opiate abuse, and not receive adequate prenatal care.

Abstinence brought about through use of opiate

COMPARISON OF OPIATE AND DEPRESSANT WITHDRAWAL

OPIATE WITHDRAWAL	DEPRESSANT* WITHDRAWAL
Anxiety and dysphoria	Anxiety and dysphoria
Craving and drug-seeking	Craving and drug-seeking
Sleep disturbance	Sleep disturbance
Nausea and vomiting	Nausea and Vomiting
Lacrimation	Tremors
Rhinorrhea	Hyperreflexia
Yawning	Hyperpyrexia
Piloerection and gooseflesh	Delirium
Sweating	Seizures
Mydriasis	Possible death
Abdominal cramping	
Hyperpyrexia	
Tachycardia and hypertension	

* Alcohol or barbiturates.

---

antagonists is called *precipitated withdrawal*. It has an immediate onset, and can be much more severe than spontaneous withdrawal. Its duration is determined by the duration of action of the antagonist (e.g., naloxone-precipitated withdrawal is shorter than naltrexone-precipitated withdrawal). In most other respects, the precipitated abstinence syndrome closely resembles the spontaneous abstinence syndrome. Because of differences in sensitivity of opioid-dependent persons to opiate antagonists, the response to small doses of narcotic antagonists should be used to diagnose opioid physical dependence before initiation of pharmacotherapy.

Cross-dependence Cross-dependence occurs with all full opioid agonists but not with some partial agonists. For someone physically dependent on heroin, opioids such as dihydromorphine, meperidine, oxycodone, and others can reverse opioid withdrawal signs, and at appropriate doses can produce a heroin-like intoxication. Even less efficacious opioid agonists such as codeine and dextropropoxyphene show cross-dependence with heroin. Herein lies one of the major problems physicians face in prescribing opioids for outpatients. Heroin abusers often convincingly exhibit symptoms that require analgesics as a means of obtaining opioids to treat their withdrawal symptoms.

Mixed opioid agonist/antagonists and partial opioid agonists such as pentazocine, butorphanol, nalbuphine, and buprenorphine have considerably less potential for abuse than full opioid agonists, although each offers a slightly different profile of abuse potential. With the exception of buprenorphine, these drugs show little cross-dependence with heroin and can exacerbate withdrawal; thus they offer little attraction for the dependent person. Buprenorphine, on the other hand, can prevent opioid withdrawal and may be used for pharmacotherapy. In addition, when these drugs are given chronically for analgesia, little if any physical dependence develops. Even when buprenorphine is substituted in dependent heroin abusers, the eventual discontinuation of buprenorphine may not be accompanied by significant withdrawal signs, perhaps because of its very slow rate of dissociation from the opiate receptor.

On the other hand, pentazocine, a widely prescribed analgesic, and related mixed agonist/antagonists have some ability to produce positive reinforcing effects and may be abused. One should be aware of possible nonmedical use of these drugs and of the abuse potential. Pentazocine, taken with the antihistamine tripelennamine, is referred to as *Ts and blues,* but this abuse problem has been substantially reduced by reformulation of pentazocine in combination with naloxone. The dose of naloxone is intended to block the positive reinforcing effects of pentazocine if the combination is injected IV.

Sympathomimetic Stimulants

Administration Among the sympathomimetic stimulants are cocaine, the amphetamines, and non-amphetamine stimulants such as methylphenidate and phenmetrazine.

The hydrochloride salt of cocaine is a bitter-tasting, white, crystalline material called *flake* that is generally inhaled nasally, injected IV, or infrequently taken orally. Cocaine salts are often diluted (cut) with local anesthetics, similar in appearance, taste, and local anesthetic effects. Recently abuse of free base cocaine, known as *crack,* has become common. Crack becomes volatile at a lower temperature than does the salt, so that crack can be inhaled after heating it in a pipe. It is usually sold as small hard pieces or rocks and is readily available and relatively inexpensive.

The IV or inhalation use of cocaine (see Figure 32-6) produces a rapid onset intense rush with positive reinforcing effects. Abuse by nasal insufflation may lead to irritation of the nasal mucosa, sinusitis, and perforated septum.

Initial Effects Cocaine and other stimulants activate both central and autonomic sympathetic nervous systems. Central effects include increased alertness, feelings of elation and well-being, increased energy, feelings of competence, and increased sexuality. Athletic performance enhancement has been demonstrated, particularly in sports requiring sustained attention and endurance. Although the "amphetamine margin" is small, it can provide a significant advantage in competitive sports. Thus all sympathomimetic drugs, including over-the-counter medications such as pseudoephedrine and phenylpropanolamine, are banned by most athletic associations.

Stimulant overdose results in excessive sympathetic nervous system activation with the resulting tachycardia and hypertension capable of producing myocardial infarction and cerebrovascular hemorrhage, particularly in susceptible individuals. Cocaine may also cause coronary vasospasm and cardiac arrhythmias. Other symptoms include anxiety, feelings of paranoia and impending doom, and restlessness. Patients become unpredictable and sometimes violent. Catecholamine receptor blockers are effective pharmacological antagonists, although many patients do not require medication.

An important component of stimulant intoxication is the let-down that occurs as the drug effects subside. Dysphoria, tiredness, irritability, and mild depression often follow immediately after a stimulant intoxication episode.

Abuse Patterns, Dependence, and Psychosis A dangerous pattern of stimulant abuse is that of extended, uninterrupted sequences referred to as *runs.* Runs result from attempts to maintain a continuous state of intoxication, both to extend the pleasurable feeling and to postpone the postintoxication crash. Acute tolerance can occur, particularly with IV use, resulting in a need for increasingly larger doses. This spiral of tolerance and dosage increases is often continued until drug supplies are depleted or the individual collapses from exhaustion. During runs, drug-taking and drug-seeking take on a compulsive character that make intervention difficult.

Another typical abuse pattern begins with self-medication. Stimulants are used in certain occupations to achieve sustained attention (e.g., by long-distance truckers or students) or to make some tasks appear easier (e.g., anorectics for overweight individuals). These patterns can lead to increased dosage and frequency, producing tolerance and further dosage escalation. Alcohol or depressant drugs may be used to counteract the resultant anxiety and insomnia, establishing a cycle of "uppers and downers."

In animal models repeated cocaine or amphetamine administration does not produce physical dependence like that seen with opioids and depressant drugs, but extended periods of uninterrupted high-dose self-administration do occur. Thus stimulant dependence must involve psychological dependence. Animals that undergo repeated stimulant administration also experience long-term changes in brain chemistry.

In humans, mood and behavior changes have been described when drugs are discontinued, possibly reflecting neurotoxicity. Fatigue and depression, sleep disturbances, hyperphagia, and EEG abnormalities have also been noted during stimulant cessation. Although it is still controversial whether these abstinence effects represent a true withdrawal syndrome, the psychological sequelae are important in the maintenance of abuse and are significant targets of treatment interventions.

Personality changes commonly occur in stimulant abusers and include persecutory delusions, preoccupation with self, hostility, and suspiciousness. With severe abuse, a toxic psychosis can result. Often difficult to differentially diagnose from paranoid schizophrenia, amphetamine and cocaine psychoses resulting from stimulant abuse require psychiatric management. Antipsychotic medication may be used with some success (see Chapter 23).

Cocaine use during pregnancy is associated with complications that include abruptio placentae, lower gestational age at birth, lower birth weight, and neurobehavioral impairment of the newborn.

Pharmacotherapy of Stimulant Abuse No standard pharmacotherapy is used to treat cocaine or amphetamine abuse. As mentioned, antipsychotic medications are useful in the management of stimulant overdosage and toxic psychoses. Because of the presumed long-term alterations in dopaminergic regulation resulting from cocaine abuse, which may be a factor in relapse, research is focused on the possible use of dopaminergic agonists such as amantadine or bromocriptine, and to antidepressants such as desipramine, which may ameliorate the abstinence depression and reduce craving.

CNS Depressants The dose-response curves for abused CNS depressant drugs are essentially the same as for ethanol except for more shallow slopes (Figure 32-8). Blood concentrations of 0.02% to 0.05% result in mild intoxication, anxiety reduction, and

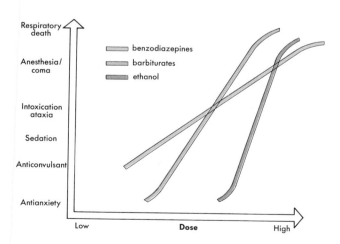

FIGURE 32-8   Comparison of dose-effect relationships for acute effects of ethanol, barbiturates, and benzodiazepines (see text).

muscle relaxation, while 0.03% to 0.07% may produce drowsiness. A concentration of 0.07% impairs motor activity and performance and higher concentrations (0.25% to 0.35%) produce loss of consciousness. In contrast, with benzodiazepines, gram quantities may not be lethal, resulting in a dose-effect curve that covers a much wider dose range. Barbiturates and nonbarbiturate sedatives produce similar dose-effect relationships, but with curves much steeper than for benzodiazepines.

Abuse of depressant drugs usually is to (1) produce ethanol-like intoxication or (2) self-medicate anxiety and/or insomnia.

Barbiturates and nonbarbiturate sedatives, such as methaqualone, glutethimide, and meprobamate, can produce an ethanol-like intoxication and are sometimes abused for this purpose. The more rapidly acting barbiturates such as secobarbital and pentobarbital are used rather than those with a slower onset, such as phenobarbital.

In overdosage with depressant drugs pupils are sluggish and miotic, respiration shallow and slow, deep tendon reflexes absent or attenuated, and patients are unresponsive. There are no known antagonists for barbiturates or nonbarbiturate sedatives, whereas competitive benzodiazepine antagonists (e.g., flumazenil) are under development. Although benzodiazepines are rarely lethal, they enhance the effects of other depressants, including alcohol, which may have been taken concurrently.

Repeated use of depressant drugs produces physical dependence, and cross-dependence occurs among barbiturates, nonbarbiturate sedatives, benzodiazepines, and alcohol. Signs and symptoms of depressant withdrawal are often opposite to the acute pharmacological effects of these drugs. They include dysphoria, anxiety and restlessness, hyperreflexiveness, insomnia and EEG abnormalities, muscle weakness, and tremor. The occasional appearance of convulsions and delirium make depressant withdrawal a medical emergency.

Hallucinogenic Compounds

Most of the hallucinogenic compounds have no recognized medical use. Nearly all hallucinogens produce varying degrees of sympathomimetic effects often evident as tachycardia, pressor effects, psychomotor stimulation, or euphoria. For substituted amphetamines, these effects may predominate, particularly at higher doses, probably resulting from enhanced catecholaminergic neurotransmission. However, the most prominent effects are on subjective experience, believed to result from modulation of serotonergic neurotransmission, possibly at the 5-HT$_2$ receptor. These effects include (1) lability of mood, (2) altered thought processes, (3) altered visual, auditory, or somatesthetic perception, (4) experience of having enhanced insights into events and ideas, and (5) impaired judgment. Mood swings can range from profound euphoria to anxiety and even terror. Panic states (bad trips) are the symptoms that most commonly lead abusers to seek medical assistance. Bad trips generally are not the result of overdoses, although larger doses are more likely to produce this result; rather, they result from the propensity of the hallucinogen drug experience to undergo rapid transformation. For this reason, the nature of hallucinogenic drug intoxication is highly dependent upon the environment. Unexpected or frightening events can transform the experience dramatically. Bad trips usually respond to calm reassurance and removal from the threatening environment until the drug effect wears off. Medication is rarely needed except when excessive sympathomimetic stimulation may indicate treatment with antipsychotics.

Although acute overdose is not a common problem with hallucinogenic compounds, a number of other dangers are present. The most significant is the risk of injury caused by impaired judgment. Psychiatric illness may be precipitated by even an occasional encounter with hallucinogenic compounds in subjects with a predisposition. With repeated use, this problem is exacerbated. Another potential danger, suggested by animal experiments, is neurotoxicity from severe depletion of dopamine or serotonin, accompanied by neuronal degeneration, most clearly shown with certain substituted-phenethylamine hallucinogens (e.g., methylenedioxymethamphetamine). Whether this occurs in abusers is presently unknown. Finally, the effects on fetal development are poorly understood, with conflicting evidence from in vitro and animal studies.

Another poorly understood aspect of hallucinogen abuse is *flashbacks,* where users reexperience aspects of hallucinogen intoxication while drug-free. Flashbacks also may occur with marihuana or other drug use. They can be no more than reviewing something already seen, or they can be a frightening episode that may reflect an emerging psychopathology, since hallucinogenic drug abuse may be an important etiologic factor in the development of psychoses.

The antimuscarinics, especially atropine or scopolamine (Chapter 9), are the most notable nonclassical hallucinogens. Certain Indian tribes in North and Central America practiced ritual use of these plants because of their ability to produce profound alteration in consciousness. Signs of anticholinergic poisoning occur, which can be quite dangerous, with hyperpyrexia that can produce neuropathology. The appropriate treatment is the acetylcholinesterase inhibitor physostigmine. Patients who claim hallucinogenic drug overdose should be carefully examined for signs of anticholinergic crisis. Strychnine, at sublethal doses, and other CNS poisons also occasionally appear in street samples of hallucinogens.

Others

Phencyclidine Phencyclidine (PCP) is no longer used clinically but produces dissociative anesthesia similar to that of ketamine (Chapter 30) although with less troublesome side effects. PCP shows respiratory and cardiovascular depression, and in PCP overdose, a hypertensive crisis may be produced. PCP-intoxicated individuals may exhibit some sympathomimetic stimulation.

It was not until smoking and insufflation became the routes for PCP administration that the PCP abuse epidemic began; this allowed users to better titrate the dose. PCP is generally sprinkled onto plant material (e.g., dried parsley or marihuana) and used as crude cigarettes, sometimes known as *crystal joints* or *killer weed*. PCP itself is often referred to as *angel dust* or just *dust*. Although PCP is the major drug abused in this class, many other analogs of PCP produce similar effects. Ketamine also has PCP-like abuse potential.

PCP combines the actions of sympathomimetic stimulants, barbiturates, and hallucinogens. The subjective experience of PCP intoxication is unlike that of classical hallucinogens (Table 32-1). The perceptual effects are not as profound and relate more to somesthesis. Distortions of body image are common, and a strong motivation for PCP abuse is to enhance sexual experience, hence the street name *love boat* and *lovely*.

Bizarre, and sometimes violent, behavior may result. PCP intoxication often includes motor incoordination, and at high doses, cataleptic behavior ac-

Table 32-1 Signs and Symptoms of PCP Intoxication	
Abuse Effects	**Untoward Side Effects**
LOW DOSE	
Dreamy, carefree state	Impaired judgment
Mood elevation	Mood swings, panic
Heightened or altered perception	Partial amnesia
MODERATE DOSE	
Inebriation	Ataxia, motor impairment
Dissociation, depersonalization	Confusion, disorientation
Perceptual distortions	Preoccupation with abnormal body sensations
Diminished pain sensitivity	Amnesia
	Exaggerated mood swings, panic
HIGH DOSE	
All of the above, hallucinations	Catatonia, "blank stare," delirium, drooling, severe motor impairment, psychotic behavior, hypertensive crisis, amnesia

companied by nystagmus and a blank stare. Amnesia for events during high-dose PCP intoxication is common. After smoking PCP, intoxication typically lasts 4 to 6 hours.

The major dangers with PCP abuse are production of risk-taking behavior and development of progressive personality changes that culminate in a toxic psychosis. PCP overdosage is rarely lethal, but may require careful management because of the severe incapacitation of the subject. There is no PCP antagonist available. Benzodiazepines may help calm anxiety, but the use of antipsychotic medications in mild PCP intoxication is controversial. PCP is a weak base (pKa of 8.5) whose elimination can be increased somewhat by aggressive acidification of the urine (pH less than 5.5).

Although some tolerance can develop during long-term PCP abuse, dramatic dosage escalation is uncommon. The dependence produced by PCP has not been very well characterized, but clearly it does not have the physical dependence potential of opioids and depressants.

Schizophrenic patients or individuals with schizophrenic tendencies are particularly at risk for PCP psychosis, and there is some evidence that PCP exacerbates schizophrenia. PCP psychosis shares many features of schizophrenia and may respond to antipsychotic medication.

Cannabis Marihuana, of which THC is the main psychoactive cannabinoid, is generally consumed by smoking hand-rolled cigarettes or *joints,* or by using other smoking paraphenalia. A typical user will smoke a portion of a joint, often shared with other users. After smoking, the onset of peak intoxication is delayed 15 to 30 minutes, making dosage titration more difficult than with some other drugs. The effects generally last 4 to 6 hours.

Except with very high doses, marihuana intoxication is considerably less intense than intoxication with hallucinogens or PCP. Users exhibit mood lability including euphoria, anxiety, fear, and even panic attacks. Users identify improved experiences of music, movies, sexual behavior, and other activities as strong motivation for their usage. Thought processes, judgment, and time estimation are altered. Marihuana has little direct effect on psychomotor coordination except that altered perception and judgment can impair task performance, including driving. Marihuana often produces drowsiness, particularly 1 to 2 hours after smoking. Physiological effects include tachycardia and infection of the conjunctiva.

Major dangers of marihuana abuse include harmful effects of impaired performance, preoccupation with marihuana use to the exclusion of other activities, and the development of personality changes and psychopathology. Acute overdose deaths with cannabinoids are extremely rare. The most extreme intoxication results from oral administration of plant products or extracts, but bad trips from intoxication generally respond well to reassurance and removal of patients from threatening environments. Because of the frequency of marihuana use, accidents and injury during intoxication are important concerns. Cannabinoids can be detected in urine many days after marihuana use and urinalysis can be used to establish marihuana use, but such detection cannot establish intoxication or impairment, which generally lasts only a few hours after acute use.

Inhalants Many volatile chemicals and gases produce CNS effects and can be subject to abuse. Relatively little is known about the psychopharmacology of these compounds. These chemicals are considered in the following three broad groups: (1) gases such as nitrous oxide, (2) volatile liquids, and (3) aliphatic nitrites.

Nitrous oxide, a clinically used general anesthetic agent (Chapter 30), produces a short-lived mild intoxication that is characteristic of the early onset of anesthesia. Abuse of nitrous oxide is largely confined to health professionals.

Volatile liquids subject to abuse include anesthetics, organic solvents, freons, and petroleum products. Some of the more popular abused agents are (1) toluene-containing paint thinners, correction fluids, and plastic glues, (2) other alkyl-benzene solvents and cleaners, benzene and xylene, (3) chlorinated hydrocarbon cleaners and degreasers such as methyl chloroform and methylene chloride, and (4) general anesthetics. Particularly dangerous are products containing freons, ketones, organic metals, and n-hexane. Some of these compounds are suspected carcinogens, some are cardiotoxic, some produce well-defined neuropathies, while still others produce hepatotoxicity. The problem of identifying specific toxic effects is very difficult since few of the chemicals are abused in pure form.

The intoxication produced by inhaling these materials is poorly understood. In animals, toluene, methyl chloroform, and halothane produce alcohol-like behavioral effects, and abusers seem to seek an alcohol-like intoxication with these agents. Motor performance deficits similar to those produced by alcohol and depressant drugs occur with solvent abuse.

Aliphatic nitrites are volatile liquids. Amyl nitrite used medically to treat angina is supplied in ampules, which are broken open and the contents inhaled. These "poppers" are subject to abuse; however, more recently other aliphatic nitrites, such as butyl nitrites, have been made available in specialty stores as room "odorizers." Since aliphatic nitrites are smooth muscle vasodilators, intoxication with dizziness and euphoria probably results from hypotension and cerebral ischemia secondary to peripheral venous pooling. Nitrites are often abused in conjunction with sexual activity and are popular among homosexual males for their claimed ability to enhance orgasms, probably the result of penile vasodilatation. Nitrite use can result in accidents related to syncope.

Nicotine Nicotine self-administration is the basis of most tobacco use and it is clear that nicotine is the component in tobacco that causes dependence. Although the psychological effects of smoked nicotine are fairly subtle, they occur reliably and include mood changes, stress reduction, and some performance enhancement.

The nicotine withdrawal syndrome emerges soon after smoking cessation, peaks in 24 to 48 hours, and may last for 10 days or more, with tobacco craving continuing in many persons for years after stopping tobacco use. The major symptoms are dysphoria, irritability, anxiety, difficulty in concentrating, fatigue, and sleep disturbances. Observable signs include decreased heart rate, increased caloric intake, and weight gain. The most persistent symptom is tobacco craving. Nicotine-containing gum may be used to treat the withdrawal syndrome while patients are participating in a smoking cessation program.

Caffeine Caffeine, together with other methylxanthine stimulants, is present in beverages made from coffee beans or tea leaves. A typical cup of brewed coffee contains 85 to 150 mg caffeine, and mugs of strong coffee can have upwards of 200 mg per cup. Caffeine is also present in various over-the-counter medications, including analgesic preparations, stimulants, and weight-control products, with 100 to 200 mg caffeine per capsule typical. Excessive consumption of any of these products or combined consumption can result in well over 1 g/day caffeine intake. Patients receiving theophylline for bronchodilation may be especially sensitive to caffeine due to additive effects.

The acute active oral dose of caffeine in nontolerant individuals is 85 to 200 mg. Effects are increased alertness, loss of fatigue, and a greater capacity for activities requiring sustained attention. These effects can be demonstrated in well-controlled laboratory studies. Higher doses (>about 150 mg) can produce nervousness, restlessness, and tremors, while very high doses of methylxanthines can result in convulsions. Caffeine consumption late in the day can result in insomnia, and the anxiety and nervousness associated with caffeine consumption can be misdiagnosed as an anxiety disorder. It is obviously important to obtain a reliable history of *total* methylxanthine intake when patients complain of nervousness or insomnia.

The nature of methylxanthine dependence is controversial with few good studies. Evidence exists for tolerance and dependence in heavy users. Heavy coffee drinkers who omit their morning coffee report irritability, inability to work effectively, nervousness, restlessness, lethargy, and headache. This syndrome has an onset of 12 to 24 hours, peaks at 20 to 48 hours, and has a duration of about 1 week. Two neurochemical actions of methylxanthines are thought to be relevant (see Chapter 57); (1) methylxanthines, particularly caffeine and theophylline, inhibit cyclic nucleotide phosphodiesterase resulting in increased concentrations of cAMP, although there is doubt whether the modest changes in cAMP produced by therapeutic concentrations of methylxanthines can produce all of these effects and (2) methylxanthines are also antagonists of adenosine, possibly as receptor blockers (see Chapter 57). Caffeine is very effective in blocking the depressant effects of adenosine analogs. Since adenosine can inhibit adenylate cyclase, its inhibition by caffeine would facilitate formation of cAMP.

ABUSE THERAPY AND PATIENT REHABILITATION

Opiates

Medications play an increasing role in the treatment of opiate abuse, but they are only adjuncts to psychosocial and educational considerations. Detoxification of patients receiving opioids for pain relief is accomplished by tapering the dose of prescribed opioid or by substituting methadone or another longer-acting medication. Only rarely does such iatrogenic dependence lead to illicit opioid use.

Simple detoxification of dependent opioid abusers by itself is rarely sufficient to prevent relapse. Most heroin abusers have undergone detoxification numerous times, either medically or as a result of interrupted drug supply or incarceration. Detoxification can be unmedicated, and certain types of treatment approaches prefer this method. The withdrawal syndrome, while more intense, terminates in about a week. Medicated withdrawal generally relies on the principle of cross-dependence. Dependent heroin abusers can be stabilized on a long-acting oral medication, such as methadone, which postpones the onset of withdrawal by about 24 hours. The dose of methadone is then gradually decreased; commonly about a 20% dose reduction per week for 5 weeks is used. Withdrawal signs are mild but the patient will be uncomfortable for most of the withdrawal period. As mentioned earlier, buprenorphine may have some advantages over methadone for detoxification, although it has not yet been approved. Another approach for detoxification is to stop the use of opioids and treat the signs and symptoms of the withdrawal. Since many of the signs and symptoms reflect stress and sympathetic nervous system activation, medications such as clonidine have been used successfully, particularly in mildly dependent subjects. Antianxiety agents may also be useful in alleviating the fear and stress of withdrawal.

Maintenance therapies also are based on cross-dependence, the most common being with methadone. Methadone is the drug of choice because of its good oral bioavialability and long duration of action. Methadone maintenance patients receive single, daily oral doses chosen to prevent withdrawal signs but not large enough to produce significant intoxication. Urinalysis for continued illicit drug use is also an important feature of most methadone maintenance programs. Although methadone maintenance of opiate abusers is somewhat controversial, it has many proven benefits. It breaks the destructive pattern of continued IV drug abuse and crime, is attractive to many abusers who would not otherwise seek treatment, provides the opportunity for other therapeutic interventions, and the dependence-producing properties help ensure continued patient participation. Take-home medications and other clinic privileges can be used to reinforce changes in positive behavior.

In theory, opiate antagonists could also be used for treatment of opiate abuse. Following a sufficient oral dose of naltrexone, positive reinforcement from opiates can be prevented for up to 24 hours, and oral naltrexone has been approved for use as an antagonist to block opioid effects. However, its role in treatment differs considerably from that of methadone. Patients given naltrexone must be detoxified or else precipitated abstinence will occur. Naltrexone does not produce dependence, thus patient compliance is less assured. On the other hand, the patient must plan ahead to use opiates, breaking the spontaneity of a relapse episode.

Stimulants

No standard pharmacotherapy is used to treat cocaine or amphetamine abuse. As mentioned, antipsychotic medications are useful in treating stimulant overdoses and in the management of toxic psychoses. Because of the presumed long-term alterations in dopaminergic regulation resulting from cocaine

abuse, which may be a factor in relapse, research is focused on the possible use of dopaminergic agonists such as amantadine or bromocriptine, and to antidepressants such as desipramine, which may ameliorate the abstinence depression and reduce craving. However, further research is needed to establish their effectiveness.

Rehabilitation

The life-style of the physically dependent heroin abuser, probably the minority of heroin users, fits the stereotype of the "street addict." To prevent withdrawal, multiple daily injections of heroin are needed and tolerance often develops, leading to escalating dosage. Because injections are required every 6 to 8 hours, the individual awakes in the morning needing an injection. Forced out into the streets in the morning, usually feeling ill and without money for drug purchases, the abuser often turns to criminal behavior. The social and economic cost to society resulting from the crimes, including larceny, prostitution, and drug dealing, is enormous. This is true despite the relatively low incidence of heroin addiction, estimated at about one half million persons in the United States. It is this cycle of heroin use and crime that is the major focus of rehabilitation of the hard-core heroin or other drug addict.

REFERENCES

Balster RL: Abuse potential evaluation of inhalants, Drug Alcohol Depend 49:7, 1987.

Balster RL: The behavioral pharmacology of phencyclidine. In Meltzer HY, editor: Psychopharmacology: the third generation of progress, New York, 1987, Raven Press.

Brody SL and Slovis CM: Recognition and management of complications related to cocaine abuse, Emerg Med Reports 9:41, 1988.

Cregler LL and Herbert M: Medical complications of cocaine abuse, N Engl J Med 315:1495, 1986.

Gawin FH and Kleber HD: Abstinence symptomatology and psychiatric diagnosis in cocaine abusers, Arch Gen Psych 43:107, 1986.

Goldberg SR and Stolerman IP, editors: Behavioral analysis of drug dependence, Orlando, 1986, Academic Press.

Goldstein A: Heroin addiction and the role of methadone in its treatment, Arch Gen Psych 26:291, 1972.

Grabowski J, Stitzer ML, and Henningfield JE, ed: Behavioral intervention techniques in drug abuse treatment, National Institute on Drug Abuse Research Monograph No 46, DHHS Publication No (ADM) 84-1282, Washington, DC, 1984, US Government Printing Office.

Griffiths RR and Woodson PP: Caffeine physical dependence: a review of human and laboratory animal studies, Psychopharmacology 94:437, 1988.

Hollister LE: Health aspects of cannabis, Pharmacol Rev 38:1, 1986.

Hughes JR and Hatsukami D: Signs and symptoms of tobacco withdrawal, Arch Gen Psych 43:289, 1986.

Jaffe JH: Pharmacological agents in the treatment of drug dependence. In Meltzer HY, ed: Psychopharmacology: the third generation of progress, New York, 1987, Raven Press.

Kreek MJ: Multiple drug abuse patterns and medical consequences. In Meltzer HY, ed: Psychopharmacology: the third generation of progress, New York, 1987, Raven Press.

Schuster CR and Pickens R: AIDS and intravenous drug abuse. In Harris LS, ed: Problems of drug dependence 1988, National Institute on Drug Abuse Research Monograph No 90, DHHS Publication No (ADM) 88-1605, Washington, DC, 1988, US Government Printing Office.

US Department of Health and Human Services: The health consequences of smoking: nicotine addiction. A report of the surgeon general, DHHS (CDC) Publication No 88-8406, Washington, DC, 1988, US Government Printing Office.

CHAPTER 33

Drugs for Sleep Disorders

<table>
<tr><th colspan="2">ABBREVIATIONS</th></tr>
<tr><td>DR2</td><td>class II antigen of major histocompatibility complex</td></tr>
<tr><td>EEG</td><td>electroencephalogram</td></tr>
<tr><td>GABA</td><td>γ-aminobutyric acid</td></tr>
<tr><td>NREM</td><td>non-rapid eye movement</td></tr>
<tr><td>REM</td><td>rapid eye movement</td></tr>
<tr><td>$t_{1/2}$</td><td>half-life</td></tr>
</table>

 THERAPEUTIC OVERVIEW

Sleep disorders are a frequent patient complaint. In the United States about 30% of adults have difficulty sleeping and about 6% complain of excessive daytime sleepiness. Medication to treat symptomatic sleep disorders is both widely used and abused by patients and extensively prescribed by physicians.

A classification system that is currently helpful in the diagnosis and treatment of sleep disorders consists of four major categories: (1) DIMS, disorders of initiating and maintaining sleep, termed the insomnias; (2) DOES, disorders of excessive sleep or sleepiness, the hypersomnias; (3) DAWS, changes in the awake-sleep schedule, circadian rhythm disturbances caused by shift work changes or jet lag, and (4) dysfunctions associated with sleep, its various stages, or partial arousals, called parasomnias. The use of pharmacological agents to treat categories 1 and 2 are discussed in this chapter. Category 3 symptoms are usually transitory and alleviate in a few days

THERAPEUTIC OVERVIEW

SLEEP DISORDERS

Insomnias (trouble sleeping—DIMS)
Hypersomnias (excessive sleep—DOES)
Awake-sleep cycle problems (DAWS)
Parasomnias (sleep dysfunctions)

TREATMENT

Insomnias with CNS depressants
Hypersomnias with CNS stimulants
Both types of drugs have potential for abuse (especially stimulants)

once a new schedule is established without the use of medications, and category 4 is a group of miscellaneous disorders without specific drug therapies.

Insomnia and daytime sleepiness are symptoms and not specific diseases. Many diseases have symptoms of insomnia; treating insomnia with drugs provides symptomatic therapy only, and if given for an extended period, dramatically alters the normal sleep cycle and may lead to pharmacologically induced sleep disturbances. Hence, hypnotics should be used temporarily, but how long is controversial. Clearly, sleep medication for insomnia should not be used indiscriminately without a thorough analysis of what goal is being accomplished.

Sleep-promoting drugs act as CNS depressants and include the benzodiazepines, barbiturates, and other diverse compounds. For the opposite effect, namely treatment of excessive sleepiness, CNS stim-

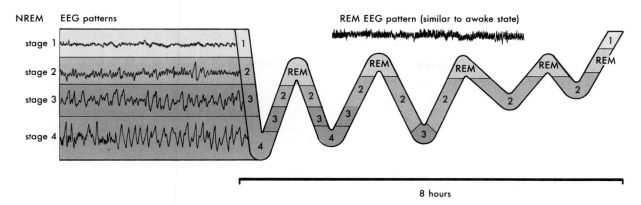

FIGURE 33-1   Characteristic EEG patterns for different stages of human sleep. The EEG pattern for stage REM sleep resembles that for the awake state (see text).

ulants are used, many of which have potential for abuse (Chapter 32).

The therapeutic aspects of sleep related drugs are summarized in the box.

MECHANISMS OF ACTION

Sleep Cycle

Sleep is a normal, readily reversible physiologic state, distinguished by relative quiescence and unconsciousness, decreased responsiveness to sensory stimuli, characteristic posture, and reduced activity of most voluntary muscles. It occurs approximately every 24 hours and varies in duration depending on age, normal physiology, and the presence of pathology. Infants and children require more sleep than do adults. The average normal adult sleeps about 8 hours, although there are considerable individual differences. Older normal adults tend to have more fragmented sleep.

The two major forms of sleep are characterized by distinct behaviors, dreams and their recall, and polygraphic (brainwave, electromyograph, eye movement), metabolic, and temperature changes. These forms are REM (rapid eye movement) and NREM (non-rapid eye movement) sleep. Both states differ behaviorally from wakefulness in terms of sensation and perception, thought progression, and movement control.

Sleep in humans can be subdivided into five stages, of which stages I-IV characterize NREM sleep

and one of REM sleep. Different stages of sleep result in different wave patterns in the electroencephalogram (EEG). During the awake state, a rapid, low-amplitude rhythm prevails (α and β waves). As sleep deepens, the wave pattern becomes progressively slower and much larger in amplitude. The α rhythm is diminished and replaced by β and occasional τ waves (stage I), sleep spindles (stage II), and ultimately high-amplitude slow δ waves (stages III and IV). The δ waves are characteristic of relatively deep sleep (Figure 33-1). REM sleep results in desynchronization of the EEG and a wave pattern closely resembling the waking stage accompanied by episodes of rapid eyeball movement. Generally, it is most difficult to arouse individuals from REM sleep.

The normal sleep cycle of adults shifts dramatically (minute to minute) between the different stages of sleep, with REM episodes occurring approximately every 90 to 100 minutes with longer durations later in the sleep period. In contrast, the duration of stage IV (NREM) sleep is longer during the early part of the sleep period. When a patient has been awake for 24 hours and is allowed to sleep, the brain spends much more time first in stage IV and then in stage REM sleep in an attempt to recoup the lost sleep especially of those two stages. In a normal adult about 4 to 5 short sleep cycles of NREM (average 95 min each) are interspersed with periods of REM sleep to give 6 to 8 hours of total sleep. Vivid, illogical, and bizarre dream recall occurs when a person is aroused from REM sleep and if unpleasant, these are called nightmares. Night terrors (present especially in children) and sleep walking occur during REM sleep and are not recalled by the individual. However, some are remembered after NREM sleep but lack detail and vividness.

As patient age increases, stages III and IV (NREM) become less prominent; geriatric patients also spend less time in these stages. Patients with dementia and serious mental diseases such as schizophrenia and depression have marked sleep disturbances, especially in stage III and (NREM) with an earlier onset of REM sleep than do normal subjects.

Sleep-Wakefulness: Neurotransmitters

The neurochemistry of sleep and wakefulness is still not understood, and it is not known whether two separate systems exist in the brain for these two behavioral states. Wakefulness is mediated by the arousal or activating system that is located in the brainstem reticular formation and hypothalamus. Neurons from these structures innervate wide areas of the neocortex (via the diffuse thalamic projection system) and the paleocortex or limbic system (via the hypothalamus). The neurotransmitters implicated in wakefulness are acetylcholine, catecholamines (in-

cluding dopamine and norepinephrine), histamine, and glutamic acid. Acetylcholine and norepinephrine are thought to play important roles in REM sleep. Both REM and NREM sleep involve similar brain areas. Serotonin and GABA are the most important neurotransmitters in NREM sleep. Peptides are also apparently involved in NREM, but like many of the other neurotransmitters, their precise role has not been established.

Because such a large variety of neurotransmitters are involved in sleep, many drugs acting on these diverse neurotransmitters affect wakefulness as well as the different stages of sleep. From a practical therapeutic point of view, the most widely used sleep-promoting medications are certain benzodiazepines and barbiturates that act on different sites of the GABA type A receptor in the brain. The benzodiazepines and barbiturates promote inhibitory presynaptic or postsynaptic actions of GABA by acting allosterically on GABA type A receptors. The role of GABA neurotransmitters in anxiety is discussed further in Chapter 25. The molecular actions of the GABA type A receptor are described in greater detail in Chapters 2 and 25.

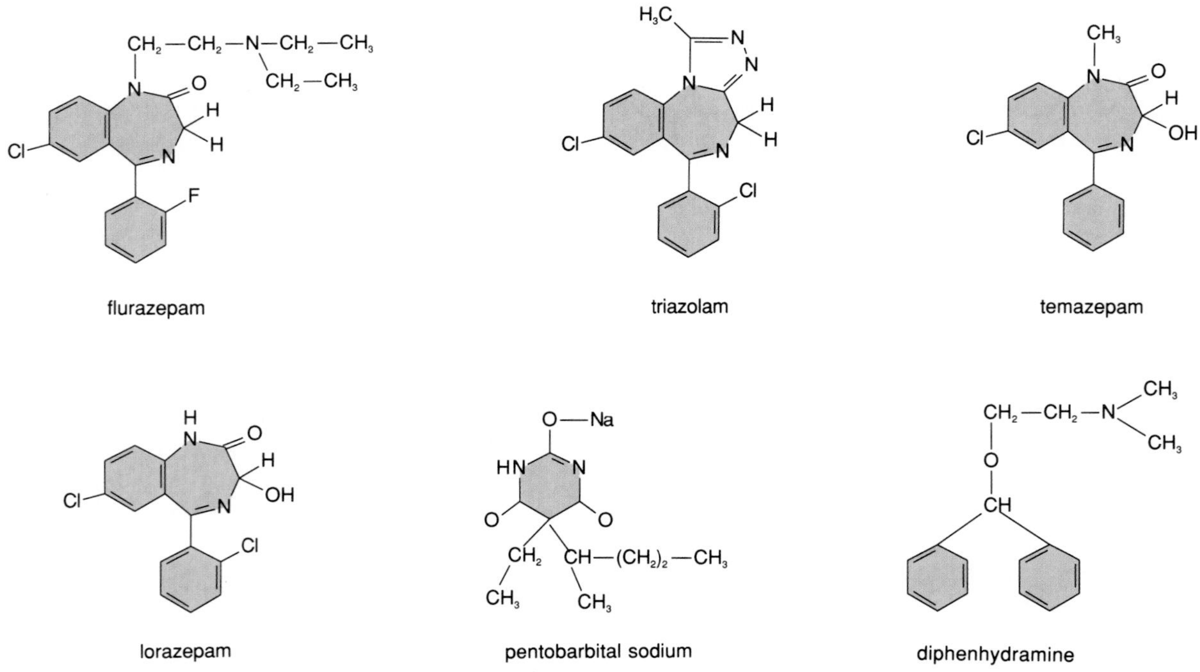

FIGURE 33-2   Chemical structures of frequently used drugs for promotion of sleep.

Specific Drugs

The primary sleep-promoting drugs are benzodiazepines, barbiturates, and a miscellaneous group. The chemical structures of these compounds are shown in Figures 33-2 and 33-3.

Although the barbiturates and the benzodiazepines act upon the same GABA system, the benzodiazepines produce relatively shallow dose-response curves, while the barbiturates have steeper dose-effect properties (see Figure 32-8). Clinically, this is very important. Therefore the benzodiazepines are much safer compared to barbiturates and other sleep-promoting agents if taken in overdosage. The molecular mechanisms of action of chloral hydrate and paraldehyde resemble those of ethyl alcohol (Chapter 31) and involve actions on cell membranes to increase fluidity. The detailed molecular mechanisms of action of many of the other hypnotics are not well studied but may involve actions on other sites of the GABA type A receptor.

Other sleep-promoting medications include muscarinic cholinergic antagonists such as scopolamine, now used chiefly as a preanesthetic agent to promote sleep and reduce secretions before surgery. Over-the-counter nonprescription preparations often contain as a sedative an H_1 antihistaminic, of which diphenhydramine and doxylamine are frequently used examples. Diphenhydramine has some muscarinic anticholinergic properties as well. Its chemical structure is shown in Figure 33-3. In view of the role of serotonin (Chapter 25) in sleep, one of its precursors, L-tryptophan, was used to promote sleep but has been withdrawn from this use because of possible contaminant toxicity. However, pure L-tryptophan may be made available in the future. Many antipsychotic drugs, and especially antidepressants, promote sleep especially

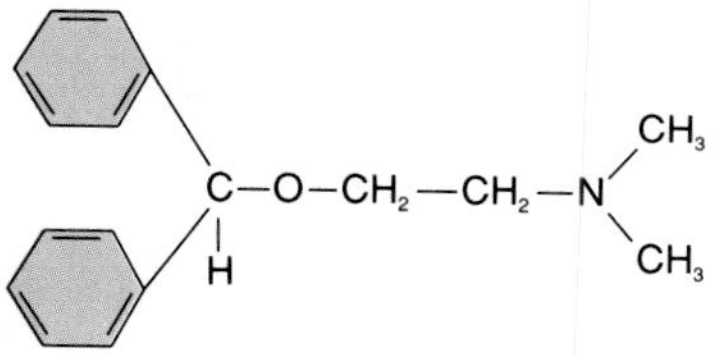
diphenhydramine

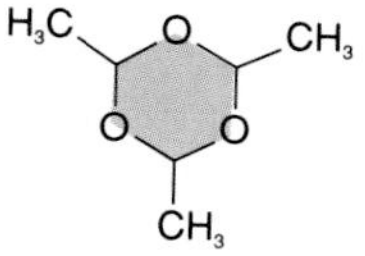
paraldehyde

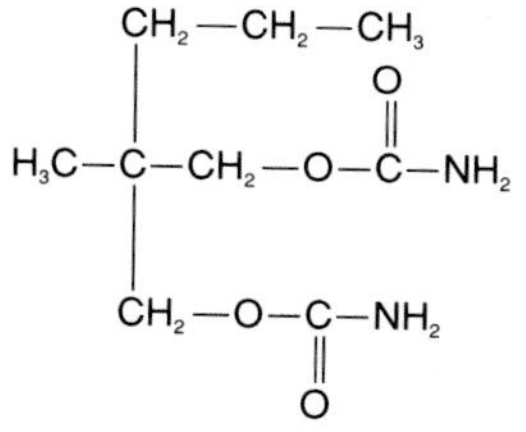
meprobamate

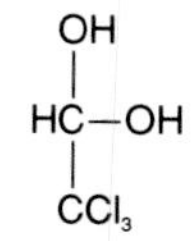
chloral hydrate

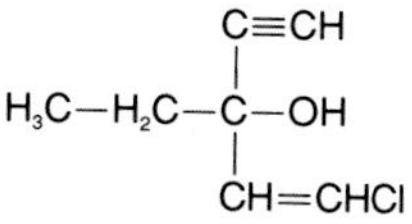
ethchlorvynol

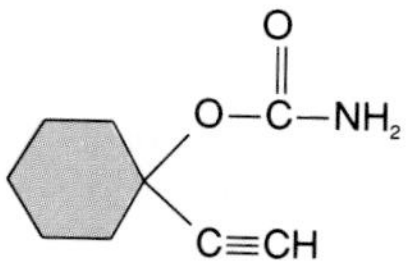
ethinamate

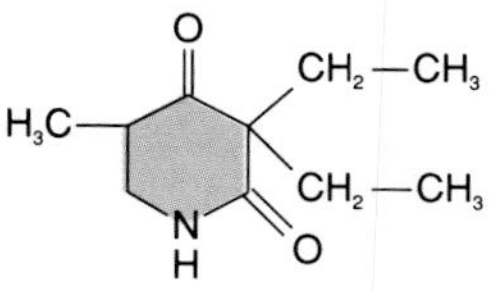
methyprylon

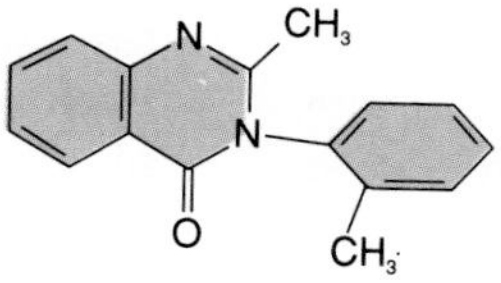
methaqualone

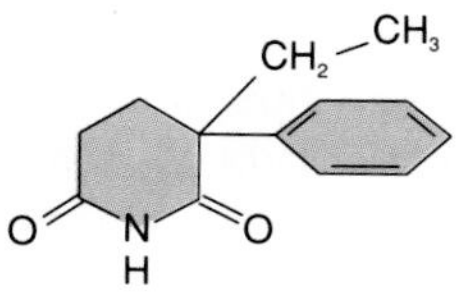
glutethimide

FIGURE 33-3 Chemical structures of less frequently used drugs for promotion of sleep.

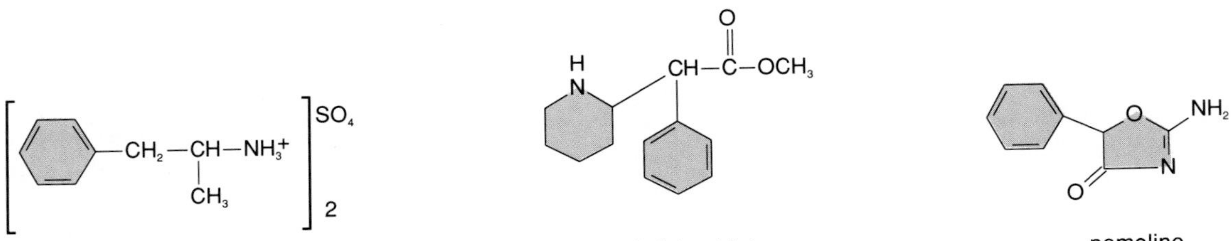

dextroamphetamine sulfate
(dextro isomer)

methylphenidate

pemoline

FIGURE 33-4   Chemical structures of stimulants used to reduce excessive sleep.

when given at bedtime, but these drugs are used primarily to treat the specific mental disease causing the disturbance of sleep (see Chapters 23 and 25).

CNS stimulants used to treat excessive sleep include the amphetamines (Chapter 32), methylphenidate and pemoline. The structures of these compounds are shown in Figure 33-4.

PHARMACOKINETICS

The pharmacokinetic parameter values for these drugs are listed in Table 33-1. All of the benzodiazepine hypnotics now in clinical use are reasonably well absorbed following oral administration and reach peak blood and brain concentrations within 1 to 2 hours. Their duration of action varies considerably, and the formation of active metabolites further contributes to their effects. Flurazepam is a long-acting prodrug that undergoes conversion to desalkylflurazepam, a long-acting active metabolite. Relatively little flurazepam and desalkylflurazepam are excreted unchanged in the urine and undergo further biotransformation in the liver. Hence, their elimination half-life in young adults is long (Table 33-1) and increases even further in older patients and in patients with liver disease. Temazepam has an intermediate elimination half-life, while triazolam has the shortest. Triazolam is an especially potent benzodiazepine that produces significant amnesia. Jet travelers have been known to take triazolam, go to sleep, wake up, and act normal but have no memory of that part of their trip. After nighttime use, some patients report rebound anxiety and confusion the next day, especially with triazolam. This drug should be used cautiously, particularly in the elderly.

Lorazepam is used as an hypnotic and an antianx-iety drug (see Chapter 25) and quazepam, which also is converted to an active metabolite, is almost exclusively used for its sleep-producing effects.

Barbiturates are weak acids, and those listed in Table 33-1 are well absorbed. Only pentobarbital is still widely used as a hypnotic. The barbiturates (Table 33-1) undergo biotransformation in the liver, where they are metabolized by the microsomal enzyme oxidative system and conjugated with glucuronic acid for excretion by the kidneys. Rapid tolerance occurs to the sleep-promoting effects of these barbiturates so that treatment is recommended for a maximum of 2 weeks. Their duration of action is about 4 to 6 hours but their elimination half-lives are much longer. Phenobarbital, which is not considered here, earlier had wide use as a sedative-hypnotic, but is now used almost exclusively as an anticonvulsant. The ultrashort-acting barbiturates are used as IV anesthetic agents and are discussed in Chapter 30.

Chloral hydrate is an irritating liquid also available as a less irritating sodium salt of the phosphate ester. It is converted to its active metabolite, trichloroethanol, in the liver. Trichloroethanol is conjugated with glucuronic acid and excreted into the urine. The plasma half-life of trichloroethanol is 4 to 12 hours. The effects of chloral hydrate on the sleep cycle are similar to those of barbiturates, but in low dosage, REM sleep is suppressed less.

Paraldehyde is a cyclic trimer of acetaldehyde. It is a liquid with a rather strong odor and disagreeable taste that alcoholics apparently like. Oral paraldehyde is rapidly absorbed and facilitates sleep within 15 minutes. It is biotransformed in the liver to acetaldehyde and subsequently oxidized by aldehyde dehydrogenase to acetic acid, and then to CO_2, and water. It is seldom used as a hypnotic, but has for over a century been used as a sedative in a variety

Table 33-1 Pharmacokinetic Parameters

Drugs	Administered	$t_{1/2}$ (hr)	Disposition
BENZODIAZEPINES			
lorazepam	Oral	8-25	M (main)
flurazepam	Oral	50-98	M (main)*
temazepam	Oral	9.5-12.4	M (main)
triazolam	Oral	1.5-5.5	M (main)
BARBITURATES			
amobarbital	Oral	16-40	M (main)
pentobarbital	Oral	15-50	M (main)
secobarbitol	Oral	15-40	M (main)
MISCELLANEOUS			
chloral hydrate	Oral	4-9.5	M (main)*
ethchlorvynol	Oral		M (main)
ethinamate	Oral	2.5	M (main)
glutethimide	Oral	10-12	M (main)
methyprylon	Oral	4	M (main)
paraldehyde	Oral	3.4-9.8	M (main)
NONPRESCRIPTION ANTIHISTAMINICS			
diphenhydramine	Oral	3.7-4.5	—
doxylamine	Oral	4-12	—

M, Metabolized.
*Active metabolites.

of psychiatric and medical management situations.

The remaining hypnotics vary in duration of action and elimination half-lives. All are biotransformed in the liver to less active metabolites. Most of these hypnotics alter the sleep cycle in a fashion similar to the benzodiazepines and barbiturates with minor differences.

The two drugs widely used as over-the-counter hypnotics are the sedative H_1 antihistamines diphenhydramine and doxylamine. Diphenhydramine has a shorter half-life than doxylamine (Table 33-1). Tolerance rapidly develops to the sedative effects of both. Good systematic sleep cycle studies with these agents, especially in the small doses approved, are lacking, in spite of their widespread use in nonprescription preparations.

RELATION OF MECHANISMS OF ACTION TO CLINICAL RESPONSE

Drugs that reduce the activity of the brain and spinal cord are termed CNS depressants, and de-

pressants used clinically to promote sleep are sometimes termed hypnotics, or less commonly, soporifics. The term hypnotics for sleep promotion should not be confused with hypnosis, which is a mental state induced in a susceptible individual in response to suggestion. Although sensory perception, mood, memory, and motor performance appear to be altered in the hypnotized state and hypnotic suggestion usually involves statements that the person is "very tired and sleepy," the hypnotic state is quite different from true sleep.

Almost all of the drugs used to alter the sleep cycle act on normal as well as ailing subjects. REM sleep, which at one time was considered the most important type of sleep, is supressed by drugs such as barbiturates and scopolamine. In addition, stages III and IV of NREM sleep are also reduced by the barbiturates. Tolerance to REM suppression occurs, but REM rebound with intense dream recall and nightmares on drug withdrawal is especially marked (Figure 33-5). Benzodiazepines also suppress REM sleep to various degrees, as well as stages III and IV of NREM sleep. The latter effect is useful in treating patients

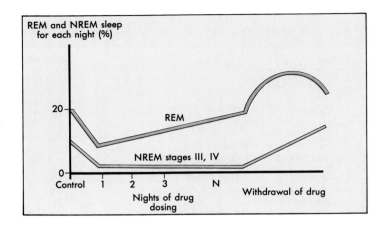

FIGURE 33-5 Typical REM and NREM effects; tolerance and excessive rebound to barbiturate hypnotics. Benzodiazepines produce similar but less pronounced effects (see text).

with night terrors, which are related to those stages.

All hypnotics alter the normal sleep cycle to suppress REM sleep, decrease stages III and IV of NREM sleep and produce tolerance on continued use. They may or may not cause REM rebound on withdrawal. Thus, the key issue is whether temporarily some sleep with side effects is better than no sleep (insomnia). For short periods (days to a few weeks) some sleep is clearly better than none; however, over a period of a few weeks, months, and especially years, patients with insomnia who take sleep medications nightly develop marked drug-induced abnormalities of their sleep cycle. *Hence, hypnotics must be prescribed for short-term use only.* Unfortunately, in patients with severe insomnia most other treatments are not very successful. Such patients frequently pressure their physicians to continue prescribing medication indefinitely. This situation ultimately markedly alters the patient's sleep cycles detrimentally. Such patients must be weaned from all sleep medications and their primary problems treated in some other fashion, preferably without drugs.

Anesthesia should not be confused with sleep. General anesthesia involves a loss of consciousness. It persists as long as the anesthetic agent is present at sufficient partial pressure in the brain (see Chapter 30).

The disorders associated with excessive sleep or hypersomnias can be divided into about 10 categories of which the most common is narcolepsy (etiology unknown). It is characterized by excessive daytime sleepiness, disturbed nocturnal sleep, and especially pathological REM sleep. This syndrome is characterized by early onset REM periods and other REM pat-

terns that cause cataplexy (extreme muscle weakness induced by emotional activity) and sleep paralysis, both day and night. Although the etiology of narcolepsy has not been established, there is a link between DR2, the class II antigen of the major histocompatibility complex, and narcolepsy. The majority of narcolepsy patients are DR2 positive, suggesting an association with or an involvement of the immune system.

The drugs used to treat the symptoms of excessive daytime sleep are CNS stimulants, of which amphetamines, methylphenidate, and pemoline are most frequently used. Dextroamphetamine is the most efficacious, but also produces more side effects such as irritability, tachycardia, tolerance, and drug dependence. Methylphenidate is effective, while exhibiting fewer side effects. Pemoline has a longer duration of action than the other two agents. The tricyclic antidepressants are also used as adjunctive therapy and may control certain symptoms of the disorder. The abuse potential and other side effects of the CNS stimulants are described in Chapter 32.

SIDE EFFECTS, CLINICAL PROBLEMS, AND TOXICITY

The therapeutic goal in using hypnotic agents is to promote sleep, with their use in treating insomnia only symptomatic. All of the drugs used alter the normal sleep cycle and should be administered for only days or weeks and almost never for months or years. The rate of tolerance development varies with the chemical class, individual compound, and dosage. With the barbiturates two types of tolerance occur,

---

CLINICAL PROBLEMS OF SLEEP DRUGS

PROMOTE SLEEP (TREAT INSOMNIAS)

Greater toxicity problems with barbiturates, limit treatment cycles to days to a few weeks

Drugs used for symptomatic treatment only

DEPRESS SLEEP (TREAT HYPERSOMNIAS)

CNS stimulants

Produce irritability, tachycardia, tolerance, and drug dependence and have significant abuse potential

---

TRADENAMES

In addition to generic and fixed combination preparations, the following tradenamed materials are available in the United States.

BENZODIAZEPINES

Ativan, lorazepam
Dalmane, flurazepam
Dormalin, quazepam
Halcion, triazolam
Restoril, temazepam

BARBITURATES

Amytal, amobarbital
Nembutal, pentobarbital
Seconal, secobarbital

MISCELLANEOUS

Doriden, glutethimide
Noludar, methyprylon
Placidyl, ethchlorvynol
Valmid, ethinamate

---

pharmacokinetic and cellular. In the first type, barbiturates have the well-known property of stimulating their own metabolism by induction of the P-450 system enzymes (see Chapter 5). In cellular tolerance, their effect upon the CNS is decreased. Daytime residual sleepiness or hangover may be a problem with some of the longer-acting compounds. Rebound anxiety and rebound REM sleep also occur with some of the compounds. Both psychological and physical dependence are very common with most classes of hypnotics. Physical withdrawal signs and symptoms resemble alcohol withdrawal and may include convulsions misdiagnosed as epilepsy. All substances may produce allergic and idiosyncratic reactions in addition to side effects that are extensions of their normal pharmacology. Major side effects of the hypnotics include excessive sedation, dizziness, additive, or in some cases potentiating action with alcohol, coma, respiratory depression, and death. The lethal effects are especially prominent with barbiturates and have led to marked reduction in their use, concomitant with an increase in the use of benzodiazepines. Benzodiazepines are less toxic but can produce serious toxicity in combination with ethyl alcohol. Abuse of hypnotic agents is possible in susceptible individuals and can lead to substance dependence and withdrawal problems similar to that of ethyl alcohol. Cross tolerance and cross dependence to alcohol are the rule for most hypnotics.

These agents are capable of crossing the placenta and therefore can cause depression in the neonate. Withdrawal symptoms can occur in the newborn if the mother is dependent on any of these drugs.

Barbiturates are contraindicated in intermittent porphyria, since they can induce the enzymes responsible of porphyrin synthesis. Glutethimide overdosage is especially very difficult to treat and hence the drug is now seldom prescribed.

The clinical problems with sleep drugs are summarized in the box.

REFERENCES

Borbey A and Valtax JL, eds: Sleep mechanisms, Experimental Brain Research, Suppl 8, Berlin, 1984, Springer Verlag.

Gillin JC and Byerley WF: The diagnosis and management of insomnia, N Engl J Med 322:239, 1990.

Kelly DD: Sleep and dreaming. In Kandel ER and Schwartz JH eds: Principles of neurosciences, ed 2, New York, 1985, Elsevier Publishing Co, Inc.

Kelly DD: Disorders of sleep and consciousness. In Kandel ER and Schwartz JH, eds: Principles of neurosciences, ed 2, New York, 1985, Elsevier Publishing Co, Inc.

Kryger MH, Roth T, and Dement WC, eds: Principles and practices of sleep medicine, Philadelphia, 1989, WB Saunders Co.

Williams RL and Karacan I, eds: Pharmacology of sleep, New York, 1986, John Wiley & Sons.

ENDOCRINE SYSTEMS: HORMONES AND RELATED COMPOUNDS

The endocrine system can be defined classically as a diverse group of glands that secretes on demand chemical substances called *hormones* directly into the bloodstream. The secreted hormones are transported via the bloodstream to organs or cells where they regulate organ and cellular activities. The hypothalamus-pituitary, thyroid, parathyroid, pancreas, adrenals, ovary, testes, and sometimes placenta and intestinal mucosa are considered to be the main endocrine glands producing hormones.

The endocrine hormones affect the activities of most organs and many types of cells. These actions occur via extremely intricate pathways, including positive and negative feedback control loops and sequences involving hormones from endocrine glands that act to control hormonal secretions from other glands. A given hormone typically exerts multiple actions, and a given function typically is influenced by several different hormones. After synthesis, an endocrine hormone is packaged in the endocrine gland and stored for later release as needed. Special releasing hormones often bring about the secretion of the stored, packaged hormone.

The endocrine hormones can be divided into two chemical structural types: (1) the peptides and amino acid derivatives and (2) the cholesterol-based steroid compounds. The typical plasma concentrations for endocrine hormones range from 10^{-7} to 10^{-9} M for steroids and usually range much lower (10^{-9} to 10^{-11} M) for peptide hormones. The half-lives of a number of endocrine hormones are quite short (5 to 30 minutes). The steroid hormones can be grouped into six classes: glucocorticords, mineralocorticords, estro-

gen, progestin, androgen, and vitamin D.

Pharmacological intervention in the treatment of endocrine malfunction or disease state generally takes one of three approaches: (1) replacement or supplementation of the natural hormone, (2) use of the hormone to obtain a specific response, or (3) use of drugs to modify the concentration or action of a specific hormone.

A list of the major endocrine hormones and the glands most responsible for their synthesis and secretion is given in Table V-1, see following page. The chapter in which each hormone is discussed is also indicated, but only for those hormones that are involved in pharmacological intervention. Endocrine hormones that are not utilized in therapeutics are not discussed, since their pharmacological roles remain to be established. Most of the diagnostic uses of endocrine hormones also are not included, unless the results are utilized in some way to formulate a pharmacological therapeutic approach.

The endocrine hormones act at target organs and cells through specific receptors. The receptor mechanisms are the same in many respects to the mechanisms of the central or peripheral neurotransmitter systems, already discussed in Chapter 2 and developed further in the peripheral autonomic and central nervous system sections (Chapters 8 to 10 and 22). Because receptors play a key role in the mechanisms of action of endocrine hormone systems, the next chapter contains a summary of the key receptor concepts pertinent to endocrine systems, with special emphasis on the unique features for the endocrine receptors.

Table V-1 Major Endocrine Hormones

Hormone	Secreted by	Chapter
Peptide or Amino Acid Derivative		
insulin	pancreas	39
glucagon	pancreas	39
somatostatin	pancreas	39
pancreatic polypeptide	pancreas	39
thyroid hormones	thyroid	38
antidiuretic hormone (ADH)	pituitary	41
oxytocin	pituitary	41
adrenocorticotropic hormone (ACTH)	pituitary	41
thyroid stimulating hormone (TSH)	pituitary	41
luteinizing hormone (LH)	pituitary	41
follicle-stimulating hormone (FSH)	pituitary	41
growth hormone (GH)	pituitary	41
prolactin	pituitary	41
gonadotropin-releasing hormone (GnRH)	pituitary	41
luteinizing-hormone releasing hormone (LHRH)	pituitary	41
thyrotropin-releasing hormone (TRH)	pituitary	41
prolactin inhibiting factor (PIF)	pituitary	41
parathyroid hormone	parathyroid	42
calcitonin	thyroid	38
catecholamines	adrenals	8,10
Steroid		
estrogens	ovary, adrenals	36
progesterone	ovary, testes, adrenals	36
testosterone	testes, ovary, adrenals	37
cortisol (glucocorticoid)	adrenals	35
corticosterone (glucocorticoid)	adrenals	35
aldosterone (mineralocorticoid)	adrenals	35

CHAPTER 34

Hormone Receptors and Signaling Mechanisms

ABBREVIATIONS

βARK	β-adrenergic receptor kinase
CSF-1	colony stimulating factor-1
CURL	compartment of uncoupling of receptor and ligand
DNA	deoxyribonucleic acid
EGF	epidermal growth factor
ER	endoplasmic reticulum
HRE	hormone responsive element
IGF-1	insulin-like growth factor-1
MAP	microtubule-associated protein
PDGF	platelet-derived growth factor
RNA	ribonucleic acid
raf	a serine-threonine protein kinase oncogene
RNA Pol II	ribonucleic acid polymerase II
T3	triiodothyronine
TSH	thyroid-stimulating hormone

Hormones that are secreted by the endocrine glands exert their profound control on cellular and organ activities primarily through binding to receptors in the target organ or target cells. The inclusion of receptors as a component of the endocrine hormone intercellular communication chain thus is well established, and a number of the molecular level mechanistic details are known.

From the classical standpoint, the definition of the endocrine transfer of information requires that the transfer occur between distant organs and that a hormone be carried from its site of production to its target through the blood. However, from the point of view of the responding receptor on the target cell, it makes little difference where the hormone molecule originated. The hormone may (1) be carried via the blood from a classical hormone secreting gland (endocrine), (2) be secreted by a neighboring cell or tissue and travel by diffusion through the intercellular fluid (paracrine), or (3) be secreted by the same cell that responds to the hormone (autocrine). These three communication schemes are outlined in Figure 34-1. When the target cell is a neuron whose receptor responds to a chemical mediator (neurotransmitter) secreted into a synaptic cleft, the process can be viewed as a special case of paracrine stimulation.

In all three of the above receptor-based pathways of cellular stimulation, the biochemical and cellular mechanisms are quite similar whether the receptor is part of a classical endocrine system hormonal control loop, the autonomic nervous system, or a component of the central nervous system (CNS). In the classical sense, the term "hormone" is restricted to those endogenous compounds secreted by the endocrine glands and that participate in "endocrine stimulation." However, in the practical sense, the term hormone is used more broadly today to encompass an endogenous compound secreted by a producer cell, which triggers a response in a target cell. In this book the term hormone is restricted to the classical endocrine definition for simplicity.

The importance of receptors in pharmacology is evident from the repeated references to receptor-based mechanisms of action throughout this book. The major characteristics of receptors are described

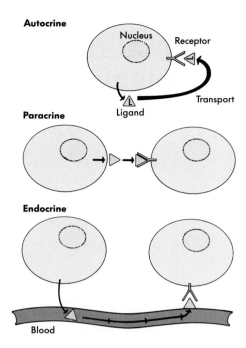

Autocrine

Nucleus   Receptor

Transport

Ligand

Paracrine

Endocrine

Blood

FIGURE 34-1   Three types of cellular stimulation: autocrine, paracrine, and endocrine. Secretion of ligand L is followed by transport and then binding of L to a receptor (shown in the shape of Y).

in Chapter 2. The applicability of receptors to specific areas of body function are covered in Chapters 8 to 10 for the autonomic nervous system, Chapter 22 for the central nervous system, Chapters 22 and 25 to 27 for cardiovascular agents, and now this and other chapters for various endocrine hormones. In all cases the receptors (1) recognize the presence of a specific ligand (i.e., the secreted compound or the hormone), and (2) trigger a set of biological responses. In addition, most receptors have some means of modulating the biological response to ligand stimulation so as to keep the stimulation appropriate to the integrated status of the cell.

ENDOCRINE HORMONE RECEPTORS

Classification

The endocrine systems incorporate a broader scope of receptor families (see the box) than do the nervous or cardiovascular systems, at least from a pharmacological viewpoint. Two general classes of

---

RECEPTOR FAMILIES

MEMBRANE RECEPTORS

Coupled to GTP-binding proteins
   Activate adenylate cyclase
   Inhibit adenylate cyclase
   Activate phospholipase C
   Affect ion channels
Tyrosine kinases
Unclassified membrane receptors

NUCLEAR RECEPTORS

Receptors for steroids, sterols, and triiodothyronine

---

receptors include the membrane receptors and the intracellular and nuclear receptors. The membrane receptors are made up of several subclasses. One class of receptors is coupled to GTP binding proteins with effects to activate or inhibit adenylate cyclase or to activate phospholipase C. Another subclass contains tyrosine specific protein kinases as integral elements. The intracellular and nuclear receptors act to control nuclear-related events including DNA and RNA function and gene expression. The tyrosine kinase family of receptors and the cell nucleus transcriptional regulating family of receptors are unique to the endocrine systems for pharmacological purposes.

General Properties

All of the hormone receptor systems carry out the molecular recognition process through noncovalent binding, in the same manner as with nonhormone receptors. Since many of the hormones are present in intercellular fluids at nanomolar or lower concentrations, a receptor with an equilibrium binding constant of 10^{-9} M^{-1} would have 50% of the sites occupied at a concentration of unbound hormone of 1 nM. The high degree of specificity required to prevent interference by related molecules arises from the high degree of complementarity between the surface of the hormone and the surface of the receptor and the ability of the two surfaces to move in a concerted fashion. The specificity, however, is not absolute. At sufficiently high concentrations, molecules that do not normally bind will sometimes bind to a receptor. This is particularly true for closely related hormones.

For example, insulin and insulin-like growth factor I are structurally related polypeptide hormones. Approximately 40% of their amino acids are identical, although each has its own receptor to which it binds with high affinity. Each also will bind to the other's receptor, but with about a 100-fold lower affinity. Normally this cross-reactivity is not significant, since physiological concentrations of the hormones are not sufficiently high. However, in certain pathological conditions, when very high concentrations of the hormone are used pharmacologically, or when synthetic analogs of the hormone are used that may have less specificity, cross-reactivity can be a problem.

The manner in which a cell responds to a hormone varies depending on its past history and present state. For example, when a cell is exposed to a hormone it will gradually become desensitized to it. Not only can a hormone affect the way a cell responds to itself (homologous effects), it can affect the way a cell responds to other hormones (heterologous effects). For example, exposure to estrogen is required to sensitize many cells to the effects of progesterone. Modulation of hormone responsiveness frequently occurs at several levels including the receptor level. Receptor responsiveness can be altered by a number of mechanisms. The number of receptors can change, either by altering their rate of synthesis and degradation, or by sequestering them to an inactive compartment of the cell. Their hormone binding affinity can change. The efficiency by which the occupied receptor transduces a response can change. Although the precise changes and the mechanisms that produce them vary from receptor to receptor and will be discussed further in later sections, receptor phosphorylation is frequently involved.

The majority of known hormone receptors are located in the cell membrane. Those few that are found intracellularly in the cytoplasm (or nucleus) are receptors for lipid-soluble hormones (e.g., steroids and thyroid hormone), which can readily pass through the cell membrane.

Receptor Internalization and Recycling

The cell membrane is a very dynamic structure, being constantly degraded and reconstituted. Its components are rapidly exchanged with those of other intracellular membrane compartments. This is particularly true for membrane receptors. The processes involved provide some of the primary mechanisms for regulating the number of cell membrane receptors (Figure 34-2), although the details may differ for different receptors and even for the same receptor in different tissues; the overall processes appear to be similar.

In the absence of hormone, most receptors are not localized to any particular region of the cell membrane. When hormones bind, they rapidly migrate to coated pits, which are specialized invaginations of the membrane where receptor-mediated endocytosis occurs. These are so termed because they are surrounded by an electron dense cage formed by the protein clathrin. Membranes within the coated pits rapidly pinch off to form intracellular vesicles rich in receptor ligand complexes. These vesicles then fuse with tubular-reticular structures called CURL (compartment of uncoupling of receptor and ligand). The internal pH of CURL is maintained at about 4.5 to 5 by an ATP-dependent proton pump. The low pH favors the dissociation of hormone and receptor making it possible for them to be sorted independently. In most cases, dissociated hormone is incorporated into vesicles that fuse with lysosomes and is thus degraded by lysosomal enzymes, while dissociated receptor recirculates to the cell surface. However, a fraction of internalized hormone may be recirculated to the cell surface along with receptor and released there, a process termed retroendocytosis. Free receptor in CURL may recirculate to the cell surface or may temporarily be sequestered in an intracellular membrane compartment or may be transported to lysosomes where it is degraded. The latter two cases will result in a net decrease in cell receptor number by a redistribution of surface receptors to an intracellular compartment or by an increase in degradation. These are ways in which hormone binding results in the down regulation of cell surface receptors.

A few important points should be stressed. First, throughout these processes the receptor remains embedded in the membrane; and the receptor orientation with respect to the membrane remains constant. Those domains of the receptor that faced the cytoplasm on the cell surface continue to face the cytoplasm after vesicles pinch off from the cell surface or fuse with other intracellular membrane structures. Similarly, those domains that faced extracellularly on the surface before vesicle formation now face the interior fluid trapped within the vesicle lumen after the pinch off or fusion is completed. Although internalized hormone may dissociate from the receptor and exist

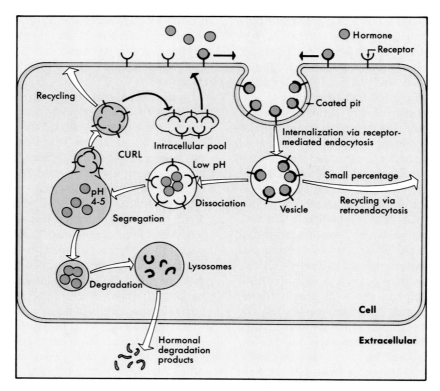

FIGURE 34-2   Pathways of receptor internalization and recycling. *CURL*, Compartment of uncoupling of receptor and ligand.

free in the lumen of vesicles, internalized hormone does not cross the membranes, and therefore does not have access to the cytoplasmic compartment. Second, it should be reiterated that there are major quantitative differences in the relative importance of these pathways for different hormones and different tissues. Thus, some receptors have a cryptic intracellular pool that far exceeds the number of receptors on the cell surface, while others have virtually no intracellular pool. Some receptors recirculate several times without being degraded in lysosomes, thus delivering several molecules of hormone to the lysosomes during their lifetime. For other receptors, almost every receptor molecule that is internalized is degraded. Third, other factors besides hormone binding may regulate receptor internalization and distribution within membrane compartments. For most receptors, phosphorylation is particularly important.

There are several possible functions for receptor internalization and redistribution. It is clearly one of the important ways that the number of cell surface receptors, and thereby sensitivity of the cell to a hor-

mone, is regulated. Since hormones that have receptors on the cell surface frequently regulate processes that occur at intracellular loci (e.g., gene expression in the nucleus), receptor-mediated hormone internalization may be a means of bringing either the hormone or the activated receptor to the site where these processes occur, or that a fragment of the hormone or receptor generated intracellularly could serve as a second messenger. Currently, however, no conclusive experimental evidence has been generated to support such hypothetical roles.

MEMBRANE HORMONE RECEPTORS

Hormone Receptors Coupled to GTP-Binding Proteins

The largest family of membrane receptors, and the one to which most hormone receptors of clinical interest belong, are those receptors that are coupled to GTP-binding proteins (Table 34-1). These include re-

Table 34-1   Hormone Receptors that Are Coupled to GTP Binding Proteins

Receptor	G-Protein	Effect
epinephrine (β_1 and β_2)	G_s	Stimulate adenylate cyclase
glucagon	—	—
vasoactive intestinal polypeptide	—	—
gastrin	—	—
secretin	—	—
corticotropin	—	—
thyrotropin	—	—
leutinizing-hormone/HCG	—	—
follicle-stimulating hormone	—	—
growth hormone-releasing hormone	—	—
corticotropin-releasing hormone	—	—
parathyroid hormone	—	—
calcitonin	—	—
vasopressin (V_2)	—	—
epinephrine α_2	G_i	Inhibit adenylate cyclase
somatostatin	—	—
angiotensin	—	—
oxytocin	—	—
opiate peptides	G_O	Inhibit calcium channels
epinephrine (α_1)	G	Stimulate phospholipase C
thyrotropin-releasing hormone	—	—
gonadotropin-releasing hormone	—	—
vasopressin (V_1)	—	—
angiotensin	—	—

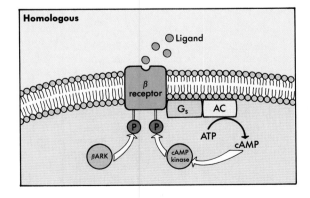
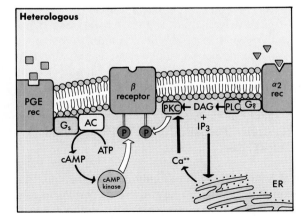

FIGURE 34-3   Phosphorylation is important in receptor desensitization. Pathways of stimulation of β-adrenergic receptor kinase *(βARK)*, cAMP-dependent protein kinase in homologous desensitization, and cAMP protein kinase and protein kinase C *(PKC)*, in heterologous desensitization by α-adrenergic receptor *(α₂ rec)* and prostaglandin PGE receptor *(PGE rec)*.

ceptors that activate or inhibit adenylate cyclase, stimulate phospholipase-C, and regulate certain ion channels. Since this class of receptors is discussed extensively in Chapter 2, the material discussed in this chapter is limited to the processes involved in the regulation of the receptor sensitivity.

Mechanisms of Desensitization

Several different processes are involved in receptor desensitization. These can be classified into *homologous desensitization* and *heterologous desensitization* (Figure 34-3). They have been most extensively studied for the β-adrenergic receptor. Receptor phosphorylation by three different protein kinases play an important role. These are *β-adrenergic receptor kinase, AMP-dependent protein kinase,* and *protein kinase C*. Receptor phosphorylation by these kinases may rapidly inhibit their interaction with G-proteins and more slowly lead to a sequestration or internalization of receptors to a compartment where they cannot interact with extracellular hormone.

β-adrenergic receptor kinase is particularly important in homologous desensitization. This kinase is only capable of phosphorylating the active agonist bound form of the receptor. It is this property that makes homologous desensitization such a specific form of desensitization. Other protein kinases, for example, cAMP-dependent protein kinase, may also prefer the agonist bound form of the receptor, but not to the same extent as does the β-adrenergic receptor kinase. Although β-adrenergic receptor kinase was originally described as a kinase specific for the β-adrenergic receptor, probably β-adrenergic receptor kinase or closely related protein kinases can phosphorylate several receptors in this family when they are in an agonist bound, active state, suggesting that this kinase will have an extensive role in homologous desensitization of G-protein coupled receptors.

TYROSINE-SPECIFIC PROTEIN KINASE RECEPTORS

Although activation of many of the receptors that are coupled to GTP binding proteins results in regulation of protein kinases, this is an indirect effect. The receptors to be discussed in this section are themselves hormonally regulated protein kinases. They differ from the usual protein kinases, which

phosphorylate proteins on serine or threonine residues, in that these protein kinases phosphorylate proteins exclusively on tyrosine residues. They include endocrine hormone receptors for insulin (Table 34-2) and receptors for several growth factors. They also include proteins that, because of their structures, appear to be transmembrane tyrosine kinase receptors for yet to be identified hormones. The biological effects resulting from activation of these receptors have as a general motif stimulation of anabolic processes, growth, and differentiation. Because of the important role these receptors play in regulating growth and differentiation, somatic mutations of these receptors may result in tumor formation and abnormal forms of these receptors have been identified as oncogenes.

It is generally believed that receptor tyrosine kinase activity is responsible for transmembrane signalling. Several proteins have been identified as substrates for these receptor tyrosine kinases. However, aside from the receptors themselves, which all undergo autophosphorylation and tyrosine kinase activation, in no case has phosphorylation of a substrate been shown to result in a functional change that can explain classically recognized consequences of hormonal stimulation. Only a small percentage of most known substrates become phosphorylated even with maximal hormonal stimulation and this occurs without changes in their function. For this reason it is believed that these substrates may be only incidental and that the physiologically relevant substrates have yet to be identified. Because activation of tyrosine kinase receptors is known to also increase serine-threonine phosphorylation of a set of proteins and also

Table 34-2	Receptor Tyrosine Kinases
Endocrine hormone receptors	Insulin receptor
	Somatomedin-C (IGF-1) receptor
Growth factor receptors	Epidermal growth factor (EGF) receptor
	Platelet-derived growth factor (PDGF) receptor
	Colony stimulating factor-1 (CSF-1) receptor
Receptors for unknown hormones (oncogenes)	cNeu
	cRos
	cKit
	cMet
	cTrk

to stimulate dephosphorylation of another set of proteins, the possibility has been considered that some serine-threonine protein kinase or some protein phosphatases could be a relevant tyrosine kinase substrate. Recently, raf, a serine-threonine protein kinase oncogene, has been shown to be a substrate for the PDGF and EGF receptor tyrosine kinases, and MAO kinase has been shown to be a substrate for the insulin receptor tyrosine kinase or a kinase phosphorylated by the insulin receptor tyrosine kinase. Since control of gene expression is a relatively proximate effect of stimulation of this class of receptors, other possible candidates for phosphorylation are trans-activating factors. Attempts to identify physiologically important substrates for receptor tyrosine kinases are an active and important area of current research.

Failure to identify substrates for receptor tyrosine kinases that could readily explain their biological functions has lead to the consideration of other possible mechanisms by which these receptors could initiate a response. Activation of several members of the tyrosine kinase family of receptors leads to the hydrolysis of PIP_2 leading to the formation of the second messengers IP_3 and diacylglycerol. This has been best documented for the PDGF receptor. Recently, an isoenzyme of PIP_2 phospholipase C has been shown to be a substrate of the PDGF and the EGF receptor tyrosine kinases. Activation of the insulin receptor stimulates a novel phospholipase C, which does not hydrolyze PIP_2, but which has as a substrate a complex phosphoglycolipid or protein-bound glycophospholipid whose hydrolysis generates a phosphoinositol-containing glycan that can mimic many of the actions of insulin and has been postulated to be a second messenger for insulin. Whether activation of these phospholipases occurs through interaction with

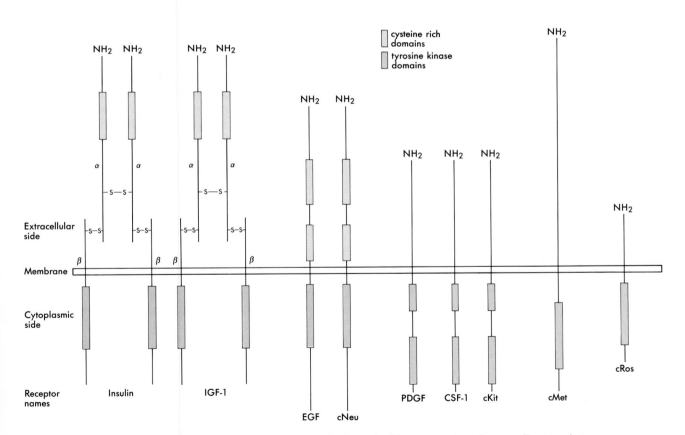

FIGURE 34-4 Comparative structures of several tyrosine kinase receptors shown as linear amino acid sequences and illustrating cysteine rich domains and tyrosine kinase domains. Many of these receptors belong to three subfamilies. Note that the tyrosine kinase domain may be present as one segment or as two divided segments. *cNeu, cKit, cRos, cMet*, Oncogenes.

a G protein and if so whether it is independent or somehow a consequence of the receptor tyrosine kinase activity remain important but unanswered questions.

Receptors in this family, characteristically have a single membrane spanning α helix that divides the receptor into an extracellular hormone binding amino-terminal portion and a cytoplasmic carboxy-terminal portion that contains a tyrosine kinase domain (Figure 34-4). Receptors for insulin and IGF-I vary slightly from this arrangement. Although their genes code for a protein with these characteristics, this protein, early in its biosynthesis, forms a disulfide linked homodimer that is subsequently cleaved to produce a disulfide-linked tetramer. The extracellular portions of receptors in the tyrosine kinase family vary widely, although there are subfamilies in which varying degrees of similarity exist. Some receptors have regions of cysteine rich sequences, which are imperfectly repeated several times. The EGF-Neu receptor family has two regions of such cysteine rich repeats, while the insulin-IGF-I receptor family has one per α subunit. It is believed that most of the cysteines in this region form disulfide bonds, creating a rigid manifold to which the hormone binds. The tyrosine kinase domain is the most highly conserved region, particularly between members of different subfamilies. There is a well-defined ATP binding region near the amino-terminal end of the kinase domain. The variable regions that flank or in some receptors interrupt the tyrosine kinase domain may have a role in substrate binding, thereby accounting for the differing substrate specificity of different members of this family.

Deletion of the extracellular hormone binding domain of several tyrosine kinase receptors has resulted in mutant receptors with constitutively active tyrosine kinases. Thus it appears that the hormone binding domain is an inhibitory regulator of tyrosine kinase, and that this negative regulation is relaxed by hormone binding. In confirmation, selective proteolysis by trypsin of the hormone binding domain of the insulin receptor disinhibits the tyrosine kinase activity.

Tyrosine Specific Protein Kinase Receptor Regulation

As with G protein coupled receptors, the tyrosine specific protein kinase receptors undergo homologous and heterologous regulation that is mediated by several different mechanisms. As with G protein coupled receptors, receptor phosphorylation has a well studied and important role. In general tyrosine phosphorylation of the receptor tends to stimulate its activity while serine or threonine phosphorylation tends to inhibit it.

Upon binding hormone, receptors are rapidly internalized by an endocytic process and may be sequestered or degraded. The net effect is to decrease the total number of cell surface receptors. Tyrosine kinase activity may contribute to this process, but is probably not essential because some receptor mutants with inactive tyrosine kinase are internalized normally. This is probably one of the most important mechanisms accounting for homologous desensitization following prolonged exposure to high concentrations of hormone.

Hormone binding stimulates tyrosine phosphorylation of the receptor. This results from autophosphorylation and is directly mediated by the receptor tyrosine kinase activity. Autophosphorylation, in turn, has been shown to stimulate the tyrosine kinase activity of several receptors and may possibly prolong or augment the hormone signal.

Hormone binding also stimulates serine-threonine phosphorylation of many of these receptors, which may result in receptor desensitization. This phosphorylation is mediated by extrinsic protein kinases. The identity of these kinases and whether they are somehow activated as a consequence of the receptor tyrosine kinase activity or whether they recognize the hormone bound receptor as is the case with β-adrenergic receptor kinase is not completely clear. In the case of the EGF receptor, protein kinase C, stimulated as a consequence of phosphoinositol breakdown may mediate the serine-threonine phosphorylation, and inhibit receptor function in three ways. It decreases the affinity of EGF binding, decreases tyrosine kinase activity, and causes receptor internalization.

Receptor phosphorylation also is important in heterologous regulation of tyrosine kinase receptors. Some tyrosine kinase receptors are themselves substrates for other tyrosine kinase receptors. For example, the insulin receptor has been shown to phosphorylate the IGF_1 receptor. This would presumably lead to activation of tyrosine kinase of the target receptor and result in positive heterologous regulation. Several tyrosine kinase receptors are substrates for cAMP-dependent protein kinase and protein kinase C. Activation of receptors coupled to adenylate cyclase or phospholipase C would generate second messengers that would activate these kinases and thereby inhibit the activity of tyrosine kinase receptors. Thus in adipocytes, β-adrenergic agonists inhibit the insulin receptor, and in hepatocytes, vasopressin inhibits the EGF receptor.

INTRACELLULAR AND NUCLEAR HORMONE RECEPTORS

Several hormones exert their effects by binding to intracellular receptors (see the box). These receptors

HORMONES WHOSE RECEPTORS ARE TRANSCRIPTIONAL REGULATORS	
Steroid hormones	Sterols-vitamin D
cortisol	Thyroid hormone
aldosterone	Retinoic acid
estrogens	
progesterone	
androgens	

belong to a closely related family of proteins that controls specific gene expression by the hormone-dependent regulation of transcription. Regulation can either be positive or negative as exemplified by T_3 stimulation of growth hormone expression and repression of TSH expression.

Although it is clear that receptors in this family exert their action in the nucleus, their subcellular localization in the basal state is currently debated. For years it was believed that in the basal state, these receptors were localized to the cytoplasm, and only when activated by hormone binding were they translocated to the nucleus. More recent evidence suggests that they may be localized in the nucleus at all times. The hormones that activate these receptors are lipophilic. These hormones freely diffuse through the cell membrane to reach the receptor. However, cell membrane binding sites with different binding affinities have been described for some of these hormones that could play a role in their transport into the cell.

A model of how these receptors are thought to regulate gene expression is presented schematically in Figure 34-5. First, the receptor is activated by binding of hormone. Activated receptor next binds to a specific region of DNA called the *hormone response element* (HRE) that is located near the promoter of a

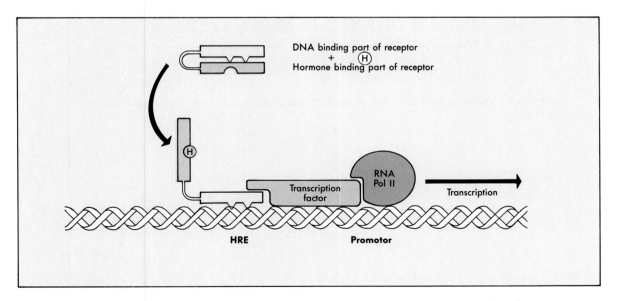

FIGURE 34-5 Nuclear receptors bind to DNA at the hormone response element (HRE) and facilitate (or inhibit) formation of an "active transcription complex" at the promotor. *RNA Pol II*, RNA polymerase II.

target gene. In the case of some steroid receptors, activation is thought to be caused by the dissociation of a heat shock protein that serves as an inhibitory subunit.

Binding of the receptor to the HRE regulates gene expression by either stabilizing (positive regulation) or interfering (repression) with the binding of accessory transcription factors that are necessary for RNA polymerase II to tightly bind to the promoter and initiate transcription. Thus, whether and to what extent a specific gene will respond to one of these hormones depends on the presence of an HRE and on the specific promoter, since different promoters appear to have different requirements for accessory factors. HREs for several receptors in this family have been identified. They are short stretches of DNA. The HREs of different target genes for the same receptor may have slight differences in their sequence, but there is usually a strong consensus. Surprisingly, there is usually considerable flexibility in the position and in some instances the orientation of the HRE with respect to the promoter. These are also properties of viral enhancers that function in a similar manner.

All receptors in this family are homologous and have a similar overall architecture (Figure 34-6). All are single polypeptide chains that contain two particularly highly conserved regions. The most highly conserved is the DNA-binding region. It is rich in cysteines and contains two hypothetical zinc-binding "fingers," which have also been identified in a number of other DNA-binding proteins (Figure 34-7). The carboxyterminal portion of the receptor contains the hormone binding domain. Within this domain is the second highly conserved region. It is particularly well conserved in closely related receptors, for example, those for steroid hormones. The hypervariable aminoterminal region and the hinge region between the two conserved regions are not essential for DNA binding, but they may modify it. In addition, they may contain regions that interact with transcription factors and target the receptors to the nucleus.

Under basal conditions, the unoccupied hormone binding domain inhibits DNA binding. When hormone binds, this inhibition is relieved, resulting in an active receptor. The receptor then binds to DNA and regulates transcription. This was revealed by creating deletion receptor mutants lacking the hormone binding domain. These were constitutively active. Figure 34-5 schematically illustrates this by showing that in the absence of hormone, the hormone-binding domain covers the DNA-binding domain. However, inhibition may result by altering the conformation of the DNA binding domain. Therefore, the nuclear receptors are similar to the tyrosine kinase receptors in

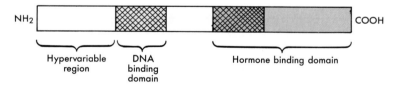

FIGURE 34-6   Structure of the nuclear receptors: cross-hatched areas are particularly highly conserved.

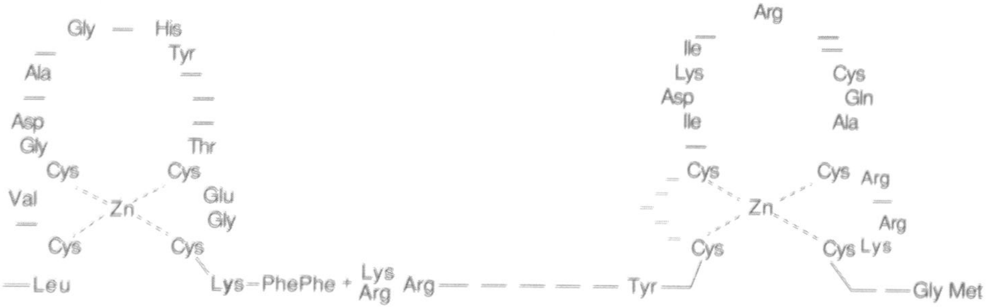

FIGURE 34-7   Hypothetical "zinc fingers" in the DNA binding domain of nuclear receptors. Amino acid residues, for which a strong consensus exists, are indicated. If no consensus exists, residues are indicated by a dash.

that the hormone binding domain inhibits receptor activity, and this inhibition is relieved by hormone binding.

SUMMARY

Much of the early work on the isolation and characterization of receptor proteins was carried out on endocrine hormone receptors. However, many questions are unanswered about the structures, mechanisms of action, and receptor regulation schemes that are relevant for an in-depth understanding of the molecular pharmacology of these systems. The tyrosine kinase receptor system for insulin and the intracellular gene regulation receptors for the adrenal steroid, sex steroid, and thyroid hormones function by mechanisms that differ markedly from those for the cholinergic, adrenergic, ligand-gated ion channel, and many of the other hormone or ligand receptors listed in Table 34-1 or in Table 2-1 in Chapter 2. The diversity of the hormone receptors is demonstrated further by noting the large number of hormones (Table 34-1) that function via G-protein secondary messenger systems. Understanding the molecular basis for the endocrine hormones is particularly important since supplementation or replacement of the endogenous hormone is a pharmacological mode of therapy that is particularly unique to the treatment of endocrine disorders.

REFERENCES

Maxwell BL, McDonnell DP, Conneely OM, et al: Structural organization and regulation of the chicken estrogen receptor, Mol Endocrinol 1:25, 1987.

Sibley DR, Benovic JL, Caron MG, et al: Regulation of transmembrane signaling by receptor phosphorylation, Cell 48(6):913, 1987.

Yarden Y and Ullrich A: Growth factor tyrosine kinases, Ann Rev Biochem 57:443, 1988.

35

Glucocorticoids and Other Adrenal Steroids

THERAPEUTIC OVERVIEW

GLUCOCORTICOIDS
Replacement of cortisol in adrenal insufficiency
Antiinflammatory and immunosuppressive agents
Myeloproliferative diseases
Brain edema

MINERALOCORTICOIDS
Replacement of aldosterone in adrenal insufficiency

 THERAPEUTIC OVERVIEW

The adrenal cortex produces cortisol (hydrocortisone, compound F), which is the main endogenous glucocorticoid in humans. Cortisol is necessary for maintenance of life, and because of this pivotol role, cortisol synthesis and secretion are tightly regulated. The hypothalamic-pituitary-adrenal axis is very sensitive to negative feedback by circulating cortisol or synthetic glucocorticoids. High plasma concentrations of glucocorticoids suppress hypothalamic-pituitary-adrenal activity by decreasing normal endogenous production of cortisol, sometimes for prolonged periods of time. Thus an abrupt cessation of a chronically administered glucocorticoid can result in the simultaneous lack of both endogenous and exogenous glucocorticoids. This situation is potentially life-threatening and may result in serious morbidity and in mortality. Gradual reduction in exogenously administered glucocorticoids may require extended

periods of time, since the hypothalamic-pituitary-adrenal systems may need up to a year to adjust and secrete cortisol at a normal rate in the absence of exogenous glucocorticoids.

The key mineralocorticoid aldosterone is also synthesized and secreted by the adrenal cortex and serves as a primary regulator of extracellular fluid volume and a major determinant of potassium metabolism.

The main therapeutic uses of glucocorticoids and mineralocorticoids are (1) replacement of cortisol for adrenal insufficiency (i.e., inadequate endogenous production of cortisol); (2) short- or long-term antiinflammatory/immunosuppression; (3) part of a multiregimen treatment of myeloproliferative diseases, other malignancies, or brain edema; and (4) replacement of aldosterone for adrenal insufficiency. The key therapeutic uses of the glucocorticoids and mineralocorticoids are summarized in the box.

MECHANISMS OF ACTION

Adrenal Glands

The adult human adrenal gland is composed of two parts: the cortex or outer part, which represents 90% of the weight, and the medulla or center part of the gland. The cortex is made up of three zones: the zona glomerulosa (outermost), the zona fasciculata (middle), and the zona reticularis (innermost, next to the medulla). Glucocorticoids are synthesized mainly in the zona fasciculata (which constitutes 75% of the weight of the adrenal gland) and mineralocorticoids in the zona glomerulosa.

Synthesis of Glucocorticoids and Mineralocorticoids

Most of the cholesterol utilized by the adrenal gland in the synthesis of cortisol or aldosterone is taken up from the blood rather than synthesized *de novo* in the adrenal cortex, although the cortex has the ability to synthesize cholesterol. Blood cholesterol is carried by both low-density and high-density lipoproteins, and the adrenal cortex has receptors for these lipoproteins. In humans, low-density lipoprotein is the major source of adrenal cholesterol. The uptake of circulating cholesterol and the *de novo* synthesis of cholesterol are interchangeable as the source of cholesterol, so that blockade of one or the other causes no significant decrease in cortisol or aldosterone biosynthesis.

In the adrenals, cholesterol is esterified and stored inside cytoplasmic lipid droplets. Activation of a cytoplasmic cholesterol ester hydrolase causes the transport of cholesterol into the mitochondria by a sterol carrier protein, where it is converted to pregnenolone. This reaction series requires NADPH and oxygen and involves removal of a portion of the side chain from carbon-17 and addition of carbonyl oxygen at position 20. The structures and synthesis pathways are outlined in Figure 35-1.

In the zona fasciculata pregnenolone is transferred from the mitochondria to the smooth endoplasmic reticulum where most of it is hydroxylated by the 17α-hydroxylase enzyme into 17α-hydroxypregnenolone, which in turn is converted to 17α-hydroxyprogesterone through replacement of a 5,6 double bond by a 4,5 double bond. The latter reaction is catalyzed by the 3β-hydroxysteroid dehydrogenase/Δ^5-isomerase

enzyme complex. A small percentage of pregnenolone is first converted by this enzyme complex to progesterone and then hydroxylated at the 17 position to 17α-hydroxyprogesterone. 17α-Hydroxyprogesterone is a strategically located steroid. In the zona fasciculata, this compound undergoes two successive hydroxylations. First, it is hydroxylated at position 21 by the 21-hydroxylase enzyme (located in the endoplasmic reticulum) resulting in 11-deoxycortisol (also called compound S). Compound S is then hydroxylated at position 11 by the 11β-hydroxylase enzyme (located inside the mitochondria) to cortisol (also called compound F). In the zona reticularis 17α-hydroxyprogesterone follows the pathway leading to the synthesis of adrenal androgens. In contrast to the above two zonae, zona glomerulosa has no 17α-hydroxylase enzyme and thus all pregnenolone is transformed to progesterone, which in turn follows the pathway for the synthesis of the mineralocorticoid, aldosterone. Cortisol and aldosterone are the major components of these synthesis pathways as carried out in the adrenal cortex.

The regulation of cortisol synthesis and secretion is by the pituitary hormone corticotropin (ACTH). ACTH is synthesized and secreted by the corticotrophs of the adenohypophysis, as discussed in Chapter 41. Pituitary ACTH is secreted in the peripheral circulation and reaches ACTH receptors located on the surface of the adrenocortical cells. ACTH interacts with these receptors and initiates a cAMP-dependent increase of the transcription of almost all enzymes involved in cortisol biosynthesis, which results in the acute increase of both cortisol production and secretion. In addition, ACTH acts as a growth factor on the adrenal cortex so that a decrease of plasma ACTH results not only in a decrease of cortisol synthesis and secretion, but also in the gradual atrophy of the adrenal cortex. Pituitary production of ACTH is very sensitive to suppression by exogenous glucocorticoids. Manipulations of this system for therapeutic purposes should be approached with the utmost care, since chronic administration of exogenous glucocorticoids represents a potentially life-threatening situation.

Most ACTH is released as a series of secretory episodes followed by an equal number of bursts in cortisol concentration in plasma. These secretory episodes of ACTH and cortisol are characterized by a sharp rise of plasma concentrations followed by a slower decline. In a 24-hour period approximately 15

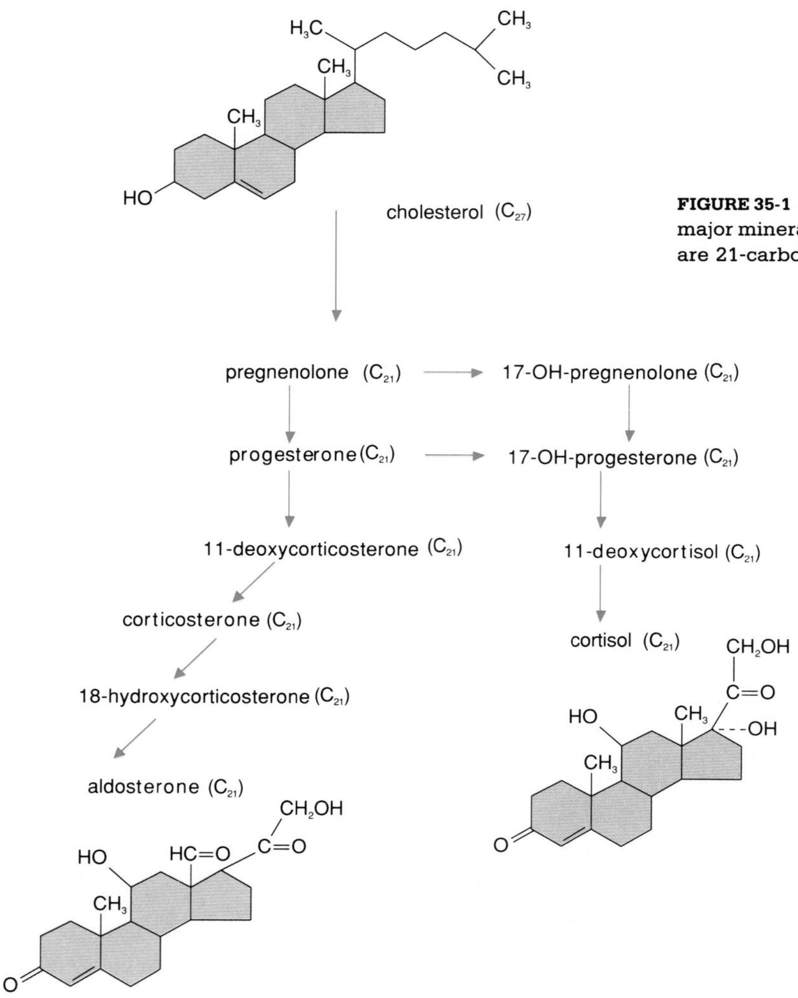

FIGURE 35-1   Synthesis of major glucocorticoid (cortisol) and major mineralocorticoid (aldosterone) by adrenal cortex. Both are 21-carbon steroids derived from cholesterol.

to 20 such ACTH and cortisol peaks occur (Figure 35-2). A circadian periodicity in the frequency and the magnitude of these secretory episodes is present, with generally greatest frequency during the early morning hours and less frequency in the late afternoon.

Glucocorticoid Receptor

All natural and synthetic glucocorticoids act by binding to a specific cytoplasmic glucocorticoid receptor. This receptor is a protein of about 800 amino acids and can be divided into three domains (see Chapter 34). The glucocorticoid binding domain is located near the carboxy-terminus region of the molecule and is where the ligand binds. The DNA-bind-

ing domain is located in the middle of the protein and contains nine cysteine residues. This region folds into a "two-finger" structure stabilized by zinc ions connected to cysteines to form two tetrahedrons. This part of the molecule binds to specific sites on DNA, called glucocortoid-responsive elements, which regulate glucocorticoid action of glucocorticoid-regulated genes. The zinc-fingers represent the basic structure by which the DNA-binding domain recognizes specific nucleic acid sequences. The amino-terminus domain of the receptor is highly antigenic, but its exact function is unknown. It may confer further specificity to the glucocorticoid–glucocorticoid receptor complex.

The inactive forms of the glucocorticoid receptors are located in the cytoplasm as polymers bound with

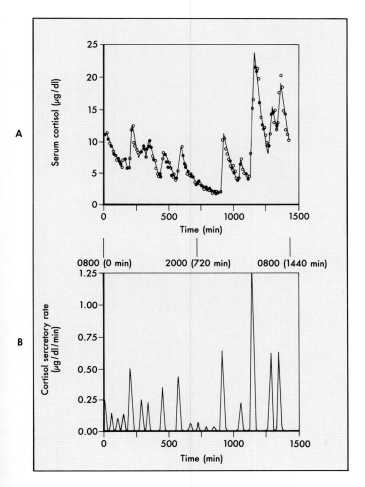

FIGURE 35-2   Serum cortisol concentrations in a healthy man. Serial blood samples collected at 10-minute intervals were assayed for serum cortisol concentrations. **A,** Concentrations plotted, with continuous line calculated using a special multiple parameter model of combined secretion and clearance of cortisol. **B,** Calculated rates of cortisol secretion as a function of time. Zero minutes = 0800 = start of experimental period. (Modified from Veldhuis JD, Iranmanesh A, Lizarralde G, and Johnson ML, Am J Physiol 257:E6, 1989.)

other proteins, one of which is the heat shock protein 90. These polymers are unable to exert any effect. Binding of a glucocorticoid to its receptor activates the receptor by changing the spatial conformation of the inactive protein. Activations include dissociation of the receptor from the heat shock on other carrier protein and a change in conformation of the hormone-binding domain. The activated glucocorticoid ligand-receptor complex then enters the nucleus (translocation) where its hormone-binding domain binds to DNA glucocorticoid-responsive elements and alters the transcription of specific genes.

Aldosterone Release and Action

Aldosterone is the main mineralocorticoid produced by the renal cortex. It acts mainly at the distal portion of the convoluted renal tubule, where it causes a decrease in the urinary elimination of Na^+ ions while allowing K^+ ions to be excreted. Aldosterone promotes the reabsorption of Na^+ (see Chapter 19 for extensive discussion). The release of aldosterone is controlled by (1) the renin-angiotesion system, (2) the concentration of K^+ ions, and (3) the concentration of ACTH, as discussed earlier.

Clinically Used Glucocorticoids and Mineralocorticoids

Structures of the principal clinically used agents are given in Figures 35-1 and 35-3.

 PHARMACOKINETICS

The pharmacokinetic parameter values for most of the clinically used glucocorticoids and mineralocorticoids are summarized in Table 35-1.

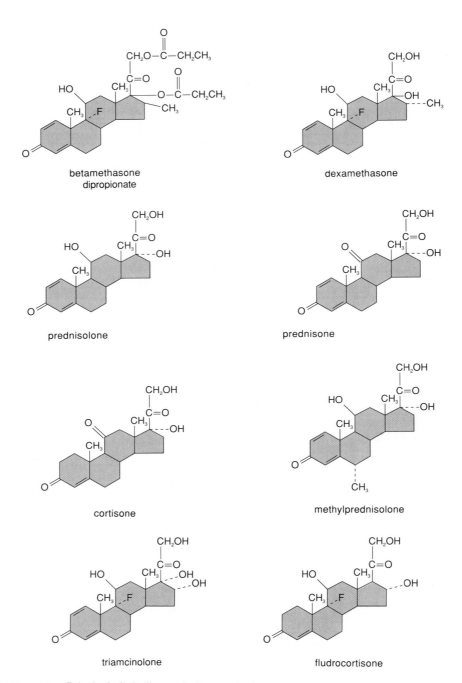

FIGURE 35-3   Principal clinically used glucocorticoids and mineralocorticoids (see also Figure 35-1).

Table 35-1 Pharmacokinetic Parameters

Drugs	Administration	$t_{1/2}$	Disposition
GLUCOCORTICOIDS			
cortisol*	IM, IV, oral +	Short	M
cortisone	Oral, IM, IV	Short	M
prednisone	Oral	Intermediate	M
prednisolone	IM, IV	Intermediate	M
methylprednisolone	IM, IV, oral †	Intermediate	M
dexamethasone	IM, oral,† topical, IV	Long	M
betamethasone	Oral, topical	Long	M
triamcinolone	Intraarticular, topical	Long	M
MINERALOCORTICOIDS			
fludrocortisone	Oral	Intermediate	M
aldosterone (for reference)	—	Short	M
desoxycorticosterone acetate	IM	Long	M

Short, 10-90 minutes; *intermediate*, several hours; *long*, 5 hours or more. M, Metabolism.
*Same as hydrocortisone.
†Intralesional, intraarticular.

The most important pharmacokinetic factors affecting the therapeutic activity of the various glucocorticoids are (1) the absorption rate from the site of application (digestive tract, skin, inhalation), (2) the plasma half-life (which is affected by binding to the plasma cortisol-binding globulin and its rate of metabolism by liver enzymes), and (3) its bioavailability. Glucocorticoids are active only if they have a hydroxy group at carbon-11. Thus cortisone and prednisone must undergo in vivo hydroxylation to cortisol and prednisolone, respectively, to become active.

Most glucocorticoids are rapidly and readily absorbed from the gastrointestinal tract, but absorption through the skin varies among preparations. In most cases skin absorption of glucocorticoids is slow enough to limit significant systemic accumulation of drug.

In plasma, 75% of the circulating cortisol is reversibly bound with high affinity to cortisol-binding globulin, 15% to albumin, with approximately 10% in the free unbound form. Bound cortisol is inactive. Conditions such as pregnancy or estrogen therapy that may lead to altered concentrations of plasma cortisol-binding globulin can alter total plasma cortisol concentrations. Thus pregnancy and estrogen therapy are associated with elevated total plasma cortisol concentrations. Cortisol-binding globulin also binds other endogenous steroids such as progesterone, deoxycortisol, and deoxycorticosterone and to a lesser degree synthetic steroids such as prednisone and prednisolone but not dexamethasone. This means that close to 100% of a given concentration of circulating dexamethasone is in the free form.

The liver and kidneys are the major sites of glucocorticoid inactivation by metabolism. The pathways leading to inactivation include reduction of the double bond at position 4-5, reduction of the keto group at carbon-3, and hydroxylation at carbon-6. About 30% of the inactivated cortisol is conjugated to form the tetrahydrocortisol- and tetrahydrodeoxycortisol-glucuronides and the conjugated products excreted in the urine.

Another important cortisol inactivation pathway takes place in the kidneys and involves oxidation to cortisone by the 11-ketosteroid reductase/11β-dehydroxysteroid dehydrogenase enzyme complex. Cortisone does not bind to the kidney mineralocorticoid receptor and thus does not exert a salt-retaining effect, although a newly described syndrome has been observed in which this enzyme complex appears not to function efficiently, resulting in salt retention, hypokalemia, and hypertension.

RELATION OF MECHANISMS OF ACTION TO CLINICAL RESPONSE

Glucocorticoid Effects

The primary therapeutic application of glucocorticoids is in replacement for adrenal insufficiency, for actions on the immune system and for antiinflammatory effects. Mineralocorticoids also may be needed to overcome adrenal insufficiency, particularly in Addison's disease. Since glucocorticoids regulate such a large number of physiological processes and affect almost every type of tissue, the differences between normal physiological responses and unwanted side effects from exogenous glucocorticoids appear to be quantitative rather than qualitative in nature. Thus an otherwise physiological effect of a given glucocorticoid is potentiated if this hormone is given in pharmacological doses or over prolonged periods of time.

Glucocorticoids affect the immune system at multiple levels: (1) neutrophil traffic, (2) antigen processing, (3) eosinopenia, and (4) lymphatic atrophy. Within hours after administration of glucocorticoids the number of circulating neutrophils increases as a result of alterations on their trafficking dynamics. The neutrophilia may result from glucocorticoid-induced decrease of neutrophil adherence to vascular endothelium and the inability of neutrophils to egress toward bone marrow or inflammatory sites. They inhibit antigen processing by the macrophages, suppress T-cell helper function, inhibit synthesis of cellular mediators of the inflammatory response (i.e., interleukins and other cytokines and prostanoids), and inhibit phagocytosis. Glucocorticoids in addition stabilize lysosomal membranes and induce eosinopenia and lymphopenia. These latter effects may be due to modification of production, distribution, and/or cell lysis and are more profound on T rather than B lymphocytes. They may explain the beneficial effect of glucocorticoids in the treatment of certain leukemias such as acute lymphoblastic leukemia of childhood. Chronic administration of glucocorticoids results in a reversible atrophy of the lymphatic system, including spleen and thymus.

Therapeutically, the most important effect of glucocorticoids is their inhibitory effect on accumulation of neutrophils and monocytes at sites of inflammation and suppression of their phagocytic, bacteriocidal, and antigen-processing activity. These effects compromise the immune system and predispose the patient to several common and/or uncommon pathogens. This represents the single most dangerous complication of chronic glucocorticoid treatment.

Other Glucocorticoid Effects

Although pharmacological doses of glucocorticoids may decrease the secretion of growth hormone from the anterior pituitary, children on chronic glucocorticoid therapy have normal plasma growth hormone and somatomedin C concentrations, while their growth is impaired. It now appears that this action of glucocorticoids may be due to inhibition of the effects of somatomedin C directly or to release of somatomedin C inhibitors by the liver.

Glucocorticoids influence the conversion of norepinephrine to epinephrine, as carried out in the adrenal medulla. The adrenal cortex surrounds the chromaffin-containing adrenal medulla. Postnatally, most of the chromaffin cells degenerate except for those that remain to form the adrenal medulla. Most of the plasma epinephrine and some norepinephrine derive from the adrenal medulla. The latter receives the adrenocortical venous effluent and thus, is normally exposed to high concentrations of endogenous cortisol. The cortisol in the adrenocortical venous effluent regulates the enzyme phenylethanolamine N-methyltransferase (see Chapter 8), which catalyzes the conversion of norepinephrine to epinephrine and which is located exclusively in the adrenal medulla and the organ of Zuckerkandl.

Mineralocorticoid Effects

The various glucocorticoids exhibit different affinities towards the mineralocorticoid receptor. Glucocorticoid-induced activation of the mineralocorticoid receptor causes elevation of blood pressure, sodium retention, and potassium and hydrogen ion excretion from the kidneys. In severe cases, patients develop hypertension and hypokalemic alkalosis. Cortisol and indirectly cortisone have the highest mineralocorticoid activity. Dexamethasone and betamethasone have minimal mineralocorticoid activity while prednisone and prednisolone have very limited activity.

Selection of Drugs

Cortisol and cortisone are used only for replacement therapy in patients with adrenal insufficiency (i.e., diminished production of endogenous glucocorticoids). They have no role in any antiinflammatory therapeutic regimen because of their high mineralocorticoid activity versus their relatively low antiinflammatory activity.

Prednisone, prednisolone, and methylprednisolone, on the other hand, have good antiinflammatory activity, intermediate plasma half-lives, and relatively low mineralocorticoid activity. These characteristics make them first choice drugs for chronic antiinflammatory/immunosuppressant therapeutic regimens. Indeed, prednisone and its derivatives are the most commonly used glucocorticoids for the treatment of a number of autoimmune diseases, such as (1) collagen diseases (systemic lupus erythematosus, polymyositis-dermatomyositis, and rheumatoid arthritis; (2) vasculitis syndromes (polyarteritis nodosa, giant cell arteritis, and Wegener's granulomatosis; (3) gastrointestinal inflammatory diseases (Crohn's disease or ulcerative colitis); and (4) renal autoimmune diseases (glomerulonephritis and nephrotic syndrome). Intermediate action glucocorticoids are also used in the treatment of bronchial asthma and chronic obstructive pulmonary disease.

Dexamethasone and betamethasone exhibit minimal mineralocorticoid activity, maximal antiinflammatory activity, prolonged plasma activity, and marked growth-suppressing properties. They represent the best choice in cases where a maximum antiinflammatory therapy is needed acutely (e.g., in cases of septic shock or brain edema). Because of their long duration of activity (i.e., prolonged suppression of hypothalamus and anterior pituitary) and because of their growth suppression and bone demineralization properties, dexamethasone and betamethasone are not first choice drugs for chronic antiinflammatory treatment.

Alternate-day glucocorticoid administration presents both advantages and problems. The antiinflammatory effect of intermediate duration of action glucocorticoids persists longer than the suppressive effect on the hypothalamic-pituitary axis and growth rate. Therefore by administering prednisone or prednisolone every other day, suppression of the hypothalamus and anterior pituitary can be lessened and growth suppression can be avoided, while an acceptable and beneficial antiinflammatory effect can be achieved. However, there are two potential problems. In some patients the antiinflammatory effect of an alternate-day glucocorticoid therapeutic regimen may not be sufficient to control the inflammation, and

an abrupt switch from a daily dose of glucocorticoids to an alternate day regimen may cause symptoms and signs of clinical hypocortisolism (sense of being tired, nausea, vomiting, or hypotension) on the days that no dose of glucocorticoid is taken.

For replacement therapy to supply mineralocorticoid, aldosterone is not used because the rate of degradation in the circulation is too rapid. Instead, a 9-fluorocortisol is used because this binds to the mineralocorticoid receptor in the renal tubule and also has a prolonged duration of action, as compared to aldosterone.

SIDE EFFECTS, CLINICAL PROBLEMS, AND TOXICITY

The primary clinical problems in the therapeutic use of glucocorticoids and mineralocorticoids are listed in the box.

Glucocorticoid Side Effects on Calcium Metabolism

One of the major side effects of glucocorticoids, especially if given in pharmacological doses and for prolonged periods of time, is their detrimental action on bone. Glucocorticoids cause osteoporosis by dis-

---

CLINICAL PROBLEMS

Side effects caused mainly by high (pharmacological as compared to physiological) concentrations and for long times

Most common side effects:

Development of Cushingoid habitus (trunkal obesity, moon facies, buffalo hump), salt retention, and hypertension (i.e. iatrogenic Cushing's syndrome)

Suppression of the immune system (rendering the patient vulnerable to common and opportunistic infections)

Osteoporosis (rendering the patient vulnerable to fractures)

Peptic ulcers (resulting in gastric hemorrhages and/or intestinal perforation)

Suppression of growth in children

Behavioral problems

Reproductive problems

Prolonged suppression of the hypothalamic-pituitary-adrenal axis after drug discontinuation

rupting the regulation of calcium metabolism at several levels. They do this by (1) decreasing absorption and renal reabsorption of calcium, (2) a direct action on bone, and (3) blockade of calcitonin effects.

Although the mechanism is not clear, glucocorticoids block vitamin D-mediated calcium intestinal absorption and renal reabsorption. Glucocorticoids increase the plasma concentration of the active vitamin D form by promoting the 1α-hydroxylation of the 25-hydroxy vitamin D to the active metabolite 1,25-dihydroxy vitamin D. The combination of decreased intestinal absorption and decreased renal reabsorption of calcium results in a glucocorticoid-induced tendency for hypocalcemia. The parathyroid gland responds to hypocalcemia by increasing the secretion of parathyroid hormone, which catabolizes bone to release calcium into the circulation. This is performed (1) by stimulating the acute removal of bone calcium by osteocytes (cells deriving from osteoblasts) and the acute bone "reabsorption" from preexisting osteoclasts (i.e., cells that secrete enzymes that remove both calcium and organic matrix from bones), (2) by stimulating the differentiation of precursor cells into osteoclasts, and (3) by inhibiting the synthesis of bone matrix (i.e., collagen biosynthesis) by osteoblasts. Glucocorticoids appear also to act directly on bones. They inhibit osteoblastic activity as documented by the low concentrations of osteocalcin, a protein produced by osteoblasts, and stimulate osteolysis by increasing the number of osteoclasts (i.e., increasing the transformation of precursor cells to osteoclasts). This increase in the number of osteoclasts results in increased bone resorption, as documented by the increased concentrations of urine hydroxyproline, an index of increased bone collagen catabolism. Finally, glucocorticoids block the bone-sparing effects of calcitonin, a 32-amino acid peptide synthesized by the parafollicular cells of the thyroid gland that inhibits osteoclastic bone resorption (see Chapter 42).

Patients with the highest risk of developing glucocorticoid-induced osteoporosis are children and postmenopausal women. This osteoporosis involves the trabecular part of the bones since these are the most metabolically active sites, and bones rich in trabecular areas (e.g., the vertebrae) are the most vulnerable to glucocorticoid effects. Interestingly, glucocorticoid-induced osteoporosis in young individuals can be reversed after discontinuation of the medication.

Glucocorticoid Side Effects on CNS, Gastrointestinal Tract, Glucose Metabolism, and Hypothalamic-pituitary Suppression

The main acute CNS action of glucocorticoids is stimulation of arousal and provision of a multidirected negative feedback system responsible for harnessing the stress response. High plasma concentrations of glucocorticoids affect the electrical activity of the brain as documented by alterations of the electroencephalogram. Although the earliest manifestation of high plasma glucocorticoid concentrations is euphoria, chronic hypercortisolism is accompanied by depression, sleep disturbances, and, in some cases, true psychotic ideation.

Chronic administration of high doses of glucocorticoids increases the incidence of peptic ulcers. The exact mechanism is unknown but glucocorticoids inhibit the synthesis of mucopolysaccharides that protect the gastric mucosa from acid and increase gastric acid output response to histamine. Because even short (less than a month) administration of glucocorticoids may be ulcerogenic, some physicians routinely prescribe antacid or cimetidine treatment when they administer glucocorticoids (see Chapters 58 and 59).

Glucocorticoids obtained their name from the profound role on glucose metabolism. Glucocorticoids increase plasma glucose by (1) increasing gluconeogenesis and glucose secretion by the liver, (2) increasing the sensitivity of the liver to the gluconeogenic action of glucagon and catecholamines, (3) decreasing glucose uptake and utilization by peripheral tissues, and (4) increasing substrates for gluconeogenesis, by increasing proteolysis and inhibiting protein synthesis in muscles.

Suppression of the hypothalamic-pituitary-adrenal axis is the most common side effect of chronic glucocorticoid therapy. The suppressive effect of glucocorticoids on the hypothalamic-pituitary-adrenal axis appears within days after starting glucocorticoid treatment. Any patient who has received glucocorticoid doses equivalent to more than 5 mg of prednisone daily for more than 2 weeks should be considered to have a suppressed hypothalamic-pituitary-adrenal axis. The time needed for the axis to recover depends on the type of glucocorticoid given, the dose and frequency of administration (i.e., daily versus alternate days), and the length of treatment. In cases of prolonged glucocorticoid administration, recovery may take a year or longer. Chronic suppression of the hypothalamic-pituitary-adrenal axis is primarily a result of defective corticotropin-releasing hormone secretion.

Pharmacological doses of glucocorticoids also act on the hypothalamic-pituitary-gonadal axis by inhibiting the secretion of gonadotropins, suppressing the effect of gonadotropins on the gonads, and affecting the action of sex steroids on their target tissues. In men, chronic treatment with pharmacological doses of glucocorticoids produces some degree of hypogonadism associated with decreased plasma testosterone. In women, glucocorticoids may cause ovulation disturbances and thus dysfunctional uterine bleeding and/or oligoamenorrhea.

TRADENAMES

In addition to generic and fixed combination preparations, the following tradenamed materials are available in the United States.

Aristocort, Kenalog, triamcinolone
Carmol HC, Cortogen, Hydrocortone, Cortril, Cortef, Hydrocort, hydrocortisone and cortisol and related esters
Decadron, Hexadrol, dexamethasone
Deltasone, prednisone
Fluorinef, fludrocortisone
Maxivate, Celestone, Diprolene, Betatrex, betamethasone
Methapred, Depo-Medrol, methylprednisolone and esters

REFERENCES

Evans RM: The steroid and thyroid hormone receptor superfamily, Science 240: 889, 1988.

Taylor AL and Fishman LM: Corticotropin-releasing hormone, N Engl J Med 319: 213, 1988.

CHAPTER 36 Estrogens, Progestins, and Oral Contraceptives

ABBREVIATIONS	
CBG	cortisol binding globulin
DNA	deoxyribonucleic acid
FSH	follicle stimulating hormone
GI	gastrointestinal
GNRH	gonadotropin-releasing hormone
LDL	low density lipoprotein
LH	luteinizing hormone
RBA	relative binding affinity
RNA	ribonucleic acid
SHBG	sex hormone binding globulin
HDL	high density lipoprotein

THERAPEUTIC OVERVIEW

The two major classes of female sex hormones are the estrogens and the progestins. Together they serve important functions in the development of female secondary sex characteristics, the control of pregnancy, the control of the ovulatory/menstrual cycle, and the modulation of many metabolic processes.

Estrogens

There are three natural human estrogens: 17β-estradiol, the principal ovarian estrogens; estriol, the principal placental estrogen; and estrone, a metabolite of 17β-estradiol and a major ovarian and postmenopausal estrogen.

Estrogens coordinate the systemic responses during the ovulatory cycle, including regulation of the reproductive tract, pituitary, breasts, and other tissues. They also play a role in progression of some tumors. The target organs for hormone action are shown in Figure 36-1, with the hypothalamic/pituitary/ovarian organs shown in Figure 36-1, *A* and the target tissues for estrogen and progesterone shown in Figure 36-1, *B*.

Estrogens are also responsible for the development of secondary sex characteristics when a female enters puberty, including the progressive development of the fallopian tubes, uterus, vagina, and external genitalia. With estrogen stimulation, fat deposition increases in the breast, buttocks, and thighs, leading to the characteristic female habitus. Estrogens also (1) initiate breast development by increasing ductal and stromal growth, (2) contribute to accelerated growth at puberty, (3) stimulate closure of the epiphyses in the shafts of the long bones, (4) stimulate synthesis and secretation of prolactin from pituitary lactotrophs, (5) produce increased cellular proliferation of uterine endometrium and stroma, in the absence of progesterone as occurs in the follicular phase of the menstrual cycle, (6) induce RNA and protein synthesis in cells, (7) generate thickening of vaginal mucosa and thinning of cervical mucus, (8) aid in maintaining bone mass, as evidenced by substantial but preventable (with estrogen replacement therapy) bone loss in postmenopausal women, (9) stimulate hepatic production of sex hormone-binding globulin, thyroid-binding globulin, blood-clotting factors (VII to X) plasminogen, and high density lipoprotein (HDL) but inhibit antithrombin III and low density lipoprotein (LDL) formation.

Estrogens also increase retention of sodium and

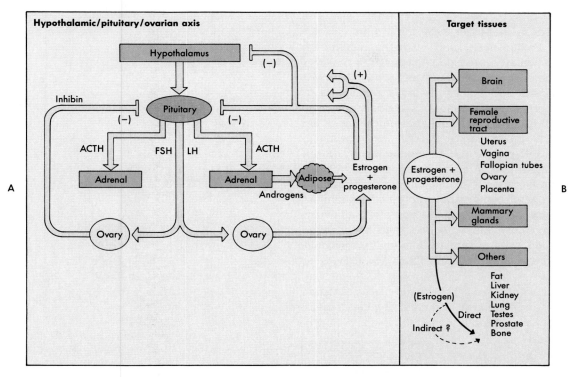

FIGURE 36-1   Feedback loops and target tissues. **A**, Schematic diagram demonstrating negative and positive feedback action of estrogens and progesterone on the hypothalamic/pituitary/ovarian axis. **B**, Other target tissues for these steroid hormones. *GnRH*, Gonadotropin-releasing hormone.

water, occasionally causing edema and decreasing bowel motility.

Estrogens may play a direct role in the progression of some endometrial tumors, and estrogen or antiestrogen therapy is used in the treatment of breast cancer and some prostate tumors. Continuous exposure of the uterus to unopposed estrogen results in abnormal endometrial hyperplasia with episodes of breakthrough bleeding and increased incidence of endometrial cancer.

Progestins

The important natural progestin is progesterone, but 17α-, 20α-, and 20β-hydroxyprogesterone have weak progestational activities. Progesterone is partially responsible for glandular development and may play a role in ductal growth. Progesterone concentrations rise rapidly in the luteal phase of the menstrual cycle, resulting in modulation of estrogen's action on

the uterus. Under the influence of progesterone, the estrogen-primed uterus initiates secretory changes in preparation for embryo implantation. Without estrogen, progesterone receptor concentrations are low and estrogen priming is necessary for progesterone receptor induction in almost all progesterone-responsive tissues, including the uterus. Progesterone is responsible for increased basal body temperature observed in the luteal phase. In the absence of pregnancy, plasma progesterone concentrations fall, resulting in sloughing of the endometrial lining. A variety of disorders of the menstrual cycle are treated with estrogens, progestins, or a combination of both.

Progesterone also (1) aids in the maintenance of pregnancy, (2) inhibits uterine contraction, (3) can alter carbohydrate metabolism, (4) may lead to decreased HDL and increased LDL concentrations, and (5) increases sodium and water elimination through competition with aldosterone for binding to mineralocorticoid receptors.

Combined Effects

There are several other ways these hormones act together. Progesterone and estrogen coordinate events associated with the luteal phase of the ovulatory cycle and pregnancy. In primary hypogonadism, estrogens and progestins are administered to optimize normal development of secondary sex characteristics. An important pharmacological use of estrogens and progestins is as oral contraceptives. Estrogens and progestins act predominantly to decrease the production of the gonadotropins, follicle-stimulating hormone (FSH), and luteinizing hormone (LH) at the pituitary-hypothalamic axis. This inhibits the midcycle LH surge and thereby prevents ovulation. Interestingly, antiestrogens have been developed that aid in the treatment of infertility by inducing an increase in circulating FSH, which leads to ovulation.

A summary of the major therapeutic uses of steroid hormones, antihormones, and steroidogenesis inhibitors is shown in the box.

THERAPEUTIC OVERVIEW

FERTILITY CONTROL

Combination oral contraception (estrogens, progestins)
Progestin-only contraception (progestins)
Postcoital contraception (estrogens, progestins)
Contragestation (antiprogestins)

HORMONE REPLACEMENT THERAPY

Menopause (estrogens, progestins [?])
Osteoporosis (estrogens, progestins [?])
Ovarian failure (estrogens, progestins)
Dysfunctional uterine bleeding (progestins, estrogens)
Luteal phase dysfunction (progestins)

OVULATION INDUCTION

Infertility (clomiphene citrate)

CANCER CHEMOTHERAPY

Breast cancer (estrogens, progestins, antiestrogens, steroidogenesis inhibitors)
Endometrial cancer (progestins, antiestrogens [?])
Prostate cancer (estrogens)

OTHERS

Endometriosis (danazol, progestins GNRH)
Diagnostic use (progestins)

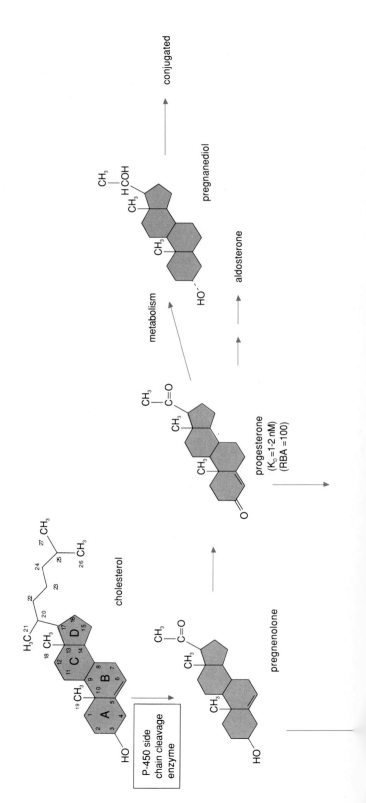

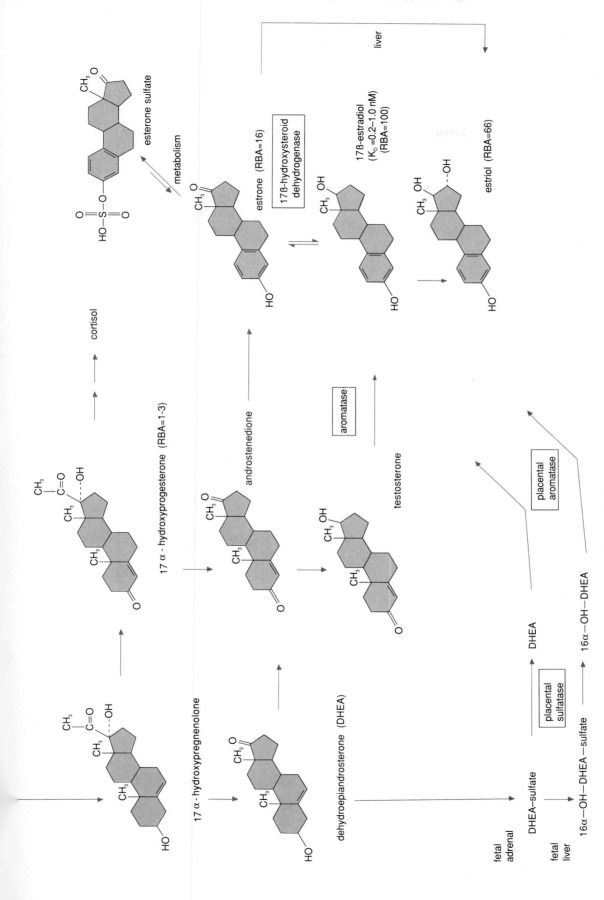

FIGURE 36-2 Steroidogenesis. Biosynthetic pathways of progesterone and the natural estrogens are illustrated. Included are the absolute binding affinities of progesterone and estradiol for their respective receptors and the relative-binding affinities (RBA) of estrone and estriol when that of estradiol is set at 100%. Also shown are important metabolites of progesterone and the estrogens. Illustrated in the boxed area is the pathway of estrogen production in the fetal-placental unit. Natural estrogens and progestins are highlighted.

MECHANISMS OF ACTION

Ligand Structure

Estrogens can be classified as either steroidal or nonsteroidal, with steroidal estrogens further divided into natural and synthetic compounds. The natural estrogens and progestins are steroids with structures derived from cholesterol. The most common natural human estrogens and some of the most frequently used synthetic ligands are shown in Figures 36-2 and 36-3.

The natural estrogens include estradiol, estrone, and estriol. They have 18 carbon atoms with an aromatic A ring, a methyl group at C13, a phenolic hydroxyl at C3, and a ketone or hydroxyl group at C17. Natural estrogens have low potency when administered orally, as they are poorly absorbed and rapidly inactivated by the liver. Estradiol is the most potent of the three.

The conjugated estrogens are coupled at C3 pre-

Steroidal agonists

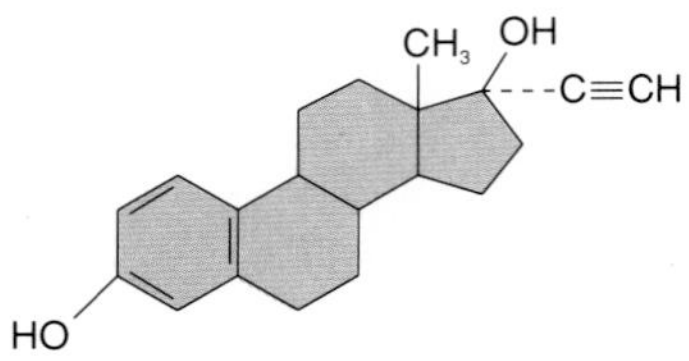

ethinyl estradiol
(RBA = 158)

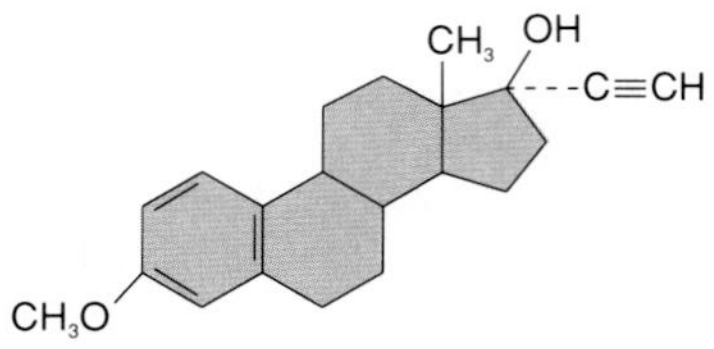

mestranol
(RBA=0.7)

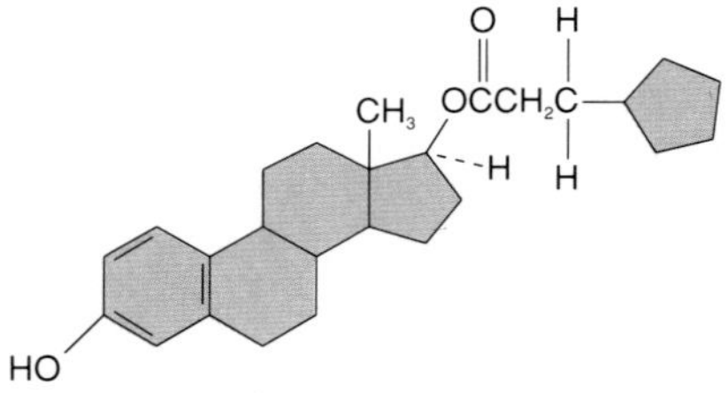

estradiol cypionate

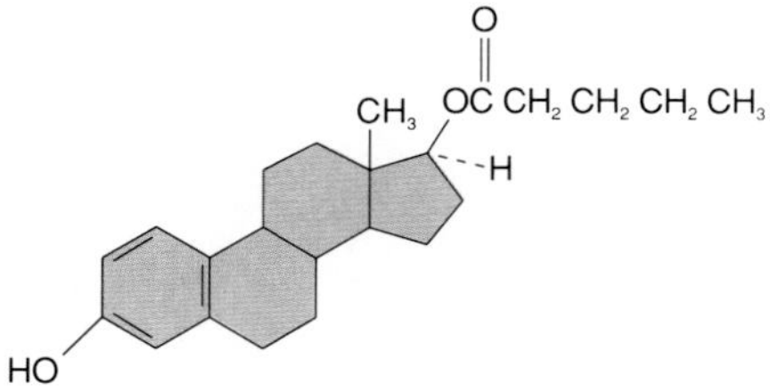

estradiol valerate

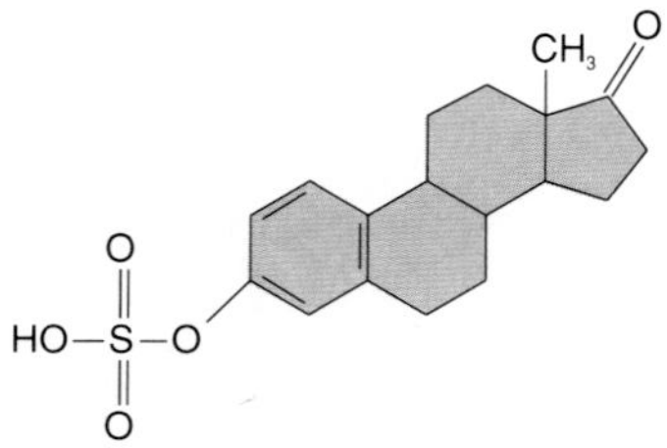

estrone sulfate

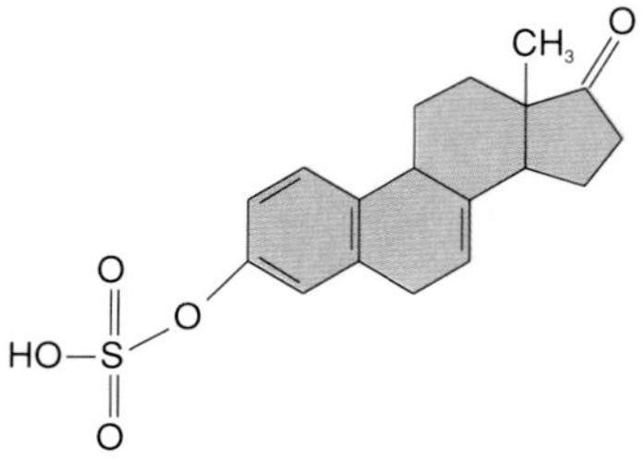

equilin sulfate

FIGURE 36-3   Commonly used estrogens and antiestrogens. Structures for a number of ligands for the estrogen receptor are shown. The relative binding affinity (*RBA*) for the ligand to the estrogen receptor, as compared to estradiol, is also shown (RBA for estradiol, 100%). Mestranol is converted to ethinylestradiol. Esterified estrogens are hydrolyzed and converted to active species.

dominantly to sulfate, but occasionally to glucuronic acid. Conjugated estrogens are prepared directly from pregnant mare's urine to give estrogen and equilin sulfates—equilin is an estrogen found in horses but not in humans—and they can also be synthesized to give estrone sulfate contents of 80% to 85% and are often referred to as esterified estrogens. Water-soluble conjugated estrogens have virtually no estrogenic activity and must be activated (hydrolyzed at C3) to be able to bind to the estrogen receptor.

The synthetic steroidal estrogens include orally active ethinyl estradiol and mestranol, used predominantly in combination oral contraceptives. Ethinyl estradiol and mestranol have an ethinyl group at C17 that protects against inactivation by the liver. Mestranol is inactive until converted to ethinyl estradiol in the liver. Other orally active synthetic steroids include estropipate and quinestrol.

The parenteral synthetic steroids include estradiol cypionate, estradiol valerate, and polyestradiol phos-

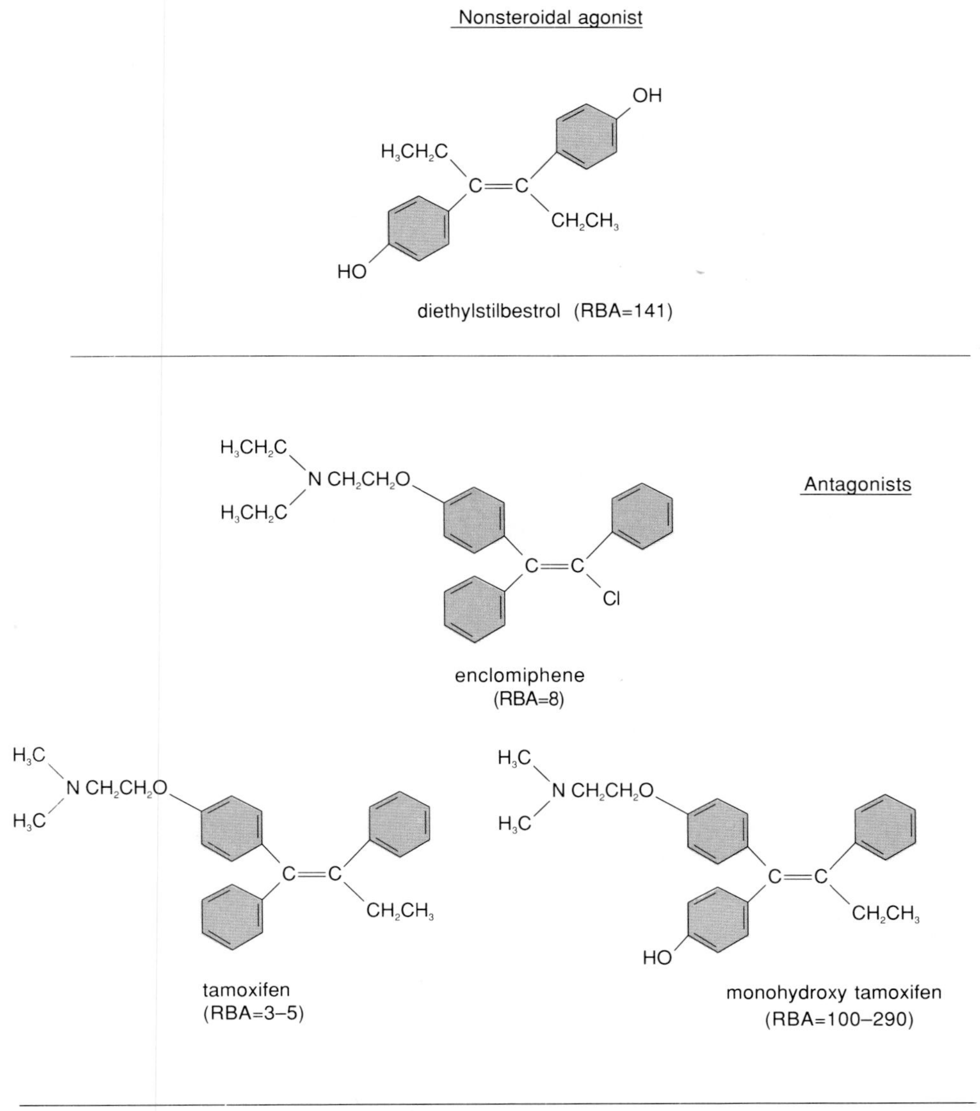
Nonsteroidal agonist
OH
H3CH2C
C=C
CH2CH3
HO
diethylstilbestrol (RBA=141)
Antagonists
H3CH2C
N CH2CH2O
H3CH2C
C=C
Cl
enclomiphene
(RBA=8)
H3C
N CH2CH2O
H3C
C=C
CH2CH3
tamoxifen
(RBA=3–5)
H3C
N CH2CH2O
H3C
C=C
CH2CH3
HO
monohydroxy tamoxifen
(RBA=100–290)

FIGURE 36-3, cont'd

phate. The synthetic, nonsteroidal estrogens include diethylstilbestrol, chlorotrianisene, and dienestrol.

The antiestrogens used clinically include tamoxifen and clomiphene citrate (see Figure 36-3). Clomiphene citrate is a racemic mixture of two stereoisomers and has both estrogenic and antiestrogenic properties. Tamoxifen is a nonsteroidal triphenylethylene derivate structurally similar to clomiphene. The trans isomer of tamoxifen is thought to produce the antiestrogenic properties.

The most common naturally occurring progestins in humans and several important synthetic progestins are shown in Figures 36-2 and 36-4. Progestin derivatives can be classified based on positions C21 or C19 (19-nortestosterone).

The C21 derivatives include the natural progestins, progesterone, and 17α-hydroxyprogesterone, which utilize the same carbon backbone as pregnenolone, from which they are derived. The other C21 compounds are derivatives of 17α-hydroxyprogesterone and include medroxyprogesterone acetate, megestrol acetate (6,7 double bond to medroxprogesterone), and

C_{21} Agonists

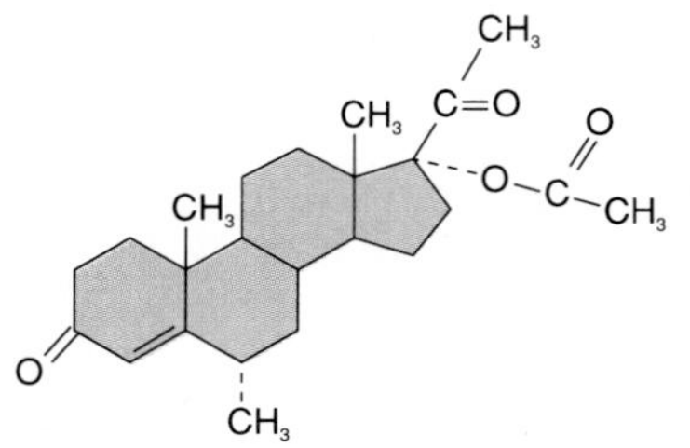

medroxyprogesterone acetate
(RBA=78)

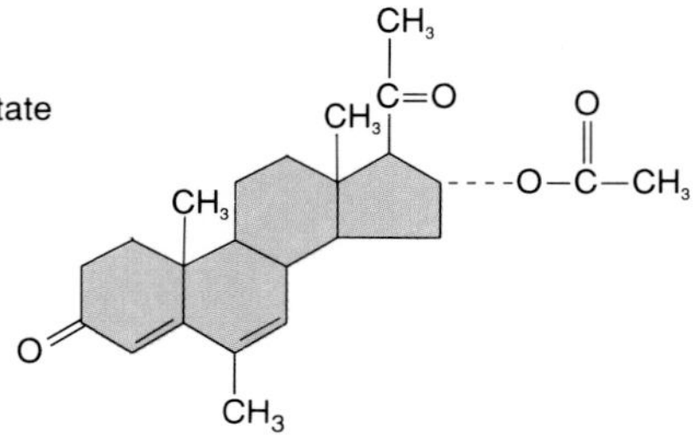

megestrol acetate

Antagonist

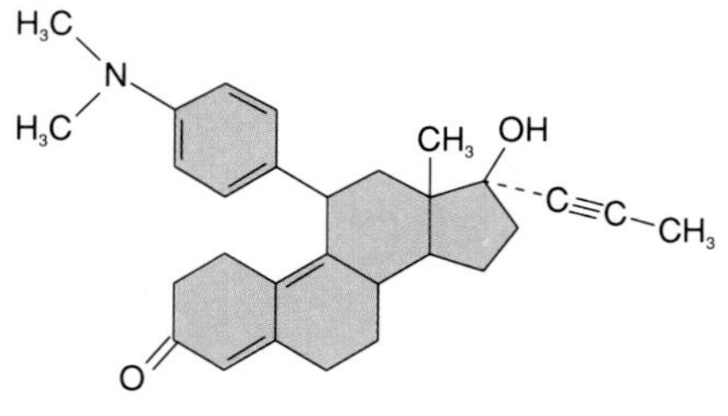

mifepristone (RU 486)
(RBA=530)

FIGURE 36-4 Commonly used progestins and antiprogestin. Structures for a number of ligands for the progesterone receptor are shown. Relative binding affinity (RBA) for the ligand to the progesterone receptor, as compared to progesterone, is also shown (RBA for progesterone, 100%).

hydroxyprogesterone caproate (6-methyl deleted and 17-acetate replaced by 17-caproate from hydroxyprogesterone acetate). Alteration to an acetate ester in medroxyprogesterone acetate and megestrol acetate helps protect these compounds from inactivation in the liver and allows their oral use.

The 19-nortestosterone derivatives are similar to testosterone, but lack the C19 methyl group. They include synthetic levonorgestrel and norgestrel, a ra-

cemic mixture of active levonorgestrel and the inactive stereoisomer. Therefore, on a weight basis, levonorgestrel is twice as potent as norgestrel.

The other synthetic progestins include norethindrone, norethindrone acetate, norethynodrel (norethindrone with C—H instead of C—CH at C17), and ethynodiol diacetate. Norethindrone acetate and norethynodrel are metabolized to the active progestin norethindrone. These synthetic compounds are orally

C_{19} Agonists

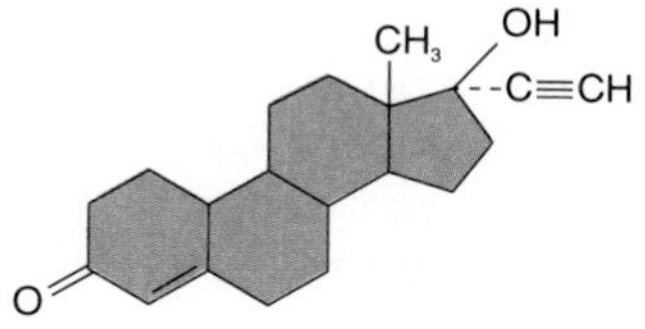

norethindrone
(RBA=85)

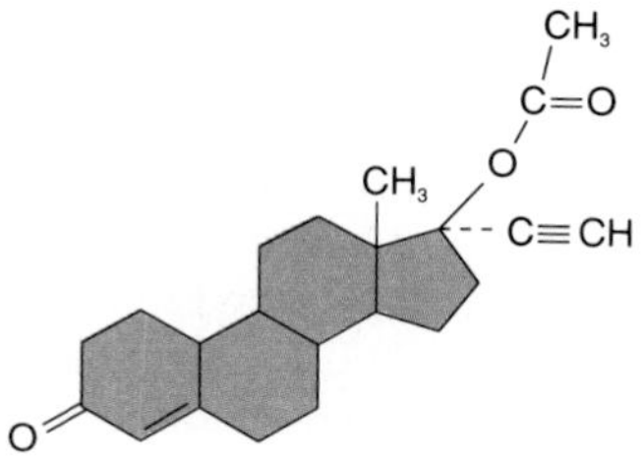

norethindrone acetate
(RBA=6)

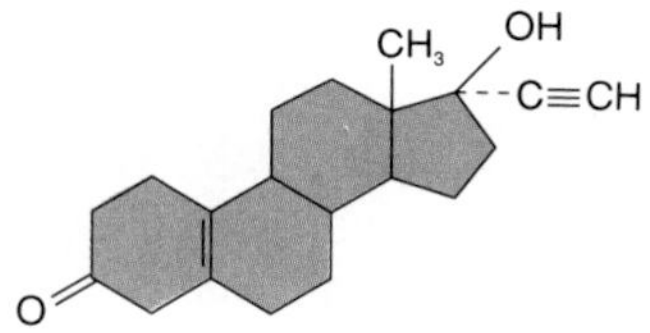

norethynodrel
(RBA=5)

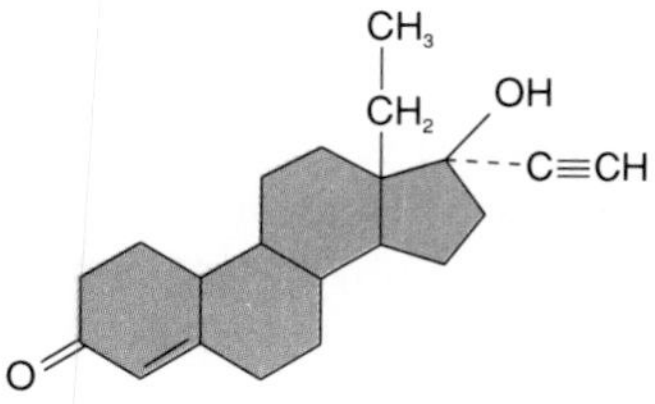

(dl) norgestrel
(RBA for levonorgestrel-95)

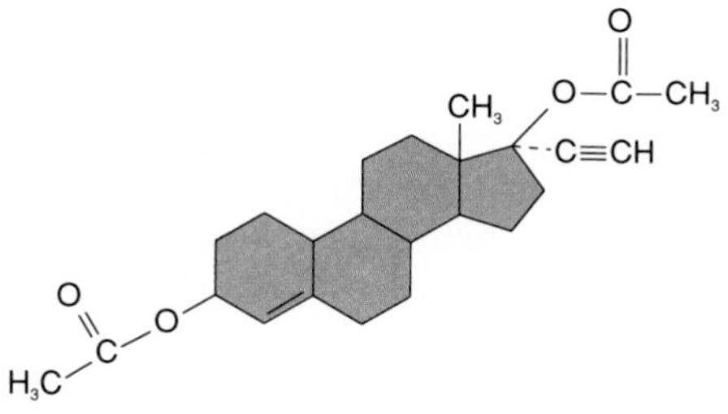

ethynodiol diacetate
(RBA =5)

FIGURE 36-4, cont'd

active with an ethinyl group at C17 to slow inactivation in the liver.

In general synthetic progestins are more potent than C21 derivatives when administered orally. Norgestrel is 5 to 10 times more potent than the same dose of norethindrone. Synthetic progestins can also display some estrogenic and androgenic activity, with progesterone and C21 derivatives showing less androgenic and no estrogenic properties.

Biosynthesis of Estrogens and Progestins

Estrogens and progestins are produced by steroidogenesis in various tissues. In nonpregnant premenopausal women, the ovary is the predominant source. During pregnancy the fetal-placental unit produces large amounts of both steroids. A significant amount of estrogen is also produced by skeletal muscle, liver, and adipose tissue via conversion of circulating androgens to estrone. Certain brain areas in males and females may produce estrogens by conversion of circulating androgens. Small amounts of estradiol are produced in the male testes.

In the biosynthesis of natural estrogens and progestins (see Figure 36-2), the rate-limiting step in ovarian production of steroid hormones is the conversion of cholesterol to pregnenolone by cytochrome P-450 side chain cleavage enzymes. Most cholesterol derives from the blood LDL form, but it can also be synthesized in the cell from acetyl-CoA. Pregnenolone can then be directly converted to progesterone or 17α-hydroxypregnenolone. Two pathways lead to androgenic steroids, androstenedione and testosterone. These androgens can then be converted to estrone and 17β-estradiol, respectively, by the aromatase enzyme. The aromatase in the ovary and peripheral tissues is responsible for aromatization of the A ring and loss of the C19 methyl group, producing a molecule with estrogenic properties.

Estriol can be produced in the liver as an oxidation product derived mainly from estrone; some estriol is also made from estradiol. During pregnancy, estriol can be synthesized in the fetal-placental unit.

Although progesterone is readily made in the placenta, direct placental conversion of cholesterol to estrogen cannot occur. Maternal cholesterol is converted to dehydroepiandrosterone-sulfate in fetal adrenals and then hydroxylated to the 16α-hydroxy derivative in fetal liver. In the placenta, which is rich in sulfatase and aromatase enzymes, the 16α-hydroxy derivative is converted to estriol, whereas dehydroepiandrosterone sulfate is converted to estrone.

The quantities of the various steroids produced in the adrenals, testes, ovaries, and placenta are probably regulated by the enzymic activity at each step of steroidogenesis in particular cell types.

During the menstrual cycle estrogen and progesterone are synthesized and released from the ovary under regulation of pituitary gonadotropins FSH and LH. Pulsatile release of hypothalamic gonadotropin-releasing hormone regulates FSH and LH synthesis and release. Gonadotropin-releasing hormone concentrations are regulated through negative and positive feedback by the steroid hormones. Estrogens and progestins also act directly on the pituitary gonadotrophs to decrease FSH and LH concentrations. In addition, an ovarian protein, inhibin, negatively affects FSH synthesis. A schematic representation of the pathways for integrated control of hormone concentrations is shown in Figure 36-1.

A normal ovulatory/menstrual cycle lasts 25 to 35 days. The steps in the ovarian and endometrial cycles are shown in Figure 36-5. The ovarian cycle is divided into the follicular (preovulatory) phase, which is predominantly concerned with the maturing follicle, and the luteal (postovulatory) phase, which is controlled by the corpus luteum. The follicle is the basic reproductive unit of the ovary and consists of the oocyte surrounded by granulosa cells, which are separated by a basement membrane from the theca cells. During follicular development both the cell layers and a follicular cavity containing fluid (the antrum) enlarge. Following ovulation the remnants of the antral fluid, granulosa, and theca cells make up the corpus luteum.

At the beginning of a menstrual cycle, several follicles increase their rates of maturation under FSH stimulation. FSH binds to its cell surface receptor on granulosa cells, leading to increased enzymatic activity to aromatize androgens to estradiol. One follicle becomes dominant while the others undergo atresia. By days 8 to 10, FSH concentrations are falling, but the dominant follicle has an increased number of FSH receptors and thereby becomes more sensitive to circulating gonadotropin concentrations. LH concentrations rise slightly during this time.

In the late follicular phase blood estrogen concentration rises rapidly and peaks at 0.3 to 0.7 ng/ml, initiating the midcycle LH surge (16 to 24 hours before ovulation) through positive feedback to the hypotha-

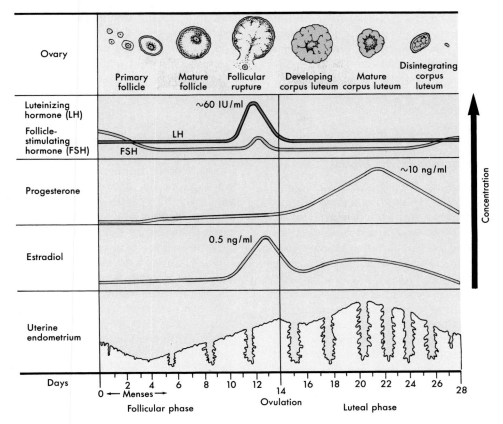

FIGURE 36-5   Ovulatory and menstrual cycle. Schematic presentation of ovarian and uterine changes that occur with the cyclical hormonal changes during the normal human menstrual cycle.

lamic/pituitary axis. The LH surge leads to follicular production of progesterone, prostaglandin $F_{2\alpha}$, and proteolytic enzymes and to follicular rupture and ovulation.

The length of the follicular phase can vary, but the luteal phase is consistently about 14 days. The corpus luteum then produces predominantly progesterone, which rises through the first half of the luteal phase (peak concentrations of 10 to 20 ng/ml). The estrogen concentrations reach 0.2 ng/ml. These high steroid concentrations feedback negatively to the hypothalamic/pituitary axis to keep the concentrations of FSH and LH low. Unless pregnancy occurs, the progesterone and estrogen concentrations fall and luteolysis occurs, leading to menses (steroid withdrawal bleeding) and the beginning of a new cycle. The negative feedback effect of high concentrations of estrogens and progestins is exploited by oral contracep-

tives to inhibit the FSH and LH peaks and thereby prevent follicular maturation and ovulation.

In the event of pregnancy, the placenta secretes chorionic gonadotropin into the maternal circulation. The chorionic gonadotropin concentration rises rapidly after implantation and peaks about 6 to 8 weeks into pregnancy. Chorionic gonadotropin maintains the corpus luteum and stimulates progesterone production, which helps maintain pregnancy. The human placenta eventually becomes the major source of circulating progesterone and estrogens, especially estriol, sometime after the fifth week of pregnancy.

As women age, the number of follicles present in the ovaries diminishes, predominantly because of atresia. Eventually, no follicles remain and the normal menstrual cycles cease (menopause). The lack of follicles means estradiol and progesterone can no longer be made in the ovary. Without these two steroid hormones to feed back on the hypothalamic/pituitary axis, FSH and LH rise to very high concentrations. Adrenal androgens, predominantly androstenedione, are still produced and can be converted by aromatase to estrone in peripheral tissues. However, because these concentrations are low, women experience a number of symptoms related to the absence of estrogens during this time.

Transport of Hormones in the Blood

Before estrogen or progesterone can lead to a response it must be secreted into the blood and transported to a target tissue. The steroid hormones are transported in the blood complexed with proteins. Estrogens are bound by sex hormone-binding globulin and progesterone by corticosteroid-binding globulin. These are relatively high-affinity, low-capacity interactions. Clearly the concentration of these binding globulins in relation to hormone determines the concentration of free hormone available to target tissues. The free concentration of hormone (not bound to serum proteins) represents the true hormone concentration available to elicit a response. The concentrations of these proteins are hormonally regulated. Estrogen administration leads to increased production of both transport proteins. Serum albumin also can bind estrogens and progesterone, but the amount of albumin in the blood is unaffected by these hormones. These are low-affinity, high-capacity interactions. Synthetic ligands show variable affinities for the serum proteins.

Receptor Mechanisms

All steroid hormones appear to act by a similar mechanism. After delivery to the target tissue, free hormone passively diffuses into the cell and through the cytoplasm and binds to a specific receptor protein in the nucleus in the case of estrogen and progesterone receptors. If a particular receptor molecule is present, the target tissue produces a response to the hormone. Different tissues can respond differently to the same hormone, although probably only one estrogen receptor protein species exists in target tissues. Therefore factors other than the receptor alone must determine the type and magnitude of response by a target tissue. The binding of estrogen or progesterone to its particular receptor in the nucleus is a high-affinity interaction. Each binds tightly to its

own receptor but weakly to the other receptor. However, progesterone crossreacts with glucocorticoid and androgen receptors. Although progesterone binds with higher affinity to its own receptor, this crossreactivity may have mechanistic importance since some progestins can elicit androgenic responses.

Cellular receptor concentrations are strongly influenced by hormonal environment. Progesterone receptors are expressed in direct response to estrogen exposure of the target tissue. High concentrations of progesterone decrease estrogen receptor concentrations, which in turn lead to decreased progesterone receptor concentrations. Furthermore, each hormone can directly regulate its own receptor concentration (down or up) in some circumstances.

The ultimate response to estrogen in the uterus and breast is increased cellular proliferation, whereas that to progesterone in these same estrogen-primed tissues is decreased cellular growth and increased cellular differentiation. The events that occur between a hormone binding to its receptor and the final expression of cellular responses remain unclear. One step by which steroid hormones promote metabolic changes in target tissues is by increasing the rate of target gene transcription. These metabolic changes eventually lead to increased DNA synthesis and cell division. The hormone-receptor complex may also elicit cellular responses by repression of gene transcription or stabilization of mRNA.

Binding of ligand to its receptor induces a conformational change in the protein, allowing the receptor to modify specific genes expression and probably involves interaction between the steroid-receptor complex and specific DNA sequences or other nuclear proteins involved in regulating transcription. This specific DNA sequence is termed a *hormone response element* and is often found upstream from the target gene (see Chapter 34 for further discussion).

Regulation of the tissue's ability to respond in a particular way to a specific hormone occurs at a minimum of three levels. First, the cell must express the appropriate receptor. Second, the gene must have a hormone response element to be a target for the hormone. Third, the target gene must have an appropriate array of chromatin proteins and transcription factors for transcription to be regulated in that tissue.

The receptor-steroid complex turnover is not completely understood. The half-life for the estrogen receptor is 2 to 4 hours, with or without bound ligand.

Possibly the receptor is processed by proteolysis, although dissociation of estradiol from the receptor may also occur.

The molecular basis for hormone action, including estrogen and progesterone, is summarized in Chapter 34. Considerable progress has been made in understanding molecular mechanisms of steroid hormone action; active research continues on the role of hormones in receptor function, the variable response of target genes, the mechanism by which receptors modulate gene transcription and mRNA stabilization, and the role of the steroid hormones in fetal development.

Antihormone action is produced by competitive binding of ligands to hormone receptors, directly blocking binding of the hormone. Antiestrogens bind to the estrogen receptor with relatively high affinity, preventing estrogen access to the binding site. The antiestrogen-receptor complex may still bind to the hormone response element, but does not initiate increased transcription of the target gene. Other genes may be directly activated by the antiestrogen-receptor complex. Interestingly, some antiestrogens have partial agonist (estrogen-like) properties in some tissues while displaying antagonist activities in other tissues. This tissue-specific action of the same compound is under active investigation.

 # PHARMACOKINETICS

Pharmacokinetic parameter values for these agents are summarized in Table 36-1.

Estrogens

Estrogens are rapidly absorbed from the GI tract, skin, and mucous membranes and after parenteral injection. The unconjugated, natural estrogens are rapidly inactivated in the GI tract and liver if taken orally; therefore other modes of delivery (transdermal, vaginal, nasal, or intramuscular) are warranted. Micronized estradiols, steroidal estrogens that contain an ethinyl group at C17, the conjugated estrogens, and nonsteroidal estrogens are orally active. Once absorbed, these drugs are rapidly metabolized in the liver. Chlorotrianisene and quinestrol have prolonged durations of action because of storage in and slow release from adipose tissue.

Estrogens are distributed to most body tissues with selective uptake by target and adipose tissues. Estradiol is tightly bound to sex hormone-binding globulin and somewhat to albumin, whereas estrone and estriol bind mainly to albumin. The conjugated estrogens bind weakly to albumin only.

Table 36-1 Pharmacokinetic Parameters

Drug	Administration	Absorption	$t_{1/2}$	Plasma Protein Binding	Disposition
estradiol	Oral (esters, IM, topical, suppository	Rapid if micro-nized	~30 min	50%-80% SHBG; 18%-48% albumin	M (main)*, R
ethinyl estradiol	Oral	Rapid	~6-20 hr	98% albumin	M (main)*, R
progesterone	IM	Poor	5 min	50% CBG; 48% albumin	M, R
levonorgestrel	Oral	Rapid	11-45 hr	80% SHBG	M
norethindrone	Oral	Rapid	5-14 hr	60%-70% SHBG; 30%-35% albumin	M
clomiphene citrate	Oral	Rapid	4-10 hr (trans), >18 hr (cis)	—	M
tamoxifen citrate	Oral	Slow	7 days	Albumin	—
RU486	Oral	<25%	10-24 hr	95% albumin	R (10%)
aminoglutethimide	Oral	Rapid	10-15 hr	20%-35%	R (35%-50%)
danazol	Oral	Rapid	~15 hr	—	M

SHBG, Sex hormone-binding globulin; *CBG*, corticosteroid-binding globulin. *M*, metabolism; *R*, renal.
*Enterohepatic cycling.

Estrogens are excreted primarily as polyhydroxylated forms conjugated at C3 with sulfate or glucuronic acid. Free estrogens are distributed to the bile, reabsorbed in the GI tract, and recirculated to the liver (enterohepatic recirculation). About one fifth of the estrogen is excreted in the feces and the remainder in the urine. Estradiol is rapidly cleared from the blood. In the liver estrone is converted to estrone sulfate, which is then excreted or hydrolyzed back to estrone. The serum half-life for estrone sulfate is about 12 hours. The common synthetic steroidal estrogens, ethinyl estradiol and mestranol, are metabolized slower than estradiol because of the ethinyl group at C17. Brain tissue can metabolize 17β-estradiol to form catechol estrogens, structurally similar to catecholamines but of unclear function in the brain. The synthetic nonsteroidal estrogens may be excreted as glucuronide or sulfate conjugates.

Progestins

Oral progesterone is almost completely inactivated in the liver, so synthetic modification is necessary to produce the orally active progestins listed in Figure 36-4. Progesterone can be given parenterally but has an elimination half-life of only a few minutes. It is converted in the liver to pregnanediol, conjugated with glucuronide at C3, and the conjugate excreted mainly in urine. The 19-nortestosterone derivatives are all orally active. Medroxyprogesterone acetate can be used orally or IM, whereas megestrol acetate is only used orally. The C21 derivatives and the 19-nortestosterone compounds all have longer plasma half-lives than progesterone. Most of these compounds are metabolized in the liver, conjugated to glucuronide, and the conjugates excreted in the urine.

Combination Oral Contraceptives

The low doses of estrogens and progestins in current combination oral contraceptives decrease side effects, but further decreases without altering contraceptive effectiveness are unlikely because of metabolic variations in women. First-pass losses in the liver limit the bioavailability and rate of metabolism of these steroids. The dosage of estrogens and progestins in oral contraceptives must be high enough to produce biologically active serum concentrations in virtually 100% of users, so the minimal effective dose to ensure prevention of pregnancy is limited.

Antiestrogens

Clomiphene citrate is orally administered and readily absorbed from the GI tract. It may enter the enterohepatic circulation with about 50% excreted in the feces within 5 days, but the half-life is shorter than this. Both enclomiphene and zuclomiphene reach peak plasma concentrations within 3 to 6 hours after an oral dose. However, enclomiphene has a shorter plasma elimination half-life (4 to 10 hours) than zuclomiphene (greater than 18 hours).

Conjugated metabolites after oral tamoxifen are primarily excreted via the biliary route into the feces. Enterohepatic recirculation of the metabolites, binding to serum albumin, and high-affinity binding to tissues all contribute to the long half-life. The major metabolites of tamoxifen include N-desmethyltamoxifen, which binds only weakly to the estrogen receptor but is present in greater concentrations than tamoxifen itself, and 4-hydroxytamoxifen, which binds much more tightly to the estrogen receptor than tamoxifen but is present in low concentrations. The antiestrogen action of tamoxifen may be aided by its metabolites.

Steroidogenesis Inhibitors

Aminoglutethimide is rapidly absorbed following administration, with maximum circulating concentrations reached in 1.5 hours. From 20% to 35% of the drug is bound to plasma proteins, and 35% to 50% is excreted unchanged in the urine, whereas 4% to 15% is excreted as acetylaminoglutethimide. None of the observed metabolites block adrenal steroidogenesis.

Oral danazol is rapidly absorbed and metabolized, but takes 7 to 14 days to reach a steady-state concentration. There are several metabolites excreted in both urine and feces (Figure 36-6).

 ## RELATION OF MECHANISMS OF ACTION TO CLINICAL RESPONSE

Fertility Control

Combination Oral Contraception The most common use for administered estrogens and progestins is oral contraception. Oral contraceptives are the most effective reversible method for preventing pregnancy in the United States. The failure rate is less than 0.7 per 100 women-years for users of combina-

aminoglutethimide

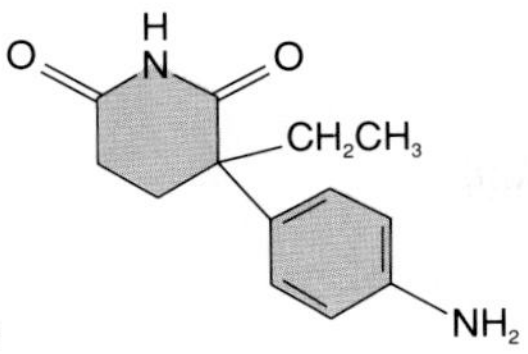

danazol
(progesterone receptor RBA=5-20)
(androgen receptor RBA ≅ 40)

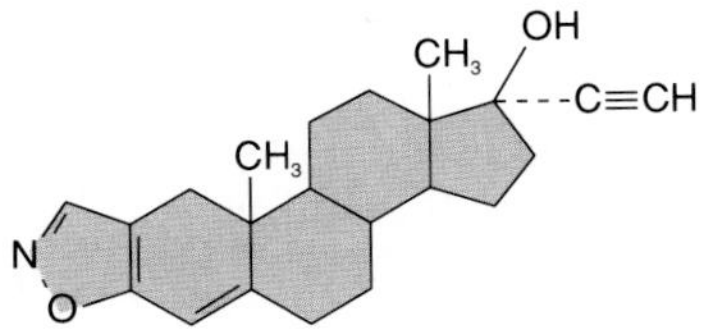

FIGURE 36-6   Structures of aminoglutethimide and danazol. Relative binding affinity (RBA) for danazol to the progesterone or androgen receptors, as compared to progesterone (RBA, 100%) or dihydrotestosterone (RBA, 100%), is shown.

tion oral contraceptives. The only method of birth control with a lower failure rate is sterilization.

Oral contraceptives available in the United States consist of progestin alone (the so-called minipill) or a combination of one of two synthetic estrogens with one of five synthetic progestins (the combination pill). The estrogen component is either ethinyl estradiol or mestranol, with mestranol slightly less potent. The progestins include norethindrone, norethindrone acetate, and ethynodiol diacetate, as well as norgestrel and its active isomer, levonorgestrel.

The present low dose estrogen contraceptives have decreased the incidence of adverse side effects and have still prevented pregnancy at rates equal to earlier higher dose estrogen formulations. The most commonly used oral contraceptives consist of a combination preparation taken for 21 days followed by 7 days without any steroids to induce withdrawal bleeding, but other dosing regimens also may be used to reduce side effects.

Combination oral contraceptives prevent pregnancy by inhibiting ovulation, presumably as a result of gonadotropin suppression induced by the estrogen and progestin effects on the hypothalamic/pituitary axis. The increased early follicular phase FSH concentrations and midcycle peaks of FSH and LH are not observed in patients taking combination oral contraceptives. The lower concentration of FSH results in decreased ovarian function with minimal follicular development. In addition, lower concentrations of en-

dogenous steroid are secreted during both phases of the menstrual cycle.

Oral contraceptives also act directly on the cervix and uterus. The cervical mucus of oral contraceptive users is usually thick and in lower quantity than is seen in a normal postovulatory phase. This may also aid in preventing pregnancy by inhibiting sperm penetration. Also the endometrium may be inhibited from developing into the appropriate state for implantation. Missing two or more doses during a cycle substantially increases the risk of pregnancy, so a high compliance rate is needed to ensure adequate contraception, especially with low concentration ethinyl estradiol preparations.

Oral contraceptives provide several well-documented health benefits beyond the control of fertility, most commonly, decreased incidence of ovarian and endometrial cancers. Although ovarian malignancy carries a relatively high mortality, long-term oral contraceptive users (more than 5 years) have a relative risk of 0.6 compared to 1.0 for nonusers. This protective effect continues for 10 to 15 years after discontinuing oral contraceptives. Endometrial cancers have relatively low mortality, but occur fairly commonly in women. A causal link between increased incidence of endometrial cancer and use of sequential oral contraceptives led to cessation of their use in 1976 (sequential oral contraceptives consisted of estrogen alone for 14 to 16 days, then 5 to 6 days of estrogen plus progestin, then 7 days without steroid).

Many studies on the association between combination oral contraceptive use and the development of endometrial cancer show a protective effect of the contraceptives. Users have a relative risk of 0.5 compared to 1.0 for nonusers. This effect appears after as little as 1 year of use and lasts 10 to 15 years after discontinuing the contraceptive. It is postulated that the mechanism is related to the use of daily progestin to oppose the proliferative actions of the synthetic estrogens on the endometrium.

Other benefits of long-term oral contraceptive use include a 50% decrease in fibroadenomatous and fibrocystic breast disease, 10% to 70% reduction of acute pelvic inflammatory disease, and decreases in other less critical problems.

Progestin-only Contraception Progestin-only formulations were developed to avert the adverse side effects of estrogens in oral contraceptives. Major problems with this approach are a slightly higher failure rate of 2 to 3 per 100 woman-years and a much higher incidence of irregular menstrual bleeding, often leading to discontinuation of the medication.

Progestin-only medication suppresses FSH and LH concentrations and ovulation to variable degrees, however, these actions cannot be the only explanation for the observed 97% to 98% success rate. Continuous progestin alone leads to scant, thick cervical mucus, endometrial atrophy (which could prevent implantation), and often quite variable length and duration of bleeding.

Medroxyprogesterone acetate is approved in 80 countries as a contraceptive, but because of increased incidence of breast tumors in beagle dogs is not approved in the United States for contraception, but only for use in the treatment of advanced endometrial and renal carcinomas and endometriosis. Its mode of action is similar to other progestin-only contraceptives. Three new progestin oral contraceptives used in Europe (desogestrel, norgestimate, and gestodene) are not available in the United States.

Postcoital Contraception Large doses of estrogens alone or in combination with progestins may prevent pregnancy following unprotected coitus but must be used within 72 hours of coital exposure to prevent pregnancy and are currently recommended only in cases of rape, incest, failure of a barrier method, or unprotected intercourse. The preparations probably act by preventing implantation because the endometrium is made nonreceptive to the blastocyst by high-dose hormone treatment.

Contragestation Mifepristone (RU 486) (see Figure 36-4) is a synthetic potent antiprogestin with 50 times less antiglucocorticoid than antiprogestin activity, which is under intensive investigation in Europe. It binds to the progesterone receptor, preventing binding by endogenous progesterone, while avoiding the usual hormone response. It also binds weakly to the androgen receptor and tightly to the glucocorticoid receptor (affinity greater than dexamethasone).

Replacement Therapy

Menopause Menopause, the natural cessation of menses, results from ovarian failure following the depletion of functional ovarian follicles. This produces decreased estrogen and progesterone production and causes various physiological and psychological changes. Vasomotor symptoms, genitourinary atrophy, osteoporosis, and cardiovascular disease in postmenopausal women can be substantially decreased if estrogen replacement therapy is begun during menopause. Controversy remains, however, regarding patient selection, treatment regimens, addition of progestin, and possible adverse effects.

An additional benefit of estrogen replacement therapy is reduced risk of cardiovascular disease, especially coronary artery disease. Women have a lower incidence of coronary artery disease before menopause than men of the same age, but after menopause the incidence increases with age and eventually parallels that in males. Estrogen replacement therapy provides a 50% to 70% reduction in the risk of arteriosclerotic cardiovascular disease in postmenopausal women. This may be related to changes in lipoprotein profile since after menopause HDL concentrations fall and LDL concentrations rise in women; and in males these changes have been correlated with increased risk of coronary artery disease. Estrogen replacement therapy increases HDL and lowers LDL concentrations and may thereby provide a protective effect. The presence of estrogen receptors in several large arteries and the direct effects of estrogen on endothelial or smooth muscle cells of coronary arteries may contribute to the protection.

The best time to initiate estrogen therapy to treat menopausal symptoms is as promptly as menopause begins. Estrogen is more effective in preventing osteoporosis, genitourinary atrophy, and cardiovascular disease than in reversing them once they have occurred. The beneficial changes in the lipoprotein profiles can be negated by the addition of progestins to the regimen. Several progestogens, especially the 19-nortestosterone derivatives, create a dose-dependent decrease in HDL and increase in LDL. The C21 progestins such as medroxyprogesterone acetate have less of an effect on lipoproteins. It is important to choose a progestin carefully and to use as low a dosage as possible to minimize the adverse effects on the lipoprotein profile.

The use of progestins with estrogen replacement therapy remains controversial.

Other Dysfunctions Other clinical dysfunctions in which estrogen replacement therapy is useful include osteoporosis, primary hypogonadism, dysfunctional uterine bleeding, and luteal phase deficiency.

Osteoporosis represents reduced bone mass per volume. Bone loss occurs naturally in both males and females with age and accelerates in women in the perimenopausal period. This involves primarily travecular (spongy) bone, but cortical bone is also lost.

Estrogen replacement therapy can decrease the rate of bone loss as well as the incidence of vertebral, wrist, and hip fractures in postmenopausal women.

Estrogen therapy initiated near the time of puberty may help stimulate normal sexual development and may be used to treat female primary hypogonadism. Concurrent treatment with androgens is discussed in Chapter 37.

Dysfunctional uterine bleeding consists of irregular menstrual cycles often characterized by prolonged bleeding. High-dose progestin therapy can be used to stop an episode of prolonged bleeding but should be followed by long-term cyclic therapy with an oral progestin to ensure occurrence of regular withdrawal bleeding.

Luteal phase deficiency results from insufficient progesterone. Ovulation is normal, but the corpus luteum functions subnormally with insufficient progesterone production to maintain pregnancy. The most popular method of treatment is natural progesterone supplementation.

Ovulation Induction

About 20% to 30% of infertility may be due to an anovulatory condition. Agents that induce ovulation in these patients include gonadotropins, gonadotropin-releasing hormone, and clomiphene citrate. Clomiphene citrate (see Figure 36-3) is used to treat ovulatory failure in patients desiring pregnancy whose mates are fertile and potent. These agents may act as antiestrogens at the hypothalamus and relieve estrogen-induced negative feedback on gonadotropin-releasing hormone release.

After clomiphene administration, pulse frequency (but not amplitude) of LH release rises significantly from increased pulse frequency of gonadotropin-releasing hormone release. Clomiphene functions best in women with normal concentrations of estrogen before therapy, and is not useful in patients with primary ovarian or pituitary dysfunction.

Cancer Chemotherapy

Approximately one third of patients with advanced breast cancer show tumor regression or prolongation of disease-free survival with therapy that decreases estrogen production or action. Early trials with high-dose progestins, androgens, glucocorticoids, and estrogens resulted in 10% to 40% response due to unknown mechanisms, but with adverse side effects. More recently the antiestrogen tamoxifen has produced an overall response of 30% to 40% with fewer adverse effects. Tamoxifen is discussed further in Chapter 43.

Reduction of estrogen production in postmenopausal women for prevention of breast cancer is discussed also in Chapter 41 and can be aided by adrenalectomy. To avoid such surgery, adrenal steroidogenesis inhibition may be used. Aminoglutethimide (shown in Figure 36-6) inhibits a cholesterol side-chain cleaving enzyme, which converts cholesterol to pregnenolone, and the aromatase enzyme, which converts adrenal androstenedione to estrone and testosterone to estradiol (see Figure 36-2). Patient supplementation with glucocorticoid replacement therapy is needed mainly to inhibit the compensatory rise in ACTH, which can override the action of aminoglutethimide. Hydrocortisone is used because aminoglutethimide stimulates the metabolism of dexamethasone. Aminoglutethimide plus hydrocortisone replacement can also reduce circulating concentrations of estrogens. Other aromatase inhibitors are under investigation.

Endometrial cancer formation is enhanced with long-term unopposed estrogen therapy, but can be treated with progestins. Progestational therapy is used as adjunctive and palliative treatment with approximately one third of advanced cases of metastatic endometrial carcinoma showing a favorable response.

Medroxyprogesterone acetate often is used and likely acts through the progesterone receptor to down regulate the estrogen receptor, to induce formation of 17β-hydroxysteroid dehydrogenase to increase estradiol metabolism. In addition, it may have direct cellular actions leading to decreased cell division. High progesterone receptor concentrations in the tumor correlate with increased survival.

High doses of estrogens such as diethylstilbestrol are used to treat advanced prostate cancer. Newer therapies decrease the high incidence of cardiovascular deaths, which are predominantly thromboembolic in nature, associated with these high doses of estrogen.

Ovarian cancer may or may not demonstrate hormonal dependence. Some studies suggest that estrogen use increases the risk of developing ovarian cancer, although some conflicting results indicate the usefulness of determining estrogen and progesterone receptor concentrations in predicting therapeutic response.

Others

Endometriosis results from ectopic endometrial cell implants occurring outside the uterus. These endometrial cells continue to respond to steroid hormones but may show subtle differences to estrogen and progesterone receptor concentrations and function.

The goal of therapy in endometriosis is to induce a hormone-poor environment, especially with low estrogen concentrations, to inhibit the growth of implants and thereby alleviate symptoms. The three main pharmacological agents used in the United States to treat endometriosis are danazol, progestins, and gonadotropin-releasing hormone derivatives. Gestrianone, a slightly androgenic and strongly antiestrogenic synthetic hormone, is also under investigation for treating endometriosis, but is not currently available in the United States.

Danazol, shown in Figure 36-6, effectively relieves the symptoms of endometriosis and may act by inhibiting either LH/FSH surge or the action of several steroidogenic enzymes or both. Danazol can interact with both androgen and progesterone receptors (see Chapter 35), and produces amenorrhea and pain relief without decreasing the basal concentrations of gonadotropins or estrogen. Between 80% and 100% of patients report lessened pain within 3 to 12 months of therapy.

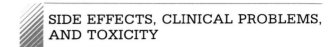

SIDE EFFECTS, CLINICAL PROBLEMS, AND TOXICITY

A brief summary of the potential problems for some of the important drugs is shown in the box.

Estrogens

Some less serious adverse effects of high-dose estrogen therapy include nausea, occasional vomiting, abdominal cramps, bloating, diarrhea, appetite changes, fluid retention, dizziness, headache, breast discomfort and enlargement, weight gain, mood changes, ocular changes, allergic rash, and changes in some serum protein concentrations, including lipoproteins (HDL increases and LDL decreases).

More serious side effects occasionally encountered include increased incidences of thromboembolic disorders, high blood pressure, gallbladder disease, and endometrial cancer.

In humans an etiological role for diethylstilbestrol in the development of clear cell adenocarcinoma of the vagina and cervix has been postulated from epidemiological data of the 1950s. Female offspring that received fetal exposure to diethylstilbesterol subsequently developed increased cancers of these types.

Progestins

The occasional and less serious side effects of high-dose progestin therapy, as it is used to treat advanced endometrial cancer or in progestin-only oral contraceptives, include breakthrough bleeding, spotting, changes in menstrual flow, amenorrhea, edema, weight changes, nausea, bloating, headache, allergic rash, mood changes, and changes in lipoprotein concentrations (HDL decreases and LDL increases). High-dose progestin results in abnormal glucose-tolerance test in 4% to 16% of women. Diabetic women or those with a prior history of glucose intolerance should be monitored after starting oral contraceptive preparations, and a progestin with as low a dose and potency as possible used.

The most common side effects of IM medroxyprogesterone acetate as a contraceptive are menstrual abnormalities, characterized by irregular bleeding early followed by amenorrhea in 50% to 70% of patients after 2 years treatment.

CLINICAL PROBLEMS

ESTROGENS

GI disturbances
Menstrual disorders
Breast discomfort
Thromboembolic disorders
Hypertension
Endometrial cancer
Decreased lactation
Drug interactions
Adverse effects on fetus (diethylstilbestrol)

PROGESTINS

GI disturbances
Menstrual disorders
Adverse changes in lipoprotein levels
Abnormal glucose tolerance
Drug interactions
Adverse effects on fetus

CLOMIPHENE CITRATE

GI disturbances
Vasomotor symptoms
Ovarian enlargement
Visual disorders
Multiple gestations

TAMOXIFEN

GI disturbances
Menstrual disorders
Vasomotor symptoms

MIFEPRISTONE (RU486) (INVESTIGATIONAL)

Menstrual disturbances (rare)

AMINOGLUTETHIMIDE (INVESTIGATIONAL)

GI disturbances
CNS disturbances

DANAZOL

Androgenic effects in women
Antiestrogen-like effects
Adverse changes in lipoprotein concentrations
Adverse effects on the fetus

Combination Oral Contraceptives

Despite over 30 years of oral contraceptive use, a great deal of controversy remains concerning the risks. Several factors must be considered: (1) many early studies that associated oral contraceptive use with specific side effects were conducted with much higher doses than present formulations; recent studies with low dose oral contraceptives show fewer adverse effects; (2) several early studies were criticized for study design in that subgroups were not identical; and (3) restricting certain high-risk patient subgroups from oral contraceptive use has decreased the association between cardiovascular side effects and oral contraceptive use.

An overview of epidemiologic studies reveals an association between oral contraceptive use and thromboembolic disease in the absence of other predisposing factors. The association between oral contraceptive use and stroke or myocardial infarction is less consistent. The death rate associated with childbirth exceeds that of oral contraceptive use for all age groups except oral contraceptive users who are more than 40 years of age and who smoke.

The risk of idiopathic venous thrombosis associated with oral contraceptive use ranges from twofold to sixfold over nonusers. These thromboembolic events are directly related to the dose of estrogen. Since the risk of thromboembolic disease rapidly returns to normal ($\simeq 1$ month) after oral contraceptives are discontinued, their use should be stopped at least 2 to 4 weeks before elective surgery and not restarted until at least 2 weeks after surgery.

An infrequent but proven side effect of oral contraceptive use is increased blood pressure over time in 1% to 5% of users. Usually the increase is small, but occasionally a rapid rise in blood pressure is observed, often within the first few months of therapy. The elevated blood pressure almost always resolves when oral contraceptives are discontinued. This increased blood pressure appears to relate to estrogen more than progestin, because women on progestin-only oral contraceptives usually do not experience the increase.

Cerebrovascular accidents are not definitively correlated with oral contraceptive use; some studies show an increased incidence of stroke while others do not. A recent large prospective study found no increased risk of stroke in oral contraceptive users. The association between oral contraceptive use and subarachnoid hemorrhage also remains controversial.

Older studies indicated an increased risk of myocardial infarction, but most of the myocardial infarctions occurred in women with other risk factors, especially older age and smoking. Nearly all new epidemiologic studies have shown no increased risk of myocardial infarction in former oral contraceptive users, and studies excluding women with other major risk factors for cardiovascular disease have shown no increased incidence of myocardial infarction or cerebrovascular accidents in oral contraceptive users over controls.

Multiple case-control studies and at least five large cohort studies published before 1987 have assessed the risk of breast cancer. The majority of studies have shown no change in the incidence of breast cancer with oral contraceptive use. A few studies showed increased risk of breast cancer with prolonged use (greater than 4 to 8 years) in women who began the medication before age 25, and three epidemiologic studies published in 1988 and 1989 showed significantly increased risk of breast cancer in long-term oral contraceptive users under 45 years of age.

Several studies have indicated increased risk of cervical dysplasia and carcinoma in situ of the cervix in long-term oral contraceptive users; however, controls for these studies were difficult to obtain. Women using oral contraceptives may be at high risk for cervical cancer if they have used these drugs for more than 5 years, and should have screening cervical cytology at least once a year.

Combination oral contraceptive formulations diminish the amount of milk produced in women who breastfeed. This effect is caused by the estrogen, even in low-dose formulations. Alternative methods of birth control (e.g., progestin-only contraceptives) should be considered for women wishing to use oral contraceptives and breastfeed. Progestins have been found in breast milk.

Oral contraceptives are contraindicated in women with a current or past history of thrombophlebitis or thromboembolic disorders, cerebrovascular or coronary artery disease, known or suspected pregnancy, undiagnosed abnormal genital bleeding, known or suspected carcinoma of the breast, uterus, cervix, vagina or other estrogen-dependent neoplasm, hepatic adenoma or carcinoma, or cholestatic jaundice of pregnancy or jaundice with prior oral contraceptive use. Oral contraceptives should be used with caution in patients with liver or renal disease, asthma, migraine headaches, diabetes, hypertension, congestive heart failure, and in patients on medication that can interfere with its effectiveness. Women who smoke and use oral contraceptives should be advised to use alternative methods of birth control after the age of 35.

Oral contraceptives are less effective with increased incidence of breakthrough bleeding when used simultaneously with rifampin, resulting from induction of hepatic microsomal enzymes. Similar interactions may occur with enzyme inducers including griseofulvin, barbiturates, carbamazepine, and phenytoin.

Estrogen Replacement Therapy

Fewer adverse effects are seen with lower physiologic dose estrogen replacement than with oral contraceptive or high-dose estrogen use because the incidence of thromboembolic disorders remains at age-appropriate levels with postmenopausal estrogen replacement therapy. Although women using exogenous estrogen can show altered coagulation profiles (i.e., elevated concentrations of factors VII, VIII, IX, and X and decreased antithrombin III concentrations) this does not lead to a functionally hypercoagulable state. Also, the synthetic estrogens (ethinylestradiol) are more likely to alter these concentrations than estradiol or conjugated estrogens used more generally in estrogen replacement therapy. Similarly, estrogen replacement therapy seems to pose little if any increased risk of hypertension or cholelithiasis.

Estrogen-only replacement therapy can increase risk of endometrial cancer, but not all women on unopposed estrogen therapy develop endometrial cancer. An adverse effect of the use of estrogen-progestin combined therapy in postmenopausal women is continued cyclic endometrial withdrawal bleeding that some women find undesirable. The association between breast cancer and postmenopausal estrogen use is less clear. Summarizing the studies to date, if estrogen replacement therapy increases the risk of developing breast cancer, it is a very small increased risk and progestins may or may not affect this risk.

Antiestrogens

With clomiphene citrate the frequency and severity of adverse effects are dose related and include hot flashes that resemble those in menopausal patients.

Visual problems occasionally occur and have been correlated with increasing total dose. Other high-dose side effects include ovarian enlargement or cyst formation, abdominal discomfort, nausea and vomiting, abnormal uterine bleeding, breast tenderness, headache, dizziness, depression, allergic dermatitis, and urinary frequency. Multiple gestations, particularly twins, occur at an incidence of 6% to 12% as compared to $\simeq$1% in the general population. Clomiphene citrate is contraindicated in patients with ovarian cysts, during pregnancy, or in patients with a past history of liver disease.

TRADENAMES

In addition to generic drugs and fixed combination preparations (other than oral contraceptives), the following tradenamed materials are available in the United States.

STEROIDAL ESTROGENS

Depo-Estradiol, depGynogen, Depogen, Dura-Estrin, Estro-Cyp, Estrofem, Estronol-LA; estradiol cypionate
Estinyl, Feminone; ethinylestradiol
Estrace, Estraderm (transdermal); estradiol
Estradurin, polyestradiol phosphate
Estroject, Estronol, Gynogen, Kestrin, Theelin, Ungen, Wehgen, estrone
Estrovis, quinestrol
Ogen, estropipate
Premarin, Estratal, Menest; conjugated estrogen
Valergen, Dioval, Delestrogen; estradiol valerate

NONSTEROIDAL ESTROGENS

DV, dienestrol
Stilphostrol, diethylstilbestrol phosphate
TACE, chlorotrianisene

ANTIESTROGENS

Clomid, Serophene; clomiphene citrate
Nolvadex, tamoxifen

PROGESTINS

Aygestin, Norlutate; norethindrone acetate
Enovid, norethynodrel
Gesterol, Progestaject-50; progesterone
Hyprogest, Pro-Depo, Duralutin, Hylutin, Prodrox; hydroxyprogesterone caproate
Megace, megestrol acetate
Norlutin, norethindrone
Provera, Cycrin, Curretab, Amen; medroxyprogesterone acetate

ANTIPROGESTINS

Mifepristone, RU 486

OTHER

Cytadren, aminoglutethimide
Danocrine, danazol

ORAL CONTRA-CEPTIVES	progestin	estrogen
Ovrette, Micronor, Nor-QD		
Progestin only	norgestrel norethindrone	
COMBINATION		
Brevicon, Nelova, Genora, Modicon, Ovcon	norethindrone	ethinylestradiol
Demulen	ethynodiol diacetate	ethinylestradiol
Levlen	levonorgestrel	ethinylestradiol
Loestrin, Norlestrin	norethindrone acetate	ethinylestradiol
Lo/Ovral	norgestral	ethinylestradiol
Norinyl, Ortho-Novum, Norethin, Nelova	norethindrone	mestranol

Side effects from tamoxifen therapy are minimal, with the most common being hot flashes, nausea, and vomiting. The possibility of using tamoxifen as long-term adjuvant treatment in some patients with breast cancer has raised questions about osteoporosis, alteration in serum lipoproteins, and increased incidence of cardiovascular disease. Preliminary results show no significant loss of bone in breast cancer patients on tamoxifen therapy for over 2 years versus controls not on tamoxifen.

Although there are no strict contraindications for use, pregnancy should be avoided while on tamoxifen therapy. Mothers should also avoid breastfeeding because tamoxifen may be present in milk and could pose a hazard to the newborn.

Other

Mifepristone (RU 486) is well tolerated with only occasional prolonged uterine bleeding. The most frequent, reversible side effects of aminoglutethimide include drowsiness, skin rash, nausea and anorexia, fever, dizziness, and ataxia, but these usually diminish with continued use.

The use of danazol is fraught with multiple antiestrogen-like and androgenic side effects, including weight gain, muscle cramps, decreased breast size, deepening of the voice, edema, amenorrhea, emotional lability, flushing, sweating, acne, mild hirsutism, oily skin and hair, altered libido, nausea, headache, dizziness, insomnia, rash, increased LDL concentrations, decreased HDL concentrations, and increased hepatic enzymes. Most of these are reversible with cessation of the drug. Also, urogenital abnormalities are possible in offspring if danazol is used during pregnancy or while breastfeeding.

REFERENCES

Baulieu EE: Contragestation and other clinical applications of RU486, an antiprogesterone at the receptor, Science 245:1351, 1989.

Beato M: Gene regulation by steroid hormones, Cell 56:335, 1989.

Clark JH and Markaverich BM: The agonistic-antagonistic properties of clomiphene: a review, Pharmacol Ther 15:467, 1982.

Jordan VC, ed: Estrogen/antiestrogen action and breast cancer therapy, Madison, Wisc, 1986, The University of Wisconsin Press.

Lindsay R: Prevention of postmenopausal osteoporosis, Ob Gyn Clin North Am 14:63, 1987.

Metzger DA and Luciano AA: Hormonal therapy of endometriosis, Ob Gyn Clin North Am 16:105, 1989.

Mishell DR: Contraception, N Engl J Med 320:777, 1989.

Robinson SP and Jordan VC: Metabolism of steroid-modifying anticancer agents, Pharmacol Ther 36:41, 1988.

Sarrell PM: Estrogen replacement therapy, Ob Gyn 72(suppl):2S, 1988.

Wharton C and Blackburn R: Lower-dose pills, Population Reports 16(3):1, 1988.

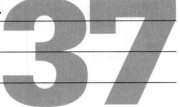

Androgens and Antiandrogens

THERAPEUTIC OVERVIEW

Androgens are produced by the testis, ovary, and adrenal glands. Testosterone, the most important androgen in males, is produced by the Leydig cells of the testis (see Chapters 35 and 36). It stimulates virilization and is an important spermatogenic hormone. Within the ovary, testosterone and androstenedione are precursor steroids for estradiol production. In both sexes, androgens stimulate body hair growth, positive nitrogen balance, bone growth, muscle development, and erythropoiesis. The mechanism of action of testosterone at its target organs is similar to that of other steroid hormones. The major use of androgens in clinical medicine is for replacement therapy in men whose production of testosterone is impaired, which is a relatively common condition. Testosterone synthesis inhibitors and antiandrogens are used to limit the effects of androgens in patients with androgen-dependent disorders, such as prostatic cancer, hirsutism, and precocious puberty.

Principal therapeutic considerations with andro-

ABBREVIATIONS	
DHT	dihydrotestosterone
DNA	deoxyribonucleic acid
FSH	follicle stimulating hormone
GTP	guanosine triphosphate
HRE	hormone responsive element
LH	luteinizing hormone

THERAPEUTIC OVERVIEW

ANDROGENS

Primary testicular insufficiency
Hypogonadotropic hypogonadism
Short stature
Osteoporosis, anemia
Testosterone and derivatives used for replacement
  therapy

ANTIANDROGENS AND ANTAGONISTS

Virilization in women
Precocious puberty in boys
Male contraceptive
Drugs used to decrease androgen synthesis or block
  androgen action

gens and related pharmacological preparations are summarized in the box.

MECHANISMS OF ACTION

Testosterone Synthesis

Testosterone, a 19-carbon atom steroid hormone is synthesized from cholesterol in the Leydig cells of the testis, the adrenal cortex, and the theca cells of the ovary following the pathways shown in Figure 37-1. In the adult gonads, the principal regulator of testicular testosterone synthesis and secretion is luteinizing hormone, which is produced by the anterior

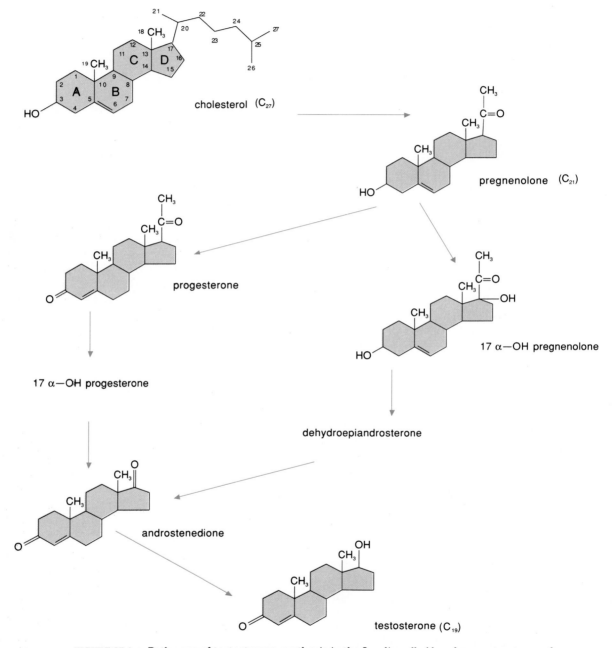

cholesterol (C$_{27}$)

pregnenolone (C$_{21}$)

progesterone

17 α—OH pregnenolone

17 α—OH progesterone

dehydroepiandrosterone

androstenedione

testosterone (C$_{19}$)

FIGURE 37-1 Pathways of testosterone synthesis in the Leydig cell. Also shown, structures of compounds and numbering system for steroid rings (A, B, C, D).

pituitary gland (see Chapter 39). In fetal testis, human chorionic gonadotropin promotes androgen formation. The precursor cholesterol is itself synthesized in the Leydig cells from acetate and stored as cholesterol esters in lipid droplets. A cholesterol ester hydrolase mobilizes free cholesterol from the lipid droplets, which in turn is transferred to the inner mitochondrial membrane. Stimulation of this transfer may represent a major action of luteinizing hormone. Whether transfer is mediated via a luteinizing hormone-responsive sterol carrier protein in vivo is not known. Mitochondrial oxidation occurs at positions C20 and C22, followed by lyase cleavage of the C-C bond between positions 20 and 22, resulting in the production of pregnenolone (Figure 37-1). These steps are catalyzed by a cytochrome P-450 enzyme system.

Pregnenolone, a 21-carbon steroid with a double-bond in the 5-6 position, is converted to a 21-carbon androgen in two steps; 17α-hydroxylation and lyase action at position 17-20, now known to be catalyzed by the same cytochrome P_{450} enzyme located in Leydig cell microsomes. Two possible pathways exist for the synthesis of testosterone from pregnenolone, as shown in Figure 37-1. One path is through 17α-hydroxypregnenolone to dehydroepiandrosterone (the Δ^5-pathway), and the second is through progesterone to 17α-hydroxyprogesterone and androstenedione (the Δ^4 pathway). Δ Refers to the position of the double bond in the A or B steroid ring. The A and B rings of pregnenolone or dehydroepiandrosterone are converted to a $\Delta^{4,5}$-keto structure by Δ^5, Δ^4 isomerase coupled to a 3β-hydroxysteroid dehydrogenase, also located within the microsomes. Finally, the microsomal enzyme 17β-hydroxysteroid dehydrogenase catalyzes the conversion of androstenedione to testosterone. Leydig cells also convert a small fraction of the testosterone produced to estradiol.

In contrast to peptide hormones, there is little intracellular storage of steroid hormones before secretion. The content of testosterone in the human testis is approximately 300 ng/g wet tissue weight. Since an adult human testis weighs about 15 g, the total testicular content of testosterone in an adult approximates 9 μg. This quantity is about 0.1% of the usual daily production of testosterone in normal adult men, (i.e., an average of 5 to 7 mg produced per 24 hours).

Fetal testosterone synthesis develops during the first trimester of pregnancy when the fetal testis is stimulated by human chorionic gonadotropin of placental origin to produce the testosterone required for male sexual differentiation. Gonadotrophs are not present in the fetal pituitary until the end of the first trimester, with luteinizing hormone and follicle-stimulating hormone secretion beginning in the second trimester. The principal stimulus to the fetal gonadotroph, as in the adult, is gonadotropin-releasing hormone. Gonadotropin secretion begins to decline late in fetal life and continues to decline in the neonate, after a prominent postnatal surge that lasts 2 to 3 months. By age 3 or 4 months, little testosterone is secreted. There is presently no explanation for this transient postnatal surge and subsequent attenuation in these secretions.

At puberty, gonadotropin secretion rises and re-awakens the Leydig cell to produce testosterone. Gonadotropin secretion exhibits a striking diurnal rhythm in early puberty, with elevated concentrations of luteinizing hormone and testosterone at night. In adult men it is more difficult to demonstrate a diurnal rhythm for luteinizing hormone, although testosterone concentrations are approximately 25% higher in the early morning hours compared to late afternoon. There are also fluctuations in luteinizing hormone secretion in adults that occur every 1 to 2 hours as a result of intermittent stimulation of gonadotrophs by gonadotropin-releasing hormone from the anterior hypothalamus. Gonadotropin-releasing hormone release episodes in turn are coupled to the excitatory discharges of an incompletely identified neural oscillator system. Intermittent gonadotropin-releasing hormone secretion is required for the pituitary to function normally, but whether pulsatile gonadotropin secretion is needed for normal testicular function remains to be clarified. However, testosterone is released into the circulation in a pulsatile fashion in response to the pulsatile stimulation of Leydig cells by luteinizing hormone. Follicle-stimulating hormone release is less clearly pulsatile in the circulation. Glycoprotein hormone α subunit secretion is also pulsatile and coupled to gonadotropin-releasing hormone stimulation, whereas free β gonadotropin subunits do not appear to be released in measurable quantities into the circulation from the pituitary.

Androgen Production by the Adrenal Glands and Ovaries

The adrenal glands secrete dehydroepiandrosterone, androstenedione, and testosterone, as well as some dehydroepiandrosterone sulfate and estrone.

Glucocorticoids and mineralocorticoids are physiologically the principal products of the adult adrenal gland. The concentrations of dehydroepiandrosterone, dehydroepiandrosterone sulfate, and androstenedione in the circulation rise between ages 7 to 10 years; this process has been termed adrenarche, to distinguish it from puberty or gonadarche, which refers to the onset of adult gonadal function. Although adrenocorticotropin stimulates the adrenal to secrete sex steroids, some additional mechanisms may be responsible for adrenarche, since there is no concomitant increase in cortisol secretion in children at this age. Adrenal androgen secretion also declines in the elderly and in individuals who are ill.

Control of Testosterone Synthesis and Secretion

The major regulator of testosterone synthesis and secretion is luteinizing hormone. Leydig cells contain cell surface receptors for luteinizing hormone, which are coupled to adenylate cylase and to specific GTP-binding proteins. The steroidogenic response also requires intracellular calcium ions and the calcium-binding protein calmodulin. Like other protein hormones, luteinizing hormone action may also involve activation of phospholipase C, which produces diacylglycerol and inositol trisphosphate from membrane phosphoinositides (see Chapter 2). Diacylglycerol can activate protein kinase C, which phosphorylates membrane and intracellular proteins. Other hormones that may influence testosterone synthesis include prolactin, cortisol, insulin, insulin-like growth factors, estradiol, and inhibin. There is a growing awareness that multiple incompletely characterized factors produced within the seminiferous tubules by germ cells and Sertoli cells and/or peritubular myoid cells can also regulate testosterone synthesis. Together these factors maintain the concentration of testosterone in adult men at 300 to 1000 ng/dl (10 to 30 nM).

Sertoli cells are somatic cells within the seminiferous tubules. Tight junctions between these cells the base of seminiferous tubules form a blood-testis barrier. Sertoli cells secrete a large number of proteins, some of which enter the tubular lumen and are important in spermatogenesis, whereas other proteins are secreted through the basal end of the cell and enter the circulation. Among these Sertoli cell proteins are androgen-binding protein, transferrin,

and inhibin. Follicle-stimulating hormone is the major regulator of Sertoli cell function. The follicle-stimulating hormone receptor is membrane bound and acts through the second messengers cAMP and calcium. Insulin and insulin-like growth factors, testosterone, vitamin A, and β-endorphins also appear to influence Sertoli cell function.

The hormones of the hypothalamus, pituitary, and testes form an internally regulated unit (Figure 37-2), which is discussed further in Chapter 41. Not only are the testes stimulated by pituitary gonadotropins, but also the testes regulate luteinizing and follicle-stimulating hormone secretions through negative feedback mechanisms (Chapter 41). Testosterone suppresses gonadotropin secretion by slowing the pulsatile release of gonadotropin-releasing hormone. A secondary action of testosterone limits pituitary responsiveness to gonadotropin-releasing hormone. Although estradiol inhibits gonadotropin release at both the hypothalamic and the pituitary levels, its exact mechanism of action depends upon gonadal status, dose, and duration of steroid exposure. Inhi-

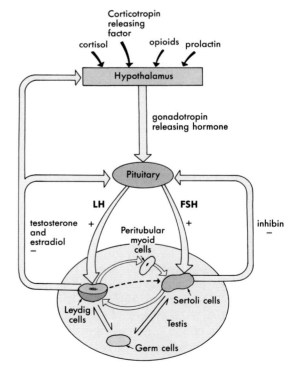

FIGURE 37-2　Hormonal control of testicular function (see text for discussion).

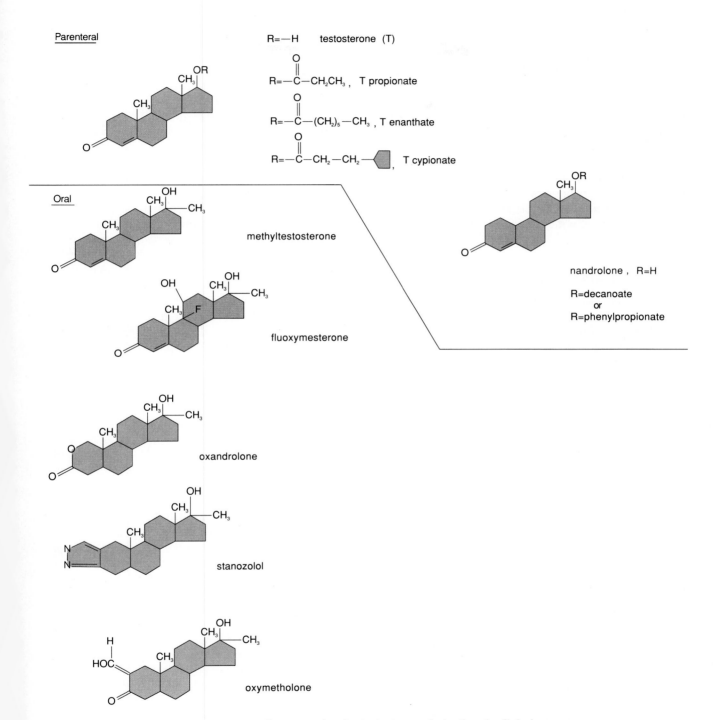

FIGURE 37-3   Structure of major testosterone derivatives in clinical use.

bin, a heterodimeric glycoprotein produced by the Sertoli cells of the testis, reduces follicle-stimulating hormone synthesis and secretion and limits both luteinizing hormone and follicle-stimulating hormone release by antagonizing the action of gonadotropin-releasing hormone.

Normal women produce approximately 0.25 mg of testosterone per day, compared to the 5 to 7 mg/day for adult men. The majority of testosterone circulating in women is derived from the peripheral conversion of androstenedione secreted by the ovary as well as the adrenal. Benign and malignant tumors of the adrenal and ovary, congenital steroidogenesic enzyme defects, and disturbances of gonadotropin secretion can be associated with increased androgen production in women.

Androgen Action

Circulating endogenous testosterone or exogenous testosterone derivatives (Figure 37-3) are transported to the target tissues, where testosterone or the exogenous androgen derivatives enter the cells.

Circulating testosterone is bound tightly to a serum glycoprotein of hepatic origin, called sex hormone-binding globulin, and weakly to albumin. Less than 1% to 2% of the circulating testosterone is thought to be unbound. However, binding to albumin is of such low affinity that it is functionally equivalent to unbound testosterone. Together the free and weakly bound testosterone, which account for approximately 50% of the testosterone found in adult male serum, can enter target tissues. The sex hormone-binding globulin is a heterodimer of molecular weight 88,000 daltons, identical in sequence to the androgen-binding protein produced by Sertoli cells; however, the two androphilic binding proteins differ in carbohydrate content. There is recent evidence to suggest that sex hormone-binding globulin binds to or enters the androgen target cells, so the transport proteins may also play a role in the action of testosterone. Estrogens and thyroxine increase, and androgens decrease sex hormone-binding globulin production, so that the concentrations of this hormone are twofold to threefold greater in women than in men. They rise further in hyperthyroidism. Through unknown mechanisms, obesity in humans is associated with low concentrations of sex hormone-binding globulin.

Once the androgens enter the target tissue cell, they may be enzymatically converted to another compound that shows greater or less androgen activity, or they may act directly with androgen receptors (Figure 37-4). When testosterone, the prototype, as well as endogenous androgens enter target tissues such as the prostate gland, testosterone can be metabolized to 5α-dihydrotestosterone, but in other target tissues such as muscle and kidney testosterone remains unchanged. There is no clear explanation for the presence of testosterone 5α-reductase in only certain androgen target tissues. However, the clinical syndrome of ambiguous genitalia in patients who lack normal testosterone 5α-reductase activity underscores the importance of the latter enzyme in the normal development of the external genitalia in human males. Dihydrotestosterone binds with slightly higher affinity to the androgen receptor than does testosterone. This difference reflects the slower kinetics of dissociation of dihydrotestosterone from the receptor. In this way 5α reduction appears to amplify the actions of testosterone in target cells.

Intracellular receptor binding of androgens and the postreceptor events are similar to those of other steroid hormones. Androgen receptors have been purified and shown to be proteins with molecular weights of approximately 120 kilodaltons with synthesis guided in humans by genes on the X chromosome. The steroid-binding monomer (4.4S) is present in cells bound to receptor-associated protein and to small molecules producing a 9S inactive oligomer. Testosterone or dihydrotestosterone binds to a hormone-binding site near the carboxy terminus of the receptor, thereby activating the receptor complex so it can bind to a nuclear DNA acceptor site, known as the hormone response element (HRE). Receptor activation involves the disaggregation of the macromolecular complex with the release of an accesssory protein exposing the DNA binding site on the 4.4S receptor. This region of the protein is rich in cysteines and is highly homologous with suggested DNA-binding domains of other steroid hormone receptors (see Chapter 34). Binding of the receptor to DNA is followed by the transcription of mRNAs for tissue-specific proteins, which constitutes the hormonal response.

Androgen regulation of target tissues may not only be positive, as in the stimulation of androgen-dependent proteins within the prostate, but also negative, as in the inhibition of gonadotropin-releasing hormone release by the hypothalamus. The molecular mechanisms for the inhibitory action of androgens are unknown.

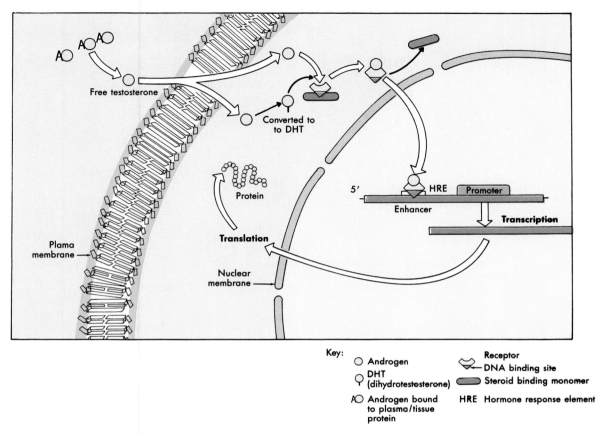

FIGURE 37-4   Schematic diagram of androgen action at target cells. (See text.)

Antiandrogens and Antagonists

The mechanism of action of antiandrogens is to block the synthesis of endogenous testosterone, while antagonists bind to the androgen receptor or otherwise block androgen action. Several drugs, including spironolactone and ketoconazole decrease testosterone production by reducing the activity of cytochrome P-450 in testicular microsomes responsible for conversion of progesterone to androstenedione through 17 α-hydroxylation and C17-20 lyase cleavage. These drugs are substrate analogs, which compete with the natural substrates for binding to the active site of the enzyme. They are also used in the treatment of other diseases. Their structures are shown in Figure 37-5.

Finasteride, an investigational 5 α-reductase inhibitor, blocks the conversion of testosterone to 5 α-dihydro-testosterone in tissues containing this enzyme, including prostate. This drug decreases pros-

tate size in rats and dogs and could be used to treat benign prostatic hyperplasia.

Spironolactone, a synthetic steroid, also acts as an androgen antagonist by binding to the androgen receptor, as do the nonsteroidal compounds flutamide and cimetidine. The latter compound is a relatively weak antiandrogen with limited clinical usefulness, whereas flutamide is used clinically, together with GnRH agonists, to treat prostate cancer.

 PHARMACOKINETICS

Pharmacokinetic parameter values for clinically used androgens and spironolactone are listed in Table 37-1, p. 525. See Chapter 52 for values for ketoconazole, Chapter 58 for cimetidine, and Chapter 19 for spironolactone pharmacokinetics.

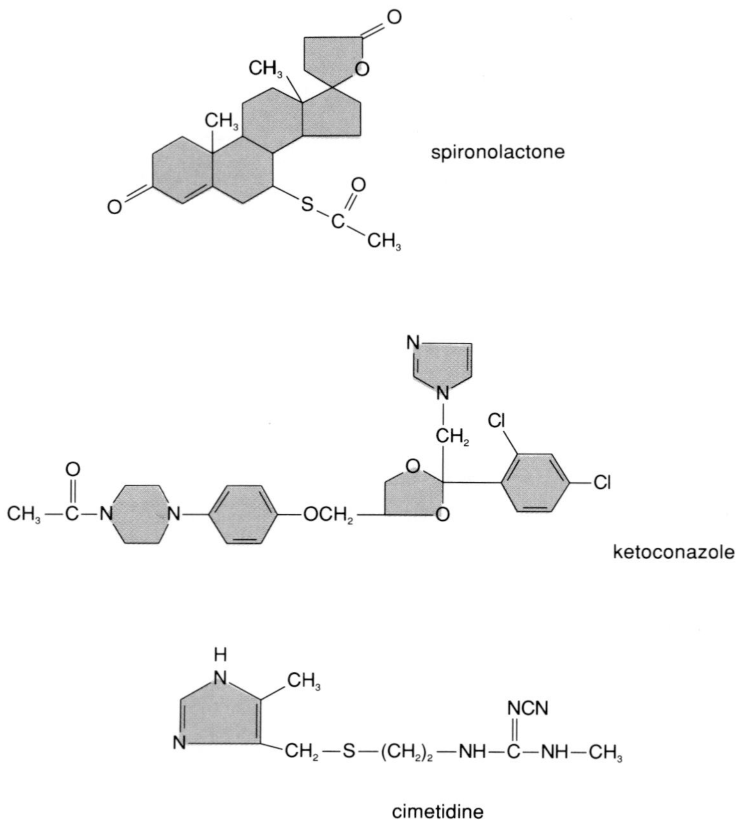

FIGURE 37-5   Structures of antiandrogens and antagonists.

Testosterone Metabolism

The metabolism of testosterone is summarized in Figure 37-6. Metabolism in liver is primarily to the 17-ketosteroids (5α) androsterone and (5β)-etiocholanolone. However, these compounds form only a small fraction of the 17-ketosteroids found in urine. The majority of the 17-ketosteroids in urine are the metabolites of androstenedione and dehydroepiandrosterone produced by the adrenal gland. Testosterone is also conjugated to sulfuric and glucuronic acids and excreted in the urine and bile.

The conversion of testosterone to estradiol via the enzyme complex aromatase occurs in the testis, adipose stroma, skin, and brain. A portion of the feedback regulation of gonadotropin secretion at the level of the gonadotropin-releasing hormone pulse generator may involve the local conversion of testosterone to estradiol. Other physiological actions of estradiol in males remain incompletely defined.

Androgen Preparations

Androgens are available for clinical use in oral and parenteral forms (see Figure 37-3 and Table 37-1). Natural testosterone taken orally or injected IM is rapidly cleared by the liver, rendering these routes ineffective for clinical use. Testosterone esterified at the 17-hydroxyl position is used for IM injection in an oil suspension. Esterification increases the lipid solubility of testosterone and prolongs its action. Testosterone propionate has a relatively short duration of action, 1 to 2 days. The more commonly used enanthate or cypionate esters can be given by deep IM injection every 2 to 3 weeks. The esters are converted to free testosterone in the circulation. Subcutaneous pellets containing testosterone have been used in Europe and Asia, but have achieved little popularity in the United States.

Transdermal delivery of testosterone has been accomplished in an effort to produce stable physiolog-

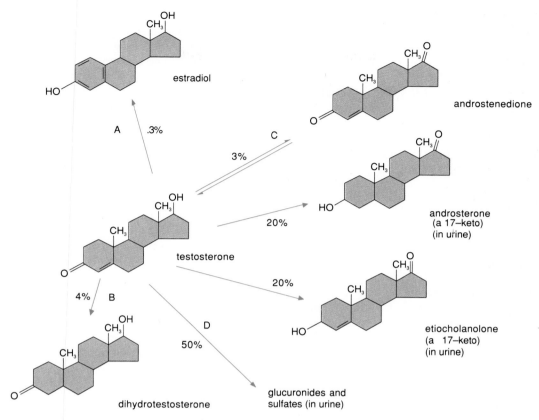

FIGURE 37-6   Metabolism of testosterone. Enzymes are: **A,** Aromatase. **B,** 5α-reductase. **C,** 17β-hydroxysteroid dehydrogenase. **D,** Hydroxylases and transferases.

Table 37-1   Pharmacokinetic Parameters

Drug	Administration	$t_{1/2}$	Disposition
methyltestosterone	Oral, buccal	Short-acting, daily	M
testosterone cypionate	IM	Long-acting, (depot)	M
testosterone enanthate	IM	Long-acting (depot) q 2-3 weeks	M
fluoxymesterone	Oral	Short-acting, daily or twice daily	M
danazol	Oral	Short-acting, daily	M
nandrolone	IM	Long-acting (depot)	M

M, Metabolized.

ical drug concentrations. A thin, flexible self-adhering polymer is applied to the scrotal skin, since absorption through this surface is considerably greater than through thicker epidermis elsewhere.

Several testosterone derivatives are available for sublingual or oral use. Alkylation produces androgens that are slowly metabolized by the liver but without testosterone as a metabolite. These derivatives interact directly with the androgen receptor. However, their androgenic potency is difficult to determine, since the end point upon which to base normal androgen action is uncertain. The pharmacokinetics of these compounds are not well established.

Danazol is only weakly androgenic and interacts with progesterone as well as androgen receptors. It inhibits pulsatile release of gonadotropins with a subsequent decline of serum concentrations of estradiol and estrone in women. A half-life of 4.5 hours has been reported.

 ## RELATION OF MECHANISMS OF ACTION TO CLINICAL RESPONSE

Replacement Theory

Testosterone is required for the normal development of male external genitalia during the first trimester of fetal life. Therefore when fetal synthesis of androgen is insufficient (e.g., an inborn enzymatic error), or there is an ineffectiveness of androgen action at its target tissues (e.g., a receptor defect), the genital phenotype may be female or ambiguous. These individuals are known as pseudohermaphrodites. In contrast, true hermaphrodites have both ovaries and testes.

At puberty in males, an increase in circulating androgens stimulates the expression of adult secondary sex characteristics. The scrotum darkens and become rugated; beard and body hair growth are stimulated; sebaceous glands are stimulated; phallus, prostate, seminal vesicles, and larynx enlarge; and the voice deepens. There is an increase in muscle mass, skeletal development, and linear growth. Finally, androgens affect the brain to stimulate libido. These processes are incomplete if androgen synthesis or actions are impaired.

Testosterone is also an important spermatogenic hormone. Both Sertoli and myoid cells contain intracellular androgen receptors and appear to be androgen target cells. Thus androgen deficiency is associated with hypospermatogenesis, and hypogonadal men are often infertile.

Aging is associated with a decline in testicular function; for example, Leydig cell volume decreases with a fall in serum testosterone concentrations after the age of 60 years. The associated rise in serum luteinizing and follicle-stimulating hormone concentrations indicates that one or more processes are adversely affecting the testis.

Several situations can develop where androgen concentrations or synthesis rates are depressed and where replacement therapy is sometimes used.

Testosterone deficiency may result from a disorder intrinsic to the testis or from insufficient stimulation of the testes by pituitary gonadotropins. The former condition is termed primary testicular failure, and the latter syndrome is termed hypogonadotropic hypogonadism. Although testosterone treatment stimulates the expression of secondary sex characteristics in men with primary testicular failure, they remain infertile.

Androgen excess is not a clinical problem in adult men. However, the production of excess androgens in boys can elicit precocious puberty, and in women can lead to infertility, disturbed menstrual rhythms, hirsutism, and, if sufficiently severe, to the development of a male body habitus (virilization). Precocious puberty refers to the onset of sexual development in boys before 9 years of age and in girls before 8 years of age. Approximately 50% of boys with true precocious puberty have a tumor of the hypothalamus.

Androgens also are used to treat adult men with testosterone deficiency from primary gonadal failure or hypogonadotropic hypogonadism. The goal of therapy is to stimulate or restore androgenization to normal. Androgens stimulate body and beard hair growth, phallic enlargement, muscle development, voice deepening, and other phenomena. In adult men who have previously established normal sexual development, androgens may increase libido and potency. These latter end points are often difficult to quantitate and are influenced by factors other than sex steroids.

Testosterone is also used to treat congenital microphallus. Most boys with a small phallus will ultimately prove to be hypogonadal as adults. Impaired androgen production in utero or resistance to androgen action presumably explains the failure of the phallus to develop normally. Treatment is usually begun with intermittent small doses of parenteral testosterone and monitored carefully to prevent unwanted virilization.

Androgen replacement to increase the height of short children and short teenagers with constitutional delay of puberty is complex and controversial, since the role of androgens in normal growth and development remains ill-defined. Further, premature closure of the epiphyseal plates with resultant growth arrest and unacceptable virilization may occur. Normal puberty in both males and females is accompanied by an acceleration in growth rate known as the pubertal growth spurt, presumably related to the increase in sex steroid secretion. Androgens increase the daily production rate and the amplitude of spontaneous growth hormone secretory episodes. Treatment of growth hormone-deficient teenagers with growth hormone together with androgens is more effective in increasing linear height than are androgens alone. In children with normal growth hormone secretion, androgen therapy initially increases growth velocity; however, accelerated epiphyseal closure may reduce ultimate adult height. Androgens may also be used to treat boys of exceptionally tall stature to accelerate epiphyseal closure and limit final height, but this use is equally debatable.

Anabolic Steroids in Normal Men

Androgens known as anabolic steroids are used by athletes to increase muscle mass and physical performance as well as used therapeutically with children to promote linear growth. These drugs are believed to be more anabolic than androgenic. This drug classification is based on in vivo bioassays in immature male rats in which increased levator ani muscle weight was found to occur at lower doses than those that stimulated the growth of the seminal vesicles and prostate. However, the interpretation of this bioassay has been criticized because the levator ani is not a typical skeletal muscle but instead is a sexual dimorphic muscle of the reproductive tract. Whether anabolic steroids differ appreciably from androgens is controversial because the androgen receptor in skeletal muscle is not known to differ from that in seminal vesicles and prostate. However, the latter tissue contains 5α-reductase whereas skeletal muscle does not. This enzyme amplifies the action of testosterone but does not influence the potency of most testosterone derivatives, and may reduce the potency of 19-nortestosterone. Thus local metabolism may influence the potency of various androgens differently, and this effect may vary among target tissues.

Drugs commonly used for their anabolic activity include derivatives of 19-nortestosterone, oxandrolone, oxymetholone, and stanazolol.

Miscellaneous Androgen Uses

The erythropoietic effect of androgens is well established. Hemoglobin concentration is 1 to 2 g/dl higher in sexually mature men than in women or children, and mild anemia is common in hypogonadal men. Polycythemia may occur as an unwanted effect of androgen therapy. Androgens have been shown to stimulate erythropoiesis by increasing renal erythro-

poietin production (Chapter 65). There is also a direct effect of androgens on erythrocyte maturation. Since 5β-androgens (which bind weakly to androgen receptors) are more effective than 5α-androgens, the binding may constitute a novel mechanism to explain the direct effect of androgens on bone marrow cells. Androgens may be used to treat patients with aplastic anemia, and such patients occasionally respond to androgen therapy; however, responses vary. Both parenteral testosterone esters and oral androgens have been used, with the less potent androgens employed in women to limit undesirable virilization. Hypogonadism is common in both men and women with chronic renal failure. There is a mean increase in hematocrit in patients with chronic renal failure treated with androgens. Patients who need frequent transfusions and who have had bilateral nephrectomy may respond more poorly.

Danazol is an androgen derivative used for treatment of endometriosis, fibrocystic disease of the breast, and premenstrual tension syndrome (see Chapter 36). Danazol is also used to prevent attacks of hereditary angioneurotic edema, a disorder characterized by recurrent edema of the skin and mucosa. These patients lack the function of the inhibitor of the activated first component of complement, and androgens increase the serum concentration of this protein. Danazol is used rather than testosterone because it is weakly androgenic.

Other indications for the use of androgens have included inoperable breast cancer, postpartum breast pain and engorgement, and the wasting of chronic diseases and malnutrition in both sexes. The mechanism through which androgens affect the normal breast and modify the growth of breast cancer cells is uncertain. Positive responses of breast cancer, which average 30%, are less than for other hormonal therapies. Potent androgens are unacceptable in women because of virilization. Less potent androgens such as danazol have also been examined, but their efficacy is uncertain. Although androgens produce a positive nitrogen balance, clinical improvement in malnourished patients with chronic disease may reflect improved nutritional status.

Antiandrogens and Antagonists

Blockade of androgen synthesis or action is used as a treatment for female hirsutism, acne, precocious puberty in males, benign prostate tumors, and other diseases. Although the role of androgens in the pathogenesis of benign and malignant prostate disease remains uncertain, disseminated prostatic cancer is treated by decreasing testosterone production and impeding its action. The limiting of production can be accomplished by orchiectomy or by drugs, although a reduction in androgen secretion or action in adult men may reduce libido and potency and cause gynecomastia (enlargement of the male breast).

Currently available androgen antagonists exert their effects by competing for binding to the testosterone/dihydrotestosterone binding site on the intracellular androgen receptor. Nonsteroidal antiandrogens, although dissimilar from testosterone in planar structure, undergo sufficient folding to allow them to simulate the structure of androgens and bind to the receptor to form an antagonist-receptor complex that fails to undergo activation. Receptor binding to nuclear acceptor sites generally does not occur, and the biological actions of circulating androgens are blocked. This mechanism differs from that of antiestrogens, which bind to one or more classes of receptors and accumulate in target cell nuclei but are inactive biologically.

One of the antiandrogens, spironolactone, is a synthetic steroid primarily used as an aldosterone antagonist in the treatment of primary and secondary hyperaldosteronism, or as an antihypertensive agent. In addition to occupying aldosterone receptors, spironolactone interacts with androgen receptors and functions as an antiandrogen. Further, spironolactone reduces the concentrations of the cytochrome P-450 17α-hydroxylase 17 to 20 lyase enzyme complex in testicular microsomes. The result is a decline in testosterone synthesis. Progesterone concentration increases because its further conversion is inhibited. However, a decrease in serum androgen concentration in men produces an increase in gonadotropin secretion, which may return the serum testosterone concentration to normal. The rise in gonadotropin secretion may increase aromatization to estradiol, leading to impotence and gynecomastia. Because of its action to block testosterone synthesis as well as to impede androgen action, spironolactone is used in the treatment of hirsute women.

Another antiandrogen, ketoconazole, is a broad-spectrum antimycotic agent used in the treatment of systemic fungal infections (see Chapter 52). Ketoconazole inhibits the synthesis of ergosterol in fungi, resulting in altered membrane permeability; inhibits the synthesis of cholesterol; and interferes with the action of cytochrome P-450 enzyme complexes in several mammalian cell types, including Leydig cells. The result is a dose-dependent decline in circulating testosterone concentrations in adult men and a rise in serum 17α-hydroxyprogesterone concentrations, suggesting an effect on the 17 to 20 lyase. Serum luteinizing and follicle-stimulating hormone concentrations rise due to the decline in testosterone negative feedback. This action of ketoconazole has prompted its investigational use in the treatment of prostatic cancer and also in gonadotropin-independent precocious puberty in boys. However, the extent of suppression of testosterone synthesis is highly variable among men. Ketoconazole also inhibits cortisol biosynthesis, and has been used as an adjunctive therapy in patients with Cushing's syndrome. Ketoconazole-treated men may develop gynecomastia.

Androgen antagonists are used to block the actions of androgens at androgen target tissues. Hirsutism, acne, androgen-induced male pattern alopecia in women, gonadotropin-independent precocious puberty in boys, and prostatic cancer represent clinical disorders that may benefit from this treatment strategy.

The histamine H$_2$-receptor antagonist cimetidine, widely used to decrease gastric acid secretion in the treatment of peptic ulcer disease and esophagitis, acts as an antiandrogen. Thus it has been reported to produce gynecomastia when given in large dosages like those used in the treatment of patients with Zollinger-Ellison syndrome. Gynecomastia occurs in less than 1% of patients treated with dosages in peptic ulcer disease. Cimetidine interacts with the androgen receptor about 0.01% as effectively as testosterone. Cimetidine also is used to treat hirsutism in women.

Cyproterone acetate, a synthetic steroid derived from 17α-hydroxyprogesterone, is an antiandrogen that is not available for clinical use in the United States, in part because it has some intrinsic suppressive effects on the corticotropic axis. Cyproterone also binds to the androgen receptor approximately 10% as well as testosterone, and is a potent progestin. When given to women, it disrupts cyclic menstrual bleeding. The combination with estrogen suppresses gonadotropin secretion, inhibits ovulation, and reduces circulating testosterone concentrations.

Flutamide is a nonsteroidal antiandrogen now approved for clinical use in the United States. It binds weakly to the androgen receptor and requires hydroxylation for metabolic activity in vivo. Flutamide is used together with gonadotropin-releasing hormone analogs in the treatment of prostatic cancer.

Inhibitors of testosterone 5α-reductase could also be useful to treat androgen-dependent disorders of tissues in which this enzyme amplifies testosterone actions in the prostate and hair follicle. Several 5α-reductase inhibitors are undergoing clinicial testing.

SIDE EFFECTS, CLINICAL PROBLEMS, AND TOXICITY

Many side effects of androgens are dose-related and occur when target tissues are stimulated excessively. These include priapism (sustained erection), acne, polycythemia, and prostatic enlargement. Androgens should not be used in men with suspected prostatic cancer. Androgens also decrease high-density lipoprotein concentrations. However, the impact of this change (which theoretically would be atherogenic) in the pathophysiology of coronary artery disease is uncertain. Weight gain and sodium retention may occur with androgen therapy, although the mechanism is unclear. Chronic androgen treatment suppresses gonadotropin secretion, decreases testis size, and depresses spermatogenesis. For this reason testosterone has been evaluated as a male contraceptive. However, azoospermia (zero sperm output) may not occur, perhaps because of the direct stimulatory effect of testosterone on seminiferous tubules. Occasionally patients treated with testosterone develop gynecomastia. This may be from the bioconversion (aromatization reaction) of administered testosterone to estradiol. Obstructive sleep apnea has been reported to be exacerbated in susceptible men treated with testosterone.

The 17α-methylated androgens may disturb hepatic function, which appears to be an idiosyncratic response. Serum transaminase concentrations may rise, and 1% to 2% of patients develop jaundice due to intrahepatic cholestasis. Peliosis hepatitis and hepatocellular carcinoma have each been reported in a few patients treated with very high doses of alkylated androgens. Accordingly, these compounds are usually reserved for individuals in whom parenteral administration is contraindicated (e.g., bleeding dyscrasias).

Danazol may produce acne, oily skin, decreased breast size, hirsutism, and decreased high-density lipoprotein cholesterol in treated women (as noted in Chapter 36).

Spironolactone binds to the androgen receptor in cultured skin fibroblasts with approximately 50% of the affinity of testosterone. Since peak spironolactone concentrations in vivo approximate concentrations of testosterone in men, this interaction could produce clinically significant effects. Moreover, long-acting metabolites of spironolactone are also antiandrogenic. As many as 50% of men treated with spironolactone develop gynecomastia. Libido may decline and impotence may occur. Amenorrhea and breast tenderness occur in women.

Professional and amateur athletes often use multiple androgens in dosages that far exceed estimated physiological replacement amounts. These androgens, like testosterone, suppress gonadotropin section and thereby reduce testicular function, including spermatogenesis. Nonaromatizable androgens reduce high-density lipoprotein synthesis and thereby high-density lipoprotein concentrations. This may increase the risk of atherosclerosis in these men. Long-term, high-dose androgen treatment may also increase the risk of benign prostatic hyperplasia and may cause prostatic cancer when these men age. Because numerous variables impact on athletic performance and because the efficacy of pharmacological androgen treatment of normal men remains controversial and the side-effects are unequivocal, the use of these drugs has been banned by the International Olympic Committee. Legislation is currently planned to limit their availability in the United States.

The clinical problems with these drugs are summarized in the box. See Chapter 52 for ketoconazole, Chapter 58 for cimetidine, and Chapter 19 for spironolactone.

CLINICAL PROBLEMS
Masculinization in women
Priapism in men
Growth disturbances in children
Fetal masculinization during pregnancy
Jaundice
Edema
Acne

TRADENAMES

In addition to generic and fixed combination preparations, the following tradenamed materials are available in the United States.

ANDROGENS

Anadrol, oxymetholone
Anavar, oxandrolone
Android, Metandren, Estratest, Oreton, Testred; methyltestosterone
Danocrine, danazol
Deca-Durabolin, nandrolone
Depo-testosterone, Andro-Cyp; testosterone cypionate
Halotestin, fluoxymesterone
Teslac, testolactone
Winstrol, nandrolone decanoate stanozolol

ANTIANDROGENS AND ANTAGONISTS

Aldactone, spironolactone
Eulexin, flutamide

REFERENCES

Bardin CW and Catterall JF: Testosterone: A major determinant of extragenital sexual dimorphism, Science 211:1285, 1981.

Loriaux DL, Menard R and Taylor A, et al: Spironolactone and endocrine dysfunction, Ann Intern Med 85:630, 1976.

Madanes AE and Farber M: Danazol, Ann Intern Med 96:625, 1982.

Sokol RZ and Swerdloff RS: Practical considerations in the use of androgen therapy. In Santen RJ and Swerdloff RS, eds: Male reproductive dysfunction: diagnosis and management of hypogonadism, infertility, and impotence, New York, 1986, Marcel Dekker.

Sonino N: The use of ketoconazole as an inhibitor of steroid production, N Engl J Med 317:812, 1987.

Wilson JD: Androgen abuse by athletes, Endocr Rev 9:181, 1988.

Winters SJ: Clinical male reproductive neuroendocrinology. In Vaitukaitis JL, ed: Clinical reproductive neuroendocrinology, New York, 1981, Elsevier Biomedical.

CHAPTER 38

Thyroid and Antithyroid Drugs

ABBREVIATIONS	
MIT	monoiodotyrosine
mRNA	messenger RNA
$t_{1/2}$	half-life
T_3	triiodothyronine
T_4	thyroxine
PTU	propylthiouracil
TcO_4^-	pertechnetate

MAJOR DRUGS

iodides
perchlorate
pertechnetate
thioureylenes
thyroid hormones

THERAPEUTIC OVERVIEW

HYPOTHYROIDISM

Administer exogenous thyroxine (T_4) or triiodothyronine (T_3)

HYPERTHYROIDISM

Surgery
Radioactive iodine
Drugs
    thioureylenes
    β blockers
    corticosteroids
    iodide
    perchlorate (ClO_4^-)
    pertechnetate (TcO_4^-)

 ## THERAPEUTIC OVERVIEW

The thyroid, like most endocrine glands, can secrete too much or too little hormone, producing hyperthyroidism or hypothyroidism. Hypothyroidism is most commonly caused by the end stages of autoimmune thyroid disease (Hashimoto's thyroiditis), in which autoantibodies have destroyed the thyroid gland. Other causes include familial goiter and surgical removal of the thyroid. Whatever the cause, hypothyroidism can be completely corrected by pharmacological preparations of thyroid hormone, either thyroxine or triiodothyroxine.

The treatment of hyperthyroidism is more complex. The most common causes of hyperthyroidism are Graves' disease (another form of autoimmune thyroid disease) and toxic nodular goiter. In Graves' disease, autoantibodies directed to thyroid membrane receptors stimulate the thyroid to overproduce thyroid hormone. The optimal approach to therapy would be to block the immunologic stimulation, but such an approach is currently impractical. Instead, antithyroid drugs, radioactive iodine, or surgery are used to block the synthesis or effects of excess thyroid hormone. Radioactive iodine and surgery are ablative approaches that can control the hyperthyroidism defin-

529

itively when their use is sufficiently aggressive. The treatments of hypo- and hyperthyroidism are summarized in the box, p. 529.

 ## MECHANISMS OF ACTION

Thyroid Hormones

The thyroid hormones 3,5,3', 5'-tetraiodothyronine (thyroxine) (T_4) and 3,5,3'-triiodothyronine (T_3) are iodinated derivatives of tyrosine (see Figure 38-1 for structures). T_3 and T_4 are synthesized in the thyroid gland, or in the treatment of hypothyroidism, are administered for pharmacological purposes. The chemical structures are the same whether T_3 and T_4 are synthesized in vivo or prepared in vitro.

The in vivo synthesis and storage of T_3 and T_4 occurs as part of the synthesis of the large glycoprotein, thyroglobulin. The thyroid gland is unique among the endocrine organs in having an extracellular compartment, the follicular lumen, in which to store its hormone. The intrathyroidal processing steps in the synthesis thyroid hormones are outlined in Figure 38-2.

Circulating iodide is concentrated by thyroid epithelial cells via an active transport system believed to be located in basal membranes. The system, which operates against an electrochemical gradient, requires energy in the form of oxidative phosphorylation and can be demonstrated only in the intact cell. Although details of the transport mechanism remain unknown, phospholipids may serve as iodide carriers across the cell membrane. Once within the thyroid cell, iodide passes down its electrochemical gradient across the apical cell membrane and into the follicular lumen. Meanwhile the peptide chain of thyroglobulin and part of its carbohydrate moiety are synthesized within the endoplasmic reticulum. Completion of the carbohydrate units occurs as the protein passes through the Golgi. The as yet un-iodinated thyroglobulin is then transported in small vesicles to the apical cell membrane where it also is released into the lumen.

Next, iodide is oxidized, then attached to tyrosyl residues in thyroglobulin, forming the thyroid hor-

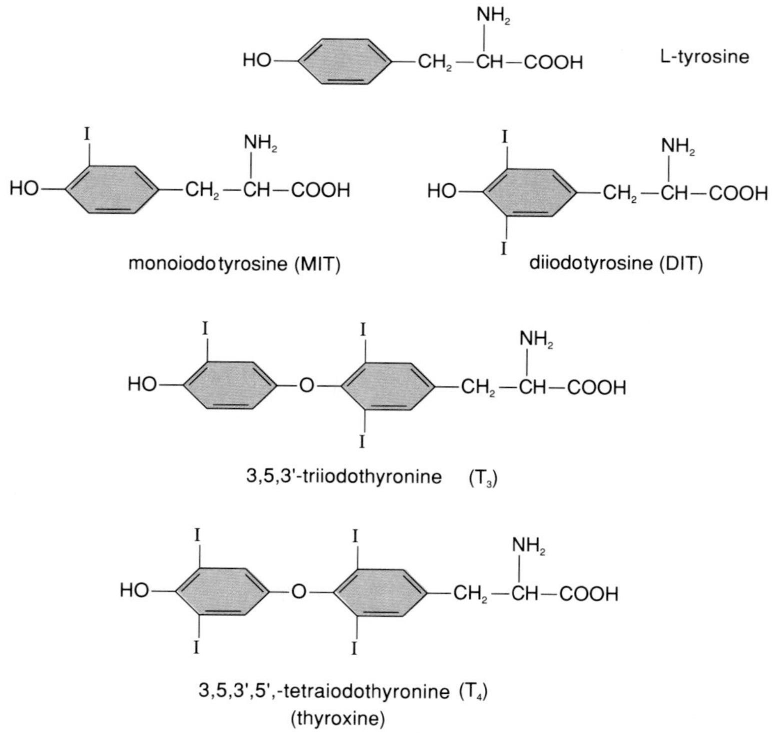

FIGURE 38-1 Structures of thyroid hormones and precursors.

mone precursors monoiodotyrosine and diiodotyrosine (see Figure 38-1). This step is mediated by a thyroid peroxidase in the presence of H_2O_2. The formation of the hormones occurs with the coupling of an "acceptor," diiodotyrosine, still linked to thyroglobulin and a "donor," diiodotyrosine or monoiodotyrosine, which loses its alanine side chain to form respectively T_4 or T_3 (Figure 38-3). This step is also mediated by thyroid peroxidase. Iodination and coupling are believed to occur at the apical cell membrane where both the peroxidase and an H_2O_2-generating source are present. Under normal circumstances, a thyroglobulin molecule contains an average of three to four residues of T_4 and zero to one residues of T_3. At least four major hormonogenic sites exist in the thyroglobulin polypeptide chains.

As thyroid hormone is needed by the body, thyroglobulin is retrieved from the follicular lumen by endocytosis in the form of either small vesicles or large colloid droplets. These endocytotic vesicles then fuse with lysosomes and undergo proteolytic breakdown of thyroglobulin, catalyzed by cathepsin D, cathepsin B, and thiol thyroglobulin hydrolase. The latter two are stimulated by thyroid-stimulating hormone and have their major activities respectively at the N- and C-termini of the thyroglobulin chain. Through the synergistic action of lysosomal endopeptidases and exopeptidases the iodamino acids are released from thyroglobulin, with T_3 and T_4 rapidly transferred intact from the lysosomes into the bloodstream by unknown mechanisms.

Most of the circulating thyroid hormones are noncovalently bound to plasma transport proteins. In humans this transport is mediated primarily by thyroxine-binding globulin and to a lesser extent by thyroxine-binding prealbumin and albumin. The affinities of each of these proteins are much greater for T_4 than for T_3. Before entry into the target cell, the hormones are released from plasma proteins. The final processing of T_4 occurs in peripheral tissues, where it is deiodinated to T_3.

The thyroid hormones exert their effects by controlling gene expression mediated via T_3 receptors located in the nucleus, and as a result of the T_3-receptor-nuclear interaction, the concentrations of selected mRNAs are altered.

Thyroid hormone receptors have been identified in all thyroid hormone-responsive tissues tested and their general physiochemical properties are identical. The receptors are nonhistone proteins capable of binding to DNA and have molecular weights of 47,000

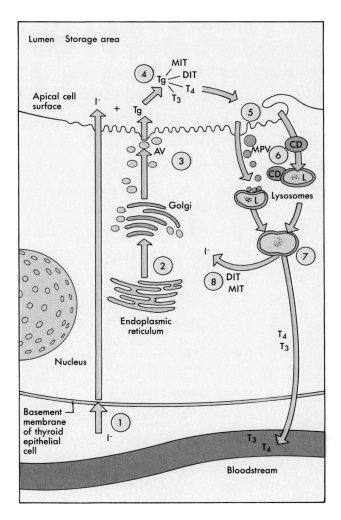

FIGURE 38-2   Intrathyroidal processing during synthesis of T_3 and T_4 hormones. *(1)*, Trapping iodide at the basement cell membrane and passage to the apical cell surface. *(2)*, Synthesis of polypeptide chains of thyroglobulin *((Tg)* including synthesis of carbohydrate units within the rough endoplasmic reticulum (rER), with completion of the carbohydrate units in the Golgi (G). *(3)*, Transport of newly formed Tg to the cell surface in small apical vesicles *(AV)*. *(4)*, Iodination of Tg, coupling of iodotyrosyl precursors to form T_4 and T_3 at the apical cell surface, and storage of iodinated Tg in the lumen. *(5)*, Retrieval of Tg by micropinocytosis into small vesicles *(MPV)* or by massive engulfment colloid droplets *(CD)*. *(6)*, Fusion of lysosomes *(L)* with *CD* and MPV, proteolysis of Tg, and release of iodinated amino acids, T_3, and T_4. *(7)*, Entrance of T_4 and T_3 into bloodstream, and *(8)*, Deiodination of DIT and MIT with recirculation of iodide.

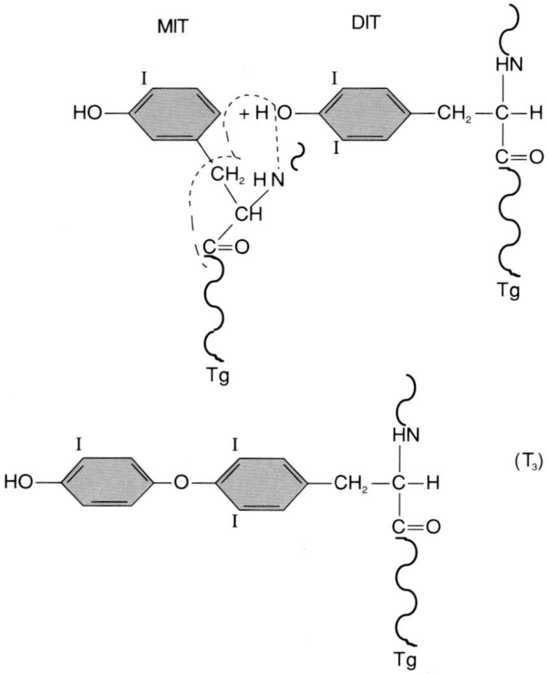

FIGURE 38-3 Formation of 3,5,3'-triiodothyronine (T$_3$) by coupling of an "acceptor" diiodotyrosine residue with a "donor" monoiodotyrosine residue with loss of the alanine side chain of the latter. T$_4$ is formed in the same manner by the coupling of two diiodotyrosine residues.

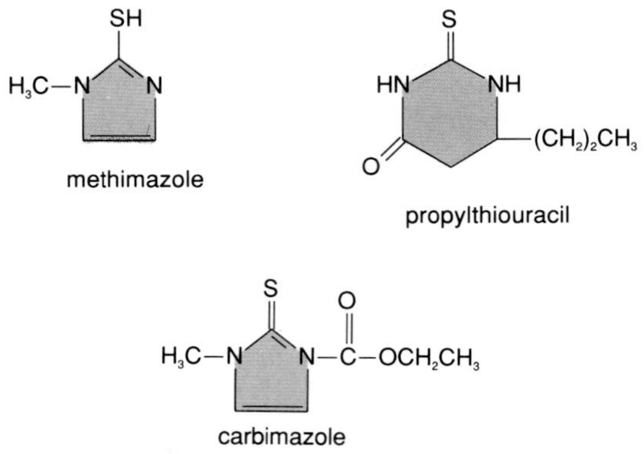

FIGURE 38-4 Structures of thioureylenes.

Table 38-1 Antithyroid Compounds

Inhibited Step (see Figure 38-2)	Compounds
Iodide concentration (Step 1)	Complex anions: ClO$_4^-$, TcO$_4^-$, SCN$^-$
Iodination (Step 2)	Thioureylenes, SCN$^-$
Coupling (Step 4)	Thioureylenes
Hormone release (Step 6)	Iodide, lithium, ClO$_4^-$
Deiodination (Step 8)	propylthiouracil
Hormone action	propranolol

to 57,000 daltons. Their identification as hormone binding sites is based on (1) their high affinity and low capacity for the thyroid hormones, (2) their relative affinities for thyroid hormone analogs that mirror the relative potencies of the biological response of each analog, and (3) the short time lapse between the formation of the thyroid hormone receptor complex and the nuclear response. Recent evidence suggests that the thyroid hormone receptor may be the product of a proto-oncogene.

Direct control of gene expression by thyroid hormones has been established in a number of systems. For some, regulation occurs primarily or exclusively at the transcriptional level. This includes the systems coding for two pituitary hormones, growth hormone (positive control) and thyrotropin (negative control). In both cases administration of T$_3$ to cultured pituitary hormone-producing cells results in rapid changes in concentrations of hormone mRNA that are commensurate with changes in transcriptional rates.

T$_3$ control of gene expression may not be directly related to transcription in all systems. An example of

this is the hepatic S14 protein. Although the function of this protein is still unknown, it appears to be associated with lipogenesis and as such may provide information on the role of thyroid hormones in controlling thermogenesis. Administration of T$_3$ in this and similar systems may act primarily to stabilize a nuclear precursor of mRNA.

Antihyperthyroid Drugs

Drugs can inhibit the synthesis of T$_3$ and T$_4$ or the action of these hormones at several steps in the synthesis sequence, as listed in Table 38-1, with reference to Figure 38-2.

Thioureylene Drugs The primary clinical drugs are the thioureylenes, propylthiouracil, methimazole, and carbimazole (not available in the United States), which inhibit the thyroid peroxidase-mediated iodi-

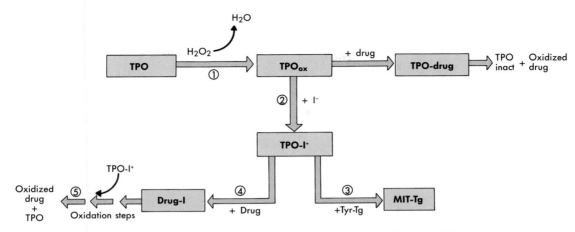

FIGURE 38-5   Inhibition of thyroid peroxidase (TPO) mediated iodination. *TPO*, Thyroid peroxidase; I^-, iodide; I^+, iodinium; T_g, thyroglobulin; *Tyr*, tyrosine; and *MIT*, monoiodotyrosine (see text).

nation and coupling steps (see Table 38-1 and Figure 38-2). The structures of these drugs are shown in Figure 38-4. Although carbimazole has a potent antithyroid activity in vitro, it probably exerts most of its in vivo effects after metabolism to methimazole.

The thioureylene drugs act in vitro either by reversibly inhibiting iodination or by irreversibly inactivating thyroid peroxidase. The scheme proposed to explain these different actions is outlined in Figure 38-5. Under normal conditions the heme group of thyroid peroxidase is oxidized by H_2O_2 (Reaction 1) and then in turn oxidizes iodide to form a complex between the enzyme and the new iodide species, depicted as the iodinium ion I^+ (Reaction 2).

In the absence of antithyroid drugs the iodide is transferred to tyrosyl residues in thyroglobulin to form monoiodotyrosine (Reaction 3). But in the presence of methimazole or propylthiouracil the drug is preferentially iodinated, depriving thyroglobulin of iodide and shutting down the synthesis of T_3 and T_4 (Reaction 4). The drug is then further oxidized by thyroid peroxidase-I^+; as the concentration of drug diminishes, more of the thyroid peroxidase-I^+ complex is used to iodinate thyroglobulin and thyroid hormone formation resumes. In the presence of sufficient concentrations of iodide, the inactivation of thyroglobulin iodination is transient, thyroid peroxidase itself is unaffected, and drug metabolism is extensive. In the absence of sufficient iodide, however, the drug reacts with the oxidized form of thyroid peroxidase, irreversibly inactivating the enzyme (Reaction 5). In the case of methimazole, the drug is believed to become

covalently linked to the heme group of thyroid peroxidase, and iodination does not resume until new enzyme is synthesized and metabolism of the drug becomes much more limited than under conditions of reversible inhibition.

Thyroid peroxidase-mediated coupling is more sensitive to inhibition than is iodination. This is in part explained by the kinetics of iodothyronine formation and in part by a direct inhibitory effect on coupling independent of the inhibition of iodination. The mechanism for this inhibition of coupling is unknown. One suggestion has been that the thioureylenes, which bind to thyroglobulin, may alter the steric configuration of this protein so that coupling between two iodotyrosine residues can no longer take place.

Propylthiouracil, but not methimazole, affects the processing of T_4 in peripheral tissues. Although the thyroid gland secretes some T_3, about 80% of the T_3 in humans originates from 5'-deiodination of T_4 in extrathyroidal tissues. Since T_3 is 10 times as active as T_4 this conversion step has considerable physiological importance. Although the relative contributions of different organs to circulating T_3 concentrations has not been established, liver and kidney are very active. The enzymes involved in 5'-deiodination have not been fully characterized. At least two different T_4-5' deiodinase systems appear to be involved. The microsomal enzyme in liver and kidney is very sensitive to propylthiouracil inhibition, while the microsomal enzyme in pituitary, brain, and brown adipose tissue is insensitive to propylthiouracil inhibi-

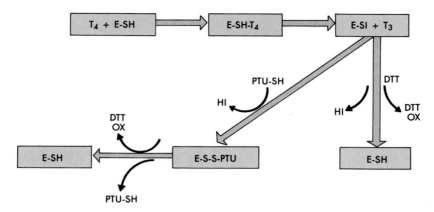

FIGURE 38-6   Pathway for liver-kidney 5'-deiodination of T_4 to produce T_3 and inhibition by propylthiouracil (PTU). DTT is dithiothreitol cofactor: E-SH is an SH group on the enzyme (see text).

tion. The latter enzyme may regulate local intracellular rather than circulating T_3 concentrations.

Propylthiouracil inhibits the liver-kidney deiodinase reaction noncompetitively with respect to T_4 and competitively with respect to the needed reduced thiol factor (Figure 38-6). In the first part of the reaction, T_3 and an enzyme-sulfinyl-iodide complex are formed. This step is unaffected by propylthiouracil; however, the drug prevents regeneration of the native enzyme by binding covalently to the enzyme, presumably at an essential SH site, forming a propylthiouracil-enzyme mixed disulfide as shown in Figure 38-6.

Other Antithyroid Drugs

Several monovalent anions block thyroid hormone sysnthesis by competitively inhibiting the active transport of iodide into the thyroid gland. Both pertechnetate (TcO_4^-) and perchlorate (ClO_4^-) have a higher affinity for the transport system than does iodide itself. Radiolabeled TcO_4^- is used clinically as a test of trapping by the thyroid. Perchlorate, in addition to inhibiting iodide uptake, also accelerates the release of iodide. This anion is effective as an antithyroid drug but is rarely used because of a high incidence of side effects, notably aplastic anemia.

Hormone secretion by the thyroid can be inhibited by excess iodide. Several mechanisms have been proposed, including inhibition of thyroglobulin endocytosis and suppression of lysosomal proteolytic activity.

PHARMACOKINETICS

Thyroxine must be converted to T_3 for its clinical effects; this provides the body some control in regulation of hormonal effect, which is probably an important benefit. The dose of T_4 varies widely among subjects; important factors influencing the dose are variability of absorption and of conversion of T_4 to T_3. The half-life of T_4 in the serum is about 5 days; thus several weeks are required to assess the affects of dose changes. The optimal dose can be gauged by clinical response and laboratory tests, particularly the concentration of serum thyroid-stimulating hormone, which should be normal when the proper dose is administered to subjects with primary hypothyroidism.

The pharmacokinetic parameter values for thyroid hormone preparations and thioureylenes are listed in Table 38-2. (See Chapter 10 for value for β-blockers and Chapter 35 for values for corticosteroids.)

RELATION OF MECHANISMS OF ACTIONS TO CLINICAL RESPONSE

Hyperthyroidism

For patients with hyperthyroidism the usual therapeutic choice is between antithyroid drugs and radioiodine. Subtotal thyroidectomy has largely been replaced by radioiodine, which is simpler, safer, and equally effective. The antithyroid drugs can be ex-

Table 38-2 Pharmacokinetic Parameters

Drugs	Administration	Absorption	$t_{1/2}$ (hrs)	Disposition	Plasma Protein Bound (%)
thyroxine (T_4)	Oral, IV	Fair (50%-80%)	5 days	M (to T_3), E	99.97
thyronine (T_3)	Oral	Good	2 days	M (conjugated)	99.70
thioureylenes					
propylthiouracil	Oral	Good	2	M (oxidized and conjugated)	82
methimazole	Oral	Good	13-18	M (oxidized and conjugated)	8
carbimazole*	—	—	—	M (to methimazole)	—

M, Metabolized; *E*, enterohepatic circulation.
*Not available in the United States.

pected to be effective in almost all patients. However, if the gland is still hyperplastic when antithyroid drugs are withdrawn, hyperthyroidism will probably recur.

Individuals with autoimmune thyroid diseases, of which Graves' disease is an example, have antibodies that stimulate the thyroid (producing hyperthyroidism) as well as antibodies that destroy the thyroid (producing hypothyroidism). The clinical status of an individual patient depends on the balance between these stimulating and destructive antibodies. Thus the natural course of Graves' disease includes a period of hyperthyroidism that is eventually replaced by euthyroidism and later hypothyroidism. Patients treated with antithyroid drugs during the entire duration of this hyperthyroid phase have no recurrence when the drugs are stopped. However, if the antithyroid drugs are withdrawn, hyperthyroidism will reappear. The clinician would like to predict how long the hyperthyroidism will last and on that basis decide whether a temporary means of treatment like antithyroid drugs is satisfactory, or whether an ablative method like radioiodine is necessary. Many attempts have been made to predict this natural course, but none are entirely successful. In general, the milder the hyperthyroidism and the smaller the thyroid gland, the shorter is the period of spontaneous hyperthyroidism. Based on these considerations many clinicians choose radioiodine for patients with large thyroids or moderately severe hyperthyroidism and reserve antithyroid drugs for those patients with small glands, mild disease, or an absolute contraindication to radioiodine, such as pregnancy.

β-blocking drugs provide a valuable adjunct to the treatment of hyperthyroidism. In contrast to the other drugs mentioned so far, the β-blockers act peripheral to the site of thyroid hormone effect rather than at the thyroid gland. The mechanism of action is not certain, but may relate to receptor inhibition in thyroxine-sensitive tissues. In addition, these drugs hinder the peripheral deiodination of T_4 to T_3. Since T_3 is the major peripheral hormone, this action also helps in the control of hyperthyroidism. The peripheral action of the β-blockers makes them useful as adjuncts because they do not interfere with the actions of the thioureylenes or radioiodine on the thyroid. Their effect is much more rapid than can be achieved by blocking thyroid hormone synthesis, as with the thioureylene drugs. Also, the β-blockers are most effective at those tissues, particularly the heart, where emergency treatment for hyperthyroidism often is needed most.

Corticosteroids are also occasionally useful in the treatment of hyperthyroidism, particularly of Graves' disease. They have no specific effect on the thyroid itself, but do have several important peripheral actions. Corticosteroids lower peripheral conversion of T_4 to T_3, have an immunosuppressive effect on thyroid-stimulating antibodies, and are antipyretic. It has not been shown convincingly that even patients with severe hyperthyroidism are truly hypoadrenal, and the emergency conditions under which this condition is usually treated make it difficult to assess the efficacy of a particular therapy such as corticosteroids. However, these steroids are used empirically when patients with severe hyperthyroidism become hypotensive and the introduction of these agents into clinical practice has coincided with improved survival of patients with severe hyperthyroidism.

Most patients show some response to thioureylene drugs within 2 weeks, although months may be needed to obtain full control. For the usual patient the duration of treatment may be a year or more. With a favorable response the gland decreases in size and the patient remains euthyroid as the dose of propylthiouracil is decreased and finally stopped. The success of treatment with antithyroid drugs varies widely with patient selection and probably with iodine content in the diet. In the United States the "success rate" has usually been well under 50%. However, in patients with mild disease, small glands, and perhaps in those with significant ophthalmopathy with Graves' disease, antithyroid drugs are a reasonable choice. If patients experience no side effects, they may remain on the drug for a number of years. However, most patients and physicians find that repeated unsuccessful attempts at withdrawal from antithyroid drugs lead them to choose radioiodine for more definitive therapy.

Hypothyroidism

Treatment of hypothyroidism is usually straightforward, involving replacement of thyroid hormone adequate for the patient's needs. Four types of preparation are available: levothyroxine (T_4), triiodothyronine (T_3), liotrix (a combination of T_4 and T_3), and desiccated thyroid or thyroid extract. Of these, T_4 is preferred and used almost universally. Desiccated thyroid is much less pure, less stable, and less predictable, although still satisfactory for most clinical purposes. Triiodothyronine is more expensive and frequently more difficult to regulate. Its chief use is in patients poor at converting T_4 to T_3, or where an effect of short duration is needed. Mixture of T_4 and T_3 is more expensive and has no clinical advantage over T_4 alone.

SIDE EFFECTS, CLINICAL PROBLEMS, AND TOXICITY

The treatment of severe, life-threatening hyperthyroidism (thyroid storm) needs special comment. Radioiodine requires several weeks to control the dis-

ease—too long for an emergency—thus, the mainstay is drug treatment. In this situation propylthiouracil is given in large doses and iodine (administered as Lugol's solution or potassium iodide) is added because of its more rapid effect. The most immediate emergency response, however, is obtained with β-blocking drugs, although these must be used cautiously in patients with coexistent heart failure. Corticosteroids are also valuable, particularly in patients with hyperpyrexia or hypotension.

Antithyroid drugs can be used in pregnancy, but should be used at the lowest dose possible because propylthiouracil and methimazole cross the placenta with ease. Fortunately, the immunosuppressive effects of pregnancy allow one to keep antithyroid drug doses to a minimum and frequently to withdraw them.

The clinical problems with these agents are summarized in the box.

CLINICAL PROBLEMS

IODIDE

Angioedema, hemorrhage, sore teeth and gums, salivation, induction of goiter and myxedema

THIOUREYLENES

Agranulocytosis, granulocytopenia, skin rash

THYROID PREPARATIONS (INCLUDING THYROXINE)

Drug interactions with warfarin, bound (T_4,T_3) by cholestyramine in GI tract

---

TRADENAMES

In addition to generic and fixed combination preparations, the following tradenamed materials are available in the United States.

Armour thyroid S-P-T; thyroid tablets
Cytomel, liothyronine (T_3)
Euthroid, Thyrolar, liotrix
Levothroid, Synthroid; thyroxine (T_4) (or thyroxine sodium or levothyroxine sodium)
Proloid, thyroglobulin

REFERENCES

Cooper DS: Antithyroid drugs, N Engl J Med 311:1353, 1984.

Hesch RD: Intracellular pathways of iodothyronine metabolism. In Ingbar SH and Braverman LE, eds: Werner's the thyroid: a fundamental and clincal text, no 5, Philadelphia, 1986, JB Lippincott.

Larsen PR, Silva JE, and Kaplan MM: Relationships between circulating and intracellular thyroid hormones: physiological and clinical implications, Endocrine Rev 2:87, 1981.

Oppenheimer JH, Schwartz JL, Mariash CM, et al: Advances in our understanding of thyroid hormone action at the cellular level, Endocrine Rev 8:288, 1987.

Samuels HH, Formanm BM, Horowitz ZD, et al: Regulation of gene expression by thyroid hormone, J Clin Invest 81:957, 1988.

Taurog A: Hormone synthesis: thyroid iodine metabolism. In Ingbar SH and Braverman LE, eds: Werner's the thyroid: a fundamental and clinical text no 5, Philadelphia, 1986, JB Lippincott Co.

Insulin and Oral Hypoglycemic Agents

 ## THERAPEUTIC OVERVIEW

The term *diabetes mellitus* encompasses a group of pancreatic endocrine-based disease states of differing etiology and severity.

Diabetes is derived from the Greek word meaning syphon, to signify the copious urine production in individuals with this affliction. Diabetes has been recognized for at least 2000 years; however, ancient physicians made no distinction between diabetes mellitus and another disease, diabetes insipidus. Both diseases involve the endocrine system and generate increased volumes of urine but are otherwise unrelated. The observation that urine from some types of diabetic patients tasted sweet (a common, if unsavory, diagnostic procedure) whereas that from other types was tasteless, led to the first distinction between diabetes mellitus and diabetes insipidus (Figure 39-1).

Diabetes insipidus results from a deficiency of antidiuretic hormone (vasopressin), a hormone necessary for the reabsorption of water in the kidney. A person lacking this hormone may produce liters of insipid urine each day. Glucose imparts the sweet taste to the urine in diabetes mellitus (*mellitus* is the Greek word for honey). In untreated disease, blood glucose rises to much higher concentrations than normal, leading to increased concentrations of sugar in the glomerular filtrate. The kidney has an active glucose transport system that normally pumps almost all the sugar out of the urine. However, with glucose concentrations of approximately 200 mg/dl (11 mM), the transport system becomes saturated and glucose spills into the urine, resulting in osmotic diuresis. Ketone bodies (discussed later) in the urine also can contribute to the diuresis.

In the early 1880s it was discovered that pancreatectomy produced symptoms of the disease in dogs, which suggested that the pancreas produces a substance that prevents the onset of diabetes mellitus. However, it was not until 1921 that Banting, Best, Collip, and McLeod successfully isolated and used insulin to treat a diabetic human. Before this, the prognosis for a patient with insulin dependent diabetes mellitus (previously termed juvenile onset) was death, usually within a few months. Life could sometimes be extended for a short time by adherence to a diet bordering on starvation. In this setting one can appreciate the impact of the discovery of insulin. Insulin was soon isolated in quantities sufficient for treating diabetes, and it became possible to reverse the course of the disease.

Diabetes mellitus has been diagnosed in approx-

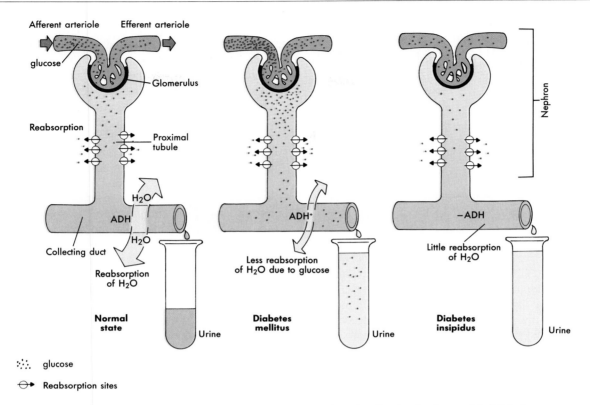

FIGURE 39-1   Schematic diagram of renal nephron functionality in the "normal," "diabetes mellitus," and "diabetes insipidus" states. Both types of diabetes produce polyuria. The three diagrams show water and small molecules, such as glucose, passing through the glomerulus into the tubule, where saturable reabsorption of glucose takes place (shown leaving the proximal tubule). In diabetes mellitus the reabsorption process cannot handle all of the glucose, so some glucose is voided in the urine (shown as the beaker contents). In the normal state, 98% to 99% of the water also is reabsorbed (shown here as water leaving the collecting duct). In diabetes mellitus less water is reabsorbed because of osmotic diuresis resulting from the elevated concentration of glucose in the collecting duct. Diabetes insipidus is characterized by a low concentration of antidiuretic hormone (ADH) necessary for reabsorption of water.

imately 3% of the general population, probably an underestimate of the true incidence. Although the widespread perception is that the disease is curable with insulin, this is far from true. Complications resulting from diabetes mellitus are among the leading causes of blindness, renal failure, cardiovascular disease, and limb amputations. Nevertheless, two groups of drugs are useful in the treatment of diabetes mellitus and are the subject of this chapter.

Types of Diabetes Mellitus

Diabetes mellitus occurs when circulating insulin concentrations decline and/or when the target cells become resistant to the hormone. Most cases can be divided into two types, which have gone by a variety of names over the past few years (Table 39-1). Juvenile onset and maturity onset were previously used. Either type can occur at either age, so that such terminology is somewhat misleading. The current preferred designations are insulin-dependent diabetes mellitus (IDDM) and noninsulin-dependent diabetes mellitus (NIDDM).

Insulin-dependent Diabetes Mellitus IDDM results from a degeneration of the pancreatic β cells, which produce insulin. It is the more serious type and accounts for approximately 15% to 20% of the total cases. There is a genetic link or predisposition, al-

Table 39-1 Nomenclature and Terminology Used to Differentiate Between the Two Major Types of Diabetes Mellitus

Insulin-dependent Diabetes Mellitus (IDDM)	Non-insulin–dependent Diabetes Mellitus (NIDDM)
TYPE I	TYPE II
ketosis prone	ketosis resistant
juvenile onset	adult onset
growth onset	maturity onset

though environmental factors must also be involved since the incidence of IDDM in homozygous twins is only about 50%. Certain viral infections increase the risk of developing IDDM, and increasing evidence indicates the disease results from autoimmune destruction of the β cells. The stimulus that prompts the immune system to attack the β cells remains a mystery. The disease has an abrupt onset clinically, although evidence now indicates that the process has been occurring slowly over a period of years, usually in childhood or early adulthood, and is associated with the symptomatic triad of polyuria, polydipsia, and polyphagia. The increased urine volume is caused by the osmotic diuresis that results from the increased concentration of glucose (hyperglycemia), and ultimately ketone bodies, in the urine. Thirst and hunger are compensatory responses to the loss of fluid and the inability to utilize nutrients. Weight loss is a hallmark of the untreated disease, as is premature cessation of growth when diabetes develops in childhood.

At the time of onset of IDDM, there may be detectable, though lower than normal, concentrations of serum insulin. However, the concentration of the hormone will decline to negligible values with the progression of the disease; and if insulin is not supplied, metabolic acidosis (ketosis) will ensue, followed shortly by diabetic coma and death. Metabolic acidosis results from the production of ketone bodies, which are synthesized from acetyl CoA in the liver. The synthetic pathway is summarized in Figure 39-2. The production of ketone bodies is an ongoing activity of the liver, which releases them into the circulation for transport to the heart, skeletal muscle, and other tissues to be used as an energy source. In the normal fed state, the concentration of ketone

bodies is relatively low because insulin stimulates the synthesis of fatty acids, a competing pathway for the use of acetyl CoA. Insulin also inhibits lipolysis, thereby decreasing the supply of fatty acids, which are a major source of acetyl CoA in the liver. Thus, when insulin concentrations are decreased, as occurs in diabetes or fasting, production of ketone bodies is favored. Severe ketosis does not develop in normal individuals because only a small amount of insulin is needed to inhibit lipolysis in adipose tissue.

The use of the term *ketone* to describe the compounds that produce ketosis is a misnomer. The term *ketone* describes the carbonyl (C=O) functional group; whereas the major ketone body produced during diabetes or fasting in humans, β-hydroxybutyrate, is not a ketone. Except for acetone, all of the diabetes ketone bodies are organic acids, explaining why decreased blood pH is associated with their production. Because acetone is volatile, it is excreted to some extent by the lungs, accounting for the "acetone breath" of individuals with severe ketosis.

The later stages of diabetic ketoacidosis are associated with severe fluid depletion, in part because of the osmotic diuresis caused by increased concentrations of glucose and ketone bodies in the urine. Fluid loss also occurs with vomiting, which is one of the ways the body attempts to rid itself of the excess acid. Unconsciousness, referred to as diabetic coma, followed by cardiovascular collapse and death, occurs if appropriate therapy is not instituted. Treatment involves administration of insulin and rehydration with careful monitoring to establish and maintain electrolyte balance.

Non-insulin–dependent Diabetes Mellitus NIDDM usually develops after 35 years of age, and most diabetics of this type are obese. In contrast to the insulin-dependent diabetic, non-insulin–dependent diabetics have significant concentrations of the circulating hormone. Indeed, the presence of insulin and the ability of sulfonylureas (discussed later) to evoke release of the hormone are indicative of NIDDM. Because only a small amount of insulin is needed to prevent ketone body formation, the non-insulin–dependent diabetic rarely develops ketosis. In some cases of NIDDM the concentrations of insulin are actually higher than normal. The apparent paradox of hyperglycemia in spite of elevated insulin is explain by the fact that the target cells are relatively insensitive to the hormone. In such resistant cells, a higher concentration of insulin is needed to elicit a

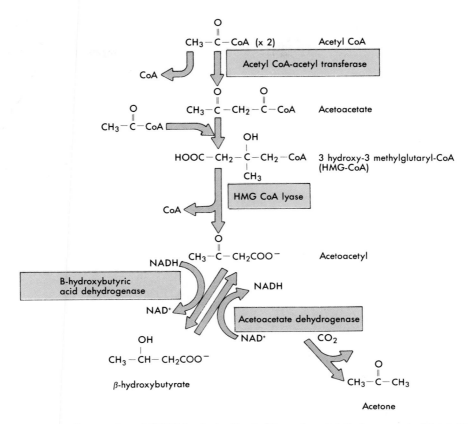

FIGURE 39-2   Progression of IDDM leads to the buildup of acetyl CoA, generated from the sequential β-oxidation of fatty acids. The excess acetyl CoA undergoes conversion to ketone bodies, some of which are acidic, and can lead to a breakdown in the control of blood pH.

response than in normal cells. In some cases of insulin resistance, concentrations of insulin receptors appear to be decreased; in others the problem seems to be distal to the receptor in the pathway of insulin action.

Diabetic coma is rarely seen in non-insulin-dependent diabetics, presumably because their endogenous insulin prevents ketosis. However, a related condition, referred to as hyperosmolar coma, can occur. It is most often observed in elderly individuals and is usually preceded by an illness or other stressful situation that increases the requirement for insulin. Under these circumstances, the insulin present becomes insufficient to prevent glucosuria. Fluid loss is compounded when vomiting is associated with the precipitating illnesss. As dehydration becomes severe, urinary output decreases in spite of the high urinary concentration of glucose. Thus, renal excretion of glucose falls, and blood sugar and serum osmolarity increase to extremely high concentrations,

leading to loss of consciousness. Like diabetic coma, hyperosmolar coma is life threatening; it is a particularly grave condition in older diabetics, who may already have compromised cardiovascular function.

Agents Used in Treatment

Insulin is still the only drug effective in treating IDDM. A class of drugs collectively referred to as oral hypoglycemic agents is now used in the therapy of NIDDM. It should be stressed that nonpharmacological methods are of the utmost importance in treating the obese non-insulin–dependent diabetic. Weight reduction and a regular program of moderate exercise, when not contraindicated by physical debilitation, should be encouraged in all obese non-insulin–dependent diabetics as proven ways of increasing insulin sensitivity. Unfortunately, poor compliance with such programs is the rule rather than the exception, and the majority of the NIDDM diabetics must be treated with insulin or oral agents to achieve adequate control.

Several classes of oral hypoglycemic agents have been identified, but only one, the sulfonylureas, are currently used in this country. The discovery of the hypoglycemic actions of sulfonylureas was made in the early 1940s during clinical trials to investigate the antimicrobial efficacy of sulfonamide derivatives. It was noted that several patients developed hypoglycemia after receiving the sulfonylurea, *p*-aminobenzene-sulfonamido-isopropylthiadiazole. More than 10 years elapsed before clinical trials established that a related compound, carbutamide, was effective in controlling blood glucose concentrations in selected NIDDM patients.

The therapeutic overview is summarized in the box.

 MECHANISMS OF ACTION

Insulin

Insulin is an acidic protein having a molecular weight of approximately 5600 (Figure 39-3). This hormone is composed of two polypeptides, termed the A and B chains, which are covalently joined by two interchain disulfide bonds. A third intrachain disulfide bridge is present in the A chain. The chains are formed by proteolysis of proinsulin, a larger single chain precursor, by removal of the intervening sequence of amino acids, referred to as the C peptide.

The conversion of endogenous proinsulin to insulin occurs in the secretory granule, where most of the insulin undergoes crystallization with Zn^{++}. Approximately equimolar amounts of insulin and C peptide are stored in the granule, along with a much smaller amount of proinsulin. When the β cell receives the appropriate stimulation, the contents of the granule are released by exocytosis. For exogenously administered insulin, granule storage is bypassed.

The amino acid sequence of insulin is highly conserved across species. Beef insulin differs from human in three amino acids. Pork insulin is more similar to the human, differing in only a single amino acid. This explains why pork insulin in less antigenic in humans than beef insulin.

The structure of insulin is similar to those of several other hormones and growth factors, including relaxin and insulin-like growth factors 1 and 2 (IGF). Conservation of the cysteine residues is of particular note, given the role of disulfide bonds in determining the tertiary structure of protein. Not surprisingly, IGF-1 and IGF-2 have some affinity for the insulin receptor; however, both growth factors have their own receptors. In some cases homologies extend to receptor structure and biological action. For example, the receptors and actions of IGF-1 and insulin are similar. In contrast, relaxin causes widening of the symphysis pubis immediately before delivery, an effect not produced by insulin.

Insulin stimulates the transport of glucose into muscle and fat cells. Since insulin does not appear to need to enter the cell to exert its effects, it can be inferred that insulin action involves an interaction with a cell-surface receptor (see Chapters 2 and 34). This interaction causes the generation of a signal that is transmitted to the inside of the cell to trigger activation of various anabolic pathways and inhibition of catabolic processes. A brief overview of current knowledge and ideas concerning the signal propagation pathway is provided in the next few paragraphs.

Insulin Receptor The first step in signal propagation begins with binding of the hormone to the receptor. The insulin receptor is a tetrameric protein complex composed to two α subunits of approximately 130,000 daltons and two 90,000 dalton β subunits (Figure 39-4; see also Chapter 32). Subsequent signal propagation appears to involve polypeptide phosphorylation alterations and a second messenger system. In the case of the cAMP system, the cyclic

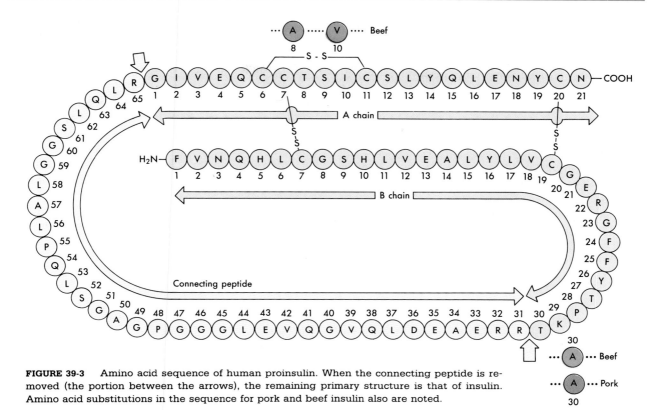

FIGURE 39-3 Amino acid sequence of human proinsulin. When the connecting peptide is removed (the portion between the arrows), the remaining primary structure is that of insulin. Amino acid substitutions in the sequence for pork and beef insulin also are noted.

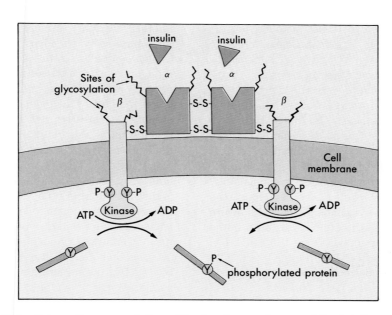

FIGURE 39-4 Schematic representation of the insulin receptor. α and β subunits and tyrosine kinase are indicated (see text).

nucleotide was found to activate a cAMP-dependent protein kinase. This kinase was found to phosphorylate glycogen synthase and hormone sensitive lipase, producing inactivation and activation, respectively, of the two enzymes. These findings provided an explanation of how epinephrine, by causing an increase in cAMP, promoted an increase in lipolysis while inhibiting glycogen synthesis. Glucagon, a hormone produced by the α cells in the islets of Langerhans, acts in the liver and fat cells by increasing cAMP. Since the actions of insulin on lipolysis and glycogen synthesis are opposite to those of epinephrine and glucagon, it is logical to suppose that insulin acts by decreasing the concentration of cAMP and the activity of cAMP-dependent protein kinase. This has been one of the most persistent hypotheses of insulin action. However, it is now clear that the major effects of insulin in cells can occur without decreases in the concentration of cAMP. Analysis of the sites on enzymes dephosphorylated in response to insulin has provided further evidence that insulin action is not mediated by decreased cAMP. For example, the sites on glycogen synthase that are dephosphorylated in response to insulin are not readily phosphorylated by cAMP-dependent protein kinase. However, it is also clear that insulin can decrease elevated cAMP concentrations. While there seems to be general agreement that insulin must act by a mechanism distinct from cAMP, what that mechanism is has not been determined. However, a set of increased and decreased polypeptide phosphorylations and the production of chemical mediators have been identified.

What may prove to be a major clue concerning the mechanism of insulin action was the discovery that the receptor is a protein tyrosine kinase. Insulin binding to the α subunit activates the kinase, which resides in the β subunit. This is described in greater detail in Chapter 34 and is only summarized here. The resulting autophosphorylation is stimulated by insulin and causes a further increase in kinase activity. Several polypeptide species have been found that are phosphorylated on tyrosines when cells are incubated with insulin, but their functions, and whether they are directly phosphorylated by the insulin receptor kinase, remain to be determined.

The homology extends to several oncogene products that are protein tyrosine kinases, such as pp60sarc, the first such kinase discovered (see Chapter 34). Interestingly, certain oncogenes are derived from growth factor receptor genes. For example, the erb B oncogene encodes a protein tyrosine kinase identical to the epidermal growth factor (EGF) receptor, except that the EGF binding domain is absent. Thus, unlike the EGF receptor, the erb B protein is not regulated by EGF and is constitutively active, presumably explaining its action on inducing uncontrolled cell proliferation. An oncogene derived from insulin receptor has not yet been discovered.

Phosphorylation Cascade or Insulin Mediator For many years it has been clear that insulin action involved changes in the phosphorylation states of enzymes in several important metabolic pathways. It was generally believed that insulin acted by promoting dephosphorylation of the proteins, as has been shown to be the case for glycogen synthase, pyruvate dehydrogenase, and hormone sensitive lipase. Recently there has been an expanding list of newly discovered protein kinases. Well over 20 are found in animal cells. It is also clear that there are multiple phosphoprotein phosphatases regulated by a variety of mechanisms. The idea that insulin must either increase the activity of a phosphoprotein phosphatase or decrease protein kinase activity is still valid. A challenge now is to determine which protein kinase(s) or phosphoprotein phosphatases are involved.

There are now good indications that insulin action also involves stimulation of protein phosphorylation. Insulin has been discovered to stimulate the phosphorylation of a relatively large number of proteins, including ATP-citrate lyase and ribosomal protein S6. So far, no change in the activity of the protein phosphorylated in response to insulin has been demonstrated. Nevertheless, finding increased phosphorylation indicates that insulin increases protein kinase activity. At least two protein serine kinases, one that preferentially phosphorylates ribosomal protein S6, and another that phosphorylates microtubule associated protein (MAP), have been shown to be increased in cells exposed to insulin. One hypothesis is that insulin binding activates the receptor tyrosine kinase, which phosphorylates and activates another kinase, perhaps a serine protein kinase, thereby setting into motion a phosphorylation cascade.

A second general hypothesis is that insulin acts by causing the generation of a unique second messenger. There is evidence that insulin promotes formation of soluble low molecular weight substances that fulfill certain criteria expected of a second mes-

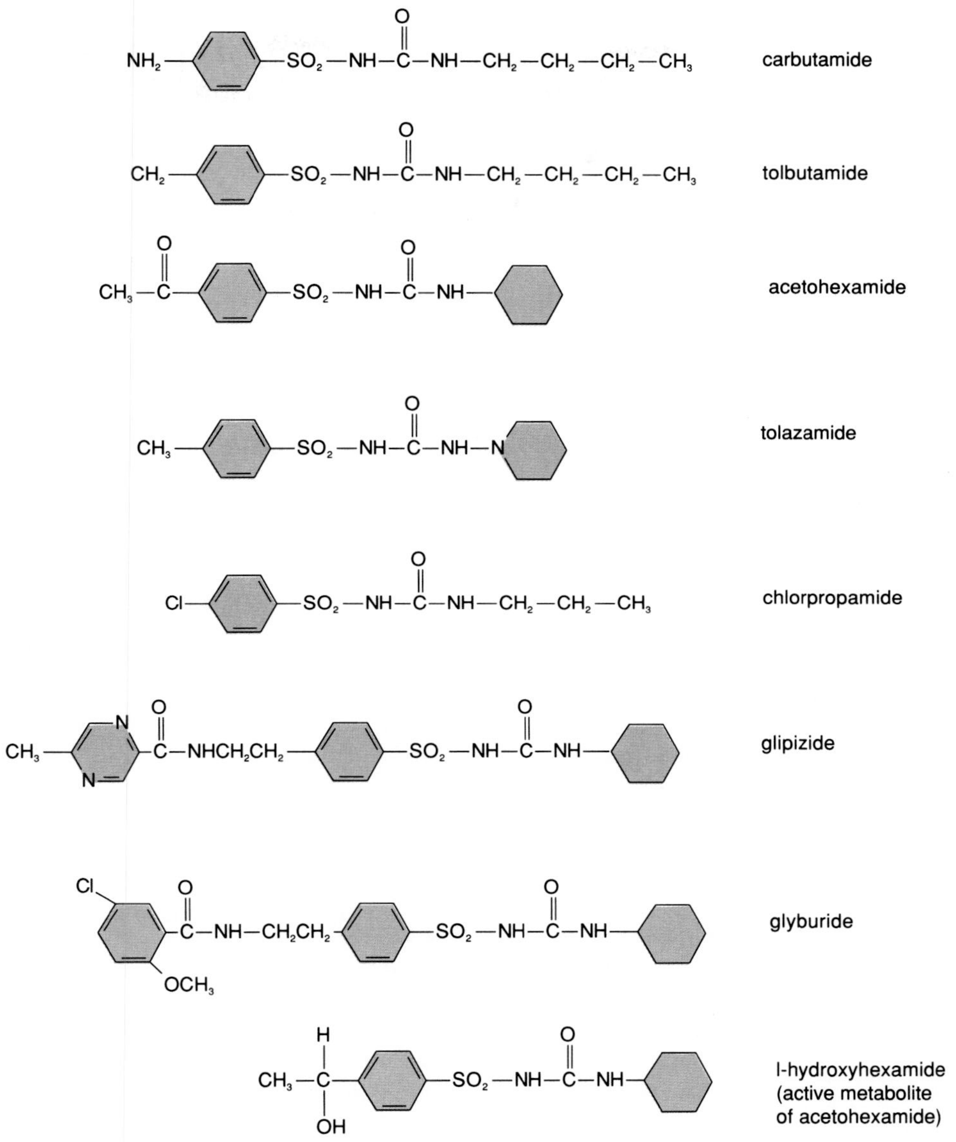

FIGURE 39-5   Structures of sulfonylurea hypoglycemic agents.

senger. For example, the substances mimic insulin when added to whole cells, and have insulin-like actions, such as activation of pyruvate dehydrogenase and cAMP phosphodiesterase, when added to cell extracts. There has been a tendency to refer to impure preparations having insulin-like activity as insulin mediators, implying that they have a role as secondary messengers. This has not yet been shown to be the case. The substances are being purified to homogeneity, but their structures remain undetermined (see also Chapter 34). However, there is reason to believe that this may change in the near future. Recent findings suggest that one such substance is an inositol phosphate glycan formed from a glycosyl phosphatidylinositol precursor found in the plasma membrane.

It should also be pointed out the second messenger and phosphorylation cascade hypotheses are not mutually exclusive. There might be two separate pathways for signal transduction or alternatively, and more likely, the two pathways may merge. For example, phosphorylation might be a step in generation of a second messenger. Alternatively second messengers may control phosphorylation state by their effects on phosphoprotein kinases and phosphatases. A third mechanism of insulin action is to redistribute glucose transporters and other proteins from an intracellular location to the cell membrane. This action is important in activating glucose transport.

Glucagon

Glucagon is a single chain polypeptide with a molecular weight of about 3500 daltons. It is processed in the α cells of the islets of Langerhans of the pancreas by cleavage of specific bonds enzymatically from a large precursor, proglucagon. A related molecule, glycentin (molecular weight about 7000 daltons), containing glucagon within it is formed from proglucagon in the stomach and GI tract.

Glucagon acts in the opposite direction from insulin to facilitate the breakdown of macromolecules. As part of its control of catabolism, glucagon acts to decrease anabolic processes in target organs. The major organ where glucagon acts is the liver, but it also produces effects in fat and in the heart. Glucagon, like insulin, interacts with a specific receptor on the outer surface of sensitive cells. The receptor is not yet as well characterized as the insulin receptor but is thought to be a single polypeptide chain of about 60,000 daltons and coupled to at least two intracellular second messenger systems. These messenger systems are the production of cAMP via activation of adenylate cyclase and the production of IP$_3$ via activation of phospholipase C.

Oral Hypoglycemic Agents

Sulfonylureas Shortly after discovery of the hypoglycemic actions in humans, it was found that these drugs also produced hypoglycemia in normal animals, but not in pancreatectomized dogs. This observation led to the suggestion that these drugs decreased blood sugar by releasing insulin from the pancreas. There is no question that the sulfonylureas promote insulin release from β cells. However, after chronic treatment with sulfonylureas, concentrations of insulin return to the pretreatment values, but the hypoglycemic effect persists. Therefore it is now clear that sulfonylureas also increase insulin sensitivity.

In isolated islet cells, sulfonylureas have little or no effect on insulin release in the absence of glucose, but in the presence of glucose, increase insulin release, sensitizing the β cells to glucose. The agents act by binding to specific receptors that are coupled to increased entry of Ca^{++} into the β cells, thus enhancing secretion. Sulfonylureas enhance the effect of insulin on stimulating glucose uptake into muscle and fat cells. Such actions can explain, at least in part, the increased insulin sensitivity.

The first generation sulfonylureas are tolbutamide, tolazamide, acetohexamide, and chlorpropamide. Glipizide and glyburide are second generation agents that have been used in Europe for the past 15 years, but only recently approved for clinical use in the United States. The structures of the first and second generation agents and the common chemical features leading to their classification as sulfonylureas are shown in Figure 39-5. The second generation drugs are effective at 10 to 100 times lower concentrations, and this difference in potency is a major distinction between the two generations of drugs.

 ## PHARMACOKINETICS

Insulin

Insulin is degraded by proteolytic systems in a variety of tissues, with the liver being the most prominent. In fact, almost half of the insulin released from the pancreas into the portal vein is destroyed by the liver before it can gain access to the general circulation. In humans, the half-life of the circulating hormone is approximately 8 minutes. The effects of insulin on glucose and lipid metabolism occur within minutes of exposing insulin-sensitive cells to the hormone. The onset of action of insulin following IV injections is very rapid, but the duration of action is short. Because of the short half-life, almost all of the hormone is cleared within an hour.

All preparations of insulin must be injected. If administered orally, most of the hormone is destroyed by the proteases in the intestinal tract before it can

Table 39-2   Pharmacokinetic Parameters

Insulin Preparation	Source	Onset (hr)	Duration (hr)
SHORT-ACTING			
Insulin injection	B, P, H	1	7
Prompt insulin zinc suspension	B, P	1	14
INTERMEDIATE-ACTING			
Isophane insulin suspension (NPH)	H, B, P	2	24
Insulin zinc suspension (Lente)	H, B, P	2	24
LONG-ACTING			
Protamine zinc insulin suspension	B, P	4	36
Extended insulin zinc suspension	B, P	4	36

H, Human; *B*, beef; *P*, pork.

be absorbed. Except in the emergency treatment of diabetic coma, insulin is administered by subcutaneous (SC) injection. Because of its relatively large size, there is some delay in absorption from the site of injection, and the duration of action is longer than seen with IV injection. Following SC injection, a soluble preparation has an onset of action of approximately 1 hour and a duration of about 6 hours. The original preparations of insulin were soluble, and multiple injections were required to maintain adequate control of blood glucose.

Insulin Preparations The pharmacokinetic parameter for insulin preparations currently available in the United States are summarized in Table 39-2. Insulin Injection is a clear solution, and is the only preparation suitable for IV use. It may be referred to as regular insulin or as crystalline zinc insulin, to denote that it was prepared by dissolving crystals of insulin-zinc. The most common use of soluble preparations is in combination with an extended action insulin, to provide a rapid rise in insulin concentrations. Several such longer-acting preparations are now available. A common property of the extended action preparations is that the insulin is in a precipitated state that can be absorbed only after it has dissolved in the interstitial fluid. Thus the prolonged duration of action is achieved by creating a depot from which the drug is slowly released, not by increasing the half-life of the circulating drug. *All long-acting preparations of insulin are suspensions, rather than solutions, and should never be injected IV.*

Two extended-action preparations are based on the interaction between insulin and protamine, a basic protein purified from salmon sperm. When insulin is mixed with protamine, a complex of insulin-protamine precipitates. Protamine Zinc Insulin Suspension is a preparation that contains excess protamine so that the insulin dissolves very slowly after injection. Consequently, the preparation has a very long duration of action (approximately 36 hours), too long to achieve good control. Regular insulin cannot be added to achieve a prompt increase in circulating hormone because the excess protamine combines with the soluble insulin, converting it to a depot form. To circumvent this problem, a second preparation of insulin was formulated that contained low concentrations of uncombined protamine. This preparation, referred to as either NPH or Isophane Insulin, has a neutral (N) pH, contains protamine (P), and was developed by the Danish scientist Hagedorn (H). Isophane denotes that the preparation contains stoichiometric amounts of insulin and protamine. The onsets and durations of action of NPH insulin are shorter than those of Protamine Zinc suspension.

The protamine-containing preparations utilized phosphate buffers. If insulin is dissolved in an acetate buffer, and excess Zn^{++} is added, the insulin precipitates as either large homogeneous crystals or as small particles. Three preparations of insulin are made from these two precipitated forms. The advantages of these preparations are that they can be mixed in any proportions without impaired activity or stability, and

Table 39-3 Pharmacokinetic Properties of Sulfonylureas

Drug	Administered*	$t_{1/2}$ (hr)	Plasma Protein Binding	Duration of Action (hr)	Active Metabolite	Elimination
tolbutamide	Oral	3-5	>90%	6-12	No	95% M, R
acetohexamide	Oral	3-11	>90%	12-18	Strongly active	60% M, R
tolazamide	Oral	7	>90%	12-14	Weakly active	90% M, R
chlorpropamide	Oral	24-48	>90%	60	Yes	90% M, R
glipizide	Oral	3-7	>90%†	24	No	90% M, R
glyburide	Oral	10-16	>90%†	24	No	50% M, R

Half-lives and durations of action vary considerably among individuals, and the values given are approximations.
Metabolite activity refers to the collective hypoglycemic action of the metabolite. *M*, Metabolism; *R*, renal excretion of metabolites.
* All are absorbed from the gastrointestinal tract.
† Not readily displaceable by other ionic-binding drugs.

they avoid allergic reactions due to protamine while retaining the desired prolonged activity.

Extended Insulin Zinc Suspension is a preparation of the large crystals. These dissolve very slowly at the site of injection so that the onset and duration of action are similar to protamine zinc suspension. Semilente insulin is a suspension of the small particles. In part because of the large surface area, the crystals dissolve rapidly and the onset and duration of action are similar to Insulin Injection. Insulin Zinc Suspension is a mixture containing 30% semilente and 70% ultralente. The onsets and durations of action are similar to NPH insulin.

Purified insulin has a specific activity of 25 to 30 units/mg. In the United States, the standard insulin preparations contain 100 units/ml, but formulations of 500 units/ml are available for patients with severe insulin resistance.

Until recently, insulin was extracted from the pancreata of slaughterhouse animals, mostly cattle and hogs. While adequate in most cases, there are some problems with these preparations, notably allergic reactions to the animal insulins. Obtaining enough of the hormone to treat all insulin-dependent diabetics worldwide was another problem. The problems may have been solved by recombinant DNA technology, which has enabled the large scale in vitro production of insulin. The recombinant human hormone is now marketed under the tradename Humulin. Another strategy is to prepare human insulin from porcine insulin by converting the alanine in position B-30 to a threonine. Human insulin prepared in this way is marketed as Novolin.

Sulfonylureas

The sulfonylurea drugs share the properties of rapid and complete absorption from the gastrointestinal tract and a high percentage of binding to plasma proteins. Most of the sulfonylurea compounds are converted in the liver to metabolites, which are excreted primarily by the kidney. Hydroxylation reactions are prominent in the metabolism of both first and second generation drugs. The hydroxylated products are less lipid soluble and therefore are more rapidly excreted in the urine than their respective parent compounds.

The pharmacokinetic parameters of the sulfonylureas are summarized in Table 39-3. Tolbutamide has the shortest half-life of the agents and is rapidly metabolized in the liver to inactive products. In some cases, the metabolites are active as hypoglycemic agents and thus extend the duration of action of the drug. Tolazamide, the most slowly absorbed, is metabolized to mildly hypoglycemic products, which are rapidly excreted. The metabolism of acetohexamide is notable in that the major metabolite, l-hydroxyhexamide (see Figure 39-5), is even more active in lowering blood glucose than the parent compound. Although extensively metabolized by the liver, chlorpropamide has the longest half-life and is administered only once daily. The half-lives of glyburide and glypizide are both approximately 24 hours, and these drugs are metabolized to inactive products by the liver. All of the sulfonylureas bind appreciably to plasma proteins; however, the first generation drugs are displaceable by other ionic binding drugs, but the second generation drugs are not readily displaceable.

RELATION OF MECHANISMS OF
ACTION TO CLINICAL RESPONSE

Insulin

The most important stimulus for release of endogenous insulin is glucose. In keeping with the function of insulin in stimulating storage of nutrients, many of the breakdown products of complex nutrient molecules also stimulate insulin release. These include amino acids, fatty acids, and ketones (Table 39-4). In addition, hormones including secretin, pancreozymin, and glucagon stimulate release. These hormones are elaborated from the intestinal tract in response to products of digestion, and their actions on the β cell explain why insulin concentrations sometimes increase after a meal before glucose concentrations rise.

In fasting humans, approximately 90% of insulin-like activity in serum is not due to insulin. This activity became known as nonsuppressible insulin-like activity (NSILA) because it was not suppressed by addition of anti-insulin antibodies to the serum. The substances responsible for NSILA have been identified as IGF-1 and IGF-2. These growth factors circulate bound to specific carrier proteins. When complexed with these proteins, the IGFs are incapable of interacting with their cellular receptors. Furthermore, unlike concentrations of insulin, IGF concentrations are not controlled by glucose. Consequently, although the actions of IGFs are similar to those of insulin, it is clear that they cannot compensate for the insulin deficit in diabetes mellitus.

Carbohydrate Metabolism

The classic action of insulin is to lower blood glucose concentration. Various effects that contribute to the uptake and storage of glucose are summarized in Table 39-5.

Insulin stimulates the transport of glucose by facilitated diffusion into muscle and fat cells. The mechanism by which insulin stimulates glucose transport is by increasing the number of transport proteins in the membrane (Figure 39-6). Insulin causes translocation of glucose transporters as well as IGF-2 receptors from intracellular compartments to the plasma membrane, indicating that translocation between cellular compartments may be a more general mechanism involved with action other than insulin.

Table 39-4   Some Factors that Control the Release of Endogenous Insulin

Stimulate	Inhibit
NUTRIENTS	
Glucose	
Amino acids	
Fatty acids	
Ketone bodies	
HORMONES	
Secretin	Somatostatin
Glucagon	
Pancreozymin	
Gastrin	
Vasoactive intestinal peptide	
Gastric inhibitory polypeptide	
Sympathetic nervous system	
PHARMACOLOGICAL CONTROL	
β-Adrenergic agonists	α-Adrenergic agonists
Cholinergic agonists	
Sulfonylureas	

Table 39-5   Actions of Insulin

Metabolism	Action
Carbohydrate metabolism	Increases glucose transport
	Increases glycogen synthesis
	Increases pentose shunting
	Increases glucose oxidation
	Decreases gluconeogenesis
Lipid metabolism	Increases fatty acid transport
	Increases triglyceride synthesis (includes fatty acid synthesis and esterification)
	Decreases lipolysis
Protein metabolism	Increases amino acid transport
	Increases protein synthesis (including mRNA transcription and translation)
	Decreases degradation

Insulin does not stimulate glucose transport in liver cells but does act on these cells to inhibit gluconeogenesis, an important action in decreasing blood sugar. Hormonal regulation of glucose production by liver and glucose utilization by muscle, fat, and other

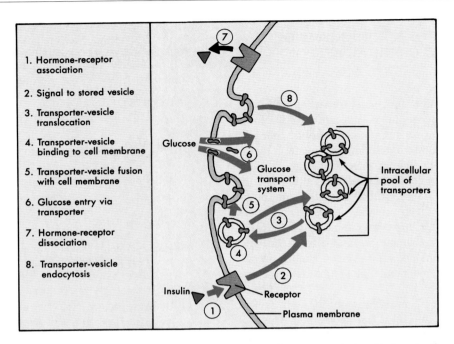

1. Hormone-receptor association
2. Signal to stored vesicle
3. Transporter-vesicle translocation
4. Transporter-vesicle binding to cell membrane
5. Transporter-vesicle fusion with cell membrane
6. Glucose entry via transporter
7. Hormone-receptor dissociation
8. Transporter-vesicle endocytosis

Glucose

Glucose transport system

Intracellular pool of transporters

Insulin

Receptor

Plasma membrane

FIGURE 39-6   Translocation of glucose transporters in response to insulin (see text).

tissues is an example of the type of dual control of synthetic and degradative pathways.

While effects of insulin on gluconeogenesis are restricted to the liver, the hormone affects the activities of a variety of intracellular enzymes involved in energy storage in all of the major insulin sensitive tissues. As a result glucose is efficiently converted to glycogene, triglyceride, and protein.

The stimulation of glycogen synthesis by insulin involves dephosphorylation and activation of glycogen synthase, the enzyme catalyzing the rate limiting step in glycogen synthesis from glucose. This effect was the first clear cut example of an action of insulin on the activity of an intracellular enzyme.

Lipid Metabolism

Insulin exerts a variety of actions to decrease the concentration of serum lipids (see Table 39-5). Because of their low water solubility, lipids are transported in blood primarily as particles composed of cholesterol esters complexed with proteins (termed lipoproteins). Before the fatty acids can be taken up into cells, the cholesterol esters must be hydrolyzed. The activity of lipoprotein lipase, the enzyme cata-

lyzing this reaction, is stimulated by insulin.

Insulin also stimulates fatty acid synthesis. Dephosphorylation and activation of two key enzymes in the synthetic pathway, pyruvate dehydrogenase and acetylCoA carboxylase, are involved in this effect of the hormone. Although synthesis is increased, the concentration of free fatty acids is decreased in response to insulin because the hormone decreases lipolysis and increases the rate of fatty acid esterification to form triglyceride. Stimulation of glucose transport into fat cells increases the supply of glycerol phosphate used in esterification. Inhibition of lipolysis involves dephosphorylation and inactivation of triglyceride lipase.

Protein Metabolism

Insulin increases protein synthesis in various cells by stimulation of a number of steps in the synthetic pathway. Control at the transcriptional level is evident by increases in specific mRNA species. Insulin also stimulates the rate of amino acid transport, increasing the precursors for protein synthesis. It has not been determined whether or not amino acid transporters are translocated to the membrane in response to in-

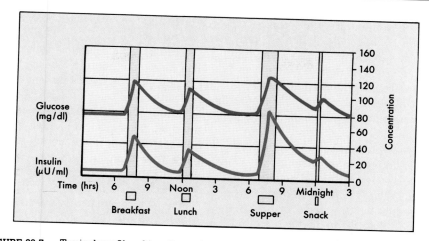

FIGURE 39-7   Typical profile of insulin and glucose concentrations in a normal individual.

sulin. Insulin also increases the rate of translation of mRNA into protein. The finding of increased phosphorylation of ribosomal protein S6 in response to insulin in some cells suggests that phosphorylation of the ribosome is involved. Finally, insulin decreases the rate of proteolysis, an action that is more sensitive to insulin than the increase in protein synthesis.

Glucagon

Glucagon is used therapeutically to increase blood glucose concentrations in patients with hypoglycemia who are unable to take oral glucose. Its chief use, however, is in radiology. When administered with a radiopaque substance, it relaxes the gastrointestinal smooth muscles, allowing better visualization of tumors and other gastrointestinal pathology.

Glucagon, which has a positive inotropic effect on the heart, can be useful in the treatment of overdosage or poisoning with β-blocking drugs.

Sulfonylureas

The relative contributions to the hypoglycemic effect of the actions of sulfonylureas on enhancing insulin sensitivity and on promoting insulin release are still being debated. However, both of these actions require the presence of insulin, either circulating or in the β cells. Thus *sulfonylureas are ineffective in treating IDDM.* Their usefulness is restricted to the therapy of some cases of NIDDM.

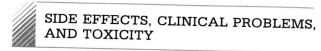

SIDE EFFECTS, CLINICAL PROBLEMS, AND TOXICITY

Problems in Achieving Good Control

The IDDM patient is absolutely dependent on administration of exogenous insulin for normal growth, and to prevent ketosis and death. In contrast, the NIDDM patient may appear to function normally without treatment of any kind. However, the disease has serious complications that are insidious in nature. Seriously impaired functioning of the renal, nervous, and circulatory systems may develop in both the IDDM and NIDDM patients. Although not yet proven, it is hoped that good control of diabetes might prevent, or at least delay, the development of long-term complications.

Maintaining glucose homeostasis with exogeneous insulin is complicated by several factors. A major problem is that control of blood sugar cannot be achieved with a fixed concentration of insulin. Blood concentrations of insulin fluctuate dramatically in normal individuals. Figure 39-7 depicts hypothetical changes in blood glucose and insulin concentrations over a 24-hour period. During a period of fasting, as occurs at night in most people, concentrations of insulin and glucose are low. Following a meal, the rise in blood glucose is attenuated because insulin concentrations also increase. Without insulin, blood sugar could increase to 500 mg/dl or higher. The pancreatic control system maintains tight control of glucose concentrations by releasing insulin in proportion to need. Thus, serum glucose concentrations are maintained within a relatively narrow range, even though food intake varies greatly. After a light snack, insulin concentrations might double, but after a large meal, the hormone concentration may increase by tenfold or more.

Any of a number of factors can cause insulin sensitivity to change, foiling even conscientious attempts at control. Exercise can markedly increase insulin sensitivity, thus decreasing the hormonal requirement. This is frequently the cause of insulin-induced hypoglycemia. Stress, pregnancy, steroid hormones or drugs, and thiazide diuretics are factors that decrease insulin sensitivity and exacerbate the signs and symptoms of diabetes mellitus.

Insulin

Delivering insulin so that it peaks in a pattern matching that seen in the nondiabetic subject is an objective that is difficult to achieve. If the insulin concentrations do not decrease as blood glucose falls, hypoglycemia ensues. In most cases multiple injections of a short-acting insulin preparation are used to produce the peaks in insulin concentrations, and an extended-action preparation is used to establish a baseline concentration.

Administering insulin with constant infusion pumps provides a means to control more precisely the concentration of circulating insulin, and there is evidence that tighter control of blood sugar is possible with these devices. Unfortunately, there is some reason to believe that simply mimicking the normal circulating insulin concentrations might not be sufficient to prevent diabetic complications. This concern arises from the relationship of the pancreas and liver in the circulatory system. Insulin is released directly into the portal vein and passes through the liver before it reaches the peripheral circulation. More than half the insulin is degraded by a single pass through the liver. Consequently, in normal individuals the hepatic tissues are exposed to insulin concentrations more than twice as high as in the vascular beds of skeletal muscle or adipose tissue. When exogenous insulin is injected in an insulin-dependent diabetic to achieve a normal blood concentration of the hormone, that concentration may be insufficient to initiate appropriate responses in the liver. Pancreas or islet

transplantation may ultimately provide a solution to this problem.

Side Effects Insulin has relatively few side effects. The most common are localized fat accumulation or atrophy, allergic reactions, and hypoglycemia.

The insulin concentration is highest at the site of injection. When the hormone is repeatedly administered at the same site, there is a tendency of the adipose tissue to hypertrophy in the surrounding region. This is presumably caused by the action of insulin to promote triglyceride accumulation in fat cells. The problem can be corrected by rotating sites of injection, a practice now routinely encouraged. Atrophy of adipose tissue at the site of injection has also been a frequent problem in the past. This is hard to explain in terms of the defined actions of insulin, and is most likely caused by stimulation of lipolysis by contaminants, possibly glucagon, in the insulin preparations. At any rate the incidence of lipoatrophy is lower with the highly purified insulin preparations now available. In fact, injection at the atrophic sites with the new purified insulin preparations has been successful in treating the atrophy.

Allergic reactions occur in a small percentage of individuals, mostly those receiving beef insulin. This occurs because this insulin differs from the human hormone (see Figure 39-3), and is recognized as a foreign substance by the immune system. In some cases, the antibodies are produced in sufficient quantity to increase the concentration of insulin needed therapeutically. Fortunately, the problem associated with allergic reactions can be corrected by changing from beef to porcine insulin, which is closer to the human hormone, or to recombinant human insulin.

Hypoglycemia is a serious complication and results when circulating insulin concentrations are too high. Among the causes are mistakes in calculating the dosage or in injecting the hormone, changes in eating patterns, or a reduction in insulin requirement. The brain and nervous tissue have an absolute requirement for glucose. When severe, hypoglycemia can cause loss of consciousness, convulsions, brain damage, and death. Therefore the physician and associates of the diabetic patient must be able to recognize the signs and correct the cause of hypoglycemia.

Symptoms of hypoglycemia are generally attributable either to increases in epinephrine and/or to abnormal functioning of the CNS. When the fall in blood glucose is rapid, epinephrine is released as a compensatory measure to stimulate hepatic glucose production and mobilization of energy reserves. Rapid heart rate, headache, cold sweat, weakness, and trembling are characteristic responses to the catecholamine. The extent to which these symptoms are observed varies considerably, depending on the individual and the rate of fall of the blood sugar concentration. Impaired neural function leads to blurred vision, an incoherent speech pattern, and mental confusion. At this point, an experienced diabetic might be capable of recognizing his or her hypoglycemic state and taking corrective action. However, the mentally disoriented individual is likely to require assistance. *The remedy is glucose.* If the subject is able, a glucose tablet, candy bar, fruit juice, or other source of sugar may be given. Because of the likelihood of choking, administering food or drink to an unconscious individual should never be attempted. In this case glucose should be administered intravenously by a trained health care professional. Glucagon can also be administered under these circumstances to raise blood glucose.

The unconscious hypoglycemic state induced by overdosage of insulin is referred to as *insulin coma.* Unfortunately, insulin coma is sometimes confused with diabetic coma. The two conditions have opposite causes, and the therapeutic intervention strategies are fundamentally different. Diabetic coma is the result of a chain of events set into motion by an insulin deficit and ultimately involves ketoacidosis, electrolyte imbalance, and dehydration. This condition usually develops over days or weeks, whereas with insulin coma, the patient may be well one minute and seriously debilitated a few minutes later. Thus when the onset is rapid, insulin coma should be suspected, particularly if it is known that the subject has recently received an injection of the hormone.

Even when diabetic coma is suspected, it is good practice to first administer glucose. In the event of a mistaken diagnosis, a hypoglycemic patient will recover as soon as blood glucose concentrations are increased, provided there is no brain damage. It should be remembered that administering insulin to a patient in insulin coma could easily cause death; giving glucose to a patient in diabetic coma will do no harm, particularly since the subject may actually be hypoglycemic because of the depletion of energy stores. It should also be noted that treatment of diabetic coma involves much more than injections with insulin and should be attempted only in the proper clinical setting where glucose and electrolyte concentrations can be monitored and maintained at proper concentrations.

Sulfonylureas

For the past 2 decades, the use of sulfonylureas in treating non-insulin–dependent diabetes mellitus has been controversial. The controversy arose from results of the University Group Diabetes Program (UGDP), a large long-term clinical trial involving 12 university medical centers. The goal of the UGDP was to determine whether insulin therapy or oral hypoglycemic agents were of any benefit in delaying the onset of diabetic complications. Several years into the study, some subjects, notably elderly women, treated with tolbutamide appeared to be dying from cardiovascular disease at a higher rate than individuals in the control groups, and tolbutamide was withdrawn from the trial. Understandably, the UGDP has become best known for its implications concerning the safety of tolbutamide and, by association, the other sulfonylurea hypoglycemic agents.

If sulfonylureas were known to place patients at increased risk of death, then their use could not be justified, particularly since insulin affords an effective, though less convenient, alternative for treating the non-insulin–dependent diabetic. Questions have been raised that cast serious doubt on the validity of the UGDP's conclusion regarding tolbutamide. For example, it has been pointed out that only 26% of the patients assigned to the original test groups actually remained in that group throughout the study, and the patients assigned to the tolbutamide group appeared to have had more risk factors (e.g., high blood pressure or elevated serum cholesterol) to begin with. Such problems have prompted the American Diabetes Association to withdraw its support of the UGDP's stance on tolbutamide. Nonetheless, the question of the safety of tolbutamide has not been put to rest.

Side Effects Depending on the sulfonylurea being taken, the incidence of side effects of some type ranges between 3% and 66%. These side effects are usually not serious and the drugs are considered relatively safe, with the possible exception discussed above. The most frequent complication is hypoglycemia, which may be brought on by overdosage, increased insulin sensitivity, change in dietary pattern, or increased energy expenditure. If the hypoglycemic response is mild, it can be corrected by decreasing the dose of the drug. However, severe cases may

CLINICAL PROBLEMS

INSULIN

Hypoglycemia
Local or systemic allergic reactions
Visual disturbances
Peripheral edema

SULFONYLUREAS

Hypoglycemia
Gastrointestinal disturbances
Hematological disturbances
Flushing especially with concurrent alcohol ingestion
Contraindicated with hepatic or renal insufficiency
Drug interactions

TRADENAMES

In addition to generic and fixed combination preparations, the following tradenamed materials are available in the United States.

INSULIN

Short-acting
  Humulin R, Novolin R, Velosin; human insulin
  Iletin Regular, insulin
  Iletin Semilente, insulin zinc suspension
Intermediate-acting
  Humulin L, Novolin L; human insulin zinc suspension (intermediate)
  Humulin N, Novolin N; isophane insulin human
  Insulabard NPH, isophane human insulin
  Lente, insulin zinc suspension (intermediate)
  NPH Iletin, isophane insulin
  NPH insulin, isophane insulin
Long-acting
  Protamine Zinc Iletin, protamine zinc insulin suspension
  Ultralente Iletin, insulin zinc suspension (extended)

SULFONYLUREAS

Diabinase, chlorpropamide
Dymelor, acetohexamide
Glucotrol, glipizide
Micronase, DiaBeta; glyburide
Orinase, tolbutamide
Tolinase, Ronase, tolazamide

persist for days after withdrawal of the drug, and require multiple injections of glucose.

Because of the high degree of binding to serum proteins, the potential exists for interactions with other drugs (e.g., phenylbutazone or salicylates) that compete for serum binding sites. This is particularly true for the first generation drugs tolbutamide, acetohexamide, tolazamide, and chlorpropamide, which bind to serum albumin chiefly by ionic interactions and therefore can be displaced by other drugs. The second generation drugs glipizide and glyburide bind to albumin by nonionic interactions and are less readily displaced by other drugs.

Gastrointestinal disturbances, allergic reactions, dermatological problems, and transient leukopenia can be expected in a small percentage of cases. A disulfiram type of response (i.e., flushing) when taken with alcohol is sometimes a problem, particularly with chlorpropamide. This drug is the only sulfonylurea that causes fluid retention, an effect that appears to be a result of stimulation of the release of ADH.

Contraindications

Therapy is contraindicated in individuals not having a proven pancreatic reserve of insulin. Attention to the metabolism and route of excretion of the drugs is required before initiating sulfonylurea therapy in subjects with impaired hepatic or renal function. In these cases, treatment with insulin may be the best choice. Teratogenic effects of sulfonylureas have not been reported, but because of the possibility of such effects and adverse reactions in the newborn, the drugs should not be administered to pregnant or lactating females. Problems are summarized in the box.

REFERENCES

Denton RM: Early events in insulin actions, Adv Cyclic Nucleotide Res 20:293, 1986.

Larner J: Insulin signaling mechanisms, Diabetes 37:262, 1988.

Lebovitz HE: Oral hypoglycemic agents, J Primary Care 15:353, 1988.

Saltiel AR and Cuatrecasas P: In search of a second messenger for insulin, Am J Physiol 255 (Cell Physiol 24): C1, 1988.

Santiago JV: Overview of complications of diabetes, Clin Chem 32 (Suppl 10): B48, 1986.

Shank WA Jr. and Morrison AD: Oral sulfonylureas for the treatment of type II diabetes: an update, So Med J 79:337, 1986.

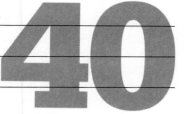

CHAPTER 40

Drugs Affecting Uterine Motility

 THERAPEUTIC OVERVIEW

Neuroendocrine mechanisms that initiate and control uterine contractility during pregnancy and parturition are complex. Regulation of myometrial (uterine) smooth muscle contraction involves changes in cell membrane function and hormone-receptor interactions.

The initiation and maintenance of uterine contractility involve an alteration in the hormonal milieu. Throughout pregnancy, the effects of high concentrations of progesterone predominate to suppress uterine smooth muscle contractility. Progesterone stabilizes the electrophysiological properties of the uterine smooth muscle membrane and prevents the release of arachidonic acid, the precursor for prostaglandin synthesis. In addition, the high concentrations of progesterone decrease the number of oxytocin and α-adrenergic receptors.

As parturition approaches, the major change in the hormonal environment is an increase in the estrogen/progesterone ratio. The increased concentrations of estrogen increase the number of gap junctions that electrically couple myometrial muscle cells. This enhances intercellular communication and raises the resting potential of the cell membrane. In addition, the number of receptors increases markedly for the following contractile agonists: oxytocin, angiotensin, and α-adrenergic agents; heightening the sensitivity of the myometrial cells to contractile stimuli. The decrease in progesterone before parturition is associated with increased prostaglandin synthesis, which also promotes uterine contraction.

Two major classes of drugs affect uterine motililty:

THERAPEUTIC OVERVIEW

UTERINE STIMULATION
Induction of labor
Augmentation of labor
Therapeutic abortion
Postpartum hemorrhage (control)

UTERINE RELAXATION
Arrest premature labor

uterine stimulants and uterine relaxants. Uterine stimulants are used to facilitate parturition, manage postpartum hemorrhage, or stimulate uterine contraction during a therapeutic abortion. Uterine relaxants (tocolytic agents) inhibit uterine contraction and are used primarily to arrest premature labor.

The therapeutic overview is summarized in the box.

 MECHANISMS OF ACTION

Uterine Contraction

The biochemical and molecular events involved in uterine smooth muscle contraction are the same as those that control other smooth muscle tissues (see Chapter 17).

Assuming that the changes previously described in the hormonal environment and in the number of the several hormone receptors on the myometrial cell membrane have taken place before parturition, the uterine smooth muscle is sensitized for contraction to occur. As with other smooth muscles, actin and myosin must interact for uterine contraction to occur, and this depends on phosphorylation of myosin light chains (MLC). This phosphorylation in turn is dependent on the activity of myosin light chain kinase (MLCK), a key enzyme in uterine contraction. Myosin light chain kinase–driven phosphorylation requires cellular Ca^{++} concentrations of 10^{-6} M or more. Additionally the enzyme is active only if associated with calmodulin, and formation of the myosin light chain kinase–calmodulin complex also is Ca^{++}-dependent.

Various hormones and drugs interact to enhance the contractile state of the uterus and are used therapeutically to induce or augment uterine contractions. In addition, these drugs may be used in the treatment of postpartum hemorrhage. The types of drugs that promote uterine stimulation are listed in Table 40-1.

Oxytocin, a nonapeptide (Figure 40-1), is synthesized in the supraoptic and paraventricular nucleus of the hypothalamus and is released from the posterior pituitary. A role for oxytocin in initiation or propagation of normal labor has been postulated for many years, but increased concentrations of oxytocin have not been demonstrated before the onset of labor. However, with an increased estrogen/progesterone ratio during labor, the number of myometrial oxytocin receptors increases markedly. The interaction of endogenous or administered oxytocin with myometrial cell membrane receptors promotes the influx of Ca^{++} from the extracellular fluid and from the sarcoplasmic

reticulum into the cell. This increase in cytoplasmic calcium stimulates uterine contraction by activation of myosin light chain kinase, as discussed previously. In addition, oxytocin acts together with prostaglandins to facilitate uterine smooth muscle contraction.

α-Adrenergic agonists used to stimulate uterine smooth muscle contraction are ergot alkaloids, ergonovine maleate and methylergonovine maleate. The mechanism involves a drug-uterine receptor interaction. The hormone receptor complex facilitates the entry of Ca^{++} into the cell, probably by opening

Table 40-1   Drugs that Promote Uterine Contraction or Relaxation

Action	Agent
Uterine stimulation	oxytocin
	α-adrenergic agonists/ergot alkaloids including ergonovine maleate and methylergonovine maleate
	prostaglandins
Uterine relaxation/tocolysis	ethanol
	magnesium sulfate
	prostaglandin synthesis inhibitors including indomethacin
	β-adrenergic drugs ($β_2$) including isoxsuprine, terbutaline, and ritodrine
	calcium channel blockers
	diazoxide
	aminophylline

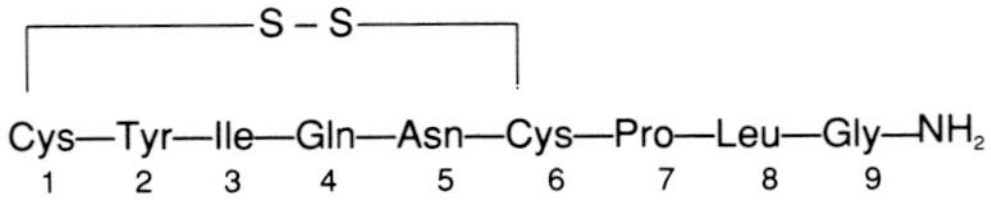

$$S-S$$

Cys—Tyr—Ile—Gln—Asn—Cys—Pro—Leu—Gly—NH₂
1   2   3   4   5   6   7   8   9

FIGURE 40-1   Structure of oxytocin, a cyclic disulfide-linked nonapeptide that stimulates uterine smooth muscle contraction.

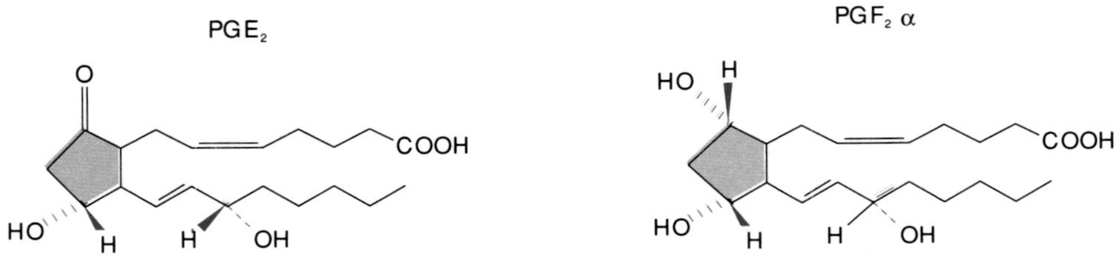

FIGURE 40-2   Structures of the uterine stimulant prostaglandins.

calcium channels through the enzymatic phosphorylation of specific membrane phospholipids. The increase in intracellular cytosolic Ca^{++} facilitates smooth muscle contraction. The sensitivity of the uterus to ergot alkaloids increases steadily during pregnancy, and the number of α-adrenergic receptors increases as the estrogen/progesterone ratio heightens at term.

Prostaglandins are the most recent addition to the list of uterine stimulants. These drugs, discussed in Chapter 18, are formed by action of several enzymes on arachidonic acid. The major prostaglandins important in pregnancy and parturition are $E_2(PGE_2)$, $F_{2\alpha}$, and (PGF_2), (Figure 40-2).

The mechanism by which prostaglandins enhance uterine contractility is poorly understood but may result from their action on cell surface receptors to increase adenylate cyclase activity and subsequent concentrations of cAMP. This increases cAMP-dependent protein kinase activity and phosphorylation of myosin light chain kinase, leading to relaxation (Chapter 17). Conversely, decreased cAMP concentrations inactivate cAMP-dependent protein kinase, increase myosin light chain kinase activity and cause contraction. In addition, prostaglandins, in conjunction with oxytocin, enhance Ca^{++} release from the sarcoplasmic reticulum into the cytosol.

In summary, the overall mechanisms by which uterine stimulants enhance myometrial smooth muscle contraction are through (1) a receptor-mediated increase in cytosolic (i.e., intracellular) Ca^{++} or (2) a reduction in the production of cAMP. For the effect of these agents to occur, the uterus must be "hormonally primed" so that concentrations of oxytocin, α-adrenergic, and prostaglandin receptors have increased above their early pregnancy values.

Uterine Relaxation

Uterine smooth muscle relaxation is modulated by two distinct regulatory pathways that utilize cAMP. The first mechanism involves inhibition of myosin light chain kinase through action of a cAMP-mediated protein kinase (see Chapter 17). In addition, cAMP promotes the accumulation of Ca^{++} in the sarcoplasmic reticulum, thus decreasing the concentration of cytosolic calcium. The concentrations of cAMP are determined by two specific enzymatic activities (i.e., synthesis via adenylate cyclase and degradation via cAMP phosphodiesterase). Stimulation of β-adrenergic receptors leads to increased adenylate cyclase activity and subsequent increases in cAMP concentration. These biochemical pathways can be modulated by pharmacological agents to promote relaxation of uterine smooth muscle (see Table 40-1) (see also Chapter 17).

The chief use of uterine relaxants or tocolytic agents is in the arrest of premature labor. Ethanol and inhibitors of prostaglandin synthesis (e.g., indomethacin) act indirectly and prevent the synthesis or release of endogenous uterine stimulants. Magnesium sulfate and β-adrenergic drugs act directly to suppress the contractile response of the myometrial smooth muscle.

Ethanol has been the most widely used tocolytic agent for inhibiting premature labor. Based on the observation that ethanol suppresses antidiuretic hormone release from the posterior pituitary gland, it has been hypothesized that ethanol could suppress oxytocin release and result in uterine relaxation. Analysis of the myometrial dose response to oxytocin before and after administration of ethanol indicates, however, that ethanol not only decreases oxytocin release but also acts directly on the myometrial cell membrane. Ethanol also may stimulate β-adrenergic receptors, which results in the production of increased concentrations of cAMP. The increased concentrations of cAMP promote relaxation of the uterus.

Prostaglandin synthesis inhibitors (e.g., indomethacin) are theoretically useful for retarding premature labor. This is based on the observation that depletion of prostaglandins prevents stimulation of the uterus by oxytocin agonists; the addition of prostaglandins restores the potency of oxytocin. It is believed that prostaglandin synthesis inhibitor drugs block spontaneous uterine contractions by reducing the amount of prostaglandins synthesized and released by myometrial cells.

The β-adrenergic drugs are the most recently added class of tocolytic agents. These drugs (i.e., isoxsuprine, terbutaline, ritodrine; structures shown in Chapter 10) are similar in structure to epinephrine. The drugs have a greater effect on B_2-adrenergic receptors (uterus and lung) than B_1-receptors (particularly the heart). The β-adrenergic drugs bind to B_2-adrenergic receptors on the outer surface of the cell membranes of the myometrial cells, activating adenylate cyclase. ATP is converted to cAMP, which activates protein kinases to phosphorylate cellular proteins. The phosphorylated proteins act to sequester intracellular Ca^{++} within the sarcoplasmic reticulum or to inactivate the MLCK. The decrease in intracellular calcium prevents the activation of the actin and myosin elements and therefore inhibits uterine contraction.

There are three other drugs that play a less significant role as uterine relaxants but that require discussion. The calcium channel blockers (i.e., nifedipine and nicardipine) inhibit the entry of calcium into smooth muscle cells and have been shown to decrease uterine contractility in various animal studies. To date these drugs have had only limited use in human pregnancy because potential negative effects on the fetus still need to be clarified. Diazoxide, a potent vasodilator agent known to inhibit uterine activity, is administered to treat hypertensive crises during pregnancy. The mechanism for tocolysis may involve a direct effect on uterine smooth muscle or may involve stimulation of the release of catecholamines. This drug has major side effects that limit its usefulness as a first-line tocolytic agent.

Aminophylline, a xanthine derivative, is used to treat asthma during pregnancy. Aminophylline may inhibit cAMP phosphodiesterase or block the adenosine receptor. The inhibition of this enzyme or blockade of this receptor results in the accumulation of cAMP, promoting uterine relaxation. Therefore aminophylline indirectly inhibits uterine smooth muscle contraction.

Parenteral administration of magnesium sulfate inhibits uterine contraction. The mechanism of action results from ionic magnesium antagonizing the action of Ca^{++} in myometrial cells. The drug may exert its effect by: (1) decreasing the frequency of myometrial muscle cell action potentials; (2) uncoupling the excitation and contraction of the uterine smooth muscle cells; or (3) directly relaxing the contractile elements.

PHARMACOKINETICS

Uterine stimulants often are administered by slow IV infusion to maintain control of the response. Oxytocin undergoes hydrolytic cleavage in the GI tract if given orally. Ergonovine maleate and its methyl analog both are well absorbed when administered orally. Disposition of oxytocin, ergonovine, and PGE_2 or $PGF_{2\alpha}$ is mainly by metabolism to inactive compounds. The plasma half-life, disposition, and other pharmacokinetic parameters for uterine stimulants are summarized in Table 40-2.

Some of the uterine inhibitors are also discussed in other chapters: ethanol in Chapter 3; indomethacin in Chapter 18; terbutaline, isoxsuprine, and ritodrine in Chapter 10. The disposition, mode of administration, half-life, and other pharmacokinetic factors for these drugs are presented elsewhere. Magnesium sulfate, usually is administered IV.

Both the uterine stimulants and uterine inhibitors are titrated to obtain the desired therapeutic response according to the clinical condition of the patient.

RELATION OF MECHANISMS OF ACTION TO CLINICAL RESPONSE

Not all uterine smooth muscle stimulants should be used for induction of labor for term or near-term pregnancies. The ergot alkaloids, for example, cross the placenta and can cause deleterious effects to the fetus; these compounds also have the potential to generate sustained, rather than intermittent, uterine contractions.

Perinatal mortality and morbidity are associated predominately with infants who undergo premature delivery. A delay of 1 or 2 weeks may often be beneficial when signs of premature labor occur. The β-adrenergic agents (especially ritodrine) magnesium sulfate, ethanol, and inhibitors of prostaglandin synthesis (indomethacin) are used clinically in the arrest of premature labor. A variety of special conditions often are encountered in patients who experience preterm labor (Table 40-3) and often must be considered during selection of the tocolytic agent. The use of indomethacin is still considered to be experimental.

SIDE EFFECTS, CLINICAL PROBLEMS, AND TOXICITY

The major side effects on the mother of the uterine stimulants (Table 40-4) include uterine rupture, cardiovascular effects, and gastrointestinal symptoms. In the fetus, if uterine contractions become too strong, the fetus can experience serious injury, hypoxia, and even death.

The major maternal side effects of the uterine relaxants (Table 40-5) are primarily associated with severe alterations on the cardiovascular system and changes in the function of the CNS. Fetal toxicities are less common.

Table 40-2   Pharmacokinetic Parameters*

Drug	Route	Absorption	$t_{1/2}$	Disposition
Oxytocin	IV, IM	Degraded	1-6 min	Metabolized in liver, kidney
Ergonovine	PO, IM, IV	Fairly well	Several hours	Metabolized in liver, bile
Prostaglandins	IV, IM, IA†, oral	—	—	Metabolized in many tissues, especially lung

0.5 mg, 1 IU for oxytocin.
* Values for uterine stimulants only; values for uterine relaxants are in other chapters (see text).
† Intraamniotic.

Table 40-3   Clinical Conditions Often Associated with Preterm Labor

Site	Condition	Site	Condition
Maternal	Acute/chronic severe systemic disease	Fetoplacental	Genetic abnormalities
	Endocrine conditions such as hyperthyroidism or hyperadrenocorticism		Fetal death
			Abruptio placenta
	Chronic hypertension		Placenta previa
	History of premature birth		Multifetal gestation
	Trauma		Premature rupture of the amniotic membranes
	Genital infection	Uterine	Multiple gestation
	Age—under 16 or over 40		Foreign body
			Infection
			Cervical incompetence or trauma
			Surgery
			Uterine anomalies

Table 40-4   Problems (Stimulants)

Drug	Maternal	Fetal	Drug	Maternal	Fetal
oxytocin	Uterine hyperactivity	Acidosis	prostaglandins	Uterine hypertonus	Death
	Uterine rupture	Hypoxia		Nausea/vomiting	
	Hypotension	Hyperbilirubinemia		Diarrhea	
	Tachycardia			Tachycardia	
	ECG changes			Headache	
ergot alkaloids	Hypertension	Serious injury to the fetus		Flushing	
	Severe headache			Fever	
	Nausea/vomiting			Seizures	
	Blurred vision				
	Convulsions				
	Death				
	Bradycardia				
	Angina				

Table 40-5　Clinical Problems (Relaxants)

Drug	Maternal	Fetal
ethanol	Tachycardia Slurred speech Restlessness Sleepiness Mood changes Dehydration Aspiration Acidosis Intoxication Aspiration	CNS depression Hiccups Excessive heat loss Intoxication Hypoglycemia Acidosis
magnesium sulfate	Skin flushing Nausea Headache Palpitations Depressed reflexes Respiratory depression Cardiac conduction problems Cardiac arrest	CNS depression (rare)
prostaglandin synthesis inhibitors (indomethacin)	Anorexia Nausea GI bleeding Headaches Confusion Allergic rashes Bone marrow depression	Premature closure of the ductus arteriosus Pulmonary hypertension Hyperbilirubinemia Coagulopathy
β-adrenergic drugs	Tachycardia Hypotension Hyperglycemia Tremors Nausea/vomiting Angina Pulmonary edema	Tachycardia Hypotension

---

TRADENAMES

In addition to generic and fixed combination preparations, the following tradenamed materials are available in the United States.

UTERINE STIMULANTS

Ergotrate, ergonovine maleate
Prostin, PGF$_2$
Syntocinon, Pitocin; oxytocin

UTERINE RELAXANTS

Brethine, Bricanyl; terbutaline
Indocin, indomethacin
Yutopar, ritodrine

REFERENCES

Caritis SN, Edelstone DI, and Mueller-Heubach E: Pharmacologic inhibition of preterm labor, Am J Obstet Gynecol 133:557, 1979.

Dawood MY et al: Oxytocin in human pregnancy and parturition, Obstet Gynecol 51:138, 1978.

Huszar G and Roberts JM: Biochemistry and pharmacology of the myometrium and labor: regulation at the cellular and molecular levels, Am J Obstet Gynecol 142:225, 1982.

Rayburn WF, DeDonato DM, and Rand WK III: Drugs to inhibit premature labor. In Rayburn WF and Zuspan FP, eds: Drug therapy in obstetrics and gynecology, ed 2, Norwalk, 1986, Appleton-Century-Crofts.

Rayburn WF and Russ JS: Uterine stimulants. In Rayburn WF and Zuspan FP, eds: Drug therapy in obstetrics and gynecology, ed 2, Norwalk, 1986, Appleton-Century-Crofts.

CHAPTER 41 Hypothalamic-pituitary Hormones

	ABBREVIATIONS
AVP	arginine vasopressin (or simply vasopressin)
cAMP	cyclic adenosine monophosphate
CRH	corticotropin-releasing hormone
DDAUP	desamino D-arginine vasopressin
FSH	follicle-stimulating hormone
GH	growth hormone
GHRH	growth hormone-releasing hormone
GnRH	gonadotropin-releasing hormone
IGF-1	insulin-like growth factor-1
LH	luteinizing hormone
SRIF	somatotropin release-inhibiting factor (somatostatin)
TRH	thyrotropin-releasing hormone
TSH	thyroid-stimulating hormone
VIP	vasoactive intestinal polypeptide

THERAPEUTIC OVERVIEW

The role of the pituitary gland in regulating hormone production by peripheral endocrine organs is well known, but the relationship between the pituitary and the hypothalamic factors that control pituitary function has been defined only recently. Peptides and biogenic amines, synthesized and secreted by specialized neurons within the hypothalamus, are transported via the hypothalamo-hypophyseal portal circulation to the anterior pituitary where, acting via specific receptors, they stimulate or inhibit hormone secretion (Figure 41-1). Anterior pituitary hormones, in turn, signal the production of hormones by peripheral endocrine organs. Hormones originating from peripheral endocrine organs subserve their own functions and provide feedback at the hypothalamic and/or pituitary level to modulate the synthesis and release of their particular trophic hormone. Thus hypothalamic gonadotropin-releasing hormone (GnRH) stimulates the secretion of luteinizing hormone (LH) and follicle-stimulating hormone (FSH) by the pituitary, which affects gametogenesis and gonadal hormone production by the testes and ovary (see Chapters 36 and 37). Thyrotropin-releasing hormone (TRH) stimulates the secretion of thyroid-stimulating hormone (TSH), which in turn, controls thyroid function. Corticotropin-releasing hormone (CRH) stimulates the secretion of adrenocorticotropin (ACTH), which promotes the secretion of hormones by the adrenal cortex. Growth hormone-releasing hormone (GHRH) and somatotropin release-inhibiting factor (SRIF) stimulate and inhibit, respectively, the production of growth hormone (GH), which has numerous effects on growth and metabolism. Hypothalamic dopamine functions to tonically inhibit the secretion of prolactin, the hormone primarily responsible for lactation. The posterior pituitary (or neurohypophysis) secretes arginine vasopressin (AVP) and oxytocin. Unlike the anterior pituitary, which is under hypothalamic control, the neurohypophysis is made up of neurons with cell bodies within the hypothalamus. These cells synthesize and secrete AVP and oxytocin that are transported by carrier proteins (neurophysins) via axons to the posterior pituitary where they are released directly into the systemic circulation.

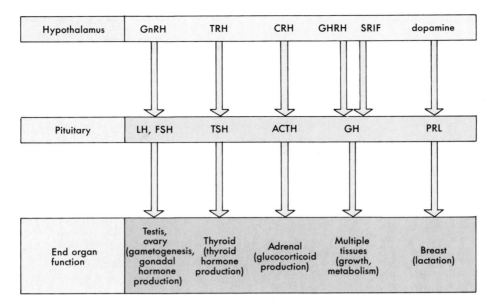

FIGURE 41-1 Relationships among the hypothalamic releasing and inhibiting hormones, the anterior pituitary hormones that the hypothalamic hormones control, and their respective target organs/tissues. *GnRH*, Gonadotropin-releasing hormone; *TRH*, thyrotropin-releasing hormone; *CRH*, corticotropin-releasing hormone; *GHRH*, growth hormone-releasing hormone; *SRIF*, somatotropin release-inhibiting factor (somatostatin); *LH*, luteinizing hormone; *FSH*, follicle-stimulating hormone; *TSH*, thyroid-stimulating hormone; *ACTH*, adrenocorticotropic hormone; *GH*, growth hormone; *PRL*, prolactin.

THERAPEUTIC OVERVIEW

HYPOTHALAMIC HORMONES

GnRH
Replacement therapy
  central amenorrhea
  idiopathic hypogonadotropic hypogonadism
Prostate cancer
Idiopathic precocious puberty
Endometriosis
Contraception
GHRH
Short stature
Dopamine agonists (bromocriptine)
Physiological hyperprolactinemia
Pathophysiological hyperprolactinemia
Acromegaly
Parkinson's disease

GHRH—cont'd
Somatostatin and analogs
Carcinoid tumor
VIP secreting tumor

PITUITARY HORMONES

LH and FSH
Infertility in women
Infertility in men with hypogonadotropic hypergonadism
GH
Short stature
AVP
Diabetes insipidus

With the exception of prolactin, each of the hypothalamic and pituitary hormones mentioned are used for diagnostic and/or therapeutic purposes. Because the major roles of TRH, CRH, TSH, and ACTH are diagnostic, these hormones are not discussed further. The hypothalamic hormones (or their analogs/agonists): GnRH, GHRH, dopamine, and somatostatin; the anterior pituitary hormones GH and LH/FSH; and the posterior pituitary hormone AVP are used therapeutically or have therapeutic potential and are discussed in this chapter. The pharmacology of oxytocin is discussed in Chapter 40. A therapeutic overview of hypothalamic hormones is listed in the box.

 ## MECHANISMS OF ACTION

Hypothalamic Hormones

GnRH Analog agonists with increased half-life and greater receptor binding and competitive antagonists have been synthesized by selective amino acid substitutions in the molecule (Figure 41-2). The majority of GnRH-positive neurons in humans are located in the medial basal hypothalamus, between the third ventricle and the median eminence. Projections from these neurons terminate in the median eminence, in close contact with the capillary plexus of the hypothalamic-hypophyseal portal circulation. These capillaries allow GnRH to be delivered into the circulation without passing through a blood-brain barrier. GnRH is formed by processing a larger prohormone, pre-pro-GnRH, transported in secretory granules to nerve terminals for storage, degradation, or release into the pituitary portal blood vessels.

At the target, GnRH binds to receptors and initiates the secretion of LH and FSH. The molecular weight of the GnRH receptor is estimated to be 136,000 daltons. Microaggregation also stimulates up-regulation of the GnRH receptor, and is followed by endocytosis-mediated internalization of the hormone receptor complex (see Chapter 34). Receptor

activation results in the influx of extracellular Ca^{++} through the opening of ligand-gated calcium channels and the hydrolysis of phosphatidylinositol 4,5-bis-phosphate (see Chapter 34).

GnRH is released in a pulsatile manner by a "hypothalamic pulse generator." This release pattern is essential for normal function. Continuous administration results in an attenuated response mediated by receptor down-regulation and postreceptor mechanisms.

Major modulators of gonadotropin secretion are inhibin (a peptide hormone synthesized by ovarian granulosa and testicular Sertoli cells) and opioid peptides. In normally ovulating women, estradiol also exerts positive feedback at the pituitary, which may be responsible in part for the preovulatory LH surge.

GHRH Growth hormone's secretion is regulated by two opposing hypothalamic hormones: GHRH and SRIF (see Figure 41-3 for regulation).

Dopamine Agonists Bromocriptine is an inhibitor of prolactin secretion (see Figure 41-4 for structure). It suppresses prolactin release by directly stimulating dopamine receptors on prolactin-secreting lactotropes in the anterior pituitary. Ample evidence implicates hypothalamically derived dopamine as the physiologically significant prolactin-inhibiting factor (see Chapter 22 for dopamine-receptor mechanisms).

Somatostatin and Analogs Somatostatin (SRIF) is a cyclic peptide containing 14 amino acids (somatostatin 14). Recently a family of somatostatin-related peptides, including an aminoterminal extended peptide (somatostatin 28), was discovered. In addition to its presence in the hypothalamus, somatostatin is widely distributed throughout the nervous system, the gut, and various endocrine and exocrine glands. It has several functions depending on its source, acting as neurohormone to inhibit pituitary GH release, neurotransmitter in the nervous system, and as an autocrine and paracrine factor outside of the nervous system.

Somatostatin 14 and somatostatin 28 have different functions, as exemplified by the greater suppressive effect of somatostatin 28 than somatostatin 14

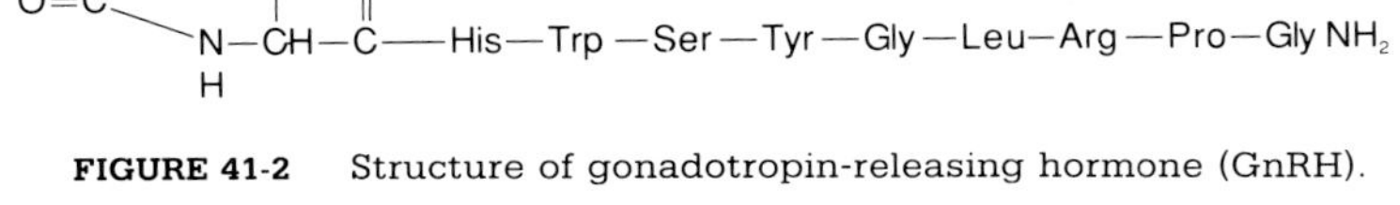

$$O=C \overset{H_2C-CH_2}{\underset{N-CH-C}{\overset{O}{\|}}}\text{---His---Trp---Ser---Tyr---Gly---Leu---Arg---Pro---Gly NH}_2$$

FIGURE 41-2   Structure of gonadotropin-releasing hormone (GnRH).

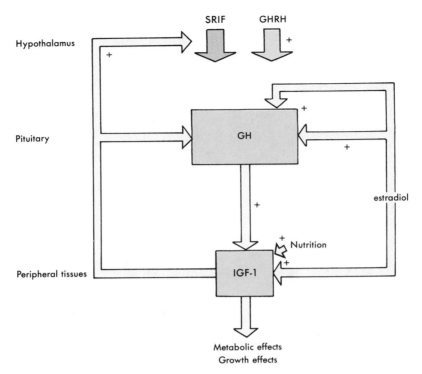

FIGURE 41-3   Schematic representation of regulation of growth hormone secretion in humans. GHRH and somatostatin *(SRIF)* are the primary stimulatory and inhibitory peptides, respectively. *IGF-1,* Insulin-like growth factor I.

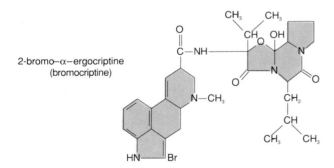

FIGURE 41-4   Structure of the prototypical dopamine agonist, 2-bromo-α-ergocriptine (bromocriptine).

on insulin secretion. Somatostatin acts via specific receptors that are present in pituitary cells, pituitary plasma membranes, brain synaptosome membranes, and pancreatic islet cells. It appears to act to decrease cytosolic Ca^{++}.

Somatostatin has a fifty-fold greater suppressive effect on glucagon than on insulin release. Its predominant effect on pancreatic islets is inhibition of glucagon-secreting cells. Somatostatin inhibits gut hormone secretion (e.g., gastrin, VIP, motilin, secretin); exocrine secretion (e.g., gastric acid, pepsin, pancreatic bicarbonate, pancreatic enzymes); and gastric emptying, gallbladder contraction, and intestinal motility. Somatostatin also decreases GI absorption and mesenteric blood flow. In the central nervous system (CNS), somatostatin has both excitatory and inhibitory influences on neurons and on neurotransmitter and neurohormone release. Its predominant role in the CNS is not established.

Pituitary Hormones

LH and FSH   LH and FSH are structurally similar glycoproteins, each consisting of two polypeptide chains linked by hydrogen bonds and with internal cross-linking by disulfide bonds. LH and FSH are composed of an identical 89 amino acid α chain and a

115 amino acid β chain unique to each hormone and responsible for specific hormonal activity. Two complex carbohydrate side-chains are attached to specific locations on the α subunit, two to the FSH-β subunit, and one to the LH-β subunit. A terminal sialic acid is found on approximately 5% and 1% of FSH and LH carbohydrate molecules, respectively. Sialic acid prolongs metabolic clearance of glycoproteins and results in a longer half-life for FSH as compared to LH. There is no evidence that other molecular forms of LH and FSH such as prohormones and fragments circulate in the plasma.

The gonadotrope secretes LH and FSH. The α and β chains are synthesized separately and appear to combine before carbohydrate addition.

Gonadotropins bind to high-affinity membrane receptors in the testes and ovary, activating adenylate cyclase. The production of cAMP signals the activation of its protein kinase and, subsequently, the phosphorylation of proteins necessary for steroidogenesis. The LH receptor has a molecular weight of approximately 180,000 daltons and binds one LH. The FSH receptor has not been characterized.

In addition to regulating estrogen production, the gonadotropins have multiple effects on ovarian follicles. FSH directly stimulates follicular growth and maturation and enhances granulosa cell responsiveness to LH. LH is essential for the breakdown of the follicular wall, resulting in ovulation, and for the subsequent resumption of meiotic division of the oocyte.

By contrast, testicular steroidogenesis requires only LH. The Leydig cells, which constitute about 10% of testicular volume, are stimulated to produce testosterone by binding of LH to surface receptors. FSH binds to Sertoli cells and, with testosterone, is essential for cellular maturation and for spermatid differentiation, the first step of spermatogenesis. The Sertoli cell is necessary for maintenance of seminiferous tubule function and germ cell development.

Growth Hormone Growth hormone is a 191 amino acid polypeptide that has 84% identity with placental chorionic somatomammotropin and marked structural homology with prolactin. Growth hormone is synthesized by somatotropes of the anterior pituitary; the major product is a 22,000 dalton peptide. The majority of circulating GH is the 22,000 dalton isoform, with 5% to 10% a 20,000 dalton isoform. GH dimers and tetramers also have been detected.

The precise mechanism by which GH exerts its

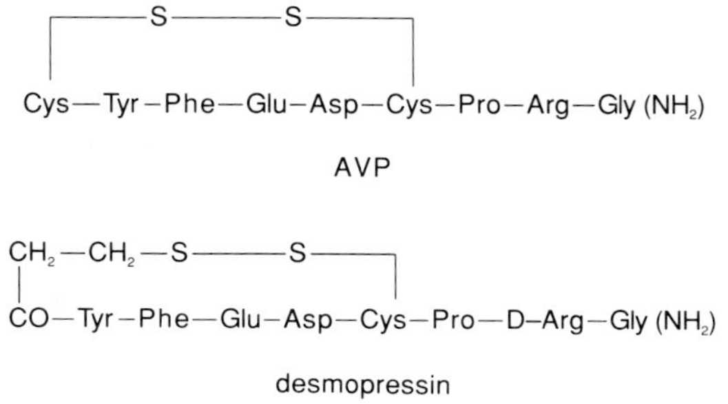

FIGURE 41-5   Amino acid sequences of arginine vasopressin *(AVP)* and an AVP analog, 1-desamino-8-D-arginine-vasopressin (desmopressin, DDAVP).

intracellular effects likely involves interaction with a specific plasma membrane receptor (or receptors). Additionally, GH binds to proteins in both cytosol and plasma. The specificity of the circulating binding protein is similar to the suggested GH receptor.

Numerous direct effects of GH on specific tissues include stimulation of RNA, protein, and IGF-I synthesis by liver; stimulation of amino acid transport and incorporation into muscle protein; and stimulation of amino acid incorporation into protein and lipolysis in adipose tissue. Additionally, GH exerts a positive influence on hematopoietic tissue.

Vasopressin AVP is a nonapeptide that functions as the primary antidiuretic hormone in humans (Figure 41-5). Synthesized primarily in the magnocellular neuronal systems of the supraoptic and paraventricular nuclei of the hypothalamus, the AVP precursor molecule contains a signal peptide, a neurophysin, and a glycosylated moiety in addition to the AVP sequence. This precursor molecule travels via neuronal axons to the posterior pituitary where granules containing cleaved and uncleaved hormone are stored. Such granules are released in response to a signal that effects Ca^{++} influx into the cell. The mechanisms that prompt the exocytosis of AVP primarily consist of osmotic signals (detected by osmoreceptors in the anterior hypothalamus) and pressure signals (detected by baroreceptors in the heart and large blood vessels). Nausea/emesis and hypoglycemia may also stimulate the release of AVP.

Of particular clinical relevance is that certain agonists (such as the desamino analog, desmopressin) (see Figure 41-5 for amino acid sequence) possess marked antidiuretic effects with minimal pressor effects (see Chapters 12 and 19 for discussion of actions of AVP).

AVP thus has reasonably well defined effects on water balance and on the cardiovascular system. Each of these actions of AVP and its effect on the production of antihemophilic factor (factor VIII) through as yet poorly understood mechanisms, has been used therapeutically.

 ## PHARMACOKINETICS

Pharmacokinetic parameters for these hypothalamic and pituitary hormones and analogs are summarized in Table 41-1.

Hypothalamic Hormones

GnRH Clinically, GnRH is administered by IV or SC routes. In hypogonadotropic patients, continuous SC infusions of GnRH result in steady-state concentrations that are one third less than those achieved with the IV route. Therefore SC administration of GnRH results in delayed and prolonged absorption of GnRH with consequently lower serum concentrations. In patients receiving pulsatile GnRH therapy,

these absorption characteristics cause the plasma GnRH concentration peaks to be significantly damped. The lack of a pulsatile GnRH concentration waveform may diminish pituitary responsiveness and explain the lower ovulation induction success rate with SC as compared to IV administration.

GnRH is metabolized, although the pathway has not been established. GnRH is not significantly bound to plasma proteins. The primary route of excretion is renal and renal insufficiency significantly lengthens the overall clearance rate. Moderate abnormalities of hepatic function do not affect GnRH clearance. Estimates of GnRH half-life are from 2 to 8 minutes, with metabolic clearance rates from 500 to 1600 ml/min. This wide range of estimates is probably caused by differences in the method of administration (single bolus versus continuous infusion) and the radioimmunoassay used to estimate concentrations.

GHRH In normal humans, GHRH (GHRH-40, GHRH-44), administered IV, SC, or intranasally, stimulates GH release in a dose-dependent fashion. The 29 amino acid GHRH analogs, $[N1e^{27}]GHRH(1-29)-NH_2$ and $GHRH(1-29)NH_2$, have similar potency and duration of action, as does GHRH 1-40.

After IV administration, the plasma half-life for disappearance of GHRH immunoreactivity is 63 minutes,

Table 41-1 Pharmacokinetic Parameter Values

Drugs	Administration	Absorption	$t_{1/2}$	Disposition
HYPOTHALAMIC HORMONES AND ANALOGS				
GnRH	IV, SC	—	2-8 min	R, M
GHRH	IV, SC Intranasal	—	63 min	M
bromocriptine	Oral	Fair (28%)	6 hr*	M (100%) B (main)
octreotide (somatostatin analog)	SC	—	80-90 min	—
PITUITARY HORMONES AND ANALOGS				
LH/FSH	IM	Good	30-60 min	M
GH	IM, SC	—	15-50 min	—
vasopressin	IM, SC	Good	3-15 min	M
vasopressin tannate	IM	(Erratic) Fair	—	M
desmopressin	IV, SC Intranasal	Good	75 min	M
clomiphene	Oral	Good	Long	B (main)

M, Metabolized; *R*, renal excretion as unchanged by drug; *B*, excreted in bile.
*90% bound to serum albumin.

with the maximal effect occurring 30 to 45 minutes after injection. Peptide degradation in the plasma occurs by removal of the first two amino terminal residues with a half-life of 6.8 minutes. There is no evidence that GHRH is bound to plasma proteins or stored in peripheral tissues.

Dopamine Agonists After oral administration, approximately 28% of bromocriptine is absorbed. Ninety percent of bromocriptine circulates bound to serum albumin. The half-life of bromocriptine is about 6 hours for the parent drug and 50 hours for metabolites. Because serum prolactin concentrations fail to be suppressed after 12 to 14 hours after bromocriptine administration, the metabolites may be pharmacologically inactive. Although the details of bromocriptine degradation are not known, it appears that the peptide aminocyclol portion of the molecule is metabolized with subsequent scission of the amide to yield bromolysergic acid derivatives together with peptide fragments. Ninety-eight percent of the drug is excreted in the feces with only trace amounts found in urine.

Somatostatin and Analogs IV administration of native somatostatin (somatostatin 14) results in a prompt decline in serum GH concentrations. The peptide is not absorbed orally and must be administered parenterally. The half-life is approximately 3 to 4 minutes, rendering it unsuitable for therapeutic use.

The 8 amino acid somatostatin analog, octreotide, has a circulating half-life of 80 to 90 minutes, but the biological effect persists for 6 to 8 hours. This analog must also be administered parenterally and is given by SC injection or continuous SC infusion.

Pituitary Hormones

LH and FSH LH and FSH are effective only if given IM. The absorption characteristics and subsequent metabolism of the gonadotropins have not been elucidated, but liver appears to be the major source of glycoprotein clearance after enzymatic removal of sialic acid. The estimated half-lives are between 30 and 60 minutes. FSH has a higher sialic acid content and consequently a longer half-life because of decreased hepatic uptake. The clearance of LH is about 30 ml/min in women and 50 ml/min in men; that of FSH is approximately 15 ml/min in women and has not been determined in men.

Growth Hormone IM and SC administration of GH to children who have a GH deficiency results in

serum concentrations that reach maximal strength 2 to 3 hours after injection and that decline progressively over approximately 15 hours. The serum half-life of GH administered both endogenously and exogenously ranges from 15 to 51 minutes. In recent studies involving stimulation of endogenous GH release with GHRH and suppression of further release with somatostatin, the half-life of endogenous GH in normal men is 19 minutes; exogenously administered synthetic GH is 15 minutes in normal men. GH is not stored in tissues and small amounts are detectable in urine.

Vasopressin Vasopressin, vasopressin tannate, and desmopressin circulate unbound to plasma proteins. All undergo metabolism in liver and kidney and may be initially inactivated by cleavage of the C-terminal glycinamide. A small amount of vasopressin (approximately 5%) is excreted as intact drug in urine.

Action durations of the three preparations are different. When administered SC or IM, vasopressin is effective for only 2 to 8 hours. After IM administration, vasopressin tannate is often absorbed erratically with a duration of action between 48 and 96 hours. Desmopressin may be given IV, SC, or intranasally. The half-life of desmopressin is consistent with the observed duration of action, in that the distribution and elimination components are 7.8 and 75.5 minutes, respectively, compared to 2.5 and 14.5 minutes for vasopressin.

 ## RELATION OF MECHANISMS OF ACTION TO CLINICAL RESPONSE

Hypothalamic Hormones

Gonadotropin-Releasing Hormone The approved and potential indications for therapy with GnRH and analogs can be divided into two categories: (1) replacement therapy in disorders characterized by isolated, abnormal function of the hypothalamic pulse generator, and (2) continuous administration (e.g., via a long-acting analog) to promote pituitary desensitization and thus effect a functional orchiectomy/ovariectomy. Although GnRH and its analogs are approved only for diagnostic use and for the treatment of advanced prostatic cancer, they will likely be used in the future as appropriate therapy for an increasing number of disorders.

Replacement therapy with GnRH or analogs is

anticipated for central amenorrhea and idiopathic hypogonadotropic hypogonadism. Central (hypothalamic) amenorrhea is characterized by abnormal function of the GnRH pulse generator. This deficiency results in inadequate gonadotropin secretion, consequent failure of ovarian follicular development, and amenorrhea. The pituitary, however, is intrinsically normal and releases LH and FSH in response to GnRH. Pulse administration of GnRH via a portable infusion pump may compensate for the underlying defect and IV administration of the hormone could result in LH, FSH, estradiol, and progesterone profiles indistinguishable from those observed in normal, spontaneous cycles. Several hundred women have been treated using IV or SC hormone delivery with results suggesting successful ovulation induction in over 90% of women treated with IV GnRH. Subcutaneous administration requires larger doses and results in a pattern of LH release that does not as closely approximate the normal cycle. The success rate is lower with SC therapy, but still more than 50% of patients achieve ovulation.

Traditional treatment of central amenorrhea includes clomiphene or human menopausal gonadotropin. These methods are clearly successful in inducing ovulation but are associated with two major complications: (1) a mild form of ovarian hyperstimulation (ovarian enlargement and abdominal pain) in approximately 15% of clomiphene cycles and 25% of human menopausal gonadotropin cycles, and (2) increased incidence of multiple pregnancies with both. Because pulsatile GnRH therapy maintains the integrity of the pituitary-ovarian axis (i.e., allows for the appropriate negative and positive feedback of gonadal hormones) and more accurately reproduces the physiology of the normal menstrual cycle, the incidence of complications may be less.

Faulty GnRH secretion in men is referred to as *idiopathic hypogonadotropic hypogonadism*. The pituitary still responds to GnRH by secreting LH and FSH. Long-term pulsatile administration of GnRH was tested in a small number of men for at least 3 months. Significant increases in serum testosterone concentrations and testicular size were noted associated with clinical manifestations of the increasing androgen concentrations. Mature spermatogenesis may be achieved in 50% of patients and, in men with unfused epiphyses, linear growth may occur. Standard treatment of this disorder included testosterone injections for masculinization and other hormones for fertility.

As more experience is gained with pulsatile GnRH for normalization of the pituitary-testicular axis and the induction of fertility, this approach may emerge as an acceptable alternative for the treatment of idiopathic hypogonadotropic hypogonadism.

The observation that orchiectomy causes regression of prostatic cancer (the second most frequent type of cancer for males in this country) leads to therapeutic approaches to decrease serum androgen concentrations in men with metastatic disease. Estrogens, acting through suppression of gonadotrope secretion and direct inhibition of androgen effects on the prostate, are also effective. Although the optimum hormonal regimen is controversial, current approaches to advanced cancer employ castration and/or estrogens. This is associated with significant side effects, including the psychological impact of orchiectomy, with thromboembolism, cardiovascular disease, and gynecomastia related to estrogen therapy. In addition, the effect on long-term survival is disappointing, with a death rate of nearly 50% at 2 years for disease with bone metastases. Partial explanations for the high failure rate may be (1) persistent production of adrenal androgen precursors that can be converted to active androgens by the prostate and (2) effective androgenic activity of very low (i.e., castrate) concentrations of testosterone.

Long-acting GnRH agonists can be used to downregulate pituitary gonadotrope receptors and suppress pulsatile LH release (Figure 41-6). GnRH therapy initially causes a temporary rise in serum testosterone concentrations, which could cause an acute exacerbation of disease symptoms, but coadministration of the antiandrogen, flutamide, can prevent this. This regimen produces side effects of hypoandrogenism (hot flashes, decreased libido) without symptoms of hyperestrogenism, and therefore appears to be better tolerated than orchiectomy/estrogen therapy. When used as the initial treatment of advanced prostate cancer, the combination of a long-acting GnRH analog and flutamide produced response rates of 95% at the initiation of treatment. After 2 years of treatment, the response rate was 70% and the death rate was 11% (as compared to 10% and 50%, respectively, with conventional modalities).

Idiopathic precocious puberty, which results in maturation of the external genitalia, accelerated linear growth, and advanced bone age, has been treated experimentally with GnRH analogs with very encouraging results.

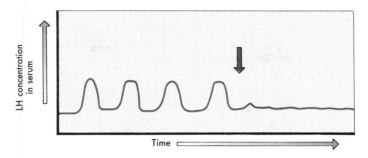

FIGURE 41-6   Schematic representation of LH serum concentration profile in a normal subject showing initial LH pulses resulting from GnRH pulse generator. Administration of a long-acting GnRH agonist at arrow down-regulates receptors and leads to decreased LH secretion.

GnRH analog therapy also is used with encouraging results in a small number of women to obtain a *medical oophorectomy* for the treatment of endometriosis.

GnRH analog therapy is being investigated as a means of female and male contraception. Preliminary studies in women are successful, but further trials are required to test for long-term side effects (e.g., osteoporosis secondary to low serum estrogen concentrations). Studies in males show failure to achieve azoospermia; therefore this approach holds little promise for further development.

Growth Hormone-Releasing Hormone GHRH is not approved for general use as a diagnostic or therapeutic agent in the United States. However, because the results of the experimental clinical trials are so compelling, certain potential applications are discussed.

Initial results of GHRH therapy in 55 children treated for up to 2 years for GH deficiency are promising. The majority of children with GH deficiency treated with the 40 or 44 amino acid peptide have an increase in growth velocity.

Dopamine Agonists The dopamine agonist bromocriptine is approved in the United States for the treatment of hyperprolactinemia (both physiological and pathophysiological), acromegaly, and Parkinson's disease.

In physiological hyperprolactinemia, circulating concentrations of prolactin, elevated during pregnancy, remain increased after delivery in preparation for lactation because prolactin plays a major role in milk secretion. If the mother does not breast feed, serum prolactin concentrations decrease and are often within the normal range by 2 weeks after parturition. However, early in the postpartum period, breast engorgement and/or mastodynia (breast pain) may occur, thus prompting efforts to suppress lactation. Treatment with bromocriptine is a highly effective approach in that it suppresses secretion of prolactin—the primary stimulus to the breast. Used in this manner, bromocriptine is as effective as estrogen in preventing engorgement. Similarly, bromocriptine is more effective than estrogen/androgen combinations in inhibiting breast engorgement and lactation. In contrast to estrogen, bromocriptine does not increase the risk of thromboembolic disease, offering a significant advantage over estrogenic preparations.

A prolactin-secreting adenoma is the common cause of pathophysiological hyperprolactinemia. The goals of treatment of these prolactinomas, as for all pituitary tumors, include reduction of tumor mass with concurrent restoration of visual fields and cranial nerve function, preservation of other anterior pituitary function, suppression of the secretion of tumor product, and prevention of recurrence/progression of the disease.

Bromocriptine lowers serum prolactin concentrations in patients with microadenomas and also lowers circulating prolactin concentrations and reduces tumor mass. Bromocriptine inhibits prolactin secretion by adenomatous cells by stimulating dopamine receptors present on these cells. Because dopamine receptor–second messenger systems seem intact in prolactinomas, a relative dopamine deficiency likely exists in patients with such tumors.

If hyperprolactinemia represents a dopamine deficiency, one would predict that withdrawal of the dopamine agonist bromocriptine would allow a return of elevated prolactin concentrations, and such is the case. Even more dramatic is the effect of bromocriptine withdrawal on tumor size. Bromocriptine shrinks prolactin-secreting macroadenomas in the majority of cases, apparently by effecting a return of the secretory machinery from a hypersecretory to a quiescent state. However, withdrawal of the agent results in a prompt reexpansion of tumor with a concurrent increase in serum prolactin concentrations. Thus the use of bromocriptine for the treatment of prolactinomas may be considered as replacement therapy, because bromocriptine corrects the relative dopamine deficiency if it is administered repeatedly.

The clinical effects attributed to therapy of prolactinomas with bromocriptine are impressive. With decreasing prolactin concentrations, galactorrhea is abolished or markedly reduced in virtually all patients. Gonadal function, frequently compromised in hyperprolactinemic subjects, is restored in the majority, although in women, normal ovulatory menstrual cycles may not return for a year. Previously infertile women achieve pregnancy rates indistinguishable from those of normal women. Signs and symptoms of intracranial tumor expansion (headache, visual field defects) show extraordinary improvement within a few days, and remain stable so long as the drug is continued. No adverse effects of chronic treatment with bromocriptine are demonstrated. Bromocriptine therapy of prolactin-secreting microadenomas and macroadenomas is a reality. Although bromocriptine does not offer a cure, it is a viable alternative to surgery.

Bromocriptine reduces (albeit rarely to normal) circulating concentrations of GH in at least 70% of patients with acromegaly, presumably via a direct effect on the adenomatous somatotropes.

For the effect of bromocriptine in Parkinson's disease see Chapter 27.

Somatostatin and Analogs Somatostatin's role in pathogenesis of disease is relatively small. The rare somatostatin-secreting tumor (usually pancreatic) is associated with mild diabetes mellitus, suppressed GH release, cholelithiasis, and GI malabsorption.

Several therapeutic uses for somatostatin are proposed, but this peptide is not available for general use in the United States. Additionally, the short half-life (3 to 4 minutes) and requirement for continuous parenteral administration limit its therapeutic usefulness. Proposed uses of this agent (or its analogs) include treatment of poorly controlled type 1 diabetes mellitus, acromegaly, GI hemorrhage, hemorrhagic pancreatitis, prophylaxis for pancreatitis in patients undergoing pancreatic surgery, and suppression of hormone secretion from a variety of hyperfunctioning endocrine tumors such as GH-secreting adenomas, insulinomas, carcinoids, glucagonomas, gastrinomas, and VIPomas.

Because the major therapeutic limitation is its short half-life, numerous analogs have been synthesized with longer durations of activity and more specific suppressive effects. The analog in current clinical use is the 8 amino acid cyclic peptide, octreotide, approved for treatment of patients with carcinoid tumors and VIP-secreting tumors. Clinical trials for treatment of acromegaly and other hypersecretory endocrine tumors and various GI disorders are in progress.

PITUITARY HORMONES

Luteinizing Hormone and Follicle-Stimulating Hormone Human menopausal gonadotropin is a purified preparation of LH and FSH extracted from urine of postmenopausal women used to treat infertility in women and men. Human menopausal gonadotropin induces follicular growth and, because of its similarity to LH and its ability to stimulate the LH receptor, is administered to induce ovulation. It successfully induces ovulation in approximately 90% of women, with subsequent pregnancy resulting in 20% to 30% who achieve ovulation. Human menopausal gonadotropin therapy directly stimulates the ovaries and bypasses the normal feedback controls of the hypothalamic-pituitary-ovarian axis. Consequently, more than one follicle may develop and ovulate with multiple pregnancies, mostly twins, occurring in about 20% of women who become pregnant in this way. A mild hyperstimulation syndrome characterized by ovarian enlargement and abdominal pain and/or distention occurs in 20% of patients. A more severe form with ascites is infrequent.

Clomiphene (Figure 41-7), with or without human chorionic gonadotropin, is commonly administered before human menopausal gonadotropin. Compared to human menopausal gonadotropin, clomiphene administration has a decreased incidence of multiple births and ovarian hyperstimulation syndrome. Human menopausal gonadotropin is reserved for women

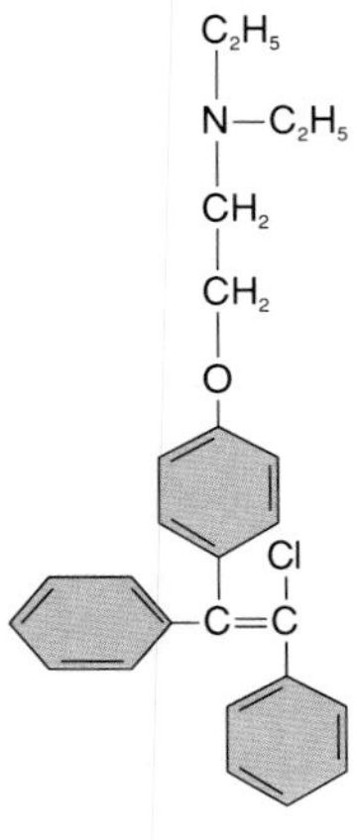

clomiphene

FIGURE 41-7   Clomiphene, a nonsteroidal stimulator of pituitary release of human gonadotropin.

in whom clomiphene therapy has failed.

Human menopausal gonadotropin therapy is indicated for inducing fertility in men with hypogonadotropic hypogonadism. Adequate sperm counts are obtained in about 75% of cases, and pregnancy results in approximately 75% of patients' wives. Occasionally, men can achieve complete spermatogenesis with human chorionic gonadotropin therapy alone.

Growth Hormone GH promotes linear growth by generation of IGF-I and influences all aspects of metabolism. This hormone is described as *anabolic, lipolytic,* and *diabetogenic.* Replacement of GH in children with GH deficiency stimulates amino acid incorporation into muscle protein, as indicated by decreased serum amino acid concentrations and decreased urinary nitrogen excretion. Treatment of GH deficiency with GH does not promote glucose intolerance or diabetes mellitus; the excessive GH in acromegaly, is associated with glucose intolerance and diabetes mellitus. The evidence that GH is lipolytic resides primarily in in vitro studies of isolated adipose tissue. Its role in the regulation of lipid metabolism in humans is unclear.

Excessive GH secretion results in gigantism or acromegaly. Gigantism occurs if GH hypersecretion is present before epiphyseal closure during puberty, and acromegaly occurs after puberty. Excessive GH secretion may cause thickening of the skin and soft tissues and result in skeletal changes such as mandibular, frontal, zygomatic bone, and acral enlarge-

ment with osseous overgrowth. These skeletal changes result in degenerative arthritis of the hips, knees, shoulders, and elbows.

Growth hormone is used therapeutically to treat children with GH deficiency. With the development of human GH using recombinant DNA technology, the supply problem for GH is resolved. Growth hormone treatment of children with GH deficiency is associated with a significant increase in linear growth rate.

Vasopressin Three forms of vasopressin are approved for clinical use: native arginine vasopressin, vasopressin tannate, and *1*-desamino-8-D-arginine vasopressin (desmopressin). Each may be employed for the treatment of diabetes insipidus.

Neurogenic diabetes insipidus is a disorder characterized by polyuria and polydipsia that results from inadequate secretion of AVP (see Chapter 39). Over 80% of the hypothalamic neuronal system responsible for synthesizing and secreting AVP must be dysfunctional before symptoms develop.

Vasopressin increases circulating concentrations of factor VIII (antihemophilic factor) (see Chapter 21), perhaps by stimulating its release from cells in the vascular endothelium. Vasopressin is used to treat mild hemophilia A and mild to moderate von Willebrand's disease. However, desmopressin, because of its relative lack of untoward side effects compared to AVP, is more often used. In patients with factor VIII concentrations greater than 5%, hemostasis may be maintained during and after surgical procedures if patients are treated 30 minutes before the procedure. In addition, desmopressin may be used in certain situations in which bleeding is a complication of trauma.

SIDE EFFECTS, CLINICAL PROBLEMS, AND TOXICITY

Clinical problems are summarized in the box, p. 572.

Hypothalamic Hormones

GnRH GnRH is generally well tolerated with the frequency of adverse reactions quite low, but occasionally nausea, lightheadedness, headache, and abdominal discomfort result from relatively large doses. Subcutaneous administration is associated with an-

GHRH Side effects of GHRH include facial flushing with higher doses given IV. Repetitive, prolonged administration may result in development of circulating antibodies but their clinical significance is not known, because the children treated demonstrate continued acceleration of linear growth. Antibodies either disappear or decrease in titer when GHRH is discontinued. No interactions with other drugs have been described.

Dopamine Agonists Adverse effects of bromocriptine may be grouped into three categories: (1) effects occurring during initiation of therapy and occasionally during chronic treatment of hyperprolactinemia and acromegaly, (2) effects occurring during treatment of Parkinson's disease, and (3) problems of teratogenicity and treatment of tumor expansion during pregnancy.

When bromocriptine is first administered, patients experience nausea with or without vomiting, dizziness, and/or postural hypotension. These effects can be minimized by beginning therapy with low doses given with food and at bedtime and gradually increasing the frequency to a full dose regimen. Most patients quickly develop a tolerance. A few patients complain of headache, fatigue, abdominal cramping, nasal congestion, drowsiness, or diarrhea, either at the onset of treatment or with chronic administration. An occasional patient will be intolerant of bromocriptine.

The treatment of Parkinson's disease with bromocriptine may result in special problems. In addition to the nausea and orthostatic hypotension commonly encountered, confusion and visual or auditory hallucinations or erythromelalgia (limb pain) may occur. Morever, in some patients their dyskinetic symptoms may worsen. These effects may represent interactions of bromocriptine with a disordered CNS. Fortunately, a substantial number of patients who manifest symptoms become tolerant of the drug, allowing treatment to continue.

The fact that infertility associated with hyperprolactinemia may be successfully treated with bromocriptine raises concerns that the drug may be teratogenic and what role to assign to bromocriptine in treating tumor expansions if it occurs during pregnancy. With regard to the former, well over 1400 bromocriptine-associated pregnancies have been described with no increased risk to the fetus. Specifically, no differences are detected in the rates of spontaneous abortion, the incidences of multiple births, or the presence of minor or severe congenital

tibody formation in a small number of patients.

Side effects from SC and IV administration of GnRH via portable infusion pumps include inflammation, infection, phlebitis, and hematoma at the catheter site. Frequency of these reactions can be significantly decreased by thorough patient education regarding aseptic technique and management of the infusion pump.

abnormalities when compared to control women not treated with bromocriptine. Although there is no evidence for teratogenicity, it is recommended that fetal exposure to bromocriptine be minimized. Fortunately, the majority of women with tumor-associated hyperprolactinemia have microadenomas and appear to have a very low rate of complications (approximately 1%) during pregnancy. The percentage of women with macroadenomas who develop headaches and visual field defects during pregnancy is significantly higher, perhaps approaching 25%. Based so far on extremely small numbers, no untoward effects on fetal development are noted when bromocriptine is administered during pregnancy.

Because bromocriptine is a dopamine receptor agonist, the concurrent administration of dopamine receptor blocking agents may negate or diminish its clinical effects. The phenothiazines (e.g., chlorpromazine) and butyrophenones (e.g., haloperidol) may modify the dopamine agonist activity of bromocriptine if used simultaneously.

Somatostatin and Analogs The adverse effects of native somatostatin are limited to suppression of insulin release. Prolonged administration results in mild hyperglycemia. Administration of the analog, octreotide, is similarly associated with mild hyperglycemia, particularly postprandially. This can be minimized by administering the drug 2 to 3 hours after meals. There are isolated reports of gallstone development during octreotide therapy, likely a result of diminished gallbladder motility. Patients usually develop acholic loose stools during the first 1 to 2 weeks of therapy but clinically significant malabsorption is not reported. No adverse effects on the cardiovascular system have been noted.

Pituitary Hormones

LH and FSH Human menopausal gonadotropin is generally well tolerated; common adverse reactions are multiple pregnancies and ovarian hyperstimulation. Gynecomastia occasionally occurs in men, and thromboembolism is a serious, but very rare, complication.

Growth Hormone Administration of human GH may promote development of anti-GH antibodies; however, only a small minority of children who received GH have impairment of growth. Pituitary derived GH is no longer available for use in the United States because several young adults developed Creutzfeldt-Jakob disease after being treated with pi-

---

> ### TRADENAMES
>
> In addition to generic and fixed combination preparations, the following tradenamed materials are available in the United States.
>
> **HYPOTHALAMIC HORMONES AND ANALOGS**
>
> Lupron, leuprolide acetate, GnRH analog
> Parlodel, bromocriptine mesylate
> Sandostatin, octreotide, somatostatin analog
>
> **PITUITARY HORMONES AND ANALOGS**
>
> A.P.L., Profasi, Pregnyl; human chorionic gonadotropin
> DDAVP, desmopressin acetate
> Pergonal, luteinizing hormone/follicle stimulating hormone
> Pitressin, arginine vasopressin
> Pitressin Tannate in Oil, arginine vasopressin tannate
> Protropin, human growth hormone
> Serophene, clomiphene citrate

---

tuitary derived GH. The currently approved human GH preparation is that produced by recombinant DNA methodology. Preliminary studies with this human GH indicate that formation of anti-GH antibodies occurs less frequently, by 10% to 20%.

A potential problem with GH resides with its misuse, particularly in the field of competitive athletics. GH use by athletes is related to its suggested anabolic properties on muscle development. Excessive, unsupervised GH administration may result in medical problems associated with acromegaly, including hyperhidrosis, arthropathy, extremity enlargement, and visceromegaly.

Vasopressin Nonspecific adverse reactions that may occur with AVP.desmopressin include nausea, vertigo, headache, and anaphylaxis. Other signs and symptoms may relate directly to specific pressor and antidiuretic effects. With regard to the former, vasoconstriction may occur and cause relatively mild problems such as skin blanching or abdominal cramping, or more serious effects such as angina or myocardial infarction. Although all preparations should be used with caution in patients with known coronary artery disease, desmopressin has lower pressor effects and may be the drug of choice. All vasopressins may cause water intoxication. Signs and symptoms of this disorder include drowsiness, listlessness, weakness, headaches, seizures, and coma. Care must be taken to closely watch for such signs and symptoms and titrate the dose appropriately.

A number of drugs, if administered simultaneously, potentiate or inhibit the effects of vasopressin. Potentiators include carbamazepine, chlorpropamide, clofibrate, urea, fludrocortisone, and tricyclic antidepressants. Conversely, inhibitors include demeclocycline, norepinephrine, lithium, heparin, and alcohol.

REFERENCES

Baylis PH: Vasopressin and its neurophysin. In DeGroot L, ed: Endocrinology, vol 1, Philadelphia, 1989, WB Saunders Co.

Conn PM: The molecular basis of gonadotropin-releasing hormone action, Endo Rev 7:3, 1986.

Evans WS, Borges JLC, Vance ML et al.: Effects of human pancreatic growth hormone-releasing factor-40 on serum growth hormone, prolactin, luteinizing hormone, follicle-stimulating hormone, and somatomedin-C concentrations in normal women throughout the menstrual cycle, J Clin Endocrinol Metab 59:1006, 1984.

Labrie F, Dupont A, Belanger A et al.: Treatment of prostate cancer with gonadotropin-releasing hormone agonists, Endo Rev 7(1):67, 1986.

MacLeod RM: Regulation of prolactin secretion. In Martini L and Gangong WF, ed: Frontiers in neuroendocrinology, vol 4, New York, 1976, Raven Press.

Moller DE, Moses AC, Jones K et al.: Octreotide suppresses growth hormone and growth hormone releasing hormone in acromegaly secondary to ectopic GHRH secretion, J Clin Endocrinol Metab 68:499, 1989.

Reichlin S: Somatostatin, N Engl J Med 309:1495, 1983.

Robinson AG: DDAVP in the treatment of central diabetes insipidus, N Engl J Med 294:507, 1976.

Vance ML, Evans WS, Kaiser DL et al. Effects of intravenous, subcutaneous, and intranasal GH-RH analog [N1e^{27}]GHRH(1-29)-NH$_2$, on growth hormone secretion in normal men: dose-response relationships, Clin Pharmacol Ther 40:627, 1986.

Vance ML, Evans WS, and Thorner MO: Bromocriptine, Ann Intern Med 100:78, 1984.

Veldhuis JD, Fraioli F, Rogol AD et al.: Metabolic clearance of biologically active luteinizing hormone in man, J Clin Invest 77:1122, 1986.

CHAPTER 42

Drugs Affecting Calcium-regulating Hormones

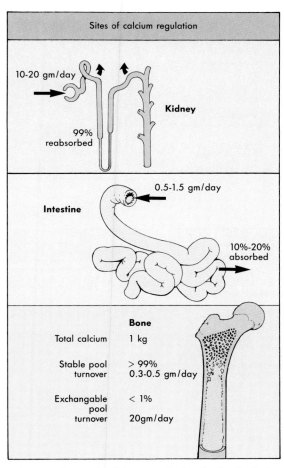

FIGURE 42-1 Sites of calcium regulation in the body (see text).

Sites of calcium regulation

10-20 gm/day

Kidney

99% reabsorbed

Intestine

0.5-1.5 gm/day

10%-20% absorbed

Bone	
Total calcium	1 kg
Stable pool turnover	> 99% 0.3-0.5 gm/day
Exchangable pool turnover	< 1% 20gm/day

THERAPEUTIC OVERVIEW

The calcium concentration in the blood is normally maintained within narrow limits, approximately 8.8 to 10.4 mg/dl. When the calcium concentrations exceed this normal range, the functions of many tissues are affected. Hypocalcemia can lead to increased neuromuscular excitability and tetany. Hypercalcemia can result in life-threatening cardiac dysrhythmias, renal damage, soft tissue calcification, and CNS abnormalities. Various disorders can cause perturbations in calcium homeostasis. These, as well as disorders that may not necessarily affect serum calcium, can lead to changes in the skeleton that interfere with its normal function of support and protection. This chapter focuses on organs that regulate calcium concentrations in plasma and extracellular fluid (i.e., bone, kidney, and intestines).

The treatment of disorders of bone and calcium metabolism involves the use not only of calcium-regulating hormones and other agents with specific effects on mineral metabolism, but also of drugs from other pharmacological categories, including gonadal and adrenal hormones, antiinflammatory drugs, diuretics, and cancer chemotherapeutic agents. The sites at which the different agents act to produce their effects on calcium metabolism include the gastrointestinal tract, the kidney, and bone (Figure 42-1). Approximately 10% to 20% of the dietary calcium is normally absorbed. Absorption is impaired in the absence of vitamin D and augmented by excess vitamin D. Renal tubular reabsorption normally recovers 99%

575

of the 10 to 20 g of calcium filtered per day. Bone is the major storehouse for calcium, containing approximately 1 kg per 70 kg human. Of this, more than 99% is in a stable pool, with a daily turnover of 0.3 to 0.5 g. Changes depend on cellular activity. An exchangeable pool of 4 to 5 g turns over at the rate of approximately 20 g/day. Turnover of the exchangeable pool is a passive physicochemical process.

Diseases associated with hypocalcemia and rickets (inadequate bone mineralization during develop-

ment) or osteomalacia (inadequate bone mineralization in the adult) are listed in Table 42-1. These disorders treated with vitamin D result from inadequate vitamin D or resistance to its action. Disorders that lead to hypercalcemia are more diverse in nature and etiology. The therapy is determined partly by the etiology of the disease, but also by severity of the hypercalcemia and the need for rapid correction. Various pharmacological approaches, including inorganic ions, diuretics, antiinflammatory agents, diuretics

Table 42-1   Disorders of Bone and Calcium Metabolism

Type of Disorder	Treatment	Examples
Disorders leading to hypocalcemia	Usually treated with vitamin D compounds and calcium	Inadequate dietary calcium and/or vitamin D Malabsorption caused by defective activation of vitamin D Malabsorption caused by end-organ resistance to vitamin D Hypoparathyroidism, pseudohypoparathyroidism Renal failure
Disorders leading to hypercalcemia	Treatments include fluids, low calcium diet, sulfate, loop-acting diuretics, glucocorticoids, calcitonin, plicamycin	Hyperparathyroidism Hypervitaminosis D Sarcoidosis Neoplasia Hyperthyroidism Immobilization
Disorders of bone remodelling	Treated with diphosphonates, calcitonin, and plicamycin	Paget's disease of bone
	Treated with estrogen (female), calcium, calcitonin, and fluoride	Osteoporosis

THERAPEUTIC OVERVIEW

VITAMIN D AND ITS METABOLITES

Rickets
Osteomalacea
Hypocalcemia
Hypoparathyroidism (10 × larger doses)
Vitamin D−resistant rickets

PARATHYROID HORMONE

Diagnostic agent for pseudohypoparathyroidism

CALCITONIN

Paget's disease of bone
Osteoporosis
Hypercalcemia of pregnancy

EDTA, FUROSEMIDE, ETHACRYNIC ACID, AND MANY OTHER AGENTS (SEE TEXT)

Hypercalcemia

CALCIUM, ESTROGEN, FLUORIDE, PARATHYROID HORMONE PLUS VITAMIN D

Osteoporosis

and anticancer agents, are employed to treat hypercalcemia. Table 42-1 also lists disorders of bone turnover not usually associated with abnormal serum calcium and phosphate, which are amenable to therapy. Paget's disease of bone is characterized by both excessive formation and resorption occurring in an irregular manner in one or more bones. In osteoporosis, there is excessive loss of bone, leading to fractures.

The therapeutic overview is summarized in the box.

 MECHANISMS OF ACTION

Vitamin D and Metabolites

Vitamin D is a secosteroid, a steroid derivative in which the B ring has been cleaved and has undergone a rearragement. Figure 42-2 shows the structures of vitamin D_2: ergocalciferol, which is synthesized from ergosterol by yeast, and vitamin D_3, cholecalciferol, synthesized from cholesterol by animals and higher plants. Vitamin D is not biologically active and first must be activated by two metabolic steps (Figure 42-3). The first step, a hydroxylation in the 25 position, occurs in the liver, predominantly in the endoplasmic reticulum. The product, 25-hydroxyvitamin D, is more potent and acts more rapidly than vitamin D. 25-Hydroxyvitamin D is further activated in the kidney to

1,25-dihydroxyvitamin D by a cytochrome P-450 enzyme-dependent hydroxylation. The 1-hydroxylation step is feedback-regulated, which is stimulated by parathyroid hormone and by low plasma phosphate concentrations. 1,25-Dihydroxyvitamin D is the most potent and most rapidly acting vitamin D metabolite.

The active vitamin D metabolites produce their effects by binding to receptors in the nucleus of the cell that initiate the synthesis of specific proteins. Among these protein products are two high-affinity calcium-binding proteins, *calbindins*, which may play a role in the stimulation of calcium transport by vitamin D, and *osteocalcin* or *bone gla protein* (BGP), a lower-affinity calcium-binding protein found extracellularly in normally and abnormally mineralized tissues. The active vitamin D metabolites have two major effects that lead to an increase in serum calcium (Figure 42-4). The first is to increase the absorption of dietary calcium and phosphate by stimulating their uptake across the GI mucosa. The effect of vitamin D on bone mineralization, the *antirachitic effect*, is an indirect result of the increased calcium and phosphate absorption. The elevated $(Ca^{++}) \times (PO_4^{3-})$ product results in the deposition of more mineral in the bone. The second action is to stimulate the release of calcium from bone. This action requires cellular activity, and the current concept (Figure 42-5) is that receptors are present on osteoblastic cells, which subsequently stimulate the activity of osteoclasts, re-

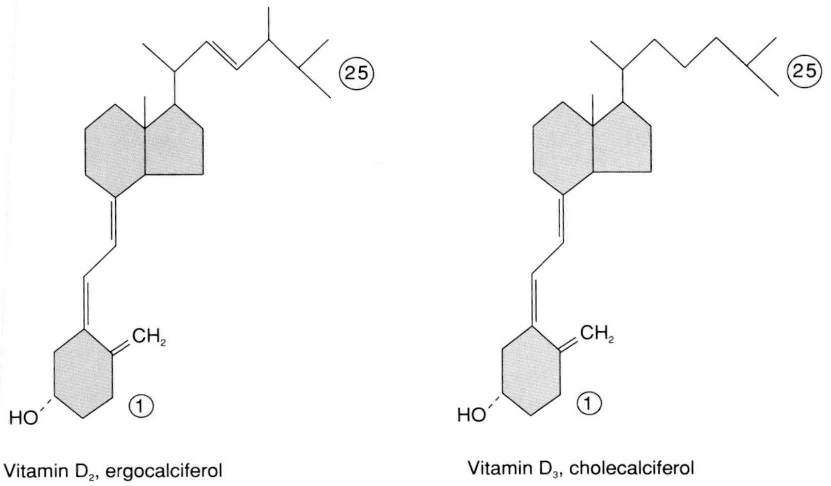

Vitamin D_2, ergocalciferol

Vitamin D_3, cholecalciferol

FIGURE 42-2   Structures of vitamin D_2 and vitamin D_3 with *1* and *25* positions indicated. Note difference in side chains.

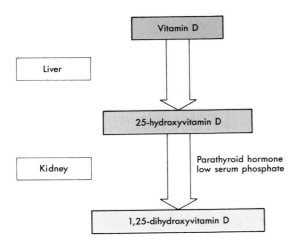

FIGURE 42-3   Vitamin D activation pathway (see text).

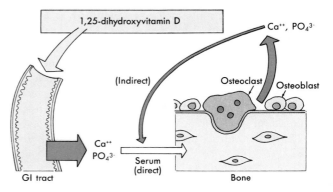

FIGURE 42-4   Major sites and effects of calcium regulation by 1,25- dihydroxyvitamin D: direct and indirect effects. Increased absorption from GI tract into serum (direct) and release from bone into serum (indirect) are shown (see text).

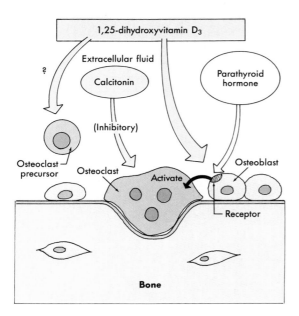

FIGURE 42-5   Cellular sites of action of calcemic hormones on bone. Hormone-osteoblast complex activates osteoclast.

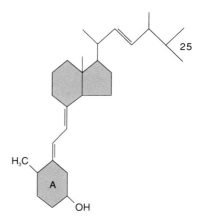

FIGURE 42-6   Structure of dihydrotachysterol. Note position of groups in A ring.

Parathyroid Hormone

Parathyroid hormone is an 84 amino acid polypeptide. It is processed from a 115 amino acid polypeptide precursor, preproparathyroid hormone (Figure 42-7) that is cleaved in the endoplasmic reticulum of the parathyroid gland to a 90 amino acid polypeptide, proparathyroid hormone. The latter is further cleaved in Golgi and secretory vesicles to an 84 amino acid polypeptide. Parathyroid hormone binds to membrane receptors in target cells and acts to stimulate protein phosphorylation. Cyclic AMP and intracellular calcium, both of which are increased by para-

leasing calcium from the bone. Effects of vitamin D metabolites on the differentiation of osteoclast precursors may also play a role. Dihydrotachysterol (Figure 42-6) is a synthetic analog of vitamin D$_2$. It is maximally activated by 25-hydroxylation and acts more rapidly than vitamin D.

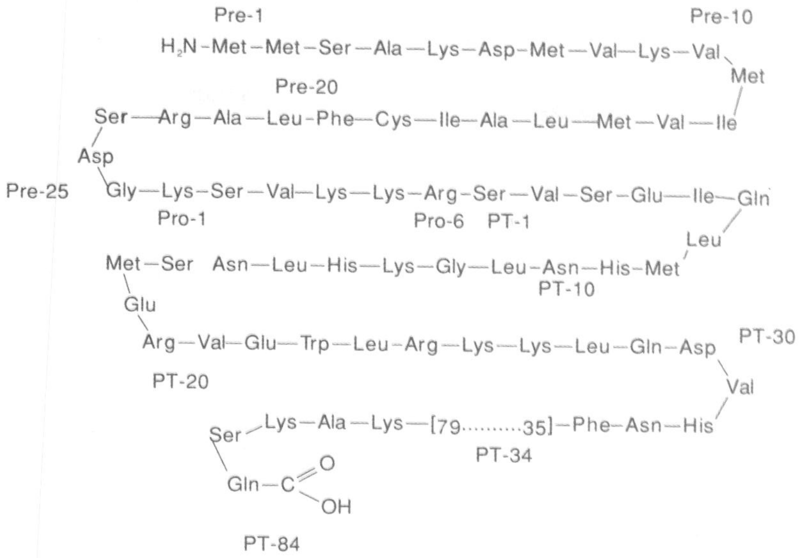

Pre-1
Pre-10
H₂N-Met-Met-Ser-Ala-Lys-Asp-Met-Val-Lys-Val
Met
Pre-20
Ser-Arg-Ala-Leu-Phe-Cys-Ile-Ala-Leu-Met-Val-Ile
Asp
Pre-25
Gly-Lys-Ser-Val-Lys-Lys-Arg-Ser-Val-Ser-Glu-Ile-Gln
Pro-1
Pro-6 PT-1
Leu
Met-Ser Asn-Leu-His-Lys-Gly-Leu-Asn-His-Met
PT-10
Glu
Arg-Val-Glu-Trp-Leu-Arg-Lys-Lys-Leu-Gln-Asp
PT-30
PT-20
Val
Ser-Lys-Ala-Lys-[79..........35]-Phe-Asn-His
PT-34
Gln-C=O
OH
PT-84

FIGURE 42-7 Preproparathyroid hormone showing 25 amino acid pre-fragment at NH_2 end, 6 residue pro-fragment in center, and 84 residue parathyroid hormone (PT) portion at COOH end; PT activity mainly in residues PT-1 through PT-34.

thyroid hormone action target tissues, are involved as second messengers. Parathyroid hormone has two major direct and one indirect site of action for mediating its effects on serum calcium and phosphate (Figure 42-8). Parathyroid hormone acts directly on the kidney to decrease renal tubular reabsorption of phosphate and to increase renal tubular reabsorption of calcium. These effects lead to an increase in serum calcium and a decrease in serum phosphate concentrations. Acting on bone, parathyroid hormone stimulates resorption and thereby increases serum calcium concentration through an effect on osteoblasts (Figure 42-5). Parathyroid hormone indirectly enhances calcium absorption by stimulating the formation of 1,25-dihydroxyvitamin D (Figures 42-3 and 42-8). Low concentrations of parathyroid hormone also have an anabolic effect on bone and increase bone formation. Analogs of parathyroid hormone that act as antagonists at the receptor have been synthesized but are not yet in current therapeutic use.

Parathyroid hormone
Ca++
Osteoclast
Ca++
Osteoblast
25-hydroxyvitamin D
Bone
1,25-dihydroxyvitamin D
Kidney
PO4 3-
Ca++
Intestine

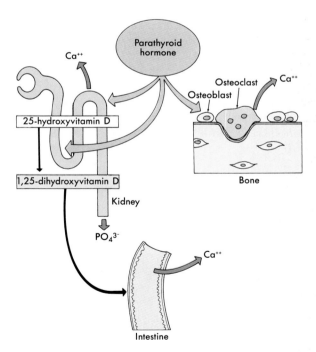

FIGURE 42-8 Direct and indirect effects of parathyroid hormone on calcium metabolism. Renal tubular reabsorption of PO_4 decreases and that of calcium increases; hormone stimulated osteoblast activates osteoclast to release calcium into extracellular fluid (see text).

Calcitonin

Calcitonin is a 32 amino acid polypeptide (Figure 42-9) secreted by the parafollicular cells of the thyroid.

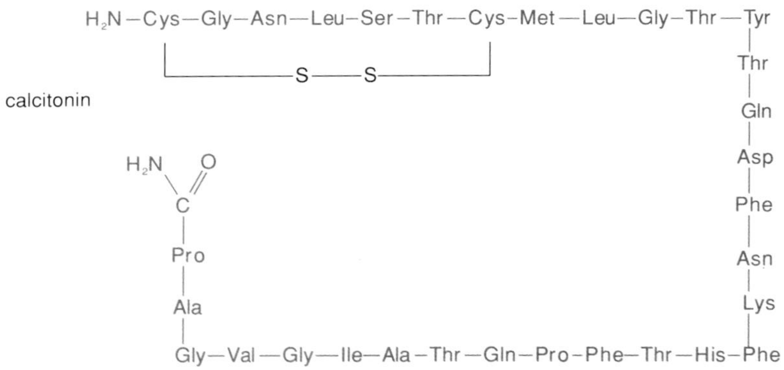

FIGURE 42-9   Calcitonin structure (see text).

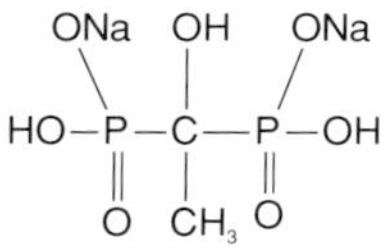

FIGURE 42-10   Etidronate disodium, showing P-C-P basic diphosphonate structure.

It decreases postprandial absorption of calcium; increases the excretion of calcium, sodium, magnesium, chloride, and phosphate; and inhibits the activity of osteoclasts (Figure 42-5). This latter action on bone is probably its most effective means of lowering serum calcium concentration. The effects of calcitonin on bone exhibit a phenomenon termed *escape*, a loss of effectiveness with continued use. This is unrelated to the formation of antibodies to the hormone and is related to a cellular event within bone itself.

Other Agents Affecting Bone and Calcium Metabolism

Phosphate salts can increase calcium deposition in bone by a physicochemical action and can rapidly lower serum calcium concentration. Sodium sulfate and EDTA form poorly dissociable calcium salts and will increase calcium excretion. Certain diuretics (specifically the loop-action diuretics, ethacrynic acid and furosemide) increase both calcium and sodium excretion. This action is not shared by the benzothiadiazides, which decrease calcium excretion. Bone resorption is inhibited by estrogens, diphosphonates, plicamycin, and glucocorticoids. The mechanism of the effect of estrogens is unknown. There is only limited evidence for the presence of estrogen receptors

initiating direct effects of estrogens in bone. Diphosphonates, such as etidronate disodium (Figure 42-10), inhibit the formation, growth, and dissolution of hydroxyapatite crystals. Their effects on crystal dissolution are likely to play a role in inhibiting resorption. Diphosphonates can also inhibit mineralization. Plicamycin, formerly called mithramycin, which inhibits bone resorption, is an antitumor agent that inhibits RNA synthesis. It has a selective effect on bone, inhibiting bone resorption at one tenth of the antineoplastic dose. Glucocorticoids can decrease the hypercalcemia elicited by vitamin D metabolites and by other factors. This effect of glucocorticoids results from decreased calcium absorption and decreased bone resorption. Glucocorticoids also decrease the synthesis of collagen and the formation of bone by decreasing protein synthesis in osteoblasts. The decreased calcium absorption and the antianabolic activity probably play a role in the effect of glucocorticoids to elicit osteoporosis. Nonsteroidal antiinflammatory agents are somewhat effective in inhibiting resorption but only that caused by increased prostaglandin synthesis. Fluoride can stimulate osteoclast activity and increase formation of bone. It is also incorporated into bone matrix, forming fluoroapatite in lieu of hydroxyapatite, making it resistant to resorption. Table 42-2 summarizes many of the effects described above.

Table 42-2 Mechanisms of Therapeutic Actions of Agents Altering Bone and Calcium Metabolism

Mechanism	Agents
Increase intestinal calcium absorption	Vitamin D metabolites
	Parathyroid hormone (indirect)
Increase renal calcium excretion	Sodium sulfate, EDTA
	Loop-acting diuretics
	Calcitonin
Increase bone resorption	Parathyroid hormone
	Vitamin D metabolites
Increase bone formation	Fluoride
	Parathyroid hormone (low concentrations)
Decrease intestinal calcium absorption	Glucocorticoids
	Calcitonin (postprandial)
Decrease renal calcium excretion	Parathyroid hormone
	Benzothiadiazide diuretics
Decrease bone resorption	Sodium phosphate
	Diphosphonates
	Glucocorticoids
	Plicamycin
	Calcitonin
	Estrogen
	Fluoride

Table 42-3 Pharmacokinetic Parameters

Agent	Route	t½	Disappearance
vitamin D	Oral*	14 days	Bile†
1,25-Dihydroxy vitamin D	Oral*	1-3 days	
parathyroid hormone	SC, IV	2-5 min	Metabolized, renal
calcitonin	SC, IM	20 min	Metabolized, renal
diphosphonate	Oral	—	Renal
fluoride	Oral or topical	—	Renal, sweat, milk, GI tract

* Bile salts needed.
† Binds to a special protein.

 PHARMACOKINETICS

Vitamin D

Vitamin D, 25-hydroxyvitamin D and 1,25-dihydroxyvitamin D are rapidly absorbed after oral administraion. Bile salts are required and absorption is impaired in biliary cirrhosis. Absorption is also decreased by steatorrhea. The vitamin D compounds circulate bound to a specific vitamin D binding protein (DBP), a slightly acidic monomeric glycoprotein of 55,000 daltons that is synthesized in liver. Metabolic fates of these compounds include conversion to the inactive glucuronide metabolites, progressive shortening of the side chain (leading to inactive calcitroic acid), and 24 and 26 hydroxylation. It has been proposed that 24,25-dihydroxyvitamin D may have unique mineralization properties, although this is not well established. Clearly, 1,24,25-trihydroxyvitamin D is a less active calcemic agent than its precursor, 1,25-dihydroxyvitamin D. 26-Hydroxylation decreases the activity of the vitamin D compounds. 1,25-Dihydroxyvitamin D has a half-life of 1 to 3 days, dihydrotachysterol has a half-life of 7 to 25 days, and vitamin D_2 has a half-life of 2 weeks. Vitamin D is stored in body tissues, including liver, fat, and muscle for long periods of time.

Parathyroid Hormone

Parathyroid hormone is rapidly metabolized in the liver and kidney to both active and inactive products. The half-life of the intact hormone in plasma is 2 to 5 minutes. The N-terminal fragment, with a molecular weight of 4000 daltons, is active, whereas the C-terminal 6000 dalton fragment is inactive. The N-terminal fragment is more rapidly eliminated. Parathyroid hormone is administered by injection for diagnostic purposes only.

Calcitonin

Calcitonin is administered intramuscularly or subcutaneously. It is weakly bound to plasma proteins. The intact molecule has a plasma half-life of 20 minutes and is rapidly metabolized to smaller fragments in the liver and kidney.

Diphosphonates

The diphosphonates are poorly absorbed (1% to 6%) following oral administration; they are not metabolized. Approximately 50% of the absorbed drug is excreted by the kidneys in 24 hours. The remainder is bound to tissue.

Fluoride

Fluoride is well absorbed following oral administration. Calcium and nonabsorbable antacids can interfere with its absorption. Fluoride is concentrated in skeletal tissues. Excretion is largely renal.

Pharmacokinetic parameters are summarized in Table 42-3.

RELATION OF MECHANISMS OF ACTIONS TO CLINICAL RESPONSE

Vitamin D and Metabolites

Vitamin D and its active metabolites are primarily used in the treatment of rickets, osteomalacia, and hypocalcemia. The actions of the vitamin D compounds to increase calcium absorption are the basis of their antirachitic activity. Effects on calcium release from bone probably contribute to the hypercalcemic effect. The use of the metabolites 25-hydroxyvitamin D and 1,25-dihydroxyvitamin D rather than vitamin D per se is logical when this disorder results from a defect in their formation. Alternatively, larger doses of the precursor can result in the production of sufficient active metabolite to bring about an adequate increase in serum calcium. Therefore doses of vitamin D more than 10 times greater than those used for simple replacement therapy are used to treat hypoparathyroidism or vitamin D-resisant rickets.

Parathyroid Hormone

Parathyroid hormone is used diagnostically. The hormone increases urinary cAMP subsequent to binding to renal receptors. This response is impaired in pseudohypoparathyroidism, a disorder in which there is resistance to the action of parathyroid hormone. In some cases, this disorder has been associated with a defective G protein in the adenylate cyclase system. Either the complete 84 amino acid polypeptide or the active N-terminal 1-34 fragment is administered intravenously in this test.

Calcitonin

Calcitonin has been used in the treatment of Paget's disease of bone to prevent abnormal bone turnover. It has also been approved to treat osteoporosis because it decreases bone resorption. Although used in the treatment of hypercalcemia of malignancy, its effects are somewhat delayed and less dramatic than those of other agents.

Hypercalcemia is also treated with sulfate, EDTA, furosemide, ethacrynic acid, glucocorticoids, and plicamycin. These agents all decrease serum calcium concentration by the effects previously described. The use of phosphate is not recommended. Recently the use of phosphate has been reported to cause death because of metastatic calcification, in many organs, particularly in the lung. Pharmacological treatment of hypercalcemia is carried out in conjunction with a low calcium diet and administration of oral and parenteral fluids. Paget's disease of bone is treated with diphosphonates and plicamycin, as well as by calcitonin. All of these agents decrease the abnormal bone turnover. Osteoporosis therapy currently attempts to prevent fractures or to limit the number of fractures by using agents that decrease bone resorption, including estrogen, and more recently, calcitonin. The NIH Consensus Conference on Osteoporosis recommended a calcium intake of 1500 mg/day for women starting about the time of menopause. Calcium per se appears to be less effective than estrogen in preventing bone loss. Calcium may act by inhibiting the secretion of parathyroid hormone. Fluoride, which can increase bone formation, is undergoing clinical trials. Another experimental approach is the use of low doses of parathyroid hormone to increase bone formation together with vitamin D to increase mineralization.

SIDE EFFECTS, CLINICAL PROBLEMS, AND TOXICITY

The problems are summarized in the box.

Vitamin D

Excess vitamin D and its metabolites can lead to hypercalcemia, a potentially fatal side effect. The immediate risk of this is greatest with 1,25-dihydroxyvitamin D, since the metabolic step that is feedback regulated, the renal 1-hydroxylase, is bypassed. However, since 1,25-dihydroxyvitamin D has the shortest biological half-life, the hypercalcemia and the possibility of cumulative effects is potentially less than with the other metabolites. There is an increased risk of toxicity in patients with impaired renal function. Serum calcium concentrations are monitored in patients on vitamin D therapy, and the drug is discontinued

---

CLINICAL PROBLEMS

VITAMIN D AND METABOLITES

Hypercalcemia
Benzothiadiazides can increase hazards of
  hypercalcemia

PARATHYROID HORMONE

Hypercalcemia (unlikely with diagnostic use)

CALCITONIN

Local hypersensitivity
"Escape" loss of effectiveness

DIPHOSPHONATES

Osteomalacia
Bone pain

FLUORIDE

GI side effects, including nausea
Musculoskeletal pain
Joint swelling
Mottled teeth enamel

TRADENAMES

In addition to generic and fixed combination preparations, the following tradenamed materials are
  available in the United States.

Calciferol, ergocalciferol, vitamin D_2
Calcimar, calcitonin
Calderol, calcifidiol, 25-hydroxyvitamin D_3
DHT, dihydrotachysterol
Didronel, etidronate disodium (a diphosphonate)
Mithracin, plicamycin (formerly called mithramycin)
Parathyroid hormone, commercial status is not
  clear (not listing diagnostic materials)
Rocaltrol, calcitriol, 1,25-dihydroxyvitamin D_3
Vitamin D is also present in a larger number of nu-
  tritional supplements

---

if hypercalcemia occurs. Benzothiadiazide diuretics can increase the hazard of hypercalcemia. Drug interactions can occur with phenobarbital, phenytoin, and glucocorticoids, all of which can interfere with vitamin D activation, as well as with the action of vitamin D metabolites on target tissues.

Parathyroid Hormone

Hypercalcemia is also a potential side effect of paraythoid hormone administration. However, this is unlikely to occur when the hormone is used diagnostically.

Calcitonin

Local hypersensitivity reactions, including skin rashes, other allergic reactions, and nausea, have been noted with calcitonin. Although calcitonin could potentially elicit hypocalcemia, this is not a common side effect. The major problem with calcitonin is the loss of effectiveness because of *escape*. Another limiting factor in the usefulness of calcitonin is its ineffectiveness when administered orally. Nasal preparations are undergoing clinical trials.

Other Agents

Some diphosphonates decrease bone mineralization, and osteomalacia and bone pain have occurred with their use. Fluoride has GI side effects including nausea. Musculoskeletal pain and joint swelling have been reported. The side effects of other agents are discussed in other chapters of this text.

REFERENCES

Fleisch H: Bisphosphonates: mechanisms of action and clinical applications. In Peck WA, ed: Bone and mineral research annual, no 1, Amsterdam, 1983, Elsevier Science Publishing Co, Inc.

Marx SJ, Lieberman UA, and Eil C: Calciferols: actions and deficiencies in action, Vitamins and hormones 40:235, 1983.

Mundy GR: Pathogenesis of hypercalcemia of malignancy, Clin Endocrinol 23:705, 1985.

Riggs BL and Melton LJ III: Involutional osteoporosis, N Engl J Med 314:1676, 1986.

Singer FR and Mills BG: Paget's disease of bone: etiologic and therapeutic aspects. In Peck WA ed: Bone and mineral research annual, no 2, Amsterdam, 1984, Elsevier Science Publishing Co, Inc.

Vernava Am, O'Neal LW, and Palermo V: Lethal hyperparathyroid crisis: hazards of phosphate administration Surgery 102: 941, 1987.

Wilson JD and Foster DW, eds: William's textbook of endocrinology, ed 7, Philadelphia, 1985, WB Saunders Co.

NEOPLASTIC CELLS: DRUGS AFFECTING CELL GROWTH AND VIABILITY

Neoplastic mammalian cells and tissues are characterized by abnormal chromosome structures and uncontrolled growth, usually accompanied by loss of cellular differentiation (anaplasia). Abnormal structural changes occur in the karyological appearance of cancer cell chromosomes, with almost all cancer cells showing some degree of aneuploidy (different than 46 chromosomes), with frequent deletions and translocations. These chromosomal changes lead to modified cellular regulation and abnormal structures of affected enzymes. The diseased cells and cell aggregates are described as tumors, neoplasms, or cancers and occur in benign (nonvirulent) or malignant (virulent) states. Malignant neoplastic cells typically are invasive in surrounding tissues, violating the basement membrane of the tissue of origin and eventually undergoing metastasis, with malignant cells released from the primary neoplasm and migrating to other tissues and organs forming metastatic tumor deposits. Over 100 types of malignant neoplasms affect humans, with classification based primarily on anatomical (organ) location and type of cell from which the neoplasm develops.

In the United States, malignant neoplasms are responsible for about 500,000 deaths per year (20% to 25% of total mortality), with about 1,000,000 new cases developing each year. Lung, large intestine, breast, and prostate neoplasms account for about 55% of both new cases and cancer deaths in the United States. Solid tumors arising from epithelial cells are termed *carcinomas,* while those generated from connective tissue and often of a fibrous nature are termed *sarcomas.* Malignancies that arise from the hemato-poietic system are termed *leukemias* or *lymphomas.*

The mechanisms by which malignant neoplasms originate in humans are still not clear. Carcinogenesis (i.e., the creation of malignant neoplastic cells) appears to be caused in several ways including activation of specific genes, called *proto-oncogenes.* Proto-oncogenes are present in many cells and, when activated to form oncogenes, initiate cellular changes such as production of modified proteins that may influence cellular differentiation/proliferation characteristic of the neoplastic state. Activation of proto-oncogenes can occur by several pathways that sometimes involve exposure of cells to specific chemicals, radiation, or viruses. Activation can result from a single point mutation. The most common oncogenes found thus far in human tumors belong to the *ras* gene family, which codes for GTP-binding proto-oncogenes. When the *ras* proto-oncogene is converted to the activated form, it can carry out cellular transformation to generate neoplastic cells. The *ras* gene is a copy of a gene found initially in a mouse sarcoma retrovirus capable of inducing tumor formation. Additional genes known as tumor suppressing genes also are present in human cells and function to suppress excessive cellular growth. Retinoblastoma (tumor of the eye) is a prototype of a malignancy caused by genetic loss of tumor-suppressing genes. Inactivation of these tumor-suppressing genes appears to be another route that leads to the formation of neoplastic cells.

Neoplastic cells traditionally are characterized by the inability to undergo differentiation yet still capable of cell division. This definition may be too simplistic,

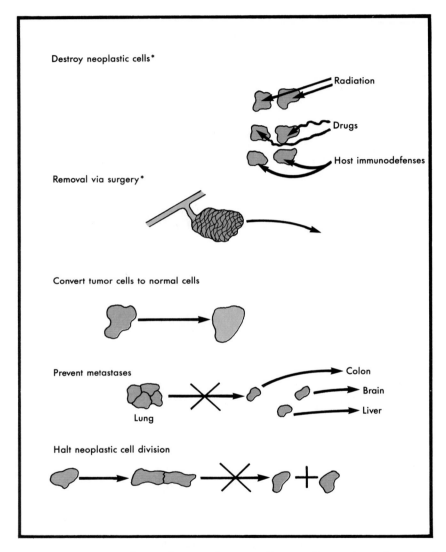

FIGURE VI-I   Major approaches to therapy of cancers. Tumor cells are shown in red and non-tumor cells in green. *, in clinical use. Others are experimental.

since some tumor cells recently have been shown to be capable of differentiation. Not all tumor cells are malignant; the stimulus that converts a neoplastic cell from the nonmalignant to the malignant state, or the reverse, is not clear. From the clinical standpoint, the primary difficulty in the successful control and treatment of malignant neoplasms is that by the time malignant cells are detected, the neoplasm often has metastasized, presenting a much more difficult therapeutic problem.

The overall approach in the therapy of neoplastic diseases (as shown in Figure VI-1) remains the removal or destruction of the neoplastic cells, while minimizing toxic effects on nonneoplastic cells. It has been a long-standing question whether drugs effective against one type of neoplasm should be effective against all types. However, clinical experience has shown a wide range of drug activities among different types (solid versus disseminated) and anatomical locations (breast, colon, lung) of tumors. Therefore interest has focused on treating each of the over 100 clinically important forms of cancer as separate disease states with development of suitable drug therapies. Some of the therapeutic approaches listed in Figure VI-1 are not available for clinical use but represent research approaches that are under study. For example, drugs that function specifically to return neoplastic cells to normal differentiating cells capable of surviving after differentiations or drugs that prevent metastases in general are not available or are highly experimental. However, drugs that stimulate the immune system to destroy those neoplastic cells not killed by antineoplastic drugs are of clinical importance and are discussed in Chapters 44 and 60.

The two chapters in this section present the mechanisms, clinical utilization, and problems associated with the clinical use of antineoplastic drugs in humans. Individual drugs are discussed in Chapter 43 and their clinical uses, usually in multiple drug protocols, are discussed in Chapter 44.

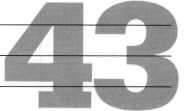

Individual Antineoplastic Drugs

MAJOR DRUGS
alkylating agents
antimetabolites
antibiotics
hormonal agents
plant alkaloids
others

THERAPEUTIC OVERVIEW

Clinically, antineoplastic agents are used in the treatment of many of the over 100 types of neoplastic diseases, with the goal of destroying neoplastic cells with minimal effects on nonneoplastic tissues. Additional drugs (discussed in Chapter 58) are used to enhance host natural defense mechanisms to eradicate those neoplastic cells not killed by the antineoplastic drugs. Although in clinical practice nearly all types of neoplastic diseases are treated using multiple drugs, in this chapter the mechanisms of action, pharmacokinetics, and side effects of the individual antineoplastic drugs are presented. The rationales for multiple drug protocols are described in the following chapter.

The effectiveness of antineoplastic drugs varies greatly with the type of cancer, the general ability of the patient to perform various functions (i.e., patient performance status), and the endpoint used to evaluate the effectiveness (e.g., tumor response, patient survival). The effectiveness of most antineoplastic agents is greater on cells that are progressing through the cell cycle (Figure 43-1), compared to cells that are resting in the G_0 phase. The "growth fraction," defined in Figure 43-1, is the fraction of cells progressing through the cycle. In addition to tumor cells that may be cycling through the cell division cycle, certain nonneoplastic cells also are undergoing cell division. In particular, the nonneoplastic cells of hair follicles, bone marrow, and intestinal epithelium are the most rapidly dividing and are especially sensitive to inhi-

FIGURE 43-1   Growth cycle for mammalian cells. In the G_o (resting) phase, the cells are dormant. A variety of stimulants, often of unknown origin in clinical situations, cause cycling of cells to begin by entry into the G_1 phase (pre-DNA synthesis). Here, precursors for DNA are formed. In the S phase, DNA synthesis occurs. This is followed by premitotic synthesis and structural developments in the G_2 phase. Mitosis occurs in the M phase to produce two cells, each of which can continue to cycle, by entry again into G_1, or can enter the resting phase, G_o. Growth fraction is total cells in the growth cycle (G_1, S, G_2, M) divided by the total cells (G_1, S, G_2, M, G_o).

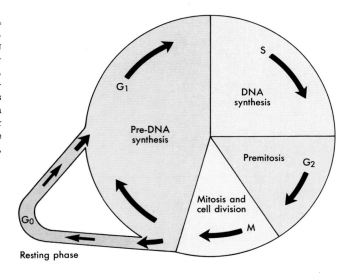

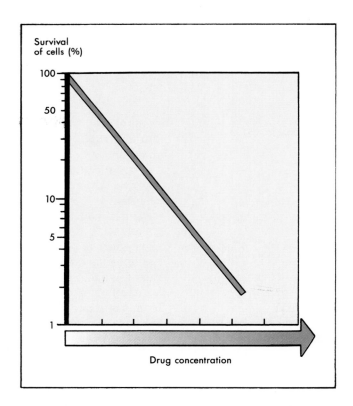

FIGURE 43-2   Decline in viable cells is first order with respect to drug concentration. Many drug-neoplastic cell combinations follow this relationship in vitro, thus establishing the principles of a fixed percentage of viable cells killed per dose of drug. This same relationship appears to apply in vivo, although the actual situation may be more complex.

bition by antineoplastic drugs. Inhibition of these nontumor cells accounts for many of the undesirable side effects with use of antineoplastic drugs.

The number of in vitro neoplastic cells that survive each dose of antineoplastic drug typically shows a first order relationship to the concentration of drug (Figure 43-2). This means that the same fraction of cells are killed with each dose of drug (log cell kill), and a series of several doses does not kill 100% of the neoplastic cells. The log cell kill hypothesis is compatible with clinical observations that a functional host immune system is needed to obtain complete kill of all neoplastic cells and thereby obtain a cure of neoplastic disease.

Of the four major types of tumors, the faster growing hematological (nonsolid) types (leukemias and lymphomas) are more responsive to treatment with drugs than are the slower growing solid types (carcinomas and sarcomas). Primary factors in this difference are the more rapid doubling times of the hematological malignancies and the greater ease of distribution of drug to leukemia or lymphoma cells as compared to carcinoma or sarcoma cells. The outer or more recently synthesized portions of many solid tumors are well vascularized and are readily accessible to drugs. However, the inner and older portions of solid tumors usually are hypoxic and often necrotic and consequently poorly accessible to the drugs. The necrotic inner cells may be dead or merely in the resting phase of the cell cycle and therefore may still be capable of returning to the cycling state. The delivery of drugs to the inner portions of solid tumors is a major unsolved problem.

Antineoplastic drugs must enter the cell to produce their desired cytotoxic effects. Some drugs can pass through the cell membrane by passive diffusion, with the concentration gradient of drug between the outside and inside of the cell driving drug uptake. Other drugs require binding to carrier proteins that then transport drug through the cell membrane and release the drug on the cytoplasmic side. Carrier-mediated transport of antineoplastic drugs is an active process that is not concentration driven, and the rate of transport often is limited by a fixed number of carrier molecules per cell.

Once the antineoplastic drug enters the cell and diffuses into the nucleus or other subcellular sites, the drug can react with target molecules to disrupt key processes that are necessary for cell viability. The target molecules and their reactions with antineo-

---

> **PRIMARY THERAPEUTIC CONSIDERATIONS WITH INDIVIDUAL ANTINEOPLASTIC DRUGS**
>
> Drug delivery problems to individual cells
> Cycling versus noncycling cells
> Log-dose kill (same fraction of cells killed per dose)
> Need for active immune system (host defenses) to eradicate remaining neoplastic cells
> Problem of central hypoxic zone of tumors

plastic drugs are described in the next section.

The main therapeutic considerations are summarized in the box.

MECHANISMS OF ACTION

Basic Approaches

A generalized summary of the basic mechanisms by which antineoplastic drugs are used for killing tumor cells is given in Figure 43-3. Only those compounds that show some selectivity for neoplastic cells are used clinically. In general, antimetabolites inhibit, or make less effective, DNA synthesis. Alkylating and intercalating agents or antibiotics damage DNA or RNA structure. Other agents, including steroids, interfere with transcription translation, and still others, including plant alkaloids, disrupt mitosis. Yet others (i.e., asparaginase) destroy essential amino acids needed for translation.

A significant number of clinically used antineoplastic drugs must undergo either chemical or enzymatic modification to generate the active cytotoxic species. The pertinent modes of activation are described later in this section.

Cellular resistance to specific antineoplastic drugs may develop in individual patients. For example, some drugs require the presence of carrier proteins for transport through the cell membrane, and those patients with neoplastic cells devoid of the carrier proteins may show a form of drug resistance. Drug resistance is discussed later in this chapter, following the discussion of the individual drugs.

The principal types of antineoplastic drugs are listed in the box, p. 592, with clinical examples of each type. Discussion of these drugs follows.

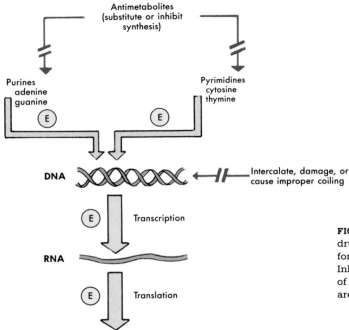

FIGURE 43-3 Basic approaches in which antineoplastic drugs are used for the selective killing of tumor cells. E stands for enzymes, some of which are inhibited by these drugs. Inhibition of DNA or RNA synthesis or replication, production of miscoded nucleic acids, and formation of modified proteins are key mechanisms of action for many of these drugs.

In the figure:

Antimetabolites (substitute or inhibit synthesis)

Purines adenine guanine — E

Pyrimidines cytosine thymine — E

DNA — Intercalate, damage, or cause improper coiling

E Transcription

RNA

E Translation

Protein — Block function in cell or on cell surface

ANTINEOPLASTIC DRUGS

ALKYLATING AGENTS

nitrogen mustards
    mechlorethamine HC1 (nitrogen mustard, HN_2 HC1)
    melphalan (L-phenylalanine, L-PAM)
    chlorambucil
    cyclophosphamide
    ifosfamide
nitrosoureas
    carmustine (BCNU)
    lomustine (CCNU)
other
    cis-diamminedichloroplatinum (cisplatin, cis-DDP)
    carboplatin (cis-dichloro-transhydroxy bis isopropylamine platinum IV [CBDCA])
    busulfan
    dacarbazine (DTIC)
    procarbazine
    triethylenethiophosphoramide (thio-TEPA)

ANTIMETABOLITES

methotrexate (MTX)
mercaptopurine (6-MP)
thioguanine (6-TG)
fluorouracil (5-FU)

ANTIMETABOLITES—cont'd

cytarabine (cytosine arabinoside, araC)
trimetrexate
2-deoxycoformycin
hydroxyurea

ANTIBIOTICS

daunorubicin (daunomycin)
doxorubicin
bleomycin
dactinomycin (actinomycin D)
mitomycin C
mithramycin (plicamycin)

HORMONAL AGENTS

prednisone
tamoxifen

OTHERS

asparaginase

PLANT ALKALOIDS

vincristine
vinblastine
etoposide (VP-16)
teniposide (VM-26)*

*Not approved in the United States.

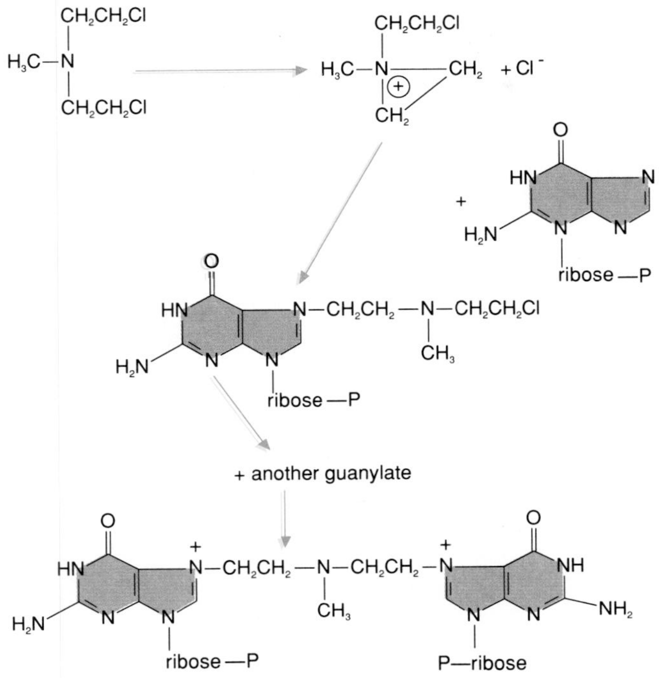

FIGURE 43-4   Alkylation of mechlorethamine, showing positively charged intermediate ion and its covalent attachment to the N-7 position of two deoxyguanylate nucleotides of DNA.

Alkylating Agents

Alkylation refers to the covalent attachment of alkyl groups to other molecules. This approach to cancer therapy came about as a result of observations on the effects of the mustard war gases on cell growth. Although the sulfur mustard war gases were too toxic for clinical use as antineoplastic agents, the related nitrogen mustard alkylating agents produced the first effective antineoplastic agents, including mechlorethamine, which is still in use today.

The process of alkylation takes place through chemical formation of a positively charged carbonium ion (also called carbocation). This positively charged group subsequently reacts with an electron rich site, particularly on DNA or RNA, to form modified nucleic acids. Some of the clinically used alkylating drugs have two alkylating groups, thus promoting the formation of covalent crosslinks between adjacent strands of nucleic acids. The crosslinks prevent subsequent separation of the dual strands of DNA during cell cycling. For maximal kill, it is important to administer the maximum tolerated dose. The alkylation sequence is shown schematically in Figure 43-4 for mechlorethamine (nitrogen mustard) coupling to the N-7 position of deoxyguanylate. In several studies with free DNA or RNA, alkylation occurred predominately at the N-7 position of the guanine base, with only minor alkylation at O-6 or N-3 of guanine, at N-1, N-3, or N-7 of adenine, or at N-3 of cytosine. With HeLa cells (named after the patient from which this cell line originated), alkylation selectivity for guanine N-7 has been shown to be 70 times that for the other unpaired ring oxygen or nitrogen atoms in the bases. In whole cells many constituents, including DNA, RNA, proteins, and membrane components, become alkylated. However, the working hypothesis is that the primary cytotoxic events occur through alkylation of DNA, especially by coupling to the N-7 position of the deoxyguanylates of either single- or double-stranded DNA.

The structures of several nitrogen mustards are shown in Figure 43-5.

Cyclophosphamide undergoes a combination of enzymatic and chemical activation to form the active phosphoramide mustard alkylating agent (Figure 43-6). Exposure of cells to cyclophosphamide and other alkylating agents can lead to carcinogenesis (i.e., the formation of neoplastic cells). For example, leukemia

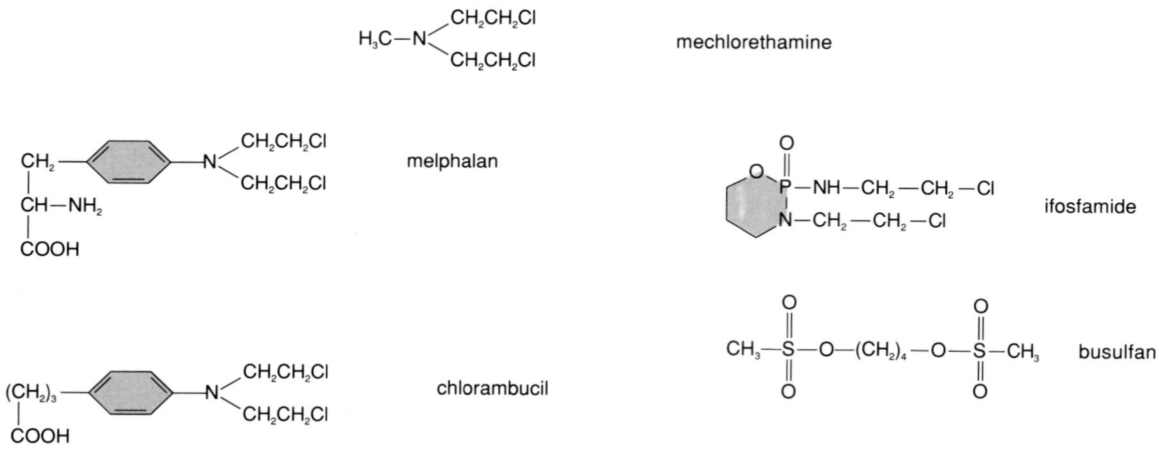

FIGURE 43-5   Structures of nitrogen mustards.

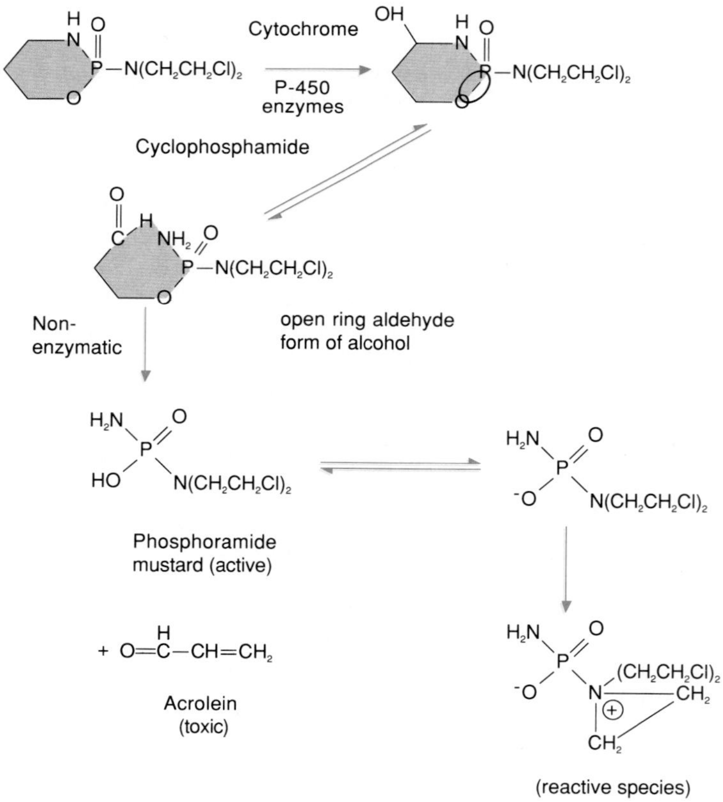

FIGURE 43-6   Mechanism of enzymatic and chemical activation of cyclophosphamide to form active phosphoramide mustard. Acrolein has some cytotoxic activity but much less than that of the phosphoramide mustard.

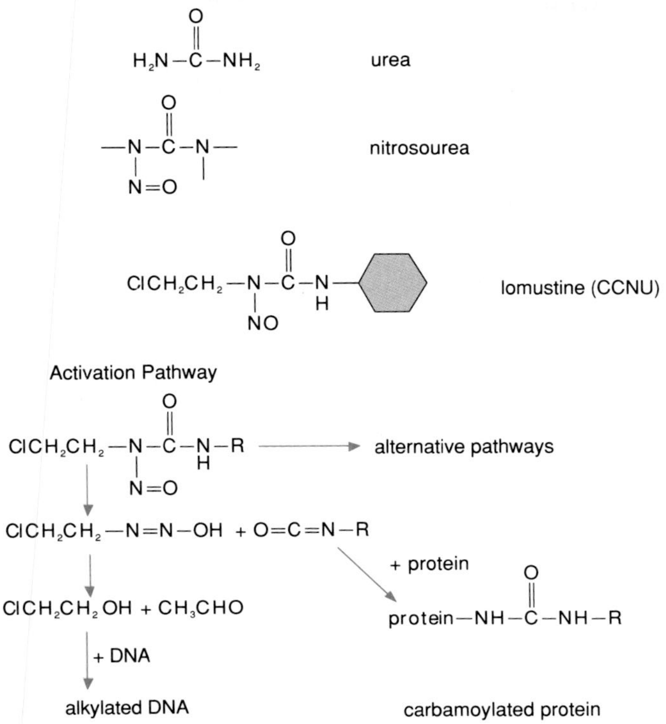

FIGURE 43-7   Structures and activation pathways for nitrosourea alkylating agents. Carbamoylation of proteins also occurs but is thought to be a lesser cause of cell cytotoxicity than is the alkylation of DNA.

is a well described long-term complication in patients treated with a regimen that includes nitrogen mustard mechlorethamine (MOPP) for Hodgkin's disease.

Another group of antineoplastic alkylating agents in clinical use is the nitrosoureas. The structures and mechanism of activation for these compounds are shown in Figure 43-7. Although alternate pathways are available by which nitrosoureas can form active alkylating species, the principal route is shown in Figure 43-7. Carbamoylation of proteins also occurs with nitrosoureas (Figure 43-7); the carbamoylated proteins may play a role in producing cytotoxicity. However, the alkylation route is thought to be the major cause of cytotoxicity during antineoplastic therapy. Nitrosoureas are lipophilic and are able to cross the blood-brain barrier. They are therefore frequently used to treat brain tumors.

Other clinical compounds that act by alkylation crosslinking of DNA are cis-diamminedichloroplatinum (II), also called cisplatin, and newer platinum analogs. For example, carboplatin in early clinical studies appears to have equal activity against ovarian and germ cell neoplasms as its parent compound, but the spectrum of its side effects is different. Cisplatin, $Pt(NH_3)_2(Cl)_2$, is a square planar complex of platinum in the plus-two oxidation state with two ammonia molecules and two chloride ions at the corners of the plane. The stereochemistry of the complex enables the cis, but not the trans, isomer to form two covalent platinum-nitrogen bonds primarily at the N-7 positions of two adjacent deoxyguanylates of DNA. This crosslink prevents replication of the DNA. Structures of cisplatin and carboplatin are shown in Figure 43-8. The detailed reaction sequence is not completely known. Chloride ions are replaced by water during formation of the platinum-nitrogen bond with DNA. The resulting DNA crosslinks are almost totally the intrastrand type. Clinically observed cytotoxicity may result in part from intrastrand crosslinking, probably on adjacent guanosine N-7 groups of DNA. Since cisplatin also inhibits DNA polymerase, the cytotoxicity may also involve inhibition of DNA synthesis.

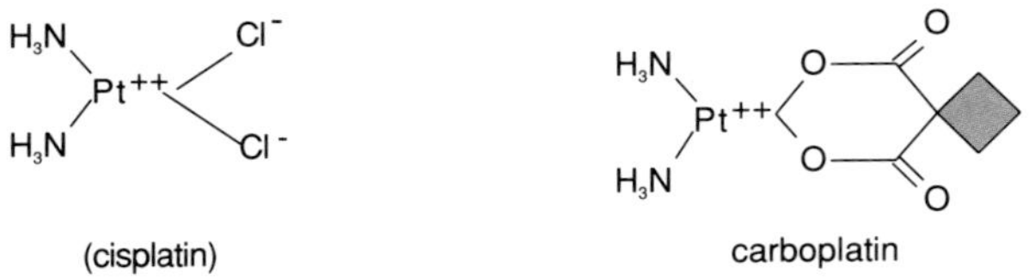

FIGURE 43-8   Square planar complex of cis-diamminedichloroplatinum (II), cisplatin, and a new platinum derivative, carboplatin.

Several other clinical alkylating agents include busulfan, dacarbazine, procarbazine, ifosfamide, and melphalan. Busulfan type compounds alkylate nucleic acid bases, primarily at N-7 of guanine, and also alkylate SH groups of glutathione or cysteine to form additional active compounds.

The specific reaction sequences by which dacarbazine or procarbazine alkylate DNA are not well understood. For dacarbazine, hydrolysis to form a reactive aryldiazonium ion, a corresponding arylcarbonium ion, or an alternative methyl carbonium ion are possibilities. In the case of procarbazine, hydrolysis to form a methyl-free radical has been proposed for the alkylation mechanism; but this is not certain. Thio-TEPA is the short name for N,N',N"-triethylenethiophosphoramide. After chemical activation thio-TEPA alkylates DNA in a manner similar to mechlorethamine. Melphelan is a phenylalanine derivative and is actively transported into the cell by the same carriers that transport leucine and glutamine. Melphelan is associated with the induction of secondary leukemias. Chlorambucil is structurally similar to melphelan and is used primarily in chronic lymphatic leukemia. Ifosfamide is similar in structure to cyclophosphamide and is activated by hepatic microsomes. Early studies with ifosfamide showed a significant incidence of hemorrhagic cystitis. Ifosfamide is now given with a systemic thiol MESNA (sodium 2-mercaptoethane sulfonate). MESNA becomes a free thiol after glomerular filtration and combines with the products responsible for the cystitis. Ifosfamide is active against a number of cancers, including small cell lung cancer, sarcomas, lymphomas, testicular carcinoma, and gynecologic cancers.

Antimetabolites

The antimetabolites are compounds that mimic the structures of normal metabolic constituents, including folic acid, pyrimidines, or purines, well enough to inhibit enzymes necessary for folic acid regeneration or for pyrimidine or purine activation for DNA or RNA synthesis in neoplastic cells. Methotrexate, 5-fluorouracil, araC, 6-mercaptopurine, and 6-thioguanine are the primary clinical antimetabolites. The antimetabolite methotrexate shows enhanced selectivity for neoplastic cells because methotrexate is selectively polymerized by tumor cells. The tetrahydrofolates act more efficiently as enzyme cofactors when present as polymers with glutamate than as monomers. Methotrexate is transported in the blood as a monomer but undergoes enzyme-catalyzed polymerization within cells and becomes trapped intracellularly as a polymer. Tumor cells have higher polymerizing enzyme activity than do nontumor cells, so a higher concentration of polymerized (more active) methotrexate is trapped within the tumor cells to act as an antimetabolite.

Folic acid is essential for enzyme-catalyzed reactions that transfer methyl groups and related groups during purine and pyrimidine synthesis. Methotrexate competitively inhibits the enzyme dihydrofolate reductase, which catalyzes the reduction of dihydrofolate (FH_2) to tetrahydrofolate (FH_4) (Figure 43-9), blocking the regeneration of FH_4 and thereby preventing the synthesis of purine and pyrimidines. Methotrexate is thus specific for cells in the S phase of the cell cycle.

Cellular transport of methotrexate is a carrier-mediated process. To overcome the limitations of carrier uptake and to enhance entry of drug into the cells by passive diffusion, up to 16 gm/day of methotrexate are infused IV over several hours. It is mandatory that the methotrexate infusion be followed by a "rescue process." Leucovorin (citrovorum factor or N^5-formyl-FH_4), a substitute for FH_4, is administered and apparently enters the cells and enables the purine and pyrimidine reaction synthesis to proceed. However, the clinical efficacy of this high dose methotrexate-leucovorum rescue approach is still being debated.

Another antimetabolite, 5-fluorouracil (5-FU) (Figure 43-10) acts by inhibiting pyrimidine synthesis (and thus DNA formation) as exemplified in Figure 43-9. Fluorouracil undergoes metabolism to the 5-fluoro analog of deoxyuridylic acid, which in turn inhibits thymidylate synthase by covalent coupling to the enzyme. Modulation of the activity of 5-FU with folinic acid, α-interferon, and the anthelminthic levimasole has been a major area of clinical investigation. Response rates of colorectal cancer are significantly in-

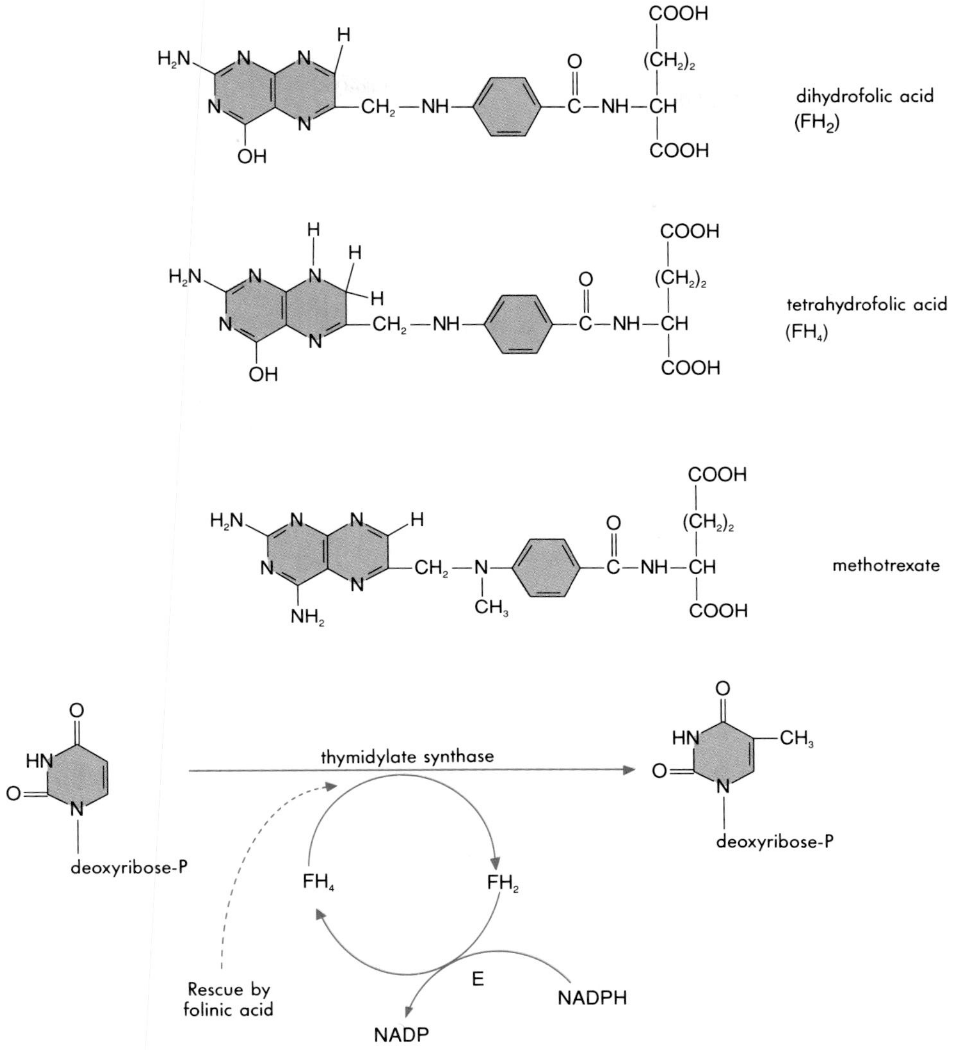

FIGURE 43-9   Structures of tetrahydrofolic acid (FH₄) and methotrexate. The reaction shown is a pyrimidine synthesis (thymidine monophosphate from deoxyuridylic acid) catalyzed by the thymidylate synthase and requiring FH₄ as cofactor. E is dihydrofolate reductase, which is reversibly inhibited by methotrexate, thus preventing regeneration of FH₄ from FH₂. The rescue path is discussed in the text. The pyrimidines are needed for DNA formation.

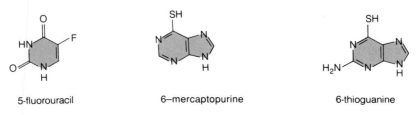

FIGURE 43-10   Structures of prototype pyrimidine antimetabolites.

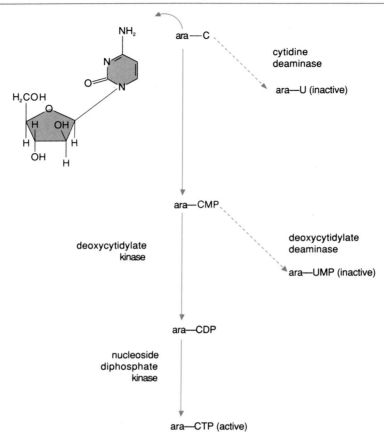

FIGURE 43-11   Competing activation and deactivation pathways for conversion of ara-C (cytosine arabinoside) to the active form that inhibits DNA polymerase.

creased when folinic acid or α-interferon is given with 5-FU. Folinic acid enhances the activity of 5-FU by stabilizing the ternary complex of thymidylate synthase. Therefore, less thymidylate synthase is available to convert d-UMP to d-TMP, and DNA synthesis is reduced. The mechanism by which α-interferon enhances activity of 5-FU is unknown. Recent trials have shown a significant benefit in the combined use of 5-FU and levamisole for colorectal cancer with lymph node involvement.

Cytosine arabinoside (araC) also acts to inhibit pyrimidine synthesis, but through a more complex pathway (Figure 43-11). The drug must undergo enzymatic conversion to the cytosine triphosphate derivative (ara-CTP), which is the active form and binds competitively to inhibit DNA polymerase. In some patients cytidine deaminase activity is high and deoxycytidine kinase activity is low, resulting in inactivation of considerable drug before its conversion to its active form.

The purine analogs 6-mercaptopurine (6-MP) and 6-thioguanine (6-TG) (Figure 43-10) also must undergo activation to form nucleotides, which then act as competitive inhibitors of several enzymes in purine synthesis pathways. The adenosine deaminase inhibitor, 2-deoxycoformycin, is highly active against hairy cell leukemia.

Hydroxyurea acts to inhibit ribonucleoside diphosphate reductase, which reduces ribonucleotides to deoxyribonucleotides required for DNA synthesis. It presumably complexes with non-heme Fe required by the enzyme for activity. It is therefore an S phase-specific agent.

Antibiotics

Several antibiotics of microbial origin are very effective in the treatment of certain tumors. These antibiotics include especially doxorubicin/daunorubicin and bleomycin, and also actinomycin D and

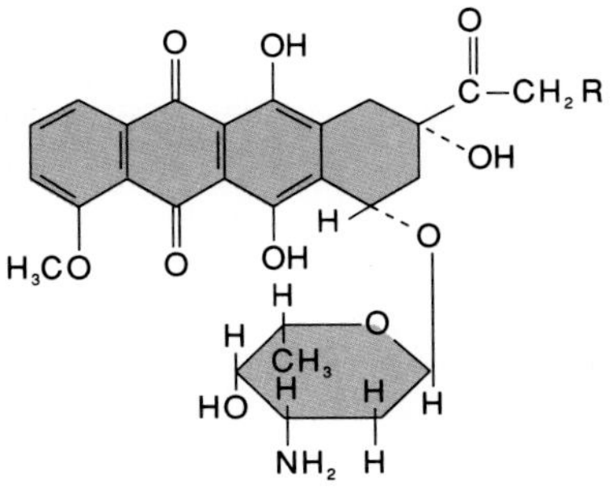

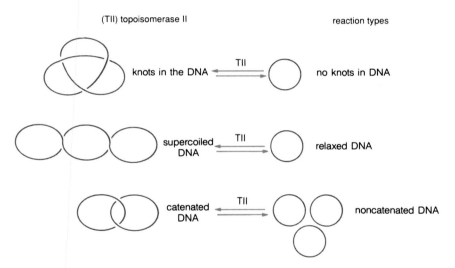

R = H daunorubicin

R = OH doxorubicin

FIGURE 43-12   Structures of daunorubicin and doxorubicin.

(TII) topoisomerase II   reaction types

knots in the DNA ⟷ TII ⟶ no knots in DNA

supercoiled DNA ⟷ TII ⟶ relaxed DNA

catenated DNA ⟷ TII ⟶ noncatenated DNA

FIGURE 43-13   Topoisomerase II mechanisms of action inhibited by the anthracyclines such as doxorubicin and other agents.

mitomycin C. The anthracycline structure of doxorubicin is shown in Figure 43-12.

Bleomycin is a mixture of several relatively high molecular weight basic glycopeptides with the one called A_2 predominating. Bleomycin forms a complex with oxygen and Fe (II), which undergoes reduction to an active form that causes DNA strand scission. This action is specific to DNA; RNA is not affected. Mithramycin (plicamycin) lowers serum Ca^{++} and is active against testicular carcinoma. Doxorubicin is the single most active agent against breast cancer, while daunorubicin is used to treat leukemias.

Doxorubicin and daunorubicin are anthracyclines that act (1) through intercalation between the bases in double-stranded DNA, (2) by inhibition of topoisomerase II, and (3) possibly by an action on the cell membrane. The topoisomerase action is summarized schematically in Figure 43-13. DNA topoisomerase II catalyzes the uncoiling and breakage of both strands of double-stranded DNA to modify the number and the types of linkage twists. The enzyme is inhibited by doxorubicin and daunorubicin by stabilizing a covalent complex of an enzyme-DNA intermediate, preventing the DNA breaks from rejoining, thereby leading to cell death. Inhibition of topoisomerase II occurs also with actinomycin D, ellipticines, etoposide (VP-16), and teniposide (VM-26).

Actinomycin D intercalates in DNA binding to deoxyguanosine. It prevents the synthesis of RNA and also inhibits topoisomerase II. Mitomycin C first undergoes chemical activation within cells resulting in the formation of a derivative that acts by crosslinking DNA via alkylation.

Plant Alkaloids

The primary compounds in this group, vincristine and vinblastine, block microtubule formation and thereby disrupt mitotic spindle formation during the M phase of the cell cycle. Etoposide (VP-16) is a semisynthetic derivative of podophyllotoxin that is prepared from the mandrake plant (May Apple) and is used to treat warts. VP-16 has significant activity against small cell cancer of the lung and testicular carcinoma and is used in most first line regimens for these diseases. Recently, reports have appeared that the dosing schedule is important. Low dose 21 day oral VP-16 has been reported to have activity against small cell carcinoma of the lung previously resistant to the drug.

Hormonal Agents

Steroids act by passing through the cell membrane and binding to cytoplasmic receptors, which then enter the nucleus and interact with chromatin to induce the synthesis of special mRNAs. The latter code new proteins that may alter physiological or biochemical reactions, leading to desired beneficial effects. However, most of the new proteins have not been identified and characterized.

Treatment strategies for breast cancer have included (1) attempts to eliminate estrogen production by the adrenals and (2) blockade of estrogen receptors using antiestrogen drugs. In postmenopausal subjects, complete elimination of adrenal-produced estrogens is not always possible because the adrenals secrete androstenedione, which undergoes peripheral conversion to an estrogen (estrone) or to testosterone. Estrone in turn undergoes conversion to estradiol.

About 70% of all postmenopausal patients whose breast tumors show the presence of estrogen receptors respond favorably to antiestrogen therapy, while only about 10% of those that show a negative receptor assay respond to antiestrogen therapy. Tamoxifen is the main antiestrogen used clinically and acts by binding to the estrogen receptors and blocking cells in the G_1 phase. By blocking the binding of estrogens, tamoxifen (see Chapter 36 for structures) decreases estrogen stimulation of the production of the α form of transforming growth factor (TGF) and secretion of associated proteins.

In metastatic prostate cancer, like breast cancer, objective responses are frequent, with hormonal manipulations consisting of either orchiectomy or pharmacologic castration. Testosterone concentrations can be reduced by the estrogen diethylstilbestrol via suppression of the pituitary gonadotropic axis. Leuprolide and goserlin (Zoladex) are analogues of gonadotropic-releasing hormones that inhibit release of gonadotropins and result in castrate testosterone concentrations. Both agents are available in depot form and can be given monthly. Both are partial agonists as well as antagonists of LHRH. They produce an initial rise in gonadotropin concentrations, followed by a decline in 2 to 3 weeks.

Flutamide is an antiandrogen that inhibits androgen binding to receptors in the nucleus. Unlike other agents discussed, it leads to increased concentrations of testosterone. The testosterone is ineffective because flutamide blocks the action of testosterone. There has been recent interest in achieving total androgen blockage (both testis and adrenal) with the concurrent use of flutamide and LHRH analogues.

Others

L-Asparaginase is administered to hydrolyze asparagine, required for growth in tumor cells in higher amounts than in normal cells. This depletes asparagine concentrations to well below 10 μM, thereby shutting off protein and eventually nucleic acid synthesis. This approach is selective for those neoplastic cells devoid of asparagine synthetase and thus unable to synthesize the essential asparagine.

Targeting the Antitumor Drugs (see also Chapter 6)

Extensive side effects produced by the actions of antitumor drugs on nonneoplastic cells have resulted in efforts to develop procedures for targeting these drugs to tumor cells. The idea is to maximize the exposure of tumor cells to the drugs while minimizing the exposure of nonneoplastic cells. Regional infusions via intraarterial channels are used where the circulatory system of the tumor can be localized, and intracavitary infusions (e.g., into the peritoneal cavity) are employed as well. Monoclonal antibody-drug conjugates are being investigated for targeting drugs to the tumor cell surface, but the heterogeneity of tumor cell surface antigens makes this approach difficult. Encapsulation of drugs in liposomes also is an investigational technique.

Mechanisms of Resistance

Some patients initially respond favorably to antitumor drugs, but later the tumor may return and the same drugs may be ineffective. In other patients a drug protocol may show few positive results, even though the same protocol has proven beneficial with other patients. These situations all are typical of resistance either present initially or developing after exposure of the patient to one or more antitumor drugs.

In resistant subjects, the reduced effectiveness can be attributed to a decreased intracellular concentration of drug, to repair of drug-induced damage, or to modified drug targets. A number of mechanisms account for these differences, as indicated in Table 43-1.

Table 43-1 Possible Mechanisms for the Development of Resistance to Antineoplastic Agents

ANTINEOPLASTIC AGENT

Decreased uptake of active agent into cancer cell
Failure of agent to be metabolized to a chemical specie capable of producing a cytotoxic effect
Enhanced conversion of agent to inactive metabolite
Increase in transport of agent from the cancer cell
Increase in concentration of sulfhydryl scavengers

CANCER CELL (DNA, TARGET ENZYME, OR OTHER MACROMOLECULE)

Repair of drug-induced DNA damage
Gene amplification; greater amount of target enzyme within the cancer cell
Reduced ability of target enzyme to bind agent

Decreased drug uptake by cells is one mechanism of resistance, especially for drugs such as methotrexate that require carrier proteins for transmembrane transport. Actinomycin D resistance is also based on decreased cellular uptake.

Enhanced cellular efflux of drug is a second mechanism. Mammalian cells possess a 1280 amino acid glycoprotein called P-glycoprotein that acts as an ATP-driven, membrane-associated transport protein. This P-glycoprotein functions to transport complex ring system, hydrophobic, positively charged antitumor drugs, as well as other compounds, out of the cell. Doxorubicin, daunorubicin, actinomycin D, etoposide, teniposide, vincristine, and vinblastine are all antitumor drugs that show resistance in cells possessing amplified genes encoding for the multidrug-resistance P-glycoprotein. It is assumed that the cells are pumping the drugs out so as to reduce the intracellular concentration, without a change in the rate of drug influx, which occurs by passive diffusion. Efforts are underway to develop compounds that will block the drug efflux action of the P-glycoprotein pumps and develop drugs that circumvent multidrug resistance. Verapamil and other calcium channel blockers deblock the P-glycoprotein pump, but unacceptably high concentrations are required.

Intracellular targets comprise a third mechanism of resistance, for which methotrexate serves as an example. In one mechanism, cells have increased intracellular concentrations of the target enzyme dihydrofolate reductase, resulting from gene amplification. In another example, an altered enzyme is present, still enzymatically active, but with a lower binding affinity for methotrexate. In a third example, methotrexate is not conjugated with polyglutamates and is therefore not retained within the tumor cell. The methotrexate-polyglutamate conjugate is less lipid soluble and therefore less likely to traverse the cell membrane. A higher unconjugated methotrexate concentration is required as monomer to inhibit dihydrofolate reductase. Thus in these examples, the enzyme is no longer inhibited to the same degree by the usual concentration of intracellular methotrexate.

Bleomycin resistance exemplifies the fourth mechanism in which cells rapidly repair the DNA breaks caused by this drug. Similar repair mechanisms may be a source of resistance for other DNA-directed antitumor drugs as well. An example could be the repair of covalent crosslinks between DNA chains.

Sulfhydryl compounds, including glutathione and metallothioneins, act as cellular protective groups, particularly against alkylating agents. Such protective compounds scavenge highly reactive compounds and represent the fifth mechanism.

A sixth mechanism involves enhanced drug metabolism either within the tumor cells or elsewhere in the body. Increased concentrations of aldehyde dehydrogenase, for example, lead to enhanced metabolism of cyclophosphamide. Numerous antitumor drugs that undergo metabolism are further examples.

 # PHARMACOKINETICS

Numerous measurements have been made to determine the plasma decay concentration curves for antitumor drugs. The standard compartment model, used to explain the plasma concentration versus time decay curves as sums of one to three exponentials, is useful in providing pharmacokinetic guidance to dosing schemes that maximize drug tumor contact while minimizing drug tissue contact. A more complex type of pharmacokinetic model, called a flow model, provides more help but is much more difficult to construct and usually unsuccessful in obtaining parameter values for individual patients. In the flow model approach, compartments are assigned to the major organs and to the tumor; the compartments are connected by blood flow rates. Then, with different drug input rates and durations of dosing, the relative exposures of tumor and nontumor tissues can be assessed. Although the flow model approach has been applied to antitumor drugs, the results are too complex to discuss here. However, there is little point to including plasma drug half-lives in the table of pharmacokinetic parameters except for bolus versus infusions. For those antitumor agents where the drug disappears rapidly from the plasma, continuous IV infusion rather than bolus injection often is needed to obtain a high enough drug concentration to obtain a suitable therapeutic effect.

The modes of administration and disposition are listed in Table 43-2.

6-Mercaptopurine undergoes enzyme-catalyzed metabolism with xanthine oxidase as the principal

Table 43-2 Pharmacokinetic Parameters

Drug	Administration	Disposition	Notes
nitrogen mustard	IV	M	
melphalan	Oral	M	
cyclophosphamide	IV, oral	M	
nitrosoureas	IV, oral	M	Lipid soluble, crosses blood-brain barrier
cisplatin	IV	R	90% protein bound
carboplatin	IV	R	3-6 hr half-life
busulfan	Oral	M	Few min half-life
methotrexate	IV	R	50% to 60% plasma protein bound
5-fluorouracil	Oral, IV	M	
cytarabine (araC)	IV	M	Few min half-life
6-MP and 6-TG	Oral	M*	Large 1st pass effect
doxorubicin	IV	M	(10 min half-life)
daunorubicin	IV	M	
bleomycin	IV	R (50%), M	
asparaginase	IV	—	
vincristine	IV	M, B	Minimal entry into CSF
vinblastine	IV	B	
etoposide (VP-16)	IV, oral	R (main), M, B	97% plasma protein bound
tamoxifen	Oral	M (main)	Enterohepatic cycling

M, Metabolized; *R*, renal excretion; *B*, biliary excretion.
* See text for drug interaction.

enzyme. Allopurinol, a drug used in the treatment of gout, also is metabolized by the same enzyme. A drug interaction occurs if the two compounds are given concurrently. A major reduction in 6-MP dosage must be instituted in patients receiving allopurinol. Coadministration of these drugs leads to slower disappearance of both. Allopurinol also lengthens cyclophosphamide half-life and increases myelotoxicity, possibly because of decreased renal elimination of cyclophosphamide metabolites. Procarbazine has an antabuse toxicity, and patients taking the drug should avoid alcohol.

The other drugs that undergo metabolism also may show interactions during multiple drug antitumor dosing, resulting in prolonged plasma concentrations of the involved drugs.

RELATION OF MECHANISMS OF ACTION TO CLINICAL RESPONSE

Most antineoplastic drugs are used in multiple agent protocols where the cytolytic effects of the different agents interact in a complex manner. The clinical use of combination chemotherapy is discussed in a separate chapter (Chapter 44).

SIDE EFFECTS, CLINICAL PROBLEMS, AND TOXICITY

Typical undesirable side effects experienced with many antitumor drugs are listed in Table 43-3. Nausea and vomiting are quite common, and strategies for ameliorating these effects are available.

Several different drugs can be used simultaneously in specific patients based on nonoverlapping, dose-limiting toxicities listed in the box.

Nephrotoxicity, peripheral neuropathy, and ototoxicity remain the major side effects with cisplatin, although the severity of the renal toxicity can be reduced through hydration of the patient and administration of mannitol. The renal damage arises from cisplatin's effect on renal tubules, resulting in decreased glomerular filtration rates and increased reabsorption. Nephrotoxicity does not develop until a week or two after treatment is begun and may be worsened by coadministration of an aminoglycoside for treatment of an infection. Cisplatin-induced neu-

Table 43-3 Typical Undesirable Side Effects with Antineoplastic Drugs in Humans*

Tissue	Undesirable Effects
Bone marrow	Leukopenia, lymphocytopenia, and resulting infections
	Immunosuppression
	Thrombocytopenia
	Anemia
GI tract	Oral or intestinal ulceration
	Diarrhea
Hair follicles	Alopecia
Gonads	Menstrual irregularities, including premature menarche; impaired spermatogenesis
Wounds	Impaired healing
Fetus	Teratogenesis (especially during first trimester)

*Many of these effects are caused by drug action on nontumor cells that usually are growing (i.e., cycling).

DOSE-LIMITING SIDE EFFECTS

bleomycin: pulmonary fibrosis ("bleomycin lung")
busulfan: pulmonary fibrosis ("busulfan lung")
doxorubicin: cardiotoxicity
cisplatin: nephrotoxicity/peripheral neuropathy
carboplatin: myelosuppression
cyclophosphamide: hemorrhagic cystitis
vincristine: neurotoxicity
cytarabine: cerebral damage

ropathy occurs mainly in large sensory fibers and results in numbness/tingling followed by loss of a sense of joint position and a disabling sensory ataxia. The toxicity is reversible after discontinuation of drug but may require a year or longer to resolve. Nephrotoxicity was observed in many patients that received cisplatin early. Dosing regimens were modified to reduce the intensity of this toxicity. Cisplatin neuropathy is a more recently observed cumulative dose-limiting side effect. Carboplatin has less neurotoxicity and nephrotoxicity but more pronounced myelosuppression than cisplatin.

Bleomycin and busulfan both result in drug-induced pulmonary fibrosis, with this side effect dose limiting. Bleomycin is excreted in the urine 50% or more as unchanged drug. Drug dose should be reduced when creatinine clearance drops below 30 ml/min (from 120 ml/min standard). Bleomycin accumulates in the lungs and skin where bleomycin hydrolase (which in other tissues actively metabolizes the drug) is present at very low activity. The continued presence of elevated concentrations of bleomycin leads to recruitment of lymphocytes and polymorphonuclear leukocytes in bronchoalveolar fluids. It is not known how this leads to fibrosis. Hypersensitivity pneumonitis also is observed with bleomycin therapy but is less frequent with methotrexate, mitomycin C, nitrosoureas, and alkylating agents.

The major side effects with cytarabine are myelosuppression and dose-limiting cerebral damage. Ocular toxicity also has occasionally been associated with higher doses. GI upset, nausea, and vomiting are seen in almost all patients receiving higher doses of cytarabine administered to overcome drug transport resistance.

Doxorubicin and other clinically used anthracyclines have a dose-limiting side effect of myocardial failure. Doxorubicin usually is discontinued when the cumulative dose reaches 500 mg/m^2 body surface area or when cardiac output shows a significant decrease. The acute cardiac effects of hypotension, tachycardia, and arrhythmias are usually not clinically significant, but long-term effects leading to cardiac insufficiency can be life threatening and necessitate discontinuing drug therapy. The chronic effects appear after weeks to months of therapy. At a cumulative dose of >600 mg/m^2, 35% of patients experience congestive heart failure, which is refractory to medical management. The detailed mechanism is complex and not well understood but appears to involve Ca^{++}, calcium-ATPase, cAMP, and lipid peroxidation. The principal metabolite of doxorubicin, doxorubicinol (carbonyl side chain converted to an alcohol), is a potent inhibitor of Na^+, K^+-ATPase, Mg^{++}-ATPase and Ca^{++}-ATPase and may contribute to this serious side effect of an otherwise highly efficacious antitumor drug. Bone marrow and GI toxicity vary with the plasma concentrations of doxorubicin.

Cyclophosphamide, which undergoes metabolism to form an active compound and other reactive metabolites (Figure 41-8), produces hemorrhagic cystitis occasionally, although this can be largely eliminated with vigorous hydration of patients during cyclophosphamide administration. As little as a single IV dose of cyclophosphamide can produce the cystitis.

The cause appears to be acrolein, which is produced as a toxic by-product of the metabolism of cyclophosphamide. This side effect is not age- or sex-related and leads to a 9 to 45 times greater risk of developing bladder cancer. The likelihood of developing bladder cancer is not as severe for oral as compared to IV administered cyclophosphamide.

With methotrexate, vinblastine, etoposide, and 5-fluorouracil the main side effect is bone marrow suppression. Vinca alkaloids such as vincristine can cause peripheral neuropathy, but this is less frequent with VP-16.

Nearly all antineoplastic drugs have side effects that are considered by the patient as very objectionable.

TRADENAMES

In addition to generic and fixed combination preparations, the following tradenamed materials are available in the United States.

Adriamycin, doxorubicin HCl
Alkeran, melphalan
BiCNU, carmustine (BCNU)
Blenoxane, bleomycin sulfate
CeeNU, lomustine (CCNU)
Cerubidine, daunorubicin HCl
Cosmegen, actinomycin D
Cytosar-U, cytarabine
DTIC-Dome, dacarbazine
Efudex, Adrucil; 5-fluorouracil
Elspar, asparaginase
Hydrea, hydroxyurea
Intron-A, interferon alfa-2b
Leukeran, chlorambucil
Matulane, procarbazine HCl
Mexate, methotrexate sodium
Mustargen, mechlorethamine HCl
Mutamycin, mitomycin C
Myleran, busulfan
Neosar, cyclophosphamide
Nolvadex, tamoxifen citrate
Oncovin, Vincasar, vincristine sulfate
Paraplatin, carboplatin
Platinol, cisplatin
Purinethol, 6-mercaptopurine
Roferon-A, interferon alfa-2a
Tabloid, thioguanine
Velban, Velsar; vinblastine sulfate

REFERENCES

Burck KB, Liu ET, and Larrick JW: Oncogenes, an introduction to the concept of cancer genes, New York, 1988, Springer Verlag.

Evans WS, Crom WR, Abromowitch M et al.: Clinical pharmacodynamics of high-dose methotrexate in acute lymphocytic leukemia, N Engl J Med 314: 471, 1986.

Kamen BA and Winick NJ: High dose methotrexate therapy: insecure rationale?, Biochem Pharmacol 37:2713, 1988.

Pratt WB and Ruddon RW: The anticancer drugs, New York, 1979, Oxford University Press.

Rose KM: DNA topoisomerases as targets for chemotherapy, FASEB J 2:2474, 1988.

Woolley PV III and TEW KD, eds: Mechanisms of drug resistance in neoplastic cells, New York, 1988, Academic Press.

CHAPTER 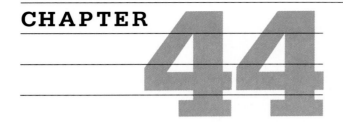 Clinical Effects with Antineoplastic Drugs

<table>
<tr><td colspan="2">ABBREVIATIONS</td></tr>
<tr><td>ALL</td><td>acute lymphocytic leukemia</td></tr>
<tr><td>AML</td><td>acute myelogenous leukemia</td></tr>
<tr><td>CGL</td><td>chronic granulocytic leukemia</td></tr>
</table>

 ## THERAPEUTIC OVERVIEW

A growing number of tumor types now respond to treatment with antineoplastic drugs. The types of clinical response to chemotherapy of advanced stage tumors in patients of various ages are listed in the box.

For children, relative 5-year survival data for the 1980s show about 90% success for Hodgkin's disease, about 85% for acute lymphocytic leukemia, and 97% for Wilms' tumor. Acute lymphocytic leukemia is the most common of the childhood neoplastic diseases, and expectations in 1990 are that about 95% should attain remission with at least one half of those being probable cures.

It is of interest to compare the list of tumor types (in the box), in which therapy has been aided greatly by antineoplastic drugs with the leading causes of cancer mortality to see if chemotherapy is effective on any of the most common forms of neoplastic diseases. Figure 44-1 summarizes the anatomical sites associated with the highest rates of cancer mortality for different patient ages. Overall, lung tumors in males and breast plus lung tumors in females are responsible for the greatest number of deaths from cancer. Some of the leukemias, lymphomas, breast

tumors, and small cell lung tumors appear in the box and Figure 44-1, indicating that these high mortality tumors are ones in which chemotherapy has proven beneficial. The small cell lung tumors represent only about 20% of lung neoplasms, with squamous cell carcinoma, adenocarcinoma, and great cell carcinoma making up another estimated 60% of lung neoplasms. Thus in spite of progress there is still a great need for more effective chemotherapy for the major neoplastic diseases.

DRUG SELECTION AND PROBLEMS

Primary Versus Adjuvant Chemotherapy

One of the difficulties in treating neoplastic diseases is that the tumor burden often is excessive by the time the diagnosis is made. This is shown schematically in Figure 44-2, where the number of cells in a typical solid tumor is shown versus time. With 10^9 cells roughly equivalent to a volume of 1 cubic centimeter in size and representing the minimum size for usual detection, the large number of cells already established at detection becomes readily evident. An upper limit of 10^{12} to 10^{13} tumor cells leads to the death of the patient. Thus by the time a tumor is detected, it has at least 10^9 to 10^{12} cells and has undergone many doublings. For acute lymphocytic leukemia, the cell doubling time during log phase (first order) growth is 3 to 4 days, whereas for lung squamous cell carcinoma it is estimated to be about 90 days. Thus in roughly 100 days, two lymphocytic leukemia cells in theory could keep doubling and reach 10^9 cells. Such a cell burden is extremely large to treat

RESPONSES OF CANCERS TO CHEMOTHERAPY

CANCERS IN WHICH COMPLETE REMISSIONS TO CHEMOTHERAPY ARE COMMON, AND CURES ARE SEEN EVEN IN ADVANCED DISEASE*

Acute lymphocytic leukemia (adults and children)
Hodgkin's disease (lymphoma)
Choriocarcinoma
Testicular cancer
Acute myelogenous leukemia
Burkitt's lymphoma
Ewing's sarcoma
Wilms' tumor
Small cell lung cancer
Ovarian cancer
Hairy cell leukemia

CANCERS IN WHICH OBJECTIVE RESPONSES ARE SEEN, BUT CHEMOTHERAPY DOES NOT HAVE CURATIVE POTENTIAL IN ADVANCED DISEASE

Multiple myeloma
Breast cancer
Head and neck cancer
Colorectal carcinomas
Chronic lymphocytic leukemia
Chronic myelogenous leukemia
Transitional cell carcinoma of bladder
Gastric adenocarcinomas
Cervical carcinomas
Medulloblastoma
Soft tissue sarcoma
Neuroblastoma
Endometrial carcinomas
Insulinoma
Osteogenic sarcoma

CANCERS IN WHICH ONLY OCCASIONAL OBJECTIVE RESPONSES TO CHEMOTHERAPY ARE SEEN

Non-small cell lung cancer
Melanoma
Renal tumor
Pancreatic carcinomas
Hepatocellular carcinoma
Prostate carcinomas

*Depending on tumor type, complete remission may result in cure of tumor.

only with drugs and is cited here to emphasize the difficulty of the therapeutic task under a typical diagnostic timetable.

In carrying out chemotherapy against a specific tumor type in an individual patient, the objective may

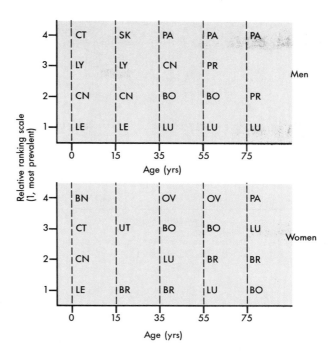

FIGURE 44-1   Leading sites of cancer mortality in 1986. *LE*, Leukemia; *BR*, breast; *LU*, lung; *BO*, colon/rectum; *CN*, central nervous; *PR*, prostate; *CT*, connective tissue; *UT*, uterine; *LY*, lymphoma; *BN*, bone; *OV*, ovary; *PA*, pancreas; *SK*, skin; *KY*, kidney.

be (1) curative, to obtain complete remission and cure the patient (e.g., Hodgkin's disease); (2) palliative, to improve symptoms but with little expectation of complete remission or cure (e.g., carcinoma of the esophagus with chemotherapy used to improve dysphagia); or (3) adjuvant, to improve chances for cure or to increase the period of disease-free survival when no detectable cancer is present, but subclinical numbers of neoplastic cells are suspected (e.g., chemotherapy for breast cancer after surgical resection of tumor).

Selection of Drug Regimen

Although choriocarcinoma (gestational trophoblastic disease) and hairy cell leukemia are treated using single drugs, nearly all other neoplasms are treated with drug combinations.

The choice of drugs and dosing schedule for multiple drug therapy has been and remains largely empirical, even though there are continuing efforts to

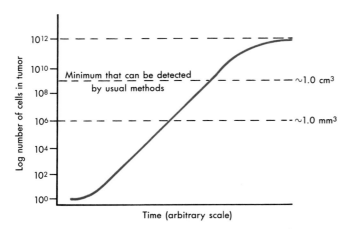

FIGURE 44-2   Typical tumor growth curve indicating roughly 10^9 cells needed for usual diagnosis.

try to understand why some combinations are more effective than others for certain tumor types. In spite of the empirical approach, several guidelines still need to be appreciated in selecting a combination of drugs. These guidelines are as follows:

1. Use drugs that show activity against the tumor type being treated. The rationale is that only rarely will a compound that shows no activity alone have an effect when used in combination.

2. Use drugs that have minimal or no overlapping toxicities. This requirement may broaden the range of the undesirable side effects of the drug combination. However, the goal of this guideline is to *reduce* the possibility of encountering life-threatening side effects that act in concert. For that reason, the side effects of the drugs selected should be diverse and not centered on the same organ system.

3. The dosing schedule for each drug should be optimal, and the doses should be given at consistent times. In establishing how often to repeat a dosing sequence, it is usual to allow sufficient time between the sequences to allow the most sensitive tissues (often bone marrow) to recover. Two weeks between sequences is often allowed for recovery.

4. Evaluate the degree of success of the combination chemotherapy on the basis of clinical effectiveness.

Many more scientific approaches have been used to select the drugs and dosing schedules for combination chemotherapy, but the results have been disappointing and usually not as good as those obtained with the empirical approach with clinical effectiveness as the evaluation criterion. Some approaches include drugs that have different mechanisms of action, in hopes that one mechanism would succeed where the others fail. Another goal of the multiple mechanism approach has been the hope of finding synergistic combinations. Several combinations are synergistic when tested against cultured tumor cells in vitro, including sequential methotrexate-5-fluorouracil; doxorubicin-cyclophosphamide; and cisplatin-VP16. A major problem of this approach is that the observed in vivo clinical results often do not correlate with the in vitro data.

The relative sequence of drugs and the timing of drug administration may play a significant role. Most of these drugs are more effective against tumor cells that are cycling than cells resting in the G_o phase, but in vivo, cells may be in any part of the cycle. The effectiveness of some drug combinations may be in part due to activation of cells from G_o to start cycling or to cycle more rapidly and thus place a greater number of cells in those portions of the cell cycle where the antineoplastic drugs can exert their cytotoxic actions. Because of this possibility, it is important that multidrug dosing schedules be followed accurately. Although existing antitumor drugs may affect the cycling of cells, the timing and sequence of drug combination administration and cellular results remains largely empirical.

Antineoplastic drugs are used as the primary mode of therapy when the tumor is known to be sensitive or when the feasibility for surgical removal or radiation destruction of the main tumor mass is poor. A more difficult situation is presented when the patient fails to respond to first line regimen of chemotherapy and alternative options are poor, thus suggesting that other chemotherapy approaches should be tried. Such patients are difficult to treat because the tumor volume may be large, the cells may be resistant to one or more of the usual drugs, and the general health of the patient is likely to be poor. An easier situation is the patient in which drugs can be used as an adjuvant following surgical and/or radiation removal of the primary tumor, such as in breast cancer.

Some examples of popular combination drug regimens are given in Table 44-1.

A trend exists toward the use of high-dose protocols with other drugs besides methotrexate to try

Table 44-1 Current Combination Drug Regimens

Terminology	Cancer	Drugs
MOPP	Hodgkin's	mechlorethamine, vincristine, procarbazine, prednisone
ABVD	Hodgkin's	doxorubicin, bleomycin, vinblastine, dacarbazine
CMF	Breast	cyclophosphamide, methotrexate, fluorouracil
CAF	Breast	cyclophosphamide, doxorubicin, fluorouracil
—	ALL	vincristine, prednisone, asparaginase later methotrexate, mercaptopurine
—	AML	cytarabine, daunorubicin
—	CGL	busulfan or hydroxyurea
—	Wilm's	actinomycin D, vincristine, doxorubicin
PACE	Small cell	cyclophosphamide, doxorubicin, cisplatin, etoposide
VIP	Germ cell cancers	etoposide, ifosfamide, cisplatin
BIP	Cervical cancer	bleomycin, ifosfamide, cisplatin
M-BACOD	Lymphoma	methotrexate, bleomycin, adriamycin, cyclophosphamide, vincristine (Oncovin), dexamethasone

ALL, Acute lymphocytic leukemia; *AML*, acute myelogenous leukemia; *CGL*, chronic granulocytic leukemia.

to push higher concentrations of drug into the tumor site and into the tumor cells. This trend is also being used with those drugs that undergo rapid degradation in plasma (e.g., cytarabine). In most cases the detailed studies needed to substantiate the efficacy of the higher dose protocols are missing or the conclusions are controversial. Therefore the use of high-dose protocols in some instances is questionable.

Special Clinical Problems

Two problems are particularly troublesome: (1) the risk of the patient developing leukemia (or other neoplastic condition) as a result of chemotherapy and (2) the frequent nausea and vomiting side effects with many of these drugs.

Several retrospective studies have been carried out to try to define the specific variables that increase the risk of leukemia developing in patients treated initially for Hodgkin's disease and others for ovarian tumors. From the roughly 30,000 patients with Hodgkin's disease, 163 developed leukemia between 1 and 10 years after being diagnosed with Hodgkin's disease. Many of them received MOPP (Table 44-1) for chemotherapy of the Hodgkin's disease. Because this rate of leukemia formation is much higher than would ordinarily be explained, the conclusion is reached that chemotherapy for Hodgkin's disease greatly increases the risk of leukemia and the data suggest that it occurs in a dose-dependent manner. However, this is a chilling conclusion because, without the MOPP pro-

TENDENCY OF ANTINEOPLASTIC DRUGS TO INDUCE NAUSEA OR VOMITING

STRONG TENDENCY

cisplatin, dacarbazine, mechlorethamine, cyclophosphamide, doxorubicin, CCMU, BCNU

MODERATE TENDENCY

daunorubicin, actinomycin D, catarabine, procarbazine, methotrexate, mitomycin C, etoposide

LOW TENDENCY

chlorambucil, vincristine, tamoxifen, vinblastine, bleomycin, hydroxyurea, fluorouracil

tocol treatment, these patients would have faced almost certain death. The increased leukemia risk must be put into perspective along with the clinical benefit. The risk of leukemia from chemotherapy is also an argument for not using high-dose chemotherapy unless the efficacy has been substantiated. Similarly, from 99,000 patients with ovarian tumor, 114 developed leukemia in about 1 to 10 years after being diagnosed with ovarian cancer. Chemotherapy (not radiotherapy or surgery) was associated with the higher incidence of leukemia, with the risk greatest with chlorambucil and melphalan and less with cyclophosphamide and thio-TEPA. The increased leukemia risk was also enhanced with higher doses of these drugs. It should be noted that not all chemotherapeutic drugs are associated with increased risk of leukemia. The increased risk is mainly with the use of alkylating agents.

Nausea and vomiting can be expected in about 70% of the patients receiving antineoplastic drugs. This figure remained the same based on observations of groups of patients in 1978, 1983, and 1987. Some of the drugs that are most and least likely to trigger this response are listed in the box, p. 609. Although clinical management of nausea and vomiting can become a serious problem, great strides have been made in its management. Some practical suggestions for controlling nausea and vomiting include the use of oral phenothiazine or dexamethasone as a first step, followed by oral or IM butyrophenone or oral/IV metoclopramide and diphenhydramine, and sedation with benzodiazepines if necessary.

BIOLOGICAL-RESPONSE MODIFIERS

Biological-response modifiers are a class of agents that stimulate the human immune system to destroy tumor cells. The α and β human interferons are efficacious in hairy cell leukemia and in certain skin cancers and may become aids for treating chronic myelogenous leukemia and non-Hodgkin's lymphoma. Interleukin-2 is another endogenous compound that has possibilities for applications in treating lung, renal, colorectal, and several other tumor types. Still other compounds include tumor necrosis factor, human growth factors, and monoclonal antibodies. These compounds are discussed in detail in Chapter 60 on immunopharmacology.

REFERENCES

Bannasch P, editor: Cancer therapy: New trends, Heidelberg, West Germany, 1989, Springer Verlag Inc.

Casciato DA and Lowitz BB: Manual of clinical oncology, ed 2, Boston, 1988, Little, Brown & Co.

Chabner BA and Collins JM, editors: Cancer chemotherapy: principles and practice, Philadelphia, 1990, JB Lippincott Co.

Foon KA: Biological response modifiers: the new immunotherapy, Cancer Res 49:1621, 1989.

Morrows GR: Management of nausea in the cancer patient. In Rosenthal S, Carignan JR, and Smith BD, editors: Medical care of the cancer patient, Philadelphia, 1987, WB Saunders Co.

Williams C: Cancer biology and management: an introduction, Chichester, 1990, John Wiley & Sons.

INVADING ORGANISMS: AGENTS THAT KILL INVADERS

Viruses, bacteria and other unicellular microorganisms, and multicellular organisms that exist in the environment also can live within the human body. This invading organism-host relationship can produce desirable, as well as undesirable biological responses within the host. In a healthy individual, bacterial flora of the gastrointestinal (GI) tract produce beneficial responses by assisting in the production of vitamins and in the breakdown of foodstuffs. However, when pathogenic organisms enter the GI tract, the human host may experience deleterious host-pathogen responses. The entry of pathogenic organisms can occur during oral ingestion, pulmonary inhalation, trauma, surgical procedures, and at any opening into a body compartment. These unwanted host-pathogen responses (termed *infections*) can occur directly through the release of toxins or antigens or indirectly through the generation of inflammation, invasion of tissues, or induction of disease states. Infections that arise from parasitic organisms gaining entry to the human host are the largest cause of morbidity and mortality worldwide. The infections often develop secondary to noninfectious primary disease states that diminish the natural defenses of the host.

Table VII-1 lists the types of pathogenic organisms that invade the human body and cause unwanted biological responses. The therapeutic approaches to the treatment of the infectious diseases, inflammation, toxins, or other responses generated by these invasions are twofold: (1) destruction or removal of the invading organisms and (2) alleviation of the symptoms. The availability of pharmacological agents that can successfully eradicate the invading organ-

Table VII-1 Invading Pathological Organisms That Can Live in a Parasitic Invader-Host Relationship in Humans, Listed in Order of Increasing Complexity

Cellular	Type	Typical Size (nm)
Acellular	Viruses	20–200
Unicellular	*Chlamydia* (P)	1000
Unicellular	Mycoplasmas (P)	1000
Unicellular	*Rickettsia* (P)	1000
Unicellular	Bacteria (P)	1000
Unicellular	Fungi: yeasts (E)	3000–5000
Unicellular	Protozoa (E)	
Multicellular	Fungi: molds (E)	2000–10,000 and larger
Multicellular	Helminths (E)	

P, Prokaryotes (no nuclear membrane); *E*, eukaryotes (with a nucleus).

isms varies considerably with the type and anatomical location of the organisms within the human host.

The only acellular organisms known to induce infectious disease states in humans are viruses. Other acellular proteinaceous agents called *prions* and small molecular weight acellular nucleic acids called *viroids* can exist in humans but probably do not contribute to human disease states, although the viruses that transmit dementia and kuru may be prions in disguise.

Viral infections are one of the major causes of temporary disabilities and work loss in humans, and some types of viral infections are fatal. Only a few effective pharmacological agents are available to halt the proliferation of or eliminate clinically important viruses.

611

The development of effective antiviral drugs has been hindered by the lack of rapid assay techniques for identifying the virus responsible for the infection in individual patients. Identification must be made early in the progression of the disease so that pharmacological therapeutic intervention can be started before the virus has widely disseminated or has caused its noxious effects. For some viral infections, prophylactic use of pharmacological agents may be the more effective strategy. The available pharmacological approaches and antiviral drugs are described in Chapter 51.

There are many unicellular pathogenic microorganisms—*Chlamydia*, mycoplasmas, *Rickettsia*, and bacteria—that are a major cause of human morbidity and mortality. The mycoplasmas, *Chlamydia* and *Rickettsia*, have only a few species that infect humans; however, there are many different bacteria that cause infectious diseases, and the pathogenicity of a bacterial species may change with time. Progress made in other areas of medicine has caused microorganisms that once were considered only commensal to be known as serious life-threatening invaders. An example of such organisms are the coagulase-negative staphylococci.

Many chemical and pharmacological approaches have been utilized in devising drugs to destroy specific bacteria, while producing minimal adverse effects on the human host. The many antimicrobial drugs and the vast variety of infectious unicellular microorganisms may seem overwhelming to the embryonic clinician. However, by noting common aspects in the mechanism of action or chemical structure of different drugs and by noting further that some drugs are more efficacious in certain anatomical regions than in other regions, it is possible to organize this topic into an easier to understand and easier to master outline. Note that the specific microbial strains of clinical relevance change with time. New strains of microorganisms appear, existing strains develop resistance to previously highly efficacious antimicrobial drugs, old strains disappear, and new problems develop with old, relatively benign strains. This further complicates the use of drugs in treatment and demands that the clinician stay informed.

The organizational scheme for drugs used to treat bacterial and related infections and some principles specific to the use of antimicrobial drugs are discussed in Chapter 45. A large group of agents act by inhibiting the synthesis of bacterial cell walls (Chapter 46). Another large group of agents act at the ribosomal level to inhibit bacterial protein synthesis (Chapter 47). Drugs that act on the bacterial tetrahydrofolate cofactor system are described in Chapter 48, and bacterial DNA replication inhibitors, along with drugs that create openings in bacterial membranes, are discussed in Chapter 49. Guidelines for the use of antibacterial drugs are summarized in Chapter 50. Chapter 51 is reserved for the special drugs used to treat mycobacterial infections, which are the cause of tuberculosis and leprosy.

The bacteria are characterized as unicellular, nonnuclear organisms. Higher orders of size and complexity are found in unicellular, nucleated fungi (which include yeast and filamentous forms) and in protozoa. The major differences are the addition of a membrane-enclosed nucleus and mitochondria within the cell. More complex fungi are found in the multicellular, nucleated molds. Still higher orders of parasitic invading organisms are the helminths (worms), estimated to infect 40% to 60% of the world population and are a medical problem in industrialized, as well as developing, countries. Drugs used in the treatment of infections resulting from these more complex invading organisms are discussed in separate chapters for fungi (Chapter 52), protozoa (Chapter 54), and helminths (Chapter 55). Although antiseptics and disinfectants are not used as drugs, these compounds are important for cleansing the skin and preparing instruments and materials used during surgery and are described in Chapter 56.

The term *chemotherapy* was coined in the 1950s to indicate the use of complex chemicals for the treatment of microbial infections (i.e., administering chemicals that inhibited or killed the invading microorganisms). Since then the term has been used in a broader context to include the use of drugs to kill any type of cell, microbial or mammalian. Therefore the term no longer is applied only to the treatment of infections caused by invading organisms but also in the treatment of neoplastic diseases, as mentioned in Chapters 43 and 44.

45

Principles of Antimicrobial Use

The era of modern microbial chemotherapy stems from the work in the early 1900s of Paul Ehrlich, who suggested that antimicrobial drugs might be found that would be chemically allied to molecular sites of action on parasitic organisms. He suggested further that this approach would be most useful if these parasitic sites of action were not present in the organs and tissues of the human host. Ehrlich defined the selective drug action of chemotherapeutic agents, beginning with the use of arsenic compounds, which subsequently led to the development of the sulfonamides. These compounds illustrated that the activity of some agents could be predicted from their physical-chemical structures.

The next breakthrough was the 1929 discovery in Great Britain of penicillin by Fleming, who demonstrated the ubiquitous nature of these agents and that antimicrobial substances could be found in molds and other microorganisms that exist in the soil. Although thousands of potential antimicrobial agents have been found in nature or synthesized chemically in the past 60 years, only a very small percentage of these have proven to be effective, nontoxic agents when used therapeutically.

The term *antibiotic* traditionally refers to substances produced by microorganisms to suppress the growth of other microorganisms. The term *antimicrobial agents* is broader in meaning since it encompasses agents synthesized in the laboratory as well as those natural antibiotics produced by microorganisms. Many agents used clinically today are produced industrially by chemical synthesis, even if orginally produced by microbial fermentation. Many agents are semisynthetic, that is, the key portion of the compound is produced industrially by microbial fermentation, and various moieties are synthetically attached. Thus the distinction between the terms "antibiotics" and "antimicrobials," or "antimicrobial agents," has little meaning today.

Antimicrobial agents can be *bactericidal* (i.e., the organisms are killed) or *bacteriostatic* (i.e., the organisms stop growing) (Figure 45-1). Both bacteriostatic and bactericidal agents are effective as chemotherapeutic drugs, but both also rely upon host defenses to aid in eliminating the pathogens. In some clinical conditions, the lack of host defenses, such as complement or antibody, makes it mandatory that bactericidal agents be used. A given agent may show bactericidal actions under certain conditions but bacteriostatic actions under other conditions, depending on the concentration of drug and the target bacteria.

Antimicrobial agents can be classified into five ma-

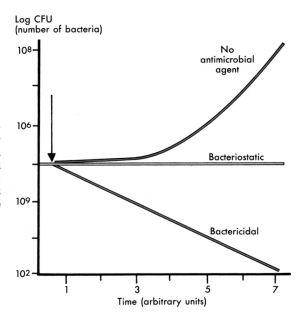

FIGURE 45-1 Bactericidal versus bacteriostatic antimicrobial agents. A typical culture is started at 10^5 colony forming units (CFU) and incubated at 37° C for various times (time in arbitrary units). With no antimicrobial agent, there is cell growth. With a bacteriostatic agent added, no growth occurs, but neither are the existing cells killed. If the added agent is bactericidal, 99.9% of the cells will be killed during the standardized test time.

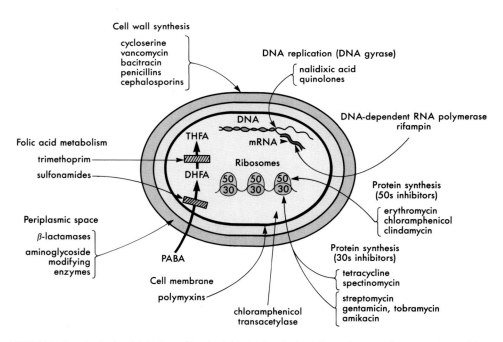

FIGURE 45-2 Antimicrobial sites of bactericidal or bacteriostatic action on microorganisms. The five general mechanisms are: (1) inhibit synthesis of cell wall, (2) damage outer membrane, (3) modify nucleic acid/DNA synthesis, (4) modify protein synthesis (at ribosomes), and (5) modify energy metabolism within the cytoplasm (at folate cycle).

Table 45-1 Classification of Antimicrobial Agents by Mechanism of Action

Mechanism of Action	Agent	Discussion in Chapter
Inhibition of synthesis or damage to cell wall	penicillins	46
	cephalosporins	46
	monobactams	46
	carbapenems	46
	bacitracin	46
	vancomycin	46
	cycloserine	51
Inhibition of synthesis or damage to cytoplasmic membrane	polymyxins	49
	polyene antifungals	52
Synthesis or metabolism of nucleic acids	quinolones	49
	rifampin	51
	nitrofurantoins	49
	nitroimidazoles	55
Protein synthesis	aminoglycosides	47
	tetracyclines	47
	chloramphenicol	47
	erythromycin	47
	clindamycin	47
	spectinomycin	47
	mupirocin	47
Modification to energy metabolism	sulfonamides	48
	trimethoprim	48
	dapsone	51
	isoniazid	51

jor groups according to the point in the cellular biochemical pathways at which the agent exerts its primary mechanism of action (Figure 45-2). These groups are (1) inhibition of synthesis and damage to the peptidoglycan cell wall, (2) inhibition of synthesis or damage to the cytoplasmic membrane, (3) modification in synthesis or metabolism of nucleic acids, (4) inhibition or modification of protein synthesis, and (5) modification in energy metabolism. The agents that inhibit synthesis of cell walls include the β-lactams, such as penicillins, cephalosporins, and monobactams, and others such as bacitracin and vancomycin. Inhibitors of cytoplasmic membranes include the polymyxins. In fungi the cell wall is damaged by the polyene antifungal agents or by the imidazoles. Inhibitors of nucleic acid synthesis include the quinolones, which inhibit DNA gyrase, and the RNA polymerase inhibitor rifampin. Protein synthesis is inhibited by aminoglycosides, which are bactericidal, and by tetracyclines, chloramphenicol, erythromycin, and clindamycin, which are usually bacteriostatic, depending on the microorganism involved. Finally,

folate antagonists such as sulfonamides and trimethoprim interfere with cell metabolism. The five major types of antimicrobial drugs according to their mechanisms of action are listed in Table 45-1.

SELECTION OF DRUG FOR INDIVIDUAL PATIENTS

Major factors that need to be considered in the selection of antimicrobial agents for therapy of individual patients are outlined in the box. If the desired procedure of identifying the organism and demonstrating susceptibility to a specific antimicrobial agent is followed, then the expectation for successful therapy is high. Unfortunately, the practical use of antimicrobial agents is more complex, because the initial antimicrobial therapy is often begun empirically without precise identification of the pathogen.

Each of the factors in the box is discussed in the following pages. The goal is to provide an overall perspective of the relative importance of each of the

---

> ## FACTORS FOR SELECTION OF ANTIMICROBIAL AGENTS FOR THERAPY IN INDIVIDUAL PATIENTS
>
> Identification of organism
> Antimicrobial susceptibility of organism
> Bactericidal versus bacteriostatic
> Host status
>   Allergy history
>   Age
>   Pharmacokinetic factors
>   Renal function
>   Hepatic function
>   Pregnancy status
>   Genetic factors
>   Anatomical site of infection
>   Host defenses, white cell function

factors before launching into the description and discussion of individual antimicrobial agents in subsequent chapters. When reference is made to individual antimicrobial agents in the present chapter, the points are reiterated in the chapters on the individual agents. Because of the importance of microbial resistance to drugs, this topic is discussed in a separate section in the latter part of this chapter and in the chapters on the individual antibacterial drugs. Clinical guidelines for the selection of antibiotics are given in Chapter 50.

Identification of Organisms

Before initiating antimicrobial therapy, it is highly desirable to determine the possible pathogen(s) in the infection site. Several direct techniques are available to identify the microorganisms.

The Gram's stain is the fastest, simplest, and most inexpensive method to identify bacteria and fungi. Any body fluid that normally is sterile should be gram stained. However, wound exudates, sputum, and fecal material can provide only preliminary information concerning the infecting microorganisms.

In addition to Gram's staining, agglutination, immunoelectrophoresis, and direct immunofluorescence techniques can be used for detection of some organisms. When it is not possible to obtain a specimen, knowledge of the most commonly infecting organisms can be used to direct therapy. For example, cellulitis can be caused by group A streptococci or by *Staphylococcus aureus*. Knowledge that these two species could be present, combined with knowledge of the resistance of staphylococci to certain antimicrobial drugs, should influence the choice of antimicrobial agent. Otitis media is primarily caused by *Streptococcus pneumoniae*, *Haemophilus influenzae*, or *Moraxella catarrhalis*. Knowledge of the incidence of β-lactamase positive *Haemophilus* isolates in a community should influence the selection of the antimicrobial agent.

Antimicrobial Agent Susceptibility of Infecting Microorganisms

The susceptibility of bacteria to specific antimicrobial agents can be determined by several methods, but the results of these tests generally are not available until 18 to 48 hours after an initial culture sample has been obtained.

One of the most common methods for determining bacterial susceptibility to antibiotics is the disk diffusion method. This is simple to perform, inexpensive, and provides data within 18 to 24 hours; however, this method is only semiquantitative and is not useful for many slow-growing or fastidious organisms. In the disk test, the surface of an agar plate is inoculated with a swab moistened with a dilution of the unknown culture. Paper disks of standard size impregnated with an antimicrobial agent are placed on this "lawn" of bacteria and incubated for 18 to 24 hours at 37° C. The test drugs diffuse from the disk into the agar, with the concentration of antibiotic diminishing at further distances from the disk. The amount of drug impregnated in the disk is selected to provide an inhibitory zone around the periphery of the disk for susceptible organisms. The diameter of the inhibitory zone is related linearly to the logarithm of the concentration of drug. The test procedure and typical results are shown schematically in Figure 45-3. Results from the disk test are provided as susceptible, resistant, and intermediate for the tested drugs. For example, an ampicillin disk may contain 10 μg of ampicillin. A zone of inhibition ≥ 14 mm indicates the organism is susceptible, whereas a zone ≤ 11 mm indicates the organism is resistant. A susceptible zone of inhibition correlates with the serum and urine concentrations that can be achieved using recommended doses of a particular agent in most patients.

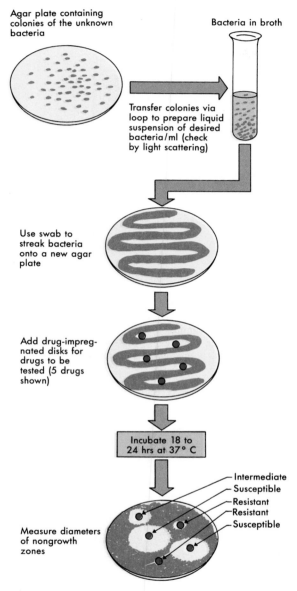

Agar plate containing colonies of the unknown bacteria

Bacteria in broth

Transfer colonies via loop to prepare liquid suspension of desired bacteria/ml (check by light scattering)

Use swab to streak bacteria onto a new agar plate

Add drug-impregnated disks for drugs to be tested (5 drugs shown)

Incubate 18 to 24 hrs at 37° C

Intermediate
Susceptible
Resistant
Resistant
Susceptible

Measure diameters of nongrowth zones

FIGURE 45-3 Disk diffusion method for testing bacteria for susceptibility to specific antimicrobial agents (see text).

Quantitative data on the antibiotic susceptibility of microorganisms can be determined by methods using broth or agar dilution. These methods detect the lowest concentration of antimicrobial agent that prevents visible growth after an 18-to 24-hour incubation. This concentration is referred to as the *minimal inhibitory concentration* (MIC). The agar or broth contains antibiotics in serial twofold dilutions that encompass the concentrations normally achieved in humans. The technique is described schematically in Figure 45-4. Deciding whether the results show the organisms to be susceptible or not requires an understanding of the pharmacokinetics of the antimicrobial agent. The plasma half-life of many antibiotics is short, so for a typical dosing schedule of 3 or 4 times per day, each dose is eliminated before the next dose is administered. This results in a plot of plasma concentration of drug versus time as in Figure 45-5, shown for IV administration to minimize the complexity of the curve. In general an organism is considered susceptible to the drug when the MIC is one fourth or less of the readily obtainable peak plasma concentration. This same test procedure can be extended further to determine the *minimal bactericidal concentration* (MBC) or minimal concentration that kills 99.9% of the microbial cells. Samples are removed from the antibiotic-containing tubes in which there is no visible microbial growth and plated on agar that contains no additional antibiotic. The lowest concentration tube from which bacteria do not grow on the agar is the MBC (see Figure 45-4). MBC determinations are necessary in only a few clinical situations, such as endocarditis or some cases of osteomyelitis or meningitis.

Because of the large number of antimicrobial agents available, it is difficult to test routinely all antimicrobial agents against an isolate. Laboratories often use one compound as representative of a group of compounds. For example, cefazolin is used as the prototype for all first-generation cephalosporins. However, marked differences in pharmacokinetics and in vitro activity have prevented finding a prototype agent for second-generation cephalosporins. It is important to recognize that susceptibility tests require interpretation. Furthermore, certain organisms such as methicillin-resistant *S. aureus* may appear susceptible to cephalosporin antibiotics, but these would not be eradicated by such drugs. Susceptibility tests may also fail to identify a resistant subset population. This may be of importance if the mechanism of resistance to an antimicrobial agent results from an effect on an enzyme that is normally repressed in the absence of the antimicrobial agent, and the sample under test does not reflect this subpopulation. This occurs with bacteria such as *Enterobacter* tested with cephalosporins or with staphylococci tested with clindamycin.

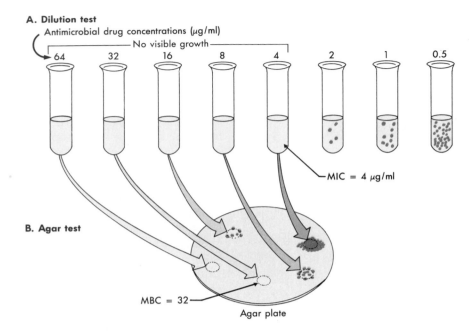

A. Dilution test
Antimicrobial drug concentrations (μg/ml)

No visible growth

| 64 | 32 | 16 | 8 | 4 | 2 | 1 | 0.5 |

MIC = 4 μg/ml

B. Agar test

MBC = 32

Agar plate

FIGURE 45-4 Dilution/agar tests for determination if MIC and MBC for a given drug and microorganism. **A,** Dilution test: each tube contains 5×10^5 colony forming units (CFU) of bacteria, plus antibiotic at the concentration indicated. The MIC is the minimum drug concentration at which no visible growth of bacteria is observed (4μg/ml in this example). **B,** Dilution/agar test: each tube in **A** that showed no visible growth is cultured on a section of the new agar plate (no additional antibiotic is added to the agar plate). The MBC is the lowest concentration where no growth occurred on the agar (32 μg/ml in this example).

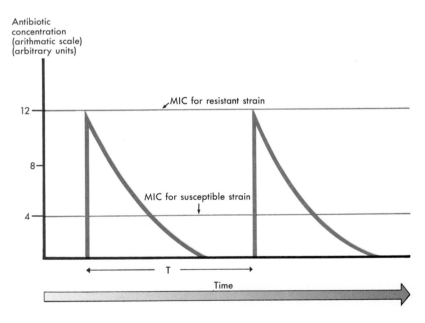

Antibiotic
concentration
(arithmatic scale)
(arbitrary units)

MIC for resistant strain

12

8

MIC for susceptible strain

4

T

Time

FIGURE 45-5 Plasma concentration of antibiotic versus time for IV administration. Drug from each dose is eliminated before next dose is administered. *T* is the dosing interval (see chapter 4). Resistant organisms require too high a concentration to be treated successfully with this drug at the doses used to obtain the peak concentrations shown. *MIC,* Minimum inhibitory concentration.

Bactericidal Versus Bacteriostatic Drug

One of the first decisions that must be made in antimicrobial therapy is whether a bactericidal therapy is required. In uncomplicated infections a bacteriostatic agent often is adequate, since the host defenses will contribute to the eradication of the microorganism. For example, in pneumococcal pneumonia, tetracyclines, which are bacteriostatic agents, suppress the multiplication of the pneumococci; however, destruction of the pneumococci is achieved by the interaction of alveolar macrophages and polymorphonuclear leukocytes. For a neutropenic individual, such a bacteriostatic agent might prove ineffective and a bactericidal agent would be necessary. Thus the status of the host influences the selection of either a bactericidal or bacteriostatic agent.

In some infections, bactericidal antimicrobial agents are necessary. Effective therapy of bacterial endocarditis requires bactericidal agents. Treatment with bacteriostatic antibiotics such as tetracyclines or erythromycin has an unacceptably high failure rate in contrast to cure rates in excess of 95% with bactericidal agents such as penicillin. Meningitis is another illness where bactericidal therapy is necessary. In meningitis, concentrations of an antimicrobial agent 8- to 10-fold above the MBC must be achieved within the spinal fluid to affect a cure. Thus susceptibility is not the only criterion for efficacy, but a drug must achieve concentrations 4-to 16-fold above the inhibitory concentration to be effective. Cefamandole inhibits *H. influenzae* and will cure pneumonia caused by *Haemophilus* organisms, but it will not cure most patients with *Haemophilus* meningitis, since CSF concentrations of the drug are usually inadequate. Unless peak serum concentrations are 8- to 16-fold above the MIC in neutropenic patients, there is a predictable high rate of failure.

Host Status

Allergy History A history of any previous allergic reaction is important in selecting an antimicrobial agent because a similar reaction to other members of the same drug class may occur. Allergy to penicillins is an important factor. Anaphylactic reactions to any penicllin compound preclude the subsequent use of penicillins. However, a rash after use of ampicillin in a patient with mononucleosis may not indicate true allergy to all penicillins, and in special situations penicillin could be used if the patient does not have a

Table 45-2 Antimicrobial Agents to be Avoided During Pregnancy

Agent	Toxicity
ANTIBACTERIAL	
aminoglycosides	Possible VIII nerve damage
chloramphenicol	Gray baby syndrome
erythromycin estolate	Cholestatic hepatitis
metronidazole	Possible teratogenic
nitrofurantoin	Hemolytic anemia
sulfonamides	Hemolysis in newborn with G6PD deficiency; increased risk of kernicterus
tetracyclines	Limb abnormalities, dental staining, inhibition of bone growth
trimethoprim	Altered folate metabolism
quinolones	Abnormalities of cartilage
vancomycin	Possible auditory toxicity
ANTIFUNGAL	
griseofulvin	Teratogenic in animals
ketoconazole	Teratogenic in animals
ANTITUBERCULOSIS	
isoniazid	Use with caution
rifampin	Use with caution
ANTIVIRAL	
amantadine	Teratogenic

positive skin test. Patients allergic to one sulfonamide are allergic to all sulfonamides. Allergy to aminoglycosides is rare. However, cutaneous eruptions ranging from urticaria to exfoliative dermatitis have been reported with every class of antiobiotics.

Age Factors Many antibiotics are removed from the body by renal elimination, which may undergo change with age. The pH of gastric secretions also is affected as part of the aging process and may influence selection of a drug. Certain antibiotics should not be given to children. For example, tetracyclines that bind to developing teeth and bone and that cross the placenta will affect the fetus and are to be avoided (Table 45-2). Similarly, sulfonamides should not be given to newborns because they displace bilirubin from serum albumin and can produce kernicterus (i.e., CNS disorder).

Pharmacokinetic Factors The administration of antimicrobial agents is usually via the oral, IM, or IV routes. Although absorption can occur following topical or rectal administration, these routes of drug delivery are uncommon. Most antimicrobial agents yield peak serum concentrations 1 to 2 hours after oral administration. Peak concentrations may be delayed when antimicrobial agents are ingested with food or in patients with delayed intestinal transit such as sometimes occurs with diabetics. After IM injections, peak plasma concentrations occur in 0.5 to 1 hour; following IV infusions of 20 to 30 minutes, the peak occurs at the end of the infusion.

The amount of antimicrobial agent that reaches the extravascular tissues and fluids, where the infection is usually present, depends on the concentration gradient between plasma and target tissue, the degree of drug binding to plasma and tissue proteins, molecular size, degree of ionization and lipid solubility of the drug, and rate of elimination or metabolism of the agent. Considerable variation exists in each of these factors among the many diverse types of chemical compounds that make up the list of clinically useful antimicrobial agents.

Renal Function Many antimicrobial agents are eliminated from the body by renal filtration and/or secretion. Since renal function changes with patient age, some antimicrobial agents can accumulate in the body and cause serious toxic reactions without a proper adjustment in dosing regimen. Toxicity may be to the kidney or to other organs. Dosage adjustments for these agents eliminated by glomerular filtration usually can be estimated on the basis of age, body size, and serum creatinine.

Aminoglycoside and certain penicillin, cephalosporin, carbapenem, and quinolone dosing schedules need to be adjusted to compensate for diminished renal function. Decreased renal function promotes hypoalbuminemia caused by poor nutrition and produces substances in blood that decrease binding of drugs to albumin to give greater concentrations of free drug. Decreased renal function also leads to increased ototoxicity from aminoglycosides, some interference with platelet function by penicillins, and neurotoxicity from penicillins, imipenem, quinolones, and polymyxins.

Hepatic Function Antimicrobials that are metabolized in the liver include chloramphenicol, erythromycin, rifampin, nitroimidazoles, and some of the quinolones. Reduction in dosage may be necessary to avoid toxic reactions in patients with impaired hepatic function. Chloramphenicol toxicity in newborns is related to failure to convert the drug to an inactive, nontoxic glucuronide. In combined hepatic-renal disease the half-life of some drugs, such as ticarcillin, increases significantly.

Pregnancy Pregnant patients or nursing mothers pose important problems in the use of antimicrobial agents, since most of these drugs cross the placenta to some degree. One must consider both the teratogenic and toxic potentials of these drugs on the fetus (Table 45-2). Certain agents such as metronidazole are teratogenic in lower animals and therefore may have this effect in humans. Other agents such as rifampin and trimethoprim may have teratogenic potential and should be used only when alternative agents are unavailable.

Use of tetracyclines in pregnancy should be avoided because they alter fetal dentition and bone growth. Tetracyclines have also been associated with hepatic, pancreatic, and renal damage in pregnant women. Streptomycin has been associated with auditory toxicity in children of mothers treated for tuberculosis. Sulfonamides should not be used in the third trimester of pregnancy because they may displace bilirubin from albumin binding sites and cause CNS toxicity in the fetus.

Many antibiotics are excreted in breast milk and can distort the newborn's microflora or act as a sensitizing agent to cause future allergy.

Genetic Factors Genetic abnormalities of enzyme function may affect the potential for toxicity of certain agents.

Hemolysis in glucose-6-phosphate dehydrogenase (G6PD) deficient individuals can be provoked by sulfonamides, nitrofurantoin, pyrimethamine, sulfones, and chloramphenicol. Individuals who do not acetylate drugs well may not inactivate isoniazid adequately and can develop peripheral neuropathy unless treated with pyridoxine. Since 50% of the U.S. population are slow acetylators, pyridoxine usually is prescribed with isoniazid.

Anatomical Site of Infection The site of infection often determines not only the antimicrobial agent but also the dose, route, and duration of drug administration. The desired peak concentration of drug at the site of infection should equal at least four times the MIC. However, if host defenses are adequate, then the peak concentration of antibiotic may be much lower and even equal to the MIC and still be effective. When host defenses are absent or inoperative, then peak concentrations of antibiotic 8- to 16-fold above the MIC may be required.

Antimicrobial agents readily enter most body tissues and compartments with the exception of the spinal fluid, brain, eye, and prostate. Concentrations adequate to treat infections of the pleural, pericardial, and joint spaces can be obtained by using the parenteral route. Antibiotics, however, may not be active in abscesses because of the low pH and the reservoir of pus and necrotic debris.

Infected heart valves provide an example of a problem associated with the infection site. Bacteria trapped in a fibrin matrix divide at a slow rate and many antibiotics are effective only on growing microorganisms. Antibiotics used in endocarditis therefore must be bactericidal, administered at high concentrations, and administered for prolonged periods so that diffusion of the antibiotic into the matrix is achieved and all bacteria are killed.

Meningitis is a difficult problem because many antimicrobial agents do not cross the blood-brain or blood-CSF barriers very well. Lipid-soluble agents such as chloramphenicol easily enter the CSF, as do agents like rifampin and metronidazole; however, aminoglycosides do not cross the CSF barrier even in the presence of inflammation. Penicillins, aztreonam, cephalosporins, and imipenem enter the CSF in the presence of meningitis to variable degrees depending upon the compound. Quinolones such as ciprofloxacin also enter the CSF at concentrations adequate to kill some microorganisms.

Osteomyelitis is an infection where an extended duration of therapy is required. Less than 4 weeks of drug administration usually results in high rates of failure to eradicate the infections. The concentration of antibiotic in bone is often low, and the bacteria are sequestered and thus prevented from coming in contact with the antibiotics.

Antimicrobial drug therapy frequently is ineffective in the presence of a foreign body such as an indwelling urethral catheter, an artificial joint, or a prosthetic heart valve. In the presence of the foreign body, microorganisms accumulate on the foreign surface and become covered with a glycocalyx coating. Large numbers of microorganisms growing at a slow rate in a sessile form are present on the foreign body, and they are protected by the coating from attack by leukocytes and most importantly from destruction by antimicrobial agents.

Microorganisms also persist in abscesses. The impairment of circulation in an abscess reduces the delivery of antibody, complement, and leukocytes.

Moreover, complement is destroyed in abscesses and cannot potentiate destruction of bacteria by leukocytes, and because of the absence of adequate oxygen and the acidic environment in an abscess, leukocytes function less effectively. Bacteria in an abscess frequently grow at a much slower rate than at other infection sites and are not killed by antimicrobial agents that easily kill them when they are rapidly dividing. In some situations the antimicrobial agent is destroyed by enzymes induced by the microorganisms or by enzymes released when the microorganisms are killed by the antibiotic that penetrates into the abscess. Antibiotic therapy can rarely cure established abscesses, lesions containing foreign bodies, or infections associated with excretory duct obstruction, unless these sites are drained surgically or by placement of catheters that drain the abcess.

Some infections are caused by microorganisms that are not destroyed when they are ingested by polymorphonuclear phagocytes or macrophages. Common pathogenic organisms such as *S. pneumoniae* or *S. aureus* are readily killed by antimicrobial agents that do not enter phagocytic cells. However, subinhibitory concentrations of antimicrobial agents can alter the surface properties of these bacteria so that when ingested, the microorganisms are more rapidly destroyed by the phagocytic cells. In contrast, some *Mycobacterium*, *Legionella*, and *Salmonella* species, for example, can survive within phagocytic cells, and antimicrobial agents that do not penetrate into the phagocytic cells often are not successful in eradicating infection caused by these organisms. The success of compounds such as isoniazid and rifampin in the treatment of *Mycobacterium tuberculosis* is because these agents enter mononuclear cells in which tubercule bacilli survive and the antimicrobial agents cause the death of the bacilli within the phagocytic cells.

Agents that do not readily enter phagocytic cells can still be effective in curing infections resulting from intracellular organisms such as *Listeria* if the antimicrobial agent is administered for a long enough period of time. Ampicillin can be used to cure an infection due to *Listeria* if the antibiotic is administered for a long time; ampicillin kills the extracellular bacteria and also alters their surface properties, increasing their destruction by macrophages. Individuals with diseases of the lymphoid system, such as chronic lymphocytic leukemia or acquired immune deficiency syndrome (AIDS), can have recurrent relapses of infection such as from *Salmonella* organisms because of inadequate white cell function and therefore reduced capacity to use the modified bacterial surface properties for phagocytic destruction of the microorganisms.

Bacterial infections associated with obstructions of the urinary, biliary, or respiratory tracts tend to persist despite antibiotic therapy. Antimicrobial agent penetration into these areas is poor, and bacteria present within the obstructed regions are in a quiescent state from which they emerge when antimicrobial therapy is discontinued since most agents do not kill resting bacteria.

Host Defenses   Absence of white cells predisposes a patient to serious bacterial infection, and in such cases bacteriostatic agents are inadequate to protect these neutropenic hosts. The critical white cell count is between 500 and 1000 mature polymorphonuclear cells/mm³. Other host defects that require use of bactericidal agents are agammaglobulinemia or asplenia, which predisposes to pneumococcal or *Haemophilus* infection, or the absence of complement components C7 to C9, which protect against *Neisseria* species. Knowledge of the organisms most frequently causing infections in patients with defects of white cells, complement, T-cells, or immunoglobulin production will aid in the selection of bactericidal antimicrobial agents to be used when such patients develop fever.

PROPHYLAXIS WITH ANTIMICROBIAL AGENTS

Prophylaxis should be directed at preventing a specific bacterial infection. This means that a particular species or several species have been shown to produce the infection, that an effective antimicrobial agent is available, and that the risk of the infection outweighs the hazard of using the antimicrobial agent. The antibiotic must be delivered to the site of probable infection at an appropriate time so that the agent will inhibit bacteria that would colonize the area and subsequently produce an infection. The use of the antimicrobial agent must be of limited duration to avoid toxicity and prevent selection of resistant bacterial flora by elimination of normal flora.

Prophylaxis can be considered in both medical and surgical situations. Medical conditions include the prevention of meningococcal meningitis, *Haemophi-*

lus meningitis, recurrent rheumatic fever, postsplenectomy infections, cellulitis complicating lymphedema, recurrent lower urinary tract infections, tuberculosis, and bacterial endocarditis. A special medical problem is the prevention of infection in the neutropenic patient. Many surgical problems require prophylaxis, including upper gastrointestinal surgery, cholecystectomy, colon surgery, appendectomy, head and neck surgery, cardiac surgery, prosthetic hip and other joint surgery, hysterectomy, and Cesarean section. The optimal agent for each condition has not been established.

An important prophylactic use of antibiotics is to prevent bacterial endocarditis. Individuals with valvular or structural lesions of the heart, where endocarditis is common, should receive antibiotic prophylaxis at the time of surgical, dental, or other procedures that may produce a high degree of bacteremia. Prophylaxis is administered just before the procedure. This method prevents the selection of resistant bacteria, reduces the number of organisms that could lodge on the valvular tissue, and alters the surface properties of the microorganism so they have reduced affinity for cardiac tissue. Since viridans group streptococci from the mouth or intestine, enterococci from the intestine or genitourinary tract, and staphylococci from skin have the greatest propensity to cause endocarditis, prophylaxis should be directed against these organisms.

The use of oral antibiotics to reduce aerobic fecal flora of neutropenic patients is controversial. A number of studies indicate that aerobic Gram-negative bacterial infections in neutropenic patients are caused by passage of bacteria across the intestinal wall with resultant bacteremia. The use of agents that eliminate aerobic bacteria but do not destroy anaerobic and streptococcal flora reduces the incidence of bacteremias in the neutropenic patient.

Prophylaxis can also be effective without eradication of all bacteria. Topical application of silver sulfadiazine to a burn wound will reduce the number of bacteria in the burn eschar to less than 10⁵ per gram of tissue and prevent burn wound sepsis.

For the prevention of postoperative wound infections, the antimicrobial agent must be present at the probable site of infection when the area may be exposed to the bacteria. The antibiotic must be given immediately preoperatively or during the operation and should inhibit the most common and important bacteria likely to produce infection.

Prophylaxis should also be used in procedures in which contamination is probable. The surgical procedures that require prophylaxis are those in which there is insertion of a foreign body, such as a heart valve or an orthopedic prosthesis. In these situations if infection develops, the consequences are so drastic that the short use of antibiotics is a minor risk.

There are disadvantages to the prophylactic use of antibiotics. Toxic or hypersensitivity (allergic) reactions may occur and superinfection with a more resistant flora can develop. Infection may be temporarily masked or there may be alteration of the ecology of the hospital flora, leading to the selection of more resistant bacteria.

MONITORING ANTIMICROBIAL THERAPY

It is critical that serum or plasma drug concentrations be determined for some antimicrobial agents to ensure that therapeutic but not toxic concentrations are attained. This is particularly important in patients with diminished renal function who are receiving antibiotics that undergo renal elimination.

The measurement of serum bactericidal titers to monitor antimicrobial therapy has primarily been used in treatment of bacterial endocarditis. Although guidelines have been developed for the size of bacterial inoculum, composition of the bacterial growth medium, amount of serum added, etc., results of this test are subject to great variability even in the most trained hands. A peak serum bactericidal titer greater than 1:8 has been correlated with successful outcomes in osteomyelitis, septic arthritis, and empyema, and peak titers ≥1:64 have been correlated with bacteriological "cures" of bacterial endocarditis. However, results of this test have not been predictive of bacteriological failure in endocarditis.

ANTIMICROBIAL COMBINATIONS

Many infections can and should be treated with a single antimicrobial agent. The combination of two or three antimicrobial agents may result in one of three responses (Figure 45-6): (1) indifferent, (2) synergistic, or (3) antagonistic.

Antimicrobial combinations are considered to elicit *indifferent* effects if the activity in combination equals the sum of separate independent activities.

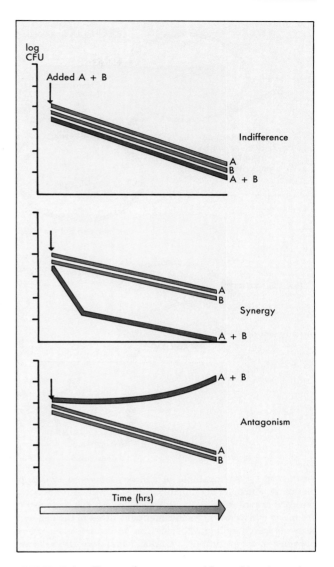

FIGURE 45-6 Types of responses with combinations of antimicrobial agents A and B given concurrently to a patient at time indicated by arrow.

Synergism is present if the activity of the combined antimicrobial agents is greater than the sum of the independent activities. Synergism is frequently defined as a fourfold or greater reduction in the MIC or MBC for both agents. For example, the MBC of ampicillin against *enterococcus faecalis* is 64 μg/ml and the MBC of gentamicin is 64 μg/ml. In combination, the MBCs are 4 and 0.5/μg/ml, respectively. Each is reduced by at least a factor of four, and thus the

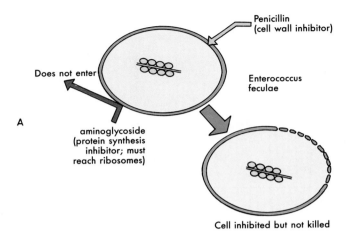

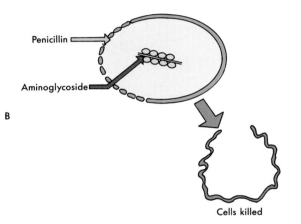

FIGURE 45-7   An example of synergy between two antibiotics. **A,** Penicillin or aminoglycoside is given, but not both; the cells are inhibited only. **B,** Penicillin and aminoglycoside are given concurrently; penicillin opens holes in the cell wall through which aminoglycosides can enter and reach the ribosomes and halt protein synthesis; therefore the cells are killed.

> **REASONS FOR CONCURRENT USE OF MORE THAN ONE ANTIMICROBIAL AGENT IN A PATIENT**
>
> To treat a life-threatening infection
> Treatment of polymicrobial infection
> For synergy of the drugs (obtain enhanced antibacterial activity)
> Prevent emergence of resistant bacteria
> Permit use of a lower dose of one of the antimicrobial agents

vival in *Pseudomonas* sepsis. The major disadvantages to combination therapy in serious infections are the added cost and the possibility of toxicity. However, if therapy is modified within 24 to 48 hours, the risks of toxicity are minimal.

Combination therapy for polymicrobial infections, such as occur at intraperitoneal and pelvic sites, has been used for years. Recently, single agents have become available that are effective in the therapy of many intraperitoneal and pelvic infections, and combination therapy is used less for such infections. Other examples of polymicrobial infections are brain abscesses often caused by a *Bacteroides* species and anaerobic and microaerophilic streptococci. Penicillin is excellent for suppressing the streptococci but may fail with the *Bacteroides* species. Metronidazole is excellent for the *Bacteroides* species but may not adequately control the streptococci. As a further example, many acute pelvic inflammatory infections are treated with two agents because one is necessary to treat the chlamydial component that may be present and the other is needed to treat aerobic or anaerobic Gram-negative and Gram-positive bacteria that may also be involved.

The prevention of emergence of resistance has been well-studied in the treatment of tuberculosis. When the mycobacteria are in a cavity, the organisms are sheltered from contact with drugs and some of the bacteria in a cavity are intrinsically resistant to the drug. Therefore the use of two drugs prevents the resistant organisms from surviving.

The use of combinations of antimicrobials to achieve a synergistic effect has been documented for three types of interactions: (1) combination of an inhibitor of cell wall synthesis with an aminoglycoside

drugs are synergistic against this organism (Figure 45-7). Combinations of antibiotics are *antagonistic* when the activity of the combination is fourfold less than the sum of the activities of the independent agents.

The reasons to use combinations of antimicrobial agents are listed in the box.

The evidence that combination antimicrobial therapy is of value in life-threatening infections has been shown for those infections occurring in neutropenic patients. Combination of an antipseudomonas penicillin and an aminoglycoside have yielded better sur-

antibiotic, (2) combination of agents acting on sequential steps in a metabolic pathway, or (3) combination of agents in which one (such as an inhibitor of β-lactamases) inhibits an enzyme that inactivates the other compound, for example, clavulanate plus amoxicillin.

Penicillins affect enterococci in a bacteriostatic fashion, with a large difference between the inhibitory and bactericidal concentrations. Aminoglycosides would inhibit enterococci if the drug could get inside the bacteria, but this does not occur at readily achievable concentrations. Because uptake of aminoglycosides by enterococci is enhanced by penicillins (see Figure 45-7), the use of both drugs enables the aminoglycoside to enter the bacterial cell. This synergism can be demonstrated in the treatment of endocarditis in humans.

Additional discussions on synergism with two antibiotics are found in the chapters on the individual agents.

BACTERIAL RESISTANCE

Bacteria have proven adept at developing resistance to new antimicrobial agents and such developments likely will continue in the future. There are several pathways by which bacterial resistance becomes apparent and several routes by which the resistance is propagated (Figure 45-8). The purpose of this section is to summarize the problem and the mechanisms, with details amplified in subsequent chapters on specific drugs.

Early studies of bacterial resistance focused on single-step mutational events, chromosomal in origin, with sulfonamide resistance an early example. Resistance to streptomycin soon followed. With the discovery of penicillin, and even before enough penicillin G had been produced on an adequate scale to treat patients, the Oxford group reported an enzyme in *Bacillus coli* (now known as *Escherichia coli*) that inactivated penicillin G. By 1944, it was shown that some *S. aureus* strains also were capable of inactivating penicillin G.

Although resistance to the tetracyclines and chloramphenicol was noted in the 1950s, it was the Japanese who found that some strains of *Shigella dysenteriae* had become resistant not only to sulfonamides but also to tetracyclines, chloramphenicol, and streptomycin. This resistance turned out not to

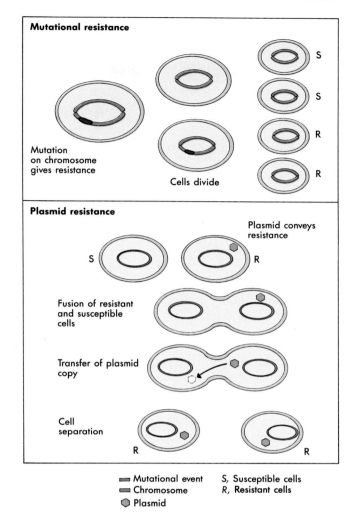

FIGURE 45-8   Propagation of resistance by chromosome versus plasmid mechanisms.

be caused by chromosomal change but to come from a transmissible, extrachromosomal piece of DNA now referred to as a *plasmid*.

Resistance-conferring plasmids have been identified in virtually all bacteria (see box, p. 626) and are widely dispersed in nature. Resistance also is present in the form of genes on transposons, and can be transferred to plasmids or become integrated into chromosomes. Chromosomal genes that code for resistance also can be transferred in the reverse direction and become attached to transposons and the resistance transferred by plasmids.

Antimicrobials are a major selective factor for the

PLASMIDS THAT CONFER RESISTANCE TO ANTIMICROBIAL DRUGS ARE KNOWN TO EXIST FOR THESE MICROORGANISMS OF CLINICAL INTEREST

Staphylococcus aureus
*Staphylococcus epider-
  midis*
Enterococcus faecalis
Clostridium species
Bacteroides species
Haemophilus influenzae
Neisseria gonorrhoeae
Acinetobacter species
Aeromonas species

Enterobacteriaceae
  E. coli
  Klebsiella species
  Proteus species
  Providencia species
  Serratia marcescens
  Many others
*Pseudomonas aerugi-
  nosa*

Table 45-3 Mechanisms of Microbial Resistance to Antimicrobial Agents

Mechanistic Type	Drugs
MODIFICATION OF TARGET ENZYME OR RECEPTOR	
PBP (penicillin binding protein)	β-lactams
RNA polymerase	rifampin
DNA gyrase	quinolones
Methylated 23S RNA	erythromycin, clindamycin
Dihydropterate synthetase	sulfonamides
Dihydrofolate reductase	trimethoprim
Altered sterol synthesis	amphotericin B
PREVENTION OF ACCESS TO TARGET RESULTING FROM DECREASED UPTAKE OR INCREASED EFFLUX OF DRUG	
Altered porin channels	β-lactams, quinolones
Membrane energy source lacking	aminoglycosides
Efflux of drug	tetracyclines
Altered sugar transport	fosfomycin
Modified aminoglycoside	aminoglycosides
Loss of transport enzyme	5-flucytosine
INACTIVATING ENZYMES	
β-Lactamases	β-lactams
Chloramphenicol transacetylase	chloramphenicol
REDUCTION IN IMPORTANCE OF TARGET	
Penicillin binding proteins	β-lactams
Folate pathway	sulfonamides, trimethoprim
FAILURE TO METABOLIZE DRUG	
Anaerobes, Candida	metronidazole, 5-flucytosine

development of both chromosomal and plasmid-mediated bacterial resistance. The use of antibiotics, whether in an individual patient or in a hospital with its special environment and catalog of microorganisms, will destroy antibiotic-susceptible bacteria and permit the proliferation of bacteria intrinsically resistant or that have acquired extrachromosomal resistance. From an epidemiological point of view, plasmid resistance is most important, since resistance in this form is transmissible and may be associated with other properties that enable a microorganism to colonize and invade a susceptible host.

The basic mechanisms of microbial resistance to antimicrobial agents are (1) the development of altered receptors or enzymes that interact with the drug, (2) a decrease in the concentration of drug that reaches the receptors (by altered rates of entry or removal of drug), (3) enhanced destruction or inactivation of drug, (4) synthesis of resistant metabolic pathways, and (5) failure to metabolize the drug. These are summarized in Table 45-3. Microorganisms can possess one or all of these mechanisms simultaneously.

Resistance Based on Altered Receptors for Drug

Examples are altered proteins to which β-lactams, penicillins, and cephalosporins bind as a key step in the action of these antibiotics as inhibitors of bacterial cell wall synthesis. In 1977 *S. pneumoniae* microorganisms resistant to penicillin G were encountered in South Africa. These organisms had altered penicillin-binding proteins (PBPs) that had decreased affinity for penicillins. Resistance of *S. pneumoniae* to penicillins, because of altered PBPs, has been increasing, and there are relatively resistant isolates in many parts of the world. This is discussed further in Chapter 46.

Erythromycin and clindamycin resistance in clinical isolates of staphylococci and streptococci is discussed in Chapter 47.

Resistance to rifampin has been found based on altered DNA-directed RNA polymerase. A change of one amino acid in the β subunit of the DNA-directed RNA polymerase alters the binding of rifampin.

The presence of an altered or new dihydropteroic synthetase that binds paraaminobenzoic acid better than do the sulfonamides is the basis for sulfonamide resistance (see Chapter 48).

Decreased Entry of Drug

Tetracycline uptake by Enterobacteriaceae is a biphasic process with an initial energy independent rapid phase thought to represent binding of the drug to cell surface layers with passage by diffusion through the outer layers of the cell wall. The second phase of uptake is energy dependent as tetracycline crosses the cytoplasmic membrane, probably with energy supplied by a gradient. Resistance occurs as a result of a drug efflux pathway and a reduced rate of influx.

Destruction or Inactivation of Drug

Many Gram-positive and Gram-negative bacteria, including some *H. influenzae,* are resistant to chloramphenicol because they possess the enzyme chloramphenicol transacetylase. Acetylated chloramphenicol binds poorly to the ribosome, and protein synthesis, which otherwise is inhibited by this drug, continues normally.

The most widely recognized example of bacterial drug resistance is that of the β-lactamases. β-lactamase enzymes catalyze the hydrolysis of penicillins and cephalosporins to produce inactive products; those bacteria that contain significant concentrations of these enzymes are resistant to many penicillins and cephalosporins. The β-lactamases are discussed in Chapter 46.

Synthesis via Resistant Metabolic Pathway

Some thymidine-requiring streptococci are not inhibited by trimethoprim and sulfonamides because the microorganisms fail to undergo the thymineless death that occurs normally when bacteria are exposed to these agents. The resistant bacteria produce adequate concentrations of thymidine nucleotides by an alternate pathway and as a result survive exposure to these drugs.

Failure to Metabolize Drug

Anaerobic bacteria such as the rare *Bacteroides fragilis* do not metabolize the nitroimidazole, metronidazole, to the active metabolite which causes DNA damage, so these bacteria are not killed by metronidazole. In addition, *Candida* species that fail to metabolize 5-flucytosine to 5-fluorouracil are not inhibited by this drug, since it is the 5-fluorouracil that causes the inhibition through an abnormality in RNA synthesis.

REFERENCES

Kaiser AB: Antimicrobial prophylaxis in surgery, N Engl J Med 315:1129 (1986).

Pratt WB, and Fekety R: The antimicrobial drugs, New York, 1986, Oxford University Press.

CHAPTER 46

Bacterial Cell Wall Inhibitors

ABBREVIATIONS

CSF	cerebrospinal fluid
MIC	minimal inhibitory concentration
OMP	outer membrane protein
PBP	penicillin-bound protein

 ## THERAPEUTIC OVERVIEW

A large group of antimicrobial agents act by inhibiting synthesis of bacterial cell walls. Included are the β-lactam antibiotics, vancomycin, and bacitracin. The discovery and development of the β-lactam antibiotics is one of the milestones of medicine, since these agents encompass the widely used penicillins and cephalosporins in addition to newer structures. The discovery of penicillin in 1929 and the development of methods for its large-scale manufacture via fermentation in the early 1940s led to the demonstration that penicillin could be used for effective clinical therapy for a large number of infections. This new therapy revolutionized the treatment of infectious diseases and added years to the life span of the population. The cephalosporins, carbapenems, and monobactams are added classes of β-lactam agents that differ chemically from the general structure of the penicillins.

Vacomycin is also a bactericidal cell wall inhibitor but not of the β-lactam family. It came into prominence as a result of (1) the occurrence of methicillin-resistant staphylococci and *Clostridium difficile*, (2) the presence of pseudomembranous colitis caused by

THERAPEUTIC OVERVIEW FOR BACTERIAL CELL WALL INHIBITORS

INHIBITOR ANTIBIOTICS

β-Lactam Agents

Bactericidal
    Inhibit many Gram-positive and many Gram-negative organisms
Agents differ by
    Organism inhibited
    Pharmacokinetics
    Bacterial resistance encountered
Agents include
    penicillins
    cephalosporins
    carbapenems
    monobactams
    β-lactamase inhibitors

Vancomycin

Bactericidal
    Inhibits methicillin-resistant staphylococci
    Inhibits *C. difficile*

Bacitracin

Topical use only for Gram-positive bacteria

C. difficile, and (3) increasing numbers of infections, which are not inhibited by the present β-lactams. Bacitracin, another cell wall active agent, is limited to topical use because of severe renal toxicity when administered parenterally.

Since the initial clinical use of penicillin, strains that previously were inhibited by penicillin G and related agents have become "resistant" to inhibition by these drugs. The development of resistance to the β-lactams is an ongoing clinical problem. Much of the resistance to the β-lactam antibiotics is caused by β-lactamase hydrolytic enzymes in the resistant microorganisms, and "β-lactamase inhibitor" drugs are now available to limit the hydrolytic deactivation of β-lactam antibiotics.

β-lactam agents are bactericidal but may be bacteriostatic under some conditions. Many of these agents can be used effectively against Gram-positive and Gram-negative organisms. The clinically used β-lactam antimicrobial agents differ in (1) the organisms against which they are effective, (2) their pharmacokinetics, stability, and suitable modes of administration, and (3) the type and extent of resistance encountered with specific bacterial strains.

The inhibition of cell wall synthesis normally leads to death of the bacteria. The osmotic pressure in the cytoplasm is high, and the cytoplasmic membrane often does not remain intact when the outer rigid cell wall is damaged, or filamentous growth (which also is lethal) may occur. Because these agents act by inhibiting cell wall synthesis, drug activity is maximum on microorganisms that are growing. A therapeutic summary of the cell wall inhibiting antibiotics is listed in the box

Because the β-lactams constitute a large number of drugs, they are discussed in their entirety before inclusion of the mechanism and clinical factors for vancomycin and bacitracin. The chemical structural variations of the different β-lactam drugs and the mechanisms of action and resistance are discussed later.

β-Lactam Drugs and β-Lactamase Inhibitors

 ## MECHANISMS OF ACTION

Mechanism of Therapeutic Effects

All β-lactam antimicrobial agents have the β-lactam ring structure (Figure 46-1). A lactam is a cyclic amide, similar to the more familiar cyclic ester (lactone). The β indicates that the amine group used to form the amide is on the second carbon from the carbonyl (C = O). Thus the β-lactam structure is a four-membered ring. Such a small ring normally is a strained structure of inherent low stability. This explains why some of the penicillins readily undergo acid or base hydrolysis and are not effective when given orally, as a result of the high acidity of the stomach.

The general structures of penicillin and cephalosporins are shown in Figure 46-2. Both classes of compounds have a second ring in addition to the β-lactam ring. Many variations are possible through addition of different R-groups. Monobactams have a single ring, and carbapenems have an unsaturated ring with the sulfur external to the ring. The sulfur of cephalosporins can be replaced by an oxygen to produce oxycephems.

The β-lactam antibiotics interfere with bacterial cell wall synthesis. The cell wall of bacteria is assembled in a series of steps, originating within the cytoplasm of the bacteria and ending outside the cytoplasmic membrane. The outer cellular coverings of Gram-positive and Gram-negative bacteria differ (Figure 46-3), but both classes have a rigid cell wall composed of a cross-linked peptidoglycan matrix. In aerobic and anaerobic Gram-negative bacteria, an outer membrane of lipopolysaccharide is located exterior to a few layers of peptiglycan. In Gram-positive bacteria the lipopolysaccharide layer is missing and many more (15 to 30) layers of peptidoglycan are present. It is at the final cross-linking step, during the cellular synthesis of this rigid peptidoglycan matrix, that the β-lactam antibiotics exert their action.

The glycan part of the peptidoglycan matrix is composed of repeating disaccharide units of N-acetylglucosamine and N-acetylmuramate connected through β-1, 4-linkages. The muramate group is composed of lactic acid [CH_3-CH(OH)-COOH] coupled to position 3 of the N-acetylglucosamine through an ether linkage (Figure 46-4). A pentapeptide is attached to the glycan (see Figure 46-4). This peptidoglycan monomer uses 20 to 25 enzymes for its synthesis.

The synthesis of the cross-linked peptidoglycan

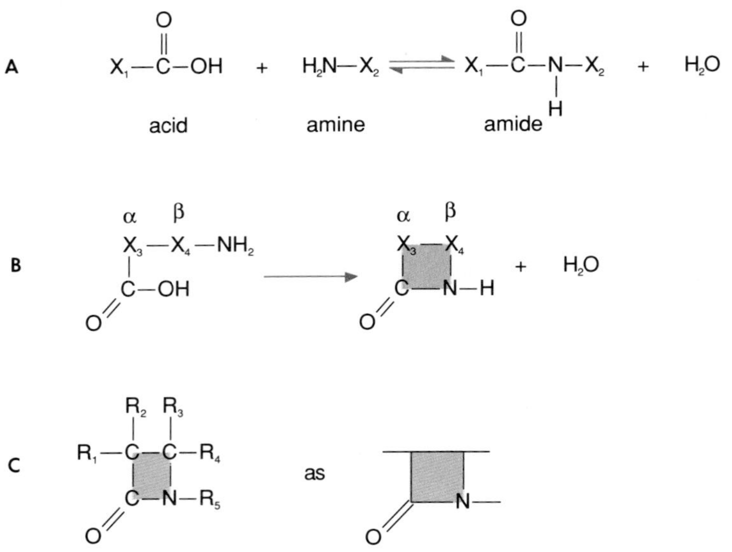

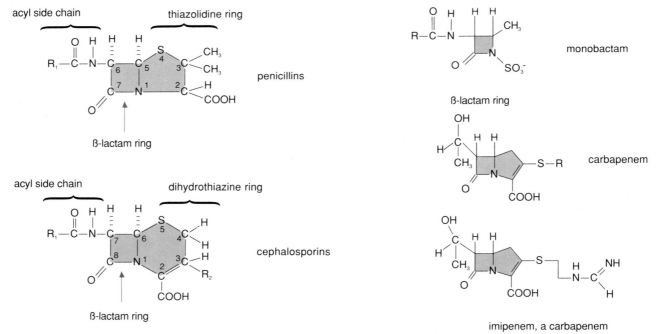

FIGURE 46-1   Description of β-lactam ring structure. **A,** Typical reaction to form an amide. In **B,** the product is a cyclic amide, called a *lactam;* X_3 and X_4 are carbons with side groups with the amine on the second or β carbon from the acid end. **C,** β-Lactam ring structure with the five R-groups that can be varied and in the skeletal form are R_2 and R_3 hydrogens. For many β-lactam drugs, R_1 is an acyl side chain and R_4/R_5 are components of a second ring.

FIGURE 46-2   General structures of the two main classes of β-lactam antibiotics. Additional variations are possible at some of the non-R group positions. The arrow points to the bond that is broken during β-lactamase catalyzed hydrolysis.

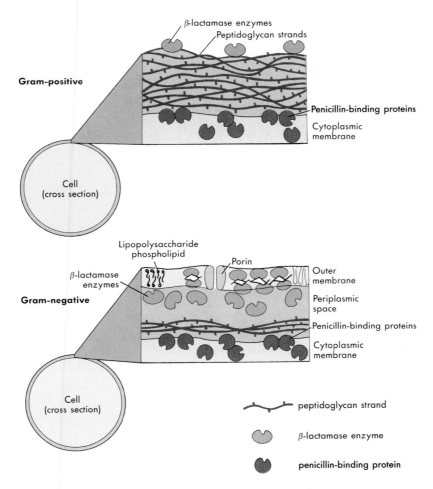

FIGURE 46-3   Outer coating of Gram-positive (20 to 30 strands) and Gram-negative bacteria showing thinner (3 to 5 strands) rigid peptidoglycan structure but added outer membrane for Gram-negative cells. β-Lactam drugs act by inhibiting the synthesis of the rigid peptidoglycan part of the cell wall.

matrix is divided into four stages. In the first stage, which occurs in the cytoplasm, uridine nucleotide precusors are synthesized, using uridine triphosphate, to make UDP-N-acetylmuramyl-peptide and UDP-N-acetylglucosamine. The muramyl pentapeptide has D-alanine-D-alanine as a terminus. This is produced by racemization of L-alanine, followed by condensation using alanine racemase and synthetase enzymes. In the second stage, in the cytoplasmic membrane the nucleotides are displaced by a membrane carrier lipid that is a 55-carbon isoprenyl alcohol phosphate. The carrier lipid brings about the translocation of N-acetylmuramyl-peptide and N-acetyl-

glucosamine across the cytoplasmic membrane. In the third part, the saccharide units are linked in sequence to form chains of alternating disaccharides (Figure 46-4) of 10 to 50 or more repeating units. The fourth step in the formation of the rigid peptidoglycan cell wall is cross-linking between chains to form continuous 2-dimensional sheets. This occurs outside of the cytoplasmic membrane but is accomplished using cytoplasmic membrane enzymes. During the cross-linking reaction, release of the membrane carrier lipids also occurs.

The cross-linking reaction is catalyzed by transpeptidase enzymes, and it is through inhibition of

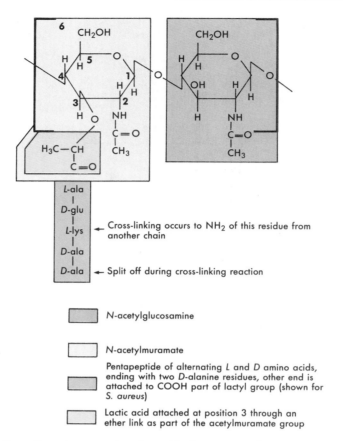

L-ala
|
D-glu
|
L-lys   ← Cross-linking occurs to NH₂ of this residue from
| another chain
D-ala
|
D-ala   ← Split off during cross-linking reaction

N-acetylglucosamine

N-acetylmuramate

Pentapeptide of alternating *L* and *D* amino acids, ending with two *D*-alanine residues, other end is attached to COOH part of lactyl group (shown for *S. aureus*)

Lactic acid attached at position 3 through an ether link as part of the acetylmuramate group

FIGURE 46-4   Repeating glycan portion of peptidoglycan matrix (shown as n units), consisting of the disaccharide *N*-acetylmuramate plus *N*-acetylglucosamine connected through β-1, 4-link, and with the lactyl and pentapeptide attached as shown.

these enzymes that the β-lactam antibiotics exert their action. In this reaction (Figure 46-5), the third amino acid from the muramyl end of the pentapeptide (chain X) of a disaccharide chain is coupled between the two terminal alanines of the pentapeptide of an adjacent disaccharide chain (chain Y). In this process, the terminal alanine is released. The thickness of the peptidoglycan cell wall varies from 1 to about 50 cross-linked sheets in different bacteria. The biochemical pathways for cell wall synthesis and the points of antibiotic attack are summarized in Figure 46-6.

The multiple β-lactam–sensitive transpeptidase enzymes in bacterial cytoplasmic membranes are called *penicillin-binding proteins* (PBPs), since they covalently bind radiolabelled penicillin G. Some of the PBPs are cross-linking enzymes that are inhibited by

the β-lactams. The PBPs in a given organism are numbered in order of decreasing molecular weight. The PBPs of Gram-negative and Gram-positive bacteria differ, with usually five PBPs in Gram-positive and six PBPs in Gram-negative organisms. However, the particular numerical designations are not the same protein in different organisms. For example, PBP-3 from one organism is not the same as PBP-3 from a different organism. Specific PBPs vary considerably in their relative abundance; all the PBPs make up about 1% of the total membrane protein in a bacterial cell. The PBPs differ between Gram-negative and Gram-positive bacteria, as shown in Table 46-1. In addition to transpeptidase action, some of the PBPs show carboxypeptidase or endopeptidase activity and function as β-lactam hydrolytic enzymes.

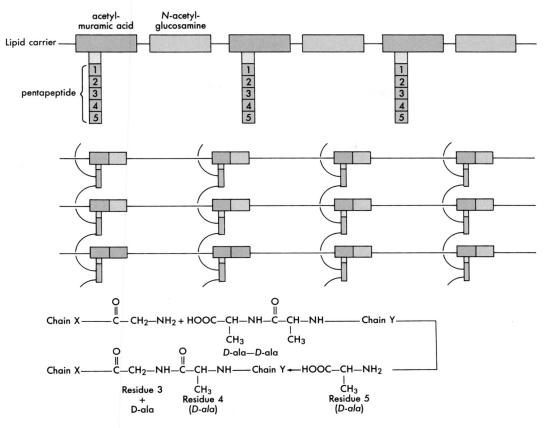

FIGURE 46-5 Cross-linking reaction to join strands and to form sheets of peptidoglycan and at the same time displace carrier.

Table 46-1 Penicillin-binding proteins

PBP Number	Molecular Weight (daltons)	Relative Amount in Bacteria (%)	Effect if Inactivated	Function of PBP
GRAM-NEGATIVE BACTERIA				
1A	90,000	6*	None unless 1B absent	Compensates for loss of 1B
1Bs†	87,000	2*	Rapid cell lysis	Cell elongation
2	66,000	<0.5*	Oval cell formation	Maintains rod shape
3	60,000	2*	Long filaments form	Septation
4	49,000	4‡	None	May increase cross linkage
5	42,000	65‡	None	—
6	40,000	21‡	None	Regulate cross linkages
STAPHYLOCOCCI (GRAM-POSITIVE) BACTERIA				
1	80,000	10	Contributes to lethality	—
2§	70,000	80	Death of bacteria	—
3	60,000-70,000	80	Death of bacteria	—
4	46,000	10	Not essential	—

*Transpeptidases.
†Several proteins.
‡Carboxypeptidase.
§Production of new PBP-2, i.e., PBP-2a, results in resistance to β-lactam antibiotics.

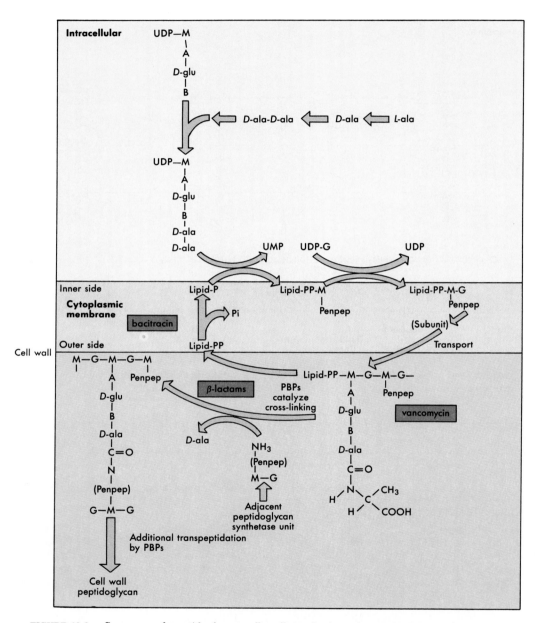

FIGURE 46-6   Summary of peptidoglycan cell wall synthesis and transport showing where in the sequence the cell wall inhibitor drugs act. Details in the intracellular portion are shown in Figure 46-4. *UDP,* Uridine diphosphate; *M,* acetylmuramate with lactyl group; *ala,* alanine; *D-glu,* D-glucose; *B,* another amino acid (lysine in Figure 46-4, can vary with the organism); *UMP,* uridine monophosphate; *G,* N-acetylglucosamine; *P* and *PP,* phosphate and pyrophosphate; *penpep,* pentapeptide of A-Glu-B-ala-ala; *A,* L-alanine; *UDP-G,* uridine-diphospho-*N*-acetyl glucosamine.

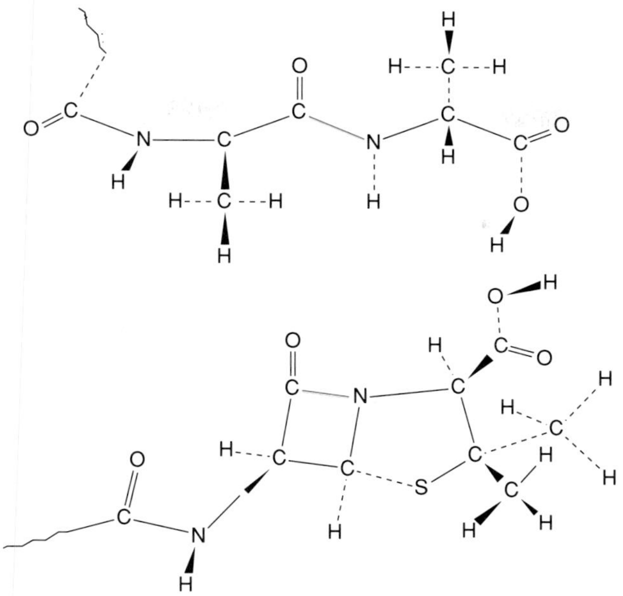

FIGURE 46-7   Molecular models. **A,** D-ala-D-ala portion of pentapeptide of peptidoglycan synthesis as compared to model of β-lactam ring portion of penicillin **(B)**. Both **A** and **B** have similar shapes and thus can bind to the penicillin-binding proteins (PBPs) that catalyze the cross-linking reaction during peptidoglycan cell wall synthesis.

During the cross-linking reaction to connect the peptidoglycan chains, the D-ala-D-ala terminus of the lactyl peptapeptide reacts with a transpeptidase enzyme to displace the final D-ala and form an acylenzyme intermediate along with the remaining free D-ala. The acylenzyme intermediate is reactive and readily couples to the free amino group of the third residue of the pentapeptide of an adjacent chain, thus completing the cross-linking and also regenerating the enzyme. Molecular modeling shows that penicillins and cephalosporins can assume a conformation that is very similar to that of the D-ala-D-ala peptide, with the reactive β-lactam ring in the same position in which the PBP acylation site is thought to sit (Figure 46-7). Therefore β-lactam antibiotics undergo acylation, with the β-lactam ring forming a covalent compound with a PBP. It is thought that the β-lactam ring opens and reacts with the OH group on a serine residue at the active site of the enzyme. This drug-PBP compound is not subject to further reaction, as is the D-ala-D-ala-PBP intermediate. Thus with the drug, the PBP enzyme is inactivated and the cross-link to the peptidoglycan chains is not carried out. The resulting morphological effects depend on the bacterial species and the PBP on which the β-lactam drug is bound. Some bacteria swell rapidly and burst. Some develop into long filamentous structures that do not divide but eventually fragment with disruption of the organism. Others show no morphological change and cease to be viable. The lysis of bacteria treated with β-lactams may be related to murein hydrolyases, which are normally involved in the synthesis of the new wall when cells divide. Some bacteria may lack these autolysins and hence be only inhibited, not killed, by β-lactam antibiotics.

The structures of common penicillins, cephalosporins, and other β-lactam antimicrobial agents are given in Figure 46-8. The structure of moxalactam has a nucleus that is not naturally occurring; the sulfur at position 1 is substituted by an oxygen.

Mechanisms of Bacterial Resistance to β-Lactams

There are three major mechanisms of resistance to β-lactam antibiotics. These include (1) destruction by β-lactam enzymes, (2) failure to reach the target PBP, and (3) failure to bind to the target PBP (Figure

Text continued on p. 641.

Penicillins

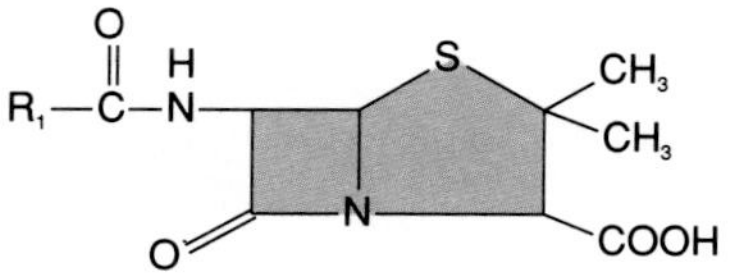

Name	Group R_1
penicillin G (benzylpenicillin)	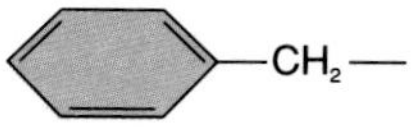
penicillin V	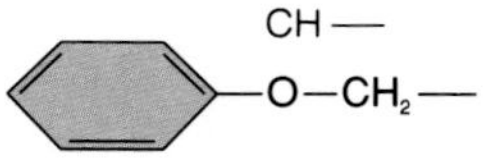
methicillin	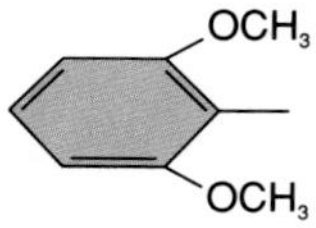
oxacillin	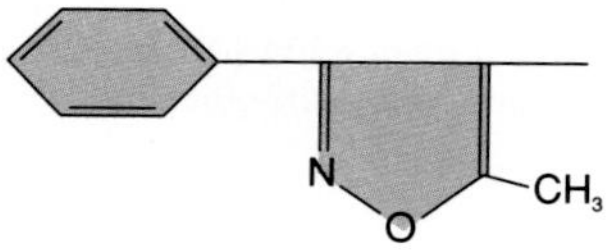
cloxacillin	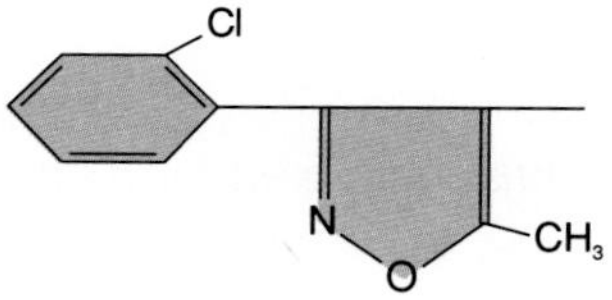
dicloxacillin	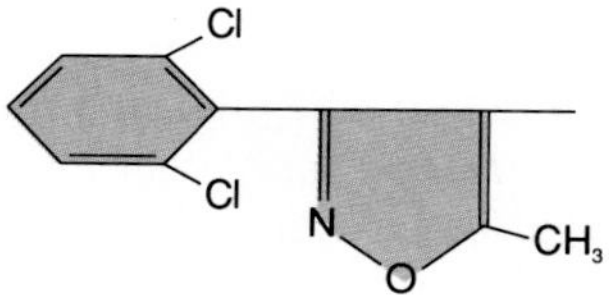
nafcillin	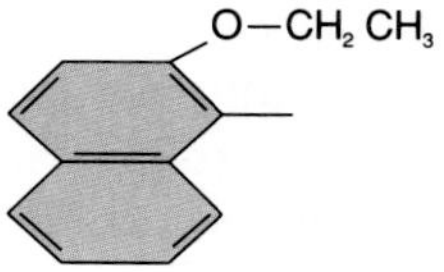
ampicillin	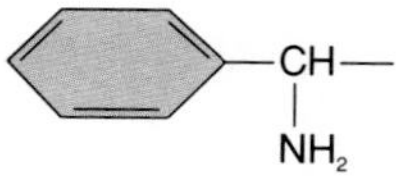

FIGURE 46-8   Structures of β-lactam antibiotics of clinical interest, including penicillins, cephalosporins, carbapenems, monobactams, and β-lactamase inhibitors.

amoxicillin

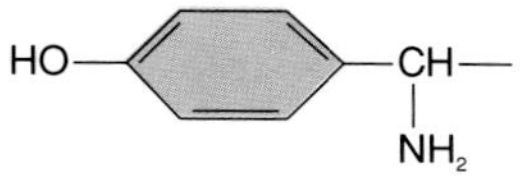

carbenicillin

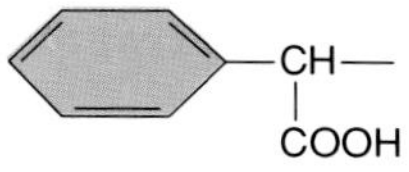

ticarcillin

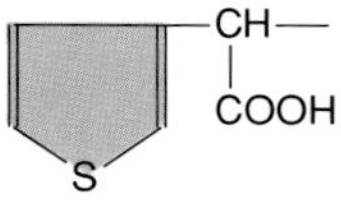

azlocillin

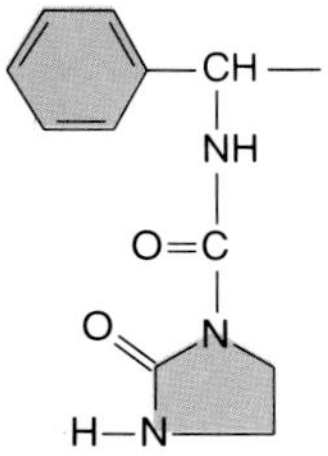

mezlocillin

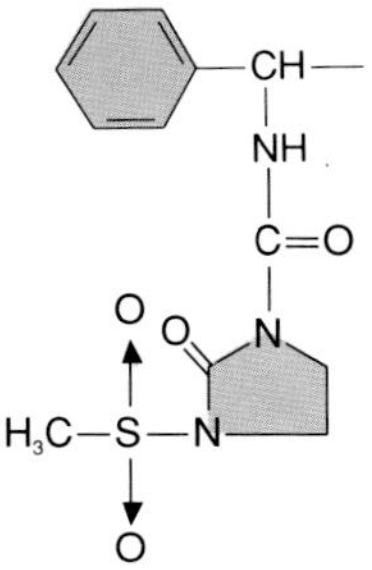

piperacillin

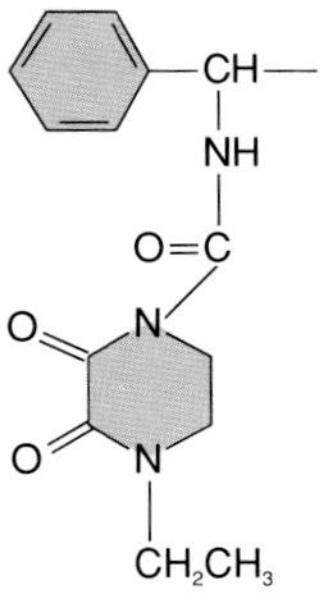

amdinocillin

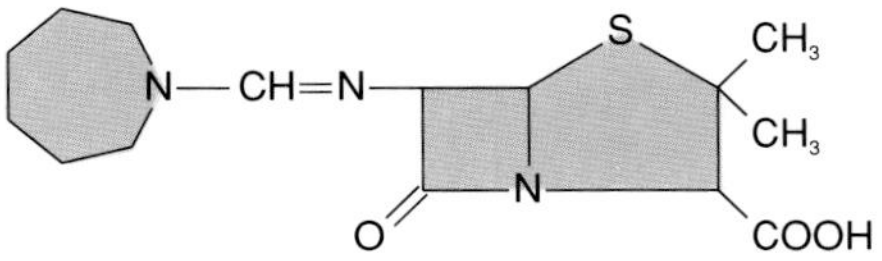

Continued.

Cephalosporins

Name	R_1	R_2
cephalexin		$-CH_3$
cephalothin		$-CH_2-O-\overset{\overset{O}{\|\|}}{C}-CH_3$
cefaclor		$-Cl$
cefazolin		$-CH_2-S-$ (thiadiazole ring) $-CH_3$
cephradine		$-CH_3$
cefadroxil		$-CH_3$
cefamandole		$-CH_2-S-$ (tetrazole ring) CH_3
cefuroxime		$-CH_2\,OCONH_2$
cefonicid		$-CH_2-S-$ (tetrazole ring) $CH_2\,SO_3\,H$

FIGURE 46-8, cont'd   For legend see p. 636.

Cephalosporins—cont'd

Name	R_1	R_2
cefoxitin		$-CH_2\,OCONH_2$
cefotetan		
cefotaxime		$-CH_2\,OCOCH_3$
ceftriaxone		
ceftazidime		
cefixime		$-CH=CH_2$
cefoperazone		
ceftizoxime		$-H$

Continued.

cefotetan

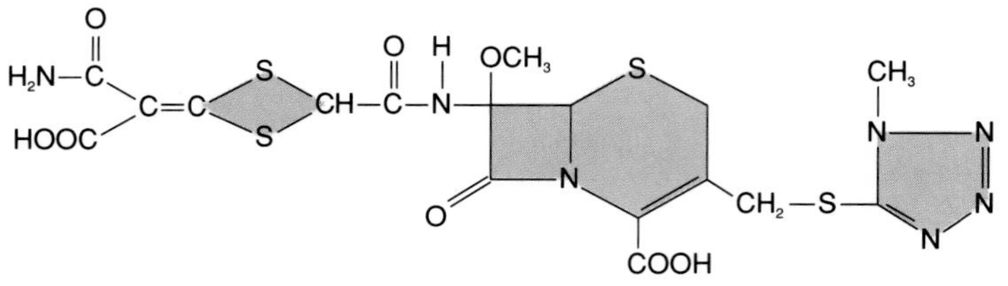

moxalactam

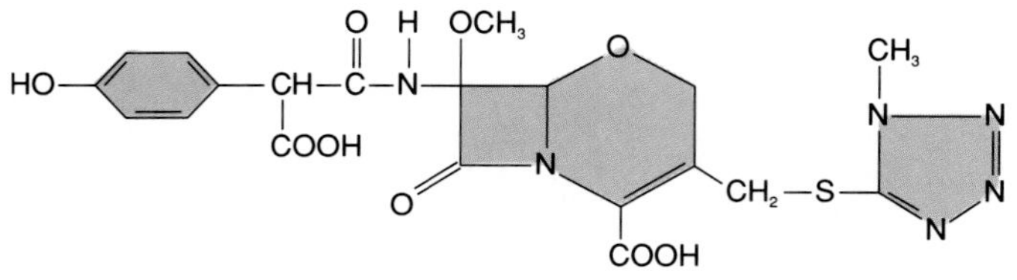

Carbapenems
imipenem

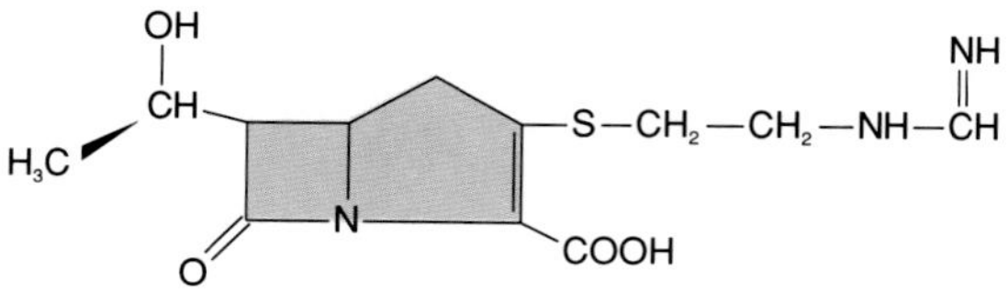

Monobactams
aztreonam

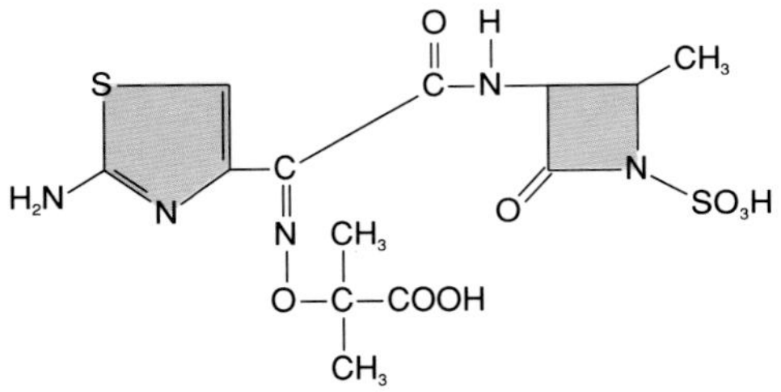

ß-Lactamase Inhibitors
clavulanate

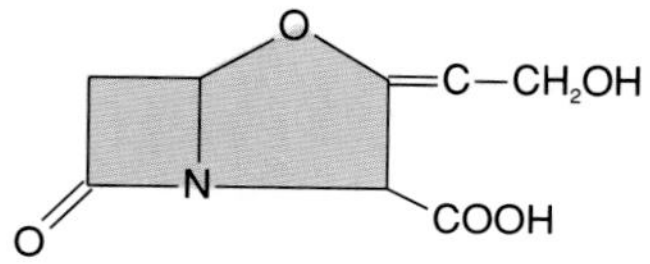

sulbactam

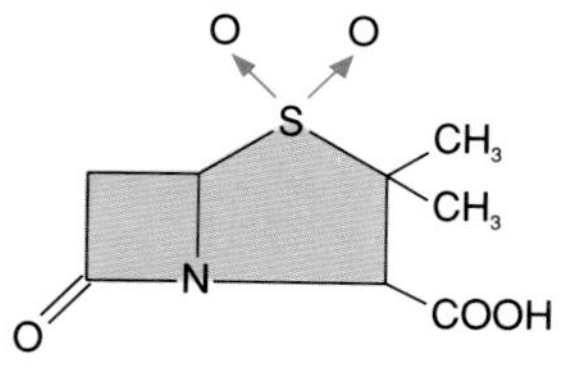

FIGURE 46-8, cont'd   For legend see p. 636.

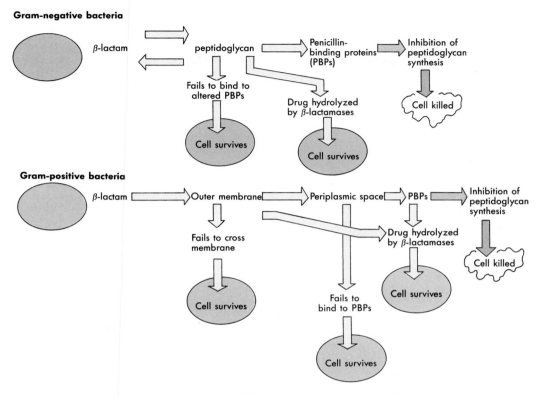

FIGURE 46-9 .Mechanisms by which resistance to β-lactam antimicrobial agents takes place. *PBPs,* Penicillin-binding proteins.

46-9). Another possibility, increased production of a PBP, was created in the laboratory but so far has not been detected clinically.

The major forms of resistance of Gram-positive bacteria to β-lactam drugs are from β-lactamases or from altered PBPs (see Figure 46-9). Within a few years of the initial widespread use of penicillin G, most *Staphylococcus aureus* demonstrated resistance to the drug, resulting in major problems for hospitals, where this microorganism is usually present. Over 90% of staphylococci are penicillin G and ampicillin resistant. The resistance occurs by spread of a plasmid-mediated β-lactamase, which acylates the β-lactam ring to produce inactive drug. In Gram-positive species, such as staphylococci, the β-lactamases are induced by penicillin and secreted into the environment as exoenzymes.

The presence of an altered PBP confers resistance to β-lactams, especially in Gram-positive organisms, and results in failure of a particular drug to bind to a key PBP. The important clinical example is the meth-

icillin resistance of staphylococci, with methicillin-resistant *S. aureus* posing a serious hospital problem. These staphylococci are not inhibited by any of the currently available β-lactams due to the poor affinity of PBP-2a (see Table 46-1), induced by β-lactam drugs for β-lactams. The failure to bind to PBPs is also the reason cephalosporins do not inhibit enterococci, such as *Enterococcus faecalis* and *E. faecium.* Aztreonam (see Figure 46-8) also does not inhibit Gram-positive species, since it fails to bind to the PBPs.

In Gram-negative bacteria, the common forms of resistance are the presence of β-lactamases and failure of the drug to reach the PBPs in the periplasmic space adjacent to the outer lipopolysaccharide membrane (see Figure 46-9). The synthesis of β-lactamases of Gram-negative bacteria can be by chromosomal-directed routes or by plasmid-directed routes. A wider variety of β-lactamases are produced by Gram-negative bacteria than by Gram-positive bacteria, with the Gram-negative organism enzymes produced constitutively or by induction. There are

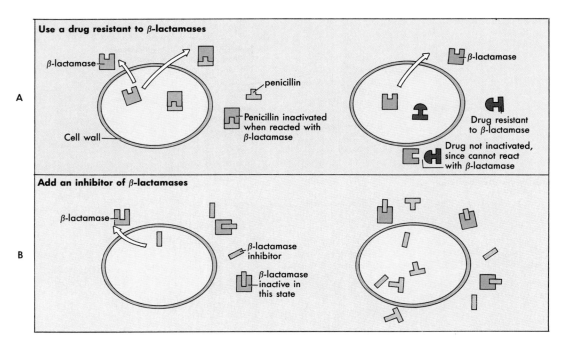

FIGURE 46-10   Alternative strategies for successful inhibition of organisms that produce β-lactamases.

many different lactamase enzymes and their classification is beyond the scope of this book.

Gram-negative bacteria have an outer lipid membrane through which β-lactam drugs must pass to reach the PBPs located on the cytoplasmic membrane (see Figure 46-3). Channels, referred to as *porins* or *outer membrane proteins* (OMP), allow β-lactams to pass through this membrane. Changes have been observed that reduce the amount of drug reaching the PBPs via porin proteins. Some β-lactam antibiotic structures are extremely stable to β-lactamases but do not readily pass through porins of Gram-negative outer membranes and thus fail to inhibit these bacteria. *Pseudomonas aeruginosa* can lose its outer membrane proteins (OMP F) and become resistant to imipenem (see Figure 46-8), which is extremely β-lactamase stable. Also, if less drug crosses the membrane to reach the enzyme and the concentration of β-lactamase is large, resistance may occur, since small amounts of even very stable agents can be destroyed, but compounds that have poor affinity and high stability for β-lactamases can inhibit the resistance (Figure 46-10, *A*).

Amino acid sequence data suggest that there are three classes of β-lactamases: classes A and C in-

clude serine enzymes and Class B includes metalloproteins. The molecular weights of the β-lactamases range from 12,000 to 32,000 daltons. The β-lactam compounds, clavulanic acid and sulbactam, (see Figure 46-8) act as strong inhibitors of class A, but not of classes B or C, β-lactamases. Coadministration of a β-lactamase inhibitor with a β-lactam antibiotic (Figure 46-10, *B*) is an alternative approach to the use of the β-lactam antibiotics that are inherently resistant to β-lactamases.

PHARMACOKINETICS

Penicillins

Penicillins differ markedly in their oral absorption, binding to serum proteins, metabolism, and renal excretion. Most penicillins are excreted as unchanged drug via renal tubular mechanisms, and adjustment of dosage is necessary in the presence of severely depressed renal function.

In general, penicillins are well distributed to most areas of the body, achieving therapeutic concentrations in some abscesses and in ear, pleural, perito-

Table 46-2 Pharmacokinetic Parameters of Penicillin

penicillin	Oral	IV	$t_{1/2}$(hr)	Protein Bound (%)	Elimination
penicillin G	*	Yes	0.5	55	R(main), M
penicillin procaine G	No*	Yes	12 hours	55	R(main)
benzathine penicillin G	No*	Yes	14 days	55	R(main)
penicillin V	Yes	Yes	1.0	60	R(main)
methicillin	Poor	Yes	0.5	35	R(main), M
oxacillin	Yes	Yes	0.4	92	R(main), M
cloxacillin	Yes	Yes	0.4	94	R(main), M
dicloxacillin	Yes	Yes	0.6	97	R(main), M
nafcillin	Poor	Yes	0.5	90	R(some); mainly B
ampicillin	Yes	Yes	1.0	15	R(some); some B
amoxicillin	Yes	Yes	1.0	15	R(main)
carbenicillin	No*	Yes	1.2	50	R(main), M
ticarcillin	No*	Yes	1.2	50	R(main), M
azlocillin	No	Yes	0.8	30	R(some); some M
mezlocillin	No	—	1.0	50	R(main), M
piperacillin	No	—	1.3	50	R(main), M
amdinocillin	No	Yes	1.0	20	R(main), M

M, metabolism; *B*, biliary; *R*, renal.
*Poor acid stability.

neal, and synovial fluids. Distribution to eye, brain, and prostatic fluid is low, whereas urinary concentrations generally are high. Concentrations of penicillins in cerebrospinal fluid are less than 1% of plasma values in uninflamed meninges and rise to 5% of plasma concentrations during inflammation. Penicillins do not enter phagocytic cells to any major extent, since the drug that enters is extruded by an anion pump.

Pharmacokinetic parameters for specific penicillins of clinical interest are summarized in Table 46-2.

Penicillins G and V and β-Lactamase Resistant Penicillins

Penicillin G is not acid stable and is rapidly hydrolyzed in the stomach when injested with food. Absorption is rapid, primarily in the duodenum and is enhanced in persons with achlorhydria. Unabsorbed penicillin is destroyed by bacteria in the colon. In contrast, penicillin V is acid stable and well absorbed even if ingested with food.

After IM injection of penicillin G, a peak plasma concentration is achieved in 15 to 30 minutes but falls quickly, because the drug is rapidly removed by the kidney. The half-life is 30 minutes. Repository forms of penicillin are available as procaine or benzathine salts. Procaine penicillin is an equimolar mixture of procaine and penicillin that delays the peak concentration by 1 to 3 hours. Serum and tissue concentrations of penicillin G are present for up to 12 hours after 300,000 units, and for several days after doses of 2.4 million units.

Benzathine penicillin is a combination of 1 mol of penicillin and 2 mols of the ammonium base that is slowly absorbed and produces a detectable plasma concentration for up to 15 to 30 days.

Penicillin G is widely distributed throughout the body, with a volume of distribution equivalent to that of extracellular fluid. In the presence of inflammation, cerebrospinal fluid (CSF) concentrations reach approximately 5% of peak plasma values, and penicillin secretion from the CSF can be blocked by probenecid.

Approximately 10% of penicillin G is eliminated by glomerular filtration and 90% by tubular secretion. Renal clearance is equivalent to renal plasma flow, with a maximum rate of approximately 3 million units eliminated per hour. The excretion of penicillin can be blocked by probenecid, prolonging the plasma half-life. Renal elimination of penicillin is markedly lower in newborns because of poorly developed tubular function; half-life of penicillin G is 3 hours in newborns compared to 30 minutes in children 1 year of age. As age increases, renal tubular excretory ability declines, with a corresponding increase in drug half-life. In the presence of anuria, the half-life is approximately 10 hours. In general, adjustments in dosage are not necessary until renal clearance decreases below 30 ml/min. Hepatic metabolism to penicilloic acid can inactivate penicillin G to some extent when renal function fails; thus with combined renal and hepatic failure, serious accumulation of drug can occur if dosing is not reduced.

Hemodialysis will remove penicillin G from the body, but peritoneal dialysis is less efficient. A small amount of penicillin is excreted in human milk and saliva, but it is not present in tears or sweat.

Considering the β-lactamase–resistant penicillins, only methicillin is not acid stable and must be administered IV, although rapid absorption occurs after IM injection. Its plasma half-life, distribution, and excretion are similar to those of penicillin G.

β-Lactamase–resistant oxacillin, cloxacillin, and dicloxacillin are absorbed when administered orally, but absorption is decreased by the presence of food. Oxacillin is least well absorbed, with cloxacillin absorbed twice as well and dicloxacillin four times as well as oxacillin. Peak plasma concentrations are achieved approximately 1 hour after ingestion. All of these drugs are highly bound to plasma albumin (>90%). Elimination is primarily via the kidney with some biliary excretion and some liver metabolism. These drugs are minimally removed from the body by hemodialysis. Oxacillin is more effective when administered IM or IV than when used orally.

Nafcillin is erratically absorbed when ingested orally, with or without food, and plasma concentrations are low after IM injection; thus the preferred route is IV. Elimination is primarily by excretion in bile and, to a much lesser extent, via kidney. It enters the CSF in concentrations adequate to treat staphylococcal meningitis or brain abscesses.

Aminopenicillins, Carboxypenicillins, and Ureidopenicillins

Ampicillin is moderately well absorbed after oral administration, but absorption is decreased and peak plasma concentrations are delayed by food. The half-life can be prolonged by coadministration of probenecid. Ampicillin is well distributed to most body compartments and achieves therapeutic concentrations in pleural, synovial, and peritoneal fluids. CSF concentrations in the presence of inflammation are ad-

equate to treat meningitis. Ampicillin is excreted in bile and undergoes enterohepatic recirculation. Urinary concentrations remain high until renal function is markedly reduced (creatinine clearance <15 ml/min).

Amoxicillin is better absorbed after oral ingestion than ampicillin and is not influenced by food. Distribution is similar to ampicillin.

Bacampicillin is an inactive ester of ampicillin that undergoes hydrolysis in the intestinal mucosa and plasma to yield ampicillin.

Carbenicillin and ticarcillin are not absorbed from the gastrointestinal tract and are therefore administered parenterally. They are rarely used by the IM route, since plasma concentrations are inadequate for treatment of *Pseudomonas* species tissue infections. Both are secreted by renal tubules. Distribution is extensive except for inadequate concentrations in CSF for treating *Pseudomonas* meningitis.

Because none of the ureidopenicillins are orally absorbed, administration is limited to IV or IM. These drugs have nonlinear pharmacokinetics with peak plasma concentration, and area under the drug versus time curve is not proportional to dose.

Amdinocillin

Amdinocillin has IV pharmacokinetics similar to those of ampicillin. It is not absorbed orally, but as a pivaloyl ester it is absorbed and hydrolyzed to yield active drug. In the United States, amdinocillin is available only for parenteral use.

Cephalosporins

Many of the cephalosporins can be administered only by the parenteral route, because IM administration is painful for some. Although cephalosporins are distributed widely into body compartments, only third-generation agents penetrate the CSF to yield sufficient concentrations to treat meningitis. All of the cephalosporins, including those eliminated primarily by hepatic mechanisms, provide high enough urinary concentrations to treat urinary tract infections. In the absence of common duct obstruction, biliary concentrations of cephalosporins exceed the plasma concentrations for all agents. Most third-generation cephalosporins penetrate the aqueous humor.

Cephalosporins with an acetoxy side-chain undergo metabolism to yield a desacetyl compound.

Table 46-3 Pharmacokinetic Parameters of Cephalosporins

cephalosporin	Oral	IV	$t_{1/2}$ (hr)	Protein Bound (%)	Renal Elimination	Metabolized
FIRST GENERATION						
cephalothin	No	Yes	0.5	70	Yes, T	Yes
cefazolin	No	Yes	2.0	85	Yes, T	No
cephalexin	Yes	No	1.0	15	Yes, T	No
cephradine	Yes	Yes	0.5	18	Yes, T	No
cefadroxil	Yes	No	1.5	20	Yes, T	No
cefaclor	Yes	No	1.0	25	Yes, T	Yes
SECOND GENERATION						
cefamandole	No	Yes	0.7	70	Yes, T	No
cefuroxime	Yes	Yes	1.7	35	Yes, T	No
cefonicid	No	Yes	3.5-4.0	>90	Yes, T	No
cefoxitin	No	Yes	0.8	70	Yes, T	No
THIRD GENERATION						
cefotaxime	No	Yes	1.0 (1.6 metabolite)	50	Yes, T	Yes (active)
ceftizoxime	No	Yes	1.8	30	Yes, T	No
ceftriaxone	No	Yes	6-8	90	Yes, T	No; bile (60%)
moxalactam*	No	Yes	2.0	60	Yes, G	No
cefotetan	No	Yes	3.5-4.0	85	Yes, T	No
cefixime	Yes	No	3.0-4.0	75	Yes, T	No
ceftazidime	No	Yes	1.6-2.0	15	Yes, G	No
cefoperazone	No	Yes	2.0	85	Yes, T	No; bile (75%)

G, glomerular; *T*, tubular.
*Bleeding problem.

Some are inactive; the desacetyl metabolite of cefotaxime is less active than the parent compound, but more active than most first- and second-generation drugs.

Cephalosporins are eliminated by renal mechanisms with varying degrees of tubular secretion and glomerular filtration. Accumulation of the agents depends on the status of renal clearance mechanisms. Cefoperazone and ceftriaxone are excreted to a major degree via the biliary route.

Pharmacokinetic parameters for the cephalosporins of clinical interest are listed in Table 46-3.

First-generation Cephalosporins

Cephalothin is not absorbed orally and is extremely painful when administered IM; therefore it must be administered IV. Because of the short half-life, it is not used much today. Cephalothin is metabolized to a less active desacetyl derivative.

Cefazolin can be administered IM or IV and is widely distributed but does not adequately penetrate into the CSF. Clearance is by glomerular filtration and tubular secretion with no metabolism.

Cephalexin is extremely well absorbed orally to give wide distribution in body tissues, including bone. This drug is not metabolized, with elimination by glomerular filtration and tubular secretion, and renal failure requires adjustment of the dosing regimen. Another orally administered agent, cefaclor, undergoes metabolism to inactive fragments in addition to renal elimination by glomerular filtration and tubular secretion.

Second-generation and Third-generation Cephalosporins

Cefamandole is not absorbed orally, is not metabolized, and is eliminated primarily by tubular secretion. Parenterally administered cefuroxime also is not

Table 46-4   Pharmacokinetic Parameters of Other β-Lactams and β-Lactamase Inhibitors

	Oral	IV	$t_{1/2}$(hr)	Protein Bound (%)	Renal Elimination	Metabolized
OTHER β-LACTAMS						
imipenem	No	Yes	1.0	20	Yes	Yes*
aztreonam	No	Yes	1.5-2.0	45-60	Yes	No
β-LACTAMASE INHIBITORS						
clavulanate (with amoxicillin or ticarcillin)	Yes (amox)	Yes (ticar)	1.0	20, 65	Yes	Yes (minor)
sulbactam (with ampicillin)	Yes	Yes	1.0	15	Yes	No

*Prevented by cilastatin.

metabolized, with renal elimination by glomerular filtration and tubular secretion.

Administration of cefoxitin is limited to IV or IM with good distribution in the body except for inadequate CSF concentrations. Elimination is similar to the other cephalosporins.

Third-generation cefotaxime, ceftriaxone, ceftizoxime, and moxalactam enter the CSF and can be used to treat meningitis. Cefotaxime is partially metabolized to a desacetyl derivative, which has antibacterial activity less than that of cefotaxime but greater than that for most first-generation or second-generation cephalosporins. The metabolite acts synergistically with cefotaxime against many microorganisms. Elimination is by tubular secretion and is blocked by probenecid; half-lives of the parent drug and the metabolite are increased in renal failure.

Ceftriaxone differs from other cephalosporins by its long plasma half-life of 6 to 8 hours. In addition, its plasma protein binding (90%) is concentration-dependent, with a greater fraction of free drug present at higher total concentrations. This is relevant for selection of dosing schedules of the drug. Ceftriaxone is not metabolized, with 60% excreted in the bile and the remainder eliminated by the kidney. Dosage must be adjusted in the presence of combined hepatic-renal dysfunction.

Other β-Lactam Drugs

Pharmacokinetic parameters of clinical interest are summarized in Table 46-4 for imipenem, aztreonam, and the β-lactamase inhibitors.

Imipenem   Imipenem is not absorbed orally because of its instability at gastric pH. In the United States, it is administered only IV and is widely distributed, but enters CSF only in the presence of inflammation, although it is not used to treat meningitis. Imipenem is eliminated by glomerular filtration and tubular secretion and undergoes hydrolysis by a dihydropeptidase in the renal tubules. To overcome this hydrolysis, imipenem is combined with a renal dehydropeptidase inhibitor, cilastatin (see Figure 46-8 for structure). Cilastatin has no antibacterial activity and does not affect the antibacterial activity or pharmacokinetic properties of imipenem, except to prevent its hydrolysis. In the absence of cilastatin, less than 25% of imipenem is recovered in the urine, with the breakdown products of imipenem nephrotoxic. With cilastatin, 70% of imipenem is recovered as parent compound and 25% as metabolites. Minimal amounts of drug are excreted in bile, although biliary concentrations are adequate for treatment of biliary tract infections.

The serum half-life of imipenem increases as creatinine clearance falls, reaching 4 hours in individuals with creatinine clearances <10 ml/min. The plasma half-life of cilastatin increases in patients with renal insufficiency, reaching 19 hours in anuria.

Aztreonam   Aztreonam is not absorbed after oral ingestion but can be administered IV or IM. It is widely distributed to all body sites and compartments, including the CSF.

Aztreonam is removed from the body by glomerular filtration and tubular secretion. In neonates of less than 2.5 kg body weight, the half-life is two to four times longer (5 to 10 hours). The half-life increases from 1.6 to 6 hours when the creatinine clearance falls below 10 ml.

β-Lactamase Inhibitors Clinically, clavulanate, combined with amoxicillin or with ticarcillin, is available. Clavulanate is moderately well absorbed from the GI tract, with peak plasma concentrations occurring 1 hour after ingestion. Combining clavulanate with amoxicillin does not alter the pharmacokinetics of either agent. Food, milk, and antacids do not affect its absorption.

When clavulanate is combined with ticarcillin and administered IV, it is rapidly distributed. Accumulation occurs when creatinine clearance is <10 ml/min. Clavulanate enters most body compartments with therapeutic concentrations in middle ear fluid, tonsillar tissue, sinus secretions, bile, and the urinary tract.

Sulbactam is combined with ampicillin for parenteral use. It will also be combined with cefoperazone. Sulbactam has pharacokinetic properties similar to those for ampicillin and is widely distributed in the body, including the CSF in the presence of meningitis. It is not metabolized, and 75% of a dose is found in the urine. The half-life is increased in renal failure to 6 hours in adults and in newborns.

RELATION OF MECHANISMS OF ACTION TO CLINICAL RESPONSE

β-Lactam Penicillins and Cephalosporins

Antibacterial Activity of Penicillins Penicillins are classified by their main antibacterial activities, as follows:

1. Penicillin G and V are active against Gram-positive and Gram-negative cocci, except β-lactamase–producing organisms (penicillinase)
2. β-lactamase (penicillinase)–resistant agents (methicillin, oxacillin, nafcillin, cloxacillin, and dicloxacillin) inhibit staphylococci and are less active than penicillin G against streptococci
3. Aminopenicillins (ampicillin and amoxicillin) are active against Gram-positive and Gram-negative organisms, and also inhibit β-lactamase–free strains of *Haemophilus influenzae*, *N. gonorrhoea*, *Escherichia coli*, *Proteus mirabilis*, and *Salmonella* species

4. Carboxypenicillins (carbenicillin and ticarcillin) inhibit *P. aeruginosa* and some *Enterobacter* and *Proteus* species
5. Ureidopenicillins (azlocillin, mezlocillin, and piperacillin) inhibit ampicillin-susceptible organisms and *Pseudomonas* and some *Klebsiella* organisms (mezlocillin and piperacillin)
6. Amdinopenicillins inhibit some aerobic Gram-negative bacteria, but not Gram-positive species or anaerobes

Penicillins G and V and β-Lactamase–resistant Penicillins The clinical uses of penicillins G and V are summarized in Table 46-5. Penicillin V is less effective than penicillin G against Gram-negative species, such as *Neisseria* and *Haemophilus*, and some anaerobic species. Penicillin G inhibits most hemolytic streptococci, but most *S. aureus* and coagulase-negative staphylococci show β-lactamase resistance. *S. pneumoniae* is susceptible in the United States but not in some European countries, and although *N. meningitidis* remains highly susceptible, many strains of *N. gonorrhoeae* are resistant through plasmid-mediated β-lactamase production, altered penicillin-binding proteins, or altered outer-membrane proteins.

Most anaerobic species, except the *Bacteroides fragilis* group, are susceptible to penicillin G, but aerobic Gram-negative *Enterobacteriaceae* and *Pseudomonas* species are resistant.

The β-lactamase–resistant penicillins include methicillin, oxacillin, nafcillin, cloxacillin, and dicloxacillin. These drugs are not destroyed by most β-lactamases of staphylococci (note that the early discovered β-lactamases were originally called *penicillinases*). Although some staphylococci contain altered penicillin-binding proteins and may show resistance to these agents, these penicillins are still used principally to treat staphylococcal infections, although they do not inhibit many streptococcal and pneumococcal isolates as well as other drugs. These agents are less active against oral-cavity anaerobic species than is penicillin G and show no activity against Gram-negative bacilli.

The term *methicillin-resistance* originally designated strains of staphylococcus that showed resistance only to methicillin, but now the term is used to indicate resistance of staphylococcus species to all β-lactams. As discussed later, vancomycin is preferred for treating infections by such organisms.

Table 46-5 Summary of Clinical Uses of Penicillins G and V

Disorder or Organism(s)	Therapy
Streptococcus pyogenes (pharyngitis)	penicillin V orally, procaine salt parenterally, or single benzathine injection; to reduce potential for rheumatic fever
S. pyogenes Less common serious types of pneumonia, arthritis, meningitis, or endocarditis	penicillin G
Streptococcal sinusitis and otitis	penicillin V orally
S. agalactiae, group B (meningitis or septicemia in newborns)	penicillin G, ampicillin
Viridans streptococci as *S. mutans* or *S. mitis* (cause bacterial endocarditis)	penicillin G; add aminoglycoside to penicillin G for some species
Pneumococcal infections (from otitis, sinusitis, and pneumonia to meningitis and other suppurative pneumococcal infections)	penicillin G; large IV doses for meningitis, endocarditis, septic arthritis, and pericarditis; lower doses for pneumonia
Anaerobic infections Oral area and chest	Frequently penicillin
Intraabdominal and gynecological	Other agents preferred
Meningococcal	penicillin G, but it will not eliminate carrier state and not effective prophylactically
Gonococcal infections	procaine penicillin plus probenecid with low incidence of β-lactamase producing *Neisseria**
Disseminated forms of gonococcal infection	penicillin G
Syphilis	penicillin G main drug; for primary, secondary or latent (<1 year) syphilis use single dose IM of benzathine penicillin; for latent syphilis (>1 year) use IV doses for central nervous system syphilis
Others	penicillin G excellent for clostridial infections such as gas gangrene from *C. perfringens* or fusospirochetal, *Listeria* organisms, or *Pasturella* organisms from bites
Prophylaxis	penicillins G or V will reduce recurrence of rheumatic fever in susceptible individuals. After exposure to gonorrhea or syphilis, administrations of penicillin parenterally will prevent development of disease. Individuals with cardiac lesions that predispose to endocarditis should receive prophylaxis during dental procedures with amoxicillin

*Increase in β-lactamase–producing *N. gonorrhoeae* has reduced effectiveness of penicillin G. Clavulonate and sulbactam add to amoxicillin, ampicillin, or ticarcillin for *Staphylococcus aureus*, coagulase negative staphylococci, *Haemophilus influenzae*, *Moraxella catarrhalis*, *Neisseria gonorrhoeae*, *Escherichia coli*, *Klebsiella pneumoniae*, *Proteus vulgaris*, *Acinetobacter* species (sulbactam only), and *Bacteroides* species.

Methicillin is used infrequently because of serious interstitial nephritis.

Aminopenicillins, Carboxypenicillins, and Ureidopenicillins The aminopenicillins, ampicillin, amoxicillin, and bacampicillin (which undergoes in vivo conversion to ampicillin), are inactivated by β-lactamases of Gram-positive and Gram-negative bacteria. The antibacterial activity of all three compounds is similar, with two to four times more activity than penicillin G against enterococci and *Listeria monocytogenes*.

Ampicillin and amoxicillin are excellent agents for treatment of upper respiratory tract infections, provided the infection is not caused by a low level of β-lactamase–producing *Haemophilus* organisms. Ampicillin and amoxicillin are used effectively to treat urinary tract infections; both agents are effective against typhoid fever.

The antibacterial activity of the carboxypenicillins (carbenicillin and ticarcillin) and that of three ureidopenicillins (azlocillin, mezlocillin, and piperacillin) differ in some important aspects. These agents inhibit *P. aeruginosa* but not β-lactamase–producing *S. aureus*, although they inhibit streptococcal and enterococcal species to varying degrees. All five antibiotics are inactivated by the β-lactamases of both Gram-positive and Gram-negative bacteria.

The ureidopenicillins (azlocillin, mezlocillin, and piperacillin) are ampicillin derivatives that have activities similar to ampicillin against streptococcal species. Azlocillin and piperacillin are 8 to 16 times more active than carbenicillin against *P. aeruginosa*. Mezlocillin and piperacillin have moderate activity against anaerobes and are similar to ticarcillin in activity against *Enterobacter*, *Serratia*, and *Providencia* species. These extended-spectrum penicillins were originally developed to treat infections of *P. aeruginosa* and, less commonly, *Proteus* and *Providencia* species but in recent years have been used to treat many other infections. Azlocillin continues to be used primarily for treatment of known or suspected *Pseudomonas* infections. In some situations, these drugs are not used as single agents because of their β-lactamase susceptibility but are combined with aminoglycosides or with β-lactamase inhibitors. They act synergistically with aminoglycosides to inhibit *P. aeruginosa*.

Amdinocillin Amdinocillin, which is also called *mecillinam*, differs from other penicillins in that it has poor activity against Gram-positive bacteria, *Haemophilus* and *Neisseria* species, and anaerobes. It binds to only one penicillin-binding protein (PBP-2) and, because of this selectivity in PBP binding, acts synergistically with other β-lactams against some bacteria.

Antibacterial Activity of Cephalosporins The cephalosporins were discovered in 1945 from a fungus, *Cephalosporium acremonium*, in sea water samples obtained near a sewage outlet in Sardinia (see Figure 46-2 for structure). Specific drug structures are listed in Figure 46-8. Compounds that possess a methoxy group at position 7 often are called *cephamycins*, but for practical purposes, these agents can be considered cephalosporins. Similarly, agents in which the sulfur at position 1 has been replaced by an oxygen are oxycephems, but microbiologically and pharmacologically they are considered to be cephalosporins.

Like penicillins, the morphological effects of cephalosporins on bacteria depend on the penicillin-binding proteins to which the drugs bind. Resistance of bacteria to cephalosporins is caused by the same mechanisms that account for resistance to penicillins (see Figure 46-9), that is, hydrolysis by β-lactamases, failure to pass through the outer wall of Gram-negative bacteria, or failure to bind to the penicillin-binding protein. Cephalosporins are more β-lactamase stable than are penicillins, in part because the ceph-

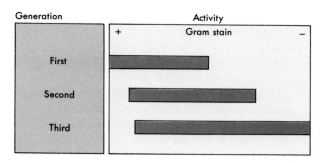

FIGURE 46-11   Summary of inhibitory activity of cephalosporins towards bacteria, based on Gram stain of the microorganisms.

alosporin structures are more resistant to β-lactamases.

Cephalosporins are classified by generations based on antimicrobial activity (Figure 46-11). First-generation cephalosporins have relatively good activity against Gram-positive organisms and moderate Gram-negative activity, inhibiting many *E. coli*, *P. mirabilis*, and *Klebsiella pneumoniae*. Some second-generation compounds have increased activity against *Haemophilus* and inhibit more Gram-negative organisms and show less activity than first-generation agents against staphylococci. Third-generation cephalosporins have less antistaphylococcal activity and more activity against streptococci, *Enterobacteriaceae*, *Neisseria*, and *Haemophilus* species. Some third-generation agents also inhibit *P. aeruginosa*.

First-generation Cephalosporins First-generation cephalosporins are cephalothin, cephradine, cefazolin, cephalexin, and cefaclor. The spectra of activity are similar, with cephalothin inhibiting most Gram-positive cocci (with the exception of enterococci), *E. coli*, *Klebsiella*, and *P. mirabilis*. Most other *Enterobacteriaceae* are resistant, and *Pseudomonas*, *Bacteroides*, and *Haemophilus* species are not inhibited. First-generation cephalosporins are used to treat respiratory, skin structure, and urinary tract infections and are also used as prophylaxis before surgery on the heart or before orthopedic prosthesis procedures.

Cephalexin and cefaclor show less activity than the other first-generation drugs against staphylococci, but cephalexin is more β-lactamase stable. Cefaclor shows greater intrinsic activity towards *H. influenzae*, but less β-lactamase stability than cephalexin. It is used to treat upper respiratory tract infections in children.

Several other first-generation cephalosporins (cephapirin, cephradine, and cefadroxil) are similar to cephalothin in antibacterial properties but differ in pharmacokinetic properties.

Second-generation Cephalosporins Second-generation cephalosporins include cefamandole, cefuroxime, cefonicid, and cefoxitin. Cefamandole and cefonicid are more active than the first-generation agents against gram-negative *Haemophilus* species, some *E. coli*, *Klebsiella* species, and other Enterobacteriaceae. They have adequate activity against Gram-positive species but do not inhibit *Pseudomonas* or *Bacteroides*. Similarly, cefuroxime inhibits Gram-positive organisms and also shows excellent activity against Gram-negative *Haemophilus* and *Neisseria* species and greater β-lactamase stability than cefamandole.

Cefoxitin is less active against Gram-positive organisms than are first-generation agents, but its high β-lactamase stability and inhibition of many β-lactamase–producing enterobactericae (but not *Enterobacter* or *Citrobacter*) species and inhibition of 85% of anaerobic bacteria make it useful. In addition, it is not hydrolyzed by the plasmid-mediated β-lactamases that destroy cefotaxime, ceftriaxone, and ceftazidime. It is used to treat aspiration pneumonitis, intraabdominal, and pelvic infections.

Third-generation Cephalosporins Third-generation cephalosporins include cefotaxime, ceftizoxime, ceftriaxone, moxalactam, cefotetan, cefixime (oral agent), and two agents with activity against *Pseudomonas* species, ceftazidime and cefoperazone.

Cefotaxime has excellent activity against Gram-positive streptococcal species, including *S. pneumoniae*, and Gram-negative *Haemophilus* and *Neisseria* species. A metabolite acts synergistically with cefotaxime, and the two compounds have better activity against *Bacteroides* species than the parent compound. Ceftizoxime and ceftriaxone have similar activity to cefotaxime. These agents are used to treat nosocomial respiratory infections, urinary infections, skin structure infections, osteomyelitis, and meningitis.

Moxalactam antibacterial activity differs from the above mentioned agents with less activity against streptococci and staphylococci, but excellent activity against the Enterobacteriaceae, including β-lactamase–producing isolates and against *Haemophilus* and *Neisseria*. It also inhibits most *Bacteroides*

species and about 50% of *P. aeruginosa*. It is no longer used in the United States.

Cefotetan is less active against staphylococci and streptococci but inhibits most Enterobacteriaceae and most anaerobic species. It is used to treat intraabdominal and pelvic infections.

Ceftazidime and cefoperazone have good activity against *P. aeruginosa*. Ceftazidime inhibits most streptococci at low concentrations, has good activity against *Haemophilus* and *Neisseria*, and inhibits β-lactamase–producing isolates of these species and most of the enterobacteriaceae. It does not inhibit *Bacteroides* species. Cefoperazone is less β-lactamose stable than the other agents.

Cefixime is an oral agent that inhibits streptococci, *Haemophilus* species, *Neisseria* species, *Moraxella* bacteria, and many enterobacteriaceae. It does not inhibit staphylococci, *Pseudomonas* species, or *Bacteroides* organisms. It is used to treat respiratory infections.

Other Beta-lactams and Beta-lactamase Inhibitors

This section includes the prototype carbapenem, imipenem, the prototype monobactam, aztreonam, and the β-lactamase inhibitors clavulanate and sulbactam.

Imipenem Imipenem has structural chemical features that differentiate it from other β-lactams (see Figure 46-8 for structure). It inhibits most Gram-positive organisms such as the hemolytic streptococci, *S. pneumoniae*, viridans group streptococci, enterococci, and *S. aureus*. The majority of Enterobacteriaceae, *Haemophilus* species, *Branhamella*, *Neisseria* species, and *P. aeruginosa* also are susceptible to inhibition by imipenem. Imipenem has extensive activity against anaerobic organisms, inhibiting most *Bacteroides* species. Filamentous bacteria are also successful targets for this drug. Imipenem has a high affinity for critical penicillin-binding proteins in a wide variety of organisms.

Imipenem shows an interesting postantibiotic effect on many Gram-positive or Gram-negative bacteria. After the concentration of drug falls below inhibitory concentrations, the bacteria that have not been killed do not resume growth for another 2 to 4 hours. The resistance of methicillin-resistant staphylococci to imipenem is the result of the induction of new binding proteins with poor affinity for all β-lactams. Imipenem is not hydrolyzed by β-lactamases of Gram-positive or Gram-negative bacteria, with the exceptions of β-lactamases from *Pseudomonas maltophilia* and several rare organisms. Resistance to imipenem usually is attributed to lack of an outer membrane porin protein (OMP F) that is necessary to transport imipenem into the periplasmic space. It is used to treat mixed infections (aerobic and anaerobic), *Enterobacter* infections, and particularly organisms that are multiply drug resistant.

The combination of imipenem-cilastatin is used to treat bacteremias and respiratory, intraabdominal, gynecological, bone and joint, and urinary tract infections that arise primarily from bacterial resistance to penicillin, cephalosporins, and aminoglycosides. It is used also in the treatment of aerobic or anaerobic bacterial infections, in which imipenem can be used as a single agent.

Monobactams

Aztreonam Aztreonam is the main monobactam of clinical interest (see Figure 46-8 for structure). The acyl side-chain provides high affinity for penicillin-binding proteins of certain Gram-negative bacteria.

Aztreonam inhibits only aerobic Gram-negative bacteria, by binding, for example, to PBP-3 of Enterobacteriaceae and *P. aeruginosa* to produce long filamentous bacteria that ultimately lyse and die. It does not bind to the PBPs of these species. It is stable against attack by chromosomal β-lactamases, but may undergo hydrolysis by plasmid β-lactamases, for example, from *K. oxytoca, P. maltophila,* or bacteria containing cefotoxime-ceftazidime hydrolyzing plasmid enzymes. Aztreonam is effective in the treatment of bacteremia, respiratory and urinary infections, osteomyelitis, and skin structure infections. It can serve as a replacement for aminoglycosides and can be combined with clindamycin, semisynthetic penicillins, metronidazole, or vancomycin to treat mixed bacterial infections.

Beta-lactamase Inhibitors

Clavulanate Clavulanate is an inhibitor of β-lactamases of *S. aureus* and of many Gram-negative bacteria, including plasmid-mediated common β-lactamases in *E. coli, Haemophilus, Neisseria, Salmonella,* and *Shigella* species. It also inhibits β-lactamases that deactivate extended spectrum cephalosporins such as cefotoxime and ceftazidime and the chromosomally mediated enzymes that occur in *Klebsiella* species.

Clavulanate has a β-lactam ring (see Figure 46-8 for structure), but has only minimal antibacterial

activity, since it binds poorly to the penicillin-binding proteins of most species. It binds to serine at the active site of β-lactamases in an irreversible manner, resulting in inactivation of the enzyme. Thus clavulanate acts as a suicide inhibitor.

Clavulanate does not inhibit chromosomally mediated β-lactamases in *Pseudomonas, Enterobacter,* and *Serratia* species. Combinations of clavulanate with amoxicillin or ticarcillin are used clinically. The amoxicillin-clavulanate combination is used to treat otitis media in children and sinusitis, bacterial exacerbations of bronchitis, and lower respiratory tract infections in adults. It is also effective in skin structure infections, particularly when anaerobic as well as aerobic organisms are present. Human and animal bite wounds, gonorrhea, and lower tract urinary infections also can be treated with this combination. The ticarcillin-clavulanate combination is effective in treating hospital-acquired respiratory, intraabdominal, obstetric-gynecological, and skin structure infections, and osteomyelitis when mixed bacteria are present.

Sulbactam Sulbactam is a penicillanic acid derivative (see Figure 46-8 for structure) that has extremely weak antibacterial activity against Gram-positive cocci and Enterbacteriaceae and inhibits several other organisms at elevated concentrations. Sulbactam acts as an irreversible inhibitor of the β-lactamases that are inhibitied by clavulanate. Sulbactam is slightly less potent than clavulanate as an inhibitor of β-lactamases and enters the periplasmic space of some bacteria less effectively than does clavulanate. Sulbactam is available clinically as an ampicillin-sulbactam combination.

SIDE EFFECTS, CLINICAL PROBLEMS, AND TOXICITY

Problems in the clinical use of the β-lactam antibiotics are summarized in the box, p. 652.

Penicillins

Adverse reactions with penicillins fortunately are few: hypersensitivity, which can be life-threatening, is the most important. Hypersensitivity includes anaphylaxis or less severe skin eruptions. Penicillins act as haptens to produce antigens that combine with proteins to evoke IgE-mediated antibody reactions. Penicillins also can undergo partial degradation to

CLINICAL PROBLEMS OF β-LACTAM AGENTS

penicillin G
- IgE antibody allergic reaction (anaphylaxis or early urticaria)
- Neutropenia

ampicillin
- Delayed hypersensitivity and contact dermatitis
- Idiopathic; skin rash and fever
- Diarrhea
- Enterocolitis

oxacillin
- Elevated serum glutamic oxalacetalate transaminase
- Neutropenia

piperacillin
- Neutropenia

methicillin
- Interstitial nephritis

nafcillin
- Elevated serum glutamic oxalacetalate transaminase

carbenicillin
- Platelet dysfunction
- Elevated serum glutamic oxalacetalate transaminase

carbenicillin—cont'd
- Sodium overload
- Hypokalemia

moxalactam
- Platelet dysfunction
- Antabuse reaction
- Prothrombin abnormality

amoxicillin-clavulanate
- Diarrhea

cephalosporins
- Idiopathic; skin rash and fever
- Phlebitis, false positive Coombs or glucose tests

cefixime
- Diarrhea

cefoxitin
- Enterocolitis

cefoperazone
- Antabuse reaction
- Prothrombin abnormality

ceftriaxone
- Precipitation in gall bladder
- Diarrhea

compounds that have varying allergic potential. The major determinants of penicillin allergy are penicilloyl acid derivatives (Figure 46-12), but minor components of benzylpenicillin and benzylpenicilloate are important mediators of anaphylaxis. Anaphylactic reactions to penicillins are uncommon, occurring in 0.2% of 10,000 courses of treatment. In contrast, a morbilliform skin eruption type allergy occurs in 3% to 5% of patients receiving penicillin.

Skin testing with benzylpenicilloyl polylysine, benzylpenicillin G, and sodium benzylpenicilloate (see Figure 46-12) has a 95% chance of identifying individuals likely to have an anaphylactic reaction if given penicillin. Failure to have a positive skin test does not exclude later development of a skin rash.

Anaphylactic reactions to penicillins should be treated with epinephrine. There is no evidence that antihistamines or corticosteroids are beneficial. Although desensitization is possible, use of a different type of antibiotic is more practical.

Although hematological toxicity to penicillins is uncommon, neutropenia may occur from suppression of granulocyte colony stimulating factor. All penicillins, particularly high concentrations of carbenicillin and ticarcillin, alter platelet aggregation by binding to adenosine diphosphate receptors on the platelets. However, significant bleeding disorders are infrequent.

Penicillins can cause renal toxicity. Interstitial nephritis is uncommon, occurring most generally with methicillin and producing fever, macular rash, eosinophilia, proteinuria, eosinophiluria, hematuria, and eventually anuria. Anatomical changes include interstitial infiltration by mononuclear and eosinophilic cells to produce tubular damage. Discontinuation of penicillin results in return of normal renal function.

Metabolic problems with penicillins occur often with the carboxypenicillins, since large doses of drug are used (18 to 30 g) causing a major load of nonre-

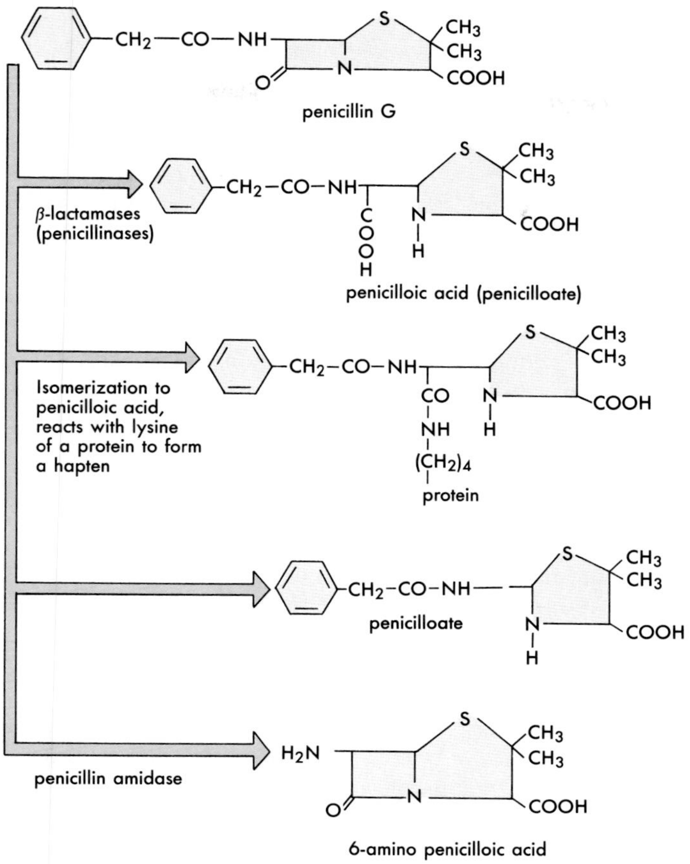

FIGURE 46-12   Some of the breakdown products of penicillin G in the presence of different enzymes and conditions.

sorbable anions in the distal tubule, thereby altering hydrogen ion exchange and ultimately loss of potassium and hypokalemia. Carbenicillin, for example, contains 5 mEg Na$^+$ per g and can produce congestive heart failure. Ticarcillin can be used at lower doses and has largely replaced carbenicillin in the United States.

GI disturbances after oral penicillins occur most often with ampicillin. The most serious problem is pseudomembranous enterocolitis arising from the toxin of *C. difficile*. This organism is inhibited by ampicillin and amoxicillin, but these antibiotics are degraded by *Bacteroides* species in the colon, thereby allowing the *C. difficile* to survive and produce its toxin. Distortion of normal intestinal flora by penicillins can produce alteration in bowel function and col-

onization with resistant gram-negative bacilli and/or fungi such as *Candida*. The addition of clavulanate to amoxicillin and ticarcillin has not increased the adverse reactions to these compounds, although an increase in diarrhea is noted with the oral preparation compared to the use of amoxicillin alone.

Hepatic function abnormalities such as elevation of serum transaminase or alkaline phosphatase concentrations often follow use of high dose of antistaphylococcal penicillins or extended spectrum antipseudomonal agents. In general, hepatic function rapidly returns to normal when agents are discontinued.

Central nervous system (CNS) based seizures occur only in patients possessing eliptogenic foci, receiving large doses of penicillin G or other penicillins, and with impaired renal function. Penicillins do not cause vestibular or auditory toxicity. Procaine penicillin can produce cardiac and nervous system sensations if the procaine inadvertently enters directly into the bloodstream.

Cephalosporins

Allergic reactions are common adverse effects with cephalosporin use, although they occur less frequently than with penicillins. Cephalosporins can produce anaphylaxis but the incidence is extremely low. It is estimated that less than 5% of individuals who have an anaphylactic reaction with a penicillin will have an anaphylactic reaction with a cephalosporin. However, a cephalosporin should not be administered to a patient who has had a severe immediate hypersensitivity reaction to a penicillin. Patients who have had skin reactions to penicillins in the form of a rash are at low risk to develop a similar rash to cephalosporins. However, maculopapular and morbilliform eruptions may occur with cephalosporin use.

About 1% of cefaclor-treated patients have a reaction that produces fever, joint pain, and local edema. All of the cephalosporins sometimes produce fever with or without rash.

GI adverse effects are uncommon, although cefoperazone, because of its high intestinal secretions and ceftriaxone, may cause diarrhea. Enterocolitis from *C. difficile* occurs with all of the cephalosporins.

Although Coombs positive reactions occur with the use of high doses of cephalosporins, they rarely cause hemolytic anemia. Neutropenia and granulocytopenia occur infrequently; platelet function is altered by moxalactam but not by other cephalosporins. Agents such as cefoperazone and moxalactam can cause disulfiram reactions when patients consume alcohol and can produce hypoprothrombinemia from alteration in prothrombin synthesis. Because of bleeding problems, moxalactam is rarely used in the United States.

Interstitial nephritis is uncommon but may occur with any cephalosporin. Neurological side effects also are rare. Cephalosporins are moderately irritating to the veins and some cephalosporins produce false positive Benedict's reactions when testing for glucose in the urine.

Other β-Lactam Drugs

Imipenem can cause allergic reactions similar to those produced by the penicillins and should not be administered to patients who have had anaphylactic

Table 46-6   Frequency of Side Reactions by β-Lactams

Reaction Type	Frequency (%)	Typical Drugs	Reaction Type	Frequency (%)	Typical Drugs
IgE antibody allergy (anaphylaxis)	0.004-.4	penicillin G	Platelet dysfunction	3	moxalactam
Delayed hypersensitivity and contact dermatitis	4-8	ampicillin*	Elevated hepatic Serum glutamic oxalacetate transaminase	1-4	oxacillin nafcillin
Idiopathic, rash	4-8	ampicillin and cephalosporins	Interstitial nephritis	1-2	methicillin
Gastrointestinal	2-5	only oral	Antabuse reaction, phlebitis	Some	cefoperazine moxalactam
Diarrhea	25	ampicillin, cefixime, ceftriaxone, cefoxitin	Hemolytic anemia, serum sickness, cytotoxic antibody, hyperkalemia, neurologic seizures, hemorrhagic cystitis	Rare	any agent
Enterocolitis	1	ampicillin			
Abnormal prothrombin (vitamin K correctable)	25	moxalactam			

*Can occur with any β-lactam.

reactions to penicillins or cephalosporins. Cutaneous eruptions can occur also. Diarrhea is infrequent, and pseudomembranous colitis is rare. Rapid infusion of imipenem-cilastatin can produce nausea and emesis, but this combination is free of hematological and renal toxicities. Imipenem alone is converted to metabolites that cause renal abnormalities in experimental animals but appear safe in humans. Imipenem binds to brain tissue with greater avidity than does penicillin G to cause seizures, which constitute the most serious toxic reaction with imipenem. Seizures have occurred in individuals with decreased renal function and an underlying seizure focus. As a result, imipe-

nem should not be used to treat meningitis.

Unlike other β-lactams, aztreonam does not cross-react with antibodies directed against penicillin and penicillin derivatives. It can be used in patients with known hypersensitivity to penicillins and cephalosporins, with low occurence of skin rashes.

There are no unusual reactions noted for the ampicillin-sulbactam combination or clavulanate-amoxicillin or clavulanate-ticarcillin combinations. The incidence of rash and GI reactions are similar to those with ampicillin used alone. The frequency of specific side reactions for β-lactam drugs is shown in Table 46-6.

Vancomycin and Bacitracin

 ## MECHANISMS OF ACTION

Vancomycin and bacitracin are two cell wall inhibitors that are structurally quite different from the β-lactam compounds and function by different mechanisms.

Vancomycin is a glycopeptide antibiotic of molecular weight 1450. It contains three substituted phenylglycines, glucose, and a unique amino sugar, vancosamine, *N*-methyl-leucine, and aspartic acid. Three different structures have been proposed for this compound with the definitive configuration still open to some question. Vancomycin inhibits cell wall synthesis in susceptible bacteria by binding to the free car-

boxyl end of the pentapeptide (see Figure 46-6). This sterically interferes with elongation of the peptidoglycan backbone. The specificity of interaction of vancomycin with D-alanine-D-alanine partially explains the minimal resistance observed to this antibiotic.

One pathway by which bacterial resistance to vancomycin could develop may require major alterations in the structure of the peptidoglycan. Such changes would involve multiple mutations to produce the necessary new enzymes, not detected so far. Resistance to vancomycin is reported for *Enterococcus* and *E. faecalis* by another pathway, namely, from a plasmid that produces a protein that interferes with the binding of vancomycin to its normal receptor. Thus far,

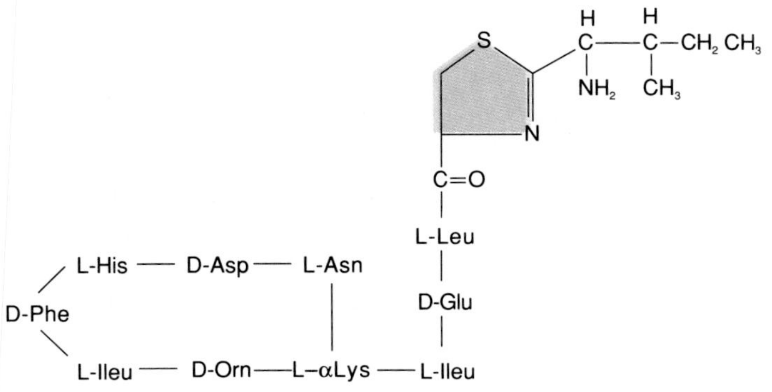

FIGURE 46-13   Structure of bacitracin.

this has occurred only in enterococci and *S. hemolyticus.*

Bacitracin is a polypeptide bactericidal antibiotic (Figure 46-14). It inhibits bacterial cell wall synthesis by interfering with dephosphorylation of the lipid carrier, the C^{55} isopreynyl pyrophosphate that moves the early cell wall components through the membrane (see Figure 46-6).

 # PHARMACOKINETICS

Vancomycin is not absorbed by the oral route and is irritative by the IM route. It should be administered by IV only, except for treatment of *C. difficile* toxin colitis, when it is administered orally but is not absorbed. Vancomycin enters many body fluids, including bile, pleural, pericardial, peritoneal, and synovial and crosses the meninges during inflammation.

Vancomycin is eliminated by glomerular filtration, with no metabolism. About 90% of the drug is eliminated in the urine, but concentrations of 100 ug/ml or more can be found in the stool of some patients after IV administration. Dosage must be adjusted based on creatinine clearance for renal-compromised patients. This drug is not removed by hemodialysis or peritoneal dialysis. Monitoring of vancomycin plasma concentrations is necessary to assure therapeutic concentrations and to avoid toxicity in patients with depressed renal function.

Bacitracin is too toxic for parenteral use, is used only topically, and is not absorbed.

The pharmacokinetics of vancomycin and bacitracin are summarized in Table 46-7.

Vancomycin should be used primarily in serious infections. It is appropriate for therapy of staphylococcal infections for penicillin-allergic patients, and is the drug of choice for methicillin-resistant staphylococcal infections. Pneumonia, endocarditis, emphysema, osteomyelitis, and wound infections respond to vancomycin. It is also useful for treating infections of coagulase-negative staphylococci, which cause prosthetic valve endocarditis, and for infections of indwelling devices such as CSF shunts and Broviac and Hickman catheters that are used in patients who have neutropenia. It is also useful for treating *Corynebacterium* infections of prosthetic valves and catheters.

Vancomycin is useful against serious streptococcal infections such as viridans group endocarditis in penicillin-allergic patients, and is the agent of choice when combined with an aminoglycoside to treat enterococcal infections.

Orally, vancomycin is used in therapy of pseudomembranous enterocolitis caused by *C. difficile;* since IV therapy is inadequate, metronidazole should be used for patients who cannot take oral medication.

Vancomycin is an appropriate prophylaxis for endocarditis in penicillin-allergic patients with valvular heart disease undergoing dental or surgical procedures.

Bacitracin. Gram-positive cocci and bacilli and some *Neisseria* and *Haemophilus* organisms are inhibited, but enterobacteriaceae and *Pseudomonas* species are resistant.

Topical bacitracin is used in many situations but has no proven value in treatment of furunculosis, pyoderma, carbuncles, or cutaneous abscesses. It is combined in several preparations with neomycin (see Chapter 45) or polymyxin (see Chapter 47) or both, but whether these topical preparations prevent infection or improve healing is questionable.

Table 46-7   Pharmacokinetic Parameters of Vancomycin and Bacitracin

	Administration	$t_{1/2}$ (hr)	Plasma Protein Bound (%)	Disposition
vancomycin	IV, oral*†	6 hr (5-9 days in anuric patients)	55	R (100%)
bacitracin	topical	—	—	—

*Not absorbed.
†Used to treat intestinal infection.

RELATION OF MECHANISMS OF ACTION TO CLINICAL RESPONSE

Vancomycin

Gram-positive but not Gram-negative bacteria are inhibited because the antibiotic cannot penetrate the outer membrane that surrounds Gram-negative species. Vancomycin is bactericidal; it inhibits staphylococci, including methicillin-resistant *S. aureus* and methicillin-resistant coagulase negative staphylococci. Hemolytic streptococci such as *S. pyogenes* (group A), *S. agalactiae* (group B), and viridans group streptococci and *S. pneumoniae*, including penicillin-resistant strains, are inhibited. Enterococci, *E. fae-*

calis, and *E. faecium* are inhibited, and bactericidal effects are not obtained. A combination of vancomycin with aminoglycosides is bactericidal against enterococci. Other species that are inhibited include *Bacillus*, *Actinomyces*, lactobacilli, *Clostridium*, and *Corynebacterium* (diptheroids), the latter possibly involved in prosthetic valve endocarditis.

SIDE EFFECTS, CLINICAL PROBLEMS, AND TOXICITY

Problems in the use of vancomycin and bacitracin are summarized in the box, p. 658.

Many of the original problems associated with the use of vancomycin no longer occur, because improved

---

TRADENAMES

In addition to generic and fixed combination preparations, the following tradenamed materials are available in the United States.

PENICILLINS

Amoxil, amoxicillin
Azlin, azlocillin
Betapen K, penicillin V
Coactin, amdinocillin
Dynapen, dicloxacillin
Geopen, carbenicillin
Mezlin, mezlocillin
Nafcil, nafcillin
Omnipen, ampicillin
Pathocil, dicloxacillin
Pentids, penicillin G
Pen-Vee, K penicillin V
Pfizerpen, penicillin G
Pipracel, piperacillin
Polycillin, ampicillin
Polymox, amoxicillin
Principen, ampicillin
Prostaphlin, oxacillin
Staphcillin, methicillin
Tegopen, cloxacillin
Ticar, ticarcillin
Trimox, amoxicillin
Unipen, nafcillin
Veetids, penicillin V
Wymox, amoxicillin
Wycillin, penicillin G procaine

CEPHALOSPORINS

Ancef, cefazolin
Anspor, cephradine
Ceclor, cefaclor
Cefadyl, cephapirin
Cefizox, ceftizoxime
Cefotan, cefotetan
Cefobid, cefoperazone
Ceftin, cefuroxime
Claforan, cefotaxime
Duricef, cefadroxil
Fortaz, ceftazidime
Keflin, cephalothin
Keflex, cephalexin
Kefurox, cefuroxime
Kefzol, cefazolin
Mandol, cefamandole
Mefoxin, cefoxitin
Monocid, cefonicid
Moxam, moxalactam
Rocephin, ceftriaxone
Suprax, cefixime
Tazicef, ceftazidime
Tazidime, ceftazidime
Ultracef, cefadroxil
Velosef, cephradine
Zinacef, cerfuroxime

CARBAPENEMS

Primaxin, imipenem-cilastatin

MONOBACTAMS

Azactam, aztreonam

β-LACTAMASE INHIBITORS

Augmentin, amoxicillin-clavulanic
  acid
Timentin, ticarcillin-clavulanic acid
Unasyn, ampicillin-sublactam

OTHER CELL WALL INHIBITORS

Vancocin, vancomycin
Vancoled, vancomycin
Vancor, vancomycin

CLINICAL PROBLEMS OF VANCOMYCIN AND BACITRACIN

vancomycin
  Ototoxicity
  Injection site irritation
  Rash, chest pain, hypotension
  Nephrotoxicity when combined with aminogly-
    cosides
bacitracin
  Nephrotoxic if enters systemic circulation (thus
    limited to topical use)

---

purification of the commercially available drug and the early history of toxicity have been overcome. Vancomycin can produce hypersensitivity reactions with macular skin rashes. Infusion of the drug often produces a "red man" syndrome with head and neck erythema and hypotension caused by histamine release.

The important side effect is ototoxicity, which occurs with high plasma concentrations and is rarely seen at concentrations below 30 ug/ml. Ototoxicity is increased by aminoglycosides and ethacrynic acid.

Nephrotoxicity is uncommon in patients receiving the drug alone, but is noted in patients who also receive aminoglycosides (Chapter 45). Phlebitis, which is common, can be avoided by use of dilute solutions and slow infusion.

With bacitracin, hypersensitivity rarely occurs after topical use. Parenterally, bacitracin causes severe nephrotoxicity by damaging renal tubule cells.

REFERENCES

Cooper GL and Given DB: Vancomycin: a comprehensive review of 30 years of clinical experience, New York, 1986, John Wiley & Sons, Inc.

Donowitz GR and Mandel GL: Beta-lactam antibiotics, N Engl J Med 318:419 and 490, 1988.

Neu HC: Beta-lactam antibiotics: structural relationships affecting in vitro activity and pharmacologic properties, Rev Infect Dis 8:237, (suppl 3): 1986.

Neu HC: The penicillins. In Mandell GL, Douglas Jr RG, and Bennett JE, eds: Principles and practice of infectious diseases, ed 3, New York, 1990, Churchill-Livingstone.

Tipper DJ, ed: Antibiotic inhibitors of bacterial cell wall biosyntheses, Oxford, 1987, Pergamon Press.

Waxman DJ and Strominger JL: Penicillin-binding proteins and the mechanisms of action of beta-lactam antibiotics, Ann Rev Biochem 52:825, 1983.

Inhibitors of Bacterial Ribosomal Actions

<table>
<tr><td colspan="2" align="center">**ABBREVIATIONS**</td></tr>
<tr><td align="right">tRNA</td><td>transfer ribonucleic acid</td></tr>
<tr><td align="right">mRNA</td><td>messenger ribonucleic acid</td></tr>
<tr><td align="right">IM</td><td>intramuscular, intramuscularly</td></tr>
<tr><td align="right">$t_{1/2}$</td><td>half-life</td></tr>
<tr><td align="right">IV</td><td>intravenous, intravenously</td></tr>
<tr><td align="right">CSF</td><td>cerebrospinal fluid</td></tr>
<tr><td align="right">ATPase</td><td>adenosine triphosphatase</td></tr>
<tr><td align="right">G6PD</td><td>glucose 6-phosphate dehydro-
genase</td></tr>
</table>

MAJOR DRUGS

aminoglycosides
spectinomycin
tetracyclines
chloramphenicol
erythromycin
clindamycin
mupirocin
fusidic acid

THERAPEUTIC OVERVIEW

A number of antimicrobial agents act by binding to bacterial ribosomes and interfering with protein synthesis. These agents include aminoglycosides, spectinomycin, tetracyclines, chloramphenicol, erythromycin, clindamycin, and mupirocin. Some of these agents exert bactericidal and other bacteriostatic actions.

The largest number of ribosomal-binding antibiotics in clinical use in the United States are aminoglycosides, also referred to as *aminocyclitols*, of which streptomycin and gentamicin are examples. The aminoglycosides are effective against Gram-negative and Gram-positive organisms; however, toxicity and development of bacterial resistance to these drugs makes their use less common. The aminoglycosides are effective against aerobic Gram-negative bacteria, often in combination with other classes of antibiotics, but are ineffective against anaerobic organisms. Be-

cause the therapeutic index of the aminoglycosides is small and the types of toxicity can be serious, close attention must be paid to the pharmacokinetics of these drugs in individual patients. Renal function in particular must be assessed, and monitoring of plasma concentration of drug is recommended.

Another ribosome-binding agent, spectinomycin, is similar to the aminoglycosides in that both are aminocyclitols, but the structures and actions are different. Whereas the aminoglycosides are bactericidal, spectinomycin is bacteriostatic.

The ribosomal-binding sites for erythromycin and clindamycin are on the same subunit, but the structures of the drugs and the spectrum of bateriostatic activities differ considerably. Tetracyclines bind to a different subunit and are effective against aerobic and anaerobic Gram-positive and Gram-negative organisms. In spite of a wide spectrum of activity, serious side effects and development of bacterial resistance limit clinical use of the tetracyclines to selected sit-

THERAPEUTIC OVERVIEW

aminoglycosides
    Small therapeutic index
    Toxicities to patient can be serious: renal, otic
    Pharmacokinetics are an important consideration
    Plasmid-mediated resistance is a problem
    Inhibit Gram-negative aerobes
tetracyclines
    Broad spectrum of organisms are inhibited
    Serious toxicities to patient
    Resistance by bacteria
chloramphenicol
    Kills major meningitis pathogens
    Serious toxicity in patient
erythromycin
    Relatively safe
clindamycin
    Inhibits Gram-positive cocci and anaerobic species
    Pseudomembranous enterocolitis toxic reaction

Table 47-1 Bacterial Ribosomal Binding and Resulting Overall Effect on Bacterial Viability

Drugs	Binds to Subunit	Bactericidal	Bacteriostatic
aminoglycosides	30S, 50S, 30S/50S interface	X	—
chloramphenicol	50S	—	X*
clindamycin	50S	—	X
erythromycin	50S	—	X†
mupirocin	leu tRNA	X	—
spectinomycin	30S	—	X
tetracyclines	30S	—	X

*Bactericidal for *S. pneumoniae, H. influenzae, N. meningitidis.*
†Bactericidal for *S. pneumoniae, S. pyogenes.*

uations. Chloramphenicol was widely used at one time, but serious side effects limit applications of this drug in the United States. Erythromycin, however, is a relatively safe antibiotic and is widely used, especially for the treatment of infections in children. Because of the success of erythromycin in the treatment of pulmonary *Legionella* infections, this drug continues to be used in the treatment of other respiratory infections in adults. Clindamycin displays antimicrobial activity similar to that of erythromycin, but the structures of the two compounds are different, and it is not effective for *Legionella* infections.

The final ribosomal-binding antibiotic, mupirocin, is a topical agent primarily used to treat cutaneous streptococcal and staphylococcal infection.

The therapeutic applications of these agents are summarized in the box.

MECHANISMS OF ACTION

The bacterial ribosomal subunit to which each of these drugs binds is listed in Table 47-1, with designation of the bactericidial or bacteriostatic response of susceptible bacteria to the drug. The principal steps in bacterial ribosomal synthesis of proteins, as carried out by the 70S ribosomes and relevant RNAs,

and the points at which the drugs act are summarized schematically in Figure 47-1.

Aminoglycosides

Aminoglycosides consist of aminosugars linked through glycosidic bonds to an aminocyclitol. In the aminoglycosides the aminocyclitol ring is a 1,3-diaminocyclohexitol with the amino groups in the *cis* configuration. Streptidine is the aminocyclitol in streptomycin, whereas 2-deoxystreptamine occurs in the other clinically important aminoglycosides. The structures of these two aminocyclitols and of streptomycin and gentamicin are shown in Figures 47-2 and 47-3.

The structures of the other clinically important aminoglycosides are summarized schematically in Figure 47-3. The particular amino sugars and the specific locations of the amino groups on the aminoglycosides distinguish the compounds and are important for the antimicrobial effect and toxicity. The commercial form of gentamicin consists of a mixture of types C_1, C_{1a}, and C_2 (see Figure 47-3), with little difference in the activities of the three components.

The aminoglycosides exert bactericidal action by entering the bacterial cell and inhibiting protein synthesis. The overall process consists of two main steps: (1) transport of aminoglycoside through the bacterial cell wall and cytoplasmic membrane and (2) binding to ribosomal sites resulting in inhibition of protein synthesis. However, many of the details of the mechanism are unknown.

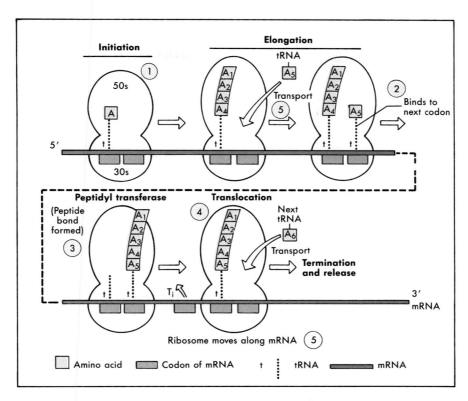

FIGURE 47-1   Bacterial protein synthesis and points where clinically used antibiotics act. The steps are as follows: (1) Streptomycin and other aminoglycosides freeze initiation, so ribosome does not progress along in mRNA and converts from polysome to monosome; (2) tetracycline and chloramphenicol prevent tRNA from binding to mRNA codon; (3) chloramphenicol and erythromycin block peptide bond formation; (4) erythromycin and clindamycin block translocation step; and (5) streptomycin and other aminoglycosides cause misreading of mRNA so that wrong amino acid is added.

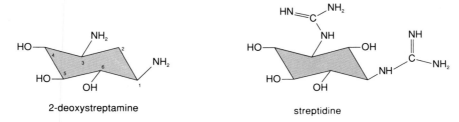

FIGURE 47-2   The two aminocyclotols found in clinically important aminoglycosides. Energetically favored chair conformations are shown.

The aminoglycosides are more effective against Gram-negative than Gram-positive bacteria. Therefore, these drugs can cross the more complex cell membrane structures of the gram-negative bacteria. A comparison of the cell membrane structures for Gram-negative and Gram-positive bacteria is shown schematically in Chapter 46 (see Figure 46-3).

The transport of aminoglycosides into bacterial cells requires several steps. Initially, there is an ionic association at the cell surface between cationic

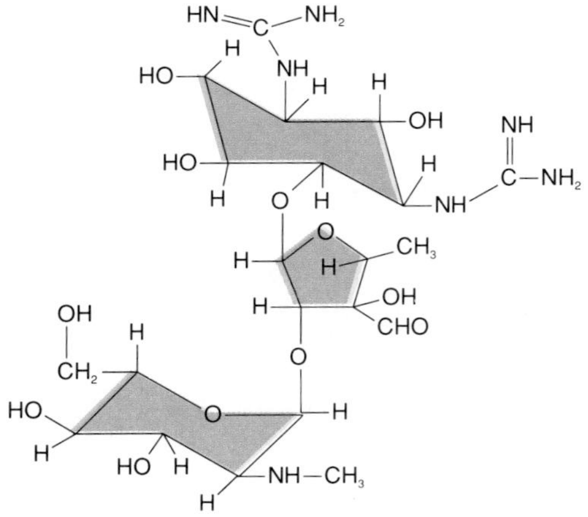

streptomycin

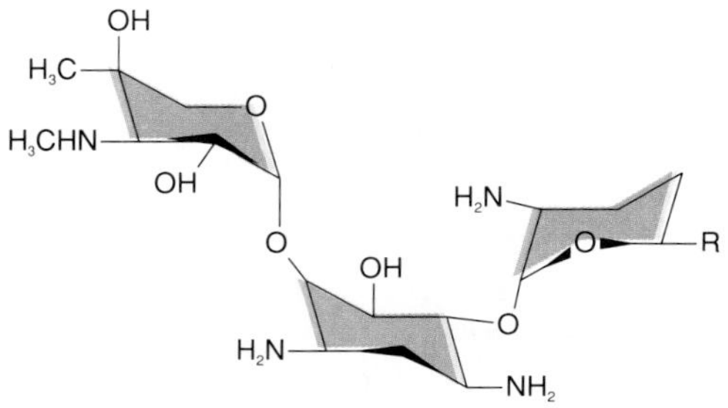

gentamicin C, R = CH(CH₃)NH(CH₃)
gentamicin C₁ₐ R = CH₂NH₂
gentamicin C₂ R = CH(CH₃)NH₂

kanamycin A: 6-aminoglucose-⬚D⬚-3-aminoglucose

tobramycin: 2, 6-diamino-glucose-⬚D⬚-3-aminoglucose

amikacin: 6-aminoglucose-⬚D⬚-aminoglucose
                   NH–CH₂–CHOH–CH₂CH₂NH₂
                          (replaces pos. 1,NH₂)

neomycin C: 2, 6-diamino glucose-⬚D⬚-ribose-2,6-diamino glucose

netilmicin: highly modified 6-carbon sugar-⬚D⬚-modified sugar
                                                    modified

FIGURE 47-3   Structures of streptomycin and gentamicin and main components of other clinically used aminoglycosides. *D*, 2-deoxystreptamine.

aminoglycosides and anionic surface charges. The aminoglycosides then penetrate the pores of the outer membrane of Gram-negative bacteria or the water-filled areas of the peptidoglycan wall in gram-positive bacteria. In the phosphate-rich Gram-negative bacteria, aminoglycosides disrupt the outer membrane and enhance their own uptake through nonporin type of channels. The aminoglycoside binds to a transport molecule that is either part of or directly linked to the electron transport chain in the cytoplasmic membrane. Movement of the drug-transporter complex across the cytoplasmic membrane occurs because of the electrical potential gradient that exists across the

membrane. The transport is an energy-requiring, aerobic step that does not occur in an anaerobic environment. After crossing the cytoplasmic membrane, the aminoglycosides bind to ribosomes. This maintains a low concentration of intracellular free aminoglycoside, which helps support the continued transfer of drug from the cytoplasmic membrane to the ribosomes to produce gradual disorganization of the membrane. There is loss of membrane integrity and eventually death of the bacteria. Calcium, magnesium, and other divalent ions inhibit the transport of aminogylcosides into the bacterial cell.

The second main step, that of binding to the ribosome, leads to inhibition of protein synthesis. This takes place on the ribosomes where mRNA acts as the template for the addition of specific activated amino acids delivered to the synthesis site attached to tRNAs. The 70S ribosomal particles (S represents the sedimentation parameter) move along the mRNA template, adding the appropriate amino acid coded by the mRNA (see Figure 47-1).

Aminoglycosides bind to several ribosomal sites, usually at the interface of the 30S and 50S subunits of the 70S bacterial ribosome, but also directly to the 30S and 50S subunits. Streptomycin, the most thoroughly studied aminoglycoside, binds to the 30S subunit near the S3 and S5 proteins. Binding depends on the amino acid sequence of the adjacent S12 protein, since alteration of one amino acid in this protein can prevent binding. Binding of the aminoglycosides interferes with protein synthesis in two ways: (1) restricting polysome formation and (2) misreading mRNA. These actions prevent normal polysome function, wherein multiple ribosomes move along each strand of mRNA to synthesize multiple amino acid chains. Instead, these drugs cause polysome disaggregation to monosomes, where only one ribosome is attached to each strand of mRNA and cannot move along the mRNA to synthesize a new peptide chain. Aminoglycosides also cause misreading of mRNA. The juncture between the 30S and 50S subunits is where mRNA and aminoacyl-tRNA interact. Binding of aminoglycosides at this site causes distortion of codon recognition, resulting in misreading to produce proteins with miscoded amino acids or polypeptide chains of abnormal length. Misreading occurs more often with deoxystreptidine compounds than with streptomycin. However, the presence of incorrect proteins does not correlate with cell death.

Bacterial resistance to aminoglycosides occurs and results from the following mechanisms: (1) altered ribosomes, (2) inadequate transport within the cell, and (3) enzymatic modification of aminoglycosides. The third mechanism is the most important clinically.

Resistance caused by altered ribosomes is relatively uncommon. Although resistance to streptomycin caused by a mutation that changes the amino acid composition of the S12 protein of the 30S ribosome has been found in enterococci, it is uncommon in Gram-negative bacteria. For ribosomal resistance to other aminoglycosides to occur, there must be multiple mutational events with alteration of several binding sites.

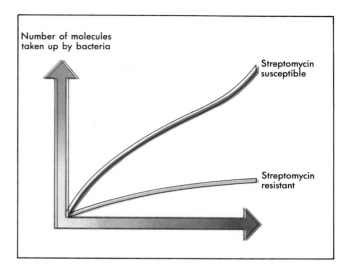

FIGURE 47-4   Resistance to aminoglycosides caused by failure of uptake as a result of enzymes that modify the aminoglycoside structure. Shown for streptomycin, which can be modified by covalent phosphorylation.

Resistance caused by inadequate transport of drug across the cytoplasmic membrane is uncommon in aerobic or facultative species, but it is seen in strict anaerobes. Mutants with alterations in the electron transfer chain and in ATPase activity have been found, but they are distinctly rare. The resistance of some *Pseudomonas* species to aminoglycosides may be related to failure of the drug to distort the lipopolysaccharide of the outer membrane, thus not allowing inhibitory concentrations of drug to enter the bacterial cell.

The common form of resistance is caused by modification of the aminoglycoside, which occurs through enzyme catalyzed phosphorylation, adenylation, or acetylation of the amino and hydroxyl groups (Figure 47-4). The genetic template for synthesis of the enzymes is located on plasmids, which means that the resistance can be spread to many different bacterial species. A large number of such enzymes have been identified. Some can inactivate only one or two compounds, whereas others can inactivate multiple aminoglycosides. For example, an enzyme that acetylates the amino group at position six of the amino hexose can inactivate kanamycin, neomycin, tobramycin, amikacin, and netilmicin, but not gentamicin or streptomycin. The altered aminoglycosides do not bind as well to ribosomes, and accelerated drug uptake is not triggered by the modified compounds.

Aminoglycoside resistance varies by location and local usage patterns. One hospital may have a low resistance to gentamicin and another hospital may have a high resistance to gentamicin. Prediction of the precise resistance mechanism is not feasible at present, and there is little evidence that restricting use of an agent will prevent resistance developing to that drug, since use of other agents may select for strains possessing enzymes that inactivate the restricted drug.

Amikacin is the most resistant of the aminoglycosides to inactivation by resistant organisms, and netilmicin is the second most resistant.

Spectinomycin

The structure of spectinomycin is shown in Figure 47-5. This compound acts by binding to the 30S ribosome subunit and inhibiting a translocation step, perhaps by interfering with movement of mRNA along the 30S subunit. Resistance to this drug is caused by the plasmid directing the synthesis of an enzyme that acetylates the compound or changes amino acids in the S5 protein of the 30S subunit.

Tetracyclines

Tetracyclines are only slightly soluble in water, but they form soluble hydrochlorides and sodium salts (see Figure 47-6 for structures). They act by binding to 30S ribosomes, thereby preventing attachment of the aminoacyl-tRNA to the acceptor site on the mRNA-ribosomal complex. This binding prevents the addition of amino acids to the peptide chain being synthesized. Unlike aminoglycosides, the tetracyclines are only weakly bound to the ribosomal proteins. Differences in the activity of the individual tetracyclines are related to their solubility in lipid mem-

branes of the bacteria. These drugs enter the cytoplasm of Gram-positive bacteria by an energy-dependent process, but for Gram-negative organisms, passage through the outer membrane is by diffusion through the porins. Because minocycline and doxycycline are more lipophilic, they can enter Gram-negative cells through the outer lipid membrane as well as through the porins. Once in the periplasmic space, the tetracyclines are transported across the inner cytoplasmic membrane by a protein-carrier system.

There are two major mechanisms of resistance to the tetracyclines. The common mechanism, which occurs in Gram-positive and Gram-negative bacteria, is plasmid-mediated and involves decreased intracellular accumulation and increased transport of drug out of the bacterial cell (Figure 47-7). Drug efflux occurs from the action of a new protein generated through induction, probably by the drug. The second mechanism appears to be alteration of outer membrane proteins secondary to mutations in chromosomal genes. Resistance to one tetracycline usually implies resistance to all of these compounds. However, some staphylococci and some *Bacteroides* species are resistant to tetracycline but susceptible to minocycline and doxycycline because of the lipophilicity of these latter agents.

Chloramphenicol, Erythromycin, and Clindamycin

Because chloramphenicol, erythromycin and clindamycin bind to the same site or sites on the ribo-

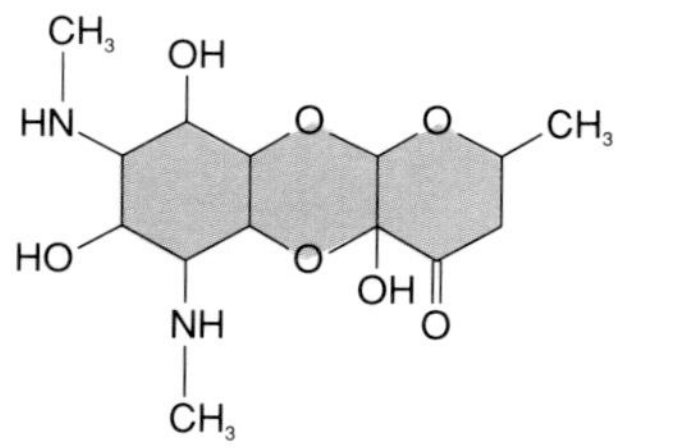

FIGURE 47-5   Structure of spectinomycin.

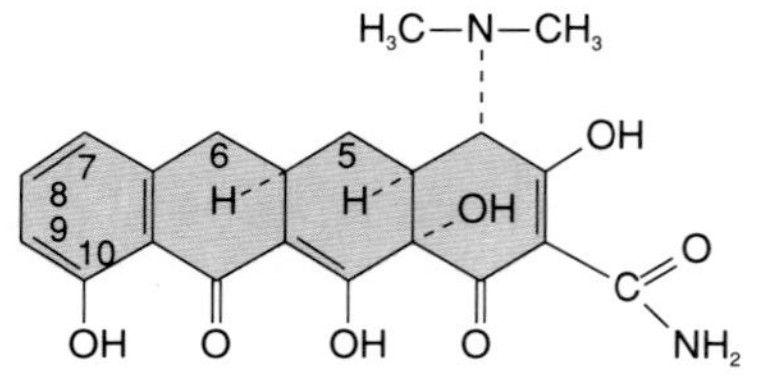

Ring position substitutions

	5	6	7
chlortetracycline	—H	—CH; —OH	—Cl
oxytetracycline	—OH	—CH$_3$; —OH	—H
tetracycline	—H	—CH$_3$; —OH	—H
demeclocycline	—H	—OH	—Cl
doxycycline	—OH	—CH$_3$	—H
minocycline	—H	—H	—N(CH$_3$)$_2$

FIGURE 47-6   Structures of tetracyclines.

somal 50S subunit, they are discussed as a group. Their structures are shown in Figure 47-8. The three bind to bacterial 70S ribosomes but not to the 80S ribosomes of fungi, protozoa, or mammalian cells.

Chloramphenicol prevents the addition of new amino acids to the growing peptide chains by interfering with binding of the amino acid-acyl-tRNA complex with the 50S subunit. This prevents association of peptidyl transferase with the amino acid and no peptide bond is formed. It is not clear whether erythromycin also inhibits the subsequent translocation step. Erythromycin inhibits binding of chloramphenicol to 70S ribosomes, but erythromycin binding is not inhibited by chloramphenicol. The mechanism of action of clindamycin is similar to that for erythromycin. Clindamycin inhibits peptidyl transferase by

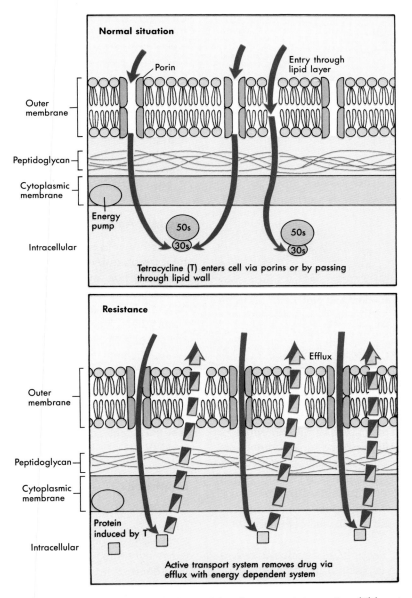

FIGURE 47-7   Major mechanism for bacterial resistance to tetracycline *(T)* (see text).

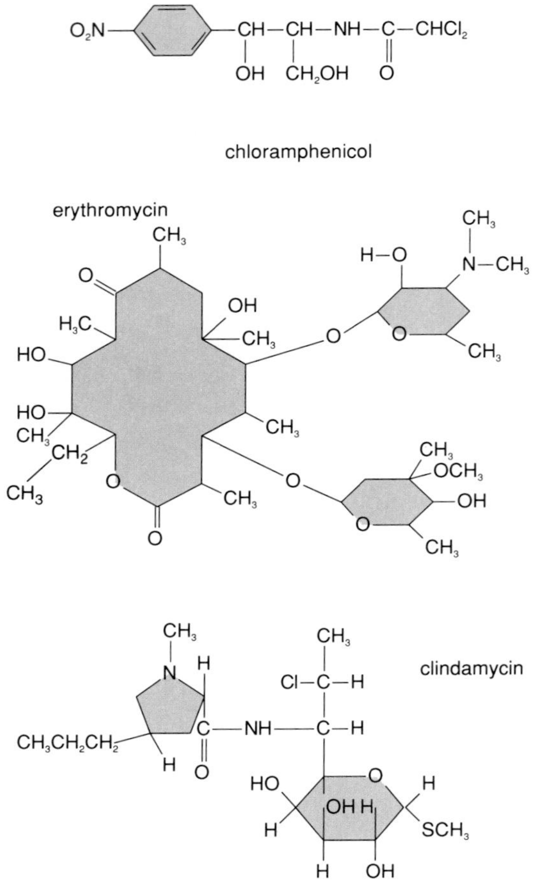

FIGURE 47-8 Structures of additional protein synthesis inhibitors, chloramphenicol, erythromycin, and clindamycin.

interfering with binding of the amino acid-acyl-tRNA. The drug does not interact with polysomes containing new peptides but binds to polysomes that are free of nascent peptides.

Bacterial resistance is observed with all three agents. The majority of resistance to chloramphenicol is caused by a circulating enzyme, chloramphenicol acetyltransferase. This enzyme catalyzes acetylation of the 3-hydroxy group of chloramphenicol, which eliminates its ability to bind to the 50S subunit. Less common mechanisms of resistance to chloramphenicol result from alterations in cell wall permeability or in ribosomal proteins.

The most important bacterial resistance to erythromycin or clindamycin is plasmid-mediated drug induction of an enzyme that methylates 23S RNA of the 50S ribosomes. The resulting dimethyladenine 23S

RNA does not bind erythromycin or clindamycin. Both drugs act as enzyme inducers, but erythromycin has greater activity. This has clinical importance because an organism resistant to erythromycin and susceptible to clindamycin can become resistant to both drugs during therapy. This is applicable to treatment of infections caused by methicillin-resistant *Staphylococcus aureus*, which is often resistant to erythromycin but may appear susceptible to clindamycin. This form of resistance is present on plasmids that can pass from enterococci to streptococci and is the basis of resistance of *S. pneumoniae* and *S. pyrogenes* to erythromycin and of some *Bacteroides* species and some clostridia to clindamycin.

Although some Gram-negative bacteria possess ribosomes that do not bind erythromycin or clindamycin, the common form of resistance is failure of the compound to pass through the outer membrane of aerobic Gram-negative bacteria. For example, the amount of erythromycin that can cross the outer membrane of Gram-negative *Escherichia coli* is 100 times less than that which crosses the membrane of *S. aureus* (Gram-positive).

Fusidic Acid

Fusidic acid is a cyclopentenophenanthene. It inhibits protein biosynthesis similarly to erythromycin by inhibiting translocation on the ribosome. It inhibits all Gram-negative cocci at concentrations of 0.03-0.12 mg/ml. It is bactericidal for many of the bacteria. Unfortunately resistance develops rapidly. It acts synergistically with other antibiotics.

Fusidic acid is well absorbed orally, but food delays absorption. Protein binding is 95%. It is well distributed in the body with high levels in bone. It is excreted in bile. It has been used to treat staphylococcal infections. It causes occasional rash and gastrointestinal upset. Jaundice has occurred when it was used IV.

Mupirocin

Mupirocin is a topical agent, previously known as *pseudomonic acid*, that inhibits Gram-positive and some Gram-negative bacteria by binding to isoleucyl-tRNA synthetase. This binding prevents isoleucine incorporation into bacterial proteins during synthesis. Because of its limited use, mupirocin is not discussed further.

Table 47-2 Pharmacokinetic Parameters

Drug	Administration	Absorption	Plasma $t_{1/2}$ (hr) Normal	Plasma $t_{1/2}$ (hr) Anuric	Disposition	Plasma Protein Binding (%)
aminoglycoside						
gentamicin	IV, IM	Poor	2	35-50	R (100)	0
streptomycin	IM	Poor	2-2.5	35-50	R (100)	35
kanamycin	IV, IM	Poor	2-2.5	35-50	R (100)	0
tobramycin	IV, IM	Poor	2	35-50	R (100)	0
amikacin	IV, IM	Poor	2-2.5	35-50	R (100)	—
netilmicin	IV, IM	Poor	2	35-50	R (100)	—
tetracyclines						
tetracycline	Oral, IM, IV, topical	75%	8	>50	R, M	55
doxycycline	Oral, IV	93%	16	20-30	R, M, B	85
oxytetracycline	Oral, IM	Good	9	Long	R (20-35), M	30
minocycline	Oral, IV	95%	16	20-30	R (5%), M	75
chlortetracycline	Oral	30%	6	>50	R, M	50
other drugs						
chloramphenicol	Oral, IV	Good	3	—	M (90%), R	50
erythromycin	Oral, IV	Usually good but variable	1.5	(4)†	M (main), R	—
clindamycin	Oral, IM, IV	90%	2.4	(6)†	M (90%), R	90
spectinomycin	IM	Poor	2.5	—	R (100%)	0

M, Metabolized; *R*, renal excretion as unchanged drug; *B*, biliary.

*Aminoglycosides have long $t_{1/2}$ values in tissue (25 to 500 hr).

†In anuric patients.

 ## PHARMACOKINETICS

The pharmacokinetic parameters for the antibiotics that act by inhibiting bacterial protein synthesis are listed in Table 47-2.

Aminoglycosides

Aminoglycosides are not absorbed by oral or rectal administration except after oral use in newborns with necrotizing enterocolitis. If there is renal impairment, even the small amount of drug absorbed by the oral route may accumulate and cause toxicity in adults. After IM injection, peak plasma concentrations occur in 30 to 60 minutes, with plasma concentrations comparable to those achieved after a 30 minute infusion. Shock decreases absorption from the IM site of injection, and thus the IM route is rarely used to treat life-threatening infections.

Topical application of aminoglycosides results in minimal absorption, except in patients with extensive cutaneous damage such as burns or epidermolysis. Intraperitoneal and intrapleural instillation produces such rapid absorption that toxicity may develop, but irrigation (of bladder), intratracheal, and aerosol delivery do not result in significant absorption. However, new techniques of aerosolization with correct particle size can produce concentrations over 100 μg/ml in the lung and 4 μg/ml in plasma.

Because of their high polarity, aminoglycosides do not enter phagocytic or other cells, the brain, or the eye. They are distributed into interstitial fluid, with a volume of distribution essentially that of the extracellular fluid. The highest concentrations of aminoglycosides occur in the renal cortex, where the drug concentrates in proximal renal tubular cells. Urinary tract concentrations are generally 20 to 100 times greater than in the plasma and remain for 24 hours after a single dose. These drugs enter peritoneal, pleural, and synovial fluids relatively slowly but achieve concentrations only slightly less than those in plasma.

Concentrations of aminoglycosides in cerebrospinal fluid (CSF) after IM or IV administration are inadequate for treatment of Gram-negative meningitis. Intrathecal administration into the lumbar space produces inadequate intraventricular concentrations, whereas intraventricular instillation yields high concentrations in both areas.

Subconjunctival injection produces high aqueous

fluid concentrations but inadequate intravitreal concentrations.

Disposition of the aminoglycosides occurs almost completely by glomerular filtration with none metabolized and less than 1% excreted via the biliary tract. A small amount undergoes reabsorption into proximal renal tubular cells. Renal clearance of aminoglycosides is approximately two thirds that of creatinine. However, these drugs can become trapped in tissue compartments to give tissue half-lives of 25 to 500 hours, and aminoglycosides can be detected in urine for up to 10 days after discontinuation of a week-long dosing schedule. The elimination of aminoglycosides depends on renal function, and corrections to dosing schedules must be made for patients who have reduced renal capacity. Because clearance of aminoglycoside is linearly related to clearance of creatinine, the latter can be used to calculate an adjusted dosing schedule. For example, a patient with a creatinine clearance of 50 mg/ml should have the total daily dose of aminoglycoside reduced by about 50% compared to the dose for normal creatinine clearance.

Aminoglycosides can be removed from the body by hemodialysis but not as well by peritoneal dialysis.

Although aminoglycosides are not metabolized and do not bind to serum proteins, they can be inactivated by certain penicillins, particularly carbenicillin and ticarcillin in patients with markedly decreased renal function.

Spectinomycin

Spectinomycin is not absorbed from the gastrointestinal (GI) tract and therefore is administered IM. Disappearance is primarily by glomerular filtration with 85% to 90% removed in 24 hours.

Tetracyclines

Some tetracyclines are incompletely absorbed and others are well absorbed when administered orally, but all attain adequate plasma and tissue concentrations. Minocycline and doxycycline are absorbed more completely and chlortetracycline is the least absorbed. Absorption is favored in the fasting state because tetracyclines form chelates with divalent metals, including calcium, magnesium, aluminum, and iron. Absorption is decreased when some tetracyclines are ingested with milk products, antacids, or iron preparations. However, food does not interfere with absorption of minocycline or doxycycline, and absorption is not reduced by histamine H_2-receptor blockers.

The tetracyclines are widely distributed to body compartments, with the apparent volume of distribution exceeding that for total body water. High concentrations are found in liver, kidney, bile, bronchial epithelium, and breast milk. These drugs can enter pleural, peritoneal, synovial, sputum, and sinus fluids; cross the placenta, and enter phagocytic cells. Minocycline displays higher concentrations than other tetracyclines in saliva and tears. Penetration into the CSF is poor and increases only minimally with meningeal inflammation; however, minocycline achieves therapeutic concentrations in brain tissue.

Tetracyclines do not bind to formed bone but are incorporated into calcifying tissue and into the dentine and enamel of unerupted teeth.

The disposition of the tetracyclines occurs by renal and biliary elimination and by metabolism. Although most of the biliary-eliminated drug is reabsorbed via active transport, some undergoes chelation and is excreted in the feces. This occurs even when the drugs are administered parenterally. Renal clearance of these drugs is by glomerular filtration. Filtration removes 20% of oral tetracycline, but this increases to 60% for IV administration. All tetracyclines, with the exception of doxycycline, accumulate in the presence of decreased renal function. Only doxycycline should be given to patients with renal impairment.

Tetracyclines are also metabolized, an important mechanism for chlortetracycline but less important for doxycycline and minocycline. Metabolism of doxycycline is increased in patients receiving barbiturates or phenytoin because these agents induce the formation of hepatic drug-metabolizing enzymes. The half-life of doxycycline decreases from 16 to 7 hours in such patients. Decreased hepatic function or common bile duct obstruction also prolongs the half-life of tetracyclines because of reduction of biliary excretion.

Chloramphenicol

Chloramphenicol is extremely well absorbed from the GI tract, with peak plasma concentrations about 2 hours after ingestion. It is also available as an inactive palmitate, most of which undergoes hydrolysis by pancreatic lipases in the duodenum with subsequent absorption of the active compound. Plasma concentrations are higher with the free compound than with the palmitate due to incomplete hydrolysis. Parenteral chloramphenicol is available as a succinate ester, which must be hydrolyzed by esterases in the liver, lungs, and kidney to the active compound. The drug should not be given IM because the plasma concentrations are unpredictable.

Because it is highly lipid soluble, chloramphenicol is well distributed throughout the body and enters pleural, ascites, synovial, eye, abscess, and CSF fluids and lung, liver, and brain tissues. CSF concentrations are 50% to 60% of those found in plasma, and this drug crosses the placenta and also enters breast milk.

About 90% of a dose of chloramphenicol undergoes liver conjugation to an inactive and nontoxic glucuronide that is filtered by the kidney. Chloramphenicol palmitate is also excreted by the kidney in the hydrolyzed or palmitate forms. The normal plasma half-life is prolonged in patients with hepatic disease but not in patients with renal disease.

Infants deficient in forming glucuronides may accumulate high concentrations of free drug. In addition, hydrolysis of the succinate may be depressed in newborns and infants. Thus, serum concentrations should be monitored if the drug is used in newborns or infants.

Erythromycin

Erythromycin in the free base form is inactivated by acid. Therefore, it is administered orally with an enteric coating that dissolves in the duodenum. Even in the absence of food, which delays absorption, peak plasma concentrations are difficult to predict, and ester forms of erythromycin are available to help in overcoming this problem. Lactobionate and glucoheptate, water-soluble forms of the drug, are available for IV administration.

Erythromycin is well distributed and produces therapeutic concentrations in tonsillar tissue, middle ear fluid, and lung. It enters prostatic fluid to yield concentrations about one third those in plasma. It does not diffuse well into brain or CSF. Erythromycin crosses the placenta and is found in breast milk, with high concentrations also observed in liver and bile.

The main routes for disposition of erythromycin are metabolic demethylation by liver and biliary excretion. Only a small percentage is excreted unchanged.

Clindamycin

Clindamycin is 90% absorbed from the GI tract. Absorption is delayed but not decreased by the presence of food. Mean peak plasma concentrations occur within 1 hour. Clindamycin is also available as a palmitate ester, which is rapidly hydrolyzed to the free drug, and a phosphate ester, the latter for IM administration.

Distribution is widespread, with clindamycin entering most body compartments and achieving adequate concentrations in lung, liver, bone, and abscesses. It enters CSF and brain tissue, but concentrations are inadequate to treat meningitis and should not be relied on to treat brain infections except toxoplasmosis. This drug enters polymorphonuclear leukocytes and alveolar macrophages and crosses the placenta.

Clindamycin is metabolized to the N-demethyl and sulfoxide, bacteriologically active derivatives, which are excreted in urine and bile. Only 10% of the dose is eliminated as unmetabolized drug in urine. The parent drug can be detected in feces 5 days after IV administration. The half-life is prolonged by severe liver disease.

 ## RELATION OF MECHANISMS OF ACTION TO CLINICAL RESPONSE

Aminoglycosides

The aminoglycosides are effective primarily against aerobic Gram-negative bacilli such as *Enterobacteriacae* or *P. aeruginosa* and have little effect on anaerobic species. Most staphylococci and streptococci are inhibited, but a few strains are resistant.

Aminoglycosides should be reserved for treatment of serious infections in which other agents such as penicillins or cephalosporins are not suitable. Aminoglycosides have no role as initial therapy of grampositive infections. They are necessary in combination with penicillins to treat endocarditis resulting from enterococci or viridans streptococci. Gentamicin is the preferred agent because streptomycin resistance is common.

Treatment of suspected septic states has been initiated with an aminoglycoside such as gentamicin or tobramycin in combination with a penicillin or cephalosporin; however, newer cephalosporins and other β-lactams such as aztreonam or imipenem have lower toxicity and can replace this use of the aminoglycosides.

Aminoglycosides are particularly effective in the treatment of urinary tract infections, probably because of their elevated concentration in the kidney. However, many other agents are available for treatment of urinary tract infections, particularly the oral quinolones. Hospital-acquired pneumonia is treated with aminoglycosides, but the effectiveness is questionable, since the pH (6.5) of the infected lung and the large amount of cellular debris present in these lungs inhibit the activity of aminoglycosides. Nonetheless, the combination of an aminoglycoside with an antipseudomonas penicillin, cephalosporin, or monobactam is usually selected when treating serious respiratory infections resulting from *P. aeruginosa*.

Another combination is that of an aminoglycoside with clindamycin or metronidazole, which is effective against anaerobic species to treat intraabdominal or gynecological infections. In addition, aminoglycosides can be combined with cefoxitin when the intraabdominal infection develops in the hospital and the potential for *Pseudomonas* infection or gentamicin-resistant *Serratia* or *Enterobacter* infection is anticipated to be significant.

Although aminoglycosides are used to treat aerobic Gram-negative osteomyelitis and septic arthritis, other agents of the β-lactam or quinolone classes are preferred. Gram-negative meningitis is more appropriately treated with third-generation cephalosporins, although intraventricular instillation of aminoglycoside may be necessary for selected *Pseudomonas* or *Acinetobacter* meningitis infections. Serious endophthalmitis can be treated with intravitreal instillation of gentamicin.

Aminoglycosides are used in combination with an antipseudomonas β-lactam to treat suspected sepsis in febrile neutropenic patients. Choice of the particular agent depends on the local susceptibility patterns. In general, gentamicin is the initial agent to use, with tobramycin reserved for *Pseudomonas* infections and netilmicin or amikacin for aminoglycoside resistance. The availability of less toxic and equally effective agents allows the aminoglycosides to be restricted to situations in which their use is undeniably expected to produce a superior outcome.

Streptomycin is used primarily to treat uncommon infections, for example, those caused by *Francisella tularensis*, resistant *Brucella* species, and resistant

tuberculosis strains or infections in patients allergic to the usual antituberculosis drugs (see Chapter 51).

Spectinomycin

Although spectinomycin inhibits a number of gram-negative bacteria, it is used to treat only infections due to *Neisseria gonorrhoeae*, especially penicillinase-producing *N. gonorrhoeae* of the genital tract, but not for pharyngeal or anal gonorrhea. Resistance is uncommon. In general, it is replaced by ceftriaxone but can be used in penicillin-allergic patients who have had anaphylactic reactions to β-lactams.

Tetracyclines

Tetracyclines are broad-spectrum agents that inhibit a wide variety of aerobic and anaerobic Gram-positive and Gram-negative bacteria and other microorganisms such as rickettsiae, mycoplasmata chlamydiae, and some mycobacterial species (see Chapter 51). The tetracyclines have many clinical uses, but increasing bacterial resistance and the development of other drugs have replaced them in some of the uses. For example, some *Streptococcus pneumoniae*, *S. pyogenes*, and staphylococci are resistant. *Haemophilus influenzae* remains generally susceptible, but many *N. gonorrhoeae* are resistant. Among the Enterobacteriaceae, resistance has increased markedly in recent years so that many *E. coli* and *Shigella* species and virtually all *P. aeruginosa* are resistant. However, tetracyclines inhibit *Pasteurella multocida*, *F. tularensis*, *Yersinia pestis*, and *Brucella* organisms. Doxycycline inhibits *B. fragilis*, but a major number of *Bacteroides* species are resistant to the other tetracyclines. Other anaerobic species such as *Fusobacterium* and *Actinomyces* are inhibited, as are *Borrelia bergdorferi* (the cause of Lyme disease) and others. *Mycobacterium fortuitum* and *M. marinum* are inhibited, and some activity is observed against *Plasmodium* species.

Tetracyclines are the preferred agents (see box) to treat rickettsial diseases such as Rocky Mountain Spotted Fever, typhus, scrub typhus, rickettsial pox, and Q fever. *Mycoplasma pneumoniae* respiratory infections respond to tetracyclines, which may be better tolerated by adults than erythromycin. Chlamydiae infections of a sexual origin such as nongonococcal urethritis, salpingitis, or cervicitis are best treated

---

THERAPEUTIC USES OF TETRACYCLINES

DRUG OF CHOICE

Ricketsial diseases: Rocky Mountain Spotted Fever,
    typhus, scrub typhus, Q fever
Mycoplasma pneumoniae
Chlamydia pneumoniae
Chlamydia trachomatous
C. psittaci
Lyme disease *(Borrelia Burgdorferi)*
Relapsing fever due to *Borrelia* organisms

ALTERNATIVE AGENT

M. pneumoniae infection
Brucellosis
Plaque
Pelvic inflammatory disease

AS TREATMENT OF SYNDROMES

Acne: low dose oral or topical
Bacterial exacerbations of bronchitis
Sinusitis
Malabsorption syndrome resulting from bowel bacterial overgrowth

---

with tetracycline or doxycycline. Tetracyclines are also effective for psittacosis, inclusion conjunctivitis, and trachoma caused by chlamydiae. Although tetracyclines inhibit many *N. gonorrhoeae*, they no longer are considered optimal therapy but are effective for syphilis if continued long enough.

As discussed under side effects, tetracyclines should not be given to pregnant women, children younger than 8 years of age, individuals with severe liver disease, or those with renal impairment.

Tetracyclines are no longer used in treating urinary tract infections, since so many other agents are available, nor are they useful as prophylaxis in viral illness to prevent bacterial infections. They have no role in the treatment of pharyngitis, and other agents are preferred against staphylococcal infections. In general, other agents should be used to treat osteomyelitis, endocarditis, meningitis, and life-threatening Gram-negative infections. Tetracycline use in intraabdominal infections, with the exception of doxycycline, is also questionable.

The only prophylactic uses of tetracycline are minocycline to eradicate the carrier state of meni-

gococci, but rifampin is the preferred agent. Doxycycline is used to prevent traveler's diarrhea, but photosensitization and resistance have decreased the value of this approach and such use is no longer recommended.

Chloramphenicol

Chloramphenicol has an extremely broad spectrum of antimicrobial activity, inhibiting aerobic and anaerobic Gram-positive and Gram-negative bacteria, chlamydiae, rickettsiae, and mycoplasmata. It is particularly active against *B. fragilis*. Although chloramphenicol is bacteriostatic for Enterobacteriaceae, staphylococci, and streptococci, it is bactericidal for *H. influenzae*, *N. meningitidis*, and many *S. pneumoniae*.

Because of its serious diverse side effects, chloramphenicol should be used only when no other drug is suitable. The major use of chloramphenicol in the United States is centered around its entry into the CSF. It is combined with ampicillin to treat meningitis in children because of the frequency of β-lactamase-producing (and thus resistant) *Haemophilus* species. However, drugs such as cefotaxime, ceftriaxone, or cefuroxime can be used as alternatives. Chloramphenicol also is used to treat brain abscesses, but metronidazole can replace it. In other serious *Haemophilus* infections, cephalosporins or trimethoprim-sulfamethoxazole can replace chloramphenicol. The same is true for its use in intraabdominal infections in which metronidazole, clindamycin, cefoxitin, and imipenem are less toxic. In the treatment of typhoid, it can be replaced by trimethoprim-sulfamethoxazole or by norfloxacin or ciprofloxacin. The later agent appears to cure carriers, which chloramphenicol fails to do.

In rickettsial diseases, chloramphenicol is appropriate for patients who cannot be treated with a tetracycline, but it should not be used for urinary tract, respiratory, or brucellosis infections because other less toxic agents are available.

Erythromycin

Erythromycin is active primarily against Gram-positive species such as staphylococci and streptococci but also inhibits some enterococci and Gram-positive bacilli (see box, p. 672). Chlamydiae, *M. pneumoniae*, some *Ureaplasma urealyticum, Legi-*

THERAPEUTIC USES OF ERYTHROMYCIN

DRUG OF CHOICE

Mycoplasma pneumoniae
Group A streptococcal infection (penicillin-allergic patient)
Legionella infection
Bordetella pertussis
Campylobacter jejuni (children)
Ureaplasma ureolyticum

ALTERNATIVE AGENT

Lyme disease
Chlamydia infection

AS TREATMENT OF SYNDROMES

Bacterial bronchitis
Otitis media (with sulfonamide)
Acne, topical

PROPHYLAXIS

Endocarditis, penicillin-allergic patient
Large bowel surgery
Oral surgery

onella and *Bordetella* species, *Campylobacter jejuni*, and most oral anaerobic species are inhibited. Most aerobic Gram-negative bacilli are resistant.

Erythromycin is used primarily as an alternative to penicillin, particularly in children, especially to treat streptococcal pharyngitis, erysipelas, scarlet fever, cutaneous streptococcal infections, and pneumococcal pneumonia. Although it can cure *S. aureus* infections, the high frequency of resistance of staphylococci does not make it an initial choice of therapy. For treating otitis media, it should be combined with a sulfonamide because of its variable activity against *Haemophilus* organisms.

Erythromycin is useful for treating sexually transmitted diseases, including ones caused by chlamydiae, and it can be used to treat chlamydial pneumonia of the newborn. It is also useful to eradicate the carrier state of diphtheria and may shorten the course of pertussis if administered early.

As a prophylactic agent, erythromycin can be used to prevent bacterial endocarditis in penicillin-allergic patients or in patients with rheumatic fever.

Clindamycin

Clindamycin inhibits most Gram-positive cocci and many anaerobes but not aerobic Gram-negative bacteria. Most enterococci are resistant, but actinomyces are inhibited.

The problem of serious diarrhea limits the use of clindamycin to specific indications. It is appropriate therapy for intraabdominal or gynecological infections in which *Bacteroides* organisms are likely pathogens but should not be used for brain abscesses when anaerobic species are anticipated. However, clindamycin is useful for anaerobic pleuropulmonary infections.

Clindamycin is an alternative to penicillin and may be preferable in certain situations in which β-lactamase-producing *Bacteroides* organisms are present. Clindamycin is also an alternative to penicillins in the treatment of staphylococcal infections but is usually not preferred to a cephalosporin or vancomycin and should not be used for endocarditis.

SIDE EFFECTS, CLINICAL PROBLEMS, AND TOXICITY

The major clinical problems for these drugs are summarized in the box.

Aminoglycosides

Aminoglycosides can produce serious side effects, of which vestibular, cochlear, and renal are the most important and most common.

Renal Toxicity Reversible renal impairment develops in 5% to 25% of patients receiving an aminoglycoside for more than 3 days. In a small number of patients the impairment can progress to severe renal insufficiency but is usually reversible. The mechanism of this nephrotoxicity appears to involve prostaglandins. In the renal cortex, aminoglycosides are transported across the luminal brush border of proximal tubular cells by binding to phosphatidylinositol in the cytoplasmic membrane and undergoing internalization by pinocytosis. Fusion with lysosomes occurs, and the aminoglycosides become trapped in the lysosomes.

Multilamellar structures, called *myeloid bodies*, also accumulate in the lysosomes (Figure 47-9), and phosphatidylinositol-specific phospholipases are in-

CLINICAL PROBLEMS

AMINOGLYCOSIDES

Nephrotoxicity
Ototoxicity
Vestibular toxicity
Neuromuscular blockade (infrequent)

TETRACYCLINES

Binding to bone and teeth: can be serious in infants or
    children under 8 years of age and during pregnancy
GI tract upsets
Hepatic and renal dysfunction
Vaginal candidiasis
Vertigo with minocycline
Photosensitivity

OTHER DRUGS

chloramphenicol: major hematological effects can be fatal
    (aplastic anemia, bone marrow suppression); grey baby
    syndrome if glucuronidation process not well developed
    (for chloramphenicol elimination); drug interactions
    with other agents that are metabolized; optic neuritis
    may result
erythromycin: relatively safe; mild GI disturbances; infre-
    quent hepatotoxicity; drug interaction with theophyl-
    line (metabolism); deafness with high doses
clindamycin: pseudomembranous colitis occurs

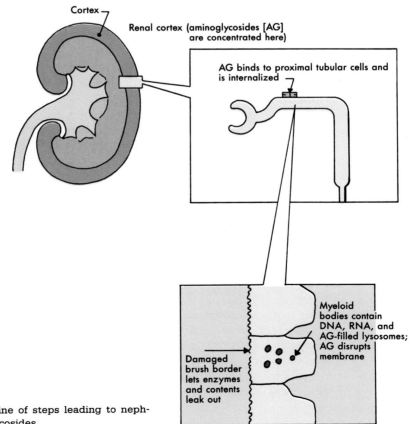

FIGURE 47-9   Schematic outline of steps leading to nephrotoxicity caused by aminoglycosides.

hibited. These enzymes are important in prostaglandin synthesis, and the initial decrease in glomerular filtration that occurs with aminoglycoside toxicity may result from inhibition of vasodilatory prostaglandins so that the angiotension II vasoconstrictor action is unopposed. Aminoglycosides also inhibit spingomyelinases and ATPases and alter mitochondria and ribosomes in proximal tubular cells.

The initial manifestation of aminoglycoside renal toxicity is increased excretion of brush-border enzymes such as β-D-glucosaminidase, alanine aminopeptidase, and alkaline phosphatase. However, it is not clinically useful to monitor the excretion of these enzymes, since fever and other factors also cause similar changes. The result is a decrease in renal concentrating ability, proteinuria, and the appearance of casts in the urine, followed by a reduction in glomerular filtration rate and a rise in serum creatinine.

Risk factors for development of renal toxicity are not completely understood despite extensive study. Toxicity correlates with total drug administered, but older age, female sex, concomitant liver disease, and concomitant hypotension appear to favor the development of the toxicity. Coadministration of aminoglycosides with vancomycin, cisplatin, cyclosporin, or amphotericin B is associated with increased renal toxicity, as is volume depletion and alkalosis.

Aminoglycosides themselves differ in their nephrotoxic potential. Neomycin is the most nephrotoxic and streptomycin is the least. However, clinical trials comparing the nephrotoxicity of the other agents yield contradictory results.

Because tubules can regenerate, renal function usually returns to normal after the drug is cleared. A small number of patients require dialysis because renal function does not return to pretreatment values.

Ototoxicity Aminoglycosides can damage either or both the auditory and vestibular apparatuses. The exact frequency of ototoxicity is unknown, but some damage probably occurs in 5% to 25% of patients, depending on the underlying auditory status and length of therapy. The mechanism of auditory toxicity is destruction of hair cells of the organ of Corti, particularly the outer hair cells in the basal turn (Figure 47-10). Inner hair cells and cells of the vascularis can also be affected. The hair cell damage is accompanied by subsequent retrograde degeneration of the auditory nerves, since the sensory cells do not regenerate. Aminoglycosides also damage hair cells of the am-

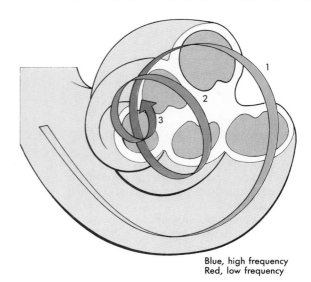

Blue, high frequency
Red, low frequency

FIGURE 47-10   Cochlea, normally lined with hair cells that are destroyed by high concentrations of aminoglycosides. Aminoglycosides produce damage to the hair cells, especially in turn No. 1 and part of turn No. 2. Hairs are shed by the damaged cells to give loss of high frequency response first (associated with turn No. 1) and low frequency loss later (associated with turn No. 3).

pullar cristae, leading to vestibular dysfunction. Aminoglycosides accumulate in perilymph and endolymph and inhibit ionic transport, the cause of cochlear cell damage. Accumulation of drug occurs when the plasma concentrations are high, and ototoxicity is probably enhanced by persistently elevated plasma concentrations of drug.

The amount of auditory or vestibular function loss correlates with the amount of hair cell damage. Repeated courses of therapy continue to damage more hair cells. An unanswered question is whether loop diuretics, such as furosemide, potentiate this ototoxicity in humans as they do in animals.

Differences in toxicity exist among the agents. Streptomycin and gentamicin cause more vestibular toxicity, and kanamycin and amikacin cause more auditory damage. Whether netilmicin is less ototoxic than other aminoglycosides is not clear. Vestibular toxicity is highest for patients who receive 4 weeks of therapy, the procedure used in the treatment of enterococcal endocarditis.

Clinical signs of auditory problems such as tinnitus or a sensation of fullness in the ears are not reliable as predictors of this toxicity. The initial hearing loss is of high frequencies outside the voice range; thus, toxicity development will not be recognized unless hearing tests are performed. Eventually the loss of hearing may progress into the auditory range.

Vestibular toxicity is usually preceded by headache, nausea, emesis, vertigo, and dizziness, so patients who are ill often have difficulty in evaluating the onset of vestibular toxicity. These patients may go through a series of stages from acute to chronic symptoms that are apparent only on standing, or the patients may achieve a compensatory state in which visual cues adjust for the loss of vestibular function.

Neuromuscular Blockade Neuromuscular paralysis is rare but appears to be caused by inhibition of presynaptic release of acetylcholine and postsynaptic receptor blockade. Aminoglycoside inhibits internalization of calcium at the presynaptic nerve terminal, thus blocking the release of acetylcholine. Presynaptic blockade is more readily caused by neomycin and tobramycin than by streptomycin, whereas the opposite order is observed for postsynaptic effects.

Neuromuscular paralysis is most likely to occur during surgery when anesthesia and neuromuscular blockers such as succinylcholine are used, but it also occurs in patients with myasthenia gravis.

Other Toxicities Reversible dose-related malabsorption is observed with oral use of aminoglycosides. It is caused by direct damage to villus cells and by binding to bile salts. Absorption of fat, protein, cholesterol, iron, and digitalis is impaired.

Spectinomycin

Spectinomycin has few adverse effects.

Tetracyclines

Tetracyclines produce adverse effects ranging from minor to life threatening. Allergy precludes the use of tetracycline. Photosensitization with a rash is a toxic rather than an allergic effect and is most often seen with demeclocycline or doxycycline.

Effects on bone and teeth preclude the use of tetracycline in children less than 8 years of age because 80% of them will develop a permanent brown-yellow discoloration of teeth if treated with tetracyclines. The effect is permanent and the enamel is hypoplastic. Binding to bone may result in depression of skeletal growth, especially in premature infants.

Tetracyclines cause dose-dependent GI disturbances including epigastric burning, nausea, and vomiting. Esophageal ulcers have been reported, but pancreatitis is rarely observed.

Hepatic toxicity is encountered most often with parenteral use but can also occur with oral administration. Pregnant women are highly susceptible to tetracycline-hepatic toxicity with development of jaundice and fatty infiltration of the liver. Tetracyclines also aggravate existing renal dysfunction.

Demeclocycline, which is used to treat chronic excessive antidiuretic hormone secretion, produces nephrogenic diabetes insipidus. Other side effects include minocycline-produced vertigo in 50% to 70% of women and 25% of men for certain dosing schedules. Superinfection caused by overgrowth of other bacteria and particularly oral and vaginal candidiasis frequently follows the use of tetracyclines.

Tetracyclines should not be used in patients receiving hyperalimentation, since they prevent new protein synthesis.

Chloramphenicol

Chloramphenicol produces serious side effects that are attributed to its action in mitochondrial membrane enzymes, cytochrome oxidases, and ATPases. Because of these adverse effects, chloramphenicol has only limited use, primarily when no other alternative treatment is suitable.

Hematological effects are the most important. Leukopenia, thrombocytopenia, marrow aplasia, and pancytopenia occurrence is 1:25,000 to 1:40,000, with a high fatality rate for those who develop an aplastic state or progress to acute leukemia. This appears to involve an idiosyncratic reaction with inhibition of stem cells and may result from a biochemical abnormality that causes formation of a toxic metabolite, possibly involving the nitrobenzene group.

Additional hematological effects include reversible erythroid bone marrow suppression, prevention of normal response to vitamin B_{12}, and hemolysis in some glucose-6-phosphate dehydrogenase (G6PD) deficient patients. The marrow suppression develops 5 to 7 days into therapy and is manifest by a decrease in hemoglobin, an increase in plasma iron, and vacuolization of erythroblasts to produce thrombocytopenia and leukopenia.

A complication known as the *grey baby syndrome* also is encountered with chloramphenicol. Neonates with excessively high plasma concentrations of drug develop pallor, cyanosis, abdominal distension, vomiting, and circulatory collapse, resulting in approximately 50% fatalities.

High concentrations of chloramphenicol are caused by inadequate glucuronidation and failure to excrete the drug by the kidneys. Children less than 1 month of age should receive only low doses of this drug, although in critical situations, excess drug can be removed by hemoperfusion over a bed of charcoal.

Chloramphenicol also can produce optic neuritis in children, GI overgrowth of *Candida* organisms, and hypersensitivity rashes.

Chloramphenicol inhibits hepatic microsomal enzymes of the cytochrome P-450 complex, leading to prolongation of the half-life of phenytoin, tolbutamide, chlorpropamide, and dicumarol; barbiturates in turn decrease the half-life of chloramphenicol.

Erythromycin

Erythromycin is one of the safest antibiotics, with GI epigastric pain, abdominal cramps, nausea, and emesis the primary side effects. Hepatotoxicity may occur with erythromycin sulfate, usually beginning 10 to 20 days into treatment and characterized by jaundice, fever, leukocytosis, and eosinophilia. The problem rapidly abates if drug administration is stopped. Erythromycin at high doses can cause reversible transient deafness.

Erythromycin prolongs the half-life of theophylline and can lead to theophylline toxicity. It also inhibits the metabolism of carbamazepine, corticosteroids, and digoxin.

Clindamycin

The most important adverse effect of clindamycin is pseudomembranous enterocolitis, estimated to occur in 3% to 5% of patients. Diarrhea may occur in up to 20% of patients. Pseudomembranous colitis is caused by the toxin produced by *C. difficile*. The illness is characterized by diarrhea, abdominal pain, and fever, with diarrhea beginning either during or

---

TRADENAMES

In addition to generic and fixed combinations of preparations that include other drugs and active compounds available as other salts, the following tradenamed materials are available in the United States.

AMINOGLYCOSIDE

Amikin, amikacin sulfate
Garamycin, gentamicin sulfate
G-myticin, gentamicin sulfate
Kantrex, kanamycin sulfate
Nebcin, tobramycin sulfate
Netromycin, netilmicin sulfate

TETRACYCLINE

Achromycin, Sumycin; tetracycline
Doryx, doxycycline
Minocin, minocycline HCl
Terramycin, Urobiotic; oxytetracycline or salt
Vibramycin calcium, doxycycline calcium

OTHER DRUGS

Chloromycetin, chloramphenicol salts
Cleocin, clindamycin salts
ERYC, Erycette, Ery Derm, Erygel, Ilotycin; erythromycin
Ilosone, erythromycin estolate
Pediamycin, Eryzole, Wyamycin; erythromycin ethylsuccinate (contains sulfisoxazole)
Trobicin, spectinomycin HCl

---

after therapy with clindamycin. Oral vancomycin or metronidazole may be needed as therapy.

REFERENCES

Davis BA, Chen L, and Tai PC: Misread protein creates membrane channels: an essential step in the bactericidal action of aminoglycosides, Proc Natl Acad Sci USA 83:6164, 1986.

Whelton A and Neu HC, eds: The aminoglycosides, New York, 1982, Marcel Dekker, Inc.

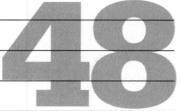

Bacterial Folate Antagonists

ABBREVIATIONS

CSF	cerebrospinal fluid
$t_{1/2}$	half-life
GI	gastrointestinal
AIDS	acquired immune deficiency syndrome
TMP/SMX	trimethoprim-sulfamethoxazole
G6PD	glucose-6-phosphate dehydrogenase

MAJOR DRUGS

sulfonamides
trimethoprim

THERAPEUTIC OVERVIEW

SULFONAMIDES

First chemotherapeutic agents
No longer urinary infection drugs of choice
    Resistant bacteria
    Side effects significant
    Other drugs available
Nocardiosis, toxoplasmosis, and burn areas: still effective

TRIMETHOPRIM-SULFAMETHOXAZOLE COMBINATION

Effective for urinary, respiratory, GI, and gonorrhea infections with many organisms and for treatment of *Pneumocystis carinii* infections and *Isospora belli*

 THERAPEUTIC OVERVIEW

The sulfonamides and trimethoprim are antibiotics that act through inhibition of the folate pathway in bacteria. The folate system serves in a donor-acceptor role for the transfer of one-carbon groups, such as methyl or methylene, and electrons in intracellular synthesis and degradation reactions. Most bacteria must synthesize their folic acid derivatives, whereas humans can rely on dietary sources. Thus inhibition of bacterial capability for the synthesis of folate can serve as a route for antibiotic development and is the common factor for the mechanism of action of the sulfonamides and trimethoprim that are described in this chapter.

The introduction of the sulfonamides into clinical medicine marks the beginning of microbial chemotherapy. In the 1930s, chemists in Germany showed that the dye, prontosil, protected mice infected with streptococci and other bacteria and that sulfonamide was the active component. A number of sulfonamide derivatives have been synthesized and tested in humans, but only a few are in clincial use. Sulfonamides formerly were preferred for the treatment of urinary tract infections. However, the development of resistant bacteria, the presence of numerous side effects, and the availability of other antibiotics have led to discontinuation of this use. These drugs remain of value in the treatment of nocardiosis, and, topically, for burn areas. The trimethoprim-sulfamethoxazole combination has many therapeutic applications. The therapeutic aspects are summarized in the box, p. 677.

 ## MECHANISMS OF ACTION

Folic Acid Synthesis and Regeneration

The bacterial synthesis of folic acid uses a multistep enzyme-catalyzed reaction sequence, summarized in Figure 48-1. Folic acid consists of p-aminobenzoic acid, pterin, and glutamic acid linked together and can undergo reduction to dihydrofolate

and further to tetrahydrofolate (see Figure 48-1). The enzymes that catalyze step A, dihydropteroate synthetase, and step B, dihydrofolate reductase, are competitively inhibited by sulfonamides and trimethoprim, respectively. Thus, these two drug types block the synthesis of tetrahydrofolate at different steps in the synthetic pathway.

Sulfonamides

The structures of many of the clinically used sulfonamides are shown in Figure 48-2. These agents are bacteriostatic. They are competitive inhibitors of p-aminobenzoic acid incorporation through a high affinity for dihydropteroate synthetase. Although competitive enzyme inhibition is the main mechanism of

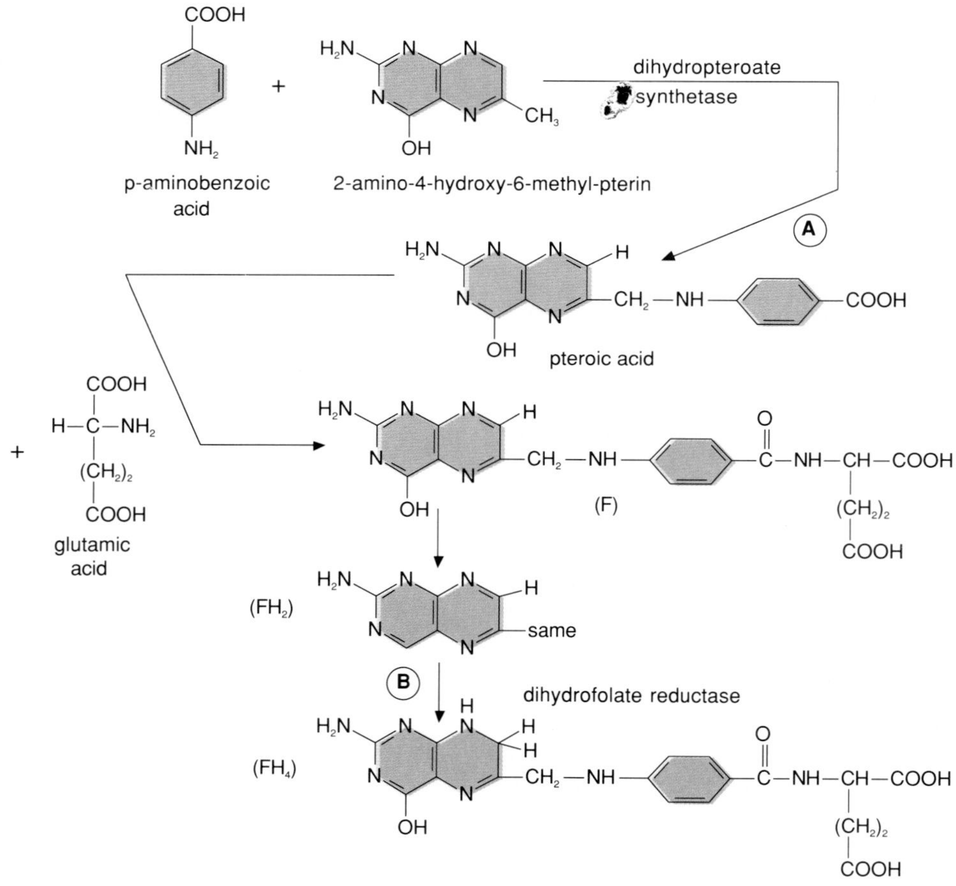

FIGURE 48-1   Bacterial synthesis of folic acid (F) and reduction to dihydrofolate (FH_2) and tetrahydrofolate (FH_4). A and B are sites of drug action.

action, the sulfonamides can function as competitive substrates for the synthetase and become incorporated into a product with pteridine, thus depleting the system of pteridine. Microorganisms cannot use preformed pteroylglutamic acid and must synthesize their own. In contrast, mammalian cells require the preformed acid. Folate metabolism is necessary for the production of thymidine, purines, and several amino acids, including methionine; therefore, when folate synthesis is inhibited, bacterial cell growth is halted. This inhibition of cell growth can be reversed by addition of purines, thymidine, methionine, and serine.

In sulfonamides the para-NH_2 group is essential for antibacterial activity and can be replaced only by groups that are converted to the free amine in vivo. Ortho and meta amino substituents are inactive. The $-SO_2NH_2$ group can be substituted, but there must be a direct sulfur-carbon link to the benzene ring.

Structural changes also have a marked effect on sulfonamide solubility. For example, sulfadiazine and sulfisoxazole are 10 and 100 times, respectively, more soluble at pH 7.5 than at pH 5.5.

Bacterial resistance to sulfonamides occurs by several mechanisms. Reduced cellular uptake of drug, which can be of chromosomal or plasmid origin, is one mechanism. Another is an altered dihydropteroate synthetase, which can result from a point mutation or the presence of a plasmid that causes synthesis of a new enzyme. Replacement of a single amino acid in the enzyme alters the affinity for sulfonamides. In enteric species, plasmid-propagated resistance is the common form. A final mechanism of resistance is production of increased amounts of p-aminobenzoic acid, which is found with some staphylococci but is not common. Resistance stemming from an altered enzyme can develop during therapy.

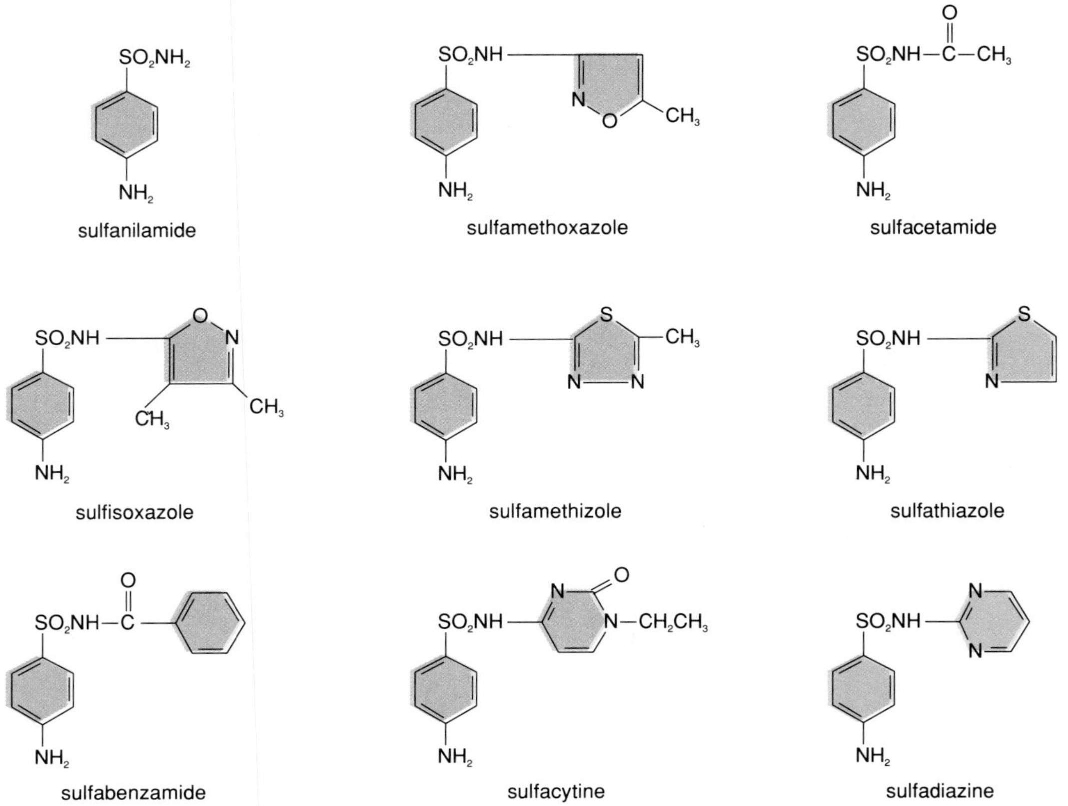

FIGURE 48-2   Sulfonamide structures.

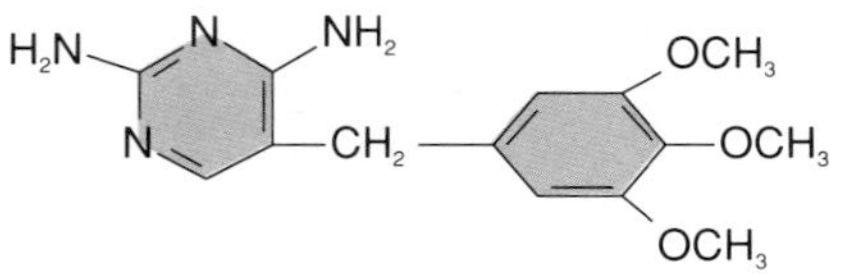

FIGURE 48-3   Trimethoprim structure.

Trimethoprim

Trimethoprim was initially used as an antimalarial drug but has been replaced by another agent that acts by a similar mechanism. The antimalarial and antibacterial actions of trimethoprim (see Figure 48-3 for structure) are based on its high affinity for bacterial dihydrofolate reductase. Trimethoprim binds competitively and inhibits this enzyme in bacterial and mammalian cells. About 100,000 times higher concentrations of drug are needed to obtain 50% inhibition of the human enzyme as compared to the bacterial. This enzyme is inhibited by methotrexate, discussed in Chapter 43. Trimethoprim thus prevents the conversion of dihydrofolate to tetrahydrofolate and thereby blocks the formation of thymidine, some purines, methionine, and glycine in the bacteria, leading to rapid death of the microorganisms.

Trimethoprim and sulfamethoxazole are used effectively in combination to give synergistic effects. The two drugs block different steps in the synthesis of reduced folic acid. Moreover, sulfonamide potentiates the action of trimethoprim by reducing dihydrofolate competing with trimethoprim for binding to dihydrofolate reductase. The combination of the two drugs is bactericidal.

Resistance to trimethoprim and to the combination of trimethoprim-sulfamethoxazole arises from permeability changes and from the presence of an altered dihydrofolate reductase. The production of this enzyme can be modified by a chromosomal mutation or by a plasmid. An increasing incidence of resistance to trimethoprim-sulfamethoxazole via the plasmid mechanism is occurring. A mutation to thymine dependence has also been found, as has overproduction of dihydrofolate reductase.

PHARMACOKINETICS

The relevant pharmacokinetic parameters are summarized in Table 48-1.

General Sulfonamides

Sulfonamides are generally well absorbed from the GI tract (approximately 70% to 95%), with the majority of absorption in the small intestine. There is minimal absorption from topical application.

Sulfonamides differ in protein binding, from a low of 35% to 50% for sulfadiazine to 80% to 99% for sulfisoxazole or sulfasalazine, with less protein binding in renal failure. The drugs enter most body compartments, including ocular, pleural, peritoneal, synovial, and CSF. Highest concentrations in the CSF are achieved with sulfadiazine, reaching 30% to 80% of simultaneous plasma concentrations. Sulfonamides cross the placenta and enter the fetal circulation.

Metabolism is a major mechanism of inactivation of sulfonamides. The agents vary in the degree of acetylation of the amino group, with the products inactive but less soluble in urine. Acetylation is increased with renal disease and decreased with impaired hepatic function. Metabolism by glucuronidation also occurs with these compounds. Sulfonamides are eliminated as metabolites. Renal elimination is by filtration, with some tubular reabsorption but only slight tubular secretion. In acid urine, some sulfonamides are poorly soluble and precipitate.

Rapid-acting Sulfonamides

Rapid-acting sulfonamides, including sulfisoxazole, sulfamethoxazole, and sulfadiazine, are rapidly absorbed and eliminated. Sulfisoxazole is acetylated, and 30% of the drug in the blood or urine is in the acetylated form. Approximately 95% is excreted in 24 hours, and urine concentrations are high. Because sulfisoxazole is highly soluble in urine, it rarely produces crystals in renal tubules. Sulfamethoxazole is similar to sulfisoxazole but is less rapidly absorbed and excreted.

Sulfadiazine is rapidly absorbed from the GI tract, with peak plasma concentrations in 3 hours. It is the most active sulfonamide, but problems of crystal formation in the renal tubules limit its use. Sulfadoxine is well absorbed and highly bound to plasma proteins, with an extraordinarily long half-life of 10 to 17 days.

Other Sulfonamides

Sulfasalazine is poorly absorbed from the GI tract and therefore can be used to treat GI infections. This

Table 48-1 Pharmacokinetic Parameters for Main Clinical Agents

Drug	Route of Administration	$t_{1/2}$ (hr)	Disposition	Plasma Protein Bound (%)
sulfacetamide	Topical	—	—	—
sulfisoxazole	Oral	6	R, M	90
sulfamethoxazole	Oral/IV	11	R, M	70
sulfadiazine	Oral/IV	17	M R	45
sulfadoxine	Oral	120-200	R, M	—
sulfamethizole	Oral	1, 5	R, M	90
sulfasalazine	Oral	6-10	R, M	99
trimethoprim	Oral	11	R (60%) M	70

M, Metabolized; *R*, renal excretion as unchanged drug.

agent is metabolized by intestinal bacteria to sulfapyridine, which is absorbed and excreted in the urine, and to 5-aminosalicylate, which is the active agent. Sulfasalazine can produce all the toxic reactions of the other sulfonamides.

Trimethoprim

Trimethoprim is well absorbed from the GI tract, with peak plasma concentrations in about 2 hours. Absorption is not influenced by sulfamethoxazole.

Trimethoprim is rapidly and widely distributed to body tissues and compartments, entering pleural, peritoneal, and synovial fluids, as well as the aqueous fluid of the eye, the CSF, and brain. Because of its high lipid solubility, trimethoprim crosses biological membranes and enters bronchial secretions, prostate and vaginal fluids, and bile. Trimethoprim and sulfamethoxazole cross the placenta.

Only 10% to 20% of trimethoprim is metabolized by oxidation and conjugation to inactive oxide and hydroxyl derivatives. It is excreted in urine with 60% of the dose excreted in 24 hours with normal renal function and a linear relationship between serum creatinine and trimethoprim half-life. The half-life of 11 hours in normal adults and children is shortened to approximately 6 hours in young children. Urinary concentrations of trimethoprim are high even in the presence of decreased renal function, and a small amount of trimethoprim is excreted in bile.

RELATION OF MECHANISMS OF ACTION TO CLINICAL RESPONSE

Sulfonamides

The antibacterial spectrum of sulfonamides varies from one community to another. Most streptococci, including *Streptococcus pneumoniae, Haemophilus influenzae*, and chlamydiae, are susceptible, and *Neisseria meningitidis, N. gonorrhoeae, Brucella* organisms, and *Campylobacter* species vary from highly susceptible to resistant. Enterococci are resistant, and some *Escherichia coli* that cause outpatient urinary tract infections are susceptible. However, most hospital strains are resistant. *Shigella* species, most staphylococci, *Bacteroides fragilis*, and *Pseudomonas* organisms are resistant. Sulfonamides inhibit *Nocardia asteroides*.

The sulfonamides are grouped into rapidly acting, intermediate acting, long-acting, poorly absorbed, and topical agents.

Sulfisoxazole, sulfamethoxazole, and sulfadiazine are the principal members of the fast-acting group.

Short-acting sulfonamides are sulfacytine, sulfamethizole, and triple sulfonamide preparations, containing sulfamerazine, sulfamethazine, and sulfadiazine in one preparation and sulfabenzamide, sulfacetamide, and sulfathiazole in another. None of these are more useful than sulfisoxazole. Sulfisoxazole is combined with phenazopyridine, a urinary analgesic, and with erythromycin ethylsuccinate for treatment of otitis media in children. Sulfamethoxazole is an intermediate-acting sulfonamide.

Sulfadiazine achieves highest concentrations in CSF and brain. When sulfadiazine is used, fluid intake must be high and/or alkalinization achieved by administration of sodium bicarbonate to reduce the risk of renal crystalluria by the drug.

The only long-acting sulfonamide used today is sulfadoxine, which is available in combination with pyrimethamine to treat malaria.

Of the poorly absorbed sulfonamides, sulfasalazine is minimally absorbed from the GI tract and is used to treat ulcerative colitis and regional enteritis. It has no effect on intestinal flora.

Sulfacetamide, a topical agent, is used in ophthalmic preparations because it penetrates into ocular tissues and fluids. Allergic reactions are rare, although it should not be used in patients with a known sulfonamide allergy.

Silver sulfadiazine is active against a large number of bacterial species, including *P. aeruginosa*, with the activity probably resulting from slow release of silver into the surrounding medium, since its action is not inhibited by *p*-aminobenzoic acid. This drug is used topically, particularly with burn patients, to reduce bacteria in the burn escher to levels low enough to prevent burn wound sepsis and to hasten wound healing. Minimal silver is absorbed, but sulfadiazine can be absorbed. Adverse reactions are uncommon. Mafenide is another sulfonamide earlier used in burn treatment that inhibits Gram-positive and Gram-negative bacteria and is not inactivated by *p*-aminobenzoic acid. It is absorbed and converted to *p*-carboxybenzene sulfonamide. It has been used to prevent burn wound colonization, but adverse reactions favor the use of silver sulfadiazine. Mafenide and its breakdown products are carbonic anhydrase inhibitors that can cause metabolic acidosis. There usually is a compensatory alkalosis caused by respiratory adjustment.

Therapeutic Uses There are few indications for use of sulfonamides because a large number of other agents are available. However, the presence of certain opportunistic infections in AIDS patients has rekindled interest in these drugs.

Sulfonamides formerly were the preferred agents for treatment of initial urinary tract infections, but acute lower tract infections now are treated with other compounds. The sulfonamides have no role in the treatment of complicated or upper urinary tract infections or in the treatment of respiratory infections, except in combination with erythromycin to treat otitis media in children. Shigellosis no longer can be treated with sulfonamides alone, and trimethoprim-sulfamethoxazole or quinolones are drugs of choice in adults.

Two additional diseases in which sulfonamides are of value are nocardiosis, which involves therapy for many months, and toxoplasmosis, using sulfadiazine or sulfisoxazole and pyrimethamine.

Although sulfonamides can be used for prophylaxis of rheumatic fever, penicillins are preferred, and in penicillin-allergic patients, erythromycin is a better alternative.

Trimethoprim

Trimethoprim inhibits many different bacteria and, with sulfamethoxazole (the TMP/SMX combination), several parasites. Trimethoprim alone inhibits most urinary pathogens, with the exception of *P. aeruginosa*. Also, it is not highly active alone against neisseriae.

The TMP/SMX combination inhibits most *Staphylococcus aureus*; coagulase-negative staphylococci, including *S. saphrophyticus*; many methicillin-resistant *S. aureus*; hemolytic streptococci; *H. influenzae*; *N. meningitidis*; *N. gonorrhoeae*; *Listeria monocytogenes*; aerobic Gram-negative bacteria such as *E. coli* and *Klebsiella*; and some more difficult species such as *Enterobacter*, *Citrobacter*, and *Serratia*. *Salmonella*, *Shigella*, *Aeromonas*, and *Yersinia* species are inhibited, but enterococci and *Campylobacter* species are resistant.

The TMP/SMX combination inhibits *Pneumocystis carinii* and *Isospora belli*, the parasitic organisms in immunocompromised patients that cause pneumonia and diarrhea, respectively.

Therapeutic Uses The TMP/SMX combination is effective in the treatment of uncomplicated urinary tract infections caused by Enterobacteriaceae. Maintaining trimethoprim in vaginal secretions is thought to contribute to reducing recurrent urinary tract infections in females. The TMP/SMX combination is also an effective therapy of prostatitis resulting from Enterobacteriaceae and in the treatment of orchitis and epididymitis due to susceptible bacteria and chlamydiae. Trimethoprim alone is effective therapy of uncomplicated and recurrent urinary tract infections in women and as a prophylaxis to prevent recurrences.

The TMP/SMX combination is also effective treatment of gonorrhea when continued over several days. It is efficacious for some chlamydial urethritis through the activity of sulfonamide. Chancroid can be treated with the combination, but not syphilis.

The TMP/SMX combination is effective treatment of acute bacterial exacerbations of bronchitis due to *H. influenzae, Moraxella (Branhamella)* species, and *S. pneumoniae.* The combination is also effective therapy of otitis media in children resulting from the aforementioned organisms but should not be used to treat streptococcal pharyngitis. Sinusitis caused by ampicillin-resistant *Haemophilus* organisms can also be treated with the combination.

The TMP/SMX combination is effective for therapy of shigellosis and for diarrhea caused by toxigenic *E. coli.* It is also useful against *Yersinia* species, systemic *Salmonella* infections, and typhoid. *Campylobacter* diarrhea is not treated.

High dose TMP/SMX is effective therapy of pneumocystis pneumonia in immunocompromised patients, equally effective to pentamidine, but adverse effects are common.

Many other infections (brucellosis, biliary tract infections, osteomyelitis, bacteremia, and endocarditis) can be successfully treated with TMP/SMX. When administered IV, it is effective treatment of *L. meningitidis* in penicillin-allergic patients.

TMP/SMX can be used successfully as prophylaxis of recurrent infection and of pneumonitis resulting from *P. carinii.* Although reductions in other Gram-negative infections may be seen in pediatric patients, the combination is less successful for such infections in adults.

SIDE EFFECTS, CLINICAL PROBLEMS, AND TOXICITY

The major clinical problems for these drugs are summarized in the box.

Sulfonamides

Sulfonamides unfortunately cause a large number of adverse reactions, the most important of which are hypersensitivity reactions. Allergic rashes are frequent, occurring in approximately 2% to 3% of pa-

---

CLINICAL PROBLEMS

SULFONAMIDES

Numerous side effects
   Hypersensitivity: rashes, fever
   Stevens-Johnson syndrome (with long-acting agents)
   Renal tubule precipitation of sulfadiazine
Drug interactions
   Protein-binding displacement
   Same metabolizing enzymes as other drugs

TRIMETHOPRIM

Side effects less pronounced
Hematological reactions
Increased serum creatinine

---

tients receiving these drugs. Rashes may be maculopapular, urticarial, or, rarely, exfoliative, as in the Stevens-Johnson syndrome. Most rashes occur after 1 week of therapy but can occur earlier in individuals previously sensitized. A serum sicknesslike illness also is seen, with fever, joint pains, and rash, which can be of the erythema nodosum type. Drug fever occurs in about 3% of individuals given sulfonamides. The patients may complain of malaise, headache, chills, and pruritus. Arteritis of a periarteritis or systemic lupus erythematosis type has also been reported.

The most serious cutaneous toxicity, that of Stevens-Johnson syndrome, is distinctly uncommon with the short-acting sulfonamides but is seen with the long-acting agents. This is the reason sulfadoxine is no longer used for malaria prophylaxis.

Several hematological toxicities are seen with sulfonamide use. These include agranulocytosis, megaloblastic anemia, aplastic anemia, hemolytic anemia, and thrombocytopenia. Agranulocytosis occurs in less than 0.1% patients and most recover, although the recovery can take up to a month. Neutropenia occurs occasionally but is rapidly resolved by stopping drug. Thrombocytopenia of a mild degree is common, but severe depression of platelet counts is rare. Hemolytic anemia can occur in G6PD-deficient individuals in which the sulfonamide serves as an oxidant. The episode usually occurs in the first week of therapy, causing an associated reticulocytosis, bilirubinemia, urobilinuria, and marked decreased of hemoglobulin concentrations. Hemolysis can also occur in patients who have normal G6PD concentrations.

Hepatotoxicity, occurring in less than 0.1% of patients receiving sulfonamides, manifests as fever, nausea, emesis, jaundice, and elevation of serum transaminases. This can rarely progress to liver failure, and the problem generally disappears with drug withdrawal. The reaction does not seem to be dose related.

Renal damage is rare with the newer sulfonamides, but sulfadiazine can precipitate in the kidneys, ureters, and bladder and lead to renal failure.

Drug interactions include potentiation of the action of sulfonylurea hypoglycemic agents, oral anticoagulants, phenytoin, and methotrexate. Mechanisms are displacement of albumin-bound drug and competition for drug-metabolizing enzymes.

Trimethoprim

Trimethoprim alone can cause nausea, vomiting, and diarrhea but rarely causes a rash. At the doses used for urinary tract infection, hematological toxicity is uncommon, although neutropenia and thrombocytopenia can occur. Trimethoprim can cause an increase in creatinine concentrations, since both compounds compete for the same renal clearance pathways.

The TMP/SMX combination has all of the complications of both agents. Hematological toxicity in the form of megaloblastic anemia, thrombocytopenia, and leukopenia occurs more often with the combination than with the single agents and can be dose related. Other toxicities include glossitis, stomatitis, and occasional pseudomembranous enterocolitis. CNS effects include headache, depression, and hallucinations.

TRADENAMES

In addition to generic and fixed combination preparations, the following tradenamed materials are available in the United States.

AVC, sulfanilamide
Bactrim, sulfamethoxazole/trimethoprim
Gantanol, sulfamethoxazole
Gantrisin, sulfisoxazole
Proloprim, trimethoprim
Septra, sulfamethoxazole/trimethoprim
Sulamyd, sulfacetamide
Thiosulfil, sulfamethiazole
Trimpex, trimethoprim

Patients with AIDS have a greater incidence of rash and neutropenia than other patients when treated with the TMP/SMX combination. The hematological toxicity can be reversed by use of folinic acid without a decrease in antimicrobial activity.

REFERENCES

Gleckman R et al: Intravenous sulfamethoxazole trimethoprim: pharmacokinetics, therapeutic indications and adverse reactions, Pharmacotherapy 1:206, 1981.

Harvey RJ: Synergism in the folate pathway, Rev Infect Dis 4:255, 1982.

Hitchings GH, ed: Inhibition of folate metabolism in chemotherapy, New York, 1983, Springer-Verlag, Inc.

National Institutes of Health Concensus Developmental Conference: Travelers' diarrhea, JAMA 253:2700, 1985.

Salter, AJ, Overview. Trimethoprim-sulfamethoxazole: an assessment of more than 12 years of use, Rev Infect Dis 4:196, 1982.

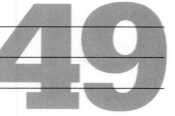

CHAPTER 49 Other Antibacterial Agents

ABBREVIATIONS	
DNA	deoxyribonucleic acid
MIC	minimal inhibitory concentration
pH	logarithm of the reciprocal of the hydrogen ion concentration
CSF	cerebrospinal fluid
$t_{1/2}$	half-life

MAJOR DRUGS

quinolones
nitrofurans
methenamine
polymyxins

THERAPEUTIC OVERVIEW

Several types of antimicrobial agents act through inhibition or damage to bacterial DNA (quinolones and nitrofurans), through disruption of bacterial cell membranes (polymyxins), or by unknown mechanisms (methenamine). The older quinolones, nitrofurans, and methenamine are used primarily to treat urinary tract infections; the newer quinolones are also effective against gonorrhea, diarrhea, selected respiratory infections, skin structure infections, and osteomyelitis (box). The newer quinolones will become increasingly important in the chemotherapy of infectious diseases.

THERAPEUTIC OVERVIEW

QUINOLONES

Urinary tract infections
Gonorrhea infections
Bacterial diarrhea infections
Respiratory infections
Skin structure infections
Osteomyelitis
Prophylaxis in neutropenic patients

NITROFURANS

Urinary tract infections

METHENAMINE

Urinary tract infections

POLYMYXINS

Mainly topical uses

MECHANISMS OF ACTION

Quinolones

These compounds include nalidixic acid, oxolinic acid, cinoxacin, and the newer fluoro-based norfloxacin and ciprofloxacin (see Figure 49-1 for structures). The fluorine at position 6 provides activity against Gram-positive organisms, and the piperazine ring in ciprofloxacin adjacent to the fluorine increases activity against Gram-negative species, particularly *Pseu-*

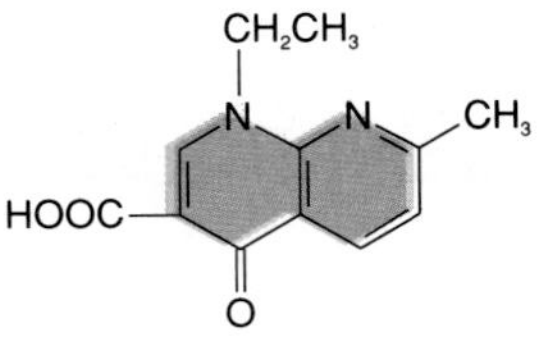

nalidixic acid

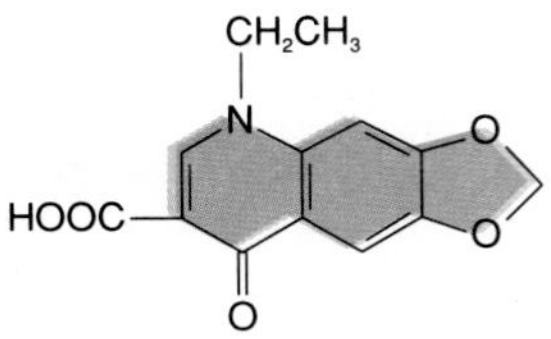

oxolinic acid

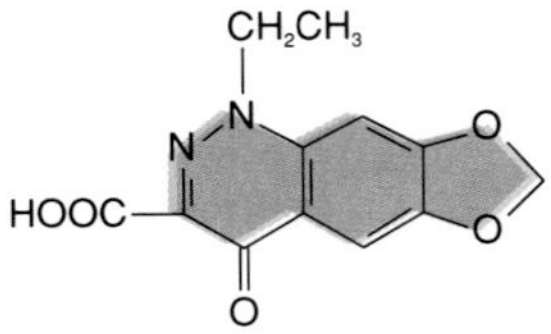

cinoxacin

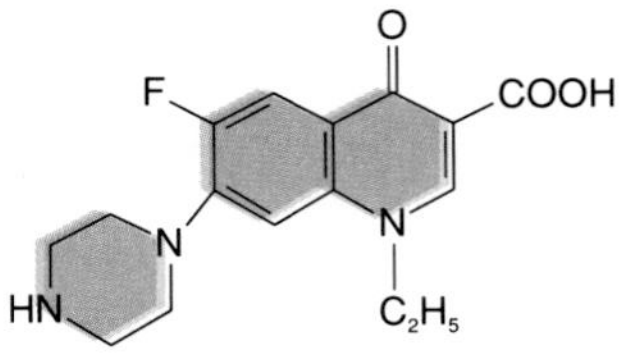

norfloxacin

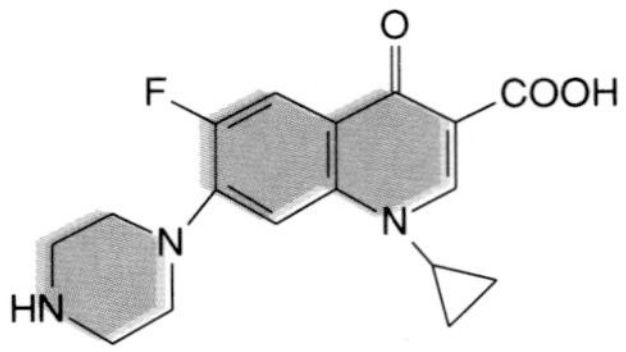

ciprofloxacin

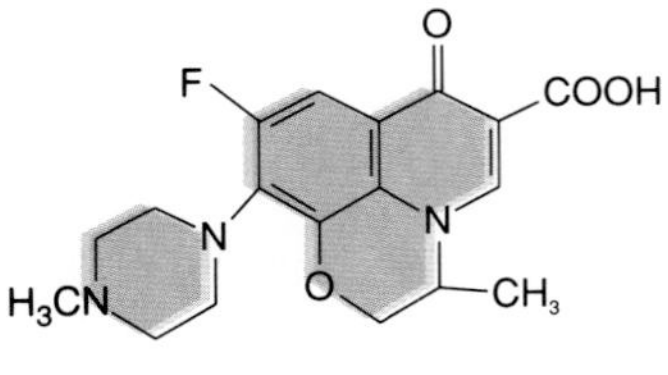

ofloxacin

FIGURE 49-1 Structures of quinolones in clinical use.

Pseudomonas aeruginosa. The keto group at position 4 and the COOH group at position 3 facilitate entry into Gram-negative bacteria by binding Ca^{++}

The quinolones act by inhibiting a bacterial DNA topoisomerase II known as DNA gyrase. The topoisomerases are enzymes that catalyze the direction and extent of supercoiling and other topological reactions of DNA chains (see Chapter 43). Bacterial DNA gyrase is the main target for the quinolones. DNA gyrases catalyze the introduction of negative spherohelical twists into closed circular DNA and the reversible joining of DNA circles. DNA gyrase consists of α and β subunits; quinolones affect the α subunit. The increased antibacterial activity of fluoroquinolones such as norfloxacin and ciprofloxacin correlates with increased inhibition of supercoiling, but the precise mechanism has not been established (Figure 49-2).

Altered DNA gyrase results in increased bacterial resistance to nalidixic acid, oxolinic acid, and cinoxacin, but the bacteria are still susceptible to inhibition by norfloxacin or ciprofloxacin. Minor increases in MICs for norfloxacin and ciprofloxacin can occur with the altered DNA gyrase α subunit, and bacteria having both the altered DNA gyrase and altered membrane permeability can become resistant to the new agents. Resistant bacteria have been found in patients treated for urinary tract infections and particularly in cystic fibrosis patients infected with *Pseudomonas* organisms and methicillin-resistant staphylococci. Most clinical Gram-negative isolates resistant to the new quinolones appear to have lost outer membrane porin proteins, which are important for transport of these agents into the bacteria, as well as possessing altered DNA gyrase. Plasmid resistance does not occur. Inhibition of topoisomerase II in mammalian cells requires much higher concentrations of quinolones than inhibition of the enzyme of susceptible bacteria.

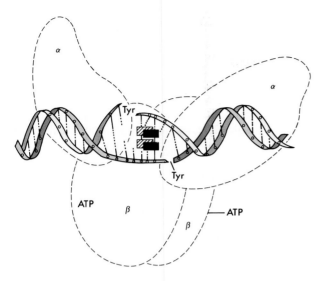

FIGURE 49-2   A model of quinolone-DNA cooperative binding in the inhibition of DNA gyrase. Illustrated are α and β subunits of the enzyme with tyrosine (*Tyr*) indicated and a drug self-assembly of four molecules of quinolone in a single-stranded DNA pocket, shown in the center of the diagram. ATP binding sites on β subunits as shown. (Reprinted with permission from Shen LE et al: Mechanism of inhibition of DNA gyrase by quinolone antibacterials, Biochemistry 28:22886, 1989. Copyright 1989 Am Chem Soc.)

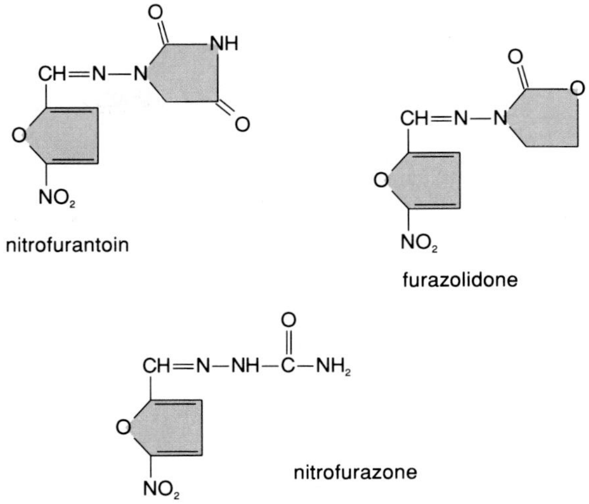

Nitrofurans

Three members of the nitrofuran group are used clinically: nitrofurantoin, furazolidone, and nitrofurazone. The structures are shown in Figure 49-3.

The precise mechanism of action of the nitrofurans is not established. They inhibit a number of bacterial enzyme systems, most probably through DNA damage. A nitroreductase enzyme converts the compounds to short-lived intermediates, including oxygen-free radicals, which interact with DNA to cause strand breakage and bacterial damage.

Resistance develops infrequently and is not plasmid mediated but appears to be caused by a mutation associated with loss of bacterial nitroreductase activity.

Methenamine

Methenamine is a hexamethylene-tetramine that undergoes hydrolysis at acid pH to produce formaldehyde and ammonia; formaldehyde is the active bacterial compound. At pH 5, 20% of methenamine is converted to formaldehyde, but at pH 7 only 6%;

FIGURE 49-3   Structures of nitrofurans.

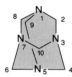

FIGURE 49-4   Methenamine structure, showing position numbers.

approximately 3 hours are needed for the reaction to go to completion at lower pH values. The caged ring structure of methenamine is shown in Figure 49-4.

Polymyxins

The polymyxins are branched-chain decapeptides of about 1000 daltons molecular weight. The structure of polymyxin B is shown in Figure 49-5. An analog with a similar structure to polymyxin E (colistin) is also used clinically.

The polymyxins are bactericidal cationic detergents. They have both lipophilic and lipophobic groups, which interact with phospholipids and disrupt bacterial cell membranes. The initial damage is to the cell wall with loss of periplasmic enzymes. The divalent cationic sites on the lipopolysaccharide component of the outer membrane of gram-negative organisms interact with the amino groups of the cyclic peptide. The fatty acid tail portion of the drug molecule penetrates into the hydrophobic areas of the

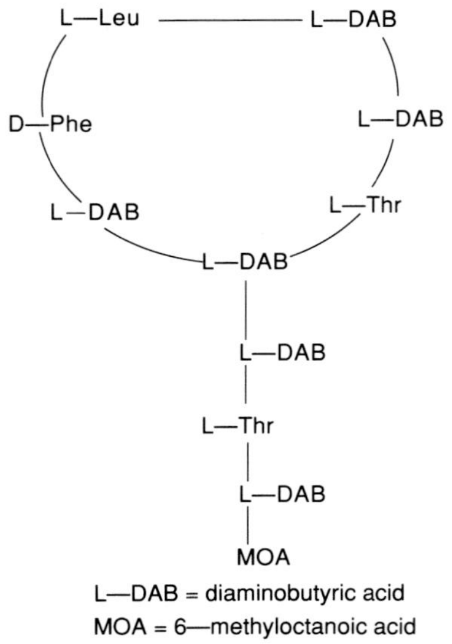

```
    L—Leu ——————— L—DAB
                          \
  D—Phe                    L—DAB
                          /
     L—DAB              L—Thr
          \            /
           L—DAB
             |
           L—DAB
             |
           L—Thr
             |
           L—DAB
             |
            MOA
```

L—DAB = diaminobutyric acid
MOA = 6—methyloctanoic acid

FIGURE 49-5   Structure of polymyxin B.

outer wall to generate holes in the membrane through which intracellular constituents leak out of the bacteria (Figure 49-6). Susceptibility is related to phospholipids in the bacteria cell wall interacting with the drug. The cell walls of resistant bacteria restrict the transport of polymyxin and prevent access of the drug to the cell membrane. Elevated concentrations of calcium or magnesium reduce the activity of the polymyxins.

PHARMACOKINETICS

The pharmacokinetic parameters for these agents are summarized in Table 49-1.

Quinolones Nalidixic acid is 95% bound to plasma proteins. It is rapidly metabolized by the liver to an active hydroxy metabolite and an inactive gluc-

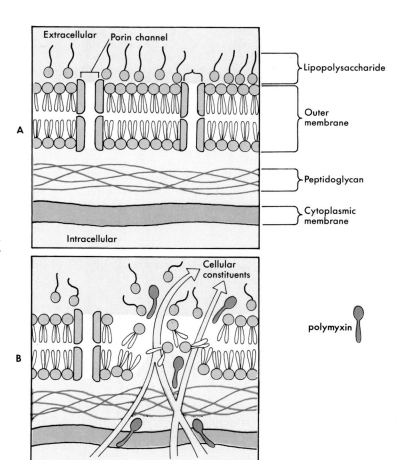

FIGURE 49-6   Mechanism of action of polymyxins. Microbial cell in **A,** absence and **B,** presence of polymyxins.

uronide. The drug is minimally distributed in the body, and only the kidney has concentrations greater than those in plasma. Nalidixic acid and the more active hydroxy metabolite are both excreted, with high concentrations achieved in urine.

Cinoxacin is metabolized to four microbiologically inactive metabolites, with 60% excreted as parent compound by glomerular filtration and tubular secretion to yield excellent urine concentrations of drug.

Ciprofloxacin is 70% to 85% absorbed orally with decreased absorption in the presence of magnesium and aluminum but not with calcium antacids and iron. Ciprofloxacin is widely distributed in the body, entering all compartments including the eye, CSF, and phagocytic cells. Concentrations in interstitial fluid equal those in plasma. High concentrations are present in salivary secretions, nasal mucosa, and bronchial epithelium, with concentrations in bile exceeding those in plasma.

Ciprofloxacin is removed primarily by glomerular filtration and tubular secretion with about 20% of a dose undergoing metabolism. There may also be some secretion by gastrointestinal cells. The half-life of ciprofloxacin is 4 hours, increasing to 10 hours in anuria. Approximately 30% of a dose is recovered in the urine. The volume of distribution is 90 to 120 L. Ciprofloxacin can be removed by hemodialysis and peritoneal dialysis.

Norfloxacin is moderately well absorbed orally, but magnesium, aluminum, and calcium antacids decrease absorption. Its volume of distribution is approximately 100 L, producing interstitial fluid concentrations equal to those in plasma, body tissues, and secretions. Norfloxacin also enters alveolar macrophages and polymorphonuclear leukocytes. It is approximately 20% metabolized to inactive oxides and glucuronides and undergoes renal elimination.

Nitrofurans Nitrofurantoin is 94% absorbed from the gastrointestinal tract, and the absorption is not altered by the presence of food. The drug exists in several crystalline forms; the macrocrystalline form is absorbed more slowly than the others. No drug accumulation occurs except in urine and bile. Disappearance of the drug is by excretion into bile, followed by reabsorption and elimination through glomerular filtration and tubular secretion to yield a brown urine. The half-life in normal individuals is 0.6 to 1.2 hours due to the rapid excretion and metabolism in tissues. As renal function declines, less drug enters the urine, so that treatment of urinary tract infections is ineffective in individuals with creatinine clearances less than 40 ml/min. In patients with severely depressed renal function, the drug accumulates and can cause neurotoxicity.

Methenamine Methenamine is absorbed from the gastrointestinal tract, but 10% to 30% is hydro-

Table 49-1	Pharmacokinetic Parameters			
Agent	**Administration**	**Absorption**	**t$_{1/2}$ (hr)**	**Disposition***
nalidixic acid	Oral	Good	8 (21 in anuria)	M R
oxolinic acid	Oral	Good	—	R
cinoxacin	Oral	Good	—	R (60%)† M
ciprofloxacin	Oral	Good (80%)	4 (10 in anuria)	R (80%) M
norfloxacin	Oral	Good	4 (8 in anuria)	R M (20%)
nitrofurantoin	Oral	Good	0.6-1.2	R M (in tissue)
methenamine	Oral	Good	4	M
polymyxin B	Topical and oral	Not absorbed in adults; absorbed by children	6 by IV	—

M, Metabolized; *R*, renal excretion as unchanged drug.
*Metabolized to active product.
†By glomerular filtration and tubular secretion.

lyzed in the stomach. Since ammonia is produced, the drug should not be used in patients with hepatic dysfunction. Methenamine is distributed widely in body fluids, crossing most membranes to enter red cells, the eye, CSF, and other body fluids. Little active compound is present because at neutral pH, only 7% of methenamine is converted to formaldehyde. Within 24 hours, 90% of a dose is excreted into the urine. Antibacterial activity is observed only in the bladder, since this is the only anatomical site in which the pH is acidic and the residence time is sufficient to enable the hydrolysis to formaldehyde to proceed. Even at a urine pH of 5, approximately 2 hours following the administration of methenamine is required to achieve a high enough formaldehyde concentration to kill bacteria. Fluids should not be forced because this reduces the concentration of formaldehyde. An available form of the drug, methenamine mandelate, should not be given to patients in renal failure, since crystalluria can occur from the mandelic acid.

Polymyxins Polymyxins are not well absorbed following either oral or topical administration. Polymyxin B has been given by oral, topical, endobronchial, IM, and IV routes and colistin by IV and oral administration. The drug may be found in urine for up to 3 days after an IV dose. Polymyxins distribute poorly to tissues and do not enter the CSF. They are excreted by glomerular filtration and accumulate to toxic concentrations, with a half-life of 50 to 70 hours in anuric patients.

Newborns can absorb toxic concentrations of polymyxin if given the drug orally. Irrigation of surfaces such as the peritoneum with solutions containing polymyxins can result in absorption of drug, leading to neurotoxicity.

RELATION OF MECHANISMS OF ACTION TO CLINICAL RESPONSE

Quinolones

Nalidixic acid, oxolinic acid, and cinoxacin have similar activities, inhibiting most Enterobacteriaceae with concentrations of drug that can be achieved in the urinary tract. However, most *P. aeruginosa* and Gram-positive organisms are resistant. These agents are used primarily for treatment of urinary tract infections, but there is little current usage because of

the availability of newer fluoroquinolones.

Ciprofloxacin and norfloxacin are effective for treatment of both uncomplicated and complicated urinary tract infections caused by Enterobacteriaceae and *P. aeruginosa*, with ciprofloxacin also active against prostatitis resulting from *E. coli*. Both compounds are used to treat gonorrhea, including the infection caused by β-lactamase–producing strains. Both agents are also efficacious for treating diarrhea caused by *Shigella* organisms, toxigenic *E. coli*, salmonellae, and typhoid. The more active ciprofloxacin is effective against respiratory infections resulting from *Haemophilus* species or *S. pneumoniae* in bronchitis and *Pseudomonas* infections in cystic fibrosis patients. Chlamydiae are inhibited, as are *Mycoplasma* and *Legionella* species, but anaerobic species generally are resistant to currently available fluoroquinolones.

Nitrofurans

Nitrofurantoin is used to treat urinary tract infections, furazolidone for intestinal infections, and nitrofurazone only for topical applications. All three agents inhibit a variety of Gram-positive and Gram-negative bacteria, including most *E. coli*, staphylococci, and many *Klebsiella* species, enterococci, neisseriae, salmonellae, *Shigella* organisms, and *Proteus* bacteria.

Methenamine

Since the rate of production of the active ingredient (formaldehyde) is difficult to control, methenamine is no longer suggested as acceptable therapy.

Polymyxins

The polymyxins are used topically to treat cutaneous *Pseudomonas* infections of the mucous membranes, eye, and ear. Oral polymyxin B or colistin can be used to prevent intestinal colonization in neutropenic patients, but adverse effects are too pronounced for systemic administration. Gram-positive and anaerobic organisms generally are resistant to the polymyxins. However, *E. coli, Klebsiella, Enterobacter, Shigella*, and several other groups of organisms are inhibited by the polymyxins. These agents can act synergistically with trimethoprim or rifampin. The mechanism appears to damage the membranes, allowing increased concentrations of drug to enter the bacteria. This has not been shown to be of clinical significance.

SIDE EFFECTS, CLINICAL PROBLEMS, AND TOXICITY

Quinolones All quinolones cause gastrointestinal reactions such as nausea, vomiting, and abdominal pain, but diarrhea and pseudomembranous colitis are rare. CNS effects are infrequent and are usually dizziness, headache, restlessness, depression, and insomnia, with occurrence of these more common in the elderly. Seizures are a rare problem. Pseudotumor cerebri, leukopenia, thrombocytopenia, hemolytic anemia, and elevated transaminase concentrations occur occasionally with nalidixic acid. Allergic reactions are uncommon, but rashes, urticaria, pruritus, and photosensitivity may occur.

Quinolones produce damage to cartilage in immature animals and therefore are not recommended for use in children, although no joint damage has been seen in children who have received nalidixic acid. Elevations of theophylline concentrations occur in patients treated with ciprofloxacin. Interstitial nephritis has occurred rarely with ciprofloxacin.

Nitrofurans The most common adverse reactions of the nitrofurans are gastrointestinal, with anorexia, nausea, and vomiting most prevalent, although they can be reduced by administering the drug with food. The nausea and vomiting seem to arise from CNS effects. Hypersensitivity reactions involving the skin, lungs, liver, or blood also occur and are often associated with fever and chills. Cutaneous effects include maculopapular, erythematous, urticarial, and pruritic reactions, which abate when drug administration is stopped.

Two major types of pulmonary reaction occur with nitrofuran use. An acute reaction, characterized by fever, cough, and dyspnea, begins approximately 10 days into the treatment. Pleural effusions and infiltrates may accompany it. This reaction appears to be immunologically mediated but resolves rapidly when drug is stopped. A second form occurs in patients receiving long-term therapy. The onset is insidious, with cough, shortness of breath, and radiological signs of interstitial fibrosis. Patients improve when the drug is stopped, but many have residual change,

which is thought to be caused by peroxidative destruction of pulmonary membrane lipids. These arise from the reactive oxygen derivatives produced by reductase action on the nitrofurans.

The nitrofurans also cause acute and chronic liver damage, including cholestatic and hepatocellular disease and granulomatous hepatitis.

Hematologic reactions include granulocytopenia, leukopenia, and megaloblastic anemia, with acute hemolytic anemia occurring in G6PD deficient patients. Several neurological reactions, including headache, drowsiness, dizziness, nystagmus, and peripheral neuropathy of an ascending sensorimotor type, are also observed. Administration of drug should be stopped if the patient notes paresthesias, indicative of peripheral neuropathy.

Methenamine Adverse effects from methenamine are uncommon and include gastrointestinal distress, painful micturition, and occasional hematuria.

Polymyxins When used topically, the polymyxins have few adverse effects. However, when used orally, large doses cause nausea and vomiting. The IV administration of polymyxins leads to serious nephrotoxicity and neurotoxicity and thus should be avoided. The polymyxins also damage mammalian cell membranes and can cause neuromuscular blockade and respiratory paralysis. They can also produce persistent blockage of acetylcholine-activated end-

---

CLINICAL PROBLEMS

QUINOLONES

Gastrointestinal effects
CNS agitation (rarely seizures)
Damage to growing cartilage (not recommended for use in children)

NITROFURANS

Gastrointestinal effects
Hypersensitivity
Cutaneous reactions
Pulmonary reactions
Liver damage hematologic reactions

POLYMYXINS

Nephrotoxicity and neurotoxicity (too serious for IV use)

plate channels, which is not reversed by neostigmine.

The mechanism of polymyxin-induced nephrotoxicity is not established but appears to result from polymyxin binding to renal tubule cell membranes. This produces proteinuria, casts, and loss of brush-border enzymes and can progress to renal failure. Renal function usually returns when the drug is discontinued.

The clinical problems of these drug groups are summarized in the box, p. 691.

REFERENCES

Hoener B and Patterson SE: Nitrofurantoin disposition, Clin Pharmacol Therap 29:808, 1981.

Shen LI et al: Mechanism of inhibition of DNA gyrase by quinolone antibacterials: a comparative drug-DNA binding model, Biochemistry 28:2886, 1989.

Wolfson JS and Hooper DC: Treatment of genitourinary tract infections with fluoroquinolones: activity in vitro, pharmacokinetics, and clinical efficacy in urinary tract infections and prostatitis, Antimicrob Agents Chemother 33:1655, 1989.

CHAPTER 50

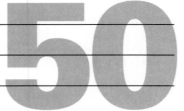

Selection of an Antibacterial Agent

ABBREVIATIONS

TMP/SMX	trimethoprim-sulfamethoxazole
CSF	cerebrospinal fluid

The basic clinical factors that need to be considered when selecting an antibiotic to treat a specific patient are described in Chapter 45, and some drugs are discussed further in Chapters 46 through 49. The extensive variety of pathogenic bacteria, the large number of available antibiotics, and the significant list of factors to be considered in arriving at a rational selection of antibiotic therapy can be confusing for the nonspecialist in infectious diseases. Since nearly all physicians use antibacterial agents, some additional guidelines for antibiotic selection are provided in this chapter.

These guidelines are as follows:

1. The strains of bacteria inhibited for each drug type and subtype
2. The bacteria most commonly associated with infections at different anatomical sites in the patient
3. The antibiotics that do or do not attain high enough concentrations at specific anatomical sites of infections for effective therapy
4. How special factors of the patient (allergy, disease states, pregnancy) and the bacteria (expectation of resistance developing) influence the selection of the antibiotic(s) and the criteria that should be used in deciding when to switch to a different antibiotic

Table 50-1 Activities of Antibiotics by Gram Stain of Sensitive Organisms

Antibiotics	Effective Against*
penicillins	Many Gram + cocci, some Gram −
cephalosporins	First generation: Gram +, some Gram −
	Second generation: more Gram −, similar Gram +
	Third generation: more Gram −, less Gram +
imipenem	Gram +, Gram −
aztreonam	Aerobic Gram − only
vancomycin	Gram + only
aminoglycosides	Aerobic Gram − bacilli
tetracyclines	Aerobic and anaerobic Gram + and Gram −
erythromycin	Gram +
clindamycin	Most Gram + cocci, many anaerobes
sulfonamides	Some Gram + and Gram −
quinolones	Some Gram + and most Gram −

*Gram +, Gram-positive; Gram −, Gram-negative.

ANTIBIOTIC ACTIVITY

The major classes of antibiotics discussed in Chapters 46 through 49 are listed in Table 50-1 along with the types of bacteria inhibited. The classifications are an oversimplification; for example, not all cephalosporins are active against all Gram-positive or Gram-negative bacteria, and several Gram-negative species are not inhibited by any of the cephalosporins. More detailed listings showing the relative activities for

Table 50-2   Susceptability of Bacteria to Antibiotics*

Organisms	A	B	C	D	E†	F†	G†	H	I	J	K	L	M	N	O	P
GRAM-POSITIVE																
Streptococcus pyogenes	4	4	4	4	4	4	4	0	0	0	3	3	4	4	4	2
Streptococcus pneumoniae	4	4	4	4	4	4	4	0	0	0	4	4	4	4	4	2
Staphylococcus aureus	0	0	0	4	4	4	4	0	2	3	2	2	3	2	4	4
Enterococcus faecalis	2	4	4	3	0	0	0	0	0	0	0	1	0	0	3	3
Listeria monocytogenes	4	4	4	4	0	0	0	0	0	0	2	1	0	0	4	2
GRAM-NEGATIVE																
Escherichia coli	0	3	3	4	3	3	4	1	3	4	2	0	0	4	4	4
Klebsiella spp.	0	0	2	3	3	3	4	1	3	4	2	0	0	4	4	4
Enterobacter spp.	0	0	2	2	0	1	2	1	3	4	2	0	0	2	4	4
Neisseriae gonorrhoeae	2	2	2	4	3	4	4	1	3	2	3	0	0	4	4	4
Pseudomonas aeruginosa	0	0	3	3	0	0	1	0	3	4	0	0	0	4	4	4
Hemophilus influenzae	1	2	2	4	1	4	4	1	2	2	2	1	0	4	4	4
ANAEROBES																
Clostridium spp.	4	4	4	4	2	3	3	0	0	0	3	3	3	1	4	0
Bacteroides spp.	1	1	2	4	0	0	1	0	0	0	1	2	4	0	4	0
Actinomyces spp.	4	4	4	4	0	1	2	0	0	0	2	3	4	0	4	0

A, penicillin G; *B*, ampicillin; *C*, pipercillin; *D*, ticarcillin-clavulanate; *E*, cefazolin (1st); *F*, cefuroxime (2nd); *G*, cefotaxime, ceftriaxone, ceftizoxime (3rd); *H*, streptomycin; *I*, gentamicin; *J*, amikacin; *K*, tetracycline; *L*, erythromycin; *M*, clindamycin; *N*, ceftazidime; *O*, imipenem; *P*, ciprofloxacin.
*Ratings based on tissue or plasma concentration expected for normal dosing schedule; *4*, >90% inhibited; *3*, >80% inhibited; *2*, 50% to 80% inhibited; *1*, 25% to 50% inhibited; *0*, <25% inhibited.
†Generation of cephalosporin.

some representative antibiotics against individual microbial species are included in Table 50-2.

BACTERIA AND ANATOMICAL SITES

It is estimated that 75% of bacterial infections treated with antibiotics receive the initial antimicrobial therapy before the pathogenic microorganisms have been identified and that for approximately 50% of treated infections, identification is never verified. It is important to realize what bacterial strains may be present at selected anatomical sites, since this may be the only meaningful information for guidance in the selection of antibiotic therapy when the locus of infection is known. Table 50-3 lists the common organisms that lead to infections at the anatomical sites indicated, and Table 50-4 groups the organisms with the anatomical locations of the infection and the drugs often used for treatment.

Numerous infections can be treated successfully with different antibiotics, so there may be more than

one correct therapy. Proponents may argue strongly in favor of a given antibiotic for treatment of a specific type of infection, but in many cases there are few verified findings to support the argument. However, there clearly are therapies that are inappropriate for a particular organism-location combination of bacterial infection.

PHARMACOKINETIC AND DRUG CONCENTRATION CONSIDERATIONS

Although an antibiotic may show high activity against the organism present at a given infection site, the drug will not be useful clinically unless the concentration of antibiotic at this site reaches a high enough value. This is especially important for antibiotics such as carbenicillin that are poorly absorbed and that do not achieve effective plasma concentrations when administered orally. Similarly, antibiotics that do not readily cross the blood-brain barrier or enter the CSF cannot be used for effective treatment

Table 50-3   Common Microorganisms Causing Infections

Body Site	Microorganisms	Gram Stain	Body Site	Microorganisms	Gram Stain
Eyes	Neisseria gonorrhoeae	−	Larynx-trachea	Respiratory viruses	
	Chlamydia trachomycetis	−		Streptococcus pneumoniae	+
	Staphylococcus aureus	+		Moraxella catarrhalis	−
	Haemophilus spp.	−	Lungs	Streptococcus pneumoniae	+
	Streptococcus pneumoniae	+		Mycoplasma pneumoniae	
	Pseudomonas aeruginosa	−		Legionella spp.	
	Fungi			Chlamydia pneumoniae	
	Herpes			Mycobacterium tuberculosis	
	Adenoviruses			Enterobacteriaceae	−
Oral cavity	Herpes			Staphylococcus aureus	+
	Candida		Bone (osteomyelitis)		
	Actinomyces	+		Salmonella species	−
	Anaerobic cocci	+		Haemophilus influenzae	−
	Fusobacteria	−		Pseudomonas aeruginosa	−
Throat	Streptococcus pyogenes	+	Urinary tract	Escherichia coli	−
	Corynebacterium diphtheriae	+		Staphylococcus saprophyticus	+
	Corynebacterium hemolyticum	+		Enterobacteriaceae	−
	Neisseria gonorrhoeae	−		Pseudomonas aeruginosa	−
	Pseudomonas spp.	−	Peritoneum (peritonitis)	Enterobacteriaceae	−
	Staphylococcus aureus	+		Bacteroides spp.	−
Lung (Abscesses)	Anaerobic spp.			Anerobic streptococci	+
	Staphylococcus aureus	+		Enterococci	+
	Mycobacterium tuberculosis			Clostridium species	+
	Fungi		Skin	Streptococcus pyogenes	+
Heart	Viridans group streptococci	+		Staphylococcus aureus	+
	Staphylococcus aureus	+		Herpes simplex	
	Enterococci	+		Clostridium perfringens	+
Meninges	Streptococcus agalactiae	+		Pseudomonas spp.	−
	Escherichia coli	−		Bacteroides spp.	−
	Streptococci pneumoniae	+		Enterobacteriaceae	−
	Haemophilus influenzae	−		Fungi	
	Neisseria meningitidis	−	Bloodstream (septicemia)	Staphylococcus aureus	+
	Listeria monocytogenes	+			
Brain (Abscesses)	Anaerobic spp.	− / +		Streptococcus pyogenes	+
	Nocardia	−		Enterobacteriaceae*	−
	Staphylococcus aureus	+		Pseudomonas aeruginosa	−
Sinuses	Haemophilus influenzae	−		Staphylococcus epidermidis	+
	Moraxella catarrhalis	−		Candida albicans	
	Streptococcus pneumoniae	+		Haemophilus influenzae	−
	Streptococcus pyogenes	+		Streptococcus pneumoniae	+
	Anaerobic streptococci	+		Neisseria meningitidis	−
	Rhinoviruses				
	Corona viruses				
Ears	Haemophilus influenzae	−			
	Streptococcus pneumoniae	+			
	Moraxella catarrhalis	−			
	Streptococcus pyogenes	+			

*E. coli, Klebsiella, Proteus, Enterobacter, Serratia species.

Table 50-4   Organisms with Common Infection Sites and Drugs of Choice

Bacteria	Infection	Drugs of Choice for Treatment	
		First Choice	Second Choice
Staphylococcus aureus (+)	Abscess	penicillin G	l-cephalosporin
	Cellulitis, bacteremia		vancomycin
	Pneumonia endocarditis	penicillin	l-cephalosporin
			vancomycin
	Meningitis	nafcillin, vancomycin	TMP/SMX
Streptococcus pyogenes (+) (Group A)	Pharyngitis	penicillin V	l-cephalosporin
	Cellulitis	penicillin V	erythromycin, clinda-mycin
Streptococcus (Group B) (+)	Meningitis	penicillin G	cefotaxime
Enterococcus faecalis	Abscesses, cellulitis, septicemia	penicillin G	l-cephalosporin
	Urinary tract	ampicillin	quinolone
	Endocarditis	ampicillin and gentamicin	vancomycin and gentamicin
	Bacteremia	ampicillin	vancomycin
Morganella morganii	Urinary tract	quinolone	TMP/SMX
Providencia spp. (−)	Urinary tract	quinolone	TMP/SMX
	Other	3-cephalosporin, aztreonam	imipenem
Pseudomonas aeruginosa (−)	Urinary tract	quinolone	aztreonam
	Pneumonia, bacteremia	antipseudomonas	ceftazidine, penicillin, ceftazidime, aztreonam, imipenem
Salmonella typhi (−)	Typhoid	TMP/SMX, ciprofloxacin	amoxicillin
Salmonella enterititis (−)	Gastroenteritis	norfloxacin, ciprofloxacin	
	Bacteremia	ampicillin	ceftriaxone
Shigella spp. (−)	Diarrhea	TMP/SMX	quinolone
Yersinia enterocolitica (−)	Diarrhea	TMP/SMX	quinolone
	Bacteremia, abscesses	3-cephalosporin	TMP/SMX
Streptococcus (Viridans Group) [+]	Endocarditis, bacteremia	penicillin G	cephalosporin
Streptococcus pneumoniae (+)	Pneumonia	penicillin G	l-cephalosporin
	Otitis, sinusitis	penicillin V	erythromycin
	Meningitis, endocarditis	penicillin G	cefotaxime
Listeria monocytogenes	Bacteremia, meningitis, endocarditis	ampicillin	TMP/SMX

+, Gram positive; −, Gram negative.

| Bacteria | Infection | Drugs of Choice for Treatment | |
		First Choice	Second Choice
Escherichia coli (−)	Urinary tract	TMP/SMX	quinolone
	Bacteremia	3-cephalosporin	TMP/SMX
Klebsiella pneumoniae (−)	Urinary tract	quinolone	cephalosporin TMP/SMX
	Pneumonia	3-cephalosporin	impenem
	Bacteremia	3-cephalosporin	aztreonam
Proteus mirabilis (−)	Urinary tract	ampicillin	TMP/SMX
Haemophilus influenzae (−)	Otitis	amoxicillin	amoxicillin-clavulate
	Bronchitis	TMP/SMX	ciprofloxacin
	Epiglotitis	cefotaxime, ceftriaxone	cefuroxime
Moraxella catarrhalis (−)	Otitis, sinusitis	amoxicillin-clavulanate	TMP/SMX
Neisseria meningitidis (−)	Carrier	rifampin	ciprofloxacin
	Meningitis	penicillin G	cefotaxime
	Bacteremia	penicillin G	ceftriaxone
Neisseria gonorrhoeae (−)	Genital	ceftriaxone	quinolone
	Disseminated	ceftriaxone	spectinomycin, amoxicillin-clavulanate
Chlamydia trachomatis	Genital	doxycycline, tetracycline	ofloxacin, erythromycin
Bacteroides spp.	Pulmonary	penicillin G, clindomycin	cefoxitin
	Sinus, oral, brain abscess	metronidazole	clindamycin
Legionella spp.	Pulmonary	erythromycin	quinolone
	Abdominal infection	metronidazole/impenem	cefotetan clindamycin
Clostridium perfringens (+)	Abscesses, gangrene	penicillin G	metronidazole
Clostridium difficile (+)	Diarrhea	vancomycin	metronidazole
Borelia burgdorferi	Lyme disease	doxycycline	ceftriaxone
Nocardia asteroides	Pulmonary, CNS	TMP/SMX	minocycline
Mycoplasma pneumoniae	Pulmonary	erythromycin, tetracycline	ciprofloxacin
Rickettsia	Typhus	tetracycline	chloramphenicol
	Rocky Mountain spotted fever	tetracycline	chloramphenical
Chlamydia psittaci	Pulmonary	tetracycline	erythromycin
Pasteurella multocida	Bite wounds	penicillin G, amoxicillin-clavulanate	doxycycline

Table 50-5   Ability of Antibiotics to Enter the CSF in Effective Concentrations

Readily Enter CSF	Enter CSF When Inflammation Present	Do Not Enter CSF Adequately to Treat Infection
chloramphenicol	penicillin G	carbenicillin
sulfonamides	ampicillin	cephalothin
trimethoprim	azlocillin	cefazolin
rifampin	mezlocillin	cefoxitin
isoniazid	piperacillin	cefotetan
metronidazole	oxacillin	erythromycin
flucytosine	cefuroxime	clindamycin
	nafcillin	tetracycline
	cefotaxime	gentamicin
	ceftriaxone	tobramycin
	ceftazidime	amikacin
	moxalactam	norfloxacin
	aztreonam	ketoconazole
	ciprofloxacin	
	vancomycin	
	ethambutol	
	pyrazinamide	
	fluconazole	

of meningeal-based infections. (See Chapter 5.) The ability of antibiotics to enter the CSF is summarized in Table 50-5.

SPECIAL FACTORS

One highly *undesirable* approach to antibiotic therapy is called "antibiotic roulette" in which the causative organism is not known and the antibiotic is changed every few days in hopes of achieving a quick cure. This action confuses the clinical situation and makes it more difficult for the follow-up physician to initiate and carry out effective therapy.

CHAPTER 51

Antimycobacterial Agents

ABBREVIATIONS

AIDS	acquired immune deficiency syndrome
RNA	ribonucleic acid
tRNA	transfer ribonucleic acid
NAD	nicotinamide adenine dinucleotide

 THERAPEUTIC OVERVIEW

Mycobacteria characteristically have a high waxy lipid content (approximately 40% of cell weight), with much of the lipid on the external surface of the cell. *Mycobacterium tuberculosis, M. avium, and M. leprae* are the pathogenic organisms that cause diseases of concern in humans, although some other nontuberculosis mycobacteria pose occasional problems.

Tuberculosis classically is a respiratory infection, and leprosy initially is primarily a disease of the skin. In both diseases the organism can and does spread throughout the body if not treated. Both diseases are chronic and require extended therapy over long periods of time.

Tuberculosis remains a serious and important infectious disease worldwide. Although the number of patients with tuberculosis in the past two decades has steadily declined, the number of new cases in inner cities has increased because of AIDS and the large number of homeless persons. An increase in tuberculosis has also been found in nursing homes. Because of the nature of the disease and the microor-

THERAPEUTIC OVERVIEW

TUBERCULOSIS

M. tuberculosis is an aerobic organism
It is a chronic disease
Combinations of drugs are used
Long-term treatment is needed
Bacterial resistance is of growing importance

LEPROSY

M. leprae is an aerobic organism
It is a chronic disease
Long-term treatment is needed
Effective drugs exist
Bacterial resistance is developing

ganism, the therapy is different than that used to treat most infectious diseases. Combination therapy is standard practice, and sometimes up to four agents are used. The desired frequency of drug administration must be considered in terms of achieving compliance, since therapy is continued for many months. Resistance is also increasingly important in determining the appropriate therapeutic program.

In the host, *M. tuberculosis* is present in three types of sites: (1) well-oxygenated extracellular cavities containing 10^7 to 10^9 organisms, (2) poorly oxygenated closed-caseous lesions containing 10^4 to 10^5 organisms, and (3) poorly oxygenated intracellular macrophages containing 10^4 to 10^5 organisms. Drugs are effective at all three sites but especially at the extracellular cavities in which the growth of the organisms is greatest.

Table 51-1   Pharmacokinetic Parameters

| | Administration | | | | |
	Route	Absorbed	t₁/₂ (hr)	Elimination Route	Plasma Protein Bound (%)
TUBERCULOSIS					
isoniazid	Oral	Good	1* 3†	M (75%)	<50%
rifampin	Oral	Good	2–4	M (active metab.) R (15%) B	75
ethambutol	Oral	Good	4	M (20%) R (main)	30
pyrazinamide	Oral	Good	10	M (main)	—
ethionamide	Oral	Good	2	M (main)	—
cycloserine	Oral	Good	10	M (35%) R (65%)	—
capreomycin	IM	Poor	3–5	R (main)	—
LEPROSY					
dapsone	Oral	Good	20-30	M (main) B	70
clofazimine	Oral	Good (70% absorbed)	7 days	M (main)	—

M, Metabolized; *R*, renal (unchanged drug); *B*, bilary.
*Rapid acetylation patients.
†Slow acetylation patients.

Leprosy is a common disease worldwide. Its epidemiology is poorly understood, but transmission appears to depend largely on the susceptibility of the individual. Children and males are most susceptible, and an incubation period of several years makes the disease difficult to detect initially. A number of agents are useful in treating this chronic infection, although problems with therapy and drug resistance have occurred. The therapeutic use of drugs in the treatment of these two major mycobacterial infections is summarized in the box.

 MECHANISMS OF ACTION

Tuberculosis Drugs

The drugs available for the treatment of *M. tuberculosis* infections are the following:

cycloserine
p-aminosalicylic acid
capreomycin
kanamycin and amikacin
fluoroquinolones

The chemical structures are shown in Figure 51-1. (See Chapter 47 for streptomycin, kanamycin, and amikacin.) The molecular mechanisms by which these drugs act on *M. tuberculosis* can be divided into three groups: protein synthesis inhibition, cell wall synthesis inhibition, and other mechanisms.

Protein Synthesis Inhibition Streptomycin, kanamycin, and amikacin act by inhibiting protein synthesis and are described in Chapter 47. Rifampin and capreomycin act similarly but at different points in the protein synthesis pathway.

Rifampin inhibits RNA synthesis by binding to the β subunit of DNA-directed RNA polymerase. Tight binding occurs only when the subunit is in its proper conformation and results in inhibition of initiation but not of ongoing RNA synthesis. Rifampin may subsequently inhibit DNA synthesis by preventing the binding of the initiated RNA molecule to the product-binding site on the enzyme (Figure 51-2). Mammalian RNA polymerases are not as sensitive as the myco-

isoniazid
rifampin
ethambutol
streptomycin
pyrazinamide
ethionamide

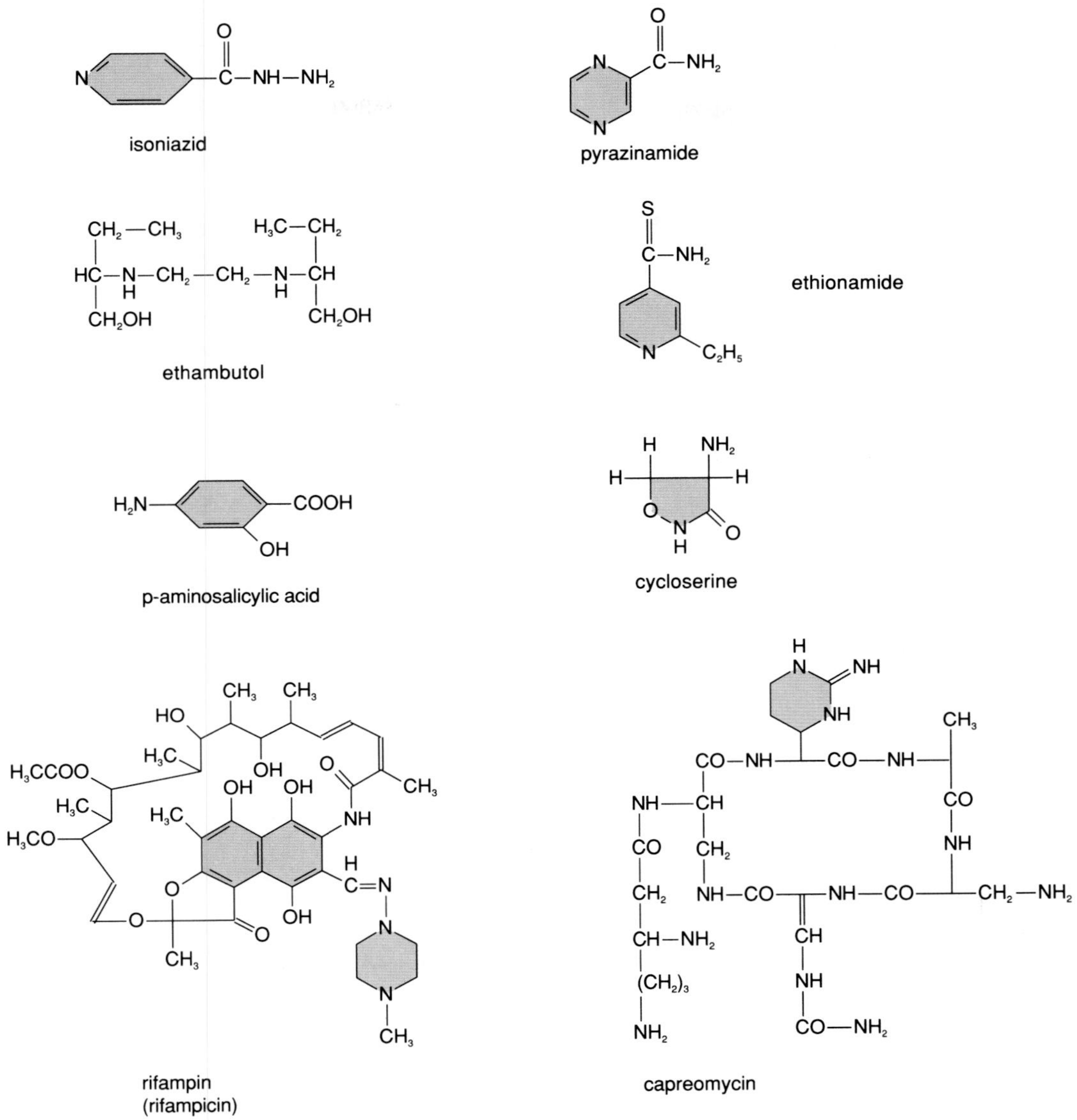

FIGURE 51-1 Structures of antituberculosis drugs.

bacterial form and are not affected by rifampin except at much higher drug concentrations. Microbial resistance is becoming more widespread and is caused by an altered β subunit of the RNA polymerase. However, the presence of organisms with an altered RNA polymerase is much lower for *M. tuberculosis* than for bacteria, particularly Enterobacteriaceae, neisseriae, and staphylococci. With staphylococci, resistance can develop with use of rifampin alone.

Capreomycin is a polypeptide that consists of four biologically active components. Its mechanism of ac-

tion is thought to be inhibition of protein synthesis by preventing translocation of peptidyl-tRNA on ribosomes.

Cell Wall Synthesis Inhibition Cycloserine acts by inhibiting two enzymes involved in the synthesis of cell walls: D-alanyl-D-alanine synthetase and alanine racemase. (See Chapter 46 for cell wall synthesis pathways.)

Isoniazid and ethionamide also act at least partly to inhibit synthesis of cell wall components, but the mechanisms of these two agents are still not clear.

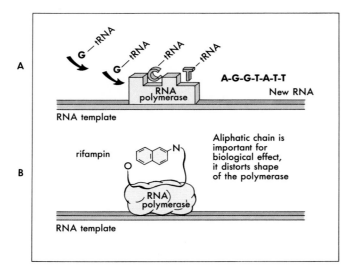

FIGURE 51-2 Mechanism of rifampin action. The drug binds to the β subunit of DNA-dependent RNA polymerase and inhibits initiation (but not ongoing) RNA synthesis. **A,** Drug is absent. **B,** Drug is bound to the polymerase and distorts the conformation of the enzyme so that it cannot initiate a new chain.

Other Mechanisms Included in this category are isoniazid, ethionamide, ethambutol, pyrazinamide, and p-aminosalicylic acid.

The mechanism of action of isoniazid is not well established. It inhibits the synthesis of mycolic acid, a major constituent of mycobacterial cell walls. Low concentrations also inhibit production of fatty acids that exceed 26 carbons in length and that are precursors of mycolic acid. Mycolic acids are unique to mycobacteria, and this may be the reason that only mycobacteria are inhibited. Isoniazid affects mycobacteria in several ways, which may contribute to its bactericidal effect on the growing cells. Isoniazid is taken up by mycobacterial cells through both active and passive transport and undergoes hydrolysis to isonicotinic acid, which is trapped within the cells at physiological pH. Uptake is reduced in some resistant cells. Isonicotinic acid reacts with the cofactor NAD to form a NAD adduct, no longer active as a coenzyme for dehydrogenase reactions. Mycolic acid formation is also inhibited. These mechanisms of action are illustrated in Figure 51-3. Which mechanism is ac-

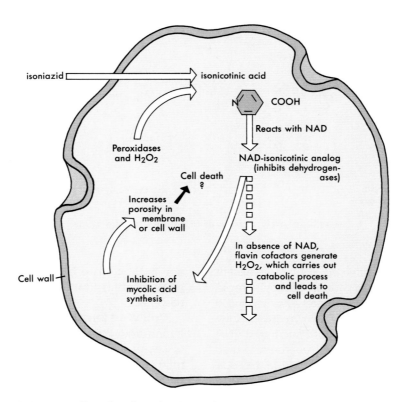

FIGURE 51-3   Postulated mechanisms of isoniazid action on *M. tuberculosis*.

tually responsible for cell death has not been determined.

The mechanism of action of ethionamide probably involves the direct inhibition of mycolic acid synthesis, possibly with cytotoxic results similar to those for isoniazid. Little is known about the details of this mechanism.

The mechanism of action of ethambutol is also not clear. It has an effect on lipid synthesis resulting in an inhibition of mycolic acid incorporation into the cell wall. Since ethambutol forms stable chelates with metal ions, it may compete with polyamines in forming reactive complexes with transfer and ribosomal RNA, thus inhibiting protein synthesis.

The mechanism by which pyrazinamide inhibits mycobacteria is not known.

p-Aminosalicylic acid acts as a competitive inhibitor of p-aminobenzoic acid in the synthesis of folate. Because aminosalicylic acid only inhibits this synthetic step in M. tuberculosis, the synthetase enzyme is distinct in tubercle bacilli, since sulfanomides do not generally inhibit mycobacteria.

Leprosy Drugs

The major drug for inhibition of M. leprae is dapsone (diaminodiphenylsulfone). The structural formula is shown in Figure 51-4.

Similar to the sulfonamides, dapsone acts as an inhibitor of dihydropteroate synthetase in the folate pathway to produce a bacteriostatic effect. Its action is antagonized by p-aminobenzoic acid.

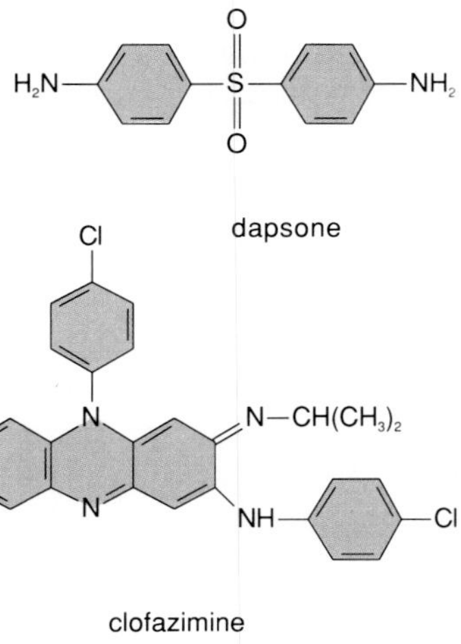

For treatment of dapsone-resistant patients, clofazimine is used. In some parts of the world, combination therapy with dapsone, clofazimine, and rifampin is recommended.

PHARMACOKINETICS

For agents in which the information is available, the pharmacokinetic parameters are summarized in Table 51-1.

Antituberculosis Drugs

Isoniazid This drug is well absorbed orally, and its absorption is decreased by aluminum antacids. Typical peak plasma concentrations are 3 to 5 μg/ml. Isoniazid enters all body fluids and compartments, with peak concentrations achieved in the pleural, peritoneal, and synovial fluids and with CSF concentrations that are 20% of those in plasma.

Isoniazid is metabolized by a liver N-acetyl transferase. The rate of acetylation determines the concentration of drug in plasma and the half-life. Slow acetylation is inherited as an autosomal recessive trait. Approximately 50% of American Caucasions and 15% of Orientals are slow acetylators. The mean half-life in rapid acetylators is 1 hour; in slow acetylators it is 3 hours. The average plasma concentration of drug in rapid acetylators is 50% of that in slow acetylators. There is no evidence that differences in acetylation are important chemotherapeutically if the drug is administered daily.

Approximately 75% of a dose is excreted in the urine as metabolites. Toxic concentrations may accumulate in renal failure in some slow acetylators.

Rifampin Rifampin is well absorbed orally and widely distributed in the body, achieving therapeutic concentrations in lung, liver, bile, bone, and urine and entering most body fluids, including pleural, peritoneal, and synovial fluids; CSF; tears; and saliva. It enters phagocytic cells and kills intracellular bacteria.

Rifampin is approximately 75% protein bound and is metabolized in the liver to a desacetyl derivative that is biologically active. The unmetabolized drug is excreted in bile and reabsorbed from the gastrointestinal tract in the enterohepatic cycle; the deacetylated metabolite shows poor reabsorption. Approx-

dapsone

clofazimine

FIGURE 51-4   Structures of drugs used against M. leprae.

imately 30% of a dose is excreted unchanged or as metabolites (50%) in the urine.

The half-life of rifampin varies during therapy from 3 to 4 hours to 2 hours after 1 or 2 weeks because of increased metabolism through induction of hepatic microsomal enzymes. No adjustment of dosage is necessary in renal failure.

Ethambutol Approximately 85% of ethambutol is orally absorbed and distributed to most body areas. CSF concentrations are 10% to 50% of plasma values. The drug crosses the placenta. Approximately 20% of ethambutol is metabolized in the liver to an aldehyde and oxidized to a dicarboxylic acid. The primary mechanism of removal involves the kidney, where the drug is both filtered and excreted. The mean half-life is 4 hours, which increases to 7 hours in renal failure. Ethambutol can be removed from the body by peritoneal or hemodialysis.

Pyrazinamide Pyrazinamide is well absorbed orally and is widely distributed in the body, readily penetrating cells and the walls of cavities. It enters the CSF if the meninges are inflamed. Pyrazinamide is metabolized by the liver to pyazinoic acid, which is subsequently oxidized to 5-hydroxypyazinoic acid by xanthine oxidase with the metabolite excreted by glomerular filtration. The half-life of pyrazinamide is approximately 6 hours.

Ethionamide Ethionamide is well absorbed orally and is widely distributed, entering the CSF to produce concentrations equal to those in plasma. It is extensively metabolized by sulfoxidation, *N*-methylation, desulfuration, and deamination to products that are excreted in the urine. It has a half-life of 2 hours.

Cycloserine Cycloserine is rapidly absorbed by the oral route and widely distributed, yielding CSF concentrations equal to plasma. About 35% of the drug is metabolized; the remainder is excreted by glomerular filtration unchanged. It accumulates in renal failure but can be removed by hemodialysis.

***p*-Aminosalicylic Acid** *p*-Aminosalicylic acid is well absorbed orally and enters lung tissue and pleural fluid. Low CSF concentrations result from active transport out of the CSF. It is metabolized in the liver by a different acetylase than the enzyme that acts on isoniazid, but it does prolong the isoniazid half-life.

Capreomycin Capreomycin is administered IM and undergoes elimination by glomerular filtration.

Aminoglycosides The aminoglycosides are discussed in Chapter 47.

Antileprosy Drugs

Dapsone is 90% absorbed from the upper gastrointestinal tract, is distributed to all body tissues, and achieves therapeutic concentrations in skin. It is approximately 70% bound to plasma proteins. Dapsone is excreted in bile and reabsorbed via enterohepatic circulation and also undergoes acetylation in the liver by the same *N*-acetyl transferase that acetylates isoniazid. The acetylation phenotype does not affect the half-life of the drug. Dapsone is excreted as glucuronide and sulfate conjugates in urine with a plasma half-life of 25 hours. The half-life is reduced in patients receiving rifampin.

Clofazimine is 70% absorbed from the gastrointestinal tract and distributed in a complex pattern with high concentrations in subcutaneous fat and the reticuloendothelial system. The half-life is estimated to be 90 days.

 ## RELATION OF MECHANISMS OF ACTION TO CLINICAL RESPONSE

Antituberculosis Drugs

Isoniazid This is the primary agent in all therapeutic and prophylactic programs for tuberculosis in which the tubercle bacilli are susceptible and the patient has no major reaction to the drug. Isoniazid is bactericidal on growing *M. tuberculosis* and bacteriostatic on resting organisms. It inhibits *M. kansasii* but not other tubercle bacilli.

The percentage of patients infected by isoniazid-resistant *M. tuberculosis* varies depending on the geographic location. It can reach 15% in some non–Asian areas, but generally is approximately 5%. Resistance in Asian countries can reach 40%. Mutants are present in most organism populations at a frequency of 10^{-6}. In cavities containing 10^7 to 10^9 organisms, some *M. tuberculosis* cells will therefore be resistant and survive therapy.

Rifampin This drug inhibits most *M. tuberculosis* at concentrations of 0.005 to 0.2 μg/ml. *M. kansasii* are also inhibited, but *M. avium-intracellulare*, *M. fortuitum*, and *M. chelonei* are usually resistant.

Rifampin also inhibits most Gram-positive bacteria such as staphylococci, streptococci, and *Steptococcus pneumoniae*, as well as many methicillin-resistant *Staphylococcus aureus*. It acts on *Listeria* organisms and enterococci, although most are inhibited but not killed, and it is extremely active against *Neisseria meningitidis* and *Haemophilus influenzae*. Rifampin inhibits many enteric species, including some *Pseudomonas* organisms, and is active against *Legionella* species, mycoplasmata, and chlamydiae. Most anaerobic species are also inhibited, including *Clostridium difficile* and *Bacteroides* organisms.

Rifampin is primarily used to treat tuberculosis, but it has a number of other uses. It is the drug of choice for chemoprophylaxis of meningococcal disease for *H. influenzae* meningitis. It is also used in combination with vancomycin to treat prosthetic valve endocarditis resulting from staphylococcal infection and can be combined with antistaphylococcal penicillins or cephalosporins to treat staphylococcal osteomyelitis. Rifampin combined with cloxacillin eliminates nasal *S. aureus* in patients with recurrent furunculosis.

Ethambutol Most *M. tuberculosis* and *M. kansasii* are inhibited by 2 μg/ml of this drug, but *M. avium-intracellulare* are not. Resistance can develop if the drug is used alone; when combined with other antituberculosis agents, the emergence of resistance is decreased but to a lesser degree than with rifampin or streptomycin. When used with isoniazid or rifampin, the inhibition of tubercle bacilli is additive.

Ethambutol inhibits only mycobacteria and is active against growing but not nonproliferating organisms to produce a tuberculostatic effect. It enters the mycobacteria by diffusion but encounters a lag time of several hours before inhibition of growth is observed.

Pyrazinamide This agent is bactericidal at acid pH of 5 to 5.5 with minimal activity at neutral pH. It enters mononuclear cells, killing the bacteria present. When it is used alone, the organisms become resistant, so it is less useful than other agents in preventing the emergence of resistance. This agent, which for years was considered a second-line drug, has recently become important as a first-line agent in multiple-drug, short-course treatment programs.

Ethionamide This is a bacteriostatic agent that inhibits *M. tuberculosis* intracellularly and extracellularly and shows no cross-resistance with isoniazid or other agents.

Cycloserine This drug inhibits *S. aureus, Escherichia coli,* Enterobacteriaceae organisms, nocardiae, and chlamydiae, as well as *M. tuberculosis* and *M. kansasii*. It shows no cross-resistance with other agents. Resistance readily develops because of re-

duced uptake of drug or altered enzymes involved in cell wall synthesis.

p-Aminosalicylic Acid *p*-Aminosalicylic acid is bacteriostatic, inhibiting most *M. tuberculosis* but is rarely used today.

Capreomycin Capreomycin only inhibits mycobacteria, and *M. tuberculosis* is only moderately susceptible. No cross-resistance is shown with isoniazid, rifampin, ethambutol, or streptomycin.

Aminoglycosides Streptomycin, kanamycin, and amikacin are aminoglycosides also active against *M. tuberculosis*. These drugs act by inhibiting protein synthesis and are described in Chapter 47.

Streptomycin was the first drug used to treat tuberculosis. It inhibits most *M. tuberculosis* and *M. kansasii,* but other tubercle bacilli are resistant. The primary incidence of resistance of *M. tuberculosis* to streptomycin is less than 5%, but resistant organisms appear if this drug is used alone. Streptomycin is not an ideal agent for tuberculosis because it does not enter the phagocytic cells in which the tubercle bacilli survive.

Amikacin also inhibits many of the atypical mycobacteria, but neither kanamycin nor amikacin are used as first-line therapy except for drug-resistant organisms.

Therapy of Tuberculosis The two major problems encountered in treating tuberculosis are the eradication of organisms that grow slowly or not at all in sheltered environments and the development of resistance in the large populations of organisms at the sites of infection. Because of these problems, therapy of tuberculosis includes the simultaneous use of two or more drugs, with treatment continued over prolonged periods. In the past, therapy of tuberculosis was continued for 18 months to 2 years with excellent results. All programs included isoniazid and a second agent to prevent the development of resistance. The problems with this approach included high cost, poor patient compliance, and risk of increased toxicity. The availability of rifampin has made it possible to use much shorter courses of therapy. Both isoniazid and rifampin are bactericidal for *M. tuberculosis,* and they enter phagocytic cells and cavities to eradicate persisting organisms. In combination, they prevent the development of resistance, which is normally extremely low for rifampin.

Current initial therapy uses isoniazid combined with rifampin for 9 months. Alternatively, both agents can be given daily for 1 month and then rifampin and isoniazid given twice weekly for 9 months. With the latter protocol, supervised administration of the drugs may be possible.

More recently, shorter programs have been developed that use intensive initial therapy with four drugs—isoniazid, rifampin, pyrazinamide, and streptomycin—which are administered daily for 2 months, followed by 4 months of isoniazid and rifampin therapy daily.

When drug resistance is probable, therapy should be started with three drugs. Risk factors include (1) the acquisition of infection in areas of the world in which resistance is high, such as southeast Asia, the Caribbean, and in certain cities such as New York, and (2) infection of patients who received previous antituberculosis drug therapy, particularly when medication was taken irregularly because this increases the possibility for development of drug-resistant organisms. Some authorities also suggest that three drugs should always be started when dealing with extensive pulmonary disease, miliary disease, or meningitis and that therapy should be adjusted when the results of susceptibility testing are available. Ethambutol or streptomycin is combined with isoniazid and rifampin in the three drug regimens.

The chemoprophylaxis of tuberculosis is directed at two different goals: prevention of infection and prevention of disease by eradication of organisms infecting the individual. Isoniazid is the most effective agent. All household contacts and close associates of a newly diagnosed patient should be treated. (This is particularly important for children younger than 7 years of age.) The second category includes individuals who have recently developed a positive skin test for tuberculosis. In these patients the risk of developing disease is highest for the first few years after the positive test results. Patients should have prophylactic therapy if (1) they have an abnormal chest x-ray and a positive tuberculin test with the length of positivity unknown; (2) they have a positive tuberculin test and a high risk of impaired cellular immunity from other agents such as prolonged therapy with glucocorticoids; (3) they are receiving immunosuppressive therapy such as azathioprine; and (4) they have a hematological malignancy, diabetes mellitus, silicosis, or a positive HIV titer. Controversy exists about whether all individuals under the age of 30 who have a positive tuberculin reaction should receive prophylaxis. Traditionally, isoniazid is administered daily for 1 year, but recent data suggest that 24 weeks may be adequate. There are no data on chemoprophylaxis for isoniazid-resistant organisms, but rifampin would be second choice.

Antileprosy Drugs

Dapsone inhibits the growth of *M. leprae* in mouse foot pads in a bactericidal manner. *M. leprae* can become resistant to dapsone, and resistance is increasing worldwide, varying from 2% to 40% in infected populations. Dapsone is administered over many years for treatment of leprosy. Recently it has been used to treat *Pneumocystis carinii* pulmonary infection in AIDS patients.

At low concentrations, rifampin is bactericidal to *M. leprae* and rapidly reduces infectivity when used with dapsone. Clofazimine is used primarily when other treatments fail or when cases become refractory to rifampin.

SIDE EFFECTS, CLINICAL PROBLEMS, AND TOXICITY

The main problems in the clinical use of these drugs for the treatment of tuberculosis or leprosy are summarized in the box.

Antituberculosis Drugs

Isoniazid Although adverse reactions are not common, a few are serious. About 2% of patients develop a rash, 1% fever, less than 1% jaundice, and only 0.2% peripheral neuritis. Approximately 15% of

---

CLINICAL PROBLEMS

TUBERCULOSIS DRUGS
  isoniazid: peripheral neuritis, hepatoxocity (elevated serum transaminase)
  rifampin: hepatitis, drug interactions
  ethambutol: retrobulbar neuritis, blindness
  ethionamide: GI disturbances
  pyrazinamide: hepatotoxicity, hyperuricemia

LEPROSY DRUGS
  dapsone: anemia, methemoglobinemia, rash
  clofazimine: discoloration of skin

patients have elevated serum transaminase concentrations. Hepatic toxicity usually occurs 4 to 8 weeks after the start of treatment and is correlated with age. It is rarely seen in patients below 20 years of age but occurs in 2.3% of patients over the age of 50. Hepatotoxicity is more common in alcoholics. Patients complain of anorexia, nausea, malaise, and fatigue. If the reaction is allowed to progress, extensive hepatocellular damage resembling viral hepatitis will develop. In many individuals, serum transaminase concentrations rise to 2 or 3 times normal; a further increase requires that the drug be discontinued. Some experts feel serum transaminase concentrations should be checked monthly in elderly patients. Whether the toxicity is caused by metabolites of isoniazid or other factors remains unclear.

Peripheral neuritis occurs in patients receiving large doses, particularly individuals with nutritional deficiency. Pyridoxine prevents neuropathy and other CNS toxicity. Other neurological toxicities include convulsions, optic neuritis, paresthesias, ataxia, and psychoses. Mental abnormalities such as transient memory impairment have been reported.

Allergic reactions such as fever, rash, and a syndrome similar to lupus erythematosus occasionally occur. Arthritic symptoms have been noted, and antinuclear antibody tests may be positive. Isoniazid can produce a sideroblastic anemia resulting from pyridoxine deficiency. The agent also potentiates the toxicity of phenytoin with possible production of nystagmus, altered gait, and signs of excessive sedation. Elevation of liver enzymes appears to increase further when isoniazid is administered with rifampin.

Rifampin This drug is generally well tolerated. It can cause gastrointestinal reactions, particularly nausea and vomiting, in 1% to 2% of individuals, but a rash is uncommon. Occasionally, patients complain of headache, dizziness, fatigue, or other CNS symptoms. Rifampin can cause hepatitis, especially in patients also receiving isoniazid or those who are alcoholics or others with previous liver disease; fulminant hepatitis is rare.

The administration of rifampin biweekly may produce a flulike syndrome with fever, chills, muscle aches, headache, and dizziness. This occurs most often after several months of therapy and begins 1 to 2 hours after a dose. The syndrome stops with daily drug administration.

Thrombocytopenia, hemolysis, and transient leukopenia have also been reported. Interstitial nephritis occurs rarely as a renal toxicity.

Rifampin interacts with many other drugs as an inducer of microsomal P-450 enzymes. It reduces the half-lives of agents such as prednisone, digitoxin, quinidine, propanolol, metoprolol, sulfonamides, clofibrate, thyroxine, dapsone, methadone, and ketoconazole. Oral anticoagulants and oral contraceptives are rendered less effective. Rifampin can stain soft contact lenses red. Since it causes teratogenic effects in rodents, it should be used in pregnancy only for severe tuberculosis.

Ethambutol Ethambutol has few adverse effects. The most important toxicity is a dose-related retrobulbar neuritis. There may be loss of central vision and color discrimination involving central fibers of the optic nerve. A less common problem is constriction of visual fields involving peripheral fibers of the optic nerve. In both cases no changes are seen on funduscopic examination, and the mechanism of the neuritis is unknown. In most patients, vision returns once administration of the drug is stopped, but recovery may take up to 6 months.

Ethambutol occasionally causes gastrointestinal upset, allergic reactions including rash, joint pains, fever, malaise, headache, and pruritus. Peripheral neuropathy develops rarely and only after many months into the treatment. This effect involves only the sensory nerves and resolves when the drug is stopped. Since ethambutol decreases the clearance of uric acid, an acute gouty attack can be precipitated, but it is rare.

Pyrazinamide Hepatotoxicity is the most serious adverse effect of pyrazinamide, and elevation of liver transaminase is the first sign of toxicity. The effect is dose related and is much less frequent with the lower doses currently being used. Hepatic necrosis and death may occur with higher doses. Serum transaminase should be determined before initiating therapy and monitored frequently. Pyrazinamide causes hyperuricemia by inhibition of renal excretion of urate. Mild arthralgias occur in approximately 70% of patients, with occasional nausea, vomiting, malaise, and fever.

Ethionamide Ethionamide produces marked gastrointestinal reactions, and many individuals cannot tolerate elevated doses. Nausea, vomiting, abdominal pain, diarrhea, a metallic taste in the mouth, and many nervous system complaints, including depression, headache, and feelings of restlessness, are typical side effects. Seizures; peripheral neuropathy; and allergic reactions with rash, purpura, stomatitis, gynecomastia, impotence, hypoglycemia, alopecia, and hypotension rarely occur. About 5% of patients develop hepatitis, which resolves when the drug is stopped.

Cycloserine Neurotoxicity is the most important side effect, but psychotic disturbances in the form of confusion, aggression, depression, and excitement also occur. Convulsions have also been noted. Cycloserine may occasionally cause rash, fever, and cardiac arrhythmias. It should not be given to patients with a prior history of seizures or psychiatric disorders.

***p*-Aminosalicylic Acid** Gastrointestinal side effects of nausea, vomiting, abdominal pain, and diarrhea occur in up to 30% of patients, with fever, malaise, joint pains, and skin eruptions found in 5% to 10% of patients.

Capreomycin The most serious adverse effect is nephrotoxicity with loss of potassium, calcium, and magnesium in the urine. The drug may also cause tinnitus, vertigo, and deafness.

Aminoglycosides The aminoglycosides are discussed in Chapter 45.

Antileprosy Drugs

Hemolytic anemia and methemoglobinemia are the common adverse effects seen with the use of dapsone. Methemoglobinemia is caused by an *N*-oxidation byproduct. Although bone marrow suppression is rare, agranulocytosis and aplastic anemia may occur. Anorexia, nausea, and vomiting are also found occasionally. Other problems include headache, insomnia, psychosis, paresthesia, peripheral neuropathy, nervousness, blurred vision, vertigo, tinnitus, fever, and skin rash.

Dapsone can provoke lepra reactions, which are exacerbations of the cutaneous manifestations of the

---

> **TRADENAMES**
>
> In addition to generic and fixed combination preparations, the following tradenamed materials are available in the United States.
>
> **TUBERCULOSIS**
>
> Capastat, capreomycin sulfate
> INH, isoniazid
> Laniazid, isoniazid
> Myambutol, ethambutol HCl
> Rifadin, rifampin
> Rimactane, rifampin
> Seromycin, cycloserine
> Trecator-SC, ethionamide
>
> **LEPROSY**
>
> Lamprene, clofazimine

---

leprosy. Fever, erythematous nodules, malaise, and joint symptoms may occur. These reactions can be controlled by using steroids.

REFERENCES

Bartmann K, ed: Antituberculosis drugs, New York, 1988, Springer-Verlag New York, Inc.

American Thoracic Society/Center for Disease Control: Treatment of tuberculosis and tuberculosis infection in adults and children, Am Rev Resp Dis 134:355, 1986.

Hastings RC and Franzblau SG: Chemotherapy of leprosy, Annu Rev Pharmacol Toxicol 28:231, 1988.

Schlossberg D, ed: Tuberculosis, ed 2, New York, 1988, Springer-Verlag New York, Inc.

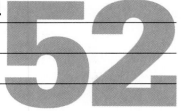

CHAPTER 52

Antifungal Agents

 ## THERAPEUTIC OVERVIEW

Fungal infections (mycoses) occur less frequently than do bacterial or viral infections but may be prevalent in some geographical locations that favor the growth of specific pathogenic fungal strains. Many fungal infections are superficial and primarily annoying, whereas others are systemic and can be life-threatening, particularly in patients with compromised host defenses, such as those receiving immunosuppressive drugs. The toxicity of many antifungal drugs limits their use, and there are, unfortunately, only a few agents that are useful in the treatment of systemic fungal infections.

Fungi are more complex organisms, compared to bacteria or viruses. For example, they have different ribosomes, cell wall components, and a nuclear membrane, as compared to bacteria. Therefore the antibacterial antibiotics are not effective against pathogenic fungi.

The two major classes of fungal infections and examples of prevalent species that are often causative organisms are summarized in the box.

THERAPEUTIC OVERVIEW

CUTANEOUS AND SUBCUTANEOUS MYCOSES

Epidermophyton spp.
Microsporum spp.
Sporothrix spp.
Trichophyton spp.
Treat with dermatological preparations

SYSTEMIC MYCOSES

Aspergillus spp.
Candida spp.
Blastomyces dermatitidis
Cryptococcus neoformans
Coccidioides immitis
Histoplasma capsulatum
Difficult to treat; available drugs often cause deleterious side effects; often need long-term therapy

 ## MECHANISMS OF ACTION

The principal antifungal drugs are polyenes, flucytosine, imidazoles, and griseofulvin.

Polyenes

The polyene (i.e., multiple double bonds) antibiotics are lactones that contain a hydrophilic hydroxylated portion and a hydrophobic conjugated double bond portion. The structures of amphotericin B, the most widely use antifungal agent, and nystatin are shown in Figure 52-1.

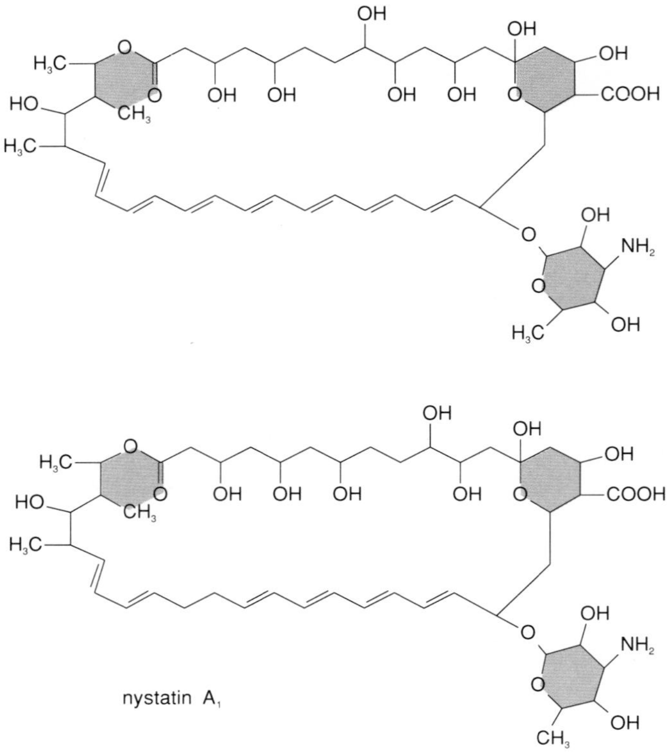

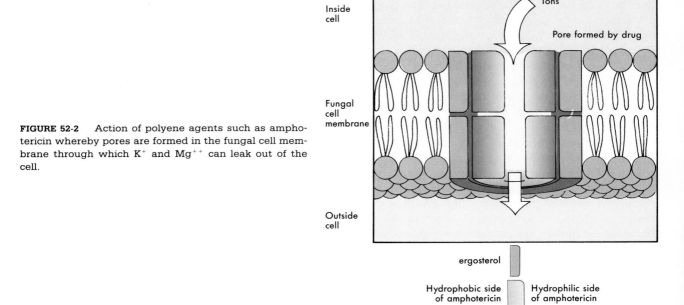

FIGURE 52-1   Structures of polyene agents.

nystatin A₁

FIGURE 52-2   Action of polyene agents such as amphotericin whereby pores are formed in the fungal cell membrane through which K⁺ and Mg⁺⁺ can leak out of the cell.

Polyenes act by binding to sterols in the cell membrane and forming channels, allowing K^+ ions and Mg^{++} molecules to leak out of the cell. The polyenes bind to the sterol and become integrated into the membrane to form a ring with a pore in the center of about 8Å diameter. K^+ leaks out of the cell through these pores, followed by Mg^{++}, and with the loss of K^+ results in derangement of cellular metabolism (Figure 52-2). It is thought that the derangement of the membrane alters the activity of enzymes in the membrane. The principal sterol in fungal membranes, ergosterol, has a stronger affinity for polyenes than does cholesterol, the principal sterol of mammalian cell membranes. Therefore the polyenes show greater activity against fungal than mammalian cells, and fungi that lack ergosterol are not susceptible to treatment by amphotericin B.

Flucytosine

Flucytosine, also called *5-fluorocytosine,* is an antimetabolite that undergoes intracellular metabolism to an active form that leads to inhibition of DNA synthesis (Figure 52-3).

Flucytosine is transported into susceptible fungi by a permease system for purines. The drug is deaminated by cytosine deaminase to 5-fluorouracil. Since cytosine deaminase is not present in mammalian cells, the drug does not undergo activation in humans. Fluorouracil, in turn, is converted by uridine phosphate (UMP) pyrophosphorylase and other enzymes to 5-fluoro-2'-deoxyuridine 5'-monophosphate, which inhibits thymidylate synthase and interferes with DNA synthesis (discussed in greater detail in Chapter 43).

Fungi can be resistant to flucytosine because they lack a permease, have a defective cytosine deaminase, or have a low concentration of the UMP pyrophosphorylase enzyme. Whether production of faulty RNA as a result of incorporation of the flurouracil contributes to the action of this agent is unclear.

Imidazoles

The structures of the principal imidazole antifungal agents are shown in Figure 52-4. Ketoconazole, miconazole, clotrimazole, and econazole are available, as is a new agent, fluconazole.

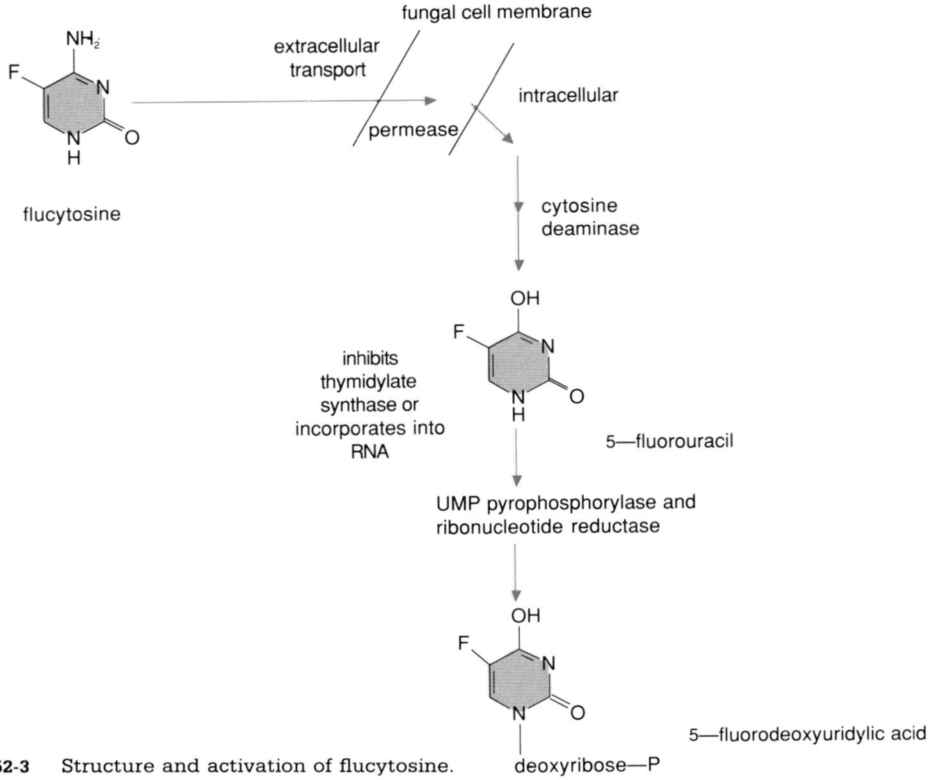

FIGURE 52-3   Structure and activation of flucytosine.

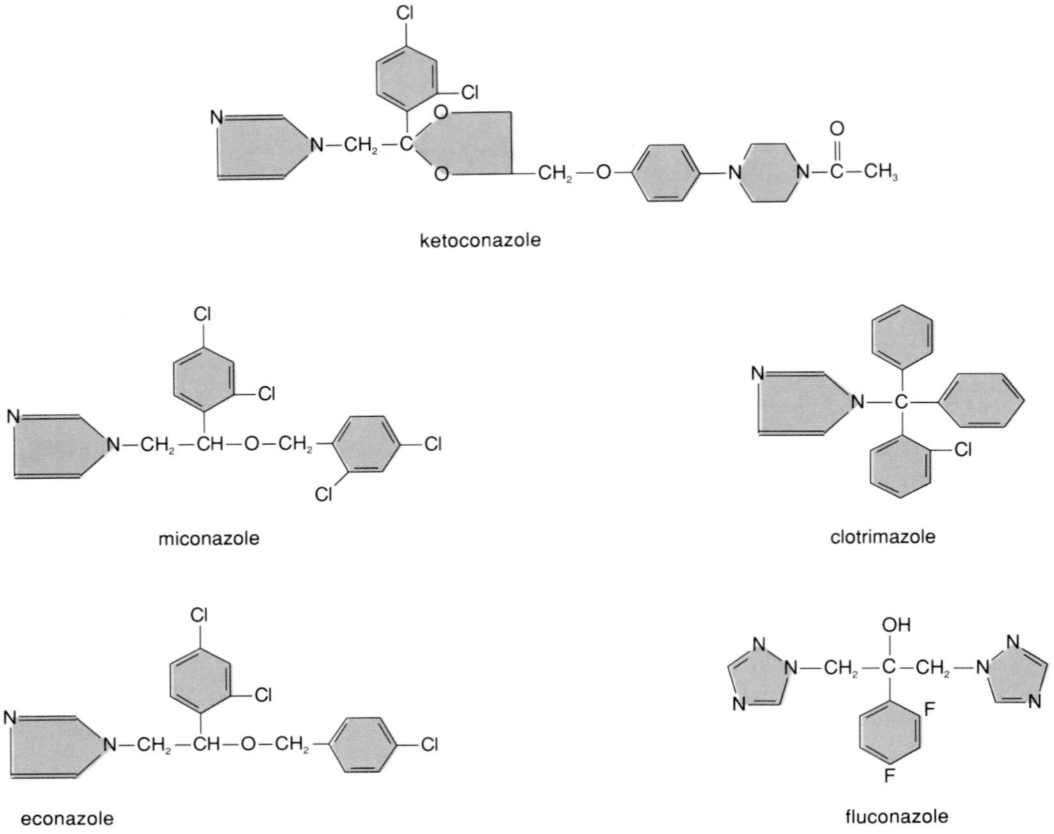

FIGURE 52-4   Structures of imidazole antifungal drugs.

Depending on the concentration of drug, imidazoles can act as fungistatic or fungicidal agents. In actively growing fungi, the imidazoles inhibit synthesis of membrane sterols by blocking the demethylation of lanosterol, so that synthesis of ergosterol is inhibited and precursor sterols accumulate in the membrane. Ketoconazole also disrupts other membrane lipids. At high concentrations, the imidazoles cause leakage of K^+ and other components from the fungal cell. Inhibition of plasma membrane ATPase is a secondary action that may contribute to or help account for the K^+ loss. Since ketoconazole inhibits fungal respiration under aerobic conditions and has an effect on fungal mitochondrial function, an alternate mechanism may be drug blockage of respiratory chain electron transport.

Griseofulvin

Whether griseofulvin is fungicidal or fungistatic is not established. It enters susceptible fungi through

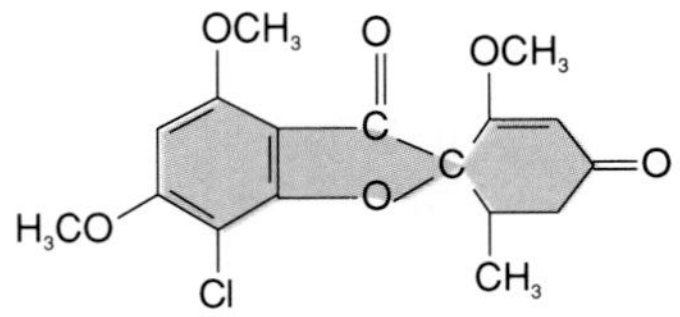

griseofulvin

FIGURE 52-5   Structure of griseofulvin.

an energy dependent transport system and inhibits fungal mitosis. It does this by binding to the microtubules that form the mitotic spindle and blocking the polymerization of tubulin into microtubules. It also binds to a microtubule-associated protein, but the role of this protein is not known. The binding site for griseofulvin on tubulin is different than that of colchicine and the plant alkaloids (see Chapter 43). This

Table 52-1 Pharmacokinetic Parameter Values for Antifungal Drugs

Drug	Administration	Absorbed	$t_{1/2}$ (hr)	Disposition	Plasma Protein Bound (%)
POLYENES					
amphotericin B	IV, topical, oral	No	24 (15 days)*	B (some) ? (main)	>90
nystatin	Topical	No	—	—	>90
ANTIMETABOLITES					
flucytosine	Oral	Good	3-6	R (85%)	<10
IMIDAZOLES					
ketoconazole	Oral, topical	Good†	8	M (95%) R (3%)	99
miconazole	Topical, IV	Poor	0.5	M (95%)	90
econazole	Topical	<1%	—	M (95%)	—
clotrimazole	Topical	<1%	—	M (95%)	—
fluconazole	IV, oral	Good	25-30 hr	R (main), M	12
GRISEOFULVIN	Oral, topical	Poor‡	20	M (main)	—

M, Metabolism; *R*, renal; *B*, biliary.
*Terminal elimination phase.
†Needs acidic pH to be absorbed.
‡Particles taken up by unknown process.

effect on microtubule assembly probably explains the morphological changes, such as curling, that are observed in the fungi. The mechanism of resistance is unknown but may be related to decreased uptake of the drug.

The structure of griseofulvin is shown in Figure 52-5.

 PHARMACOKINETICS

Pharmacokinetic parameters for the antifungal drugs are summarized in Table 52-1.

Polyenes

Amphotericin B is insoluble in water and has a large lipophilic domain in its structure, and it is not absorbed from the gastrointestinal (GI) tract. It is administered orally only to treat fungal infections of the GI tract, which sometimes develop as an aftermath of broad-spectrum antibacterial agents due to depletion of the bacterial microflora. For parenteral use, amphotericin B is combined with the detergent deoxycholate to form a colloidal suspension.

The pharmacokinetics of amphotericin B are complex, with >90% plasma protein bound, several distribution phases, and elimination phases with half-lives of 24 to 48 hours for the initial portion and about 15 days for the terminal portions. The drug can be detected in urine and serum for up to 7 weeks after a course of therapy.

Amphotericin B enters pleural, peritoneal, and synovial fluids to achieve about 50% of serum concentrations. It crosses the placenta and is found in cord blood and amniotic fluid and also enters the aqueous but not the vitreous humor of the eye. Cerebrospinal fluid (CSF) concentrations reach one third to one half those in serum. Most of the amphotericin B in the body probably is bound to cholesterol-containing membranes in tissue sites.

The principal pathway for amphotericin B disposition is not known. Some is excreted via the biliary route, and only 3% of a dose is eliminated in urine with concentrations equivalent to those in plasma. Renal dysfunction does not affect plasma concentrations of the drug, and amphotericin B is not removed by hemodialysis.

Flucytosine

Flucytosine is well absorbed from the GI tract and is widely distributed in the body, with CSF concentrations equal to 70% to 85% of those in plasma. It enters the peritoneum, synovial fuid, bronchial secretions, saliva, and bone.

Approximately 85% to 95% is excreted unchanged by glomerular filtration, with a normal half-life of 3 to 6 hours increased markedly as creatinine clearance diminishes. For special conditions, the drug can be removed by hemodialysis and peritoneal dialysis. A small fraction of the dose may be converted by intestinal bacteria to 5-fluorouracil and lead to hematologic toxicity.

Imidazoles

Ketoconazole is administered orally, since its absorption is favored at acid pH. Coadministration of antacids and histamine H_2 blocking agents reduces ketoconazole absorption. Contradictory results are reported for the effect of food on absorption of this agent. For the same dose, the plasma concentration of drug varies widely between patients.

Ketoconazole is distributed into saliva, skin, bone, and pleural, peritoneal, synovial, and aqueous humor fluids. Penetration into the CSF is poor, and effective CSF concentrations are not achieved—only 5% of the plasma concentration. The plasma concentration declines in a biexponential fashion, with a distribution half-life of about 2 hours followed by an elimination half-life of 8 hours.

Ketoconazole is extensively metabolized by hydroxylation of the imidazole and by oxidative *N*-dealkylation of the piperazine rings. It does not induce its own metabolism, as does clotrimazole. However, rifampin induces microsomal enzymes that increase ketoconazole oxidation. Only 2% to 4% of a dose is excreted in urine as active drug. Renal insufficiency does not affect plasma concentrations or half-life, but the half-life is prolonged in patients with hepatic insufficiency.

Miconazole is now used topically and rarely IV. It is minimally soluble in water and not adequately absorbed from the gastrointestinal tract. The half-life is only 30 minutes so that plasma concentrations after IV doses are low. It is metabolized by *O*-dealkylation and oxidative *N*-dealkylation but does not induce its own metabolism. Only 1% is excreted in the urine as active drug. Penetration of miconazole into CSF and sputum is poor but penetration into joint fluid is good.

Fluoconazole is rapidly absorbed after oral administration, with about 90% bioavailability and a half-life of 25 to 30 hours. Fluconazole does not require an acid environment for absorption. It does not induce the metabolism of most other agents, but it does, however, alter metabolism of oral hypoglycemic agents. About 70% of the drug is eliminated unchanged via the kidneys, with small amounts of metabolites present in urine and feces. Fluconazole is widely distributed in the body with therapeutic concentrations attained in CSF, lung, and many other areas of the body.

Griseofulvin

Griseofulvin is insoluble; however, about 50% of an oral dose passes from the gastrointestinal tract into the circulation. This uptake from the gastrointestinal tract is related to particle size and is increased when the drug is ingested with a full meal. Whether the drug diffuses through the intestinal wall or is taken up as micelles (particles of drug coated with lipid surrounded by detergent to provide a water-compatible exterior surface) is not clear. When applied topically, griseofulvin penetrates the stratum corneum, but this does not result in effective local concentrations.

Griseofulvin is widely distributed in body fluids and tissues and becomes concentrated in fat, liver, and muscle. It is deposited in the keratin layer of the skin; becomes concentrated in keratin precursor cells in the stratum corneum of the skin, nails, and hair; and is secreted in perspiration. New keratin formed during treatment with griseofulvin is resistant to fungus but griseofulvin does not destroy fungi in infected outer layers of skin. Thus a dermatophyte infection can only be cured when infected skin, nails, or hair is shed and the new keratin containing the griseofulvin replaces all of the old keratin. Skin and hair infections require 4 to 6 weeks of therapy, fingernails require up to 6 months, and toenails require up to a year.

Most of the absorbed griseofulvin is metabolized in the liver by dealkylation, and the inactive metabolite is excreted in the urine as a glucuronide. The half-life of the drug is about 20 hours.

RELATION OF MECHANISMS OF ACTION TO CLINICAL RESPONSE

Polyenes

Amphotericin B inhibits all of the fungi listed in the box on p. 709. These fungi are likely to be a cause of a systemic mycoses, including the *Mucor, Rhizopus,* and *Absidia* species that are often present as opportunistic pathogens in debilitated patients. Amphotericin B also inhibits *Sporothrix* and *Trichosporon* species, as well as some ameboflagellates and fresh water amebae, Acanthamoeba. A few fungal species show resistance, such as Allescheria boydii. Amphotericin B acts synergistically with flucytosine against *Candida* organisms and cryptococci. Synergy of amphotericin B with other agents, such as rifampin and tetracyclines, can be demonstrated in vitro, but there are no clinical studies to support the use of this or other combinations of amphotericin B and antibiotics for the treatment of fungal infections.

Nystatin has a mode of action and antifungal spectrum of activity similar to those for amphotericin B. It is too toxic for parenteral administration and is only used topically.

Flucytosine

Flucytosine inhibits *Cryptococcus neoformans,* many *Candida albicans,* and *Cladosporium* and *Phialophore* species, which cause chromoblastomycosis. Resistance of *Candida* species to this drug is extremely variable. Flucytosine does not inhibit *Aspergillus* and *Sporothrix* organisms, blastomyces, histoplasma, or *Coccidioides immitis.* This drug acts synergistically with amphotericin B against *Cryptococcus* organisms.

Imidazoles

The imidazoles inhibit many dermatophytes, yeasts, dimorphic fungi, and some phycomycetes. It is extremely difficult to interpret in vitro data on these drugs, since the results are method-dependent and do not correlate well with in vivo responses.

Ketoconazole inhibits most of the common dermatophytes and many of the fungi that cause systemic mycoses listed in the box (see p. 709). However, it is not active against *Aspergillus* organisms or phycomycetes such as *Mucor* species. The membrane actions of ketoconazole also block the formation of branching hyphae, which may aid in white cell attack on the fungi.

Since ketoconazole interferes with the synthesis of ergosterol, it probably should not be used with amphotericin B because the effect of amphotericin B would be antagonized. This has been demonstrated in vitro and in an animal model of cryptococcus infection.

Miconazole, econazole, and clotrimazole have a similar activity spectrum to that of ketoconazole. A different spectrum is observed for fluconazole, which inhibits *Candida* species, cryptococci, blastomyces, and histoplasma but not *Aspergillus* or other filamentous fungi.

Griseofulvin

Griseofulvin inhibits dermatophytes of *Microsporum, Trichophyton,* and *Epidermophyton* species. It has no effect on filamentous fungi such as *Aspergillus,* yeasts such as *Candida* organisms, or dimorphoric species such as *histoplasmata.*

Therapeutic Usage

Amphotericin B is the drug of choice to treat most serious fungal infections. Cryptococcal meningitis is treated either with amphotericin B alone or with a combination of amphotericin B and flucytosine. Systemic candidiasis is treated with amphotericin B, as are pulmonary, bone, joint, cardiac, and central nervous system (CNS) infections due to *Candida* organisms and *Coccidioides immitis* infections of the lung or meninges. Amphotericin B is the only useful agent to treat serious *Aspergillus* species and zygomyces infections. Severe acute histoplasmosis and blastomycosis are treated with amphotericin B, although ketoconazole is also useful. Other infections that respond to amphotericin B include sporotrichosis and amoebic meningoencephalitis.

Amphotericin B is also used as empiric therapy in febrile neutropenic patients who have not responded to antibacterial agents.

Fluconazole is equivalent to amphotericin in treating cryptococcal infections in AIDS patients. However, the initial response to therapy is slower than with amphotericin B, and fluconazole is preferred for lifetime maintenance therapy. It is also effective for therapy of *Candida* pharyngitis and esophagitis, and as a prophylactic agent against fungal infections in immunocompromised patients.

Nystatin is used to treat *Candida* infections of the skin, mucous membranes, and intestinal tract. It is effective for oral candidiasis, vaginal candidiasis, and *Candida* esophagitis. Although it is used prophylactically in neutropenic patients, it is ineffective except at very large daily doses.

Ketoconazole provides effective therapy for cutaneous mycoses and for oral and esophageal candidiasis in immunocompromised patients. The only systemic infection for which miconazole IV is appropriate is that caused by *Pseudoallecheria boydii*. Topically, it is comparable to clotrimazole for cutaneous candidiasis, ringworm, and pityriasis versicolor. Econazole is used topically because it can penetrate the stratum corneum.

Clotrimazole is available only for topical use. It is not used systemically because of poor absorption and induction of microsomal enzymes, which cause its inactivation. It is used topically for *Candida* infection and superficial dermatophyte (ringworm) infections. It is also effective prophylactically for oral *Candida* colonization and infection in neutropenic patients.

Griseofulvin is used only to treat dermatophyte infections of the skin, nails, or hair, with mild forms effectively handled topically.

Tolnaftate is a topical antifungal that inhibits dermatophytes such as *Trichophyton* and *Microsporum* species but not *Candida*. Its mechanism of action is unknown. It is less effective on hyperkeratotic lesions, and scalp lesions respond poorly. It has no effect on onchomycosis. Tolnaftate has no known toxic reactions.

Haloprogin is a fungicidal agent that is effective against some *Epidermophyton*, *Microsporum*, and *Trichophyton* species and inhibits *Candida* organisms. Its mechanism of action is unknown. Burning sensations and peeling of the skin are the main side effects. It is used primarily to treat tinea pedis.

SIDE EFFECTS, CLINICAL PROBLEMS, AND TOXICITY

The clinical problems and major side effects encountered with the antifungal agents are summarized in the box.

CLINICAL PROBLEMS

AMPHOTERICIN B
Fever and chills, nausea
Renal toxicity
Anemia, reduced erythropoiesis

KETOCONAZOLE
Nausea and vomiting
Hepatotoxicity

GRISEOFULVIN
Headache
Large doses are teratogenic and carcinogenic in animals

Polyenes

Amphotericin B Unfortunately, many adverse effects are associated with the IV administration of amphotericin B. The initial reactions, usually fever to as high as 40° C, chills, headache, malaise, nausea, and, occasionally, hypotension, can be controlled by antipyretics, antihistamines, antiemetics, and adrenocorticoids.

Most patients treated with amphotericin B develop some degree of renal toxicity. This is manifest by an early decrease in the glomerular filtration rate that results from vasoconstrictive action on the afferent arterioles. It may be accompanied by an effect on the distal renal tubule leading to potassium loss, hypomagnesemia due to failure to reabsorb Mg^{++}, or tubular acidosis. Drug-induced pathological changes in the kidney include damage to the glomerular basement membrane, hypercellularity, fibrosis, and hyalinization of glomeruli with nephrocalcinosis. If the serum creatinine concentration increases above 3.5 mg/dL, drug administration should be stopped for a few days. The extent of renal damage is related to the total dose of drug, and although the majority of renal function is recovered even with continued therapy, some residual damage occurs. Hydration may reduce toxicity, but mannitol infusions have not been of benefit.

Most patients who receive a normal course of therapy develop a normochromic, normocytic anemia with hematocrits of 22% to 35%. This is the result of reduced erythropoiesis due to inhibition of erythropoietin production. Red cell production returns to normal after discontinuation of therapy.

Other toxicities include rare neurotoxicity, cardiac dysrhythmias, pulmonary infiltrates, rash, and anaphylaxis. It is doubtful that amphotericin B produces liver toxicity.

Nystatin Nystatin has minimal side effects except for a bad taste when taken as an oral suspension, which in large doses can produce nausea. It is not allergenic on the skin.

Flucytosine

Occasionally patients experience nausea, vomiting, and diarrhea with flucytosine. Serious side effects are hematological: anemia, leukopenia, and thrombocytopenia. Since this drug is usually coadministered with amphotericin B, there may be reduced renal clearance of the drug. The toxicity is due to the metabolite 5-fluorouracil. Some cases of transient hepatotoxicity have been reported.

Imidazoles

Common side effects of ketoconazole, which occur in 3% to 20% of those treated, are nausea and vomiting, although nausea can be reduced if the drug is ingested with food. The most serious toxicity is hepatic, which is seen as transient elevations of serum transaminases and alkaline phosphatase in about 5% to 10% of patients. Fulminant hepatic damage is uncommon, 1 in 12,000, although a few patients develop jaundice, fever, liver failure, and even death. Thus ketoconazole use must be considered in terms of the seriousness of the infection against the risk of liver damage.

Ketoconazole can cause transient gynecomastia and breast tenderness by blocking testosterone synthesis. High doses can lead to azospermia and impotence and may block cortisol secretion and supress adrenal response to ACTH.

A principal drug interaction with ketoconazole involves interference with the metabolism of cyclosporin, which can lead to nephrotoxicity. Warfarin metabolism is not changed.

IV infusion of miconazole produces nausea and vomiting in 25% of patients. It may also cause chills, malaise, tremors, confusion, dizziness, or seizures.

Fluconazole absorption is decreased 15% to 20% by cimetidine, and warfarin-adjusted prothrombin times are altered by fluconazole.

Griseofulvin

Many patients receiving griseofulvin initially complain of headaches, but the symptom may disappear as therapy continues. Other CNS side effects include lethargy, confusion, memory lapses, and impaired judgment in routine tasks. Nausea, vomiting, bad taste in the mouth, occasionally leukopenia or neutropenia, hepatotoxicity, skin rashes, and photosensitivity also may occur. Although renal function is not decreased, albuminuria has developed. Griseofulvin administered in very large doses is teratogenic and carcinogenic in animals, but no reports of such effects in humans are available; however, griseofulvin should not be given to pregnant women.

Griseofulvin may interact and increase the metabolism of warfarin by induction of microsomal enzymes.

REFERENCES

Bennett JE, ed: Fluconazole: a novel advance in therapy for systemic fungal infections, Rev Infect Dis 12 (suppl 3):5263, 1990.

Fromtling RA: Imidazoles as important antifungal agents: an overview, Drugs Today 20:325, 1984.

Heel RC, Bragden NR, Carmine A et al.: Ketoconazole: a review of its therapeutic efficacy in superficial and systemic fungal infections, Drugs 23:1, 1982.

Janoff AS, Boni LT, Popescu MC et al.: Unusual lipid structures selectively reduce the toxicity of amphotericin B, Proc Nat Acad Sci USA 85:6122, 1988.

Stamm AM, Diasio RB, Dismukes WE et al.: Toxicity of amphotericin B plus flucytosine in 194 patients with cryptococcal meningitis, Am J Med 83:236, 1987.

53 Antiviral Drugs

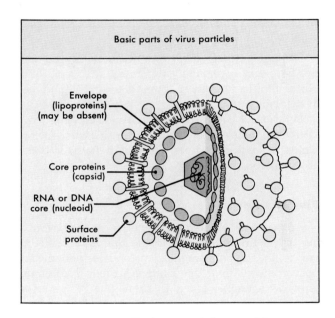

FIGURE 53-1   Basic parts of virus particles.

 THERAPEUTIC OVERVIEW

Viruses are responsible for a large proportion of the morbidity and mortality experienced worldwide. These infectious agents consist of a core genome of nucleic acid (nucleoid) contained in a protein shell (capsid) and sometimes surrounded by a lipoprotein membrane (envelope) (Figure 53-1). Viruses cannot replicate independently. They must enter cells and use cellular energy-generating, DNA- or RNA-replicating, and protein-synthesizing pathways of the host to achieve viral replication. Some viruses can integrate a copy of their genetic material into host chromosomes, achieving *viral latency,* a condition in which clinical infection can recur without reexposure to the virus.

Some genera of viruses known to cause human infections are listed in Table 53-1. Also listed is information about which genomic material—RNA or DNA—is present and examples of clinically important diseases attributed to each virus.

Viral biochemistry is not as well understood as bacterial biochemistry, so antiviral drug development has been relatively slow. The way antiviral agents act is not always known. Most currently available antiviral drugs interfere with viral nucleic acid synthesis and/or regulation; however, some agents work by interfering with virus-cell binding, interrupting virus uncoating, or stimulating the host immune system. Be-

Table 53-1 Virus Families of Clinical Importance		
Virus Genera	**Nucleic Acid**	**Clinical Examples of Illnesses**
Adenovirus	DNA	Upper respiratory and eye infections
Herpesvirus	DNA	Genital herpes, varicella, meningoencephalitis, mononucleosis, retinitis
Papillomavirus	DNA	Papillomas (warts), cancer (?)
Parvovirus	DNA	Erythema infectiosum
Arenavirus	RNA	Lymphocytic choriomeningitis
Bunyavirus	RNA	Encephalitis
Coronavirus	RNA	Upper respiratory infections
Influenzavirus	RNA	Influenza
Paramyxovirus	RNA	Measles, upper respiratory infections
Picornavirus	RNA	Poliomyelitis, diarrhea, upper respiratory infections
Retrovirus	RNA	Leukemia, acquired immune deficiency syndrome (AIDS)
Rhabdovirus	RNA	Rabies
Togavirus	RNA	Rubella, yellow fever
Hepadnaviridae	DNA	Hepatitis B

THERAPEUTIC OVERVIEW

Block uncoating of virus
Inhibit DNA polymerase of virus
Inhibit viral protein synthesis
Stimulate host immune system
Require active immune system for virus particles missed by drug
Are virustatic rather than virulytic
Include problem of viral latency
Inhibit thymidine kinase
Inhibit reverse transcriptase

cause viruses generally take over host cell nucleic acid/protein replication pathways before clinical infection is discovered, most antiviral drugs must penetrate infected cells to produce a therapeutic antiviral response. This capacity is often the source of significant toxicity to healthy cells, thus limiting a drug's usefulness.

In vitro susceptibility testing of antiviral compounds differs significantly from that for antibacterial agents. Because viruses require cells to replicate, susceptibility systems use cell cultures. In general, a greater than 50% reduction in cell plaque formation at an achievable serum concentration classifies an agent as active against a given virus. Many antiviral compounds have in vitro activity against many different viruses but are not effective clinically. Drug distribution, timing of infection, and problems with administration can limit the usefulness of many agents. Several agents become converted in the body to active compounds (acyclovir, ganciclovir) or must be present continuously to have an antiviral effect (amantadine). The various cell culture susceptibility

systems cannot be standardized for all situations.

Many antiviral agents inhibit single steps in the viral replication cycle. They are considered virustatic and do not destroy a given virus but temporarily halt replication. Optimal antiviral effectiveness requires a competent host immune system that can eliminate or effectively destroy virus replication. Patients with immunosuppressed conditions, such as leukemia, lymphoma, transplantation, and AIDS, are prone to frequent and often severe viral infections that may recur when antiviral drugs are stopped. Supportive, prolonged suppressive therapy is often necessary. Currently, no antiviral agent eliminates viral latency. Resistant strains of viruses to specific drugs can also develop.

The approaches for treatment of viral infections with drugs are summarized in the box above.

MECHANISMS OF ACTION

Viral Replication Cycle

Virions must first come in contact with an appropriate cell to initiate an infection. After contact is established, a virus penetrates the cell (Figure 53-2; step 1), disassembles (step 2), and initiates synthesis of virus components by controlling host protein and nucleic acid synthesis (step 3). Final assembly of virions (steps 4 and 5), which can be released to enter other cells and repeat the replication cycle (step 6), then occurs.

Antiviral agents have been developed that interfere with several of the steps in the virus reproductive cycle. Most are nucleic acid analogs that interfere

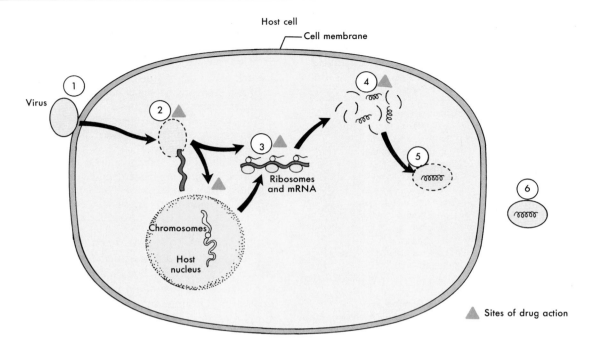

1. Attachment to host cell

2. Uncoating of virus

3. Control of DNA, RNA and/or protein production

4. Production of viral subunits

5. Assembly of virions

6. Release of virions

FIGURE 53-2   Schematic representation of virus replication. Some viruses integrate into host chromosome with development of latency (see text).

with virus DNA/RNA production and therefore inhibit virus replication. Combination antiviral therapy with multiple agents has not yet demonstrated superior clinical outcomes.

Many viruses contain unique enzymes or metabolic pathways that make them more susceptible to certain agents. Herpes simplex virus encodes a thymidine kinase that monophosphorylates acyclovir significantly better than host cell enzyme does. In this way, acyclovir, which when phosphorylated is trapped within the cell, is concentrated in infected cells, leading to greater inhibition of virus growth and fewer side effects on uninfected cells. Other members of the herpes virus family (such as varicella-zoster) are less susceptible to acyclovir. Cytomegalovirus does not encode thymidine kinase; so it is only inhibited by concentrations of acyclovir not clinically tolerated. Similarly, retroviruses all use reverse transcriptase to transcribe RNA to DNA early in their replication cycle. Inhibitors of this enzyme have been

developed and are useful in treatment of human immunodeficiency virus (HIV) infections.

Specific Drugs

Amantadine   The mechanism of action of amantadine, a symmetrical tricyclic amine (Figure 53-3), is not fully established but does not affect virus binding, absorption, penetration, or influenza virus RNA transcriptase. Amantadine is concentrated in lysosomes, increasing lysosomal pH and interfering with membrane fusion. It appears to interfere with late stage uncoating of influenza A virions, but it is not effective against influenza B, which lacks the protein (M2) to which amantadine binds in influenza A. A single amino acid change in the M2 protein results in resistance during or after therapy. The resistant virus is virulent and causes diseases in exposed individuals. Rimantadine is a related compound with similar antiviral action but different pharmacokinet-

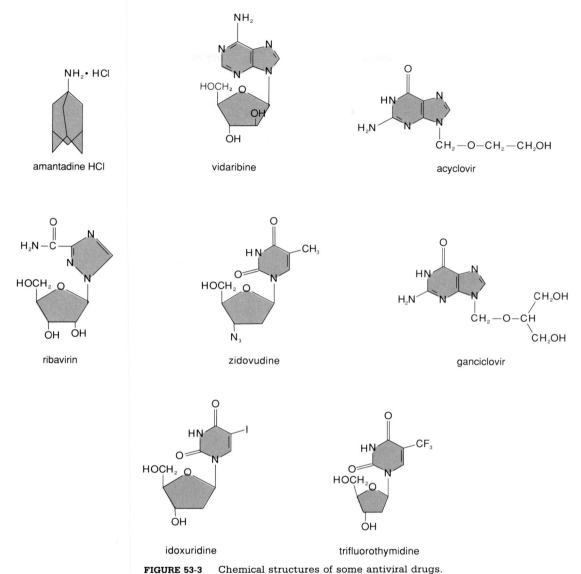

FIGURE 53-3   Chemical structures of some antiviral drugs.

ics. Resistance develops as with amantadine.

Vidarabine Vidarabine (adenine arabinoside, Ara-A) is an adenosine derivative that is converted by cellular enzymes to the triphosphate that inhibits many human and viral DNA polymerases inhibiting viral DNA synthesis (Figure 53-3). It is rapidly me-

tabolized to produce a less active compound (arabinosyl hypoxanthine) that still has an antiviral effect.

Vidarabine triphosphate formed in the cell can act as a DNA chain terminator. Since herpes simplex DNA polymerases are approximately 20 times more susceptible to this agent than host polymerases, viral

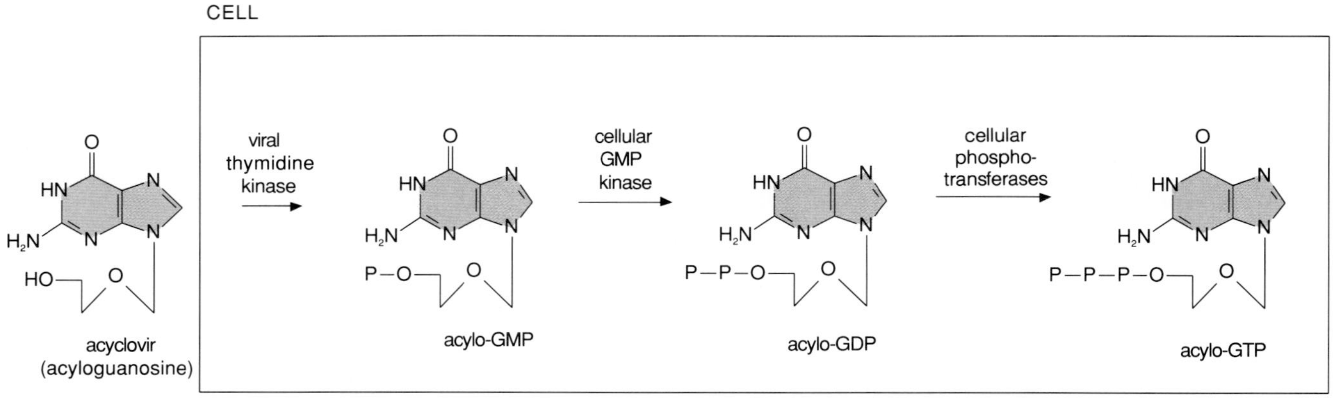

CELL

FIGURE 53-4   Phosphorylation of acyclovir. The monophosphate accumulates in the cell and is converted to the triphosphate.

selectivity is enhanced. Vidarabine triphosphate also inhibits other enzyme systems, for example, RNA polyadenylation and red blood cell transmethylation. Changes in viral DNA polymerases can result in vidarabine resistance, but this is not a common clinical problem. Use of this agent has been significantly supplanted by acyclovir.

Acyclovir (acycloguanosine) (Figure 53-3) Acyclovir is a synthetic guanosine analog that requires phosphorylation to become active (Figure 53-4). It undergoes monophosphorylation by viral thymidine kinase. Because herpes simplex types 1 and 2 viral thymidine kinases are many times more sensitive to acyclovir than host thymidine kinase, high concentrations of acyclovir monophosphate accumulate in the virus infected cells. Acyclovir monophosphate is then further phosphorylated to the active compound acyclovir triphosphate. The triphosphate cannot cross cell membranes and accumulates further. As a result, the concentration of acyclovir triphosphate is 50 to 100 times greater in infected cells than in uninfected cells.

Acyclovir triphosphate functions as a competitive inhibitor of viral DNA polymerases and inhibits virus growth. Host DNA polymerases are significantly less susceptible to acyclovir triphosphate than viral DNA polymerases. In addition, acyclovir triphosphate can act as a DNA chain terminator. Irreversible binding between the enzyme and the blocked chain occurs, causing permanent inactivation of some viral DNA polymerases.

The end result is several 100-fold inhibition of herpes simplex virus growth with minimal toxicity to uninfected cells. Altered thymidine kinase (acyclovir-resistant) herpes simplex viruses have developed. They occur primarily in patients receiving multiple courses of therapy or in AIDS patients. Changes in viral DNA polymerases can mediate resistance to acyclovir. The thymidine kinase mutants are susceptible to vidarabine and foscarnet.

Ganciclovir The structure of ganciclovir (dihydroxypropoxymethylguanine [DHPG]) is shown in Figure 53-3. It is also a synthetic guanosine analog active against many herpes viruses, and similar to acyclovir, it must be phosphorylated to become active. Infection induced kinases, viral thymidine kinase and deoxyguanosine kinase of cytomegalovirus catalyze this reaction. Following monophosphorylation, cellular enzymes convert ganciclovir to the triphosphorylated form, and the triphosphate inhibits viral DNA polymerase rather than cellular DNA polymerase. Ganciclovir triphosphate is a competitive inhibitor of GTP incorporation into DNA. Because of its toxicity and the availability of acyclovir for treatment of many herpes virus infections, its use is currently restricted to treatment of cytomegalovirus retinitis.

Ribavirin Ribavirin is a synthetic purine nucleoside analog active in vitro against a number of viruses, including some causing viral pneumonia, Lassa fever, and influenza (Figure 53-3). Ribavirin appears to undergo phosphorylation in host cells by host adenosine kinase. The 5'-monophosphate subsequently inhibits cellular inosine monophosphate formation, resulting in depletion of intracellular guanosine triphosphate.

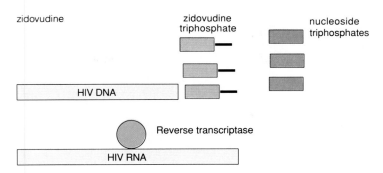

FIGURE 53-5 Phosphorylated azidothymidine (zidovudine) inhibits reverse transcriptase and is incorporated into growing HIV DNA, resulting in chain termination.

In some viruses, ribavirin triphosphate suppresses GTP-dependent capping of messenger RNA, thereby inhibiting viral protein synthesis. It also acts by suppressing viral messenger RNA initiation and/or elongation. Exogenous guanosine can reverse the antiviral effects of ribavirin in some viruses. Resistance to ribavirin has not been found.

Zidovudine Zidovudine (azidodeoxythymidine [AZT]) is a thymidine nucleoside analog (see Figure 53-3) with activity against HIV. Zidovudine becomes phosphorylated to monophosphate, diphosphate, and triphosphate forms by cellular kinases in infected and uninfected cells. It has two primary methods of action: The triphosphate acts as a competitive inhibitor of viral reverse transcriptase, and the azido group (N_3) prevents further chain elongation and acts as a DNA chain terminator. Zidovudine inhibits cellular α-DNA polymerases at concentrations approximately 100-fold greater than it inhibits reverse transcriptase, and its low degree of toxicity probably results from this disparity. Zidovudine is currently indicated as treatment for some stages of HIV infection.

Idoxuridine Idoxuridine (5-iodo-2-deoxyuridine, IUDR) is an iodinated thymidine nucleoside analog that is incorporated into DNA in place of thymidine and blocks further DNA chain elongation (Figure 53-3). In vitro, it inhibits many DNA viruses, and exogenous thymidine eliminates its antiviral effect. Idoxuridine affects mammalian cells, and its teratogenic, mutagenic, and immunosuppressive effects limit its use to topical preparations only, with special use in herpes simplex infections of the cornea. Herpes viruses resistant to idoxuridine occur clinically and generally have decreased thymidine kinase activity.

Trifluridine Trifluorothymidine is a pyrimidine analog that inhibits viral DNA synthesis by incorporation into viral DNA (see Figure 53-3). It does not require thymidine kinase for activity and is active against thymidine kinase-deficient mutants of herpes simplex virus that are resistant to acyclovir and/or idoxuridine. It is limited to topical use.

Fluorouracil The chemical structure of fluorouracil is shown in Chapter 43. As a fluorinated pyrimidine nucleoside analog it blocks production of thymidylate and interrupts normal cellular DNA and RNA synthesis. Its primary action may be to cause cellular thymine deficiency and resultant cell death. The effect of fluorouracil is most pronounced on rapidly growing cells, and its use as an antiviral agent is primarily related to destruction of infected cells (warts) by topical application.

Foscarnet Foscarnet (trisodium phosphoroformate hexahydrate) inhibits DNA polymerase and reverse transcriptase. It is active against herpes (HSV and CMV), HIV, and hepadna viruses. Resistance is due to altered viral DNA polymerase.

Interferons Interferons are naturally occurring glycoproteins produced by lymphocytes, macrophages, fibroblasts, and other human cells. There are three immunologically and chemically distinct classes: α, β, and γ. They act as antiviral agents by inhibiting viral protein synthesis and/or assembly or by stimulating the immune system. Interferons bind specific cell receptors, producing rapid change in cellular RNA. The effect results in inhibition of viral penetration or uncoating, synthesis, or methylations of mRNA, translation of viral proteins or as with retroviruses, assembly and release of virus. There is usually production of a 2′, 5′ oligo-adenylate synthetase and protein kinase that inhibit protein synthesis in

Table 53-2   Pharmacokinetic Parameters

Drug	Routes of Administration	Peak Serum Concentrations (μg/ml)	t₁/₂ (hr)	Disposition
amantadine	Oral	0.3-0.7	12-18 (doubles in elderly)	R (90%), M (9%)
vidarabine	IV, topical	0.3-0.6	minutes	M (90%), R*
arabinosyl hypo-xanthine	(See vidarabine)	3-5	3.5	R (main)
acyclovir	Topical, oral, IV	0.6-10.0	3-4	R (80%), M (20%)
ganciclovir	IV	4-6	3-4	R (90%)
ribavirin	Aerosol, oral	0.8-3.5	9 (36 hr final phase)	M (60%), R (30%)
zidovudine	Oral, IV (in trials)	0.05-1.5	0.8-2	M (75%), R (15%)
idoxuridine	Topical	—	—	M
trifluorothymidine	Topical	—	—	—
fluorouracil	Topical	—	—	—

M, Metabolized; *R*, renal excretion as unchanged drug.
*Active metabolite.

the presence of double-stranded RNA. Interferon can also prevent mRNA replication by inhibiting trans-methylation. Interferons can also protect uninfected cells from infection by mechanisms that are as yet unclear. Interferons are used for treatment of hepatitis and papilloma viruses (see also Chapter 43).

Immunoglobulins Immunoglobulins are used as antiviral agents primarily to prevent infections. Some immunoglobulin preparations have high titers against hepatitis B, herpes zoster, and rabies and are used for treatment or prophylaxis. In hepatitis A infection, standard human immune globulin is used in prophylaxis.

 PHARMACOKINETICS

For most of these agents to be active they must become concentrated within cells. Many compounds are nucleoside analogs and are rapidly metabolized to inactive compounds that are then eliminated from the body. This necessitates frequent dosing to maintain adequate drug concentrations. Some agents can only be used topically to treat certain viral infections because of severe systemic toxicity.

Because these compounds often interfere with human DNA or RNA synthesis, the use of any antiviral agent in pregnancy should be done with the utmost caution and only when the potential benefits of treatment clearly outweigh the potential risks. The pharmacokinetic parameter values for the antiviral drugs are listed in Table 53-2.

Amantadine

Amantadine is completely but slowly absorbed from the gastrointestinal (GI) tract, is 65% protein bound, and distributes well throughout the body. The volume of distribution of amantadine is between 4 and 10 L/kg. Cerebrospinal fluid (CSF) and brain concentrations are approximately 50% of concurrent serum values, and concentrations in nasal mucus equal those in serum. Amantadine is excreted in breast milk.

Serum drug concentrations vary widely with the age of the patient. Peak drug concentrations occur 2 to 4 hours after ingestion. Plasma half-life for healthy, middle-aged adults is between 12 and 18 hours. In the elderly the half-life doubles, requiring dosage reduction in these patients.

Amantadine is eliminated by kidney glomerular filtration and tubular secretion, with over 90% excreted unchanged in the urine and approximately 1% excreted unchanged in stool. Amantadine is metabolized to at least eight different compounds, with N-acetyl-amantadine as the predominant metabolite. The biological activity of these metabolites is unknown.

Vidarabine

Vidarabine is available for IV and topical application. Following infusion, it is deaminated within minutes to less active arabinosyl hypoxanthine. During infusion, vidarabine is detectable but not at concentrations expected to have significant antiviral activity. Arabinosyl hypoxanthine possesses only about 2.5% of the antiviral activity of vidarabine; however, the two compounds can act synergistically to produce antiviral effects. The metabolite distributes throughout the body, and its CSF concentrations are approximately 35% of serum values in adults and 90% in children. Vidarabine is 20% to 30% protein bound.

Serum concentrations of arabinosyl hypoxanthine during continuous infusion are between 3 and 6 μg/ml, and its serum half-life is about 3.5 hours. Arabinosyl hypoxanthine has been detected in red blood cells up to 3 weeks after vidarabine administration.

Approximately 50% of the total administered drug is excreted in the urine as arabinosyl hypoxanthine and 1% to 3% as vidarabine. About 50% of arabinosyl hypoxanthine is cleared with a 6 hour course of hemodialysis. A dosage reduction of approximately 25% is recommended for persons with renal insufficiency. A dose should be administered after dialysis.

Acyclovir

Acyclovir can be used topically, orally, or IV. Oral acyclovir is only 15% to 30% bioavailable, and food does not affect absorption. For unknown reasons, bioavailability is lower in transplant patients. Acyclovir is minimally protein bound (10% to 30%), and drug interactions through binding displacement have not been reported. The drug is well distributed, with CSF and brain concentrations equaling approximately 50% of serum values. Concentrations of acyclovir in zoster vesicle fluid are equivalent to those in plasma. Aqueous humor concentrations are 35% and salivary concentrations 15% that of plasma; vaginal concentrations are equivalent to those of plasma. Breast milk concentrations exceed those of plasma. The percutaneous absorption of topical acyclovir is low and occurs primarily when large areas are treated. Plasma concentrations of about 0.3 μg/ml have been reported in patients treated topically with this drug for herpes zoster. Peak serum concentrations following oral acyclovir average 0.6 μg/ml and occur 90 minutes after dosing, but peak serum concentrations after IV administration reach approximately 10 μg/ml.

The plasma half-life for normal adults and neonates is 3.3 and 3.8 hours, respectively. In anuric patients, it increases to 20 hours. In the urine, 60% to 90% of acyclovir is excreted unchanged, via both glomerular filtration and tubular secretion. As a result, acyclovir may interfere with the renal excretion of drugs such as methotrexate that are eliminated via renal tubules; probenecid significantly decreases the renal excretion of acyclovir. A major metabolite of acyclovir, 9-carboxymethoxymethylguanine, accounts for 10% to 20% of the total administered dose and is also excreted in urine. Acyclovir is effectively removed by hemodialysis (60%) but only minimally by peritoneal dialysis; thus supplemental doses are not given.

Ganciclovir

Ganciclovir is only used IV, since less than 5% of an oral dose is absorbed with only 1% to 2% protein bound. CSF concentrations are approximately 50% in plasma and 40% in brain tissue, with peak plasma concentrations reaching 4 to 6 μg/ml. The plasma half-life is 3 to 4 hours in persons with normal renal function, increasing to over 24 hours in patients with severe renal insufficiency. Over 90% of systemic ganciclovir is eliminated unchanged in urine, and dose modifications are necessary for persons with compromised renal function. Ganciclovir is approximately 50% removed by hemodialysis. It can be administered intravitreally with a half-life of 50 hours.

Ribavirin

Ribavirin bioavailability is about 45% and peak concentrations after IV administration are ten-fold greater than that after oral administration. It accumulates with prolonged oral use. The β phase half-life is 2 hours but the γ phase half-life is 36 hours. Ribavirin is administered via aerosol in the treatment of severe respiratory syncytial virus infections. Some ribavirin is absorbed during aerosol treatments, and after 20 hours of aerosol therapy, plasma concentrations in treated infants range from 0.8 to 3.3 μg/ml. Ribavirin concentrations in respiratory secretions are approximately 1000-fold greater.

About 3% of ribavirin accumulates in red blood cells as ribavirin triphosphate to give a prolonged serum half-life of 40 days during which the compound is slowly lost from the red cells. Concentrations in spinal fluid are about 60% those of plasma. Hepatic metabolism is the main route of elimination for ribavirin, with 30% of the drug eliminated in urine.

Zidovudine

Zidovudine is administered orally and is 60% to 65% bioavailable with 40% metabolized by first-pass. Peak concentrations occur within 30 to 90 minutes to give steady-state peak concentrations of 0.05 to 1.5 μg/ml. Zidovudine is 35% to 40% protein bound. CSF concentrations vary widely and range from 25% to 100% of serum values. It enters brain, phagocytic cells, liver, muscle, and placenta. Plasma half-life is about 1 hour. Semen concentrations are generally greater than plasma concentrations, probably due to the acidity of prostate secretions.

Zidovudine is inactivated mainly by glucuronidation (about 75% of a dose) and the 5' glucuronide has a half-life of 1 hour. Renal elimination of unchanged drug by glomerular filtration and tubule secretion accounts for another 15% of drug elimination. Drugs that can interfere with hepatic glucuronidation (such as acetaminophen) or renal tubule transport (such as probenecid) can inhibit elimination of zidovudine and should be avoided.

Idoxuridine

Idoxuridine is used only topically as a 0.1% solution or a 0.5% ointment; systemic absorption is minimal. The small amount that is absorbed undergoes metabolism to uracil and iodouracil. In vitro resistance to idoxuridine develops easily, and resistant clinical isolates have been described that may be a cause for treatment failure.

Trifluridine and Fluorouracil

Trifluridine is available for topical use only, especially as an ophthalmic preparation. Drug absorption is minimal, and no trifluridine has been detected in serum or aqueous humor from treated patients. Fluorouracil is also available as a topical preparation.

Interferons

Because interferons are glycoproteins, their pharmacokinetics are difficult to assess. Oral administration does not yield detectable concentrations. They are administered IM or SC. Simple detection of circulating compounds may not indicate clinical activity since cellular binding is necessary to effect a response and biological activity may last many days despite their clearance from serum.

Interferons are effective when injected directly into condylomata or given SC or IM. Serum concentrations peak in 4 to 8 hours and decline steadily over 1 to 2 days. Biological activity of interferons begins within an hour of injection, peaks at 24 hours, and wanes over 4 to 6 days. Interferons are distributed throughout the body and are detectable in brain and CSF. Elimination of exogenous interferon is complex. Liver, lung, kidney, heart, and skeletal muscle are capable of inactivating the compounds. Negligible amounts are found in urine.

Immunoglobulins

As antiviral therapies, immunoglobulins are given SC, IM and IV. Immunoglobulins are distributed throughout the body with only about 50% of IgG being intravascular. Following IM injection, immunoglobulin serum concentrations peak in 4 to 6 days and then decline with half-lives of 20 to 30 days. For persons with continued exposure to infectious agents such as hepatitis A, repeat immunization is often recommended every 3 to 6 months. Following exposure to rabies, infiltration of the wound with high-titer immunoglobulin to neutralize virus is recommended, with administration of the remaining immunoglobulin IM. IV gamma globulin is administered every 3 to 4 weeks to agammaglobulinemic patients. It is also given to transplant patients receiving a CMV-positive kidney or heart if the recipient is CMV antibody negative. Clearance of immune globulins is variable, with a mean half-life of 20 days.

 ## RELATION OF MECHANISMS OF ACTION TO CLINICAL RESPONSE

Human Immunodeficiency Virus and Acquired Immune Deficiency Syndrome

A retrovirus isolated in the United States and France in the early 1980s was subsequently identified and named the human immunodeficiency virus (HIV).

Acute infection by HIV often leads to acute viral illness, characterized by fever, myalgias, pharyngitis, rash, and/or headache. It generally lasts 10 to 20 days and resolves without treatment as HIV antibody develops. Some individuals acquire HIV antibody without the characteristic illness. All HIV-antibody-positive patients are considered infectious for life. In the natural history of HIV infection, the period of latency before seroconversion has not been defined.

After infection, most individuals experience a progressive decline in the number and function of infected cells (T-helper lymphocytes and macrophages) leading to progressive immunodeficiency. Other cells may also be infected. Patients are therefore susceptible to opportunistic and non-opportunistic infections and tumors. When the immune system has been so severely damaged by HIV that it can no longer counteract opportunistic infections or tumors, the diagnosis of acquired immune deficiency syndrome (AIDS) is established. Other AIDS defining conditions are the wasting syndrome and dementia.

In general, patients remain relatively asymptomatic until their T-helper cell counts fall well below the normal range. This usually takes many years, and approximately 50% of antibody-positive persons will progress to AIDS in 8 years without treatment.

As patients become more severely ill, they may require suppressive and/or prophylactic therapy with additional antiviral, antifungal, and antiprotozoal agents. Aerosolized pentamidine, trimethoprim-sulfamethoxazole, or trimethoprim-dapsone are often used to prevent pneumocystis pneumonia.

Many new agents are being evaluated as primary therapies for HIV infections. Trials with the nucleic acid analogs dideoxycytidine and dideoxyinosine are ongoing. These compounds appear to act similarly to zidovudine and can inhibit HIV in vitro. However, toxicities are somewhat different than for zidovudine, with the possibility of combination chemotherapy resulting in successful inhibition of virus growth with fewer side effects. Compounds that block binding of HIV to susceptible cells are also being tested, for example, soluble CD4 (the natural receptor for HIV surface proteins). Other approaches such as mismatched RNA, isoprinosine, and other immune stimulators are being evaluated.

Specific Drugs

Because antiviral drugs primarily inhibit viruses after infection has occurred, they are most effective when given early in the course of the infection. Many agents are limited in their use by toxicity on noninfected cells. These compounds are primarily used as topical agents.

Some drugs (e.g., immunoglobulins and interferons) can eliminate the infecting virus from the body, but these drugs are significantly less effective in immunosuppressed patients.

Amantadine Amantadine is used for the treatment and prophylaxis of influenza A infections but is ineffective against influenza B. It is most effective clinically when given before exposure or within 48 hours of development of symptoms. Clinical effectiveness has been estimated at 50% protection against infection and 60% to 70% protection against illness. It also reduces fever and palliates symptoms of influenza. Amantadine does not inhibit antibody responses to influenza, and immunity develops during amantadine therapy in persons either immunized or infected. The protective effect of amantadine is lost approximately 48 hours after stopping treatment. Groups targeted for amantadine therapy include unvaccinated persons with underlying cardiopulmonary, renal, metabolic, neuromuscular, or immunodeficiency diseases who are at increased risk for serious morbidity and mortality from influenza. Vaccination must be given since resistant mutants may develop during therapy.

Vidarabine Vidarabine was used primarily in the treatment of herpes simplex encephalitis, disseminated or CNS herpes infections in the newborn, herpes keratitis (topically), and herpes zoster in immunocompromised patients. It has generally been replaced by acyclovir.

In adults with encephalitis, vidarabine treatment improved survival from 30% to 70% and decreased long-term neurologic sequelae when compared with no treatment; however, only about 50% of surviving treated patients were neurologically normal 1 year after treatment. For the treatment of herpes encephalitis, vidarabine is inferior to acyclovir both in terms of survival and residual neurological sequelae.

Acyclovir Acyclovir can be used topically, orally, or IV. When used to treat herpes simplex, encephalitis, and most other significant herpes infections, it is more efficacious and less toxic than vidarabine.

For herpes encephalitis, acyclovir further decreases mortality to approximately 20% as compared to 50% with vidarabine. Also, about 50% of acyclovir-treated patients return to normal life as compared to about 20% with vidarabine treatment. Acyclovir should be administered as soon as possible after a diagnosis of encephalitis is made to lessen morbidity and mortality.

Systemic acyclovir is effective in reducing viral shedding, decreasing local symptoms, and decreasing severity and duration of illness when treating established mucocutaneous herpes simplex infections in immunosuppressed patients. Recurrences after termination of therapy are common. Oral acyclovir is often effective in suppressing recurrences of mucocutaneous herpes simplex infections in the immunosuppressed and is often given after systemic immune suppressive therapy.

In healthy patients with recurrent oral herpes infections, oral therapy has not proven significantly beneficial and is not generally recommended. For persons with recurrent disease who are at high risk (e.g., from sun exposure), oral acyclovir for 1 week can decrease recurrences by approximately 75%.

Topical acyclovir has no significant advantage over a placebo when treating primary genital herpes simplex infections. IV or oral acyclovir can be used to treat primary genital herpes. Both treatments decrease viral shedding, local and systemic symptoms, and time to resolution. Neither form of therapy decreases the rate or severity of recurrences.

Recurrent genital herpes is generally managed with oral acyclovir. Treatments begun within 2 days of recurrence decrease viral excretion; unfortunately, no differences in clinical symptoms are noted when compared to placebo therapy.

Approximately 75% of patients taking suppressive acyclovir will have no recurrences for 4 to 24 months, and total recurrences decrease by 90%. After discontinuation of acyclovir, recurrence rates generally return to pretreatment levels. Since recurrences of genital herpes tend to decrease in intensity and frequency with time, a 6 to 12 month suppressive trial with subsequent cessation of medication for 3 to 6 months is generally used. Herpes simplex resistance to acyclovir has been reported in persons with active lesions taking suppressive therapy. Individuals taking acyclovir are still infectious even though no lesions are visible.

Acyclovir is as effective as vidarabine in the treatment of neonatal herpes, is easier to administer, and has fewer side effects. It can also be used prophylactically with bone marrow transplant patients to prevent herpes recurrence and in renal transplant pa-

tients to decrease the incidence of cytomegalovirus infection. Therapy is most effective when begun before transplantation and continued for many weeks.

IV acyclovir is capable of limiting both varicella and zoster infections in immunocompromised patients. In zoster, it produces decreased visceral and cutaneous dissemination, shorter time to healing, and decreased duration of pain, but it needs to be given within 4 days of detection of the infection for greatest effect. With high-dose oral acyclovir treatment of zoster in immunosuppressed patients, only moderate success is noted, possibly because of poor drug absorption following oral administration. Inhibitory concentrations of acyclovir needed for varicella zoster (3 to 7 µg/ml) are about 5 times higher than those needed for inhibition of herpes simplex virus.

Acyclovir is not effective in treating cytomegalovirus pneumonia or visceral disease, Epstein-Barr mononucleosis, or chronic fatigue syndrome. However, a condition in AIDS patients known as hairy leukoplakia (a proliferation of oral epithelium related to Epstein-Barr infection) is responsive to oral acyclovir.

Ganciclovir Ganciclovir is available only for IV administration and currently is approved only to treat cytomegalovirus retinitis. After 2 to 3 weeks of treatment, over 80% of AIDS patients with retinitis improve or have no further loss of vision. Blood, urine, and throat cultures become negative or decrease 100-fold in 3 to 8 days in about 90% of AIDS patients, and clinical improvement in retinal lesions is usually observed in 10 to 14 days. After drug treatment has been completed, retinitis recurs in the majority of patients within a month if suppressive therapy is not instituted.

About 65% of AIDS patients with visceral cytomegalovirus infection have significant virological responses, but clinical improvement with ganciclovir is not as significant. Bone marrow transplant patients with cytomegalovirus pneumonia also show virological responses, but there are no differences in overall mortality with this antiviral agent.

Ribavirin Ribavirin is used in the United States as an aerosol for treatment of severe respiratory syncytial virus bronchopneumonia. When used for treating such infections, this drug is effective as shown by improved oxygenation, decreased viral shedding, and improvement of pneumonia symptoms. The aerosol particles must be of the proper size. Therefore, special generators are required for this treatment. Aerosol administration is given for 12 to 20 hours per day for 3 to 7 days and is most effective when started within 3 days of illness onset. Treatments may be effective in patients with underlying cardiopulmonary or immunosuppressive illnesses. Ribavirin is minimally effective for upper airway syncytial virus problems. Ribaviran orally or IV is the therapy of Lassa fever, an otherwise fatal disease. This is also useful in Korean and Argentine hemorrhagic fevers.

Zidovudine Zidovudine is currently the only antiviral agent approved for the treatment of HIV infection and is available in oral form.

Treatment with zidovudine in AIDS and AIDS-related complex (ARC) patients produces a significant reduction in mortality and opportunistic infections, improved physical performance (and possibly improved neurological function), and significantly improved T-helper cell counts.

For AIDS and AIDS-related complex (ARC) patients treated with zidovudine and other therapies directed at suppression of opportunistic infections, the 2 year survival is approximately 50% and 70%, respectively. This is significantly better than what was achieved retrospectively in controls.

Zidovudine-resistant virus mutants have been isolated from patients 12 to 18 months after the initiation of therapy, but worsening of clinical status has not been noted in such patients. Resistance does not appear to be associated with differences in reverse transcriptase binding.

Idoxuridine Idoxuridine can be used to treat herpes simplex keratitis and is effective for dendritic ulcers but not for deeper stromal ulcers that may develop. This agent is only used topically because of significant liver and bone marrow toxicity. It is not effective in genital herpes, localized zoster, or varicella.

Trifluridine Trifluridine is used topically to treat herpes simplex keratitis.

Fluorouracil Fluorouracil has been used topically to treat condylomata (warts) caused by human papillomaviruses, but this use is not well established. It acts primarily as an ablative agent, destroying infected and uninfected cells and can therefore be used only externally over relatively small areas. It also shows some success for treating intraurethral warts.

Interferons There are at least three classes of human interferons: alpha, beta, and gamma. These proteins are nonspecific immune stimulators that also have significant antiviral activity. The only approved antiviral use of interferon is in the treatment of condyloma acuminata. Both α- and β-interferon are effective when injected directly into lesions or administered systemically. Interferons are also effective for the treatment of Kaposi's sarcoma.

Immunoglobulins Some human immunoglobulins have high titers against specific viruses such as hepatitis B and rabies and are more efficacious against these viruses than nonspecific immunoglobulin. The viral infections for which immunoglobulins are used are listed in the box. Immunoglobulins are given IM, as close as possible to the time of exposure to the virus. In some circumstances an immunoglob-

---

VIRAL INFECTIONS TREATABLE WITH IMMUNOGLOBULINS

Cytomegalovirus	Rabies
Hepatitis A	Varicella*
Hepatitis B	Measles*

*Immunoglobulin treatment reserved for persons at high risk for complications.

Table 53-3 Summary of Principal Uses of Antiviral Drugs

Drug	Clinical Indications
amantadine	Influenza A prophylaxis and treatment
vidarabine	Significant herpes simplex and herpes zoster infections
acyclovir	Herpes simplex and herpes zoster infections; suppression of recurrent herpes simplex
ganciclovir	Cytomegalovirus retinitis, possibly systemic disease
ribavirin	Severe respiratory syncytial virus pneumonia, Lassa fever
zidovudine	HIV infection, AIDS
idoxuridine	Herpes simplex corneal infections
trifluorothymidine	Herpes simplex corneal infections
fluorouracil	Condyloma acuminatum
interferons	Condyloma acuminatum, hepatitis B, C
immunoglobulins*	Prophylaxis against hepatitis A and B, rabies, measles, varicella

*Specific immunoglobulin preparations available for some infections.

ulin should also be given in close physical proximity to the lesion (e.g., in rabies) to provide high concentrations to lymphatic tissues. In most situations, IM injection provides adequate systemic immunoglobulin concentrations to prevent the development of clinical infection. Since immunoglobulins do not provide long-term immunity, they must often be given as a series of injections together with vaccine therapy.

The use for the individual antiviral drugs are summarized in Table 53-3.

SIDE EFFECTS, CLINICAL PROBLEMS, AND TOXICITY

Because most antiviral drugs are derivatives of nucleic acids, which must penetrate cells to be active, significant toxicities to uninfected cells often occur. Most toxicities involve bone marrow suppression with resultant loss of granulocytes, platelets, and erythrocytes. In many instances, toxicities are so severe that drug administration is limited to topical use only. The clinical problems are summarized in the box.

Amantadine

The most common side effects of amantadine therapy are GI upsets and CNS side effects such as ner-

vousness, insomnia, and headache. These develop within the first week of therapy and decrease with time, despite continued treatment. Side effects are reversible after discontinuation of the drug and are markedly less if lower doses are used in the elderly. Adverse events occur in 5% to 33% of persons taking amantadine for influenza prophylaxis.

Amantadine also has anticholinergic properties that can cause dry mouth, urinary retention, ventricular arrhythmias, pupillary dilatation, and psychosis with excess dosing. Therefore, amantadine should be used with caution in patients with glaucoma or urinary retention. The anticholinergic effects of amantadine are enhanced by antihistamines and anticholinergic drugs. Amantadine is embryotoxic and teratogenic in rodents at high doses. Because safety during pregnancy and breastfeeding are not established, caution should be exercised. Physostigmine given every 1 to 2 hours in adults may temporarily reverse serious neurological reactions.

Vidarabine

Vidarabine causes mild to moderate anorexia, nausea, and vomiting in approximately 15% of patients. Bone marrow suppression, neurotoxicity with tremors, confusion, ataxia psychosis, aphasia, seizures, and coma, as well as a syndrome of intense muscle cramps lasting up to several weeks after stopping vidarabine, have been reported. Theoretically, allopurinol may increase vidarabine concentrations and subsequent toxicity resulting from blockage of vidarabine metabolism, but the clinical importance of this drug interaction is unknown. Because vidarabine is poorly soluble, large fluid volumes are administered daily and fluid and electrolytes monitored.

Topically, vidarabine can cause pain, itching, photophobia, and hypersensitivity reactions, although patients generally have fewer allergic reactions to vidarabine than to idoxuridine.

Vidarabine is teratogenic, mutagenic, and oncogenic in some animals and should not be used in pregnancy unless potential benefits outweigh potential risks.

Acyclovir

Acyclovir is well tolerated with few side effects. Because the pH of IV-administered acyclovir is 9 to 11, phlebitis is the most common side effect, occur-

CLINICAL PROBLEMS	
amantadine	GI upset
	CNS effects (nervousness, insomnia)
	Anticholinergic effects
vidaribine	Anorexia, nausea, vomiting
	Bone marrow suppression
	Muscle cramps, fluid balance
acyclovir	CNS effects (nervousness, headache)
	Decreased renal function
ganciclovir	Bone marrow suppression
	CNS effects
	Rash, fever
ribavirin	Headache, GI upset, dyspnea, teratogenic
zidovudine	Bone marrow suppression
	Granulocytopenia
	Myositis

ring in 15% of patients. Temporary elevations of serum creatinine concentrations and rash each occur in 5% of patients. About 1% of patients experience headache, confusion, nervousness, or other CNS side effects, and coma has been reported. Elevations of creatinine are more common with rapid infusions of less than 1 hour and if the patient is dehydrated. Crystalline nephropathy can occur. Coadministration of probenecid reduces renal clearance of the drug and prolongs the serum half-life. No effects on sperm motility or morphology are noted in patients undergoing long-term suppressive therapy. In comparison with placebo, topical acyclovir has the same incidence of pain, rash, and pruritus during treatment of genital herpes.

In experimental systems, acyclovir has not shown increased teratogenicity, but mutagenicity has been observed at extremely high doses. Its safety in pregnancy is unknown, and acyclovir should be given only when its potential benefits and risks are carefully evaluated.

Ganciclovir

Most clinical experience with ganciclovir is in the treatment of cytomegalovirus retinitis in AIDS patients in which the most common side effects are bone marrow suppression (up to 40%), CNS abnormalities (up to 15%), rash (6%), and fever (6%). Neutropenia (less than 1000 granulocytes/mm^3) and thrombocytopenia (less than 50,000 platelets/mm^3) are the most common manifestations of marrow suppression. These effects are most often observed in the second week of therapy but may occur after several months. Effects are usually reversible, but fatal infections during granulocytopenia can occur. Concurrent use of zidovudine increases bone marrow toxicity, with about 33% of treated patients developing CNS or bone marrow toxicities significant enough to interrupt therapy. AIDS patients who have received long-term ganciclovir therapy have significant increases in follicle-stimulating hormone (FSH), luteinizing hormone (LH), and testosterone concentrations.

Ganciclovir is teratogenic and mutagenic in several different experimental systems.

Ribavirin

Aerosolized ribavirin is generally well tolerated, but some bronchospasm may occur. In adults with chronic obstructive pulmonary disease and among asthmatics, significant deterioration of pulmonary function has been reported with aerosol therapy. Aerosols may also cause rash or conjunctivitis, but no significant effects on bone marrow have been reported. Ribavirin may be passively absorbed by employees working with patients treated with aerosols. The clinical importance of this is unclear, but pregnant women should not be exposed to the aerosol.

Ribavirin aerosols must be generated with a small particle aerosol generator approved for this purpose. Care should also be taken to prevent aerosol condensation in the delivery tubing, and ribavirin should not be given with other aerosols.

In HIV-infected patients receiving chronic oral ribavirin therapy, headaches, GI complaints, insomnia, lethargy, mood swings, and dyspnea on exertion occur. Ribavirin can cause extravascular hemolysis with resultant increases in serum bilirubin, uric acid, and iron concentrations. A dose-dependent macrocytic anemia may develop after about 2 weeks of ribavirin therapy. After administration of ribavirin has ended, a reticulocytosis is frequently noted.

Ribavirin is teratogenic or embryolethal in all species tested to date and is contraindicated in pregnant women or women who may become pregnant during exposure to the drug.

Zidovudine

The greatest problem associated with zidovudine therapy is bone marrow suppression. In the initial studies with zidovudine, therapy was reduced or temporarily stopped because of hematological toxicities in 33% of the patients. These effects were related to host status, since granulocytopenia (less than 750 cells/mm^3) developed in 50% of zidovudine recipients when their initial absolute T-helper cell counts were below 100 cells/mm^3 but developed in only 20% of recipients when initial T-helper cell counts were above 100 cells/mm^3. Similarly, transfusions were required in 40% versus 20% of persons with T-helper cell counts of less than and greater than 200 cells/mm^3, respectively.

Megaloblastic erythrocyte changes occur within 2 weeks of therapy in most recipients but do not predict the development of anemia or poor clinical outcome. Recent studies using zidovudine earlier in the course of HIV infection and with low doses have shown only 3% to 5% of patients experiencing side effects.

The most common nonhematological side effects of therapy are headache, nausea, insomnia, and myalgias. Long-term studies of zidovudine therapy suggest these symptoms usually improve despite continued therapy, but dose modification may be necessary. Severe neurotoxicity such as seizures, encephalopathy, and polymyositis can occur. Proximal muscle weakness and rhabdomyolisis can also develop. Black nail pigmentation occurs with long therapy.

Several drug interactions with zidovudine have been reported. Probenecid inhibits the renal excretion of zidovudine and may increase marrow toxicity. Agents such as acetaminophen that may interfere with drug glucuronidation should not be taken concurrently. When used with ganciclovir, zidovudine markedly increases the risk for bone marrow suppression, and concomitant dapsone use with zidovudine has been reported to cause severe anemia. Neurotoxicity has been reported with the combined use of acyclovir and zidovudine.

The teratogenicity and mutagenicity of zidovudine have not been completely evaluated. Acute overdose does not produce bone marrow toxicity but can cause coma.

Others

Idoxuridine is generally well tolerated; however, it can cause mild local irritation, headaches, and nausea. Idoxuridine is teratogenic and mutagenic and should be used only when the potential benefits outweigh the potential risks of therapy.

Adverse effects are uncommon with trifluorothymidine. Mild transient burning of the eyes occurs in approximately 5% of patients, and palpebral edema develops in about 3% of patients. Systemic trifluorothymidine has resulted in reversible bone marrow suppression when used for 3 to 5 days as an antineoplastic agent. Many topical ophthalmic agents have been used in conjunction with trifluorothymidine without interference or adverse effects. These agents include antibiotics (erythromycin, polymyxin B, gentamicin, and sulfacetamide); steroids (prednisolone, dexamethasone, and hydrocortisone); and other ophthalmic drugs (atropine, scopolamine, pilocarpine, and epinephrine). Trifluorothymidine has teratogenic and mutagenic potential and should be used in pregnancy only when the potential benefits outweigh the potential risks.

> ### TRADENAMES
>
> In addition to generic and fixed combination preparations, the following tradenamed materials are available in the United States.
>
> Cytovene, ganciclovir
> H-BIG, Hyperhep, Hyperab, VZIG; immunoglobulins
> Retrovir, zidovudine
> Roferon, interferon
> Stoxil, Dendrid, Herplex; idoxuridine
> Symmetrel, amantadine
> Vira-A, vidarabine
> Virazole, ribavirin
> Viroptic, Trifluridine; trifluorothymidine
> Zovirax; acyclovir

The most common side effects of topical fluorouracil therapy are local pain, pruritus, and irritation. Contact dermatitis with scarring has also been reported.

Intralesional interferons produce pain at the injection site and leukopenia; malaise and fever also occur. In about 10% of patients the side effects are severe enough to warrant discontinuing therapy. For patients with extensive genital warts receiving systemic interferon therapy, more significant systemic side effects are reported.

Immunoglobulins are well tolerated, with pain at the injection site and brief low-grade fever the most commonly reported side effects. True allergic reactions with urticaria and/or angioedema rarely occur but IV gamma globulin can activate the alternative complement pathway producing an anaphylactoid reaction.

REFERENCES

Crumpacker CS II: Molecular target of antiviral therapy, N Engl J Med 321:163, 1989.

Langtry HD and Campoli-Richards DM: Zidovudine, Drugs 37:408, 1989.

McKinlay MA and Rossmann MG: Rational design of antiviral agents, Ann Rev Pharmacol Toxicol 29:111, 1989.

Yarchoan R, Mitsuya H, Meyers CE et al: Clinical pharmacology of 3'-azido-2', 3'-dideoxythymidine (zidovudine) and related dideoxynucleosides, N Engl J Med 321:726, 1989.

54

Drugs Effective Against Parasitic Helminthic Infections

ABBREVIATIONS

CNS	central nervous system
GABA	γ-aminobutyric acid
ATP	adenosine triphosphate
DNA	deoxynucleic acid
RNA	ribonucleic acid

MAJOR DRUGS

albendazole
diethylcarbamazine
ivermectin
mebendazole
metrifonate
niclosamide
oxamniquine
praziquantel
pyrantel pamoate
suramin
thiabendazole

 THERAPEUTIC OVERVIEW

Human infections caused by helminths (worms) produce significant medical problems not only in developing countries in tropical climates but also in highly industrialized countries in more temperate climates. About 300 million people are infected with blood-dwelling flukes (*Schistosoma* spp.), and hookworms and ascariasis are among the 20 infections that cause the highest morbidity rates in much of Africa, Asia, and South America. Although their prevalence is higher in certain regions of the world, helminths have no geographical boundaries and are carried by their hosts (parasitized humans) throughout the world.

The life cycle of the helminths is often complex and plays a critical role in the spread of the organism and its infection of humans. The life cycle for schistosomes is summarized in Figure 54-1. Some organisms live in the bloodstream (portal blood) of the intestinal tract; lay approximately 300 eggs per day; and through the action of elastases, break through the intestinal wall and exit the host via the feces. In water, the eggs hatch, forming parasites that use snails as carriers (intermediate host). The parasite undergoes asexual multiplication to produce thousands of infective parasitic cercaria, and humans are infected through contact with the cercaria in infested water. In Africa, only 1 snail in 5000 harbors the parasite, but 65% to 95% of the people in nearby villages are infected when exposed to infected water. Some parasites evade the immune system of the host by coating themselves with host antigens or simply avoiding damage to their surface by shedding and repairing areas that have been damaged by the host immune system.

The helminths are divided into three groups: nematodes (roundworms), trematodes (flatworms, flukes), and cestodes (flatworms, tapeworms). These three groups, the important species within each group, and the drugs available for the treatment of the different groups are summarized in Table 54-1. Some of the helminths are potentially dangerous, such as certain tissue-dwelling larval tapeworms. The life cycle of human-infecting hookworms (nematodes) is shown in Figure 54-2.

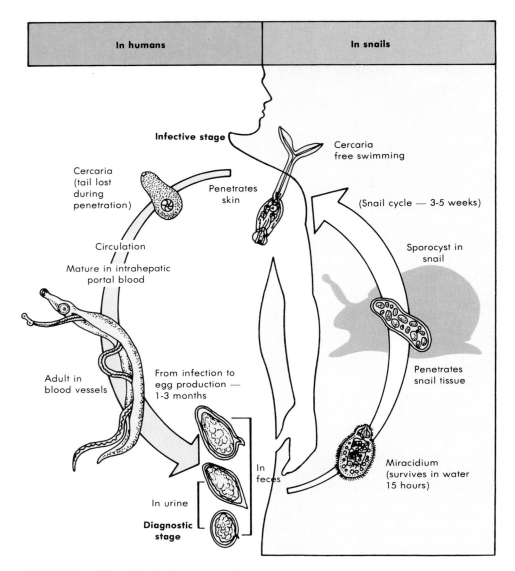

FIGURE 54-1 Life cycle of schistosomes (see text). From Murray PR, Drew WL, Kobayashi GS, and Thompson JH: Medical Microbiology, St. Louis, 1990, The C.V. Mosby Co.

 MECHANISMS OF ACTION

The strategy for the use of drugs to treat helminthic infections differs markedly from that employed in the treatment of bacterial or fungal infections. Most anthelmintic drugs are targeted at nonproliferating adult organisms, whereas with bacterial and fungi the targets are young, growing cells. The helminthic life cycle (see Figures 54-1 and 54-2) is strongly dependent on the following factors: (1) neuromuscular co-ordination for worm feeding movements and for maintaining a favorable location of the worm within the host; (2) carbohydrate metabolism as the source of energy, with glucose the primary substrate; and (3) microtubular integrity, since egg laying and hatching, larval development, glucose transport, and enzyme activity and secretion are hindered when the microtubules are modified. Most anthelmintic agents are targeted at one of these three biochemical functions in the adult organism.

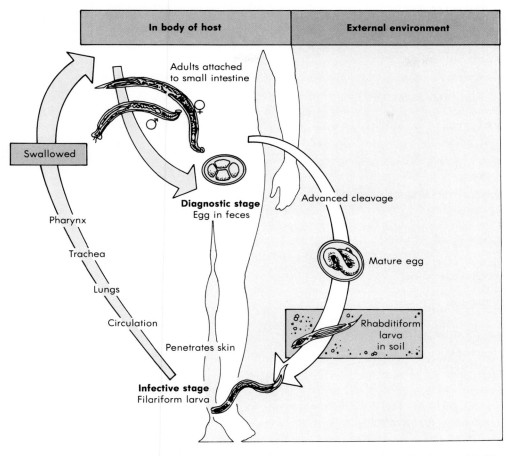

FIGURE 54-2   Life cycle of hookworms (see text). From Murray PR, Drew WL, Kobayashi GS, and Thompson JH: Medical Microbiology, St. Louis, 1990, The C.V. Mosby Co.

The structures of the primary anthelmintic agents are shown in Figure 54-3. The sites of action and the physiological effects of each of the agents is listed in Table 54-2.

Mebendazole and Thiabendazole

Mebendazole, thiabendazole, and albendazole (not available in the United States) are embryotoxic to mammals and extremely embryotoxic to helminth larval nematode development in utero *(Onchocerca volvulus)* or within the egg. In adult nematodes these compounds stop production of secretory products such as acetylcholinesterase and result in disappearance of cytoplasmic microtubules from nematode tegumental and intestinal cells. Mebendazole and thiabendazole block the assembly of tubulin dimers into tubulin polymers (Figure 54-4) in a process mimicked by colchicine, a powerful antimitotic and embryotoxic drug.

Pyrantel Pamoate

The nervous system of helminths appears to be the target for pyrantel pamoate, ivermectin, and metrifonate, since all three produce a rapid change in motor activity of the helminth. Pyrantel pamoate produces a powerful cholinomimetic effect on the nematode muscle cells by binding to cholinergic receptors, which results in cell depolarization and muscle contraction. This paralytic action on gut-dwelling nematodes leads to expulsion of the helminth from the host intestinal tract.

Text continued on p. 739.

Table 54-1 Therapeutic Overview

Helminth Infection	Drug of Choice	Alternate Drug
INTESTINAL NEMATODES (ROUNDWORMS)		
Capillaria philippinensis	mebendazole	pyrantel pamoate
Ascaris lumbricoides	mebendazole	pyrantel pamoate
Enterobius vermicularis (pinworms)	mebendazole	pyrantel pamoate
Necator americanus	mebendazole	pyrantel pamoate
Ancylostoma duodenale	mebendazole	pyrantel pamoate
Strongyloides stercoralis	thiabendazole	mebendazole
Trichinella spiralis	mebendazole	thiabendazole
Trichuris trichiura hookworm	mebendazole	pyrantel pamoate
EXTRAINTESTINAL NEMATODES (ROUNDWORMS)		
Dracunculus medinensis	thiabendazole, metonidazole	niridazole
Onchocerca volvulus (adult)	suramin†	
Onchocerca volvulus (microfilariae)	ivermectin	diethylcarbamazine
Wuchereria bancrofti (adult)	diethylcarbamazine§	ivermectin‡
Wuchereria bancrofti (microfilariae)	diethylcarbamazine§	ivermectin‡
Brugia spp. (adult)	diethylcarbamazine§	ivermectin‡
Brugia spp. (microfilariae)	diethylcarbamazine	ivermectin‡
Loa loa	diethylcarbamazine	ivermectin‡
LARVAL NEMATODES (ROUNDWORMS)		
Strongyloides stercoralis	thiabendazole*	mebendazole
Cutaneous larva migrans	thiabendazole	
Visceral larva migrans	thiabendazole	
Trichinella spiralis	thiabendazole, mebendazole	
INTESTINAL CESTODES (TAPEWORMS)		
Taenia saginata (beef tapeworm)	praziquantel	niclosamide
Taenia solium (pork tapeworm)	praziquantel	niclosamide
Diphyllobothrium latum	praziquantel	niclosamide
Hymenolepis nana	praziquantel	niclosamide
LARVAL CESTODES (TAPEWORMS)		
Taenia solium	praziquantel	niclosamide
Echinococcus granulosus	albendazole	
Echinococcus multilocularis	albendazole	
BLOOD-DWELLING TREMATODES (FLUKES)		
Schistosoma mansoni	praziquantel	oxamniquine
Schistosoma haematobium	praziquantel	metrifonate
Schistosoma japonicum	praziquantel	niridazole
INTESTINAL TREMATODES (FLUKES)		
Heterophyes heterophyes	praziquantel	
Metagonimus yokogawi	praziquantel	
LIVER TREMATODES (FLUKES)		
Clonorchis sinensis	praziquantel	
Opisthorchis spp.	praziquantel	
Fasciola hepatica	praziquantel§	bithinol
LUNG TREMATODES (FLUKES)		
Paragonimus spp.	praziquantel	bithinol

*Some success reported for ivermectin, but this drug is for investigational use only in the United States.

†The microfilaricidal drug, ivermectin, is given first, followed 2 to 3 weeks later by suramin.

‡This drug is for investigational use only in the United States.

§Effectiveness of diethylcarbamazine against these adult filariae is questionable.

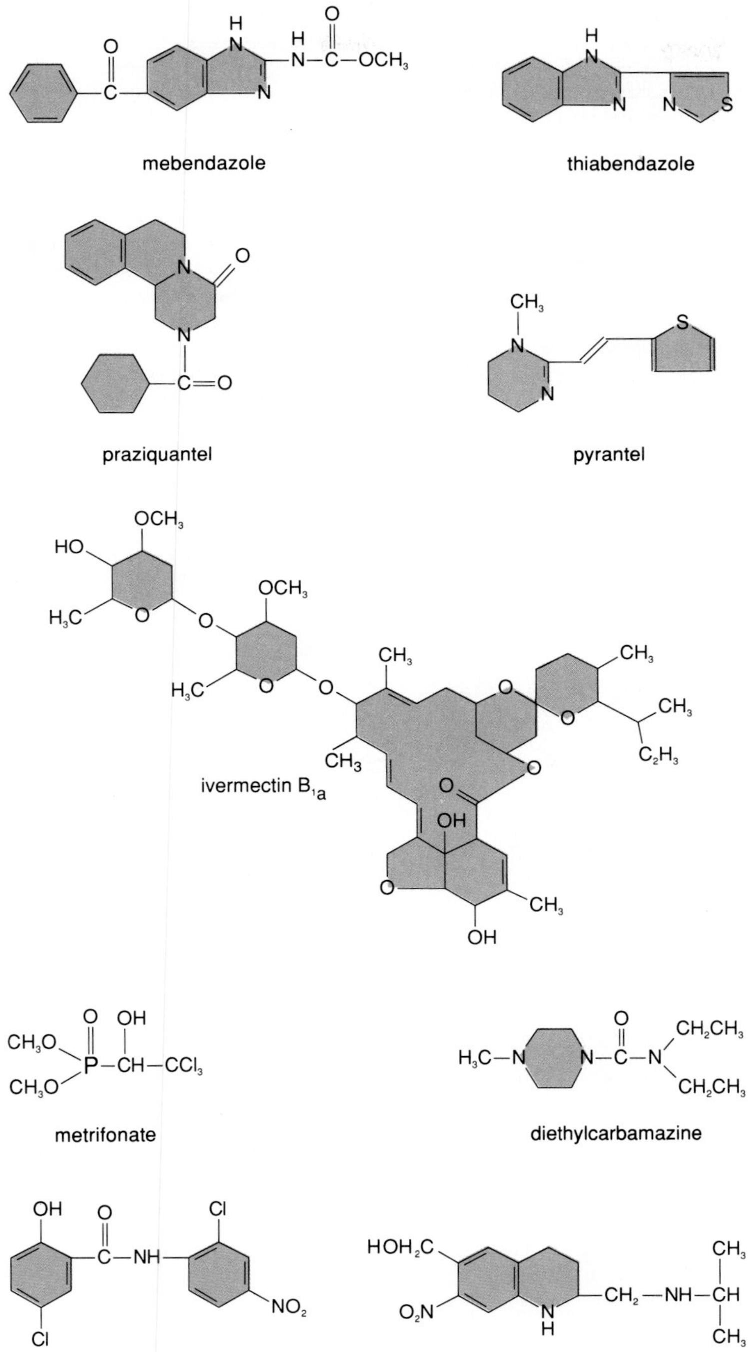

mebendazole

thiabendazole

praziquantel

pyrantel

ivermectin B$_{1a}$

metrifonate

diethylcarbamazine

niclosamide

oxamniquine

FIGURE 54-3   Structures of primary anthelmintic agents.

Table 54-2 Sites and Mechanisms for the Major Anthelmintics

Drug	Site of Action	Physiological Effect	Molecular Mechanism
mebendazole thiabendazole	Cytoplasmic microtubules in tegumental and intestinal cells of nematodes	Inhibit protein secretion and glucose transport	Binds to colchicine receptor on tubulin dimers
praziquantel	Tegument and muscle	Contracts muscle; disrupts tegument that attracts antibody and phagocytes	Change in membrane permeability; synergy with host immune system
pyrantel pamoate	Cholinergic synapse on muscle cells of nematodes	Contraction of muscle cells	Binds to cholinergic receptor
ivermectin	Uterus of female *O. volvulus*	Blocks release of microfilariae	Not known
diethylcarbamazine	Surface of microfilariae	Exposes antigens on surface that bind antibody which attract phagocytes	Not known
metrifonate	Cholinergic synapse	Causes flaccid paralysis of muscles	Inhibits acetylcholinesterase
niclosamide	Mitochondria	Gradual paralysis of muscles	Uncouples anaerobic phosphorylation
suramin	Appear to alter cells lining intestinal tract	May block absorption from intestinal tract	Inhibits many enzymes, including dehydrogenases, dihydrofolate reductase, protein kinases
oxamniquine	No particular site	Reduction in protein synthesis followed by degeneration of tegument	Alkylates parasite DNA

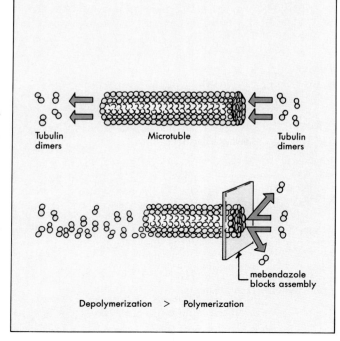

FIGURE 54-4   A, Under normal conditions, tubulin dimers are continually being polymerized on and depolymerized from the ends of the microtubule. **B,** Mebendazole or colchicine can bind a high affinity site on the tubulin dimer and prevent polymerization or assembly, leading to depolymerization or complete breakdown of the microtubule.

Diethylcarbamazine

Diethylcarbamazine shows no activity in vitro but kills the microfilariae readily in vivo (Figure 54-2), possibly altering the parasite surface membrane and thus activating the host immune system. There is a decrease in muscle activity and subsequent paralysis of the worms.

Ivermectin

Ivermectin produces rapid and marked inhibition of nematode movement by interacting with the chloride channel on the helminth GABA receptor complex. This receptor mediates inhibitory effects on nematode muscle cells. Ivermectin is used extensively to control gut-dwelling nematode infections in domestic and farm animals and because it concentrates in the hides of animals prevents insect damage. Its use in humans is limited to treating the filarial parasite *Onchocerca volvulus*. The drug has no lethal effect on the adult *O. volvulus* but dramatically acts on microfilariae produced by the female parasite. First, ivermectin alters the ability of the microfilariae to evade the host immune system, thus allowing the immune system to recognize this body as a foreign antigen. Second, ivermectin alters the reproductive

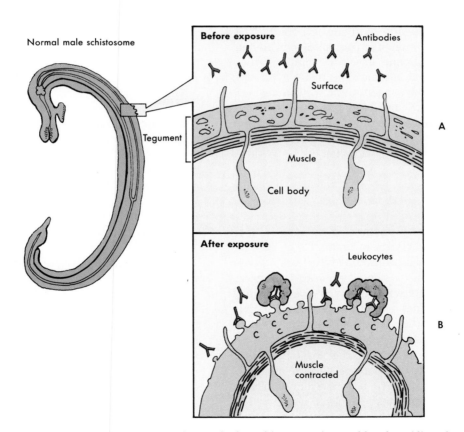

FIGURE 54-5   Before exposure to praziquantel, the schistosome is capable of avoiding the numerous antibodies directed toward surface and internally located antigens. **A,** Cross section of the dorsal surface of a normal male schistosome. Within 1 to 2 seconds after exposure to praziquantel, the muscles of the schistosome contract because of drug-induced influx of calcium ions into the schistosome tegument. **B,** The change in permeability of the schistosome surface toward external ions initiates the appearance of small holes and balloon-like structures, making the parasite vulnerable to antibody-mediated adherence of host leukocytes that kill the helminth.

system of adult female *O. volvulus* by reducing its capacity to produce microfilariae. The exact mechanism and receptor associated with this action of ivermectin on nematode reproductive function is not known.

Praziquantel

The action of praziquantel on *S. mansoni* and other schistosomes is described schematically in Figure 54-5. Synergy between the drug and the response of the humoral immune system of the host is noted. This occurs through disruption of the surface, which protects the parasite from the host immune system, to allow antibodies to attack parasite antigens not normally exposed on the surface. Irreversible damage to the parasite surface and tegument probably occurs when complement and/or host leukocytes are recruited to the sites where antibody is bound. This rapid and dramatic action of praziquantel may be due to a drug-induced change in the helminth permeability toward divalent cations. The result is an elevation of calcium ion concentration within various cells of the helminth. It has been proposed that this action initiates both the spastic contraction and damage to the tegument. The nature of the receptor or receptors mediating these events has not been identified.

Niclosamide

Niclosamide acts by uncoupling oxidative phosphorylation in mitochondria in mammals as well as parasites. The drug is absorbed by gut-dwelling cestodes but not by gut-dwelling nematodes. Cestode mitochondria generate ATP in the absence of oxygen through pathways that use other terminal electron acceptors. These novel pathways generate a hydrogen gradient across the parasite mitochondrial membrane susceptible to the action of niclosamide. Thus cestodes exposed to niclosamide cannot generate ATP. Loss of helminth ATP ultimately immobilizes the parasite within the intestine so that it is expelled with the feces.

Oxamniquine

Oxamniquine inhibits DNA, RNA, and protein synthesis in *S. mansoni*. Compounds similar to oxamniquine are highly mutagenic, although oxamniquine itself is not. The parasite may have a unique enzyme capable of esterifying oxamniquine to form a reactive metabolite whose action alkylates helminth DNA.

Metrifonate

The paralytic action of metrifonate, an organophosphate, on the motor activity of *S. mansoni* and *S. haematobium* is directly related to inhibition of parasite acetylcholinesterase. Inhibition of this enzyme elevates the concentration of the inhibitory neurotransmitter acetylcholine within the helminth. The drug is active against *S. haematobium* but not extremely active against *S. mansoni*. This may be due to differences in drug accessibility, in that adult *S. mansoni* reside within the mesenteric veins, whereas *S. haematobium* live within the veins surrounding the bladder. The paralytic action of the drug dislodges the parasites from the veins. On rare occasions when *S. mansoni* infections are located in the urinary bladder, this organism is just as susceptible to the drug as *S. haematobium*.

Suramin

Suramin inhibits numerous enzymes of filarial helminths, most notably lactate dehydrogenase, malate dehydrogenase, dihydrofolate reductase, and various protein kinases. It is a large polyanion that complexes proteins readily.

 PHARMACOKINETICS

The pharmacokinetic parameter values are summarized for the anthelmintic agents in Table 54-3.

For treatment of intestinal helminthic infections, the drugs should not be absorbed but remain in the gastrointestinal (GI) tract where the organisms are usually located. However, with the more difficult to treat extraintestinal or systemic helminthic infections, it is necessary that the drugs be absorbed and enter the systemic circulation.

Mebendazole is poorly absorbed from the intestinal tract and shows a large first pass effect. Bioavailability is increased by food. Thiabendazole is well absorbed but rapidly metabolized to 5-hydroxythiabendazole and the latter conjugated with glucuronide or sulfate and excreted in the urine.

Niclosamide is also poorly absorbed but reaches the systemic circulation because it binds tightly to albumin.

Table 54-3 Pharmacokinetic Parameters

Agent	Administration	Absorption	t½ (hr)	Disposition
diethylcarbamazine	Oral	Rapid	9–13	R (50%), pH dependent M (50%)
ivermectin	Oral	Rapid	28	M (main)
niclosamide	Oral	Poor	—	—
mebendazole	Oral	Poor* (5-10%)	0.9–1.1†	M (main) first pass
praziquantel	Oral	Rapid (80%)	4	M (90%) first pass
thiabendazole	Oral	Poor	—	M (main), R
oxamniquine‡	Oral	Rapid	1–2	M (main)
metrifonate	Oral	Rapid	1.5 (3 terminal)	M
suramin	IV	Poor	36–49	R (main), B
pyrantel pamoate	Oral	Poor	—	R (10%-20%), F

M, Metabolized; *R*, eliminated unchanged by renal mechanisms; *B*, bile; *F*, feces.
*Increased by food, bioavailability only 22% (first pass).
†2–5 hr in other studies.
‡50% bioavailability (vs IM).

Pyrantel pamoate is poorly absorbed and thus acts effectively in the GI tract. The bulk of the drug is present in the feces, with only 10% to 20% excreted in urine. Unlike drugs used almost exclusively against gut-dwelling nematodes, diethylcarbamazine is completely absorbed within 1 to 2 hours and undergoes rapid metabolism, with most of the metabolites excreted in the urine.

Similar to diethylcarbamazine, praziquantel is rapidly and almost completely absorbed, with peak plasma concentrations appearing 1 to 2 hours after administration. This drug is rapidly metabolized to a 4-hydroxycyclohexyl derivative that is then conjugated and excreted in the urine.

High concentrations of the drug are found in liver, bile, and muscle, and traces are also present in the brain and CSF. Approximately 80% is bound to plasma protein. Recent studies of ivermectin in humans show a prolonged disposition half-life, probably because of drug deposition in fatty tissue from which it slowly diffuses.

Oxamniquine and metrifonate are rapidly absorbed from the intestine, with peak plasma concentrations appearing 1.5 to 3 hours after administration. Food delays the absorption of oxamniquine and limits the concentration achieved in the plasma. The major metabolite of oxamniquine is formed in the intestine before absorption, and its concentration in the plasma can be 8 to 10 times greater than that of oxamniquine.

This metabolite is devoid of any anthelmintic activity and is excreted in the urine within 12 hours after administration of oxamniquine.

Metrifonate undergoes extensive metabolism, including spontaneous rearrangement at neutral pH to form active dichlorvos. Dichlorvos is the metabolite responsible for the antischistosomal activity associated with metrifonate. The only anthelmintic to be given parenterally—suramin—has an unusually long half-life because it binds so strongly to plasma proteins. Metabolism of suramin appears to be negligible.

Ivermectin is administered orally or intravenously. It is widely distributed in the body with concentration in liver and fatty tissue. Most is excreted in feces, with minimal amounts found in the urine. A single dose can be detected in tissues for up to 28 days.

 RELATION OF MECHANISMS OF ACTION TO CLINICAL RESPONSE

Anthelmintics for Intestinal Nematode Infections

Many nematodes reside as adults within the intestinal tract. Examples are *Ascaris lumbricoides* (large roundworm), *Enterobius vermicularis* (pinworm), *Necator americanus,* and *Anclyostoma duodenale* (the hookworms), along with *Strongyloides stercoralis, Trichinella spiralis,* and *Trichuris trichiura* (whipworm). The anthelmintic used to treat these intestinal roundworms is mebendazole, with the exception of Strongyloides infections where thiabendazole is recommended, although mebendazole may be adequate. The drug acts slowly on these helminths, so organism elimination from the intestinal tract may take 3 days following a course of therapy.

Pyrantel pamoate is also extremely effective against the major gut-dwelling nematodes and is not readily absorbed from the intestine. The drug is well tolerated with no reported toxic side effects and no contraindications. An analog, oxantel, is used in combination with pyrantel to provide effective therapy for the three major soil-transmitted nematodes: *Ascaris* organisms, hookworms, and *Trichuris* species.

Anthelmintics for Extraintestinal Nematode Infections

Adult nematodes of clinical significance also reside outside the GI tract. Infections by adult nematodes in tissues are termed *filariases,* and the larvae that are released are called *microfilariae.* Special note should be taken concerning the lack of effective drugs against the extraintestinal nematodes, a group of helminths that inflict a considerable amount of human suffering worldwide. *Dracunculus medinensis* (guinea worm) and adult *O. volvulus* along with their microfilariae live within subcutaneous tissues and are devastating parasites. Unfortunately, no effective drugs for either adult parasites exist, although treatment of *D. medinensis* with thiabendazole or niridazole (not available in the United States), allow the worm to be mechanically withdrawn from the ulcer more easily by virtue of an antiinflammatory effect. The microfilariae released by female *O. volvulus* can be destroyed by diethylcarbamazine, but the destruction increases skin (Mazzoti reaction) and eye pathology.

A new microfilaricidal drug, ivermectin, has fewer side effects than diethylcarbamazine, and a single dose can eliminate microfilariae for up to 6 months. Ivermectin has a dramatic effect on the tissue-dwelling microfilariae of *O. volvulus.* These microfilariae are responsible for widespread blindness in rural West and East Africa.

Wuchereria bancrofti and *Brugia* spp. are filarial nematodes that dwell within lymph glands, causing lymphedema of the extremities (elephantiasis). Mul-

tiple doses of diethylcarbamazine eliminate some of the adult parasites and most of the circulating microfilariae. Recent clinical trials with ivermectin suggest that this drug may be superior to diethylcarbamazine in the treatment of these filarial infections. Another less pathogenic filarial parasite that resides in subcutaneous tissues, *Loa loa,* can be effectively controlled with diethylcarbamazine.

In addition to adult nematodes, many larval forms are pathogenic. For example, larvae released by adult *S. stercoralis* can cause serious damage to the lining of the gut, and in patients with a depressed cell-mediated immune system the larvae can invade many organ systems and cause death. *T. spiralis* larvae migrate from the gut-dwelling adult to the skeletal muscles predominantly but also to the heart, lungs, and nervous system where the larvae cause myositis and trichinosis.

Thiabendazole should be used for trichinosis and visceral larval migrants, and thiabendazole and mebendazole can be considered for *S. stercoralis* or cutaneous larval migrants. These drugs may suppress the immune response more than actually destroying the tissue-dwelling larva. Antiinflammatory steroids are often coadministered in cases where the infection is intense.

Anthelmintics for Cestode Infections

Adult tapeworm infections are predominantly not symptomatic. Parasites such as *Taenia saginata* (beef tapeworm); *T. solium* (pork tapeworm); *Diphyllobothrium latum* (fish tapeworm), which can cause vitamin B_{12} deficiency; and *Hymenolepis nana* (dwarf tapeworm) live within the intestinal tract of man and can be easily eliminated with praziquantel or niclosamide.

The problem with some cestode infections arises when the larval forms take residence in an organ system. If a human ingests the eggs of *T. solium,* the hatching pork-tapeworm larvae invade various organs. The pathogenic response (referred to as *cysticercosis*) depends on the organ invaded, with the most serious effect associated with larvae invading the CNS. Praziquantel effectively eliminates cysticercosis. However, worm death causes ingress of white blood cells and cerebral edema. Patients should be treated with steroids (prednisone or dexamethazone) before and during therapy. If humans consume the egg of the tapeworm *Echinococcus granulosus* or

E. multilocularis, the resulting infection can be fatal, especially for *E. multilocularis.* The larvae from these eggs migrate principally to the liver or lung where they form small cysts that can increase in size. Treatment with mebendazole gives marginal results, but albendazole (not available in the United States) is effective.

Anthelmintics for Trematode Infections

Preeminent in medical and economic importance are the schistosomes or blood-dwelling flukes of *S. mansoni, S. japonicum,* and *S. haematobium.* They cause schistosomiasis, which is a source of morbidity in many countries of Africa and the Carribean Islands. Although oxamniquine and metrifonate are used to control schistosomiasis, praziquantel has become the drug of choice. Liver flukes (*Opisthorchis* spp.) and lung flukes (*Paragonimus* spp.) are important parasites in Asia. Other clinically troublesome flukes are intestinal flukes *Heterophyes heterophyes* and *Metagonimus yokogawai* and the liver fluke *Fasciola hepatica.* Praziquantel is now used to treat all of these trematode infections with the exception of *F. hepatica,* in which results have been mixed.

Oxamniquine is still used in some areas to treat *S. mansoni* infections. Drug resistance has been detected in Brazil.

Metrifonate, an organophosphate that is converted to the active antischistosomal compound dichlorvos, is still used for *S. haematobium* infections in some countries.

SIDE EFFECTS, CLINICAL PROBLEMS, AND TOXICITY

With some notable exceptions most of the major anthelmintics present few problems when administered to infected patients (see box). Side effects associated with diethylcarbamazine are frequent but usually not severe.

Some anthelmintic agents accumulate as a result of binding to lung tissue, as in the use of diethylcarbamazine for treating patients with *W. bancrofti* or *Brugia* spp. (organisms that dwell mainly in lymph glands). The resulting side effects include headache, weakness, joint pains, nausea, and vomiting. In heavily infected patients, effects may include small focal reactions of pain, tenderness, and inflammation in the groin and thigh, especially in *Brugia* infections.

CLINICAL PROBLEMS

DIETHYLCARBAMAZINE

O. Volvulus Infections

Intense pruritus and papular rash
Swelling of inguinal lymph nodes
Chorioretinitis and optic nerve atrophy

B. Malayi and *W. Bancrofti* Infections

Nausea
Vomiting
Pain in joints
Fever

Loa Loa Infections

Similar to *B. malayi*
Encephalitis due to *Loa* organisms should not be treated until encephalitis subsides

IVERMECTIN

O. Volvulus Infection

Similar to but milder than diethylcarbamazine
No adverse ocular effects

MEBENDAZOLE

Contraindicated during pregnancy

METRIFONATE

Avoid treating patients recently exposed to insecticides

PRAZIQUANTEL

Cerebral edema, aqueductal stenosis (prevented by steroids)

SURAMIN

Toxic compound to be used with caution especially with patients having renal insufficiency

THIABENDAZOLE

Severe hepatitis with prolonged use

Initiating therapy with a low dose and gradually increasing to a higher dose can attenuate these side effects. With *Loa Loa,* microfilariae can migrate to the CNS and produce encephalitis, which can be greatly exacerbated by treatment with diethylcarbamazine. Treatment should be delayed in favor of corticosteroid therapy to suppress encephalitis, which then allows the use of diethylcarbamazine. When diethylcarbamazine is given to patients with onchocerciasis, an intense hypersensitivity reaction associated with drug action on tissue-dwelling microfilariae may occur. Itching within minutes after dosing is followed by a fine papular rash and hyperpyrexia, tachycardia, and headache. The severity of this reaction is often proportional to the number of microfilariae. The reaction can sometimes be severe, and the patient may remain prostrate for 24 hours. In addition, diethylcarbamazine can cause eye lesions including chorioretinitis and optic nerve atrophy, along with marked increase in punctate keratitis and limbitis, an eye inflammation.

Problems associated with ivermectin treatment of onchocerciasis are fewer than with diethylcarbamazine. The pruritus is less prominent, and eye lesions are not observed. In an extremely small number of cases, a mild hypotensive response is observed.

With niclosamide, undesirable side effects include malaise, fever, abdominal discomfort or pain, and pruritus. There are no contraindications to the use of niclosamide, and it has been administered to debilitated patients and pregnant women.

Poor absorption of mebendazole is responsible for the few side effects associated with its use even in sick and debilitated patients. With high doses, alopecia and reversible neutropenia are seen. This drug is embryotoxic and teratogenic and thus should not be given to pregnant women. Thiabendazole induces anorexia, nausea, vomiting, and dizziness, and approximately 30% of patients receiving it will be incapacitated for several hours; this may increase to 50% with higher doses. Unlike mebendazole, thiabendazole is not embryotoxic or teratogenic in rats, but these toxicities in humans have not been reported. The drug can produce a severe allergic hepatitis when used for longer than 2 days, as is necessary in severe infestations of the small intestine. It may also interfere with xanthine metabolism.

The high degree of safety associated with praziquantel makes it possible to control human trematode and cestode infections. Three groups of side effects have been identified: abdominal discomfort, headache and dizziness, and skin manifestations. Most of these side effects appear within the first 12 to 24 hours after dosing. The third effect may result from antigens released by dying parasites that initiate an allergic reaction. Most patients tolerate the drug without serious side effects. Even patients with advanced schistosomiasis, Symmers' periportal fibrosis, or esophageal varices have been treated without complication.

TRADENAMES

In addition to generic and fixed combination preparations, the following tradenamed materials are available in the United States.

Antiminth, pyrantel pamoate
Biltricide, Distocide; praziquantel
Mintezol, thiabendazole
Niclocide, niclosamide
Vansil, oxamniquine
Vermox, mebendazole

Treatment of CNS lesions always requires premedication with steroids.

Side effects associated with oxamniquine and metrifonate usually are minor, and both drugs are well tolerated. Some dizziness and drowsiness has been reported along with a mild fever following the administration of oxamniquine, and patients with a history of epilepsy may experience convulsions after exposure to this drug. Oxamniquine can be used in patients with severe hepatosplenic schistosomiasis. Side effects with metrifonate include mild vertigo, colic, lassitude, and nausea. Patients receiving this drug should avoid contact with insecticides containing anticholinesterase agents.

Suramin must be used with great care. Within hours after administration of suramin, papular eruptions, paresthesias, photophobia, lacrimation, hyperesthesias of the palms of the hand and soles of the feet, and palpebral edema are commonly observed. The drug is administered parenterally and accumulates in the kidney and can induce albuminuria. In addition, hematuria and urinary casts may appear. A persistent albuminuria should be handled by altering the treatment schedule or discontinuing use of the drug if casts appear in the urine.

REFERENCES

Campbell WC and Rew RS, eds: Chemotherapy of parasitic diseases, New York, 1986, Plenum Publishing Corp.

Edwards G and Breckenridge AM: Clinical pharmacokinetics of anthelminthic drugs, Clin Pharmacokinet 15:67, 1988.

Vanden-Bossche H, Thienpont D, and Janssens PG, eds: Chemotherapy of gastrointestinal helminths. In Vanden-Bossche H, Theinpant D, and Janssens PG, eds: Handbook of experimental pharmacology, vol 77, New York, 1985, Springer-Verlag, Inc.

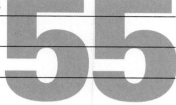

CHAPTER 55

Drugs Effective Against Parasitic Protozoal Infections

ABBREVIATIONS

AIDS	acquired immune deficiency syndrome
ATP	adenosine triphosphate
NAD	nicotinamide adenine dinucleotide
DNA	deoxyribonucleic acid
CNS	central nervous system
NADH	nicotinamide adenine dinucleotide reduced
CSF	cerebrospinal fluid

THERAPEUTIC OVERVIEW

THERAPEUTIC STRATEGIES

Control disease vector
Improve hygiene and sanitation
Vaccination attempts
Drugs

PROTOZOAL INFECTIONS ENDEMIC

INFECTION-VECTOR

Malaria—mosquito
Leishmaniasis—sandflies
Trypanosomiasis—tsetse fly
Amebiasis—food, water
Giardiasis—food, water
Toxoplasmosis—meats, cats

RESISTANCE DEVELOPS TO SPECIFIC DRUGS

 ## THERAPEUTIC OVERVIEW

Parasitic protozoa infect a significant percentage of the world population to produce malaria, leishmaniasis, trypanosomiasis, amebiasis, giardiasis, trichomoniasis, and other diseases. Protozoal diseases are more prevalent in tropical climates but are also found in the United States. International travel and immigration of persons from other countries to the United States provides opportunities for exposure of U.S. inhabitants to these organisms.

Protozoa invade host cells, multiply, and eventually destroy the host cells. Infections with these organisms typically have acute and primary phases that result in death or development of a chronic latent stage, interspersed with relapses.

Malaria is the most significant protozoal disease in terms of morbidity and mortality, with over 1 million infant deaths a year directly attributable to this disease in Africa. Other protozoal diseases, such as amebiasis, giardiasis, and trichomoniasis are widely dis-

tributed, whereas leishmaniasis and trypanosomiasis are found primarily in tropical areas. Some protozoal infections are becoming increasingly associated with immunocompromised individuals, including those with acquired immune deficiency syndrome (AIDS).

The prevention and treatment of protozoal diseases follows four strategies: control the vector, improve hygiene and sanitation, provide vaccination, and administer chemotherapy. Chemotherapeutic approaches are used effectively to treat and prevent many protozoal infections, although some agents have adverse effects or are eventually met with resistance. Thus, optimal treatment uses all four strategies.

The primary therapeutic considerations with protozoal diseases are summarized in the box.

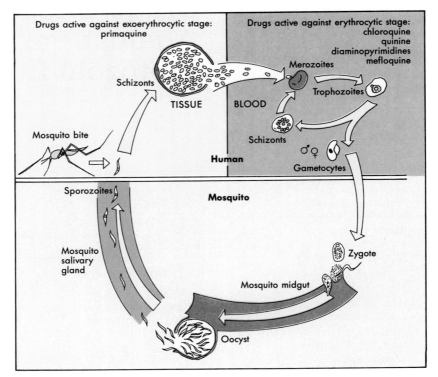

FIGURE 55-1   Life cycle of *Plasmodium* protozoa. Drugs used to treat infection are effective against either erythrocytic or exoerythrocytic stages of the parasite.

 MECHANISMS OF ACTION

Antimalarial Agents

Malaria is caused by protozoa of the genus *Plasmodium* present in the human host either in the erythrocytic *(blood)* stage or the exoerythrocytic *(tissue)* stage. The life cycle of a malaria parasite is summarized in Figure 55-1. Drug treatment chiefly involves the use of aminoquinolines, such as chloroquine, its analogs, and a number of additional drugs, for the erythrocytic stage and chiefly primaquine for the exoerythrocytic stage. Newer compounds, such as mefloquine, ginghaosu (also known as *artemisinine*), and halofantrine are also used, and several antibiotics are often administered in combination with the antimalarial agents. Older agents that have wide use include quinine and quinidine. The structures of some of the antimalarial drugs are shown in Figure 55-2.

The mechanism of antimalarial action of chloroquine and other 4-aminoquinolines is still unclear.

Several mechanisms have been proposed. In one, binding of drug to ferriprotoporphyrin IX, released from hemoglobin in infected erythrocytes, produces a complex that is toxic for plasmodial and RBC membranes. In a second, uptake and concentration of drug into the parasites raises the pH of intracellular acidic vesicles. This damages the ability of the parasite to degrade hemoglobin and causes the characteristic morphological changes seen microscopically.

The mechanisms of action of quinine and mefloquine are thought to be similar to that of chloroquine. Quinidine (see Chapter 14) also has some antimalarial properties. Both quinidine and quinine display potentially hazardous cardiac toxicity.

The diaminopyrimidines, such as pyrimethamine and trimethoprim, inhibit dihydrofolate reductase in malarial parasites. These agents are effective at concentrations far below those needed to inhibit the mammalian enzyme (see Chapter 43), so selectivity can be attained. Inhibition of parasite dihydrofolate reductase blocks the synthesis of tetrahydrofolate, a

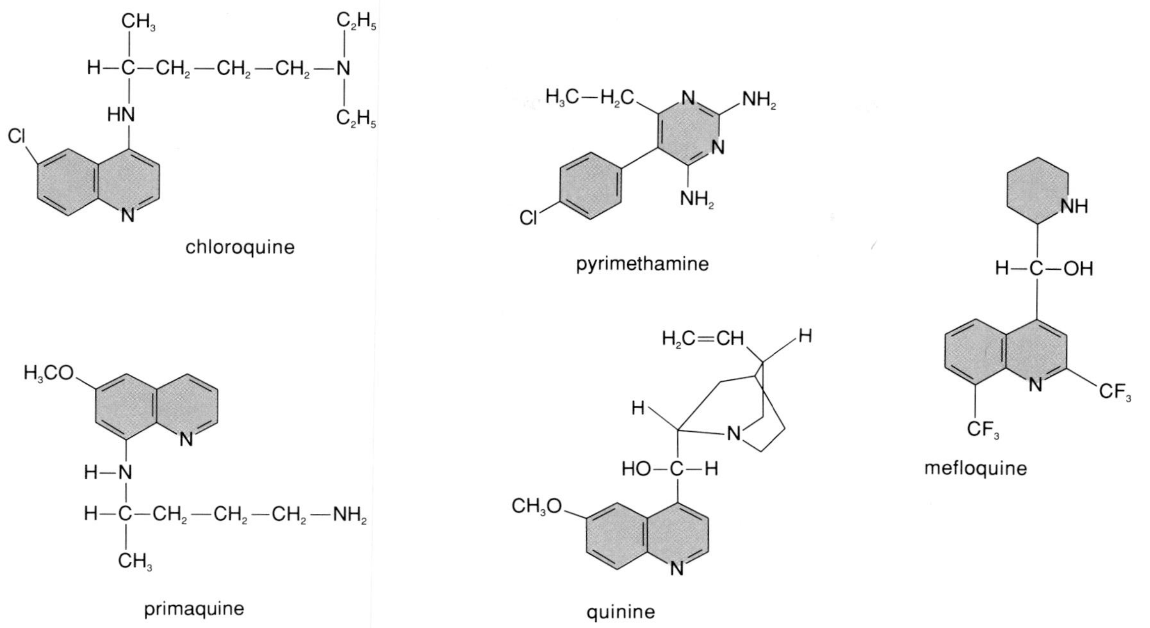

FIGURE 55-2   Structures of some drugs used in the treatment of malaria.

precursor necessary for the formation of purines, pyrimidines, and certain amino acids (see Chapter 48). Parasites exposed to these agents do not form schizonts in the red blood cells or liver. When a diaminopyrimidine is used with a sulfonamide or sulfone, a synergistic effect is achieved by blockade of two steps in the same metabolic pathway (see Chapter 48). Sulfonamide inhibits the synthesis of aminobenzoic acid to dihydropteroic acid while the diaminopyrimidine blocks the reduction of dihydrofolate to tetrahydrofolate.

Sulfonamides, tetracyclines, and clindamycin are often administered with antimalarial agents. The mechanism of action of sulfonamides is discussed in Chapter 48 and that for the tetracyclines and clindamycin in Chapter 47. The molecular mechanisms of the newer experimental ginghaosu and halofantrine are not known.

Antileishmaniasis Agents

Tissue forms of leishmania are the target for pentamidine isethionate, meglumine antimoniate, sodium stibogluconate, and amphotericin B. The structures of these drugs are shown in Figure 55-3. Meglumine antimoniate is a compound similar to sodium

stibogluconate. (See Chapter 52 for the structure and mechanism of action of amphotericin B.)

Meglumine antimoniate and sodium stibogluconate are antimonials and the drugs of first choice against leishmaniasis. They inhibit the glycolytic enzyme phosphofructokinase and certain Krebs cycle enzymes in *Leishmania* organisms. The resulting decreased energy production is parasiticidal.

Pentamidine isethionate acting against *Leishmania* species may interact with DNA or with nucleotides, or it may interfere with the uptake and function of polyamines. Amphotericin B interacts with ergosterol, an important membrane sterol in *Leishmania* protozoa, to increase membrane permeability and cause loss of low-molecular-weight carbohydrates and amino acids. Both pentamidine and amphotericin B are second-line drugs for use with leishmaniasis.

Antitrypanosomiasis Agents

African trypanosomiasis is treated with the arsenicals tryparsamide and melarsoprol and/or suramin and pentamidine. For Chagas' disease, nifurtimox and benznidazole are the agents of choice. The structures of some agents are shown in Figure 55-4.

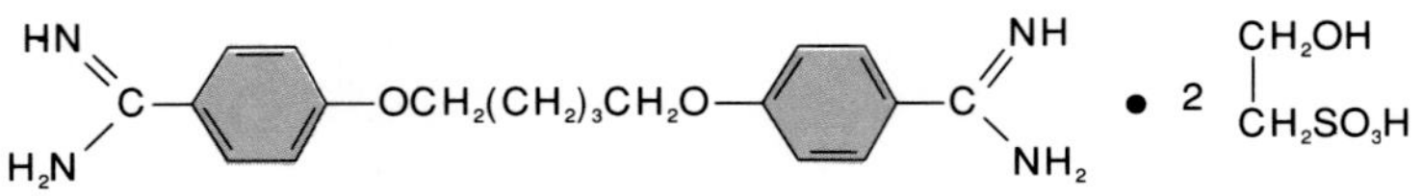

pentamidine isethionate

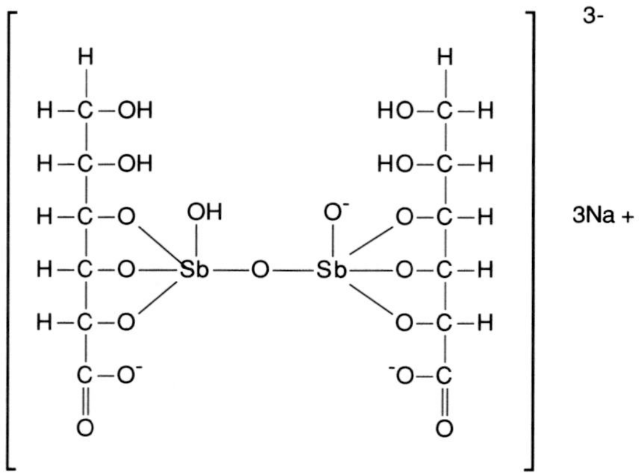

sodium stibogluconate

(shown for Sb^{5+})

FIGURE 55-3   Structures of drugs used in the treatment of leishmaniasis.

tryparsamide

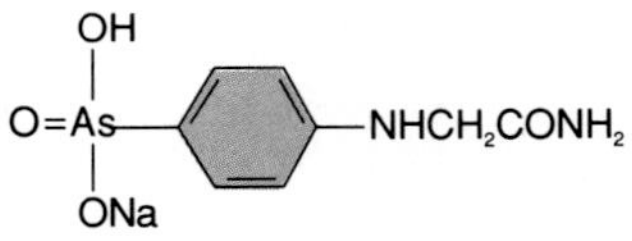

melarsoprol

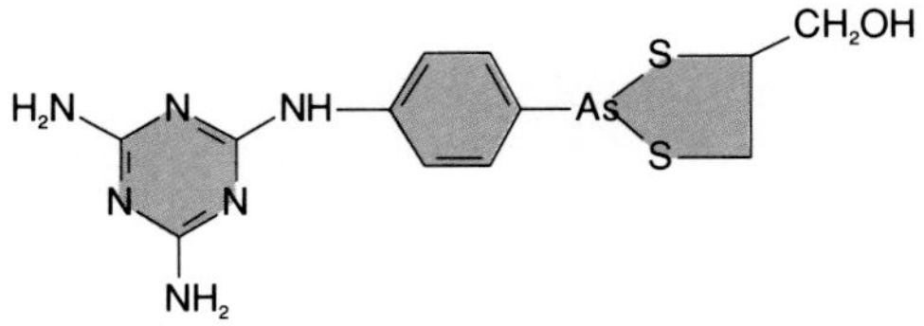

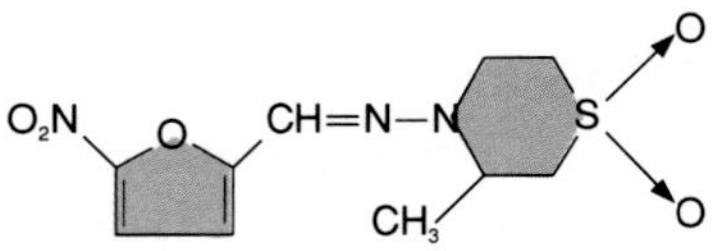

nifurtimox 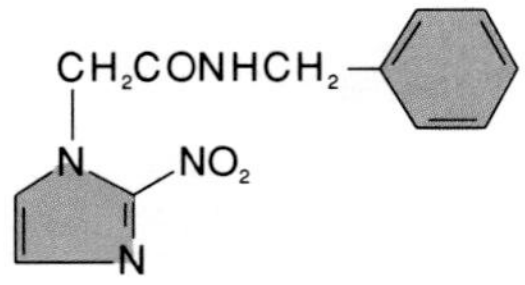   benznidazole

FIGURE 55-4   Structures of drugs used in the treatment of trypanosomiasis.

Once the infection has reached the CNS, melarsoprol or tryparsamide is the preferred drug. These arsenical drugs act on sulfhydryl groups of enzymes, which are essential catalysts in carbohydrate metabolism. Melarsoprol inhibits parasite pyruvate kinase, causing decreased concentrations of ATP, pyruvate, and phosphoenolpyruvate. These drugs also inhibit *sn*-glycerol 3-phosphate oxidase, needed for regeneration of NAD in trypanosomes but not found in mammalian cells. Inhibition of parasite metabolism at two sites produces a trypanocidal effect.

Suramin inhibits parasite *sn*-glycerol 3-phosphate oxidase and glycerol 3-phosphate dehydrogenase (Figure 55-5), causing a net decrease in ATP synthesis. An alternative to suramin is pentamidine. In trypanosomes, pentamidine may bind to the adenine- and thymine-rich regions of DNA, inhibiting DNA replication. Like suramin, pentamidine does not penetrate into the CNS and therefore is not useful in late CNS stages of infection with *Trypanosoma brucei gambiense*. Similarly, because *T.b. rhodesiense* invades the CNS so rapidly, pentamidine is effective only in the very early stages of infection.

Nifurtimox, the drug of choice for treatment of Chagas' disease, exerts its trypanocidal action by forming free radicals. The free radicals react with molecular oxygen to form superoxide anion (O_2^-), hydrogen peroxide (H_2O_2), and hydroxyl-free radical (OH·) (Figure 55-6). Trypanosomes are highly sensitive to these reactive intermediates, which cause peroxidation of lipids and DNA, because these organisms contain no catalase or glutathione peroxidase. Nifurtimox is highly toxic to human cells as well, but limited selectivity is achieved because the rates of radical formation are much decreased in human cells than in trypanosomes.

Antiamebiasis Agents

Iodoquinol, diloxanide furoate, and paromomycin are used against intestinal forms, emetine or dehydroemetine against systemic forms, and metronidazole against both forms of *E. histolytica*. The structures of these agents are shown in Figure 55-7.

Iodoquinol is the drug of choice for asymptomatic individuals who pass amebic cysts; an alternative drug, diloxanide furoate, is amebicidal; and a third agent, paromomycin, is an aminoglycoside antibiotic that is amebicidal and acts by inhibition of protein synthesis (see Chapter 47). Emetine and dehydroemetine also inhibit protein synthesis, probably by

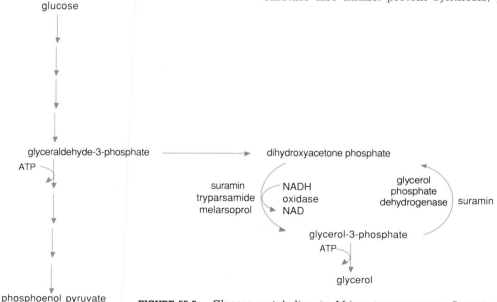

FIGURE 55-5 Glucose metabolism in African trypanosomes. Suramin inhibits *sn*-glycerol phosphate oxidase and *sn*-glycerol phosphate dehydrogenase, preventing reoxidation of NADH and decreasing ATP synthesis. The arsenicals (e.g., tryparsamide and melarsoprol) inhibit *sn*-glycerol phosphate oxidase as well as pyruvate kinase, resulting in a parasiticidal effect.

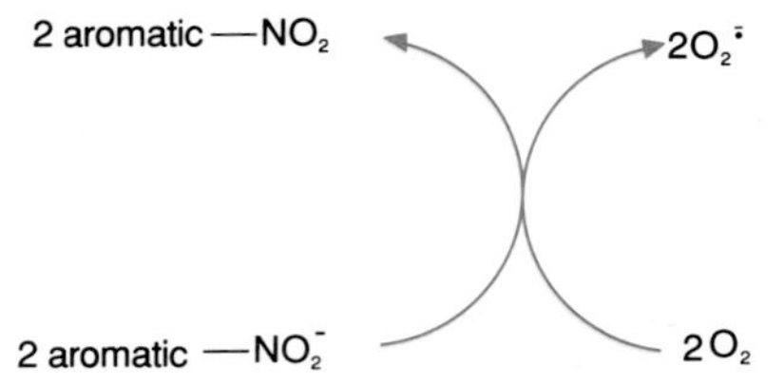

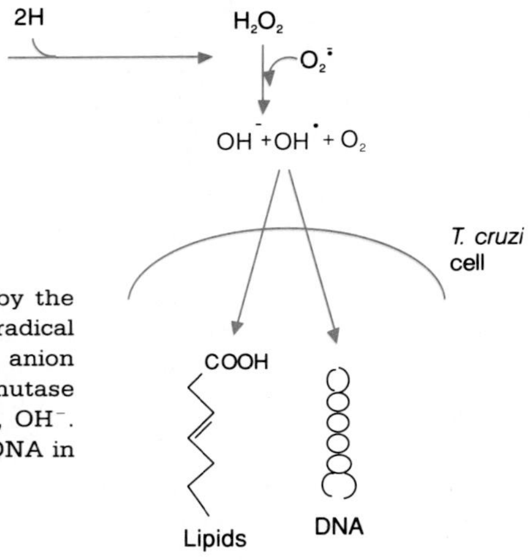

FIGURE 55-6   Generation of reactive intermediates by the aromatic nitro group of nifurtimox. The anion free radical reacts spontaneously with O_2 to form superoxide anion (O_2^-). H_2O_2 subsequently formed by superoxide dismutase can react with O_2^- to generate the hydroxyl radical, OH^-. Once formed, $OH^{\cdot}$ causes peroxidation of lipids and DNA in *T. cruzi*.

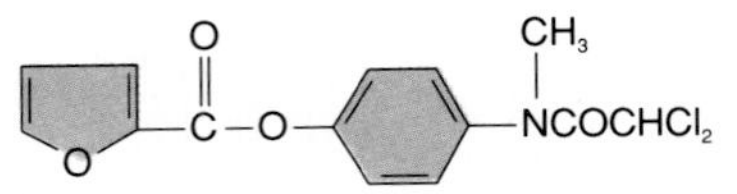

diloxanide furoate

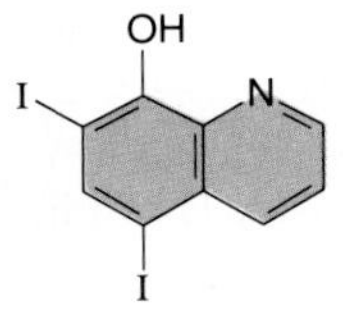

iodoquinol

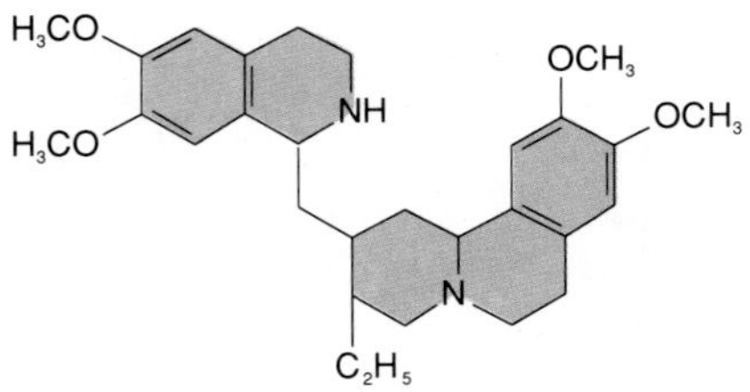

emetine

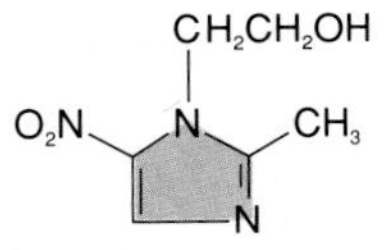

metronidazole

FIGURE 55-7   Structures of drugs used in the treatment of amebiasis.

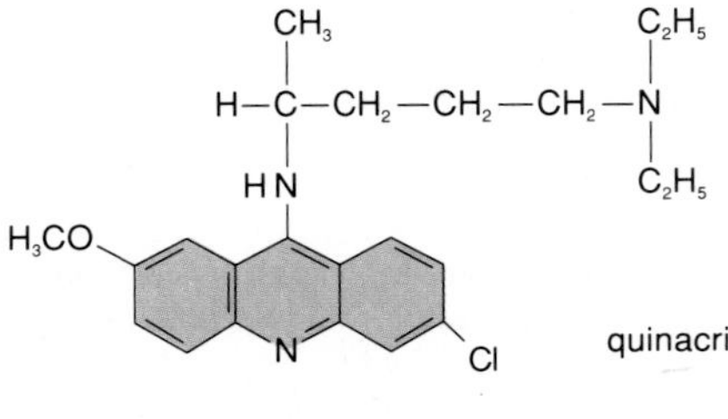

quinacrine

FIGURE 55-8   Structure of quinacrine.

blocking translocation along the mRNA of the ribosome during chain elongation.

Metronidazole interacts with amoeba DNA, destroying the ability of the DNA to serve as a template for further DNA and RNA synthesis. It covalently binds to guanine and cytosine residues, causing loss of helical structure and breakage of DNA strands.

Antigiardiasis and Antitrichomoniasis Agents

Metronidazole and quinacrine are the main drugs used to treat these infections. The structure of quinacrine is shown in Figure 55-8. It presumably acts by intercalation into parasite DNA.

Other Agents

Spiramycin, a macrolide antibiotic of the erythromycin group, inhibits protein synthesis and is used to treat cryptosporidiosis.

 ## PHARMACOKINETICS

Some of the drugs discussed in this chapter may not be generally available in the United States. The Centers for Disease Control in Atlanta should be contacted to check on availability, since it maintains stocks of some of these agents for disbursement on special request.

Pharmacokinetic characteristics of trimethoprim and sulfonamides are discussed in Chapter 48, those of tetracyclines and clindamycin are in Chapter 47, and those of suramin are in Chapter 54. The information on the pharmacokinetic parameter values for these drugs is summarized in Table 55-1.

The absorption of chloroquine is rapid and complete; food may increase bioavailability. Fifty percent is bound to protein and serum lipids, and 30% is metabolized in liver to N-deethyl-derivatives. After a single dose, the half-life is 48 hours; however, because of accumulation in liver, spleen, kidney, lung, and leukocytes, the effective half-life is 3 to 4 days. Chloroquine is detected in serum and urine up to a year after treatment. It can be administered IM but not IV.

Primaquine interferes with metabolism of chloroquine and should be administered after treatment for *Plasmodium vivax* but with a period of overlap. It is well absorbed orally and is eliminated in 24 hours. It is widely distributed, with retention in tissues, and

is converted to carboxyprimaquine. Less than 5% appears in urine.

Mefloquine is slowly absorbed from the gastrointestinal tract, and peak concentrations are not reached until 36 hours. It has a half-life of 14 days, is 99% protein bound, and undergoes extensive enterohepatic recirculation.

Pyrimethamine is completely absorbed after oral ingestion. It is slowly eliminated and has a half-life of 4 days, with suppr<!-- -->esive concentrations present in plasma for almost 2 weeks. It undergoes minor metabolism.

Pentamidine is not adequately absorbed from the gastrointestinal tract. It is administered IV or IM and is slowly eliminated from the body because of accumulation in tissues, but it is rapidly cleared from the blood. Fifteen percent is excreted in urine in 24 hours, but detectable amounts are found up to 8 weeks after a 2-week course of therapy.

Aerosol pentamidine produces sustained lung concentrations without clearance for 48 hours. Apical segments of the lungs are less well supplied than are the lower lobes.

Melarsoprol, a trivalent arsenical compound, is administered IV. Plasma concentrations decrease rapidly after administration, and no drug is detectable after a few days. It is excreted by the kidney.

Nifurtimox is rapidly absorbed and metabolized with little drug detected in plasma after 24 hours. Metabolites are excreted in the urine.

Benznidazole is rapidly absorbed orally, widely distributed throughout the body, and metabolized with metabolites excreted in urine.

Tryparsamide is administered IV. CSF concentrations are achieved within 20 hours. It is excreted unchanged in the urine.

Suramin is administered IV. It is extensively bound to serum proteins, and elimination is slow. It is distributed widely, and significant concentrations can be found in tissues up to 3 months after therapy. The drug is not appreciably metabolized, and the free drug is excreted in urine.

Sodium stibogluconate and meglumine antimoniate are administered IM or IV. Pharmacokinetics are quite complex with a three-compartment model and an initial half-life of 2 hours and terminal half-life of 30 to 35 hours after IV and over 700 hours after IM administration. Conversion of pentavalent antimony to trivalent antimony probably occurs, which may explain the toxicity. Antimonials are concentrated in reticuloendothelial cells.

Table 55-1 Pharmacokinetic Parameter Values

Drug	Administration	Absorption	t½ (hr)	Disposition	Plasma Protein Binding (%)
MALARIA					
chloroquine	Oral, IM	Good	3–4 days	M, R	50
pyrimethamine	Oral	Good	110	M (90%)	Tissue bound
quinine	Oral, IM, IV	Good	10	M (95%)	70
mefloquine	Oral	Fair	14 days	M enterohepatic cycle	99
LEISHMANIASIS					
meglumine antimoniate	IM, IV	No	2, 35†	R	Tissue bound
sodium stibogluconate	IM, IV	No	2, 35†	R	Tissue bound
pentamidine isethionate*	IV, IM	No	6–8 weeks	R	Tissue bound
TRYPANOSOMIASIS					
tryparsamide	IV	No	—	R (main)	—
nifurtimox	Oral	Good	—	M (main)	—
benznidazole	Oral	Good	—	M	
AMEBIASIS					
iodoquinol	Oral	Fair	—	M	—
diloxanide furoate	Oral	Good	—	M	—
paromomycin	Oral	Poor	—	—	—
emetine	IM	No	Long	R	Tissue bound
metronidazole	IV, Oral	Good	8	M, R	20
GIARDIASIS					
quinacrine	Oral	Good	—	R	Tissue bound

M, Metabolized; *R*, eliminated unchanged by renal mechanisms.
* Aerosol available for *Pneumocystis carinii*.
† Initial and terminal.

Diloxanide furoate is rapidly and almost completely absorbed from the gastrointestinal tract, with ester hydrolysis occurring in the intestine. It has a half-life of 6 hours and is excreted in urine as the glucuronide.

Eflornithine (DL-α-difluoromethyl-ornithine) can be administered orally or IV. Large doses of 20 g/day are necessary. It crosses the blood-brain barrier into the CSF. It is also present in lung tissue. The CSF to serum ratio is from 0.09 to 0.45.

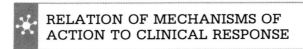

RELATION OF MECHANISMS OF ACTION TO CLINICAL RESPONSE

Antimalarial Agents

Human malaria is caused by four species of obligate intracellular protozoa of the genus *Plasmodium*. *P. vivax* is the most common, *P. falciparum* the most severe, and *P. ovale* and *P. malariae* are less common

and of intermediate severity. These parasites reproduce asexually in humans and sexually in mosquitoes of the genus *Anopheles*. In the asexual stages, the malaria parasites invade erythrocytes where they multiply and ultimately burst the cells to release a new invasive population of parasites. The pathology and symptoms of malaria are caused strictly by the asexual blood forms of malarial parasites, and many drugs have been developed that selectively target these stages. Figure 55-1 depicts the malaria life stages within the human host. Sexually differentiated forms (gametocytes), which are infective to the mosquito, are also found in the circulation and offer another site of action of certain antimalarials.

When an individual is infected from the bite of a mosquito, some parasites leave the mosquito and enter the circulation and localize in hepatic parenchymal tissue. Here, the parasites multiply and form exoerythrocytic schizonts; this is an asymptomatic stage of the disease and represents a third target for drug

Table 55-2 Drugs of Choice	
Infection	**Primary Drugs**
Malaria	chloroquine*
	pyrimethamine
	quinine, quinidine†
Leishmaniasis	meglumine antimoniate
	sodium stibogluconate
Trypanosomiasis	melarsoprol
	suramin
	nifurtimox
Amebiasis	iodoquinol, metronidazole
Giardiasis	metronidazole, quinacrine
Trichomoniasis	metronidazole

* Mefloquine is used as prophylaxis in areas where *P. falciparum* is resistant to chloroquine.
† Quinine and quinidine are used to treat *P. falciparum* malaria of the CNS.

treatment. After a period of 5 to 16 days, the exoerythrocytic schizonts rupture, releasing thousands of merozoites, the infective blood stage of the parasite, into the circulation. The rupture and reinvasion of red blood cells by the merozoite form of the parasite are responsible for the fever and clinical manifestations of the disease.

Chloroquine and related compounds remain the drugs of first choice (Table 55-2) for the treatment of susceptible malaria strains. Chloroquine has no effect against the exoerythrocyte stages of plasmodia and thus does not prevent infection; however, it is highly toxic to the asexual blood stages of all four *Plasmodium* species except *P. falciparum*. During an acute febrile attack, chloroquine lowers fever within 24 to 48 hours, and parasites are no longer visible in the blood 48 to 72 hours posttreatment. The drug completely cures chloroquine-sensitive *P. falciparum,* the most lethal of the malaria species in humans. Chloroquine is well tolerated, inexpensive, and effective orally. Unfortunately, resistance of *P. falciparum* to chloroquine is widespread in Asia, Africa, and South America, greatly limiting the use of this agent.

Quinine is only used orally to treat mild attacks and by the IV route to treat acute attacks of multidrug resistant *P. falciparum,* which causes cerebral malaria. Quinine is never used alone but is often combined with a sulfonamide or tetracycline antibacterial agent.

Pyrimethamine has been used in the past in combination with antibiotics or with sulfadoxine, a sul-

fonamide with an extremely long plasma and tissue half-life, as prophylaxis for chloroquine to treat resistant *P. falciparum* and *P. vivax* malaria. Synergism produced with a sulfonamide-diaminopyrimidine combination is desirable because lower doses of each drug can be used to obtain the therapeutic effect. However, the combination is no longer recommended for either prophylaxis or treatment since it can cause the exfoliative dermatitis reaction (Stevens-Johnson syndrome).

Mefloquine is a newer antimalarial used for the chemoprophylaxis of falciparum malaria. Resistance to mefloquine has been reported but is rare. *P. vivax* has a latent liver stage. Thus after treatment with chloroquine, it is necessary to administer primaquine for 2 weeks. In rare cases, Southwest Pacific isolates are relatively resistant to primaquine and relapse occurs. Patients are treated with larger doses for a longer period and monitored for hematologic toxicity. Ginghaosu, also called *artemisinine,* is a Chinese drug with possible antimalarial effects.

Antileishmaniasis Agents

Leishmaniasis parasites exist intracellularly in phagolysosomes of mononuclear tissue phagocytes, but infected cells are found throughout the body, including the bloodstream. The tissue forms of the parasite are called *amastigotes* and serve as the chemotherapeutic target for the treatment of the disease. Prevention or cure of leishmaniasis has been hampered significantly by both the lack of effective drugs and the toxicity associated with existing agents. Meglumine antimonate and sodium stibogluconate (antimony sodium gluconate) are first-line drugs for treatment of leishmaniasis, with pentamidine and amphotericin B alternative drugs for treatment of various forms of the disease (Table 55-2).

Antitrypanosomiasis Agents

Trypanosomiasis, caused by *T.b. rhodesiense,* leads to progressive CNS involvement and almost always death, and that from *T.b. gambiense* causes a chronic debilitation known as sleeping sickness with severe CNS involvement.

Once CNS involvement is apparent, melarsoprol and tryparsamide are the drugs of choice (Table 55-2). Both are effective for the treatment of the meningoencephalitic stage of African trypanosomiasis, but because melarsoprol acts more rapidly and causes fewer side effects, it is surpassing tryparsamide in use. Melarsoprol is also effective against tryparsamide-resistant trypanosomes. An investigational agent that exploits biochemical pathways found only in the parasite is α-difluoromethylornithine, a potent inhibitor of polyamine synthesis in *T.b. gambiense* and *T.b. rhodesiense.*

Suramin is the drug of choice for African sleeping sickness (Table 55-2). When given IV, it is active against blood forms of *T.b. gambiense* and *T.b. rhodesiense,* particularly in the early stages of the disease. Once the disease has progressed to involve the CNS, suramin cannot prevent progression since it does not penetrate the blood-brain barrier.

For the treatment of Chagas' disease caused by *T. cruzi,* nifurtimox is the drug of choice (Table 55-2), with benznidazole as an alternative that is efficacious against nifurtimox-resistant *T. cruzi.*

Antiamebiasis Agents

Amebiasis, caused by *Entamoeba histolytica,* is found throughout the world and is transmitted by the oral-fecal route following ingestion of infective cysts. The cysts change into trophozoites that reside in the colon, where they form new cysts passed into the environment to complete the life cycle. These organisms may produce amoebic dysentery and liver abscesses. The drugs used to treat amebiasis are specific for the location of the organism. For example, diloxanide furoate, paromomycin, and iodoquinol (Table 55-2) are effective against intestinal (noninvasive) forms of the parasite. Systemic amebicides include emetine and dehydroemetine, used for the treatment of severe amoebic dysentery, and metronidazole, used against both intestinal and systemic forms of the infection. Emetine and dehydroemetine are rarely used because of their serious cardiac toxicity except in the treatment of intestinal invasive amebiasis.

Metronidazole is not effective for the treatment of individuals who are asymptomatic but continue to pass cysts, although it is extremely effective for treatment of dysentery and amoebic liver abscesses.

Antigiardiasis and Antitrichomoniasis Agents

Giardia lamblia, a flagellated protozoan, causes the most common of the intestinal protozoal infections in developed countries. Giardiasis is transmitted via the passage of infective cysts, which become trophozoites after ingestion. The trophozoites are found in the duodenum, and the presence of these organisms may result in diarrhea but frequently results in non-specific bloating with passage of foul-smelling stools. Giardiasis is best treated with metronidazole or quinacrine (Table 55-2).

Trichomoniasis is a sexually transmitted disease caused by *Trichomonas vaginalis,* usually located in the genitourinary tract. Trichomoniasis is treated successfully with metronidazole, in which cure rates exceed 90% (Table 55-2).

Other Agents

Four protozoal parasites—cryptosporidia, *Isospora belli, Pneumocystis,* and toxoplasma—are particularly important sources of infection in the immunocompromised host. While clinical manifestations of these diseases are rare in immunocompetent individuals infected with these organisms, predisposing factors such as leukemia, lymphoma, and acquired immune deficiency syndrome (AIDS) can cause infection by these parasites to become fatal to these individuals. Currently, there is no treatment for cryptosporidiosis.

Pneumonias caused by *Pneumocystis carinii* occur exclusively in immunocompromised individuals and contribute significantly to the mortality associated with AIDS. These infections are always fatal if left untreated. Recommended treatment for *P. carinii* infection is initially trimethoprim-sulfamethoxazole (see Chapter 48) with pentamidine isethionate or trimethoprim-dapsone as alternative drugs. Pentamidine can be administered as an aerosol as prophylaxis against recurrence.

Toxoplasma gondii, the causative agent of toxoplasmosis, can produce systemic infection in both immunocompetent and immunocompromised individuals. Domesticated animals, particularly cats, serve as intermediate hosts for *Toxoplasma gondii,* passing infective oocysts in their feces. Treatment of toxoplasmosis is done with sulfonamides (discussed in Chapter 48) combined with pyrimethamine. However, pyrimethamine is teratogenic and should not be used in treatment of pregnant women. Alternative agents are clindamycin in the United States or spiramycin, a macrolide, in Canada and Europe.

SIDE EFFECTS, CLINICAL PROBLEMS, AND TOXICITY

Although the treatment of protozoal diseases with drugs is usually successful when the treatment is begun before the disease has reached an advanced state, these drugs have serious side effects and toxicities that need to be understood. These problems are likely to become more prevalent with the growing need to increase drug concentrations in an attempt to overcome resistances to the drugs that are developing in these organisms. The clinical problems are summarized in the box.

Antimalarial Agents

Chloroquine has little toxicity unless overdosing occurs, in which case progressive retinopathy, skin lesions, ototoxicity, cardiac depression, and heart block can occur. Pruritus, vomiting, and headache can occur with normal doses. *P. falciparum* resistance to chloroquine is widespread, thus limiting the usefulness of this relatively safe agent. Chemically related mefloquine has minimal toxicity but can cause mental confusion and seizures and is not recommended for an individual with a convulsive disorder. Primaquine has gastrointestinal side effects and, if administered to glucose-6-phosphate dehydrogenase–deficient (G6PD) patients, leads to hemolysis.

The side effects associated with quinine are many. This drug has a narrow therapeutic index, and toxicity occurs at concentrations only slightly above those needed for a parasiticidal effect. CNS effects, such as analgesia, antipyresis, and hypotension occur. Blood dyscrasias and *cinchonism*, which manifests as tinnitus, headache, nausea, and visual and hearing disturbances, are also associated with clinical use of quinine. An oral overdose or IV administration can result in cardiac depression.

Pyrimethamine is relatively free of problems at prophylactic doses but may produce a folic acid deficiency and severe leukopenia and/or thrombocytopenia, with the former reversible by administration of folinic acid. The pyrimethamine-sulfadoxine preparation used with chloroquine may produce Stevens-Johnson syndrome, which can be lethal.

Antileishmaniasis Agents

Sodium stibogluconate is relatively safe, with muscle pains, joint stiffness, and bradycardia the principal side effects. The second-line drugs for treatment of leishmaniasis must be used much more carefully. Pentamidine isethionate produces serious hypotension when administered IV; therefore care is needed during any other parenteral form of administration of this drug. Hypoglycemia and blood dyscrasias are additional side effects that may be seen. The other second-line drug, amphotericin B, may produce serious nephrotoxicity and hypokalemia. (See Chapter 50 for further discussion of side effects.)

Antitrypanosomiasis Agents

Melarsoprol is a highly toxic agent and may cause mild myocardial damage, hypertension, colic, and

---

CLINICAL PROBLEMS

ANTIMALARIAL AGENTS

Development of organism resistance to chloroquine
primaquine/chloroquine: hemolysis with use in glucose-6-phosphate-dehydrogenase deficient patients
quinine: CNS effects and cinchonism, multiple side effects
pyrimethamine-sulfadoxine in combination with chloroquine may produce Stevens-Johnson syndrome

ANTILEISHMANIASIS AGENTS

pentamidine isethionate: hypotension, pancreatic β cell toxicity
amphotericin B: serious nephrotoxicity

ANTITRYPANOSOMIASIS AGENTS

Nausea and vomiting with most agents
Impaired vision and even blindness with tryparsamide

ANTIAMEBIASIS AGENTS

metronidazole: disulfiramlike reaction to alcohol, peripheral neuropathy, metal taste, GI upset
emetine: cardiac dysrhythmias
iodoquinol: requires monitoring of thyroid function

vomiting but is less toxic than tryparsamide. Vomiting, nausea, impaired vision, and blindness are associated with long-term use of tryparsamide and thus limit extensive dosing with this agent. Suramin causes vomiting, pruritus, urticaria, photophobia, and peripheral neuropathy. Hypotension, hypoglycemia with pancreatic islet β cell destruction leading to diabetes, and blood dyscrasias are associated with pentamidine isethionate. Rarely it causes renal toxicity.

Nifurtimox and benznidazole, used in the treatment of Chagas' disease, produce GI upsets and rashes. Nifurtimox may also cause anorexia, tremors, paresthesia, and polyneuritis, and the benznidazole rash is intensified by light.

Antiamebiasis Agents

The side effects seen with diloxanide furoate, paromomycin, and metronidazole are mainly annoying and not substantive at normal concentrations. Diloxamide furoate may produce flatulence, nausea, or vomiting, and paromomycin may cause GI disturbances. Metronidazole, a widely used drug, may cause nausea, headache, and a disulfiramlike reaction with alcohol (see Chapter 19). Patients receiving iodoquinol may experience a rash, diarrhea, enlargement of the thyroid, and blindness with long-term therapy.

Considerable toxicity is associated with the use of emetine or dehydroemetine. These drugs persist in the body for prolonged times, and cardiac toxicity, especially dysrhythmias, as well as muscle weakness and diarrhea may develop. Thus these drugs need to be used with great care.

Antigiardiasis and Antitrichomoniasis Agents

Metronidazole is discussed previously; quinacrine side effects are mild but include dizziness, headache, metallic taste, GI upset, vomiting, and occasional psychosis.

TRADENAMES

In addition to generic and fixed combination preparations, the following tradenamed materials are available in the United States.

Aralen Hydrochloride, chloroquine HC1
Aralen Phosphate, chloroquine/primaquine phosphates
Atabrine, quinacrine HC1
Daraprim, pyrimethamine
Fansidar, pyrimethamine-sulfadoxine
Flagyl, Protostat, metronidazole
Pentam, pentamidine isethionate
Plaquenil, hydroxychloroquine sulfate
Yodoxin, iodoquinol

REFERENCES

Campbell WC and Rew RS, eds: Chemotherapy of parasitic diseases, New York, 1986, Plenum Publishing Corp.

Cook GC: Prevention and treatment of malaria, Lancet I:32, 1988.

Drugs for parasitic infections, Med Lett Drugs Ther 30:76, 1988.

Miller KD, Greenberg AE, and Campbell CC: Treatment of severe malaria in the United States with a continuous infusion of quinidine gluconate and exchange transfusion, N Engl J Med 321:65, 1989.

Monk JP and Benfield P: Inhaled pentamidine, Drugs 39:741, 1990.

Van Voorhis WC: Therapy and prophylaxis of systemic protozoan infections, Drugs 40:176, 1990.

CHAPTER 56

Antiseptics and Disinfectants

	ABBREVIATIONS
ATPase	adenosine triphosphatase
DNA	deoxyribonucleic acid
pH	logarithm of the reciprocal of the hydrogen ion concentration
RNA	ribonucleic acid

ANTISEPTICS CURRENTLY USED TOPICALLY (ON SKIN)

AGENT

Ethyl alcohol (70%)
Isopropyl alcohol (70%)
Tincture of iodine (2%)
Povidone iodine
Chlorhexidine
Quaternary ammonium compounds before urethral catheterization or ophthalmic surgery

 ## THERAPEUTIC OVERVIEW

Agents described in this chapter are not taken internally and are not used to treat disease but are employed to prevent infection by destroying or limiting the growth of microorganisms on foreign surfaces and on skin. In contrast to other antimicrobial agents, antiseptics and disinfectants lack specificity.

Sterility is the complete absence of all forms of microbial life. Substances, instruments, or devices that are introduced into normally sterile areas of the body must be sterile. Sterilization is best accomplished by heat—steam under pressure that provides 121° C for 15 minutes or dry heat that produces 160° to 180° C for 3 hours. Thermolabile solutions may be sterilized by passage through membrane filters that have a pore size of 0.22 microns. Optically clear solutions may also be sterilized by exposure to 254 nm ultraviolet radiation for doses of approximately 200,000 microwatt-sec/cm². Lensed instruments or prosthetic devices may be sterilized by high voltage electron or gamma radiation. More often, such materials are subjected to "cold sterilization," that is, exposure to ethylene oxide gas or immersion in solutions of glutaraldehyde or alcoholic-formaldehyde.

Antisepsis

Living tissue such as skin or mucous membranes cannot be sterilized, but the risk of infection can be minimized by reducing the number of microorganisms on such tissues. Antiseptics are applied to living tissues to inhibit microorganism growth. These agents are used in presurgical scrubs of the surgeon's hands and applied to the patient's skin before incisions or injections are made. The degerming action is only temporary; bacterial multiplication resumes after minutes or hours. Antiseptics may be used as solutions or incorporated into soaps, salves, ointments, dressings, mouthwashes, or douches. Commonly used antiseptics are listed in the box.

Disinfection

Sterility is not necessary in many clinical situations. Instruments used in anatomic locations normally inhabited by indigenous microorganisms, such as thermometers, specula, or proctoscopes, need not

Table 56-1 Disinfectants Commonly Used in Hospitals in the United States

Use	Agent
Cold sterilization of catheters, endoscopic instruments	Ethylene oxide
	Glutaraldehyde
	Alcoholic formaldehyde
	Oxidizers
For thermometers	Ethyl alcohol
Disinfection of floors, walls, and other surfaces	Phenolic compounds
	Iodophors
	Quaternary ammonium compounds
	Chlorine compounds

Table 56-2 Antiseptics and Disinfectants Listed by Mechanism of Action

Mode of Action	Agent
Oxidation	Hydrogen peroxide
	Ozone
	Peracetic acid
	Chlorine compounds
Alkylation	Ethylene oxide
	β-propiolactone
	Formaldehyde
	Glutaraldehyde
Protein denaturation	Alcohols
	Phenolic compounds
	Iodine
	Heavy metals
Surface active agent	Quaternary ammonium compounds
Cation ionization	Dyes
Membrane damage	Chlorhexidine

be sterile; they must be rendered free of microbial pathogens, however. It is often necessary to block the transfer of pathogens from patient to patient by fomites or other inanimate objects or surfaces. This process of destroying pathogens, termed *disinfection,* does not necessarily achieve complete sterility. Disinfectants kill pathogenic microorganisms and are used on inanimate objects or surfaces. Agents used as disinfectants include halogen-containing compounds, phenols, quaternary ammonium compounds, aldehydes, and oxidizing agents. Table 56-1 lists disinfectants currently in use.

Bacterial Inhibition versus Elimination

Antiseptics and disinfectants may be characterized as *bacteriostatic*—inhibiting the growth of bacteria, or *bactericidal*—and kill most vegetative forms of bacteria. Bactericidal agents are not necessarily effective against spores, *Mycobacterium tuberculosis,* fungi, or viruses unless specifically designated as sporicidal, tuberculocidal, fungicidal, or virucidal. Certain agents have been termed *sterilants,* since they can effectively sterilize inanimate objects or surfaces when used appropriately. Sterilants include ethylene oxide, glutaraldehyde, alcoholic-formaldehyde, β-propiolactone, peracetic acid, and chlorine dioxide.

 MECHANISMS OF ACTION

The mode of action of this diverse group of substances varies and, in many cases, is not well understood. Some are highly reactive oxidizing or alkylating agents and, as such, may be considered as general protoplasmic poisons. Most damage microbial cell walls or cytoplasmic membranes by denaturing proteins, lowering surface tension, or inhibiting essential enzymes. The effectiveness of these chemical agents is almost always influenced by concentration, temperature, and time of exposure. The agents are listed by their general mechanism of action in Table 56-2.

Alcohols

The commonly used alcohols are ethanol (C_2H_5OH) and isopropanol ($CH_3CH(OH)CH_3$). The bactericidal activity of aliphatic alcohols increases with increasing chain length to a maximum of 5 to 8 carbon atoms. Unbranched chains are more active than the iso configuration; tertiary alcohols are the least active. For alcohols to be effective against microorganisms, water must be present. The most effective alcohol concentrations are 60% to 70%, with the activity markedly decreasing above 95% and below 60%.

Alcohols probably act as protein denaturing agents. At low concentrations they may be used as substrates for some bacteria, but at higher concentrations dehydrogenation reactions are inhibited. Some microorganisms are lysed by alcohols.

Ethyl and isopropyl alcohols are rapidly bactericidal and are highly effective against vegetative Gram-positive and Gram-negative bacteria, tubercle bacilli, the pathogenic fungi, and many viruses, especially those with lipid coats. Alcohol has no effect on bacterial spores.

Alcohol is used alone or in combination with other agents as a surgical antiseptic. It evaporates rapidly and produces excessive dryness of the skin, but emollients can be added to reduce this effect.

Alcohol is also used as a disinfectant for clinical thermometers.

Halogens

Iodine and Iodophors Iodine precipitates proteins and oxidizes essential enzymes. It is rapidly bactericidal and tuberculocidal, and active against many viruses and pathogenic fungi at concentrations as low as 0.05%. Activity against spores requires prolonged exposure times.

Elemental iodine dissolves in aqueous potassium iodide, alcohol, or ether. It can also be solubilized by complexation with cationic or nonionic surfactants; such complexes are known as *iodophores*. Although iodine is effective over a wide pH range, more free iodine (the active form) is released at low pH values.

The mode of action of iodine is multifactorial. It reacts with NH groups of nucleotide bases and some amino acids to prevent hydrogen bonding and iodinates the ring of aromatic amino acids and of histidine. The sulfhydryl group of cysteine is oxidized to a disulfide cross-link, interfering with protein synthesis and activity. Iodine reacts with the phenolic group of tyrosine, causing steric phenolic hindrance in hydrogen bonding of the phenilic hydroxyl group. In addition, iodine interacts with the carbon-carbon double bond of unsaturated fatty acids, altering the properties of lipids and their role in membrane stabilization.

Iodine is used as an antiseptic and a disinfectant. As a skin antiseptic, Iodine Solution (2% iodine + 2.4% potassium iodide) and Iodine Tincture (2% iodine, 2.4% potassium iodine and 44% to 50% alcohol) are used. Tincture of iodine should be dated, and discarded when outdated, because the iodine concentration increases as the alcohol-water component evaporates. Concentrations of iodine in excess of 3% may produce skin blistering. Burns can result if skin treated with tincture of iodine is covered with an occlusive dressing. Tincture of iodine should always

be removed from the skin with 70% alcohol after completion of a surgical procedure.

Disadvantages of the tincture or solution of iodine are staining of skin and fabrics, skin sensitization, irritation and pain at wounds and mucocutaneous junctions, and corrosion of many metals.

Povidone iodine iodophors (Figure 56-1), prepared by complexing iodine with polyvinylpyrrolidone, are widely used. Povidone iodine is more stable than the tincture at normal ambient temperatures, much less irritating to tissues, and less corrosive to metals: fabric stains are readily removed. However, the cost is significantly higher than the tincture and the staining of some plastics is reported. Povidone iodine is toxic to exposed fibroblasts, and irrigation of open wounds with this substance may delay healing.

Surfactant iodine iodophors are used as disinfectants of floor areas, work surfaces, and food-handling utensils. Iodine is also used for disinfection of clinical thermometers and other instruments, and for the emergency disinfection of drinking water.

Mercurial Compounds Organic mercurial compounds have a weak bacteriostatic action and are less effective than alcohols. Serum reduces antimicrobial action, and skin sensation can occur. Only thimerosal is available for topical use. Mercury compounds should not be applied to large areas of denuded skin. Ingestion can cause renal failure. Dimercaprol is an effective antidote.

Chlorine and Chlorine Compounds Aqueous solutions of chlorine exhibit rapid bactericidal action. Elemental chlorine reacts with water to form hypochlorous acid, but how hypochlorous acid destroys microorganisms is not clear. It may liberate nascent oxygen, which in turn oxidizes essential components of protoplasm. Or perhaps chlorine combines with cell membrane proteins to form *N*-chloro compounds that interfere with cellular metabolism. Chlorine oxidizes the sulfhydryl groups of certain enzymes, causing irreversible inactivation.

The active free chlorine and hypochlorous acid are in pH-dependent equilibrium, with rapid bactericidal, tuberculocidal, and, in many cases, virucidal actions at concentrations of 0.2 to 2.0 parts per million of available chlorine. Pathogenic fungi are more resistant and require a minimum of 100 parts per million of available chlorine. The activity of chlorine compounds increases as the concentration of available chlorine increases; in practice, concentrations of 2000 parts per million or more of available chlorine are used.

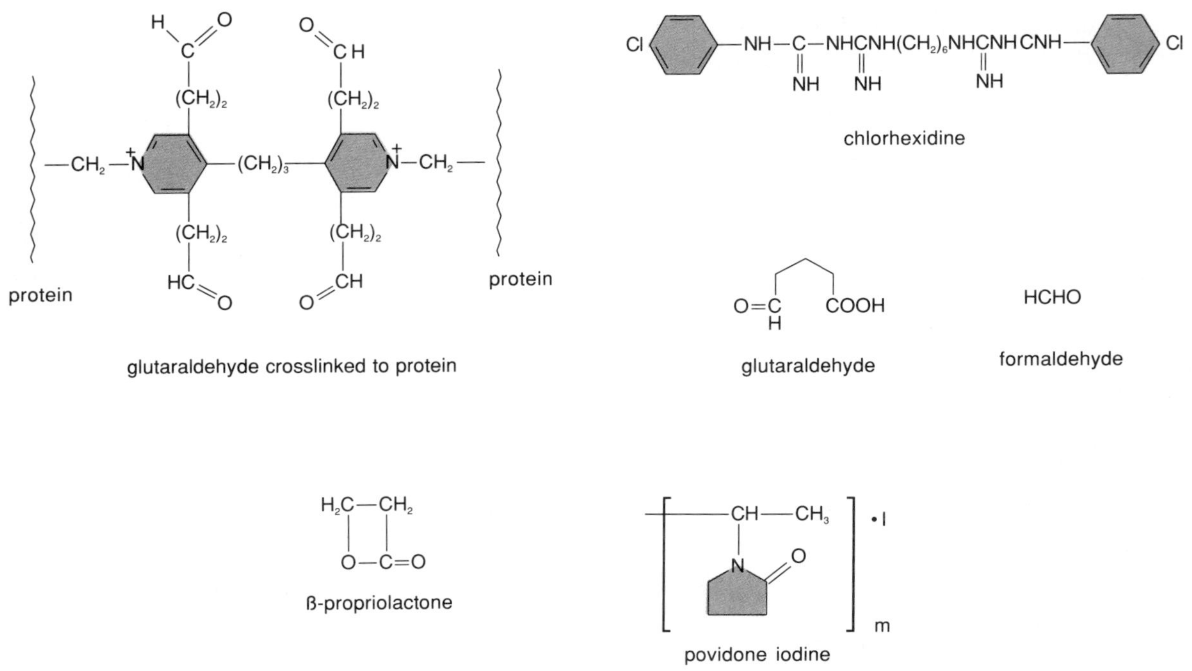

FIGURE 56-1   Structures of antiseptics and disinfectants.

With each 10° C rise in temperature, the activity of chlorine increases approximately 50%.

Chlorine is no longer used as an antiseptic because of its irritant effects and inactivation by organic matter. However, it is widely employed as a disinfectant of municipal water supplies. Its activity is quickly inhibited by dirt or extraneous material, as well as by soap or highly alkaline detergent solutions.

Widely used chlorine compounds are sodium and calcium hypochlorites, which act through nascent release of hypochlorous acid.

Chlorine dioxide is more rapidly sporicidal than hypochlorous acid, and proprietary binary systems that produce chlorine dioxide are useful as sterilants and disinfectants. Another compound, chlorite, is activated with an organic acid to chlorous acid, which slowly converts to chlorine dioxide, chloride, and chlorate ions.

Chloramines are produced by the reaction of hypochlorous acid on an amine, amide, imine, or imide. Organic chloramines are N-chloro derivatives of sulfonamides, heterocyclic nitrogen compounds, guanidine derivatives, or anilides. Various chloramine compounds have from 25% to 29% available chlorine, depending on the formulation. In general, N-chloro compounds are much slower in action than hypochlorites, but under acid conditions they are more effective bactericides.

Halazone or p-sulfondichloramidobenzoic acid is used for emergency water disinfection. A 4 mg halazone tablet is sufficient to render 1 liter of water safe to drink after 30 minutes. It will not inhibit cryptosporidium.

Aldehydes

Aldehydes act via alkylation. Even in low concentrations, exposure of bacteria to formaldehyde (see Figure 56-1) results in accumulation of 1,3 thiazine-4-carboxylic acid, an inhibitor of methionine formation. The action of glutaraldehyde may involve reaction with bacterial sulfhydryl or amino groups.

Formaldehyde   Formaldehyde is a gas that is irritating to the eyes, nose, and skin. Solutions of formaldehyde in water, known as *formalin,* contain 37% to 40% formaldehyde. At low concentrations, formaldehyde is bacteriostatic; growth of most vegetative bacteria is inhibited by 20 μg/ml. Stronger solutions, such as 8% aqueous formaldehyde (20% formalin), are bactericidal, sporicidal, tuberculocidal, and fungicidal, and inactivate most viruses. The germicidal action of formaldehyde is increased by combination with alcohol; 20% formalin in 70% alcohol can be used to disinfect metal instruments.

Glutaraldehyde Glutaraldehyde (Figure 56-1) is more potent and less irritating than formaldehyde. It is more active in an alkaline environment, but "activated" with sodium hydroxide it has a shorter useful life. It is sporicidal and viricidal, including HIV-1. Glutaraldehyde solutions are inactivated by proteins; hence instruments must be washed before use. Glutaraldehyde must be removed from instruments by sterile water immersion; otherwise it will cause burns to skin or mucous membranes.

Phenolic Compounds

Although phenol is no longer used as a disinfectant or antiseptic, it is used as a reference compound for evaluation of other germicidal compounds. Compounds are compared in a standardized manner for antibacterial effectiveness against phenol to give values known as the *phenol coefficient*.

Halogenation of phenolic compounds potentiates their germicidal effectiveness, with para substitution to the hydroxyl more effective than ortho. Bactericidal potency of halogenated phenols is further increased by introduction of aliphatic or aromatic groups into the nucleus. For example, ortho-alkyl derivatives of *p*-chlorophenol are more actively germicidal than para-alkyl derivatives of *o*-chlorophenols, and numerous synthetic phenols, such as *o*-phenylphenol, *p*-chlorobenzyl phenol, and *p*-tert-amylphenol, are used as disinfectants. These substances are not inactivated by soap or organic soil and at 2% to 3% concentrations kill vegetative bacteria, tubercle bacilli, pathogenic fungi, and most lipophilic viruses, but they are not sporicidal. Spores of *Clostridium difficile* will persist on surfaces soiled with feces. Combinations of these compounds with synthetic detergents make ideal disinfectants for cleaning and disinfection of hospital floors and other hard surfaces.

Derivatives of dihydroxy phenol or resorcinol have some germicidal activity, and hexylresorcinol is employed as a topical antiseptic. Its use is limited by hepatic and myocardial toxicity and production of burns on skin and mucous membranes.

Bis-phenols, two phenolic moieties linked together, possess high bacteriostatic activity. Similar to other phenolic compounds, halogenation increases the antibacterial effectiveness, particularly with Gram-positive bacteria. One example, hexachlorophene, is used extensively in antiseptic soaps, with a residual film on the skin being bacteriostatic primarily for Gram-positive bacteria, but such action develops only when hexachlorophene-containing soaps are used frequently and repeatedly. There is evidence that repeated use of hexachlorophene soaps causes an increase in Gram-negative flora of skin. Earlier widely used 3% emulsions of hexochlorophene for preoperative scrubs, washes for neonates, and washes for burn patients have been discontinued because of absorption from the skin into the systemic circulation, resulting in serious central nervous system toxicity, spongiform degeneration of the brain. The use of hexochlorophene in deodorant soaps and cosmetics is banned by the Food and Drug Administration.

Phenyl carbamides, salicylanilides, and carbamilides also are used in soaps and cosmetics for skin degerming. Many of these compounds have marked antifungal activity but are not sporicidal. Brominated salicylanilides and trifluoromethylated salicylanilides are effective as soap germicides, particularly in low concentrations.

Chlorhexidine

Chlorhexidine (see Figure 56-1) has marked antimicrobial activity against Gram-positive and Gram-negative bacteria and many yeasts and molds. But tubercle bacilli, bacterial spores, aspergillus (filamentous fungus), and viruses are not susceptible.

Chlorhexidine is absorbed on the cell surface, resulting in disorganization of the bacterial cytoplasmic membrane. Low concentrations promote leakage of cytoplasmic constituents. Chlorhexidine inhibits membrane-bound ATPase, and, at the higher concentrations used for antiseptic purposes, rapidly coagulates cytoplasmic constituents.

Like hexachlorophene, chlorhexidine remains on the skin to give a cumulative and continuing antibacterial effect that persists for at least 6 hours on gloved hands.

Chlorhexidine is effective in the presence of blood and organic matter, is nonirritating, and is not absorbed from intact skin or mucous membranes into the blood. A preparation of 5% chlorhexidine and 4% isopropanol is widely used in Europe as a "frequent use" alcohol-based hand wash.

Quaternary Ammonium Compounds

Quaternary ammonium compounds are cationic ammonium compounds with significant antibacterial activity when one of the four organic groups used in this class is between 8 and 18 carbons long. Representative compounds are benzalkonium chloride (alkylbenzyldimethylammonium chloride) and cetylpyridinium chloride (1-hexadecylpyridinium chloride).

Quaternary ammonium compounds are odorless, soluble in water and alcohol, and relatively nontoxic and nonirritating to tissues. Their mode of action is primarily through denaturation of cell membrane and cytoplasm components to produce release of nitrogen and potassium from the cells. Lipoprotein complexes throughout the cell are split, liberating autolytic enzymes. Quaternary ammonium compounds are bacteriostatic at low and bactericidal and fungicidal at higher concentrations, but certain organisms, such as *Pseudomonas aeruginosa, Mycobacterium tuberculosis, Trichophyton rubrum,* and *T. interdigitale,* are resistant to these agents. Indeed, *P. aeruginosa* and *P. cepacia* grow in solutions containing quaternary compounds. Viruses, in general, are more resistant than bacteria and fungi, and they are not effective against bacterial spores.

The quaternary ammonium compounds are neutralized by soaps and anionic detergents, and their activity is markedly decreased by organic matter and by dilution with hard water. They are selectively absorbed by fabrics, gauze, and cotton, so that a 1:1000 aqueous solution becomes a 1:2000 solution in the presence of cotton or gauze, permitting the growth of organisms such as *Pseudomonas.* The use of such contaminated solutions has resulted in a number of severe and fatal nosocomial infections. It is recommended that when aqueous quaternary ammonium compounds are used for antiseptics before surgical procedures they be dispensed as autoclaved solutions of 1:500 in quantities sufficient only for a single use. When used for antiseptic purposes, they are more effective as tinctures (i.e., 1:1000 diluted with 70% alcohol).

A 1% to 2% benzalkonium solution is a preferred topical agent in the treatment or prophylaxis of bite wounds from animals suspected of having rabies. However, the individual should receive rabies antiglobin and a rabies vaccine.

A final rinse of quaternary ammonium compounds is used to impregnate the fabric of hospital gowns and bed linens to assist destruction of microorganisms in the laundry process. Control of "diaper rash" is achieved by this process by suppression of disease-producing bacteria. Quaternary ammonium compounds are also used to sanitize utensils and food-processing equipment.

Oxidizing Agents

Hydrogen Peroxide The active agent of hydrogen peroxide is believed to be the hydroxyl free radical formed by the decomposition of hydrogen peroxide and possibly by the reduction of oxygen to superoxide. The hydroxyl free radical can attack membrane lipids, DNA, and other essential components of the cell.

Hydrogen peroxide (3% to 6%) is bactericidal and virucidal; higher concentrations (10% to 25%) are sporicidal.

Hydrogen peroxide is used for disinfection of plastic implants, contact lenses, and surgical prostheses.

The presence of catalase, which inactivates peroxide, limits the usefulness of hydrogen peroxide as an antiseptic. Hydrogen peroxide is toxic to fibroblasts and may delay wound healing. Cleansing of deep wounds and lacerations with hydrogen peroxide under pressure is contraindicated because this practice has resulted in subcutaneous gas formation.

(Other oxidizing agents such as ozone and peracetic acid are discussed under sterilant gases.)

Sterilant Gases

Formaldehyde Formaldehyde is available commercially in aqueous solutions containing up to 40% of the gas (see aldehyde section). It is also available as paraformaldehyde, a solid polymer that contains 91% to 99% formaldehyde. Paraformaldehyde sublimes rapidly when heated above 150° C. The action of formaldehyde is discussed in an earlier section.

Ethylene Oxide Ethylene oxide is a colorless gas at room temperature that is soluble in water and most organic solvents and readily penetrates porous materials. Ethylene oxide is flammable and explosive; thus for practical use, it is diluted with inert gases such as carbon dioxide to 10% ethylene oxide and 90% inert gas. Ethylene oxide has a high temperature coefficient, with each 10° C increase in temperature reducing the time for sterilization by about 50%. Doubling the concentration also halves the time required to achieve sterility. The lethal effect of ethylene oxide on microorganisms depends on moisture, with maximum sporicidal activity at 28% relative humidity.

Ethylene oxide acts by alkylation, especially of terminal carboxyl, amino, sulfhydryl, and hydroxyl moieties on proteins. It also alkylates nucleic acids at the N-7 position of guanine.

Ethylene oxide is effective against all types of microorganisms, including bacterial and fungal spores, vegetative cells, rickettsia, and viruses. It has a more rapid sporicidal action than formaldehyde. Its main advantage is that it can be used to sterilize medical and laboratory equipment that might be damaged by other sterilizing methods, especially those requiring elevated temperatures.

A disadvantage of the use of ethylene oxide is its slow action as a sterilant. The sterilizing time can be shortened somewhat by increasing the temperature, the concentration, and/or the pressure. The use of heat and pressure requires a special chamber. Ethylene oxide is absorbed by many materials, and plastics or instruments that may be in contact with patient skin or mucous membranes must be aerated for 24 hours or longer to remove all traces of the gas. Polycarbonates and various plastics will release products that can cause tissue damage. This has led to tracheal stenosis when ethylene-oxide–sterilized tracheal tubes were not adequately aerated before use in intensive care units.

β-Propiolactone β-Propiolactone (see Figure 56-1) is a colorless liquid at room temperature that is effective as a vapor-phase decontaminant against vegetative cells, bacterial spores, pathogenic fungi, viruses, and rickettsia.

β-Propiolactone is a strong alkylating agent and functions like ethylene oxide. Moisture is necessary and a relative humidity of 70% or greater is required for decontamination. It is more rapidly sporicidal than ethylene oxide, with a concentration of 1 to 2 mg/L to sterilize all available surfaces in a large enclosed area in 2 hours at ambient temperature, but its penetrating power is poor.

β-Propiolactone has strong lacrimator, respiratory irritant, vesicant, and weak carcinogenic properties. It is used to disinfect hospital rooms, operating rooms, military barracks, and animal housing, but it has too many detrimental properties to be suitable for general use as a hospital disinfectant.

Since the decomposition products of β-propiolactone are harmless, the compound is used to sterilize blood plasma and other biologicals for medical use.

Peracetic Acid Peracetic acid is a pungent-smelling compound that is available commercially as a 40% solution. It is unstable, slowly decomposing to acetic acid, hydrogen peroxide, water, and oxygen. Its undesirable properties include those of lacrimator, respiratory irritant, vesicant, and corrosive action on metals.

Peracetic acid is highly reactive, oxidizing many organic compounds, and may be regarded as a general protoplasmic poison. It is rapidly bactericidal and sporicidal, but like other sterilant gases, requires a high relative humidity. Peracetic acid is used primarily as a solution for disinfection but is also active in the gas phase.

Ozone Ozone, highly unstable O_3, is used primarily for water purification, showing better effectiveness than chlorine for rapidly killing bacteria, viruses, and the cysts of enteric parasites. Unlike chlorine, ozone leaves no residual taste or odor and does not produce toxic chlorinated organic products in waste water.

Little Used Materials

Silver compounds, triphenylmethane dyes, and acridine dyes are used only in special situations. Free silver ions are cytotoxic to bacteria, forming silver protein complexes that concentrate in the cytoplasmic membrane to give the "oligodynamic" effect. Silver nitrate solution is still used occasionally for routine prophylactic instillation into the eyes of newborn infants, and silver sulfadiazine cream (1%) is effective in the prevention of infection in severely burned individuals (see Chapter 49).

Triphenylmethane dyes such as crystal violet, brilliant green, and parafuchsin were formerly used as local antiseptics on wounds and burns. They were limited to bacteriostatic effects against Gram-positive organisms, and their activity was markedly decreased by serum. The acridine dyes acriflavine and proflavine differ from the triphenylmethane dyes by showing activity against Gram-negative and Gram-positive bacteria and by remaining active in the presence of serum. The acridines bind to DNA, RNA, and other proteins to inhibit DNA synthesis, with proflavin inhibiting DNA and RNA polymerases. These dyes were formerly used to treat infected wounds and act slowly against vegetative cells, but not spores. They are no longer used due to their potential carcinogenicity when activated by ultraviolet (UV) light.

TRADENAMES
In addition to generic and fixed combination preparations, the following tradenamed materials are available in the United States.
Zephiran, Ionax Scrub; benzalkonium chloride
Diaparene, methylbenzethonium chloride
Betadine, Isodine; povidone iodine
Clorpactin XCB, oxychlorosene
pHisoHex, Septisoft, hexachlorophene
Hibiclens, chlorhexidine gluconate
Cidex, glutaraldehyde

REFERENCES

Block SS: Disinfection, sterilization and preservation, ed 3, Philadelphia, 1983, Lea & Febiger.

Hugo WB, ed: Inhibition and destruction of the microbial cell, New York, 1971, Academic Press, Inc.

OTHER SYSTEMS AND SPECIAL TOPICS

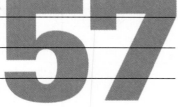

PART VIII

CHAPTER 57

Drugs Affecting Respiratory Function

ABBREVIATIONS

cAMP	cyclic adenosine monophosphate
cGMP	3′, 5′ cyclic guanosine monophosphate
$t_{1/2}$	half-life
IV	intravenous, intravenously
SC	subcutaneous, subcutaneously
COPD	chronic obstructive pulmonary disease
GI	gastrointestinal
FEV	force expiratory volume

MAJOR DRUGS

leukotrienes
cromolyn sodium
corticosteroids
β_2-agonists
theophylline
α-blockers
ipratropium bromide

THERAPEUTIC OVERVIEW

Asthma is characterized by increased responsiveness of the trachea and bronchi, to stimulation, which leads to widespread narrowing of the airways and reduced respiratory function. The severity of the reduction may be alleviated spontaneously or as a result of therapy. Reversible obstructive airway, bronchospastic, or hyperactive airway diseases are terms used interchangeably with asthma.

Asthma may also be thought of as an imbalance between the cholinergic and adrenergic branches of the autonomic nervous system, which leads to increased airway reactivity. Normal bronchial smooth muscle tone is controlled by vagal cholinergic innervation, and cholinergic activity or sensitivity is often increased in asthma. In addition, a large number of factors and suggested mediators of bronchial hyperreactivity and inflammation may initiate or aggravate bronchoconstriction.

Antihistamines have little clinical significance in the treatment of asthma, probably because histamine is not the primary mediator of bronchoconstriction in humans. Leukotriene D_4 is a potent bronchoconstrictors for humans. Compounds that block the synthesis of leukotrienes or block actions at the receptor for leukotrienes have great potential utility and are being tested as potential new drugs. Calcium channel blockers, including nifedipine and diltiazem (see Chapter 26), cause modest improvement in pulmonary function, and although unlikely to be useful for treatment of bronchospasm, they may be useful in comparison with β-adrenergic antagonists in the treatment of angina or hypertension in asthmatic patients.

The goals of asthma therapy are (1) rapid bronchodilation to improve respiratory function and (2) prevention of bronchoconstriction. The contributing factors to bronchoconstriction and the pharmacological approaches to therapy are summarized in the box.

CONTRIBUTING FACTORS TO BRONCHO-CONSTRICTION (ASTHMA)

Autonomic imbalance
  parasympathetic—irritant receptor response
  sympathetic—altered responsiveness
  nonspecific irritants—ozone, sulfur dioxide
Vasoactive/spasmogenic mediator release
  histamine
  platelet-activating factor
  prostaglandin D_2
  leukotrienes C_4, D_4, E_4
  adenosine
Chemoattractant release
  high-molecular-weight neutrophil chemotactic factor
  eosinophil chemotactic factors of anaphylaxis
  leukotriene B_4
  hydroxyeicosatetraenoic acid
  platelet-activating factor
  chemotactic factors (lymphocytes, monocytes, basophils)
Infection
Iatrogenic
  β-adrenergic blockers
  cholinesterase inhibitors
  prostaglandin synthetase inhibitors
Allergens
Environmental pollutants
Psychological
Respiratory heat loss (postexercise-induced)

Therapeutic Approaches

Use drugs to
  produce rapid bronchodilation
  prophylactally prevent bronchoconstriction
Reduce exposure to
  mediator-releasing agents
  iatrogenic agents

 MECHANISMS OF ACTION

The principal drugs and mechanisms of action are summarized in Table 57-1.

Cromolyn Sodium

Cromolyn sodium inhibits the degranulation of mast cells and prevents the release of mediators of

Table 57-1 Summary of Mechanisms of Action

Mechanism	Drugs
Increase cAMP	β-adrenergic agonists
	theophylline (?)
Antagonize adenosine	theophylline
Decrease cGMP	ipratroprium bromide
Prevent mediator release	cromolyn sodium
Block mediator effects	antihistamines
	leukotriene receptor antagonists
Multiple mechanisms	corticosteroids

bronchospasm, possibly by inhibiting cellular calcium fluxes (Figure 57-1).

However, the importance of the actions of cromolyn sodium in the prevention of bronchoconstriction has been recently questioned and alternative mechanisms have been proposed. Cromolyn sodium attenuates the ability of platelet activating factor to cause nonspecific airway hyperreactivity and increased vascular and epithelial permeability to macromolecules in bronchial tissue. This antiexudative action of cromolyn sodium may be central to its efficacy in preventing bronchospasm.

The drug has no bronchodilator activity per se. It is used only prophylactically and is most effective against extrinsic factor and exercise-induced asthma. Its structure is shown in Figure 57-2.

Corticosteroids

Prednisone and other antiinflammatory corticosteroids are the most effective antiasthmatic drugs available. The seriousness of their adverse effects, however, limits their use to the refractory cases of asthma. Corticosteroids have several actions important to their effects in asthma (see box) (for molecular mechanisms, see Chapter 33).

Corticosteroids increase the synthesis of macrocortin and lipomodulin, which inhibit the activity of phospholipase A_2, leading to inhibition of synthesis of leukotrienes, prostaglandins, and thromboxanes (see Chapter 28). A reduction in leukotriene B_4 interferes with leukocyte chemotaxis. Decreases in other leukotrienes, LC_4 and LD_4, are associated with reductions in bronchiolar smooth muscle contraction, vascular permeability, and airway mucus secretion.

Corticosteroids also restore the responsiveness of

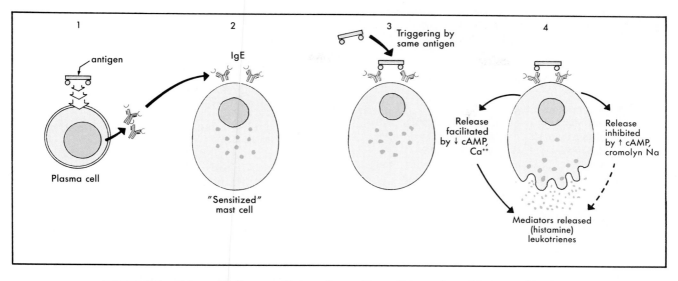

FIGURE 57-1   Schematic diagram of interactions with mediators released from sensitized mast cells in response to an allergen. Step 1, antigen stimulates plasma cells to produce IgE antibodies, which can then bind to mast cells (step 2), resulting in "sensitized" mast cells. Step 3, antigen can then bind to the IgE antibodies on the sensitized mast cells, which causes degranulation and mediator release (step 4).

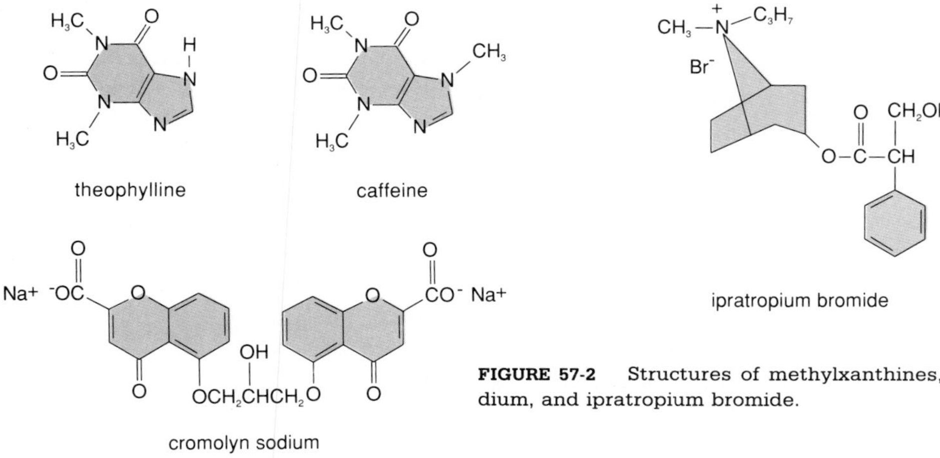

theophylline

caffeine

ipratropium bromide

cromolyn sodium

FIGURE 57-2   Structures of methylxanthines, cromolyn sodium, and ipratropium bromide.

leukocytes and bronchial smooth muscle to β-adrenergic agonists. This is an important effect because β_2-receptors tend to become refractory to β-agonists with prolonged exposure. Corticosteroids reduce the inflammatory component of asthma by the actions listed in the box, p. 770.

Theophylline

Theophylline is a methylxanthine, similar to caffeine (see Figure 57-2 for structures). For many years, it was generally accepted that theophylline caused bronchodilation by acting on smooth muscle cells to inhibit phosphodiesterase, which catalyzes the

MECHANISMS OF ACTION OF
CORTICOSTEROIDS

Increase synthesis and sensitivity of β-adrenergic re-
ceptors
Decreased mucosal edema
Decreased vascular permeability by vasoconstriction
Inhibition of cholinergic mechanisms and cyclic GMP
Inhibit the release of leukotrienes C_4 and D_4
Decreased late-phase inflammatory response (inhi-
bition of leukotriene B_4?)
Monocytes, eosinophils, and lymphocytes leave cir-
culation
Neutrophils reenter the circulation

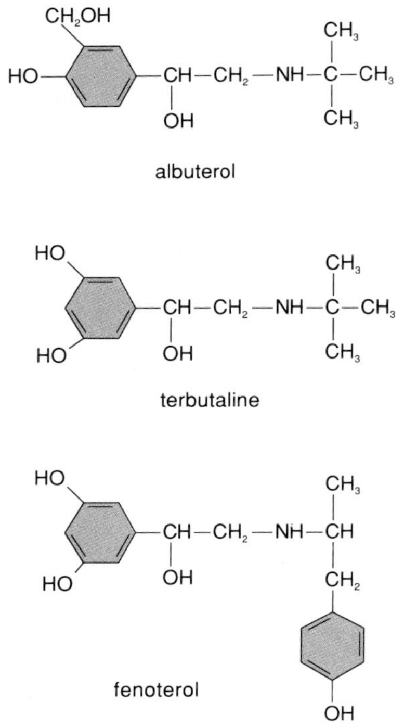

FIGURE 57-3   Structures of β-adrenergic agonists. Increased
$β_2$ selectivity requires a large substituent on the amino group,
and ring hydroxyl groups in the 3 and 5 positions confer
increased $β_2$ selectivity. Lack of one or both of the 3 and 4
hydroxyl groups increases oral bioavailability. Alternatively,
modification of the 3-OH as with albuterol increases $β_2$ selectivity and oral bioavailability. (See Chapter 10 for structures of epinephrine, isoproterenol, and metaproterenol.)

breakdown of cAMP. It is accepted that an increase
in cAMP leads to bronchodilation; however, the clinical significance of the phosphodiesterase inhibition
mechanism is doubtful, because the concentrations
required to inhibit this enzyme exceed those achieved
with usual doses of theophylline.

Theophylline is an adenosine antagonist in bronchial smooth muscle and in other tissues. Inhalation
of adenosine causes bronchoconstriction in patients
with asthma but does not affect people who do not
have asthma. It also causes contraction of isolated
airway smooth muscle and an increase in histamine
release from lung cells. This proposed mechanism,
however, does not explain why enprofylline, another
xanthine derivative but without adenosine antagonistic properties, is a more potent bronchodilator than
theophylline.

It has also been proposed that theophylline may
act by altering intracellular calcium transport, but
there is limited evidence for this mechanism at present. Thus, the molecular mechanism of action of theophylline remains unclear.

β-Adrenergic Agonists

The molecular mechanism of action of $β_2$ agonists
is well established (see Chapters 8 and 10). Interaction
of the agonists with $β_2$-receptors causes activation of
adenylate cyclase, resulting in increased cAMP and
bronchodilation. The molecular sequence of events
whereby elevated cAMP results in relaxation of bronchial smooth muscles is discussed in Chapters 8 and

10. The structural chemistry and functional groups
that lead to increased $β_2$ selectivity are illustrated in
Figure 57-3.

Anticholinergic Drugs

For centuries, stramonium and belladonna alkaloids have been smoked as a treatment for asthma.
Atropine has good bronchodilator properties but its
clinical use is limited by its systemic toxicity. Recently, ipratropium bromide, a quaternary isopropyl
derivative of atropine (see Figure 57-2) has proven to
be an effective bronchodilator with little systemic toxicity when given as an aerosol. This is due to its low
lipid solubility and poor absorption across biological
membranes.

The importance of vagal innervation of bronchial

Table 57-2   Pharmacokinetic Parameter Values for Bronchodilators

Drug	Administration	Absorption	$t_{1/2}$ (hr)	Disposition
theophylline	Oral, SC, IV	Good	8.7 (see text)	B (50%) R (10%) M
ipatropium bromide	IV, inhalation	Poor	3	In feces
cromolyn sodium	Inhalation, IV	Poor	1.3	R (60%) B
terbutaline	Oral, SC	Fair (50%)	3-4	M (60%) R
albuterol	Oral, inhalation	Good	4-5	M (60%) R (30%)

B, Biliary excretion; *M*, metabolized; *R*, renal excretion as unchanged drug.

smooth muscle is well established. Since the degree of cholinergic hyperreactivity in people with asthma is variable, the response to ipratropium bromide is also variable.

Ipratropium bromide antagonizes muscarinic receptors in bronchial smooth muscle, which leads to decreased concentrations of cGMP and resultant bronchodilation. Ipratropium bromide may also prevent mast cell degranulation through a similar mechanism. The molecular sequence of events whereby decreased cGMP results in relaxation of bronchial smooth muscle is discussed in Chapters 8 and 10.

 PHARMACOKINETICS

The pharmacokinetic parameter values for the bronchodilator drugs are summarized in Table 57-2.

Theophylline is well absorbed from the gastrointestinal (GI) tract and completely metabolized to inactive compounds in the liver. Its rate of hepatic metabolism is dose dependent and thus may deviate from first order kinetics at high serum concentrations. The wide degree of variability in theophylline clearance is attributed to a number of variables, listed in Table 57-3. The volume of distribution is relatively constant at 0.5 L/kg of body weight. The mean disappearance half-life varies from 8.7 hours in adults who do not smoke to 5.5 hours in people who smoke and 3.7 hours in children. Premature infants have a ninefold increase in half-life. The development of timed-release preparations of theophylline with half-lives of 8 to 24 hours aids theophylline therapeutics

Table 57-3   Factors Influencing the Clearance of Theophylline

	Increased	Decreased
Cigarette smoking	+	
Diet		
Charcoal broiled meat	+	
High carbohydrate		+
High protein	+	
Methylxanthines		+
Drugs		
cimetidine		+
erythromycin		+
phenobarbital	+	
Age		
Neonates		+
Children (1-16 yr)	+	
Elderly (>65 yr)		+
Disease state		
Hepatic disease		+
Congestive heart failure		+
Pulmonary edema		+
COPD		+
Acute viral illness		+

by improving patient compliance and preventing nocturnal dyspnea.

Monitoring of serum concentrations of theophylline is necessary, since the range of safe therapeutic concentrations is narrow, the interindividual variability in clearance is large, and the drug has significant dose-related toxicity. The degree to which age, other drugs, and disease states alter theophylline clearance is not predictable.

Table 57-4   Properties of β-Adrenergic Bronchodilators

Drug	β₂ Selectivity	Onset of Action (min)	Peak Effect (hr)	Duration of Effect (hr)
albuterol	+ + + +			
Inhalation		5-15	0.5-1	3-6
Oral		15-30	2-3	8
bitolterol	+ + + +			
Inhalation		3-4	0.5-1	5-8
epinephrine	0			
Inhalation		3-5	—	1-1.5
Subcutaneous		6-15	0.3	<1-4
isoetharine	+ +			
Inhalation		1-6	0.25-1	2-3
isoproterenol	0			
Inhalation		2-5	—	1-2
metaproterenol	+ + +			
Inhalation		<1	1	1-2.5
Oral		15-30	1	<4
terbutaline	+ + + +			
Inhalation		15-30	1-2	3-6
Oral		<60-120	<2-3	4-8
Parenteral		<15	<0.5-1	1.5-4

After inhalation, only about 10% of cromolyn sodium is systemically absorbed via the lungs and GI tract and apparently does not cause systemic effects. The duration of action is 4 to 6 hours. Like cromolyn sodium, ipratropium bromide is poorly absorbed and has few systemic effects. The peak effect occurs in 1 to 2 hours after inhalation, with a duration effect of 3 to 5 hours.

Since a quick onset of action is desired with bronchodilators, some of the time factors for the onset and duration with the β-adrenergic bronchodilators are summarized in Table 57-4.

Pharmacokinetic values for the corticosteroids are given in Chapter 35.

RELATION OF MECHANISMS OF ACTION TO CLINICAL RESPONSE

Theophylline

Several actions of theophylline contribute to its beneficial pulmonary effects in bronchospastic disease (see box). It relaxes bronchial smooth muscle and thus dilates both large and small airways. This effect appears to be relatively independent of the initiator of bronchoconstriction. Mucociliary clearance is improved, which may be, in part, a consequence of bronchodilation. In addition, theophylline increases the contractility of the diaphragm and its resistance to fatigue. Caffeine also has bronchodilator activity, with doses of 100 to 200 mg that may be consumed in 1 to 3 cups of brewed coffee, causing modest increases in pulmonary function.

The methylxanthines also have several cardiovascular effects. Theophylline has a positive inotropic effect and causes arteriolar and venular dilation. The increased cardiac output and vasodilation of the efferent arterioles of the kidney contribute to an increased rate of glomerular filtration and a brief diuresis. The diuresis, positive inotropic effect, and reduction in ventricular afterload contribute to the enhanced cardiovascular performance in patients with chronic obstructive pulmonary disease (COPD) after oral or intravenous theophylline.

The central nervous system (CNS) stimulation caused by methylxanthines is due to their ability to antagonize adenosine receptors. Caffeine is a more potent central nervous system stimulant than theophylline. At oral doses of 50 to 200 mg, caffeine causes cortical stimulation, increases alertness, and improves psychomotor performance in most individuals. Headache, anxiety, irritability, and insomnia may also occur.

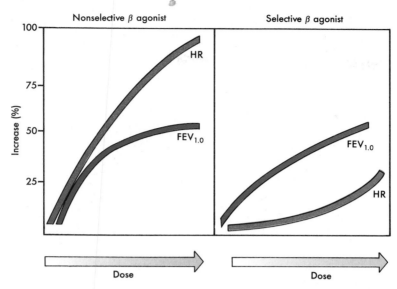

FIGURE 57-4   Dose-response curves for a nonselective and selective (i.e., albuterol) β-agonist bronchodilator. Response defined as increase in forced expiratory volume at 1 second (FEV$_{1.0}$) or increase in heart rate *(HR)*.

PHARMACOLOGIC EFFECTS OF THEOPHYLLINE

RESPIRATORY

Bronchial smooth muscle relaxation
Increased vital capacity
Increased mucociliary clearance
Increased diaphragmatic contractility and decreased fatigue

CARDIOVASCULAR

Increased heart rate
Increased ventricular ejection fractions
Decreased pulmonary artery pressure
Decreased right and left ventricular end-diastolic pressure
Decreased stroke work
Peripheral vasodilation

GASTROINTESTINAL

Increased gastric acid secretion

RENAL

Diuresis

CENTRAL NERVOUS SYSTEM

Mild cortical arousal, leading to increased alertness and deferral of fatigue
Stimulation of medullary respiratory centers
Decreased seizure threshold

β-Agonists

The pharmacological actions of the β-agonists are discussed in Chapters 8 and 10. Bronchodilation is the primary action of interest in treating asthma. Stimulation of β$_2$-receptors in skeletal muscle causes tremor and may limit dosage, but β$_2$-receptor stimulation also causes relaxation of vascular and uterine smooth muscle. Importantly, the β$_2$ selectivity of albuterol, terbutaline, and metaproterenol is only relative. Figure 57-4 illustrates that as the dose of a selective β_2-agonist such as albuterol is increased, its β_2-receptor selectivity is lost, as reflected by an increase in heart rate (which responds mainly to β_1-receptors).

SIDE EFFECTS, CLINICAL PROBLEMS, AND TOXICITY

The clinical problems with the bronchodilator drugs are summarized in the box.

Methylxanthines

Theophylline frequently causes heartburn, nausea, vomiting, epigastric pain, and CNS stimulation (irritability, insomnia, tremor). These effects may occur at subtherapeutic or therapeutic plasma concentrations and may necessitate termination of therapy. As plasma concentrations of theophylline increase above 15 to 20 μg/ml, the frequency and severity of these effects increase markedly. Tachycardia, fever, and hematemesis may occur as well. Seizures and cardiac dysrhythmias may occur and are life-threatening. Seizures may occur in the absence of other evidence of toxicity and have a reported mortality rate of 50%. Seizures and dysrhythmias are increasingly likely at plasma concentrations greater than 35 μg/ml. Ventricular dysrhythmias usually respond to lidocaine. Theophylline is considered safe in pregnancy.

In large doses, methylxanthines act at the medullary respiratory center to stimulate respiration. Theophylline is used for this effect in neonatal apnea and Cheyne-Stokes respiration, but the possibility of seizures must also be considered. The xanthines also increase the volume and acidity of gastric secretions and reduce lower esophageal sphincter tone, therefore theophylline and caffeine can exacerbate peptic ulcer disease.

β_2-Agonists

Skeletal muscle tremor is the most common side effect of the selective β_2-agonists. It may be severe enough to limit use in patients, but some tolerance develops with continued use. Tremor, anxiety, restlessness, tachycardia, and palpitations are much more likely with oral administration of the β_2-agonists. The cardiac toxicity of tachycardia, palpitations, exacerbation of angina pectoris, and dysrhythmias limit

CLINICAL PROBLEMS
theophylline
Narrow therapeutic index
Nausea, vomiting
Seizures
Cardiac dysrhythmias
β_2-agonists (terbutaline, albuterol)
Tachycardia
Tremors
cromolyn sodium
Throat irritation
Coughing
Bronchospasm
ipratropium bromide
Dry mouth

the use of parenteral and inhaled epinephrine and isoproterenol to urgent situations. All of these drugs may cause hypokalemia.

Tachyphylaxis, as reflected by subsensitivity of β_2-receptors, may develop with continued use but there is little evidence that it is of major clinical significance, although administration of corticosteroids can be used to increase the responsiveness of β_2-receptors. The cardiac effects of the agonists may be more pronounced in hyperthyroid patients.

Epinephrine and isoproterenol should be avoided in patients taking monoamine oxidase inhibitors because of the risk of a pressor response.

Cromolyn Sodium

Cromolyn sodium is relatively nontoxic, but its inhalation may cause throat irritation, coughing, and occasional bronchospasm. Inhalation of a β_2-agonist before administration of cromolyn sodium can prevent the bronchospasm. Dermatitis, gastroenteritis, and myositis may also develop (see also Chapter 58).

Corticosteroids

The adverse effects of systemic corticosteroids limit their use and are described in Chapter 33. Metered-dose inhaler preparations of corticosteroids (e.g., beclomethasone dipropionate) is a major advance, with the only significant side effects being oropharyngeal candidiasis, dysphonia, coughing, and wheezing.

Ipratropium Bromide

The common adverse effect of inhaled ipratropium bromide is local drying in the mouth and upper airways. Typical systemic atropine-like side effects occur infrequently.

Problems in Asthma Treatment

Clinical problems of asthma include occasional episodes of coughing and wheezing, the need for maintenance therapy, and severe asthmatic episodes. The occasional asthmatic attack may be managed with a β_2 agonist inhaler. Particularly when such episodes are triggered by cold, exercise, or exposure to a specific allergen such as animal dander, use of cromolyn sodium before exposure can be very effective. A combination of a β_2 inhaler and sodium cromolyn may give increased efficacy, and using the β_2 drug first can prevent bronchospasm occasionally induced by cromolyn sodium.

Several options are available when maintenance therapy is required. Regular use of β_2 agonist inhaler and/or cromolyn sodium may be sufficient. Because of the more pronounced systemic effects of the oral forms of the selective β_2 agonists, their application is limited to patients who cannot use or tolerate aerosol preparations. Maintenance therapy with theophylline is common, especially when using combinations of submaximal doses of theophylline with terbutaline or albuterol. This combination produces equivalent bronchodilation with fewer side effects compared to using maximal doses of both. Severe chronic refractory asthma requires the use of oral cortico steroids. Alternate day therapy with prednisone may reduce steroid side effects but often is not effective.

The role of bronchodilators in the treatment of chronic bronchitis and emphysema is not defined. The benefit of theophylline appears related to the degree of reversibility of the airway disease. The ability of theophylline to increase contractility, decrease fatigue of the diaphragm, and increase mucociliary

---

TRADENAMES

In addition to generic and fixed combination preparations, the following tradenamed materials are available in the United States.

Atrovent; ipratropium bromide
β-Agonists
  Alupent, Metaprel; metaproterenol
  Brethine, Bricanyl, Brethaire; terbutaline sulfate
  Proventil, Ventolin; albuterol sulfate
  Tornalate, bitolterol mesylate
Corticosteroids
  AeroBid, Nasalide; flunisolide
  Azmacort, triamcinolone
  Beclovent, Vanceril; beclomethasone dipropionate
Intal, Nasalcrom, Opticrom; cromolyn sodium
Theobid, Theo-Dur, Slo-phyllin, Theolair, Aerolate, Uniphyl, Theovent; theophylline (some)

---

clearance may be beneficial in the treatment of COPD. However, patients with this disease are more susceptible than patients with asthma to the toxic cardiovascular effects of theophylline.

REFERENCES

Gross NJ: Ipratropium bromide, N Engl J Med 319:486, 1988.

Hendeles L and Weinberger M: Selection of a slow-release theophylline product, J Allergy Clin Immunol 78:743, 1986.

Holgate ST, Mann JS, and Cushley MJ: Adenosine as a bronchoconstrictor mediator in asthma and its antagonism by methylxanthines, J Allergy Clin Immunol 74:302, 1984.

Jonkman JHG: Therapeutic consequences of drug interactions with theophylline pharmacokinetics, J Allergy Clin Immunol 78:736, 1986.

Kaliner M: Mast cell mediators and asthma, Chest 87:25, 1985.

Persson CGA: Overview of effects of theophylline, J Allergy Clin Immunol 78:780, 1986.

Spector S: The use of corticosteroids in the treatment of asthma, Chest 87:735, 1985.

CHAPTER 58

Histamine and Antihistamines

ABBREVIATIONS	
IgE	immunoglobulin E
AV	atrioventricular
MAO	monoamine oxidase
BAL	bronchoalveolar lavage-derived mast cells
FMLP	N-formyl-methionylleucylphenylalanine
SRS-A	slow reacting substance of anaphylaxis

THERAPEUTIC OVERVIEW

Histamine is an endogenous compound that is synthesized, stored, and released primarily by mast cells and after release exerts profound effects on many tissues and organs. It is one of the cellular mediators of the immediate hypersensitivity reaction and the acute inflammatory response, as well as a primary stimulant of gastric acid secretion. A central neurotransmitter role for histamine has been recently proposed.

These actions of histamine preclude its use as a drug. Its importance in medicine and pharmacology lies in its pathophysiological actions, the therapeutic usefulness of drugs that prevent its release from mast cells, and drugs that block the receptors that mediate the actions of histamine.

Because the actions of histamine have considerable species variation, it is difficult to extrapolate results from studies on experimental animals to humans. Most of this discussion is based on the results of studies with human volunteers or with organs and tissues obtained from human subjects.

The experimental IV administration of histamine to human volunteers produces dose-related effects primarily in heart, vascular and extravascular smooth muscle, and secretion of the gastric mucosa. The actions of histamine are mediated by at least 3 distinct receptors, H_1, H_2, and H_3. Of these the receptors H_1 and H_2 are the best characterized and mediate well defined responses in humans. A summary of some of the actions of histamine that are mediated by H_1-receptors and H_2-receptors is given in Table 58-1.

Responses such as bronchoconstriction are mediated by H_1-receptors and are selectively antagonized by classical antihistamines such as diphenhydramine. Responses such as facial cutaneous vasodilation and gastric acid secretion are mediated by H_2-receptors and are selectively antagonized by agents such as cimetidine or ranitidine.

The H_3-receptor has been studied only in experimental animals. This receptor is found on nerve endings and mediates inhibition of neurotransmitter release. This applies to the release of histamine from histamine-containing nerves in the central nervous system (CNS) and the release of acetylcholine from the myenteric plexus.

MECHANISMS OF ACTION

Action of Histamine

The structure of histamine is shown in Figure 58-1. The mechanism of signal transduction by histamine at receptors H_1 and H_2 differs. The contractile actions on smooth muscle and the neuronal actions that are mediated by H_1-receptors result from stimulation of the breakdown of inositol phospholipids.

Table 58-1   Selected Actions of Histamine in Humans

Organ/Tissue	Action	Receptor
Cardiovascular		
Vascular	Decrease in total peripheral resistance	H_1 and H_2
Facial cutaneous	Vasodilation	H_2
Forearm	Increased blood flow	H_1 and H_2
Gastric mucosa	Increased blood flow	H_2 (?)
Carotid artery	Relaxation	H_2
Basilar artery	Constriction	H_1
Pulmonary artery	Relaxation	H_2
	Constriction	H_1
Coronary artery	Constriction	H_1
Postcapillary venules	Increased permeability	H_1
Heart	Increased sinoatrial rate	H_2
	Increased force of contraction	H_2
	Increased atrial and ventricular automaticity	H_2
Respiratory		
Bronchiolar smooth muscle	Contraction	H_1
	Relaxation (?)	H_2 (?)
Gastrointestinal		
Oxyntic mucosa	Acid and pepsin secretion	H_2
Gastrointestinal smooth muscle	Relaxation and contraction	H_1
Gall bladder smooth muscle	Contraction	H_1
	Relaxation (?)	H_2 (?)
Cutaneous nerve endings	Pain and itching	H_1 and H_2 (?)
Adrenal medulla	Epinephrine secretion	H_1
Basophils	Inhibition of IgE-dependent degranulation	H_2

These actions have been demonstrated in human volunteers or in organs or tissues obtained from human subjects. (?) means that the response was not uniformly observed or the receptor mediating the response was not well characterized.

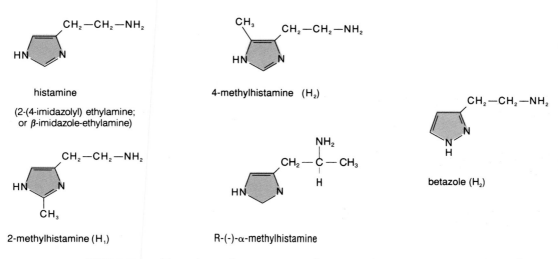

FIGURE 58-1   Histamine and some agonists (with specific receptor indicated).

However, the stimulus-response mechanism for the H_1-receptor–mediated relaxation of vascular smooth muscle is not known. Some experimental evidence suggests that the relaxant actions of histamine are indirect and may involve the synthesis and release of relaxant factor derived from endothelium.

The actions of histamine that are mediated by H_2-receptors may be due to the activation of adenylate cyclase. This occurs in H_2-receptor systems that mediate acid secretion, relaxation of vascular smooth muscle, neuronal excitation, inhibition of basophil degranulation, and increases in myocardial contractility. Such action may include H_2-receptors located at other sites.

Synthesis and Metabolism of Histamine

Histamine is synthesized in vivo by decarboxylation of the amino acid L-histidine, catalyzed by the pyridoxal phosphate-dependent enzyme, L-histidine decarboxylase (Figure 58-2). Most of the histamine in tissues is stored in an inert form at the site of synthesis. Very little preformed histamine exists in a freely diffusible form. When histamine is released from its storage site, it becomes active but is rapidly converted to inactive metabolites.

Two primary pathways exist for the catabolism of histamine (Figure 58-2). The oxidative deamination path is catalyzed by diamine oxidase and leads to the formation of imidazole acetic acid. The second path involves methylation of the telenitrogen in the imidazole ring catalyzed by histamine-N-methyl transferase and results in the formation of N methyl-histamine. As shown in Figure 58-2, these primary metabolites are subject to further metabolism. In the periphery, both pathways contribute to the metabolism of histamine, but in the CNS, the methylation pathway predominates.

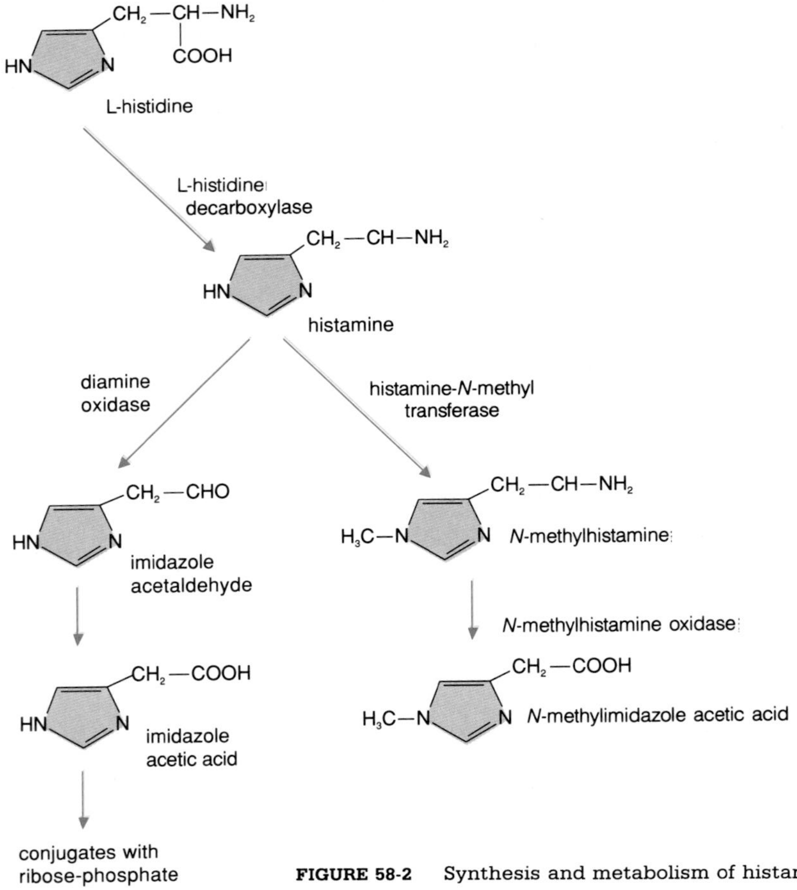

FIGURE 58-2   Synthesis and metabolism of histamine.

Storage and Release of Histamine by Mast Cells and Basophils

The major sites of histamine storage and release are mast cells. Other sites include basophils and neurons in the CNS and cells not fully characterized.

Histamine is distributed throughout the body, indicating that the sites of synthesis and storage also are widely distributed. However, the greatest concentrations of histamine occur in the skin, lungs, and gastrointestinal (GI) mucosa.

Basophils and mast cells are similar in that both have high affinity IgE binding sites on their plasma membranes and both store histamine in secretory granules. Mast cells are heterogenous and can be classified on the basis of staining properties, anatomical localization, or susceptibility to degranulation induced by a polyamine, *compound 48/80*. The anatomical classification is commonly used; the cells are donoted as *mucosal* or *connective tissue* mast cells. However, mixed populations of mast cells are in both anatomic locations, and additional heterogeneity exists within the two major classes of mast cells. Human mast cells differ with respect to the structure of the heparin proteoglycan in storage granules, the type of proteoglycan, the types of neutral serine proteases in the storage granules, the relative amounts of prostanoids and leukotrienes that are synthesized and released on degranulation, and the inhibition of antigen-induced degranulation by cromolyn sodium. Properties of mast cells isolated from human tissues are shown in Table 58-2.

Histamine exists in mast cell granules as an ionic complex with a proteoglycan, chiefly heparan sulfate, but also chondroitin sulfate E. Histamine in basophils also is stored in granules as an ionic complex, predominantly with the proteoglycan chondroitin monosulfate. The release of histamine and many other mediators from mast cells and basophils is common during allergic disorders but also can be induced by drugs and endogenous polypeptides to produce pseudoallergic reactions. This is shown schematically in Figure 58-3. The participation of mast cells in the immediate and delayed hypersensitivity reactions, as well as possible participation of mast cells in the pathology of nonallergic disorders, provides the therapeutic rationale for the use of agents that antagonize histamine and agents that prevent mast cell degranulation.

The release of histamine from mast cells and basophils occurs by two general processes of degranulation: noncytolytic and cytolytic. The cytolytic release of histamine from mast cells occurs when the plasma membrane is damaged. This type of release is energy-independent, does not require intracellular Ca^{++}, and is accompanied by the leakage of cytoplasmic contents. Cytolytic release can be induced by a variety of substances, including phenothiazines, histamine H_1-antagonists, and some of the narcotic analgesics. The concentrations of these agents that are required to produce a cytolytic release are in considerable excess over those required for therapeutic effects.

Table 58-2   Some Properties of Isolated Human Mast Cells and Basophils

Tissue of Origin	Mast Cell Type	Histamine Release Evoked by			Inhibition of IgE-dependent Release by			IgE-dependent Release of	
		48/80	Morphine	FMLP	Cromolyn	Theophylline	β-Agonists	PGD$_2$	LTC$_4$
Skin	CT	+ + + +	+ + +	−	−	+	+ + + +	+ + +	+
Lung									
Parenchyma	M	−	−	−	+	+	+ + + +	+ + +	+ + +
BAL	M	−			+ + +	+	+ + + +	+ + +	+ + +
Intestinal mucosa	M	−	−	−	+	+	+ + + +	+ +	+ + +
Basophils		−	−	+ + +	−	+	+ + + +	−	+ + +

BAL, Bronchoalveolar lavage-derived mast cells; *CT*, connective tissue; *M*, mucosal; *FMLP*, N-formyl-methionylleucylphenylalanine (a chemotactic tripeptide). The intensity of the event is given qualitatively, (−) for no response to (+ + + +) for a marked response. PGD$_2$ is a prostaglandin (see Chapter 18) and LTC$_4$ is a leukotriene. Effect of theophylline refers to clinically nontoxic plasma concentrations.

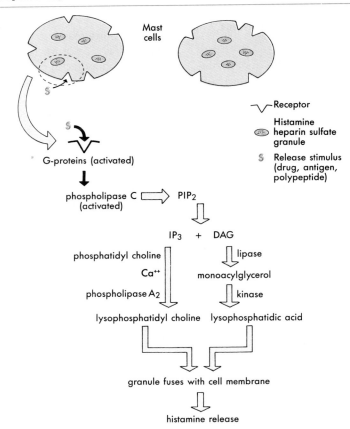

FIGURE 58-3   Release of histamine from mast cells. PIP_2 is phosphatidylinositol-4,5-bis-phosphate; IP_3 is inositol 1,4,5-tris-phosphate; DAG is 1,2-diacylglycerol. (See Figure 58-4 and Chapter 2 for more details.)

Noncytolytic release can be induced by a variety of compounds. It is generally thought, though not unequivocally established, that noncytolytic release is evoked as a consequence of specific binding of a ligand to a receptor in the plasma membrane of the mast cell or basophil. In contrast to cytolytic release, noncytolytic release requires ATP for energy, depends on changes in free intracellular Ca^{++}, and is not accompanied by leakage of cytoplasmic contents. Noncytolytic release is characterized by exocytosis of the secretory granules. The classical example is the degranulation of sensitized mast cells or basophils induced by cross-bridging adjacent IgE molecules bound on the membrane surface of the cell. The cascade of biochemical events that begins with the interaction of antigen and IgE molecules and culminates in the degranulation of human mast cells and

basophils is summarized in Figure 58-4. In addition to histamine, other constituents of the storage granules are released. These include heparin, eosinophil and neutrophil chemotactic factors, neutral protease, and other enzymes. Also newly synthesized mediators such as prostaglandin D_2, leukotriene C_4 and D_4 (SRS-A, slow reacting substance of anaphylaxis), leukotriene B_4, and platelet activating factor are released.

Noncytolytic release also is produced by nonimmune mechanisms. A variety of agents can produce degranulation independently, without prior exposure. In general, such histamine liberators are basic in nature. Examples of polybasic substances are the polyamine 48/80 and basic polypeptides such as bradykinin, substance P, N-formyl-methionylleucylphenylalanine, protamine, the anaphylatoxins (C3a, C4a, and C5a), and the mast cell degranulating pro-

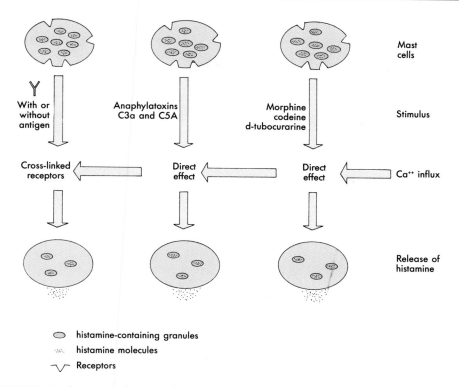

○ histamine-containing granules

histamine molecules

‿‿‿ Receptors

FIGURE 58-4   Summary of mast cell release of histamine. Some stimuli act indirectly through F_c receptors and some act directly on mast cells.

tein present in bee venom. With the exception of protamine, a heparin antagonist, none of these agents has any therapeutic use. Compound 48/80 is used extensively in experimental studies on mast cells. The remaining agents listed may be pathological stimuli for mast cell and basophil degranulation.

Noncytolytic degranulation can be induced by several drugs, including *d*-tubocurarine, heroin, morphine and codeine, doxorubicin, and guanethidine.

Histamine release in vivo may also be produced by some plasma expanders, notably those based on cross-linked gelatin, and by radiocontrast media, especially those of high osmotic strength. The mechanism of release is not elucidated, but is thought to occur via degranulation.

The receptors mediating the noncytolytic degranulation induced by the paucibasic agents have not been characterized. These receptors are not the ones associated with the desired therapeutic actions of these drugs. In general, problems with histamine release by these drugs occur readily after IV adminis-

tration of the drugs. Usually, this does not result in a serious pseudoallergic reaction; however, serious life-threatening reactions can occur.

Inhibitors of Mast Cell and Basophil Histamine Release/Degranulation

Because many mediators are released from mast cells and basophils during noncytolytic degranulation, agents that can prevent the degranulation reaction and subsequent release of mediators are of therapeutic value.

Drugs that inhibit mast cell and basophil degranulation are used in the treatment of reversible bronchospastic disorders (see Chapter 55). Methylxanthines, such as theophylline, and β_2-selective agonists, such as albuterol, can inhibit the degranulation of mast cells and basophils. Both classes of drugs do so by increasing intracellular concentrations of cAMP; methylxanthines possibly by inhibition of phosphodiesterase, and β_2-selective agonists by activation of adenylate cyclase. The ability to produce bronchodilation and stabilize mast cells may contribute to the actions of β_2-selective agonists. However, for the methylxanthines, bronchodilation is their major action rather than stabilization of mast cells. The concentrations of theophylline required to inhibit degranulation correspond to plasma concentrations usually associated with systemic toxicity.

Only one agent, cromolyn sodium (see Chapter 55 for structure), has stabilization of mast cells and prevention of noncytolytic degranulation as its primary action.

The mechanism by which cromolyn prevents noncytolytic mast cell degranulation is not known. Cromolyn has no effect on binding of IgE or the interaction between bound IgE and antigen. Nor does it have any effect on the binding of nonimmunological agents that produce degranulation. Its action occurs independently of changes in the cellular content of cAMP (discussed in Chapter 55).

Histamine H₁-Receptor Antagonists

Agents referred to as antihistaminics are those that antagonize the actions of histamine mediated by H_1-receptors. Agents referred to as histaminics stimulate gastric acid secretion and blushing that are mediated by the H_2-receptor.

Before the advent of selective antagonists for the H_1-receptor, histamine was thought to be the primary mediator of immediate hypersensitivity reactions. Although the early H_1-antagonists blocked the histamine-induced hypotension and bronchoconstriction, they were not very effective in histamine-induced anaphylaxis. The clinical ineffectiveness of the older and the current H_1-antagonists to control anaphylaxis is due in part to the lipid mediators released during mast cell degranulation that are the primary cause of hypotension and bronchoconstriction.

The present histamine H_1-antagonists have little structural resemblance to histamine (see Figures 58-1 and 58-5 for structures). A common structural

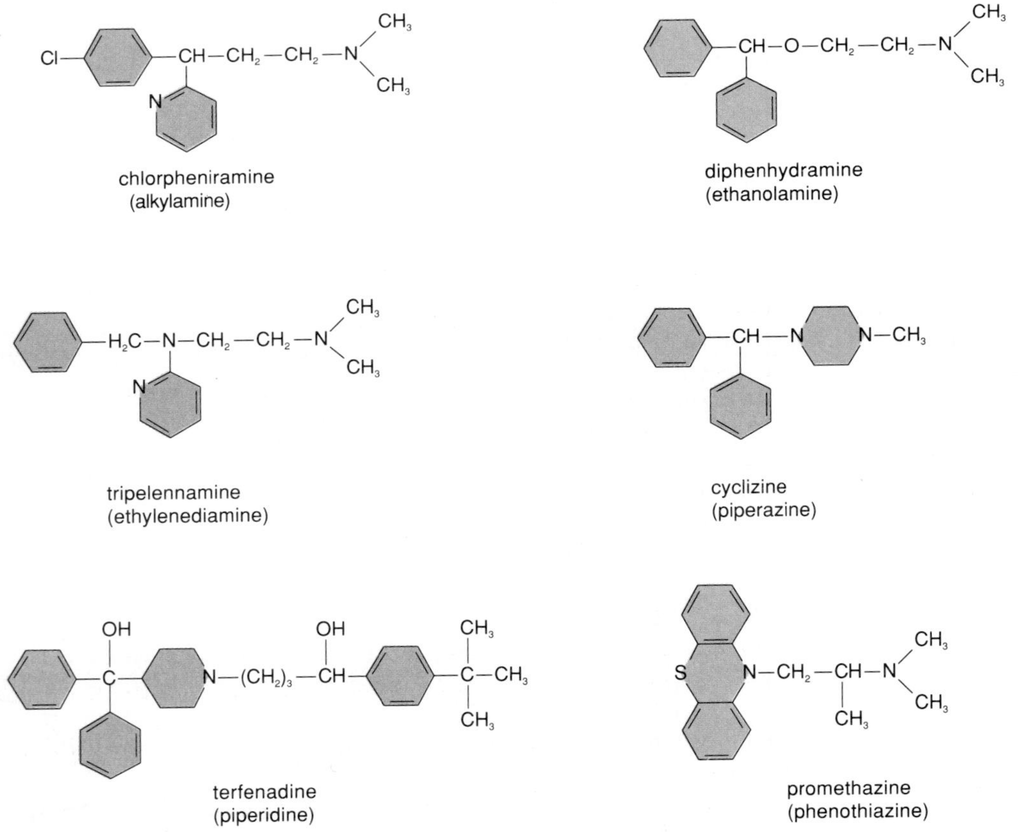

FIGURE 58-5   Some histamine H₁-receptor antagonists with chemical classification.

feature is a substituted ethylamine containing a nitrogen atom in an alkyl chain or a ring.

These agents are usually classified according to the chemical group containing the substituted ethylamine. The groups and representative drugs are alkylamine (chlorpheniramine), ethanolamine (diphenhydramine), ethylenediamine (tripelennamine), piperazine (cyclizine), piperidine (terfenadine), and phenothiazine (promethazine). In addition, there are other compounds that exhibit antihistamine activity.

The antihistamines act via competitive antagonism of histamine at H_1-receptors with the exception of terfenadine and astemizole, which act in a noncompetitive (i.e., insurmountable by added agonist) manner. Thus the ability of most of these agents to antagonize endogenously released histamine depends on the local concentration of histamine and that of the antagonists. The latter is limited by adverse effects of the antagonists from actions at other receptors. However, these non-H_1-receptor−actions may contribute to the limited usefulness of these agents in the treatment of allergic disorders.

Many of the actions of these antagonists are due to blockade of histamine H_1-receptors and are predictable based on the actions of histamine mediated by H_1-receptors. Differences are the result of pharmacokinetic properties that govern tissue distribution and duration of action and to actions at sites other than the H_1-receptor. In addition to blocking H_1-receptors, all of these agents exhibit weak to marked blockade at muscarinic receptors, and some block additional receptors. For example, cyproheptadine is a fairly potent antagonist of serotonin, and promethazine exhibits weak α-adrenergic receptor and moderate dopamine D_2-receptor blocking. Terfenadine and astemizole differ in that, at therapeutic doses, they exhibit very little blocking activity at sites other than the H_1-receptor.

Histamine H_2-Receptor Antagonists

The mechanism of action of these drugs to inhibit gastric acid secretion is also discussed in Chapter 59. The histamine H_2-receptor antagonists revolutionized the medical management of peptic ulcer disease. It was known for many years that the conventional H_1-receptor antagonists did not significantly inhibit histamine-induced gastric acid secretion. A deliberate effort was therefore made to develop drugs that would block parietal cell histamine receptors and provide a new approach to pharmacological regulation of acid secretion. The primary approach was systematic modification of the histamine molecule to generate H_2-receptor−selective antagonists. Whereas the H_1-receptor antagonists do not require a histamine-like nucleus, an imidazole-like nucleus is required for recognition by H_2-receptors. However, the histamine imidazole ring can exist in two tautomeric forms, only one of which is recognized by the H_2-receptor. Addition of 4-methyl (see Figure 58-1) substitution provided the appropriate tautomer for recognition, and 4-methylhistamine is relatively selective as an agonist at the histamine H_2-receptor. Side-chain substitution led to the therapeutically useful antagonist, cimetidine. Recently introduced H_2-receptor antagonists contain furan or thiazol rings (see structures in Chapter 59).

The H_2-receptor antagonists inhibit food-, gastrin-, and acetylcholine-induced gastric secretion of acid, as well as acid secretion induced by histamine. As expected, the H_2-receptor antagonists are especially effective in blocking the secretory effects of histamine or selective H_2-receptor agonists.

PHARMACOKINETICS

Pharmacokinetic parameter values for the H_1-receptor antagonists are given in Table 58-3. Values for cromolyn sodium are in Chapter 55 and values for H_2-receptor antagonists are in Chapter 59. For a discussion of cromolyn sodium pharmacokinetics, see Chapter 57.

H_1-Antagonists

The H_1-antagonists are well absorbed after oral administration and have onsets of action of about 30 minutes to an hour. Most have durations of action between 3 to 6 hours in adults. Notable exceptions are astemizole, which has an active metabolite with a half-life of about 100 hours. Other exceptions are meclizine with a duration of 12 to 24 hours, and terfenadine and mequitazine with durations of 12 hours. The ability of most antihistamines to block the triple response after intradermal injection of antigens or histamine can persist for 1 to 2 days after cessation of therapy.

There are two subclasses of these agents with respect to body distribution. The older antihistamines distribute throughout the body and readily penetrate

Table 58-3 Pharmacokinetic Parameter Values for H_1-Receptor

Drug	Administered	Absorbed	$t_{1/2}$ (hr)	Disposition
chlorpheniramine	Oral	Good	20	M
diphenhydramine	Oral	Good	4-8	M
tripelennamine	Oral	Good	—	M
cyclizine	Oral	Good	7-24	M
terfenadine	Oral	Good	16-22	M
promethazine	Oral	Good	7-15	M
astemizole	Oral	Good	24	M

M, Metabolized.

the CNS. Agents recently introduced, such as astemizole and terfenadine, or agents currently in clinical trials, such as loratidine, mequitazine, and temelastine, do not readily penetrate the CNS. The newer agents have a lower incidence of sedative effects than the older agents.

The antihistamines are extensively metabolized by the liver, and metabolites are eliminated by renal excretion. Some of the agents are substrates for monoamine oxidase (MAO). These agents can induce hepatic cytochrome P-450 enzymes and may facilitate their own metabolism and that of other drugs.

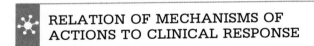

RELATION OF MECHANISMS OF ACTIONS TO CLINICAL RESPONSE

Actions of Histamine

Vascular System The effects of histamine on the systemic vasculature are complex, and different vascular beds show different outputs. Most vascular beds respond with vasodilation mediated by either or both H_1- and H_2-receptors. Other beds respond with vasoconstriction mediated by H_1-receptors and/or vasodilation mediated by H_2-receptors.

The predominant action of histamine is dose-dependent vasodilation resulting from relaxation of arteriolar smooth muscle, precapillary sphincters, and muscular venules. A decrease in systemic blood pressure generally occurs only at doses of histamine higher than those required to produce vasodilation of cutaneous vessels. At the lower doses needed for cutaneous vasodilation, a moderate and transient hypertensive response is frequently seen. The mechanism for this response is not known, but may be due to constriction of large vessels.

Histamine acts at H_1-receptors of endothelial cells in all postcapillary venules to produce contraction of muscle cells and exposure of permeable basement membrane. This results in edema from the loss of fluid and plasma protein to the surrounding tissue.

A synopsis of the actions of histamine on the vasculature is seen in the triple response that follows the intradermal injection of histamine. Initially, a small red spot is produced at the site of injection that is slowly surrounded by a flushed area. A wheal appears at the original red spot in a few minutes. The red spot and the erythema are caused by vasodilation, with the red spot resulting from the direct actions of histamine on the cutaneous vasculature and the erythema-axon reflexes that produce vasodilation. These vasodilatory responses are mediated by both H_1-receptors and H_2-receptors, with the major contribution by the H_1 component. The wheal occurs from edema formation. Histamine also stimulates nerve endings to produce pain, when injected intradermally, and itching, when administered into the epidermis. The extrapolation of the local vascular reactions of the triple response to systemic effects of large doses of histamine is one way in which cardiovascular shock can occur.

Heart

Histamine exerts direct and indirect actions on the human heart. Indirectly, histamine produces an increase in heart rate and force of contraction that results from greater sympathetic tone from baroreceptor discharge in response to a decrease in blood pressure. The direct actions of histamine on the human heart are mediated primarily by H_2-receptors. The actions are a positive chronotropic response that is due to an increase in the rate of spontaneous depolarization of sinoatrial nodal cells, an increase in atrial and ventricular automaticity, and an increase in myocardial contractile force. Modest tachycardia, which is sensitive to blockade by cimetidine, occurs at doses of histamine that produce very little change in systemic pressure. The lower doses of histamine decrease systemic blood pressure; its indirect actions override its direct actions on the heart.

Other cardiac actions of histamine that may have clinical importance have been demonstrated in experimental animals. Histamine acts at H_1-receptors to decrease the rate of atrioventricular (AV) conduction and at H_1-receptors and H_2-receptors to decrease fibrillation thresholds. The actions of histamine on the electrical properties of cardiac tissue and its ability to produce coronary vasoconstriction account for the dysrhythmic actions of this compound. The actions of histamine may be clinically important in provoking cardiac shock that arises in anaphylaxis and dysrhythmias produced by drugs known to cause histamine release in vivo, such as doxorubicin.

Respiratory System In most species, including humans, histamine produces contraction of airway smooth muscle. This occurs after the administration of histamine by inhalation or IV injection. Bronchoconstriction is mediated by H_1-receptors and is the major response of airway smooth muscle to histamine. In healthy humans, histamine is not especially potent; however, the airway smooth muscle of people with asthma is hyperreactive to histamine, as well as to other spasmogens. Previously, aerosolized histamine was used as a provocative test for bronchial reactivity to assist in the diagnosis of asthma. Inhalational histamine is rarely used for this purpose now but is used in the clinical pharmacological evaluation of new antihistamines.

Histamine produces a modest relaxation of contracted bronchial smooth muscle by a presumed action on H_2-receptors. Because patients with asthma tolerate agents that block H_2-receptors, it is doubtful that this action of histamine has any major physiological significance.

In addition to actions on airway smooth muscle, histamine acts on H_1-receptors to increase airway fluid and electrolyte secretions. Although not demonstrated in human tissues, it is likely that histamine can produce pulmonary edema by similar processes. The actions of histamine on the respiratory system can contribute to bronchial obstruction in extrinsic asthma (see Chapter 57).

Gastrointestinal System A well-known physiological function of histamine is its role as a primary mediator in the secretion of gastric acid. This is discussed in Chapter 59.

Histamine exhibits relaxant and contractile activities on smooth muscle in the alimentary canal. This has been demonstrated in human tissues on isolated smooth muscle preparation obtained from the large intestine and gallbladder. In the former, a biphasic effect of histamine was mediated by H_1-receptors. In the latter, the contractile response was mediated by H_1-receptors and occasional relaxant responses by H_2-receptors. The physiological significance of these actions is not established.

Other Actions In addition to the major actions discussed previously, headaches, nausea, and vomiting are also experienced by human volunteers receiving histamine. In high doses, histamine stimulates the release of catecholamines from the adrenal medulla, an effect for which individuals with pheochromocytoma are more sensitive.

Histamine in the Central Nervous System The role of histamine in the CNS is largely inferred from the results of studies on experimental animals. Postulated roles for brain histamine include thermal regulation, regulation of water balance, modulation of nociception, regulation of blood pressure, and arousal. The central effects involve H_1-receptors and H_2-receptors and may also involve H_3-receptors.

Histamine Agonists

Several compounds are available that selectively bind to and activate H_1-, H_2-, or H_3-receptors (see Figure 58-1). These compounds are useful research tools and rarely are used clinically. H_1-selective agonists have no clinical uses. The H_2-selective agonist betazole is used occasionally as a gastric secretagogue in diagnostic tests for acid secretion. Because its selectivity for H_2-receptors is moderate, it produces systemic actions as a result of activation of H_1-receptors. Pentagastrin is a preferred gastric secretagogue because it produces fewer systemic effects than betazole. The H_3-selective agonists are not used clinically.

Inhibitors of Mast Cell Degranulation

Cromolyn sodium is the only agent presently available that inhibits noncytolytic degranulation of mast cells, with others under development. Cromolyn is effective against mucosal mast cells, particularly

Table 58-4 Properties of Representative Histamine H_1-Antagonists and Drugs Possessing H_1-Antagonist Properties

Chemical Class/Agents	Comments

alkylamines
  brompheniramine
  chlorpheniramine
  dexchlorpheniramine
  triprolidine
	Very little sedative, moderate antimuscarinic, no antiemetic, and no antimotion sickness actions

ethanolamines
  clemastine
  dimenhydrinate
  diphenhydramine
	Significant antimuscarinic and antimotion sickness actions; also marked sedative actions; diphenhydramine in many over the counter preparations

ethylenediamines
  pyrilamine
  tripelennamine
	Mild to moderate sedative actions; very little antimuscarinic or antimotion sickness actions at usual doses

piperazines
  cyclizine
  hydroxyzine
  meclizine
	Varying degrees of antimuscarinic, antimotion sickness and sedative actions; cyclizine and meclizine, least sedative and antimuscarinic actions, used primarily in treatment of motion sickness and vertigo; hydroxyzine, marked sedative and antimuscarinic actions, as well as marked antimotion sickness action, used primarily as sedative and mild anxiolytic agent

piperidines
  astemizole
  cyproheptadine
  phenindamine
  terfenadine
	Low sedating and no antimotion sickness and little to moderate antimuscarinic activities; phenindamine, more likely to produce stimulation than other antihistamines; cyproheptadine, marked antiserotonin activity.

phenothiazines
  methdilazine
  promethazine
  trimeprazine
	Marked antimuscarinic, antiemetic, and antimotion sickness activities; sedation is common, especially with promethazine

those in lung tissue in close contact with the alveoli. Cromolyn has no effect on the connective tissue mast cells or on basophils.

Cromolyn exhibits no antagonist activity toward mediators released from mast cells. Nor does it have direct relaxing actions on bronchial smooth muscle. Its major effect is to prevent immunological and non-immunological induced noncytolytic degranulation of mast cells. It is of value only when used prophylactically. Unlike β_2-selective agonists, it is ineffective against an ongoing degranulation.

Cromolyn is indicated in the prophylactic management of reversible bronchospastic disorders, extrinsic asthma, and exercise-induced asthma that do not respond well to treatment with methylxanthines or sympathomimetic bronchodilators. All patients with asthma can benefit from cromolyn therapy, although young patients respond best. Cromolyn is useful in the prophylaxis of allergic rhinitis and allergic conjunctivitis. Cromolyn also can prevent bronchial pseudoallergic reactions caused by aspirin-like drugs and environmental pollutants.

Clinical effectiveness of cromolyn requires at least 4 weeks of therapy. If an individual does not respond after 4 weeks, it is doubtful that cromolyn will be of any benefit. It is effective only if used before a challenge that can produce degranulation of mast cells. To maintain protective effects that can last for hours, cromolyn must be administered frequently. Cromolyn is not effective in the treatment of an acute asthma attack or in the treatment of status asthmaticus (see Chapter 57).

H_1-Antagonists

All of the H_1-antagonists have antiallergic properties. With varying degrees, they exhibit sedative, antiemetic, antimotion sickness, antiparkinsonism, and local anesthetic actions. Several antihistamines are used exclusively for one or another of these characteristics rather than for their utility in uncomplicated allergic reactions. These properties may or may not be related to the ability of these agents to block H_1-receptors.

The effectiveness of the agents in the treatment of motion sickness, extrapyramidal symptoms, and insomnia may be due to their antimuscarinic actions. However, this is not uniformly accepted, and it has been proposed that sedation is due to the blockade of central H_1-receptors. The antiemetic activity is largely confined to the phenothiazine class and probably results from blockade of dopamine D_2-receptors. The local anesthetic actions are due to blockade of sodium channels in excitable membranes. Thus the actions of antihistamines at sites other than the H_1-receptor can contribute to therapeutic uses, as well as to adverse effects. A summary of the pharmacological properties of representative H_2-antagonists is given in Table 58-4.

The release of histamine from mast cells and basophils is accompanied by the release of many other mediators of the immediate hypersensitivity response. Drugs that antagonize histamine are only useful as monotherapy in mild pseudoallergic or true allergic reactions and as adjunctive agents in the treatment of severe reactions. The treatment of severe allergic reactions requires the use of a physiological antagonist such as epinephrine that will reverse the hypotension, laryngeal edema, and bronchoconstriction produced by the mast cell mediators.

The H_1-antihistamines are used in the symptomatic treatment and prevention of allergic disorders. Their effectiveness is limited to symptoms due mainly to the actions of histamine and not other mediators. The allergic reactions that respond best to treatment with H_1-antagonists are seasonal, but also include perennial allergic rhinitis, conjunctivitis, and itching associated with acute and chronic urticaria. Antihistamines are of some value in the treatment of atopic dermatitis and contact dermatitis. The choice of a nonsedative or sedative H_1-antihistamine in treating these disorders depends on whether sedation is desirable. Tolerance may develop to the sedative properties within a few days.

The older H_1-antagonists are not beneficial in the treatment of bronchial asthma. As previously noted, this is due to the role of mediators other than histamine and, possibly, because local concentrations of the H_1-antagonists are too low relative to the local concentrations of histamine to produce effective blockade.

Tolerance to the antihistamines occurs. Frequently, switching to a different agent results in restoration of the desired therapeutic effects. It is not known if the tolerance is due to the induction of drug-metabolizing enzymes or changes at the receptor. Experimentally, attempts to demonstrate an up-regulation of H_1-receptors after chronic treatment with antagonists have been disappointing.

H_1-antihistamines that distribute to the CNS are used in the prophylactic treatment of motion sickness. Promethazine and diphenhydramine are the most potent but also produce a high incidence of sedation. Promethazine is effective as an antiemetic in reducing vomiting from a variety of causes. Meclazine, cyclizine, and dimenhydrinate, a salt of diphenhydramine, are used in over-the-counter preparations for prevention of motion sickness. However, none is as effective as scopolamine in preventing nausea and vomiting associated with motion. These agents also are used in the symptomatic treatment of vertigo.

H_2-Antagonists

The H_2-antagonists presently used clinically are cimetidine, famotidine, nizatidine, and ranitidine. All act as competitive antagonists at histamine H_2-receptors and are used primarily in the management of peptic ulcer disease. Their pharmacological actions are described in detail in Chapter 59.

SIDE EFFECTS, CLINICAL PROBLEMS, AND TOXICITY

Clinical problems with cromolyn sodium and the H_1-antagonists are listed in the box. Clinical problems for H_2-antagonists are given in Chapter 59.

Cromolyn Sodium

Because cromolyn sodium is not well absorbed, systemic toxicity is rare. Many patients use cromolyn for several years without adverse effects or the de-

---

CLINICAL PROBLEMS

CROMOLYN SODIUM
Airway irritant
Bad taste
Headache

H_1-RECEPTOR ANTAGONISTS
Antimuscarinic actions
Sedative effects
Some CNS depression (in older drugs)
Topical use allergic reaction

velopment of tolerance. The aerosolized powder has irritant effects that can cause coughing, wheezing, bronchospasm, and pharyngeal discomfort. The irritant properties can worsen bronchoconstriction during an acute attack. Adverse effects associated with the nasal solutions occur in about 2% of patients. Frequent adverse effects are nasal irritation, bad taste, and headache. The common adverse reaction associated with the ophthalmic solution is a transient ocular stinging or burning on instillation. The ophthalmic solution contains benzalkonium chloride and should not be used with soft contact lenses. Hypersensitivity reactions are rare.

H$_1$-Antagonists

The majority of H$_1$-antagonist adverse effects are due to the antimuscarinic and sedative actions of the antihistamines. With the older agents, central depressant effects are common untoward reactions and occur in about 50% of patients. Antihistamines with antimuscarinic activity may cause dryness of the mouth, blurred vision, dysuria or urinary retention, constipation, and other symptoms attributable to blockade of muscarinic receptors. Additional central effects include insomnia, nervousness, tremors and euphoria. Paradoxical excitation can occur in children. Nausea, vomiting, diarrhea and epigastric distress are reported.

The major signs of acute overdose are similar to those caused by classical antimuscarinic agents and are treated accordingly (see Chapter 9).

The incidences of central depression and antimuscarinic effects are less for the newer agents such as astemizole and terfenadine. With these agents, the incidences of CNS depression and antimuscarinic effects are comparable to those produced by placebo.

The incidence of true allergic responses is low with systemic administration. However, allergic responses are relatively common after repeated topical use; therefore topical use is discouraged.

Teratogenic effects produced by piperazine derivatives are observed in experimental animals. Although there is no evidence that this occurs in humans, this class of antihistamines, as well as all others is not recommended during pregnancy.

The centrally acting H$_1$-antihistamines can potentiate the actions of other central depressant agents: hypnotic sedatives, narcotic analgesics, general anesthetics, and alcohol. Similarly, their antimuscarinic actions are additive with those produced by other agents. MAO inhibitors can potentiate the antimuscarinic actions of antihistamines.

REFERENCES

Armang JM, Garbag M, Lancelot JC et al: Highly potent and selective ligands for histamine H$_3$-receptors, Nature 327:117, 1987.

Ganellin CR and Parsons ME: Pharmacology of histamine receptors, Bristol, 1982, John Wright and Sons.

Ganellin CR and Schwartz JC: Frontiers in histamine research, Oxford, 1985, Pergamon Press.

Green JP, Prell GD, Khandalwal JK et al: Aspects of histamine metabolism, Agents Actions 22:1, 1987.

Pearce FL: On the heterogeneity of mast cells, Pharmacology 32:61, 1986.

Robert A: Effect of drugs on gastric secretion. In Johnson LR, ed: Physiology of the gastrointestinal tract, New York, 1987, Raven Press.

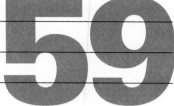

CHAPTER 59 Gastrointestinal Drugs

ABBREVIATIONS

GI	gastrointestinal
cAMP	cyclic adenosine monophosphate
H^+, K^+-ATPase	hydrogen-potassium-adenosine triphosphatase

MAJOR DRUGS

- antacids
- cimetidine
- diphenoxylate
- H_2-receptor antagonists
- loperamide
- propantheline
- proton pump inhibitors

THERAPEUTIC OVERVIEW

The gastrointestinal (GI) tract stores, digests, and absorbs nutrients and eliminates wastes. Regulation of the GI organs results from control by intrinsic nerves of the enteric nervous system, neural activity in the central nervous system (CNS), and by an array of GI hormones. These processes are summarized in Figure 59-1.

The pharmacologically treatable impairments to the normal motility, digestion, secretion, and absorption functions of the stomach and intestinal tract are peptic ulcers, inadequate propulsion of solid wastes in the colon and rectum, diarrhea, infections, or inflammation. In each case, potential beneficial effects must be carefully considered against potential adverse effects.

Peptic ulcer is a benign lesion of gastric or duodenal mucosa occurring at a site where the mucosal epithelium is exposed to acid and pepsin. There is constant confrontation in the stomach and upper small bowel between acid-pepsin aggression and mucosal defense. Usually, the mucosa can withstand the acid-pepsin attack and remain healthy. That is, a mucosal "barrier" to back-diffusion of acid is maintained. However, an excess of acid production or an intrinsic defect in the barrier functions of the mucosa can allow the defense mechanism to fail and ulcers to result. Peptic ulcers can be produced by excess acid or a mucosal defect, and the therapeutic strategy for management of peptic ulcer disease may be directed at reduction of acid exposure of the mucosa or improvement in the integrity of the mucosal barrier.

Many patients with duodenal ulcer disease have an elevated mass of gastric parietal cells and elevated gastric acid secretion. Patients with gastrin-secreting tumors (gastrinoma, Zollinger-Ellison syndrome) secrete excess amounts of acid and almost invariably develop duodenal ulcers. In gastrinomas, excess acid production clearly overwhelms the mucosal defense. In contrast to patients with duodenal ulcers, patients with gastric ulcers often have normal or low rates of basal and stimulated acid secretion. These patients, and some with duodenal ulcers, may encounter a primary defect in the mucosa that provides inadequate defense against acid-pepsin attack.

The role of pepsin in peptic ulcer is not known,

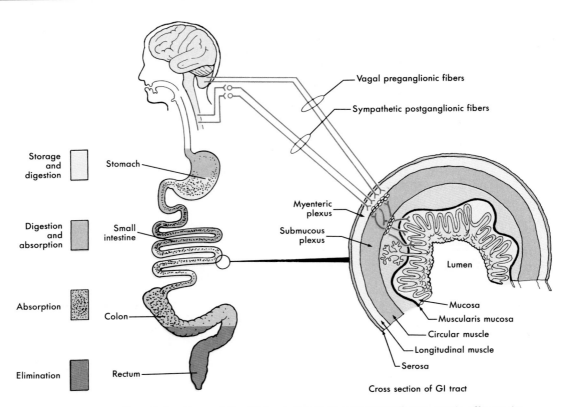

FIGURE 59-1   Overall functions of the GI tract. Extrinsic and intrinsic autonomic efferent innervation of the wall of the intestine. The enteric nervous system of the GI tract innervates smooth muscle and mucosa. Efferent and afferent neurons are organized in intramural plexuses; the most prominent plexuses are the myenteric plexus between the longitudinal and circular muscle coats and the submucous plexus between the circular muscle and the muscularis mucosa.

despite the name of the disease. Most successful therapeutic approaches to peptic ulcer are based on the adage, "no acid, no ulcer."

Frequency of defecation and the quantity and consistency of stool are subject to pharmacological regulation. However, dietary changes alone may be sufficient in many cases to restore normal bowel habits. In patients with functional intermittent or chronic constipation, treatment with a laxative may be indicated. The physician should be aware that constipation can arise from functional disorders, drug treatment, or by low-residue diets. Excess use of laxatives can lead to adverse effects, including nutritional imbalance, abdominal cramps, fluid and electrolyte disturbance, and reliance on laxatives for bowel movements.

Diarrhea is a GI problem that can be acute, often secondary to an enteric bacterial or viral infection, or chronic, often secondary to inflammatory or functional bowel disease. The best way to manage diarrhea is to remove the cause. This includes eliminating the infection, removing the secretagogue-producing tumor, or curing the inflammation. The major hazard associated with diarrhea is loss of fluid and electrolytes. Serious sequelae of diarrhea can generally be avoided simply by replacement of fluid and electrolytes by oral or IV administration, often the preferred choice in infants and in patients with self-limiting diarrheal diseases. However, many patients with trivial or serious acute or chronic diarrhea require antidiarrheal therapy for personal comfort and convenience.

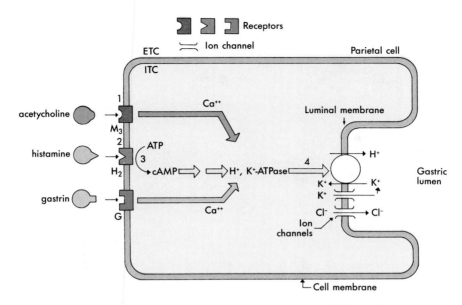

FIGURE 59-2   Diagram of the mechanisms regulating secretion of HCl by the gastric parietal cell. Receptors for acetylcholine, histamine, and gastrin interact when activated by agonists to increase availability of Ca^{++} and stimulate the H^+, K^+-ATPase of the luminal membrane. Acid secretion can be decreased pharmacologically by blockade of acetylcholine M_1-receptors *(1)*, histamine H_2-receptors *(2)*, intracellular adenylate cyclase *(3)*, or the H^+, K^+-ATPase *(4)*.

THERAPEUTIC OVERVIEW

Peptic ulcer (gastric or duodenal)
   Excess acid—neutralize, block secretion
   Mucosal barrier breakdown—repair lesions
Gastric emptying and propulsion of contents through
   intestine—prokinetic drugs
Constipation—laxatives
Diarrhea—remove source, opioid and other drugs

These disease states or disturbances of the GI tract are summarized in the box.

 MECHANISMS OF ACTION

Drugs for Treatment of Peptic Ulcers

Secretion of acid by gastric parietal cells is regulated by histamine, acetylcholine, and gastrin (Figure 59-2). Psychic stimuli (sight and smell of food) and the presence of food in the mouth or stomach stim-ulates vagally mediated gastric acid secretion resulting from acetylcholine actions on parietal cells. Acetylcholine acts at parietal cell muscarinic cholinergic receptors (M_3 in Figure 59-2) coupled to calcium channels that allow entry of extracellular calcium into the parietal cell. Gastrin is released from the antral mucosa by the presence of food that raises antral pH. The gastrin circulates through the bloodstream to act at gastrin receptors on parietal cells. Activation of gastrin receptors is thought to mobilize intracellular calcium in the parietal cell. Histamine is released from nearby mast cells to act at parietal cell histamine H_2-receptors. The histamine H_2-receptors are coupled to adenylate cyclase. Activation of histamine H_2-receptors results in formation of intracellular cAMP that ultimately activates a protein kinase. The histamine H_2-receptors, muscarinic cholinergic receptors, and gastrin receptors mutually interact to augment the secretory actions of histamine, acetylcholine, and gastrin, but of these three regulatory receptors, histamine is thought to be the most important and may serve as the "final common pathway" in regulation of gastric acid secretion. Activation of any of the three types of parietal cell receptors appears to result in increased activity of a protein kinase that activates

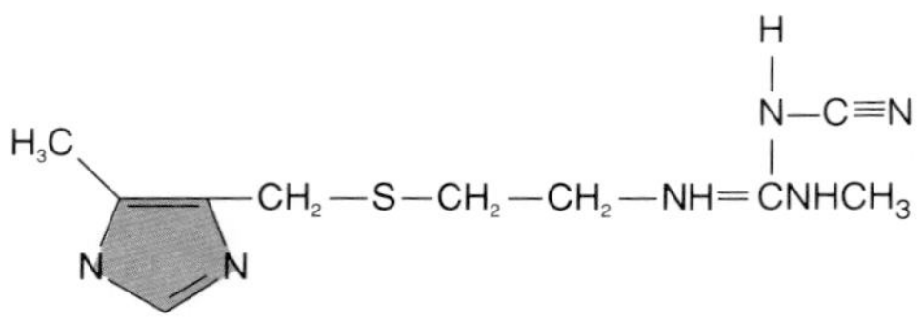

cimetidine

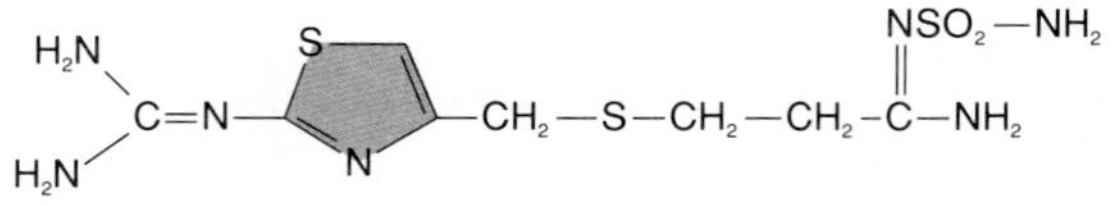

famotidine

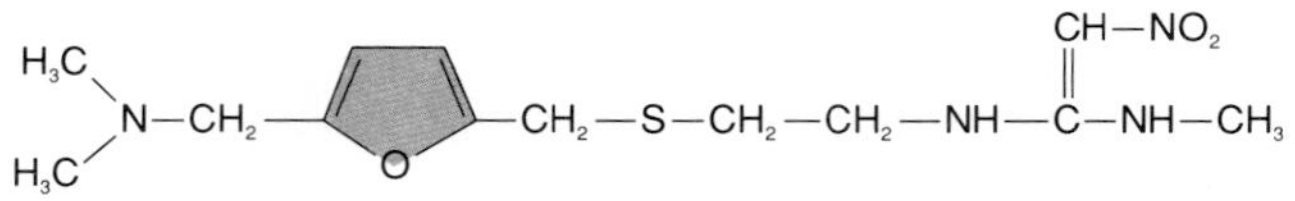

ranitidine

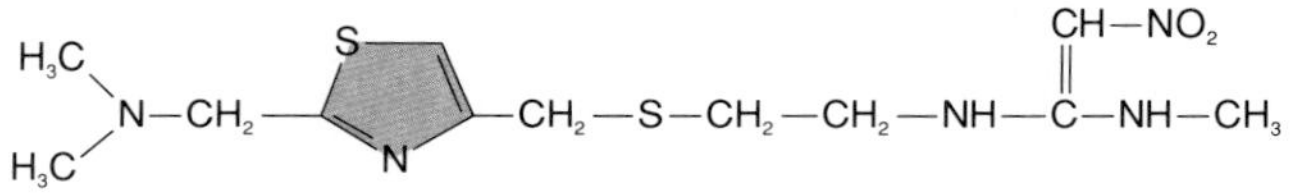

nizatidine

FIGURE 59-3 Structures of histamine H_2-receptor antagonists used in management of peptic ulcer disease.

the H^+, K^+-ATPase located at the luminal membrane of the parietal cell. The H^+, K^+-ATPase serves as the "proton pump" that secretes H^+ into the gastric lumen.

Drugs can decrease gastric acid secretion (Figure 59-2) by blocking the histamine H_2-receptors, by blocking the muscarinic M_3 cholinergic receptors, by inhibiting histamine-induced activity of adenylate cyclase, or by inhibiting activity of the H^+, K^+-ATPase of the parietal cell.

The molecular mechanism of action of histamine and antihistamines is discussed in detail in Chapter 58. A brief discussion relevant to gastric acid secretion is included here. The histamine H_2-receptor on the parietal cell mediates the stimulatory effect of histamine on acid secretion. Activation of the H_2-receptor also augments the secretory actions of gastrin and acetylcholine on the parietal cell. The only important peripheral role of H_2-receptors in humans appears to be their role in regulation of acid secretion. For this reason, H_2-receptor antagonists provide remarkably specific therapy for peptic ulcer disease. In fact, the efficacy of H_2-receptor antagonists as inhibitors of acid secretion provides strong evidence for an important role of histamine as a physiological mediator of gastric acid secretion. Histamine H_2-receptor antagonists inhibit acid secretion brought about by histamine, as well as the secretion induced by gastrin, cholinergic agents, food, and reflux vagal stimulation.

The H_2-receptor antagonists include cimetidine, famotidine, nizatidine, and ranitidine (see Figure 59-3 for structures) and act to decrease acid and pepsin secretion by competitive antagonism at parietal cell histamine receptors (Table 59-1). H_2-receptor antagonists do not block cholinergic receptors or gastrin

(1) $\quad Al(OH)_3 + 3HCl \rightleftharpoons Al\,Cl_3 + 3H_2O$

(2) $\quad Mg(OH)_2 + 2HCl \rightleftharpoons Mg\,Cl_2 + 2H_2O$

(3) $\quad Mg\,Cl_2 + Na_2CO_3 \rightleftharpoons MgCO_3\,(PPT) + 2NaCl$

(4) $\quad MgCl_2 + 2R{-}COONa \rightleftharpoons Mg(R{-}COO)_2\,(PPT) + 2NaCl$

FIGURE 59-4   Intragastric and intestinal interactions of prototype antacids. (1) Interaction of aluminum hydroxide with gastric acid to form soluble aluminum chloride. (2) Interaction of magnesium hydroxide with gastric acid. (3) Soluble magnesium chloride interaction with sodium carbonate in the lumen of the intestine to form insoluble magnesium carbonate. (4) Interaction of soluble magnesium chloride with fatty acid salts in the lumen of the intestine to form an insoluble magnesium soap. *PPT*, Precipitate.

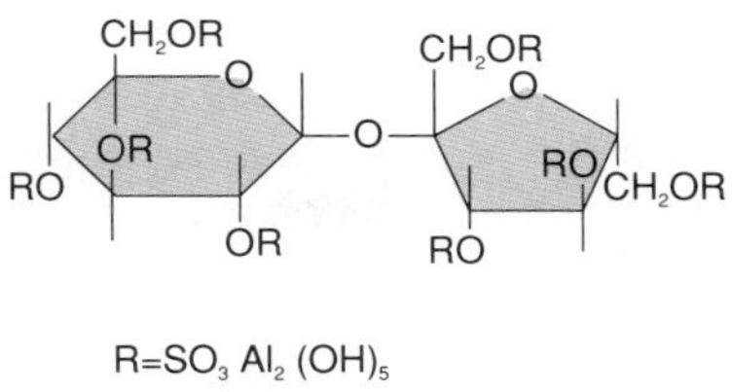

$R = SO_3\,Al_2\,(OH)_5$

FIGURE 59-5   Structure of sucralfate.

Table 59-1   Summary of Actions of Antiulcer Drugs

Category of Drug	Mechanisms of Action
H_2-antagonists	Block H_2-receptors, decrease H^+ secretion
muscarinic antagonists	Block muscarinic receptors, decrease H^+ secretion
prostaglandins	Inhibit cAMP, decrease H^+ secretion
proton pump inhibitors	Inhibit H^+, K^+-ATPase, decrease H^+ secretion
antacids	Neutralize secreted H^+
sucralfate	Protect mucosal barrier

receptors. The decrease in acid and pepsin secretion that results from blockade of H_2-receptors allows the mucosa, in particular the duodenal mucosa, to tolerate the diminished acid load presented and effectively promote healing of the ulcer. H_2-receptor antagonists increase the incidence of ulcer healing, improve the rate at which healing occurs, and prevent recurrence of ulcers.

Antacids act by neutralization of intragastric hydrochloric acid (HCl) and the cations (sodium, calcium, magnesium, aluminum) form soluble chloride salts (Figure 59-4). NaCl can be absorbed from the small intestine but the divalent ions form poorly soluble bicarbonates and carbonates that precipitate and remain in the bowel lumen to be excreted in the feces. Calcium, magnesium, and aluminum ions can also interact with fatty acids to form insoluble salts

(soaps) that also are excreted in the feces.

Another type of peptic ulcer drug is typified by sucralfate, which is a basic aluminum salt of sucrose octasulfate (Figure 59-5). Unlike the other drugs presently available for management of peptic ulcer disease, sucralfate does not decrease the concentration or total amount of acid in the gastric lumen. Instead, it acts to protect the gastric and duodenal mucosa from acid-pepsin attack. Sucralfate appears to possess three relevant actions: it complexes with proteins at the ulcer site to form a protective layer, it decreases back-diffusion of hydrogen ions, and it binds to pepsin and bile salts.

Molecular mechanisms of other drugs used in the treatment of peptic ulcers are covered in Chapter 9 (muscarinic cholinergic antagonists) and Chapter 18 (prostaglandins).

Prokinetic Drugs

The precise mechanism by which metoclopramide and related prokinetic drugs increase GI contractions is not known. The mechanism may be related to increased release of acetylcholine at the terminals of cholinergic neurons innervating GI smooth muscle, or the drug may make more effective the actions of acetylcholine at smooth muscle muscarinic cholinergic receptors. Metoclopramide possesses dopamine-receptor antagonist properties, and some portion of its antiemetic activity may result from blockade of brainstem dopamine receptors. However, several related prokinetic drugs without dopamine-receptor antagonist actions also exert antiemetic effects.

Some of the experimental prokinetic-antiemetic drugs possess significant antagonist activity at 5-hydroxytryptamine $5HT_3$ receptors, and this may be important in regulation of motility and initiation of nausea and vomiting.

Laxatives

Laxatives (also known as *purgatives* or *evacuants*) can be divided into several pharmacological categories according to their mechanisms of action: secretory, saline, emollient, or bulk-forming laxatives. Each category displays specific pharmacological characteristics. The secretory laxatives act on crypt cells of the intestinal mucosa to open chloride channels that allow movement of chloride, sodium, and water into the intestinal lumen. Chloride channels of enterocytes (cells that line the intestinal mucosa) are regulated primarily by intracellular cAMP, therefore it is thought that many secretory laxatives directly or indirectly stimulate adenylate cyclase activity, thereby increasing intracellular concentrations of cAMP in the crypt cells.

Antidiarrheal Drugs

Diarrhea results from excessive fluid in the lumen of the intestine that generates rapid, high volume flow and overwhelms the absorptive capacity of the colon. It is important to note that in most diarrheal conditions fluid and electrolyte absorption occurs at an essentially normal rate.

Diarrhea can be treated in the following ways (Table 59-2):

1. By increasing resistance to flow by increasing segmenting intestinal contractions or by increasing viscosity of luminal contents
2. By increasing mucosal absorption or decreasing secretion
3. By removal of diarrhea-producing chemicals
4. By preventing formation of diarrhea-producing chemicals

Transport of fluid and electrolytes by the intestinal mucosa is regulated by neurons of the enteric nervous system and by the chemical composition of the luminal contents. It is believed that neurons of the submucous plexus of the intestine terminate near mucosal epithelial cells and act to increase or decrease absorption by villus cells and secretion by crypt cells.

The natural opioids, morphine and codeine, and synthetic opioids such as loperamide and diphenoxylate are discussed in regard to mechanism and side effects in Chapter 28. The opioid drugs in particular can act on intestinal neural elements to promote mucosal transport from the lumen. In addition, opioids can act in the CNS to alter extrinsic neural influences on the intestine to promote net absorption

Table 59-2 Summary of Actions of Antidiarrheal Drugs

Category of Drug	Mechanisms of Action
opioids	Increase resistance to flow, decrease propulsion, decrease net fluid secretion
anticholinergics	Decrease propulsion
bismuth subsalicylate	Decrease fluid secretion
gel-forming agents	Increase resistance to flow, promote formed stools
ion exchange resins	Bind bile acids

of fluid and electrolytes. The specific neurotransmitters of submucosal neurons affected by opioids have not been identified. Although none is presently used in the management of diarrhea, adrenergic agonists with actions at α_2 receptors can promote fluid and electrolyte absorption.

 PHARMACOKINETICS

Pharmacokinetic parameter values of drugs that are used systemically are summarized in Table 59-3.

The present H_2 antagonists may be administered orally once or twice daily for management of acute phases of duodenal ulcer and once daily for maintenance therapy. The daily oral dose may be given at bedtime to minimize potential adverse side effects, such as somnolence or dizziness, and to control nocturnal acid secretion. Cimetidine, famotidine and ranitidine are also available for IV administration.

The plasma half-lives of the H_2 antagonists are relatively short, ranging from approximately 1½ hours for nizatidine to 3.0 hours for famotidine. Cimetidine, famotidine, nizatidine and ranitidine are excreted in the urine, primarily as intact drugs. However, there can be significant (up to 30%) formation of the corresponding S-oxides (cimetidine and famotidine) or N-oxides (nizatidine and ranitidine) as well. Because renal elimination is an important terminating mechanism for all of the H_2 antagonists, dosage reduction may be necessary in patients with renal insufficiency.

Sucralfate is available for oral use only. Slight absorption occurs from the intestine and most of the drug is excreted intact in the feces. The small fraction that is absorbed is excreted intact in the urine.

Table 59-3 Pharmacokinetic Parameter Values

Drug	Administered	Absorption (%)	$t_{1/2}$ (hr)	Disposition
H₂-RECEPTOR ANTAGONISTS				
cimetidine	Oral, IV	60	2	R (main), M
nizatidine	Oral	90	1.5	R (main), M
ranitidine	Oral, IV	50	2	R (main), M
famotidine	Oral, IV	45	3.0	R (main), M
OTHERS				
sucralfate	Oral	Poor	—	Excrete in feces
propantheline	Oral	7.0	2	M (main), R
metoclopramide	Oral, IV, IM	80	2	R (main), M
diphenoxylate	Oral	90	12	M (main), B, R
loperamide	Oral	Poor	11	B (main), R

M, Metabolized; *R*, renal excretion as unchanged drug; *B*, biliary excretion.

RELATION OF MECHANISMS OF ACTION TO CLINICAL RESPONSE

Drugs for Treatment of Ulcers

Histamine H₂-Antagonists Cimetidine was the first H₂-receptor antagonist and is a widely used drug. It is an effective and relatively safe agent for therapy of peptic ulcer disease. However, although it demonstrates a remarkable safety record, cimetidine may produce some potentially serious side effects under certain conditions, including antiandrogenic actions and interference with drug metabolism.

Similar to other histamine H₂-receptor antagonists, cimetidine blocks parietal cell H₂-histamine receptors and markedly inhibits basal acid secretion (including nocturnal secretion), as well as secretion induced by meals. By decreasing acid secretion, cimetidine decreases ulcer pain and promotes mucosal healing. A disadvantage is its relatively short duration of action (plasma half-life of 2 hours), requiring its administration more than one time daily during the acute phase of ulcer therapy in many patients.

Ranitidine, nizatidine and famotidine are H₂-receptor antagonists more recently introduced for treatment of peptic ulcer. As shown in Figure 59-3, ranitidine, nizatidine, and famotidine differ chemically from cimetidine in the structures of the ring and the side-chain. Ranitidine, nizatidine, and famotidine display longer durations of action than cimetidine, whereas nizatidine has a shorter plasma half-life.

None of these new drugs possesses antiandrogenic properties or interferes significantly with drug metabolism by hepatic cytochrome P-450 enzymes. The newer agents may therefore have certain advantages over cimetidine.

Gastric Antacids Antacids employed for treatment of peptic ulcer disease are weak bases that neutralize the HCl in the stomach. Antacids thus do not decrease secretion of acid; in fact, some can increase secretion. They instead neutralize acid in the lumen of the stomach to produce two desirable therapeutic effects: decrease the total acid load delivered to the duodenum and inhibit the pepsin activity. The activity of pepsin is significantly decreased at pH 5 and above. Antacid therapy that raises intragastric pH above 4 to 5 is adequate to achieve the desired therapeutic endpoint while minimizing the side effects antacids can produce.

Antacids are divided into two general categories: systemic and nonsystemic. Systemic antacids are absorbed into the bloodstream, with potential to increase blood pH and alkalinize urine. The classic example is sodium bicarbonate (baking soda). Nonsystemic antacids contain a cation (usually calcium, magnesium, or aluminum) that is poorly absorbed in the small intestine, does not alter blood pH, and does not alkalinize urine. For occasional, intermittent therapy, a systemic antacid poses no hazard. When used regularly for days or weeks, however, a systemic antacid is undesirable and a nonsystemic antacid is required.

Adequate treatment with antacids provides effective treatment of peptic ulcers, reflected in rate of healing and the incidence of healing. The major disadvantage of antacid therapy is the frequent dosing required and the attendant side effects. Most antacids have a chalk-like, disagreeable taste. Attempts are made to disguise the taste with various flavorings, but patients soon tire of antacids, and compliance with prescribed dosing is often poor. Antacids are therapeutically effective only when present in the stomach and lose their effect after gastric emptying. In addition, antacids may cause undesired or dangerous side effects. Relative safety data indicate that antacids are less safe than some alternative forms of ulcer therapy, such as histamine H_2 antagonists.

Sodium and potassium salts such as sodium bicarbonate or potassium bicarbonate have a rapid onset of action, providing almost immediate neutralization, and can briefly raise intragastric pH to 5 to 7 or even higher. However, the neutralizing effect is of short duration and, as acid secretion continues, the acidity soon returns to pH 1 to 2. In contrast, most calcium salts have a relatively rapid onset of action and a neutralizing capacity in which the pH remains elevated as long as calcium is present in the stomach. However, the pH is usually raised to only 4 to 5 (still an acceptable endpoint). Calcium salts act directly on stimulus-secretion coupling to increase the release of gastrin and also to promote acid secretion, resulting in "acid rebound" after the calcium empties from the stomach. For these reasons, calcium salts are not recommended as antacids for the treatment of peptic ulcer. Magnesium hydroxide (milk of magnesia) has a rapid onset of neutralizing action and can raise intragastic pH to 8 to 9. By contrast, magnesium trisilicate and aluminum oxide neutralize acid slowly, and these salts have a slow onset of action. The total neutralizing capacity is adequate to maintain pH at desirable levels as long as the salts are present in the stomach. However, magnesium (laxative) and aluminum salts (constipative) can affect consistency of the feces and frequency of defecation. Individual characteristics of antacid compounds have led to the formulation of various mixtures that combine ingredients to offer rapid onset and relatively long duration of action and balance laxative and constipating effects. Satisfactory antacid formulations are liquid dosage forms that allow faster and more complete interaction of the antacid with H^+ and are more effective than solid dosage forms.

Different antacid products vary in sodium content. Because patients with peptic ulcers may consume large quantities of antacid, a high sodium content could constitute a health hazard, especially for patients on restricted sodium intake. Many low-sodium antacid preparations are available.

Sucralfate Controlled trials and experience with patients indicate that sucralfate can increase the incidence and rate of peptic ulcer healing with a minimum of adverse side effects. However, the efficacy of sucralfate as an antiulcer drug is less than that achieved with histamine H_2-receptor antagonists.

Prostaglandins Several products of arachidonic acid metabolism, including prostaglandins (see Chapter 28), exert gastric antisecretory effects and cytoprotective actions on the gastric and duodenal mucosa. In most tissues, prostaglandins stimulate adenylate cyclase activity and thereby increase intracellular formation of cAMP. In parietal cells, many prostaglandins inhibit adenylate cyclase stimulation by histamine (Figure 59-2) and thereby inhibit an essential step in histamine-stimulated acid secretion.

It is expected that one or more prostaglandins will soon be available for treatment of peptic ulcer disease. Misoprostol was recently introduced for prevention of mucosal damage induced by nonsteroidal antiinflammatory drugs. Administration of misoprostol to patients who received large doses of aspirin and related antiinflammatory drugs is expected to reduce the incidence of severe mucosal damage. The likely candidates for treatment of peptic ulcer are synthetic derivatives of prostaglandin E_1 or prostaglandin E_2 and contain substitutions at positions 15 or 16 of the side chain to protect against enzymatic attack and inactivation by prostaglandin dehydrogenase. The protected prostaglandins, such as 15, 15-dimethyl and 16, 16-dimethyl prostaglandin E_2, are active orally (see Chapter 18).

Proton Pump Inhibitors Secretion of H^+ into the gastric lumen results from activity of parietal cell H^+, K^+-ATPase. Activity of the H^+, K^+-ATPase is evidently regulated by availability of free intracellular calcium and activity of protein kinase. Calcium can be made available for activation of the H^+ transport enzyme by activation of histamine, acetylcholine, or gastrin receptors. Blockade of these regulatory systems decreases H^+ secretion. However, direct inhibition of H^+, K^+-ATPase produces the most effective mechanism known to inhibit gastric acid secretion. Omeprazole has been introduced and other agents are undergoing clinical trials for the management of peptic ulcer disease. Initial results indicate that certain proton pump inhibitors such as omeprazole are extremely efficacious and can reduce acid secretion almost to zero. Drugs that inhibit the H^+, K^+-ATPase may find clinical use in patients resistant to other types of pharmacological agents and in patients with gastrinomas; however, concerns about serious side effects exist.

Prokinetic Drugs

The prokinetic drugs increase gastric emptying in the treatment of diabetic gastroparesis, show promise in increasing tone of the lower esophageal sphincter in management of gastroesophageal reflux, and are used for antiemetic effects. Metoclopramide, for example, exhibits significant antiemetic activity and is often considered the preferred antiemetic in patients receiving antineoplastic drugs.

Laxatives

Laxatives consist of secretory, saline, emollient, and bulk-forming agents. Secretory laxatives increase secretion of fluid and electrolytes into the lumen of the bowel by the intestinal mucosa, resulting in fluid accumulation and a watery luminal content that flows rapidly through the small and large intestines. The classical secretory laxative is castor oil. One of the fatty acids esterified with glycerol in castor oil is ricinoleic acid, a hydroxylated analog of oleic acid. Ricinoleic acid acts on the intestinal mucosa to allow movement of fluid into the lumen of the bowel. Liberation of ricinoleic acid requires hydrolysis of castor oil triglyceride in the stomach and small bowel. Other natural secretory agents include the anthraquinone derivatives, cascara, senna, and aloe, which are popular as lay remedies. Synthetic agents include phenolphthalein, bisacodyl, and danthron.

Saline laxatives usually contain a cation (e.g., magnesium), anion (e.g., sulfate or phosphate), or nonabsorbable sugar that carries obligatory water of hydration and is poorly absorbed from the bowel. Saline cathartics retain fluid in the lumen and promote flow through the bowel. Examples of typical saline laxatives include magnesium hydroxide, sodium phosphate, and sodium sulfate. The disadvantage of saline laxatives is that they often produce explosive, watery bowel movements. Their advantage is a rapid onset of laxative effect, often within 3 hours of administration. Lactulose is a poorly absorbed sugar that increases accumulation of fluid in the lumen of the bowel. Emollient laxatives act as nonabsorbed lubricants to enhance flow through the bowel and to soften rectal contents.

The safest and generally preferred laxatives are the bulk-forming agents, including bran, methylcellulose, and psyllium, prepared from plantago seeds. Bulk-forming laxatives consist of nondigestible cellulose fibers that become hydrated in the intestine, decrease viscosity of luminal contents to increase flow through the bowel, and swell to provide bulk to activate the defecation reflex. The bulk-forming agents are essentially innocuous, relatively inexpensive, and satisfy the psychological needs of nearly all patients.

Antidiarrheal Drugs

Opioid Agents The most effective nonspecific antidiarrheal drugs are the natural opioids, including morphine and codeine, and synthetic opioid agents, such as loperamide and diphenoxylate. Opioids increase segmenting contractions of the small and large intestines, increasing resistance to flow through the lumen. Opioids decrease secretion of fluid and electrolytes into the lumen and promote mucosal absorption. These actions result in slowed transit through the GI tract, allowing time for more complete absorption of fluid, increased segmenting activity that also increases fluid absorption, and direct inhibition of secretory processes and stimulation of absorptive processes, leading to increased viscosity of luminal content and to formed stools.

Opioids that effectively cross the blood-brain barrier, such as morphine and codeine, probably act at central sites in the brain and spinal cord to decrease transit and accumulation of fluid in the lumen of the intestine. They also act locally on neural and smooth muscle elements in the intestine to increase segmenting contractions and to reduce propulsive contractions. Opioids that do not effectively cross the blood-brain barrier, such as loperamide and diphenoxylate, act primarily by local neural and smooth muscle effects to increase segmenting contractions. The natural and synthetic opioids act on neural elements in the intestine, primarily in the submucous plexus, to inhibit secretion and promote net absorption.

The increased segmenting contractions in the proximal duodenum decrease the gastroduodenal pressure gradient required for gastric emptying, causing opioids to delay gastric emptying, and contributing to the overall antidiarrheal effect.

Diphenoxylate is available commercially as a mixture with atropine, the latter serving as a deterrent to abuse. Diphenoxylate crosses the blood-brain barrier poorly and in usual therapeutic doses does not produce CNS side effects. However, in overdose, diphenoxylate can cause respiratory depression reversed by naloxone.

Loperamide is a more recently developed opioid antidiarrheal with the advantage of poor penetration across the blood-brain barrier and therefore has virtually no CNS effects. Loperamide is essentially devoid of opioid subjective effects when taken orally and presents a very low abuse potential.

The opioid diarrheal drugs are remarkably effective in management of acute diarrhea secondary to numerous causes. Opioids with CNS activity should be used cautiously in acute diarrheal states and generally should not be used for management of chronic diarrhea. Loperamide is successful in management of chronic diarrhea secondary to inflammatory bowel disease or irritable bowel syndrome. Opioid antidiarrheal agents should not be employed in symptomatic treatment of diarrhea induced by enteric infections with invasive organisms, especially species of *Shigella* and *Salmonella*.

Bismuth Subsalicylate Bismuth subsalicylate in several clinical trials is an effective antidiarrheal agent especially useful against enterotoxigenic strains of *Escherichia coli*.

Gel-forming Substances Substances that form a semisolid gel-like consistency within the intestinal lumen increase resistance to flow through the intestine and increase firmness of stools. Typical gel-forming substances include attapulgite, kaolin, and pectin. The gel-forming substances may offer more psychological benefit than reversal of pathophysiological processes. These substances form clay-like gels when hydrated. They do not remarkably reduce the volume of fluid excreted and thus have little therapeutic benefit other than promoting formed stools.

Antifoaming Agents Small bubbles of gas, primarily air entrapped during chewing and swallowing, can lead to gastric bloating, flatulence, and uncomfortable intestinal distention. A variety of antifoaming agents, often surfactants, is used to break up gas bubbles in the stomach. The popular agent is simethicone, used alone for this purpose or present in many commercial antacid mixtures. Although si-

methicone can produce a dramatic defoaming effect in the stomach observable by endoscopy, its efficacy in pathological intestinal distention has not been demonstrated.

SIDE EFFECTS, CLINICAL PROBLEMS, AND TOXICITY

Clinical problems of drugs for treatment of ulcers are summarized in the box.

Drugs for Treatment of Ulcers

Histamine H$_2$-Antagonists The troublesome side effects of cimetidine are not directly related to blockade of H$_2$-receptors. Side effects of cimetidine include interference with the metabolism of certain other drugs and its antiandrogenic effects. Cimetidine interacts with hepatic cytochrome P-450 and slows the clearance of some drugs that require the cytochrome P-450 enzyme system for metabolism, including hydroxycoumadin, phenytoin, propanolol, diazepam, and other drugs. Interference with their metabolism by cimetidine can lead to elevated plasma concentrations and toxic responses to the other drugs.

Cimetidine can bind to testosterone receptors and thus exert antiandrogenic effects, resulting in decreased sexual libido and gynecomastia in males treated with high doses. The antiandrogenic effects have not occurred in patients treated with ordinary doses of cimetidine, but have occurred in some patients with Zollinger-Ellinger syndrome after treatment with very high doses.

CLINICAL PROBLEMS		
Peptic ulcer therapy		
cimetidine	Interferes with metabolism of other drugs	
	Antiandrogenic effect (binds to testosterone receptors)	
antacids	Constipation	
	Diarrhea	
inhibitor (omeprazole) proton pump	Gastric mucosal hyperplasia	

Cimetidine can induce mild mental confusion and disorientation in elderly or severely ill patients. This effect is thought to result from elevated plasma concentrations with conventional doses but only in patients with impaired hepatic and renal functions and possibly with openings in the blood-brain barrier for easier penetration by drugs such as cimetidine that otherwise would not readily cross this barrier. Experience with cimetidine illustrates the need to evaluate drug doses with special care, particularly for elderly patients. A number of occasional incidents of diarrhea or skin rash occur with cimetidine in a small fraction of patients.

The recently introduced H$_2$-receptor antagonists, famotidine, ranitidine, and nizatidine, do not bind significantly to cytochrome P-450 of human liver and have not been found to alter the hepatic elimination of diazepam, metoprolol, theophylline, or hydroxycoumadin. However, ranitidine reduces hepatic conjugation of acetaminophen in rats and reduces renal clearance of triamterene in humans. Similar considerations apply to the antiandrogenic effects of cimetidine. The more recently introduced H$_2$-antagonists do not bind significantly to testosterone receptors and have not been found to induce gynecomastia. All of the H$_2$-antagonists produce a small incidence of mild, reversible side effects, such as dizziness, diarrhea, constipation, and headache. Collectively, the H$_2$-antagonists appear to be remarkably safe drugs.

Gastric Antacids Antacid therapy is complicated by the failure of physicians and patients to consider antacids as actual drugs, with benefits, hazards, and therapeutic ratios. Side effects can cause problems. Although divalent and trivalent metal ions are poorly absorbed and thus serve as nonsystemic antacids, small amounts of the ions are absorbed from the lumen of the intestine. Systemically absorbed calcium, magnesium, or aluminum are apparently innocuous in small amounts in most patients after short courses of therapy. However, in patients with renal insufficiency in which the cations are not adequately excreted, sufficient cations can be absorbed to exert systemic toxicity. Calcium salts can produce systemic hypercalcemia resulting in formation of calculi (milk alkali syndrome), and excess circulating magnesium can induce muscle weakness and fatigue. Aluminum can bind phosphate in the lumen of the gut and prevent adequate absorption of phosphate, leading in time to phosphate deficiency with muscle weakness and resorption of bone. The ability of aluminum to bind phosphate in the intestine is therapeutically useful in patients undergoing hemodialysis who otherwise tend to accumulate phosphate. Common problems encountered with antacids used as therapy for peptic ulcer are constipation and diarrhea. To solve this problem, an acceptable balance in stool frequency and consistency can be achieved by mixtures of magnesium and aluminum salts or by alternating doses of magnesium- or aluminum-containing antacids.

Prostaglandins Many prostaglandins induce diarrhea because they promote secretion of fluid and electrolytes into the lumen of the bowel and may also inhibit intestinal segmenting contractions that retard flow of luminal contents. In contrast to their effects of parietal cell adenylate cyclase activity, prostaglandins stimulate cAMP production in enterocytes and thereby increase intestinal secretion leading to net accumulation of fluid in the lumen. Another potential problem with prostaglandins is uterine stimulation, especially during pregnancy.

Proton Pump Inhibitors A potentially serious adverse side effect of omeprazole and possibly other proton pump inhibitors is gastric mucosal hyperplasia, which may lead to dysplasia and gastric cancer. The hyperplasia is thought to result from excessive secretion of gastrin from the antral mucosa as a consequence of antral alkalinization associated with profound inhibition of acid secretion. Gastrin exerts trophic effects on gastric and intestinal mucosa. If the gastric hyperplasia is caused by excessive release of gastrin, then gastric hyperplasia is a theoretical side effect associated with any antisecretory drug. However, excess gastrin secretion may be associated only with extremely efficacious drugs, such as proton pump inhibitors.

Prokinetic Drugs Because of its activity as a dopamine-receptor antagonist, metoclopramide can induce dystonia or Parkinson's diseaselike side effects. More recently developed prokinetic drugs, such as cisapride, still in clinical testing, block dopamine receptors and do not produce extrapyramidal side effects. Actions at 5HT$_3$ receptors may be important components of their beneficial effects. The prokinetic drugs without dopamine-receptor antagonist actions appear to produce antiemetic effects, suggesting that local gastric actions may be important in suppression of emesis. Because emesis is associated with orally progressing intestinal and gastric contractions (reverse peristalsis), prokinetic drugs may suppress emesis by promoting abnormal moving contractions.

TRADENAMES

In addition to generic and fixed combination preparations, the following tradenamed materials are available in the United States.

HISTAMINE H₂ ANTAGONISTS

Axid, nizatidine
Pepcid, famotidine
Tagamet, cimetidine
Zantac, ranitidine

ANTACIDS

ALternaGEL, Amphojel aluminum hydroxide
Aludrox, aluminum hydroxide, magnesium hydroxide
Carafate, sucralfate
Gaviscon, aluminum hydroxide, magnesium carbonate
Milk of Magnesia, magnesium hydroxide
Mylanta, Simeco, aluminum hydroxide, magnesium hydroxide, simethicone
Mylicon, simethicone
Riopan, magaldrate

ANTICHOLINERGICS AND OTHER AGENTS USED TO TREAT PEPTIC ULCER

Bentyl, dicyclomine
Cantil, mepenzolate
Cytotec, misoprostol
Losec, omeprazole
Pathilon, tridihexethyl
Peptavlon, pentagastrin
Pro-Banthine, propantheline
Reglan, metoclopramide
Robinul, glycopyrrolate
Valpin, anisotropine

LAXATIVES

Chronulac, lactulose
Colace, ducusate
Dulcolax, bisacodyl
Modane, danthron
Neoloid, castor oil
Prulet, phenolphthalein

ANTIDIARRHEAL DRUGS

Imodium, loperamide
Lomotil, diphenoxylate
Questran, cholestyramine

REFERENCES

Bode G, Malfertheiner P, and Ditschuneit H: Pathogenic implications of ultrastructural findings in *Campylobacter pylori* related gastroduodenal disease, Scand J Gastroenterol 23(suppl 142):25, 1988.

Burks TF: Actions of drugs on gastrointestinal motility. In Johnson LR, ed: Physiology of the gastrointestinal tract, New York, 1987, Raven Press.

Daniel EE: Pharmacology of adrenergic, cholinergic, and drugs acting on other receptors in gastrointestinal muscle, Handbook of Experimental Pharmacology 59(II):249, 1982.

Gabella G: Structure of muscles and nerves in the gastrointestinal tract. In Johnson LR, ed: Physiology of the gastrointestinal tract, New York, 1987, Raven Press.

Gullikson GW and Bass P: Mechanisms of action of laxative drugs. Handbook of Experimental Pharmacology 70(II):419, 1984.

Porro GB and Petrillo M: The natural history of peptic ulcer disease: the influence of H₂-antagonist treatment, Scand J Gastroenterol 21(suppl 121):46, 1986.

Schulze-Delrieu K: Metoclopramide, New Engl J Med 305:28, 1981.

Wolfe MM and Soll AH: The physiology of gastric acid secretion, N Engl J Med 319:1707, 1988.

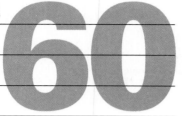

CHAPTER 60

Immuno-pharmacology

ABBREVIATIONS	
CMI	cellular-mediated immunity
CSF	cerebrospinal fluid
CSF	colony stimulating factor
CTL	cytolytic T lymphocytes
DTH	delayed-type hypersensitivity
INF	interferon
IL	interleukin
LAK	lymphokine-activated killer cell
TNF	tumor necrosis factor
MHC	major histocompatibility complex
G-CSF	granulocyte–colony stimulating factor
M-CSF	macrophage–colony stimulating factor
GM-CSF	granulocyte macrophage–colony stimulating factor
IG	immunoglobulin
APC	antigen presenting cell
HAT	hypoxanthine aminopterin thymine
HLA	histocompatibility leukocyte antigen
HPRT	hypoxanthine phosphoribosyl transferase

PHARMACOLOGICAL MODULATION OF THE IMMUNE SYSTEM

SUPPRESSION

Overcomes organ/tissue transplantation rejection
Reduces effects of autoimmune diseases

STIMULATION

Enhances activity of immune system against viruses, microorganisms, or other invading organisms
Enhances immune system activity against neoplastic cells of the host

THERAPEUTIC OVERVIEW

The immune system defends the body against invading organisms, foreign antigens, and host cells that have become neoplastic. In addition, the immune system is an active participant in autoimmune diseases, hypersensitivity reactions, and transplant tissue rejections.

The ability of the immune system to discriminate between foreign molecules and antigenic sites of foreign cells and normal endogenous molecules and cells of the host results in elimination of most diseases before an overt pathological condition is established. Moreover, after an infection or neoplasm becomes established and chemotherapy initiated, drugs kill only a fraction of the invading organisms (Chapter 45) or neoplastic cells (Chapter 43), and a functional immune system is needed to eradicate the remaining organisms or cells. This ability to recognize foreign antigens allows destruction and removal of invading organisms by various effector mechanisms of the immune system. However, in autoimmune diseases, inappropriate immune responses against host cells (self-antigens) may occur. In addition, an overt response to an antigen may result in tissue-damage reactions known as *hypersensitivity responses*.

801

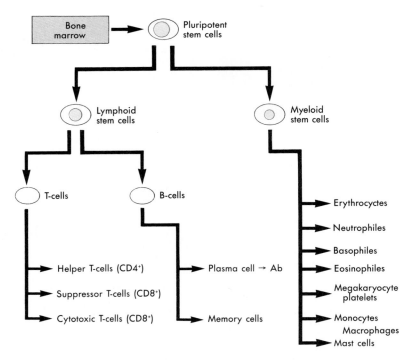

FIGURE 60-1   Terminology, sources, and interrelationships of components of the immune system. Terms in ( ) with T-cells represent names of markers. (*Ab*, Antibody.)

Pharmacological modulation of the immune system can stimulate or suppress the response, as summarized in the box.

 ## MECHANISMS OF ACTION

Immune System Components

Cell Types   The cells of the immune system are formed from pluripotent stem cells produced in bone marrow. These stem cells undergo a sequence of cellular differentiations, outlined in part in Figure 60-1, to form B lymphocytes, T lymphocytes, erythrocytes, leukocytes, monocytes, macrophages, and mast cells.

Lymphocytes are the primary cell types involved in the immune response. There are two types of lymphocytes, B and T. Both are derived from bone marrow lymphoid stem cells, but T cells go through an additional maturation process in the thymus. Although the morphology of T cells and B cells is similar, the functions of these two types are distinct. After antigen exposure, B cells develop into antibody-producing plasma cells, whereas T cells are divided into functional subtypes that possess distinct cell surface antigens.

The other major participant in the immune response is the bone-marrow−derived macrophage (see Figure 60-1). When unactivated and circulating, it is referred to as a *monocyte;* however, when it migrates into the extravascular spaces, it is known as a *macrophage.* In comparison to unactivated lymphocytes, macrophages are larger and possess a greater cytoplasmic to nuclear ratio. The macrophage contains lysosomes filled with various catabolic enzymes. The macrophage membrane possesses digestive enzymes and receptors for binding complement components and the constant or Fc region (Figure 60-2) of antibodies (immunoglobulins). The size and cytoplasmic contents are determined by the activation state. The primary functions of macrophages are phagocytosis, antigen presentation, and cytokine production. Phagocytic macrophages are distributed throughout many tissues (Table 60-1) and collectively are called the *reticuloendothelial system.* The generation of superoxide free radicals and digestive enzymes allows the macrophage to destroy other phagocytized organisms or molecules. This phagocytic process is also

Table 60-1 Cells that Constitute the Reticuloendothelial System

Tissue	Cell Type
Liver	Kuppfer cells
Brain	Microglial cells
Spleen	Macrophages
Lymph node	Macrophages
Lung	Aveolar macrophages

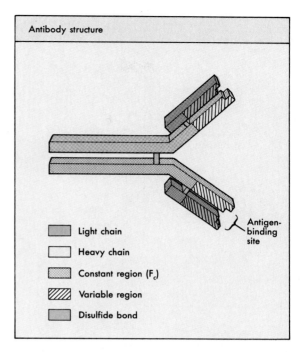

FIGURE 60-2   Antibody structure, showing light and heavy chains, variable regions, constant regions, and disulfide bonds.

important in altering and cleaving large antigen molecules before presentation to T lymphocytes (antigen processing).

Polymorphonuclear granulocytes and mast cells also participate in immune system processes. Three types of polymorphonuclear granulocytes (neutrophils, eosinophils, and basophils) originate from bone marrow and are located primarily in the vascular system. These cells constitute 50% to 60% of the total circulating leukocytes, with most being neutrophils (90%) and eosinophils (3% to 5%). Granulocytes can move out of the vascular system between endothelial cells and into tissue. Neutrophils have an important role in host resistance to microorganisms. Opsonized organisms bind neutrophils via complement and Fc receptors and are phagocytized. Although eosinophils are morphologically similar to neutrophils, they are thought to be mainly involved with reactions against parasitic infections. Basophils and mast cells are important effector cells in IgE-mediated allergic reactions. The binding of IgE to these cells stimulates the release of vasoactive amines (e.g., histamines, see Chapter 57), causing vasodilation and loss of vascular fluids into tissue (discussed in more detail in the section on hypersensitivity). Basophils and mast cells are functionally very similar but differ in that basophils may enter tissue from blood and have a polymorphonuclear nucleus, whereas mast cells are residents of connective tissue and have nuclei with a more oval mononuclear shape.

Organs and Tissues Immune system cells migrate from the bone marrow via the circulatory system to secondary lymphoid organs, lymph nodes, spleen, and mucosal tissue (gastrointestinal [GI], respiratory, urogenital). The centralization of immunocompetent cells in secondary lymphoid tissue, rather than dispersal throughout the circulatory system, provides a location where antigen may be retained and presented to lymphocytes. Moreover, activated lymphocytes may interact more readily with neighboring lymphocytes in the lymphoid tissue. These cells may then migrate out of the secondary lymphoid organs and function at distant sites in the body. Lymph nodes are distributed throughout the body and are interconnected by lymphatic vessels and the circulatory system. This allows lymphocytes to circulate between different organs and to more readily contact foreign antigens. The lymphatic circulatory system drains into the thoracic duct and then back into the vascular system. Secondary lymphoid organs are organized as reticular structures to allow cells to migrate into the lymphoid tissue where they may contact antigen and then migrate out into the periphery as mature, antigen-specific lymphocytes. Different types of immunocompetent cells are distributed in distinct regions in the tissues.

Antibodies One of the primary components of the immune response is antibodies. Antibodies are immunoglobulins secreted from B cells that have been stimulated with antigen. Antibodies produced in re-

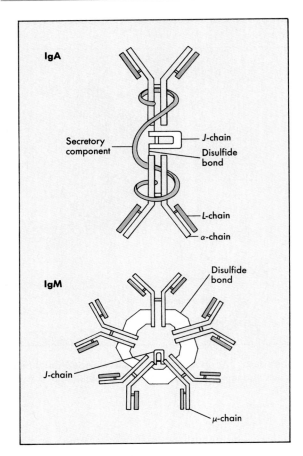

FIGURE 60-3   IgA and IgM structure. The secretory IgA is composed of two immunoglobulins connected by a J-chain and secretory component. IgM is composed of five immunoglobulin molecules joined with a J-chain. (*L-chain*, Light chain; μ*-chain*, heavy chain.)

sponse to a specific antigen bind only that specific antigen. Immunoglobulins are composed of two heavy and two light chains, as shown schematically in Figure 60-2. Antigen binds to a portion of the variable region (V) and affords specificity to the immunoglobulin. The other region is named the *constant region* (Fc). There are five classes of immunoglobulins: IgA, IgD, IgG, IgE, and IgM. The IgA and IgM immunoglobulins contain multiple immunoglobulin units joined by disulfide bonds (Figure 60-3).

Antigens, which stimulate the formation of antibodies, may be molecules of various types (e.g., proteins, carbohydrates, lipids, nucleic acids). However, many low molecular weight compounds such as drugs and environmental contaminants are not capable of inducing antibody production. If these small mole-

cules are bound to high molecular weight molecules (carriers), these compounds (called *haptens*) can become antigenic. Antibodies are produced against either haptens or hapten-carrier conjugates.

Immune defenses against infectious organisms and neoplastic cells are commonly classified as innate or acquired (also known as adaptive). Responses that are antigen-independent are considered innate, whereas acquired immunity involves antigen recognition and is characterized by an antigen-dependent action. In many host defense responses, both innate and acquired immunity occur.

Immune Response

Innate Immunity Commonly referred to as the first line of defense, innate immunity encompasses a wide variety of cell types and mechanisms of action. Microorganisms and tumor cells are phagocytized by macrophages and neutrophils after activation by cellular components of the invading organism (e.g., endotoxin) or cytokines (e.g., macrophage activating factor). Tumor cells may be lysed in an antigen non-specific manner by natural killer cells or lymphokine-activated killer cells. Another important component of the innate response is the complement cascade, in which certain components act as substrates for other enzyme components. The substrates are then activated to form enzymes that convert other components of the cascade to active enzymes. The activated complement components form complexes that are capable of lysing the invading organisms, and these complexes may be activated by cellular constituents on bacteria (alternate pathway) and thus do not require antigen recognition.

Acquired Immunity Antigen stimulation of lymphocytes may result in the development of humoral and/or cell-mediated immune responses. Humoral responses involve the participation of antibody. Macrophages and T-helper cells are required in addition to B cells in most humoral immune responses (Figure 60-4). This collaborative effort involves the production of interleukin 1 and antigen presentation to T cells by macrophages. The CD4 containing T-helper cells will only recognize antigen when associated with major histocompatability (MHC) class II antigens (Figure 6-5). The combination of antigen activation and interleukin 1 binding to receptors on T-helper cells results in the production of interleukin 2 and other interleukins. Antigens bind to specific immunoglobulin receptors on B cells. Lymphokines produced by T cells

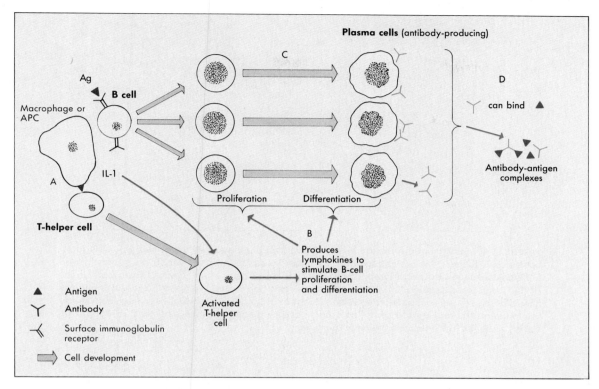

FIGURE 60-4   Generation of a humoral immune response. There are several cell types required in the generation of the antibody producing plasma cells. Antigen *(Ag)* is processed and presented to T-helper cells with class II MHC antigens *(A)* (see Figure 60-5). This results in the synthesis and secretion of lymphokines, which act on B cells, macrophages, and T-helper cells *(B)*. Antigen-activated B cells proliferate and differentiate to plasma cells *(C)*. Antibodies are produced that bind antigen *(D)*. (*IL*, Interleukin; *APC*, antigen presenting cells such as macrophages.)

stimulate the antigen-activated B cells to proliferate and differentiate into antibody producing plasma cells. Concurrent with the generation of activated T cells and B cells, antigen also induces the generation of suppressor T cells. These cells are thought to down-modulate the immune response by the secretion of suppressive factors. However, since several laboratories have been unable to characterize the factors, the area of suppressor cells remains controversial.

Cell-mediated responses also require macrophages to present antigen to T cells and produce interleukin 1 and other factors (Figure 60-5). These steps may lead to the generation of cytolytic T cells and/or activation of macrophages. In the generation of cytolytic T cells, antigen is presented to the cells, and production of interleukin 2 by the activated T-helper cells stimulates the proliferation and differentiation of cytolytic T cells to mature cytolytic T cells. Cytolytic T

lymphocytes may be produced against graft tumor (Figure 60-6) or virus-infected cells. Antigen recognition and binding of cytolytic T cells to antigen of cells results in the lysis of target. In delayed-type hypersensitivity reactions, antigen-stimulated T-helper cells secrete lymphokines, which recruit and activate macrophages. These macrophages are then capable of phagocytizing the foreign organisms or host cells in an antigen nonspecific manner. This can occur in reactions against tuberculosis and with chemicals such as urushiol from poison ivy.

Modulation of Response by Hormones and CNS   The interplay between hormones and neurotransmitters and the immune response is very important in presenting a multi-organ response to stimuli. Glucocorticoids secreted by the adrenal cortex during stress can lead to suppressed immune responses and movement of lymphocytes out of the

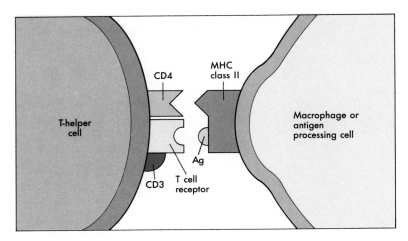

FIGURE 60-5   Molecular interaction between a macrophage and a T-helper cell. The CD4 molecules on T-helper cells act as receptors for major histocompatibility (*MHC*) class II antigens. CD8 molecules on cytotoxic T lymphocytes recognize MHC class I (*not shown*). Close association of the T cell receptor and CD4 allows for the presentation of antigen-class II antigen complex. This binding results in the transduction of a signal via the CD3 molecule. MHC class II antigens are found on macrophages, B cells, and other specialized antigen-presenting cells (APCs). MHC class I antigens are present on all somatic cells.

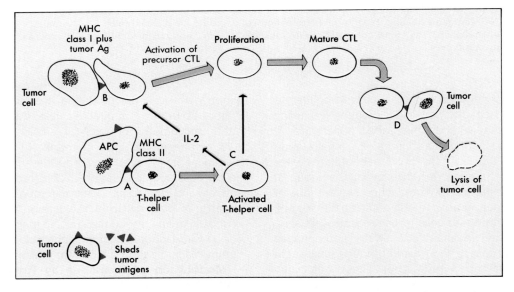

FIGURE 60-6   Cytolytic T lymphocyte (*CTL*) generation against tumor cells. Tumor antigens are processed and presented to T-helper cells in the context of MHC class II antigens (*A*). Precursor CTL are activated with antigen presented in the context of MHC class I antigens (*B*). T-helper cells secrete a variety of lymphokines that stimulate the maturation of CTL (*C*). The tumors cells are then recognized and lyzed by mature CTL (*D*). (See Figure 60-4 for key.)

vascular space. Prolactin enhances the immune response by binding to prolactin receptors on lymphocytes. Central nervous system (CNS) control of the immune response is suggested by decreased immune responses in patients bereaved by death of a spouse. Neuroanatomical studies demonstrate the presence of neurons in lymph nodes and spleen in close contact with lymphocytes. Receptors for neurotransmitters are present in lymphocytes.

Pharmacological Immunosuppression

Pharmacological approaches for immunosuppressive therapy stress selective eradication of certain cells, similar to selective killing of tumor cells during cancer chemotherapy (Chapter 43). Target immunocompetent cells must be selectively altered or deleted to prevent adverse effects on other tissues. Approaches to obtaining immunosuppression can be divided into four categories according to their relative selectivity. The least selective (category 1) approaches affect proliferating cells and include irradiation, deoxyribonucleic acid (DNA) alkylating agents, and antimetabolites. Nontarget tissues with high proliferative rates such as bone marrow and GI tract epithelium also are adversely affected. Depletion of immunocompetent cells (category 2) may be accomplished by physical removal of cells (e.g., splenectomy, thoracic duct drainage) or by use of antilymphocyte serum. A more selective method (category 3) affects only certain subpopulations of lymphocytes, such as is obtained with cyclosporine or monoclonal antibodies specifically against cell surface antigens. A still more ideal method (category 4) is selective alteration of only those antigen-specific cell populations that mediate the response. In this manner, immune responses against pathogenic organisms and tumors are not altered. Suppression of the immune response by drugs is obtained currently via categories 1 and 3. Different immunosuppressive therapies involve the use of more than one drug to obtain optimal results. Currently, numerous treatment regimens are used, many of which have been developed empirically. The primary uses of immunosuppressive drugs are in the prevention of transplant rejection and the treatment of autoimmune diseases.

The principal drugs used to obtain immunsuppression include corticosteroids, cyclophosphamide, azathioprine, methotrexate, cyclosporine, and experimental antibody, as well as experimental FK-506.

Corticosteroids Structures of the corticosteroids are illustrated in Chapter 35.

Glucocorticoids secreted by the adrenal cortex affect a wide range of normal physiological functions; the immune system is a major target. The administration of glucocorticoids to patients results in decreased numbers of circulating lymphocytes, basophils, and eosinophils over a 24-hour period, whereas the number of neutrophils increases. In addition, changes in corticosteroid concentrations during the normal diurnal cycle and in stressful situations correlate with decreases in the number of circulating lymphocytes. The lymphopenia observed in humans is attributed to the migration of cells into extravascular spaces, with a greater T-cell migration than B-cell or monocyte migration. A majority of the cells migrate to bone marrow. Some studies suggest that changes in membrane proteins produce the altered migratory behavior.

Although corticosteroid-induced lymphopenia is well documented, the importance of this effect on immunosuppression is not clear. It is apparent, however, that corticosteroids alter the immune response by directly changing immune cell function, with T-cell–mediated responses affected to a greater extent than B-cell responses. The macrophage is the primary target responsible for the decreased immune response. Exposure of macrophages to corticosteroids results in decreased IL-1 production, decreased expression of MHC class II antigens, and decreased phagocytosis of virus-infected cells, tumor cells, bacteria, and fungi.

Cyclophosphamide The structure, activation to phosphoramide mustard and acrolein, and antitumor mechanism of action of cyclophosphamide are discussed in Chapter 43.

The roles of the active phosphoramide mustard and acrolein in mediating the actions of cyclophosphamide on the immune response are unclear. The mustard is thought to alkylate DNA and mediate the antiproliferative and immunosuppressive effects. This is consistent with the hypothesis that the selective cytotoxic effects on B cells are attributable to a greater proliferative rate. However, the highly reactive, sulfhydryl-binding acrolein may also play an important but unclear role in the drug action.

Azathioprine The structure of azathioprine is shown in Figure 60-7. This drug undergoes metabolism to 6-mercaptopurine (see Chapter 43), which is further metabolized to the active antitumor

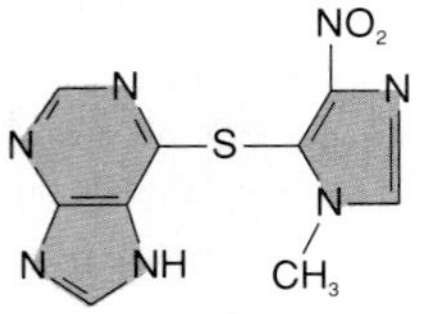

azathioprine

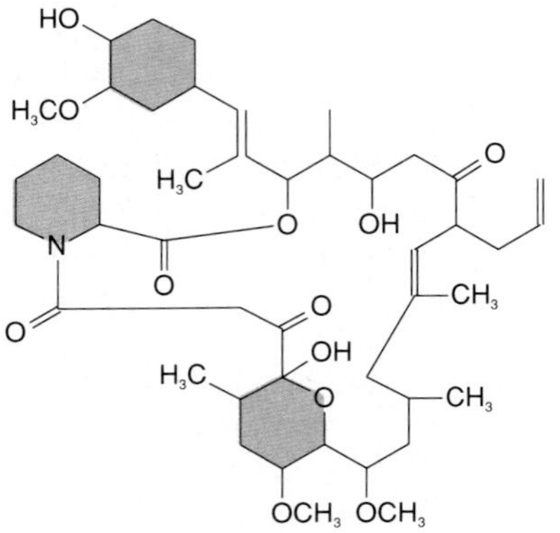

FK506

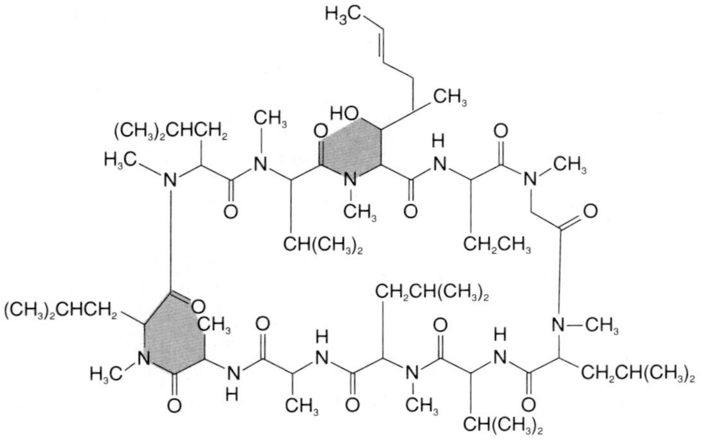

cyclosporin A

FIGURE 60-7   Structures of several immunosuppressants, including the 11 amino acid cyclosporin A.

and immunosuppressive thioinosinic acid. This inhibits hypoxanthine-guanine phosphoribosyltransferase, which mediates conversion of purines to the corresponding phosphoribosyl-5' phosphate and of hypoxanthine to inosinic acid. This leads to inhibition of cellular proliferation. The mechanism of immuno-

suppression is mediated by the antiproliferative actions. However, as with cyclophosphamide, immunosuppression by azathioprine may be mediated in part by other mechanisms. Inosine reverses the 6-mercaptopurine–induced suppression of in vitro immune response but does not reverse suppression of azathioprine.

Methotrexate Methotrexate is discussed in Chapter 43. The immunological and antitumor mechanisms are similar.

Cyclosporine Cyclosporine A is a cyclic endecapeptide purified from two strains of fungi imperfecti, *Tolypociadium inflatum* Gams and *Cyclindrocapon lucidum* Booth (see Figure 60-7).

Cyclosporine A primarily affects T-cell–mediated responses, whereas most humoral immune responses not requiring T cells are spared. The effectiveness of cyclosporine A is based on selective inhibition of T-helper cell activation and slight enhancement of T-suppressor cell activity. The major effect on T-helper cells is via inhibition of interleukin-2 production. Messenger RNA concentrations for interleukin-2 and γ-interferon are decreased. The decreased interleukin-2 production in turn leads to decreased numbers of interleukin-2 receptors and functional unresponsiveness of CTL precursor cells. Because there is positive feedback through interleukin-2 production and interleukin-2 receptors, the decreased interleukin-2 production of T-helper cells also leads to decreased interleukin-2 receptors on T-helper cells. Cyclosporine does not, however, affect the proliferative response of activated cytolytic T lymphocytes (CTL) to interleukin 2 or the lytic activity of CTL. Consistent with this is the observation that cyclosporine is effective only during the very early stages of antigen activation of T-helper cells. There is also evidence for inhibition of macrophage antigen presentation and interleukin-1 production by macrophages.

Several mechanisms of action of cyclosporine have been proposed. Cyclosporine binds to the cytosolic proteins, calmodulin, and cyclophilin. The role of calmodulin is supported by the findings that calmodulin antagonists inhibit binding of cyclosporine to cytosolic proteins and calmodulin-dependent phosphodiesterase activity is inhibited by cyclosporine. However, similar binding occurs in cells sensitive and insensitive to cyclosporine. In addition, nonimmunosuppressive derivatives of cyclosporine A also bind to calmodulin. A more current mechanism of action is through binding of cyclophilin. The binding of cyclosporine A to cyclophilin is ten times greater than to calmodulin. Cyclophilin is also found in many tissues not associated with the immune system. The structure of cyclophilin is identical to that of peptidyl-prolyl *cis-trans* isomerase, an enzyme involved in the folding of proteins. The function of cyclophilin and how cyclosporine binding to this protein can selectively alter T-helper cell activity are not clear.

Monoclonal Antibodies Antibodies have been used recently as pharmacological agents to obtain greater therapeutic specificity and fewer side effects. The generation of antibodies by injecting antigen into different animal species results in generation of numerous B-cell clones, each producing antibodies against different antigenic sites of a large molecule. However, the amount of antiserum obtained is limited, significant amounts of antigen must be purified, the quality of antibody varies between batches, and the antiserum may contain antibodies against certain unwanted determinants. The development of monoclonal antibodies allows circumvention of these problems. Fusion of antibody producing plasma cells with neoplastic myeloma cells yields a cell population called a *hybridoma,* capable of secreting a specific antibody and continually proliferating (Figure 60-8). Isolation, characterization, and cultivation of single clones of hybridomas can result in the generation of one type of antibody against a specific antigen in almost unlimited supply.

The use of antibodies with drugs can be divided into targeting drug-antibody conjugates to cell surface tumor antigens (see Chapter 6) and using antibodies as drugs against specific cell surface components important for immune response, such as antigen binding sites or lymphokine receptors. The latter is employed in immunosuppressive treatment for specific inhibition of lymphocyte function or depletion of certain cell populations. Polyclonal antilymphocyte and antithymocyte sera are successfully used in the prevention of graft rejection, with sera that is produced by the injection of human thymocytes or lymphocytes into sheep, horses, or goats. Monoclonal antibodies to lymphocyte antigens may replace the use of polyclonal sera. Monoclonal antibodies against the CD3-receptor complex on T cells and the interleukin-2 receptor are the most widely studied, and the use of anti-CD3 antibodies in the treatment of acute rejection of renal transplants has now been approved.

The anti-CD3 preparation evolved out of attempts to find monoclonal antibodies to clinically alter T cell responses. In testing antibodies of a clone that appeared to bind only T cells, it was found that the clone specifically bound to the CD3 or T3 structure on T cells. The CD3 unit is associated with the T cell antigen receptor complex involved in signal transduction to the T cell after binding of antigen to the receptor complex (Figure 60-5). Intravenous (IV) administration of anti-CD3 leads to a dramatic decrease

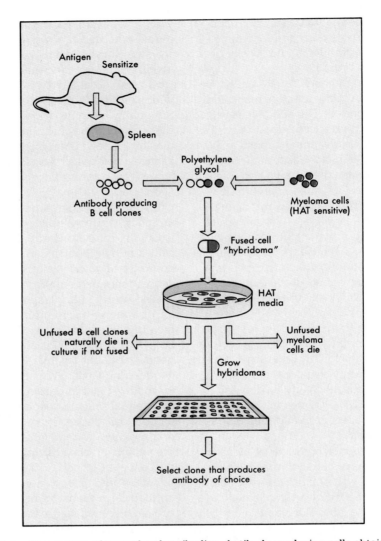

FIGURE 60-8   Preparation of monoclonal antibodies. Antibody producing cells obtained from a mouse treated with antigen are fused with myeloma tumor cells in the presence of polyethylene glycol. The fused cells are called *hybridomas*. Each hybridoma secretes antibody against one specific antigenic site and continues to proliferate. To separate the unfused lymphocytes and myeloma cells from the hybridomas, the cells are incubated in cell culture medium containing hypoxanthine, aminopterin, and thymidine *(HAT)*. Aminopterin inhibits the conversion of tetrahydrofolate to dihydrofolate (major pathway of purine synthesis). In the presence of aminopterin, normal cells survive by using xanthine and thymidine (salvage pathway). The myeloma cells lack the enzyme hypoxanthine phosphoribosyltransferase (HPRT), an enzyme required for the salvage pathway. Thus in the presence of HAT, the myeloma cells die in culture unless fused with normal B cells, which provide HPRT. These cells are grown and the antibody secreted is tested.

in T3-positive cells. Although the mechanism of T cell depletion is unknown, T cells are opsonized with anti-CD and removed by the reticuloendothelial system.

FK-506 FK-506 is a recent immunosuppressive macrolide undergoing early human trials in renal, heart, and liver transplant patients with early success. The mechanism of action may be similar to cyclosporin. The structure is shown in Figure 60-7. It inhibits the synthesis of interleukins 2, 3, and 4, granulocyte macrophage–colony stimulating factor (GM-CSF), tumor necrosis factor-α, and γ-interferon. FK-506 is roughly 100 times more potent than cyclosporine. FK-506 also binds to a protein with peptidyl-protyl *cis-trans* isomerase activity that is distinct from cyclophilin.

Pharmacological Immunostimulation

The availability of drugs that stimulate the immune response against infections and tumors is desirable, but many drugs are limited as a result of low efficacy and life-threatening toxicity. Compounds that act as general stimulators of the immune response (for example, BCG and dextran polymer) were extensively studied from the 1950s to the mid 1980s but produced only marginal effects and are seldom used today.

Lymphokines, colony stimulating and tumor necrosis factors, and interferons are new leads that may generate more potent and safe compounds for possible use in stimulation of the immune response.

Lymphokines Interleukin 2 (IL-2) is a 15,420 dalton peptide of 133 amino acids that is produced by T-helper cells. Human recombinant interleukin 2 is commercially available.

As discussed previously, IL-2 stimulates T-helper cells and CTL cells to proliferate. IL-2 stimulation of cell proliferation is dependent on expression of IL-2 receptors with prior antigen stimulation. IL-2 incubation with lymphocytes also stimulates production of lymphokine-activated killer cells that lyse tumor cells in an antigen nonspecific manner but do not affect normal cells.

Colony Stimulating and Tumor Necrosis Factors Four colony stimulating factors (CSF) (Table 60-2), named for their ability to induce the formation of certain types of colonies from bone marrow cells grown in soft agar cultures, affect bone marrow cell populations at different stages of maturity. Multi-CSF (called *interleukin-3*) stimulates the primitive progenitor cells of granulocytes, megakaryocytes, mast cells, macrophages, and erythrocytes. In contrast, more differentiated progenitor cells are stimulated by granulocyte–colony stimulating factor (G-CSF) and macrophage–colony stimulating factor (M-CSF) to proliferate and differentiate into granulocytes and macrophages, respectively. Both of these cell lineages are stimulated by GM-CSF. As cells of certain lineages mature from progenitors to more committed states, they became refractory to certain CSFs and sensitive to other subtypes. The production of CFSs by various cell types and development of drugs that stimulate or inhibit their secretion by the immune system is under intense research (Figure 60-9). After exposure to a pathogen (e.g., bacteria, virus-infected cells) T cells activate and produce IL-3 and GM-CSF, whereas activated macrophages produce M-CSF, G-CSF, and GM-CSF. Activated macrophages also produce interleukin 1 and tumor necrosis factor (TNF), which stimulate the production of GM-CSF, G-CSF, and M-CSF by endothelial cells and mesenchymal cells. In this manner, the host produces more granulocytes and macrophages to combat the invading organism. CSFs also act on mature neutrophils to increase their ability to destroy the invading organism.

The discovery of tumor necrosis factor (TNF) was based on the observation that bacterial infections in

Table 60-2   Classification of Colony Stimulating Factors (CSF)

CSF Subtype	Cell Origin	Cell Types Produced with Stimulation
CSF-multi (interleukin-3)	T cell	Granulocytes, macrophages, megakaryocytes, mast cells, erythrocytes
GM-CSF	T cell, macrophage, endothelial cell, mesenchymal cell	Granulocytes, macrophages
G-CSF	Macrophage, endothelial cell, mesenchymal cell	Granulocytes
M-CSF	Macrophage, endothelial cell, mesenchymal cell	Macrophages

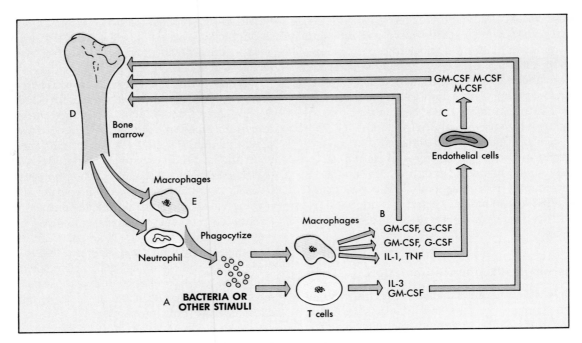

FIGURE 60-9   Secretion of colony stimulating factors *(CSFs)* in response to immune stimulation. Bacteria or other stimuli *(A)* activate macrophages and T cells to produce a variety of CSFs *(B)*, which also stimulate endothelial cells to produce CSFs *(C)*. CSFs stimulate production of macrophages and neutrophils from bone marrow *(D)*. These cells are then able to phagocytose the bacteria *(E)*. (*IL-1*, Interleukin 1; *IL-3*, interleukin 3; *G-CSF*, granulocyte–colony stimulating factor; *M-CSF*, macrophage–colony stimulating factor; *GM-CSF*, granulocyte macrophage–colony stimulating factor.)

patients with tumor were correlated with the regression of the tumors. It was later found that bacterial cell wall components stimulated the secretion of TNF by macrophages. TNF is named for its ability to produce hemorrhagic necrosis of tumors by an unknown mechanism and acts on the inflammatory process and immune response.

TNF (called *TNF-α*) is a 157 amino acid protein functionally similar to another cytokine, lymphotoxin (called *TNF-β*). Recombinant TNF is produced by several companies.

After injury or bacterial infection, a sequence of events occurs that involves TNF (Figure 60-10). In bacterial infections, granulocytes such as neutrophils migrate into the infected area and attack the microbes. These effects are potentiated by the actions of interleukin 1 and TNF on endothelial cells and neutrophils. Macrophages are also recruited, activated, and secrete interleukin 1 and TNF. Both cytokines stimulate T cells, which results in production of IL-2

and interferon. Further production of TNF by macrophages is stimulated by interferon.

Interferons   The interferons (IFN) are named after their ability to interfere with viral RNA and protein synthesis. There are three types of interferons, α, β, and γ, which are synthesized by different cell types. With viral stimulation, the α form is primarily synthesized in macrophages, and the β form in macrophages and fibroblasts. The γ form is produced in T lymphocytes after stimulation with antigen or mitogens.

Recombinant IFN is commercially available and is undergoing clinical trials. The structure of α-IFN and β-IFN are similar (30% homology), whereas there is no sequence homology between γ and the α-β types. α-IFN and β-IFN can bind to the same receptor. The human α, β, and γ forms each have molecular weights of 20 to 25 kilodaltons, and all three differ as to antigenicity.

Although all interferons show antiviral actions, α

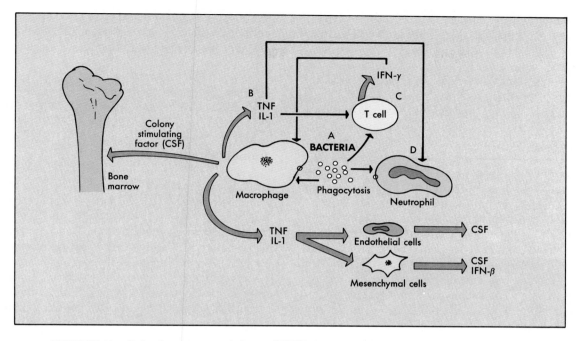

FIGURE 60-10   Role of tumor necrosis factor *(TNF)* in bacterial infections. Macrophage activation by bacteria *(A)* results in the production of TNF along with CSFs and IL-1 *(B)*. TNF and IL-1 stimulate T cells to produce IFN-γ *(C)*, which further activates macrophages. TNF and IL-1 also stimulate neutrophils and enhance phagocytosis of bacteria *(D)*. Macrophage-derived CSF also stimulates bone marrow, while macrophage-derived TNF and IL-1 stimulate endothelial and mesenchymal cells to produce CSF and IFN-β. *(IL-1*, Interleukin 1; *CSF*, colony stimulating factor; *IFN-γ*, interferon γ; *IFN-β*, interferon β.)

and β are more potent than γ. However, γ-IFN affects the immune system more than α-IFN or β-IFN. The major action of γ-IFN on the immune system is the induction of antigen expression on macrophages and B cells. This results in increased ability to present antigen and may also be a factor in induction of autoimmune responses. The differentiation of B cells to antibody producing cells is also stimulated by γ-IFN. Activation of macrophages by γ-IFN results in greater cytocidal action as a result of increased secretion of hydrogen peroxide, phagocytosis, and expression of Fc receptors. These effects on macrophages are greater than those obtainable with α-IFNs or β-IFNs.

The inhibition of viral replication by IFN may result from the induction of an enzyme that inhibits viral replication by catalyzing breakdown of viral RNA. The antitumor actions of IFN appear to be a result of reduced oncogene expression.

 PHARMACOKINETICS

Immunosuppressive Drugs

Numerous synthetic derivatives of glucocorticoids are used as immunosuppressive agents. The pharmacokinetic parameters of glucocorticoids are described in Chapter 35.

The pharmacokinetics of cyclophosphamide and methotrexate are discussed in Chapter 43.

Azathioprine is usually given IV as a loading dose on the day of transplantation with subsequent oral maintenance doses. It is rapidly absorbed from the GI tract, even to a greater extent than 6-mercaptopurine, thus providing an advantage over 6-mercaptopurine. Azathioprine is metabolized in the liver to 6-mercatopurine. However, other minor metabolites may account for the differences in the action of azathioprine and 6-mercaptopurine. Most of the metabolites are excreted in urine. The half-life of azathioprine is 5 to 6 hours.

Cyclosporine, a highly nonpolar compound, is administered orally in olive oil or in a galenic formulation or IV in a cremophor vehicle. When given orally, absorption occurs slowly and is highly variable between individuals with a mean oral bioavailability of only 30%. Because of variability, concentrations of cyclosporine must be monitored to maintain effectiveness and prevent toxicity, especially in patients with renal allografts. The nonpolar characteristics of cyclosporin result in a large volume of distribution. In the blood, 40% to 60% of cyclosporine is bound to lipoproteins. Disposition is by metabolism with a half-life of 19 hours. Metabolism of cyclosporine occurs in the liver, mediated by the cytochrome P-450 system. Some of the metabolites are immunosuppressive but are less potent than the parent compound. Metabolites are predominantly excreted via the biliary system, with only 10% excreted in the urine.

Anti-CD3 receptor complex is administered IV. Blood concentrations decline to 10% of peak values after 24 hours, but the mechanism of clearance is not known.

Immunostimulant Drugs

IL-2 can be administered IV by bolus or continuous infusion; the latter results in less toxicity. Elimination of IL-2 from serum follows a first phase half-life of 6 to 7 minutes, in which most of the IL-2 is cleared, and a second phase half-life of 70 minutes.

After IV or IM injection, serum TNF concentrations decrease rapidly within 30 minutes and then continue to slowly decrease. TNF concentrates in the liver, kidneys, spleen, and GI tract.

With interferons, the route of administration depends on the target tissue or disease, with topical, IV, IM, SC, and intranasal widely used. Because the interferons are proteins, the oral route is not effective. Most of the pharmacokinetic information on interferons is available for α-IFN. The vascular half-life is 6 to 8 hours after IM injection, but the fate of α-IFN is not known. Concentrations in the cerebrospinal fluid (CSF) are about 0.08 times that in serum. Penetration into the lung and fluid compartments of the eye are poor, and little drug crosses the placenta. Virtually no interferon is recovered in urine, and blood concentrations are not altered in renal deficiency. Neutral-

izing anti-α–IFN antibodies are produced in some patients and may present a problem. Development of methods to monitor the generation of this antibody are under study.

RELATION OF MECHANISMS OF ACTION TO CLINICAL RESPONSE

Immunosuppression

Graft Rejections Genetically coded antigens are the determining factor in the rejection of a graft by a host.

Most human studies of transplant rejection involve renal allografts. The types of rejection processes can be classified according to how quickly the rejection occurs. Hyperacute rejection can occur within minutes and is mediated by cytotoxic antibodies already circulating in the host as a result of prior exposure to graft antigens. Cytotoxic antibodies to type ABO blood group antigens may mediate rejection in a mismatch. Accelerated rejection occurs in 2 to 5 days with the mechanism being an accelerated form of the acute process, again mediated by prior exposure to graft antigens (secondary immune response). Acute rejection occurs over 7 to 21 days and is mediated by a primary response requiring a longer time for generation of effector cells. Chronic rejection is observed after about 3 months. The immune process of graft rejection is divided into afferent and efferent stages.

Afferent Stage Initiation of the response is mediated by graft cells possessing MHC class II antigens that are incompatible with the host (bone-marrow–derived dendritic cells, Langerhans cells, certain endothelial cells of human tissue). These cells, termed *passenger cells,* drain into the lymphatics and directly stimulate T cells in lymph nodes. Contact between circulating T cells and special antigens may also occur in the graft. It is known that tissues containing a greater burden of passenger cells are more likely to be rejected (e.g., skin and bone marrow). In addition, removal of passenger cells before transplantation dramatically increases the chances of acceptance.

Efferent Stage Activation of macrophages and T cells during different stages leads to various effector mechanisms by which the host may destroy the graft: antibody, CTL, and delayed-type hypersensitivity (DTH). The involvement of CTL and antibody in transplant rejection are more clearly documented than the role of DTH. Common to all three responses is the role of T-helper cells. Special antigens on the graft can activate T-helper cells and production of lymphokines, which stimulate the activation, proliferation, and growth of T lymphocytes, B lymphocytes, and macrophages. In delayed-type hypersensitivity response, T-helper cell–produced lymphokines activate and recruit monocytes to the graft. These activated macrophages nonspecifically destroy surrounding tissue.

Autoimmune Diseases The basic mechanism by which the immune system selectively destroys infectious microbes and tumor cells is through its ability to discriminate between self and nonself antigens. A dysfunction in this ability may lead to an immune response against one's own tissue, an autoimmune disease. Although the manifestations of autoimmune diseases are well described, only within the last few years have a number of these diseases been classified as autoimmune responses (e.g., type 1 diabetes and insulin-dependent diabetes). The discovery of an autoimmune origin has led to investigation of immunosuppressive therapy for treatment. Several contributing factors may trigger or predispose individuals to an autoimmune disease. Each type of autoimmune disease may have a different etiology. There is a genetic predisposition associated with the expression of certain MHC (HLA) antigens. A greater occurrence in the elderly has also been found. Mechanisms proposed include the following:

1. Possible induction of cells that possess self-antigens to express MHC class II antigens and activate autoreactive T cells
2. Dysfunction of the suppressor T-cell system removing down-regulatory actions on autoreactive T and B cells
3. Immune response against foreign agents with similar structure to self-antigens
4. Exposure of sequestered cellular antigens not normally exposed to the immune system
5. General stimulation of the immune response by viruses and bacteria, which leads to lymphokine production and nonspecific stimulation of autoreactive B-cell clones

Autoimmune diseases are categorized as organ-specific and organ-nonspecific. In organ-specific diseases, immune responses are mounted against antigens specific for a certain organ, with manifestations of the diseases being dysfunction of the specific organ. In contrast, with organ-nonspecific diseases, immune responses are against tissue components in most cell types (DNA, cytoskeletal proteins). Examples include organ-specific (Hashimoto's thyroiditis, myasthenia gravis, Graves' disease, type 1 diabetes) and organ-nonspecific (systemic lupus erythematosus). In these five examples, the antibodies that are produced are antithyroid hormone, antiacetylcholine receptor, antithyroid stimulating hormone, antiinsulin, or antibodies to intracellular components, respectively.

Immunosuppressive Drugs

Glucocorticoids Numerous synthetic derivatives of glucocorticoids are in use as immunosuppressive agents. Only the minimal effective dose should be given if corticosteroids are to be administered over a long period (months to years) to minimize toxicity. Glucocorticoids are usually administered in conjunction with other immunosuppressive agents to treat graft rejection and autoimmune diseases. Because of their antiinflammatory actions, glucocorticoids are effective in treatment of immunological problems that are exacerbated by inflammatory reactions.

Cyclophosphamide Cyclophosphamide is used to treat autoimmune diseases and to prevent rejection of grafts. However, its use has dramatically decreased since the discovery of cyclosporine. As with other immunosuppressive drugs, cyclophosphamide is given often in combination with corticosteroids. Because of the life-threatening toxicities that may occur with cyclophosphamide, extreme care should be taken to administer the minimal dose necessary.

Humoral immune responses are more sensitive to the effects of cyclophosphamide than cell-mediated responses. However, both arms of the immune response are affected at high doses. Low doses of cyclophosphamide enhance various immune responses. These findings are attributed to the selective inhibition of suppressor T-cell generation or a selective effect on suppressor T cells. Because many tumors elicit the induction of suppressor T cells that down-regulate the immune response against foreign tumor cells, the selective elimination of suppressor T cells by low-dose cyclophosphamide may enhance the destruction of tumor cells.

Azathioprine In contrast to cyclophosphamide, the primary targets of azathioprine are cellular-mediated immunity (CMI) responses. Inhibition of in vitro immune responses is maximum during initiation of the response. This time-dependent action is consistent with the clinical findings that azathioprine is ineffective against ongoing rejection of grafts. Additional in vitro investigations indicate that azathioprine primarily effects antigen-stimulated lymphocytes, whereas unstimulated spleen cells are unaffected. Primary immune responses are suppressed with azathioprine treatment, whereas secondary responses are unaffected.

Methotrexate Although methotrexate is a potent immunosuppressive agent, its numerous adverse effects and the development of cyclosporine has limited its use in the treatment of immune-associated diseases. However, low-dose methotrexate is now used to treat rheumatoid arthritis refractory to conventional drugs. Because rheumatoid arthritis is an autoimmune disease, the immunosuppressive actions of methotrexate could account for its effectiveness. However, the low doses used may not affect the immune system and the antiinflammatory effects may be the major contributing factors that inhibit neutrophil and macrophage function. The sudden onset of action and flare-ups after discontinuation also suggest nonimmunosuppressive effects.

Cyclosporine The objective of immunosuppressive therapy is to specifically inhibit the immune response against the graft or autoantigen. However, drugs that also affect proliferating cell propulsions such as cyclophosphamide, azathioprine, and methotrexate produce life-threatening bone marrow suppression. Until the early 1980s, the use of these drugs in combination with corticosteroids was the preferred immunosuppressive therapy. Their use has largely been supplanted by cyclosporine, which usually is effective in preventing the onset of acute graft rejection (during the first 3 weeks). The absence of bone marrow toxicity makes it very beneficial in bone marrow transplants. Cyclosporine therapy may be replaced with azathioprine and prednisolone or steroid therapy alone at a later date. Cyclosporine treatment is also useful for autoimmune diseases, and trials are in progress to determine if cyclosporine in combination with other drugs may be beneficial in the treatment of insulin-dependent diabetes mellitus. Initial trials are promising, if the patient is started on cyclosporine before complete loss of the β-insulin–producing cells of the islets.

FK-506 FK-506 is effective in prolonging liver and other organ transplants and appears to act similarly to cyclosporine. FK-506 may eventually replace cyclosporine if the preliminary low toxicities hold true.

Monoclonal Antibodies A commercial anti-CD3 monoclonal preparation is used to reverse acute graft rejection of patients being administered other immunosuppressive drugs and to prevent acute graft rejections. Patients are then continued on other immunosuppressive drugs. Because the anti-CD3 antibody is a murine monoclonal antibody (different constant and variable regions), patients usually develop neutralizing antibodies after 10 days of treatment. The development of antibody against the anti-CD3 antibody, however, does not result in allergic or anaphylactic reactions. When the anti-CD3 antibody is given in conjunction with prednisolone and azathioprine, development of neutralizing antibodies is attenuated.

Immunostimulant Drugs

Lymphokines IL-2 is administered to patients with metastatic carcinomas with marginal results, and large doses of IL-2 produce severe fluid retention. Consequently, adoptive transfer of IL-2–induced lymphokine-activated killer (LAK) cells were conducted. In this time-consuming and costly procedure, patients are first administered low doses of IL-2. Then peripheral lymphocytes are isolated and cultured with IL-2 to stimulate LAK cell production. Finally, LAK cells are infused with IL-2. This approach is successful in the treatment of metastatic renal cell carcinoma, melanoma, colorectal cancer, and non-Hodgkins lymphoma and has been approved for use in treatment of renal cell carcinomas and melanomas. Although small amounts of IL-2 are used in this approach, severe fluid retention is still a problem. A recent modification involves removing tumor cells, isolating tumor-infiltrating lymphocytes, incubating them with IL-2 to activate and stimulate proliferation, injecting the patient with the added lymphocytes, and low concentrations of IL-2. The tumor-specific infiltrating lymphocytes are more effective than the LAK cells in killing tumor cells, but more importantly, much lower quantities of IL-2 are needed.

Colony Stimulating and Tumor Necrosis Factors CSFs appear to have a major potential for use as pharmacological agents without major toxicities. Patients with depressed bone marrow function undergoing cancer chemotherapy or immunosuppressive therapy, receiving bone marrow transplants, or with aplastic anemia would benefit greatly. The induction of differentiation by CSFs may be possible in the treatment of certain tumors.

The results of GM-CSF initial clinical trials are favorable. Patients with certain bone marrow dysfunctions from disease or cancer chemotherapy were administered GM-CSF intravenously over 2 weeks, with dramatic increases in neutrophils, eosinophils, and monocytes and minimal side effects.

Results of initial clinical trials to determine tolerated dose and adverse effects of TNF for use in tumor treatment indicate good tolerance. The antitumor effects of TNF have been demonstrated in animal models and are now being examined in clinical trials.

In the near future, multiple lymphokines may be administered to obtain greater therapeutic effects. Studies in experimental animals demonstrate that combined treatment with IL-2 and TNF results in synergistic enhancement of antitumor effects.

Interferons α-IFN is effective in the treatment of hematological cancers, especially hairy cell leukemia, chronic myelogenous leukemia, and T cell lymphomas related to mycosis fungoides. Because γ-IFN stimulates various cell types involved in immune destruction of tumors, there is interest in the use of γ-IFN. Initial clinical studies show that administration of γ-IFN to humans results in immunoenhancement. Whether this will lead to antitumor actions is not determined from present clinical trials.

In the treatment of viral infections, α-IFN is effective against chronic hepatitis B. Intranasal administration of α-IFN is useful in the treatment of rhinoviral infections, an especially valuable procedure in immunocompromised patients.

The activity of the IFNs is quantified by their ability to inhibit viral growth in cultured cells. Because of this, care must be used when comparing preparations for immune response or antiproliferative effects.

Additional agents are under study that induce synthesis of IFN in the body. These inducers may be grouped into viral and polyanionic polymers.

SIDE EFFECTS, CLINICAL PROBLEMS, AND TOXICITY

Clinical problems are summarized in the box.

Immunosuppressive Drugs

The side effects of the corticosteroids are discussed in Chapter 35 and those for cyclophosphamide and methotrexate in Chapter 43.

The major limiting toxicity of azathioprine is

CLINICAL PROBLEMS
corticosteroids
Electrolyte imbalance
Cushing's syndrome
Osteoporosis
cyclophosphamide
Myelosuppression
Hemorrhagic cystitis
methotrexate
Bone marrow suppression
Gastrointestinal upsets
azathioprine
Bone marrow suppression
cyclosporin
Nephrotoxicity (reduced glomerolar filtration)
Hepatotoxicity (cholestasis)
Neurotoxicity
Hypersensitivity to vehicle
Lymphokines (IL-2)
Fluid retention
Fever, chills
Interferons (IFN)
Fever, myalgia, fatigue
CSF and TNF
Fever, chills, fatigue
Possible endotoxin shock with TNF

suppression of bone marrow. Leukopenia and/or thrombocytopenia occurs after a delay and is reversible after discontinuing drug. The severe or prolonged suppression of bone marrow may predispose the patient to opportunistic infections. Liver toxicity is a common side effect. Since allopurinol inhibits azathioprine metabolism, its concurrent use is contraindicated.

One of the major advantages of cyclosporine is its relatively selective effect on T-helper cells and the absence of myelotoxicity in comparison to cyclophosphamide, azathioprine, and methotrexate. However, its use is limited by other toxicities. Nephrotoxicity with reduced glomerular filtration is a common and dose-limiting side effect, with the mechanism unknown. The incidence of hepatotoxicity with cholestasis and hyperbilirubinemia nearly doubles in patients on cyclosporine. Neurotoxicity, including tremors, is observed in about 20% of patients, and elevated concentrations of several plasma enzymes may be seen. Moderate hypertension may also occur in 50% of patients. Hypersensitivity to the drug vehicle also occurs.

The administration of anti-CD3 IV may produce flu-like symptoms with fluid retention and possible pulmonary edema. The flu-like symptoms can be effectively treated by administration of acetominophen.

Immunostimulant Drugs

IV administration of IL-2 and other lymphokines results in fever and chills. Lethargy and malaise also are observed. The major limiting toxicity of IL-2 is the dramatic increase in fluid retention caused by vascular leakage. This can lead to life-threatening pulmonary edema and ascites. The mechanism of this toxicity may be related to IL-2 activation of endothelial cells, as observed in other cell-mediated immune responses.

The common adverse effect of CSFs is bone pain, which is correlated with white blood cell counts and occurs independent of dose. Some common effects observed with IV administration of proteins (e.g., monoclonal antibodies and IL-2) are also observed: fever, chills, myalgia, fatigue, headaches, reduced appetite, and nausea.

With TNF, the induction of endotoxic shock and wasting (cachexia) observed in patients with infections of tumors was mediated in part by IL-1 and another factor produced by activated macrophages. This cytokine, termed *cachectin,* was later found to be identical to TNF. Thus one of the main concerns of TNF administration is the possible induction of endotoxic shock. Clinical studies reveal a similar non-life-threatening syndrome of effects observed with IV administration of IFN and CSF, namely, fever, chills, and malaise.

The adverse effects of IFN are dependent on source and preparation. In several human studies with partially purified recombinant α-IFN, the major side effects were fever, myalgia, headache, fatigue, and numbness of extremities. α-IFN also reportedly produces bone marrow depression.

Hypersensitivity Reactions

Drug hypersensitivities are immunological responses, which result when drugs act as antigens. Although the immune system usually plays a beneficial role, normal physiological immune responses to certain drugs may result in adverse reactions, which vary with the type of antigen and the site of contact. Hypersensitivity occurs only after previous exposure to an antigen. Another common feature is the marked interindividual difference in susceptibility, consistent with the observation that predisposition to hypersensitivity appears to be partially a heritable trait.

Drug-Induced Autoimmune Diseases

Systemic lupus erythematosis is characterized by the production of circulating autoantibodies and delayed-type hypersensitivity reactions against self-antigens (i.e., cellular DNA, basement membrane). A strong correlation between the induction of systemic lupus erythematosis signs and symptoms and exposure to certain drugs is reported for hydralazine, procainamide, isoniazid, penicillamine, anticonvulsants, chlorpromazine, lithium carbonate, β-adrenergic blockers, methyldopa, and nitrofurantoin. Symptoms disappear after discontinuation of drug treatment. These drugs may induce systemic lupus erythematosis by altering immunoregulation (i.e., suppressor T cells), binding to self-molecules and generating self-reacting antibodies, or altering self-molecules (DNA) to appear foreign. Different mechanisms may occur for different drugs.

Administration of penicillamine for long periods (months to years) is associated with induction of myasthenia gravis, characterized by acetylcholine-receptor antibodies at the neuromuscular junction. In patients treated with penicillamine, 20% possess antibodies against skeletal muscle, whereas only 0.5% possess the antireceptor antibody and symptoms.

The presence of glomerular nephritis in patients who have been exposed to mercury is correlated with deposition of complement and antibodies at the basement membrane. Administration of mercury chloride to experimental animals results in development of an-

---

TRADENAMES

In addition to generic and fixed combination preparations, the following tradenamed materials are available in the United States.

Sandimmune, cyclosporine, azathioprine, anti-CD3 receptor
Imuran, azathioprine
Muromonab, CD3; anti-CD3

tibasement membrane antibodies and induction of membranous glomerular nephropathy. The mechanism is unknown. Similar signs and symptoms are observed in a small number of patients who were administered gold for rheumatoid arthritis.

REFERENCES

Blick M, Sherwin SA, Rosenblum M et al: Phase I study of recombinant tumor necrosis factor in cancer patients, Cancer Res 47:2986, 1987.

Bonnem EM and Oldham RK: Gamma-interferon: physiology and speculation on its role in medicine, J Biol Resp Modif 6:275, 1987.

Handschumacher RE, Harding MW, Rice J et al.: Cyclophilin: a specific cytosolic binding protein for cyclosporin A, Science 226:544, 1984.

Kaplan BD: Cyclosporine, N Engl J Med 321:1725, 1989.

Paul WP: Fundamental immunology, ed 2, New York, 1989, Raven Press.

Roit IM, Brostoff J, Male DK: Immunology, St. Louis, 1985, The CV Mosby Co.

Rosenberg SA, Lotze MT, Muul LM et al.: A progress report on the treatment of 157 patients with advanced cancer using lymphokine-activated killer cells and interleukin-2 or high-dose interleukin-2, N Engl J Med 316:889, 1987.

Tocci MJ, Matkovich DA, Collier KA et al.: The immunosuppressant FK 506 selectively inhibits expression of early T cell activation genes, J Immunol 143:718, 1989.

Turk JL and Parker D: The effect of cyclophosphamide on the immune response, J Immunopharmac 1:127, 1979.

Nutritional Aspects of Pharmacology

FOODS AS DRUGS

As interest in health and disease has increased within recent years among the general population, the use of nutrients for the prevention or cure of certain medical problems has also grown. It is important that medical practitioners are aware of the usefulness of nutrients and of their possible effects on disease states, as well as their potential for abuse.

Fiber, Oat Bran, Starch Blockers

Dietary fiber has been used to treat various medical problems for the last 50 years but recently has come to increased public attention. From 1945 to the early 1970s, it was observed from studies in Africa that native diets rich in fiber and bulk correlated well with reduction in gastroenterological problems common to Western civilization. Dietary fiber has since been suggested to improve or cure various diseases or conditions, including obesity, diabetes, colon cancer, diverticulitis, hemorrhoids, hiatus hernia, heart disease, varicose veins, and gallstones. Unfortunately, firm data are lacking for most of these conditions. *Expert opinions indicate that only constipation and diverticulitis are benefited by dietary fiber.*

Dietary fiber is defined as those plant substances resistant to digestion by the human small intestine. Fiber is a collective term representing three distinct groups of carbohydrates (cellulose, hemicellulose A, and hemicellulose B) and lignin, a noncarbohydrate plant substance.

Nutritional biochemists classify fiber into four groups: cellulose, hemicellulose A, hemicellulose B, and lignin. The food industry classifies fiber into two categories: soluble and insoluble. Soluble fiber dissolves in neutral or acid detergents during extraction, and nonsoluble fiber does not (Figure 61-1). Other important properties of the various fiber types are the ability to hold water, cationic exchange properties, and antioxidant action. A summary of the physiological, chemical, and clinical aspects of fiber is presented in Table 61-1, p. 822.

The most familiar fiber is cellulose, a major constituent of plant cell walls in wheat and oat bran. Cellulose is a linear polymer of glucose, but unlike the α 1,4 linkage of glycogen and maltose, the β 1,4 linkage cannot be broken down enzymatically. Hemicellulose A fiber is heteropolymeric with linkages formed between hexose units of glucose, galactose, and man-

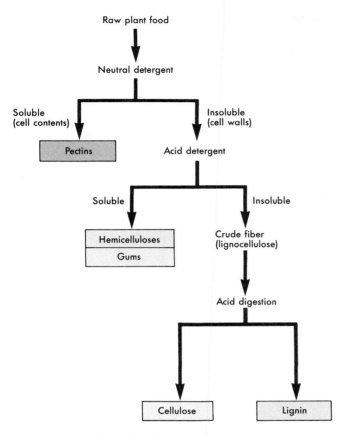

FIGURE 61-1   Classification of fiber types based on extraction procedures. Major dietary fiber groups are highlighted.

nose, as well as between pentose units such as xylose and arabinose. These agents are sometimes referred to as *gums* or *mucilages*. The consistency of fibers in this category are "gluelike" and delay gastric emptying, thereby decreasing the rate of small bowel absorption. Guar gum is an example of hemicellulose A that is often added to foods during processing to binds water and ingredients together. In the plant, guar gum prevents dehydration of the plant seed. Hemicellulose B fiber, or pectin, also retains water and binds minerals and heavy metals in the gastrointestinal (GI) tract. Lignins are the noncarbohydrate components of fiber and exist as polymers of oxygenated phenylpropane units. The resistance to degradation of the cross-linked units enables these fibers to pass undigested through the small intestine and provide bulk for the feces. Most of the hemicelluloses are degraded by bacteria in the colon and increase bulk by increasing fecal bacterial mass. Most of the cellulose

and lignin pass through the colon without degradation, thus increasing fecal bulk, which is the likely mechanism of alleviation of constipation and is useful for the treatment of diverticular disease. Increased fecal bulk reduces intraluminal colonic pressure, thus decreasing the tendency to form diverticulae.

The use of fiber for treatment of diabetes mellitus has been investigated extensively. Moderate concentrations of hemicellulose fiber (particularly the gums and pectins) in the diet of diabetic subjects reduce mean blood glucose and insulin concentrations after a meal. Long-term studies of diets high in soluble fiber demonstrate an improvement in glycemic control, reduction in glucosuria, and decreased ketonuria, although it is not clear whether this is an effect of the fiber or of the high plant-food diet. Supplements of wheat or oat bran demonstrate only modest improvement in the control of diabetes. The mechanisms of improvement with soluble fiber may be related to a delay in gastric emptying and in glucose absorption. The slower release of carbohydrates and proteins into the duodenum and their delayed absorption reduce the rise in blood glucose and insulin.

The delayed gastric emptying caused by some hemicelluloses may also be useful in treating the "dumping syndrome." Long-term studies evaluating the effectiveness of pectin for the dumping syndrome suggest that changes in the pattern of GI motility occur and may account for some of the improvement.

The popularity of fiber is enhanced by advertisements promoting its ability to lower serum cholesterol concentrations. These claims are based on data from studies in which diets high in fiber and carbohydrate reduce serum cholesterol concentrations. These studies were performed in patients with diabetes and normal blood lipid concentrations. It is not clear whether fiber results in lipid lowering or whether reduction in dietary fats or the increase in dietary carbohydrates is more important. The viscous types of fiber are the most effective for lowering cholesterol concentrations, whereas the lignins produce more variable results. Wheat bran, which is mainly cellulose, does not reduce serum cholesterol concentrations. Lignins decrease cholesterol and lower serum triglyceride concentrations by increasing fecal bile salt losses, thus binding these salts in the GI tract and preventing their reabsorption. This effect led to the development of bile salt anion exchange resins, such as cholestyramine (see Chapter 20), to reduce cholesterol. Lignins reportedly lower concentrations of low density lipo-

Table 61-1   Physiological and Therapeutic Implications of Dietary Fiber

Physicochemical Property	Type of Fiber	Physiological Effect	Potential Clinical Implication
Viscosity	Gums, mucilages, pectins	↓ gastric emptying ↑ mouth to cecum transit ↓ rate of small intestinal absorption (e.g., of glucose, bile acids)	Dumping syndrome Diabetes Hypercholesterolemia
Particle formation and water-holding capacity	e.g., Wheat bran, pentosan content, polysaccharide-lignin mixtures	↑ gastric emptying ↓ mouth to cecum transit ↓ total GI transit time ↓ colonic intraluminal pressure ↑ fecal bulk	Peptic ulcer Constipation Diverticular disease Dilute potential carcinogens
Adsorption and non-specific effects	Lignin, pectin mixed fibers	↑ fecal steroids output ↑ fecal fat and N losses (small)	Hypercholesterolemia Cholelithiasis
Cation exchange	Acidic polysaccharides (e.g., pectins)	↑ small intestinal losses of minerals (±), trace elements (±), heavy metals	Negative mineral balance, probably compensated for by colonic salvage antitoxic effect
Antioxidant	Lignin (reducing phenolic groups)	↓ free radicals in digestive tract	Anticarcinogenesis?
Degradability (colonic bacteria)	Polysaccharides (free of lignin)	↑ gas and SCFAs production, ↓ cecal pH	Flatus, energy production

From Jenkins DJA: Carbohydrate. In Shils ME and Young VR, eds: Modern nutrition in health and disease, Philadelphia, 1988, Lea & Febiger, Publishers; adapted from Am J Clin Nutr 32:365, 1979.

protein (LDL) cholesterol while maintaining high density lipoprotein (HDL) cholesterol levels, resulting in an improved LDL:HDL ratio. However, there is no general ageement on these observations. Gums and pectin are also reported to lower serum triglyceride and cholesterol concentrations more consistently and improve the LDL:HDL profile.

Because obesity is seldom observed among primitive cultures that consume diets high in fiber, the use of fiber has been recommended in weight reduction programs. Mechanisms proposed are decreased absorption of nutrients, increased satiety from bulk, calorie dilution, and production of GI factors that reduce food intake or body weight. Although fecal calorie loss increases on a high fiber diet, the difference is attributable to dietary fiber and not to malabsorption of other nutrients. Because some fiber delays gastric emptying, a feeling of fullness or satiety may occur early, which can signal the end of a meal. Several studies suggest that GI hormone secretion is altered with a high fiber diet, which may also reduce food intake. Generally, long-term studies using fiber for weight reduction have not been successful.

Other proposed nutritional treatments for obesity include *starch blockers*. Theoretically, such agents prevent breakdown of starch and reduce absorption, but most of these substances are partially digested and inactivated in the stomach before significant starch-blocking effects can occur. Controlled clinical trials have not validated claims for efficacy.

The link between fiber and gallstone formation, while tenuous, appears to have some support. Bran fiber can alter the composition of the bile salt pool, particularly chenodeoxycholic acid. Bile stone formation is reported to be reduced by bran, but further study is required to fully evaluate this action. Colon cancer is reported to be inversely correlated with fiber intake, but the relationships are not yet substantiated. Use of dietary fiber in the treatment of Crohn's disease and inflammatory bowel disease is controversial.

Overconsumption of fiber can produce adverse effects. Diarrhea and increased flatus occur; these conditions may be uncomfortable or socially unacceptable but are not dangerous. Delayed gastric emptying and increased esophageal reflux can result in irritation and pain. Whereas lack of fiber can lead to constipation and irritable bowel syndrome, fiber taken without sufficient fluids may exacerbate the problem. Mineral deficiencies caused by excessive fiber in the GI tract are rare but may be clinically important with low mineral intake. Calcium, magnesium, iron, and zinc are at highest risk.

Amino Acids

Use of specific amino acids by the general population to treat diseases has increased with the availability of purified amino acids in health food stores. Lysine and arginine are promoted as regulators of body composition and muscle growth. However, clinical studies disprove these claims and indicate that this practice is ineffective and may be dangerous.

Tryptophan, once widely used as a sleep promoter, has been temporarily withdrawn from the market by the U.S. Food and Drug Administration because of toxicity encountered with use of tryptophan on a long-term basis. Interest in tryptophan as a pharmacological agent arose after its discovery as a precursor of the neurotransmitter, serotonin. Milk, a rich source of this amino acid, was prescribed as a means to induce sleep, providing a historical background for this use. Brain tryptophan concentrations in experimental animals can be elevated by providing excess dietary tryptophan. Turnover in the brain is then increased. This diet-neurotransmitter relationship occurs with tryptophan and 5-HT because the rate-limiting enzyme for serotonin biosynthesis is tryptophan hydroxylase, an enzyme not normally saturated and therefore regulated by substrate concentrations, which are diet-dependent. Generally, high protein diets decrease tryptophan uptake into the brain because of competition from the neutral amino acids that share the transport system. The tryptophan to neutral amino acid ratio is an important dietary index of the ability of a food to alter brain tryptophan. Increases in dietary tryptophan relative to other neutral amino acids (tyrosine, phenylalanine, valine, isoleucine, and methionine) or increases in dietary carbohydrate enhance tryptophan—neutral amino acid ratios and thus uptake into the brain.

One role ascribed to tryptophan is in the regulation of food intake. Another is that tryptophan is involved in the selection of food types.

One certified function of tryptophan is as a precursor of niacin. Tryptophan was used to cure pellagra in the early 1920s, before its role as a substrate for niacin synthesis was elucidated. This disease is rare today because niacin is readily available in the American diet.

Fish Oils, Fatty Acids, Lipids

While fatty acids and lipids have important structural roles in cells and in growth, they also serve as precursors for numerous bioactive metabolites,

Table 61-2 Bioactive Compounds Synthesized from the Two Essential Fatty Acids: Linoleic and Linolenic Acids

Class of Compounds	Linoleic (n-6) Fatty Acids	Linolenic (n-3) Fatty Acids
Prostaglandins	PGE_1, PGE_2	PGE_3
Thromboxanes	TXA_1, TXA_2	TXA_3
Prostacyclin	PGI_3	PGI_2
Leukotrienes	$8,9\text{-}LTA_3$, LTA_4	LTA_5

From Myers AK: The eicosanoids: prostaglandins, thromboxane, and leukotrienes. In DeGroot LJ, ed: Endocrinology, Philadelphia, 1986, WB Saunders Co.

namely prostaglandins, thromboxane, leukotrienes, and hydroxy fatty acids (see Chapter 18). The rate of synthesis of these active metabolites is substrate dependent; therefore dietary manipulations can alter the amount and type of these compounds. The essential fatty acids, linolenic and linoleic acids, are not synthesized by man and must be supplied in the diet. Linolenic-derived fatty acids are the omega-3 (n-3) family of compounds, while linoleic-derived fatty acids are the omega-6 (n-6) family. In lipid biology the double bonds are named from the methyl end rather than the carboxyl end, thus n-3 and n-6 fatty acids have a double bond after the third and sixth carbons from the methyl end. There is a preference of the desaturase enzyme for the n-3 over the n-6 configuration.

Oils from vegetables and legumes such as soybeans, corn, peanuts, and cottonseed are rich sources of n-6 fatty acids. Flesh of deep sea fish such as halibut and salmon are high in n-3 fatty acids. A list of representative bioactive products obtained from each of these essential fatty acids is presented in Table 61-2. Linoleic acid gives rise through intermediate desaturation and elongation to dihomo-γ-linolenic acid, which can be converted to arachidonic acid by further desaturation (Figure 61-2). Arachidonic acid (20:4n-6) serves as a precursor for prostaglandin, prostacyclin, and thromboxane synthesis via the cyclooxygenase pathway (see Chapter 18) or for leukotriene and hydroxy fatty acid synthesis via the lipoxygenase pathway.

See Chapter 18 for the effects of prostaglandins and leukotrienes on the various biological systems.

Omega-3 fatty acids are also converted into biologically active compounds, but the major interme-

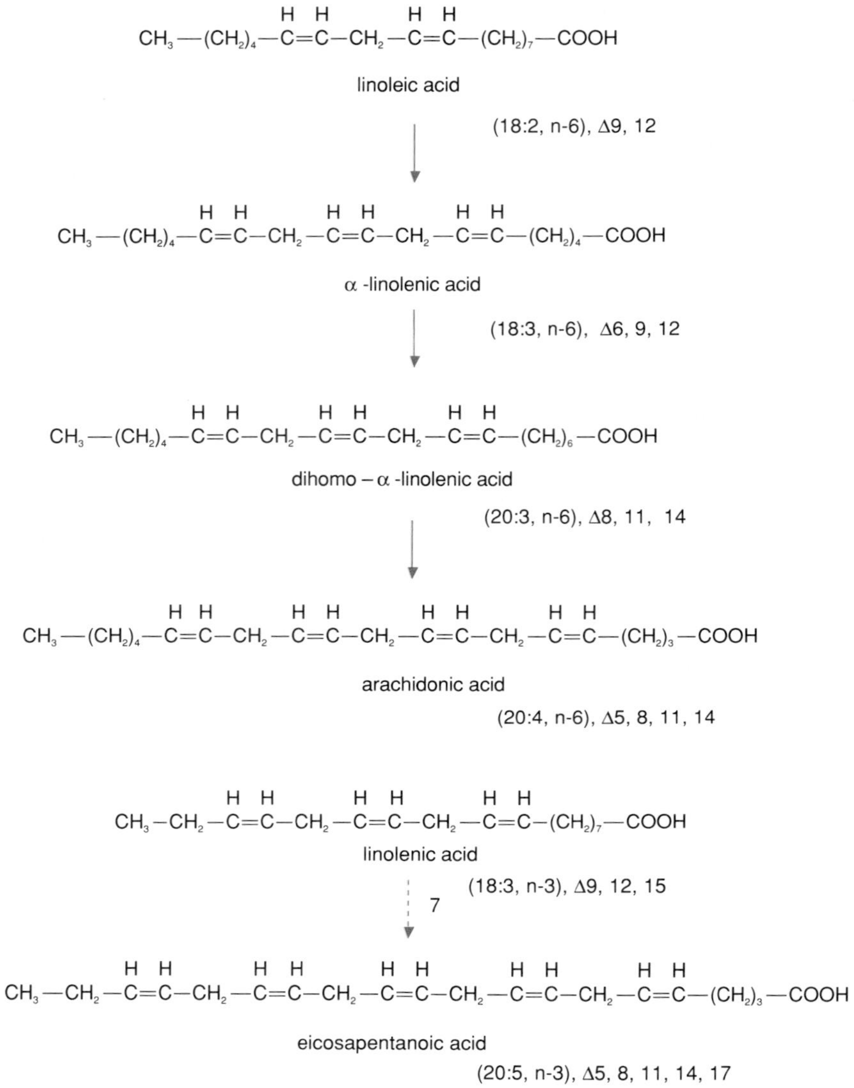

$$CH_3-(CH_2)_4-\overset{H}{\underset{}{C}}=\overset{H}{\underset{}{C}}-CH_2-\overset{H}{\underset{}{C}}=\overset{H}{\underset{}{C}}-(CH_2)_7-COOH$$

linoleic acid

(18:2, n-6), Δ9, 12

$$CH_3-(CH_2)_4-\overset{H}{\underset{}{C}}=\overset{H}{\underset{}{C}}-CH_2-\overset{H}{\underset{}{C}}=\overset{H}{\underset{}{C}}-CH_2-\overset{H}{\underset{}{C}}=\overset{H}{\underset{}{C}}-(CH_2)_4-COOH$$

α -linolenic acid

(18:3, n-6), Δ6, 9, 12

$$CH_3-(CH_2)_4-\overset{H}{\underset{}{C}}=\overset{H}{\underset{}{C}}-CH_2-\overset{H}{\underset{}{C}}=\overset{H}{\underset{}{C}}-CH_2-\overset{H}{\underset{}{C}}=\overset{H}{\underset{}{C}}-(CH_2)_6-COOH$$

dihomo − α -linolenic acid

(20:3, n-6), Δ8, 11, 14

$$CH_3-(CH_2)_4-\overset{H}{\underset{}{C}}=\overset{H}{\underset{}{C}}-CH_2-\overset{H}{\underset{}{C}}=\overset{H}{\underset{}{C}}-CH_2-\overset{H}{\underset{}{C}}=\overset{H}{\underset{}{C}}-CH_2-\overset{H}{\underset{}{C}}=\overset{H}{\underset{}{C}}-(CH_2)_3-COOH$$

arachidonic acid

(20:4, n-6), Δ5, 8, 11, 14

$$CH_3-CH_2-\overset{H}{\underset{}{C}}=\overset{H}{\underset{}{C}}-CH_2-\overset{H}{\underset{}{C}}=\overset{H}{\underset{}{C}}-CH_2-\overset{H}{\underset{}{C}}=\overset{H}{\underset{}{C}}-(CH_2)_7-COOH$$

linolenic acid

(18:3, n-3), Δ9, 12, 15

7

$$CH_3-CH_2-\overset{H}{\underset{}{C}}=\overset{H}{\underset{}{C}}-CH_2-\overset{H}{\underset{}{C}}=\overset{H}{\underset{}{C}}-CH_2-\overset{H}{\underset{}{C}}=\overset{H}{\underset{}{C}}-CH_2-\overset{H}{\underset{}{C}}=\overset{H}{\underset{}{C}}-CH_2-\overset{H}{\underset{}{C}}=\overset{H}{\underset{}{C}}-(CH_2)_3-COOH$$

eicosapentanoic acid

(20:5, n-3), Δ5, 8, 11, 14, 17

FIGURE 61-2   Synthesis of precursor fatty acids from linoleic (18:2, n-6) and linolenic (18:3, n-6) essential fatty acids.

diates are eicosapentaenoic (20:5,n-3) and docohexaenoic (22:6,n-3) fatty acids.

Dietary fatty acids determine which prostaglandins are produced by the body, since particular enzymes prefer specific substrates. Omega-3 fatty acids are preferentially incorporated into the 2-position of membrane phospholipids, where they function as cell regulators upon release. When cells are stimulated by phospholipase A_2, there is mobilization of fatty acids from the 2-position of the phospholipids, providing the substrates for entering the cyclooxygenase or lipoxygenase pathways. Certain fatty acids (18:2, n-6, 18:3, n-3, and 20:3, n-9) are competitive inhibitors for prostaglandin and leukotriene precursors (20:3, n-6, 20:4, n-6, and 20:5, n-3). Not only is there a difference between n-6 and n-3 fatty acids, but there is also a great deal of variation within these groups in determining the final bioactive product. Also, the fatty acid hierarchy for entering the cyclooxygenase and lipoxygenase pathways differs among species. Present data with fish oils do not support a role for these fatty acids in lowering serum cholesterol.

A prudent approach to reducing serum cholesterol by dietary means is to substitute the saturated fat with a mono-unsaturated fat such as olive oil. Mono-unsaturated fats lower serum cholesterol, particularly the LDL concentration. Epidemiological studies of populations consuming diets high in mono-unsaturated fatty acids show a much lower incidence of cardiovascular disease than other cultures consuming more saturated fat, even though the total fat in the diets of the two groups is comparable.

Vitamins

Dietary factors have long been used in the treatment of disease. The ancient Egyptians applied juice from cooked livers to their eyes to reverse night blindness. The Greeks consumed the liver in addition to applying the juice topically. We now recognize that the active agent present in the liver is vitamin A.

It is estimated that between 35% to 50% of the adult population in the United States supplement their diet daily with vitamins. All age groups are represented in the list of regular users of vitamins. The very young (1 to 5 years of age) and the elderly are the most frequent users on a regular basis.

Vitamin A and the Retinoids Vitamin A and the related natural and synthetic analogs are referred to as the *retinoids*. The three major effects of the retinoids studied extensively are their role in night vision, growth, and carcinogenesis. The mechanism of vitamin A action in vision is well described. Vitamin A in its *cis*-retinal form is combined with opsin to form rhodopsin during darkness or when exposed to specific phospholipids. When light reaches the rods of the eye, a cascade of events results in the breakdown of rhodopsin and the formation of activators of membrane hyperpolarization.

As plasma concentrations of vitamin A fall, there is a concurrent decrease in the amount of vitamin A in the retina and pigment epithelium, and less rhodopsin is synthesized. Night blindness occurs because dark adaptation is dependent on the amount of rhodopsin in the outer segment of the rods. Dietary supplementation of vitamin A usually reverses this condition. Zinc deficiency and protein-calorie malnutrition also decrease rhodopsin content.

The link of vitamin A to cancer is conjectural but based on its effects on cellular growth and differentiation and on drug-metabolizing enzymes. Retinoids convert keratin-producing cells into mucus-producing cells. They also stimulate differentiation of certain carcinoma cells. One hypothesis is that vitamin A directly regulates gene expression by entering the nucleus of a cell, with its binding protein, and interacts with the chromatin. As a result, new mRNA is transcribed that encodes for different cellular proteins.

Consistent with these data demonstrating that vitamin A stimulates cellular differentiation, experimental studies in animals show an antitumor effect of retinoids. In animals, resistance to pulmonary cancer (caused by administration of 3-methylcholanthrene) is conferred by vitamin A in the diet. Similarly, vitamin A can retard onset or prevent cervical, vaginal, and intestinal cancers induced in animals by 7,12-dimethylbenzanthracene. Vitamin A is postulated to have a protective effect in colon cancer and in various chemical toxicities.

A possible alternative mechanism for the anticancer effects of the retinoids is that vitamin A affects the synthesis or activity of the drug-metabolizing enzyme system and thereby alters the cell's ability to remove toxins.

Several other pharmacological uses for vitamin A and the retinoids are in the treatment of cystic acne (isotretinoin) and psoriasis (etretinate). However, excessive vitamin A intake is more common than deficiency. Yellowing of the skin occurs in people taking excessive amounts of vitamin A or β carotene. Other major symptoms of retinoid overdose are dryness of the skin, alopecia, hepatosplenomegaly, anorexia, headache, and fatigue. Massive overdoses may be fatal. Excess retinoid intake during pregnancy has been associated with birth defects.

Other Vitamins Since vitamins are so widely used and generally without physician oversight, the potential for hypervitaminosis (particularly those vitamins that are fat soluble) is present.

Niacin Pharmacological doses of niacin lower serum cholesterol in some patients. Niacin, as nicotinic acid, taken daily in 3 to 6 gram quantities produces vasodilation and flushing initially, with these side effects disappearing in a few days. Nicotinamide intake does not produce the flushing observed with nicotinic acid and dose not lower serum cholesterol.

Pantothenic Acid Pantothenic acid is important as an acyl carrier in transmitochondrial fatty acid transport and activation. Reports from the late 1940s and early 1950s claim that this vitamin can be used in wound healing and healing of skin lesions. No deficiency of this vitamin has been recognized in man on a normal diet.

Choline and Inositol Choline and inositol have structural and transmitter functions in the nervous system and in cell membranes. Phosphatidylcholine and phosphatidylinositol comprise the phospholipid component of the plasma membrane and intracellular membranes. Phosphatidylcholine is present in the membrane as a structural compound, whereas phosphatidylinositol, with the bisphosphoinositides and trisphosphoinositides, act as second messenger systems. Choline can be converted to the neurotransmitter acetylcholine, while lecithin can serve as a fatty acid dose or for esterification of cholesterol by lecithin-cholesterol acyltransferase (LCAT), be a methyl group donor in 1-carbon metabolism in lieu of methionine, and serve as a precursor for diacylglycerol formation. Preliminary studies propose a relationship between choline concentrations and memory loss in elderly patients. Large doses of lecithin or choline may reverse memory loss. The mechanism for this reversal could be an increased synthesis of acetylcholine. High choline diets increase brain acetylcholine concentrations in rats. Because of these functions, and because concentrations of acetylcholine and the phosphoinositides can be altered by diet, many physiological functions ascribed to these vitamins can be modulated by nutritional means. Although these substances have potential usefulness, adequate studies do not yet substantiate claims for these compounds. Because overconsumption of choline and lecithin causes side effects such as depression, increased sensitivity of dopamine receptors, and excessive neurotransmitter synthesis, supplements of these substances in the diet are not recommended.

Vitamin B_6/Pyridoxine Vitamin B_6/pyridoxine is extremely important because of its numerous metabolic functions, the most central of which is as a cofactor in enzymatic reactions. As such, pyridoxine participates in all transaminations, decarboxylations, dehydratase reactions, and side-chain cleavage reactions. Thus it is involved in almost all aspects of amino acid metabolism. Reported therapeutic uses of pharmacological doses of vitamin B_6 include treatment of sideroblastic anemia (when not effectively treated by folate, iron, or vitamin B_{12}) and in the improvement of muscle tone in patients with Parkin-

son's disease who receive L-DOPA. It is also useful in Huntington's chorea and in newborn infant convulsive seizures and those caused by isoniazid. Use of B_6 in the latter instances may be related to its effects to enhance GABA synthesis because low concentrations of this neurotransmitter are present in these conditions. Another reported use of pyridoxine is in the treatment of carpal tunnel syndrome, particularly in the elderly. Pyridoxine is used to treat homocystinuria and primary oxalosis. Because of its role in transamination, this vitamin is helpful in alleviating "Chinese restaurant syndrome" in which large amounts of monosodium glutamate (MSG) must be eliminated from the body. Massive doses of pyridoxine can cause a peripheral neuropathy; therefore, caution should be used in prescribing it.

Vitamin C Although historically vitamin C (ascorbic acid) was among the first nutrients used in the treatment of disease (scurvy), there are few or no established effective therapeutic uses beyond the treatment of scurvy. Its function as a reducing agent and antioxidant may be important. However, whether high doses confer health improvement is questionable. Vitamin C excess is associated with iron overload and may confound assays for glucose and mislead diabetic patients who need to calculate insulin requirements.

The use of vitamin C to treat the common cold was proposed by Linus Pauling, two-time Nobel laureate. The rationale for the use of vitamin C in cold therapy, however, is weak. Controlled studies do not document an effect of vitamin C on cold duration or severity of symptoms.

Various other therapeutic uses for vitamin C are promoted, but most of these are based on uncontrolled studies. Claims that vitamin C intake may help lower blood cholesterol, prevent artherosclerosis, or prolong life in cancer patients are not substantiated.

Food Toxicants and Additives

Naturally Occurring Food Toxicants Contrary to popular belief, food derived from plants contains far more toxicants than food of animal origin. Numerous drugs are extracted from plants and many pharmaceuticals have been developed because of medicinal effects first discovered from consuming plant products.

Protease inhibitors are common in many plants, with perhaps the most notable being soybean trypsin inhibitor. These substances inhibit growth in rats fed raw soybeans and are inactivated when soy is heated. Usually, food processing will eliminate bioactivity; therefore it is of concern mainly among health food enthusiasts who eat the raw soybeans. Recent work postulates an anticancer action for these compounds, but this has not been documented.

Hemagglutinins, or red blood cell agglutinators, in various foods are collectively referred to as *phytoagglutinins*. Legumes (soybeans, kidney beans, peanuts, etc.) in particular have high concentrations of these substances, and overconsumption of these foods may cause intravascular clotting abnormalities. Fortunately, most of these compounds are destroyed during digestion and do not present a threat to the individual eating a diversified and well-rounded diet; however, vegetarians may be at risk for excessive blood clotting if moderation is not exercised.

Mycotoxins are fungal toxins in foods of potential toxicity for humans. The ingestion of aflatoxin (the fungus produced on peanuts) has caused large scale poisonings in India and Thailand. Susceptibility to poisoning varies with nutritional state and is increased by protein malnutrition. Aflatoxin B is classified as a carcinogen by the World Health Organization and chronic exposure to this and other mycotoxins is thought to be responsible for inducing cancer throughout Africa and Asia. Signs of mycotoxin poisoning include gastrointestinal (GI) bleeding, hypertension, encephalopathy, jaundice, and death.

Hormones and Growth Promoters Diethylstilbestrol (DES), a synthetic estrogen, has been withdrawn from use after it was shown to induce ovarian and renal cancer. Most estrogens are taken up rapidly by the blood and cleared, but DES has a prolonged half-life as a result of a decreased clearance rate. The unfortunate experience with DES heightens awareness of the possibility for contamination of food products by steroids. Estrogens in feed are used to increase the growth of livestock. Estrogens therefore appear in foodstuffs and safety regarding their use has been questioned. The effects of steroids and growth promoters are described in the endocrine chapters (Chapters 34, 35, and 36).

Antibiotics Antibiotics have been used for about 50 years in agriculture to promote health and growth of livestock and poultry. Tetracyclines, penicillins, and monensin are employed for these purposes. Numerous mechanisms are proposed to account for the growth effects observed when these antibiotics are administered long-term. One theory is that they increase absorption of nutrients in the GI tract by decreasing bacterial damage to intestinal mucosa. The major concern in food production is the effect that these substances may have on humans consuming antibiotic-treated animals. This practice has led to the emergence of antibiotic-resistant bacteria in animals used for food with the potential of transfer to man. One hazard may be that of allergic sensitivity. Although the use of antibiotics in animal feed should be discouraged, there is no data currently available that treatment of food animals with antibiotics has produced adverse effects.

Methylxanthines and Tannins Coffee and tea are consumed by a large proportion of the population. Caffeine is a widely used psychoactive drug. Other caffeine or xanthine sources are diet pills, aspirin compound preparations, soft drinks, and chocolate. Because of effects on phosphodiesterase activity and cAMP concentrations, as well as interactions with adenosine, the consumption of coffee and tea and other caffeine-containing foods and drugs should be questioned by physicians during a medical history. Although many decaffeinated products exist, caffeine intake from caffeine-containing drinks is of major concern, particularly because of excessive consumption by children. Adverse effects such as cardiac dysrhythmias and CNS hyperactivity are observed when caffeine is used in excess. In children and adults, a frequent result of caffeine withdrawal after moderate to excessive consumption is headache. A cup of coffee (5 oz) contains about 80 mg of caffeine; tea has half that amount. Soft drink quantities range from 35 to 60 mg per 12 oz serving. Thus children who consume a soft drink will receive a greater dose on a body weight basis than adults who ingest a cup of coffee.

Tannins are a family of compounds of which tannic acid is the most prominent. These substances exist as natural components of foods (such as those present in teas) or they may be added during processing (as in beers and wines) where they serve as clarifying agents. Tannins inhibit absorption of iron and alter the uptake of other minerals from the intestine. Consumption of normal levels of tannins probably will not present problems. However, heavy consumption of teas, for example among the elderly, is correlated with low blood concentrations of iron.

Monosodium Glutamate MSG is a flavor enhancer used in processed food and is an important ingredient in Chinese food. "Chinese restaurant syndrome" is caused by the inability to degrade this substance. As stated earlier, pyridoxine supplementation can help prevent or reverse the flushing and weakness that result from this syndrome by stimulating transamination reactions required to detoxify this compound. Of perhaps greater concern are the unknown effects MSG may have on the CNS. MSG has been used in experimental animals to cause specific brain lesions. Whether these effects can be observed in humans is not known, but caution should be exercised. Children in particular should avoid consumption of large quantities of MSG.

Food Preservatives and Dyes The Federal Food, Drug and Cosmetic Act of 1958 describes a food additive as anything added directly or indirectly to a food preparation. This definition includes radiation treatment of foodstuffs. The Delaney clause of the amendment specifically prevents use of a food additive if it experimentally induces cancer in animals or man. The manufacturer of a food product must demonstrate that an additive is safe when used in a certain quantity in a specific manner. An exclusion of this demonstration of safety was made for products used before the Act became effective, if no problems of usage are documented or if they are considered safe by scientific judgment. Exempted materials Generally Regarded As Safe (GRAS) are listed by the Food and Drug Administration (FDA).

A GRAS list exists for chemical preservatives and includes substances such as ascorbic acid, the tocopherols, and other antimicrobials and antioxidants. It also includes butylated hydroxyanisole (BHA) and butylated hydroxytoluene (BHT). However, the use of the latter two preservatives is limited by quantity added. Total BHA and BHT concentrations cannot exceed 0.2% of the lipid content of the food. Because these substances are antioxidants, their concentrations relate to fat concentrations, whereas antimicrobials are generally regulated on a percentage of total food. BHA and BHT cause tumors in experimental animals, and acceptable limits for these compounds have been established.

Treatment of Diseases by Nutrients

Wernicke-Korsakoff Syndrome The Wernicke-Korsakoff syndrome is a neuropsychiatric disorder caused by thiamine deficiency and is often seen in chronic alcoholics. It is characterized by abnormal gait, impairment of mental function and memory, and paralysis of ocular movements. The enzyme transketolase isolated from fibroblasts of patients with the Wernicke-Korsakoff syndrome binds thiamine pyrophosphate with only one tenth the affinity of that in normal individuals. This enzyme of the pentose cycle of carbohydrate metabolism requires thiamine pyrophosphate to transfer an aldehyde unit to an aldose acceptor. Because only the affinity of this enzyme for thiamine is affected, it is possible to reverse symptoms of this disease by supplementing the diet with thiamine. Two other thiamine-dependent enzymes, pyruvate dehydrogenase and α-ketoglutarate, are normal in Wernicke-Korsakoff patients.

Glycogen Storage Diseases The enzyme deficiency responsible for a common form of this group of inherited disorders, von Gierke's disease, is glucose-6-phosphatase. Deficiency of this enzyme prevents the liver from breaking down stores of glycogen and is responsible for the enlargement of the liver that is characteristic of the disease. Hypoglycemia occurs between meals and with increased blood lactate and pyruvate from stimulation of glycolysis. There are at least seven variations of glycogen storage disease in muscle and liver that are related to specific enzyme defects and can be modulated by diet. High glucose diets should be avoided and complex carbohydrates should be used in place of monosaccharides and disaccharides. Patients should avoid acute elevations of plasma glucose, but the hypoglycemia necessitates frequent meal feedings.

Phenylketonuria Public awareness of phenylketonuria, an inherited inborn error of metabolism, has increased since the artificial sweetener aspartame, marketed as Nutrasweet, became a popular food additive. Persons with phenylketonuria are unable to convert phenylalanine to tyrosine, which results in an accumulation of phenylalanine in every tissue in the body. Aspartame, which is a dipeptide of phenylalanine and aspartic acid, taken in excess could result in harmful amounts of phenylalanine. The disease is usually caused by a defect in or the absence of the enzyme phenylalanine hydroxylase. Individuals who have this disease are usually mentally retarded and have defective myelination of the nerves and hyperactive reflexes. Life expectancy is decreased dramatically, and quality and longevity of life can be enhanced by early diagnosis and avoidance of phenylalanine.

Familial Goiter There are two inborn errors of metabolism affecting the thyroid. The first is a dehalogenase deficiency that reduces organic iodine available to the thyroid, and the second is an iodide transport defect that also results in low iodine concentrations in the thyroid. Symptoms include hypothyroidism and goiter. In both cases iodine supplementation in the diet is effective (see Chapter 38).

Gout Gout can be inherited or result from ingestion of high protein or purine diets. The problem is expressed in individuals with deficiencies in the enzymes hypoxanthine-guanine-phosphoribosyltransferase or glucose-6-phosphatase or in individuals with excessive activity of phosphoribosyl pyrophosphate synthetase. Restrictions in protein and purine intake and alcohol in combination with a high fiber diet can alleviate the problem. Weight reduction may help prevent gouty episodes.

Diabetes Mellitus Type II or non-insulin-dependent diabetes mellitus is a disease in which nutrition management is extremely important. In many cases, proper nutritional guidance can obviate the need for pharmacological intervention. Factors in diabetes treatment are discussed in Chapter 39. In general, a modest fat, high carbohydrate diet (50% to 60% of calories) with an emphasis on complex carbohydrate (approximately two thirds of total) has been proposed. However, low carbohydrate diets are also recommended by some. Artificial sweeteners can be used in moderation, and fructose is proposed as an alternative to sucrose. Potential adverse effects of fructose reported by some investigators suggest caution in its use. Fish oils were initially proposed for people with diabetes, but recent evidence suggests that they may produce an unfavorable HDL:LDL ratio; therefore supplements should be avoided. Mono-unsaturated fats are proposed as a means of decreasing artherogenic risks in people with diabetes, and some investigators suggest replacement of some dietary carbohydrate with mono-unsaturated fats. Increased insoluble fiber may be helpful, but care should be taken to avoid deficiencies in minerals or vitamins when increasing fiber intake.

DRUG-NUTRIENT INTERACTIONS

Dietary Factors Affecting Drug Efficacy

There are many ways in which drug efficacy can be altered by nutritional factors. Foods containing pectin fiber that delay food entry from the stomach to the duodenum alter (1) the time for orally administered drugs to reach the intestine and be absorbed

and (2) the nature of the duodenal contents after the drug arrives. The type of foods consumed and their transit time will affect the amount of bile released and the pH of the intestinal environment. These are all-important considerations if alterations in time or rate of drug absorption will affect treatment efficacy. Interactions of food and drugs in the intestine are frequent and should always be considered if a patient is not responding appropriately to a drug. One prominent example is the binding of calcium and tetracycline when the drug is taken with milk, decreasing its absorption.

Fats, fiber, proteins, and carbohydrates may interfere with or promote intestinal absorption of drugs. Amino acids and L-DOPA share the same transport system, so a protein meal will reduce the effectiveness of this particular drug. Nutrients in the bloodstream and the intestine may alter clearance rate of a drug. Theophylline is an example of this type of interaction. Protein increases theophylline metabolism, and infant formula or milk slows drug metabolism.

Drug Effects on Nutrient Status

Antibiotics Antibiotics may interact with nutrients by causing malabsorption and maldigestion, depending on the specific drug. Tetracycline reduces iron and calcium absorption by binding in the intestine and forming a complex that cannot be taken up by the gut. Neomycin reduces absorption of minerals, vitamin B_2, lipids, glucose, and nitrogen by affecting gastroenterological structure. Villi are shortened, the integrity of the crypt cells is disrupted, and infiltration of the lamina propria occurs with neomycin treatment at therapeutic concentrations. Enzymatic activity and micelle formation in the GI tract are also disrupted.

Other antibiotics that may interfere with nutritional status are the cephalosporins, which can cause hemorrhage of the intestine (functioning as vitamin K antagonists), and the aminoglycosides, which inhibit normal kidney function and cause excess excretion of calcium, magnesium, and potassium. The antituberculosis agent, isoniazid, is an antagonist of pyridoxine (vitamin B_1) but also can cause reduction in niacin (pyridoxine is a cofactor in niacin synthesis) and vitamin D deficiency. In the latter instance, isoniazid inhibits the L-α-hydroxylase of the kidney and the 25-hydroxylase of the liver (see Chapter 42).

Drugs that Reduce Intestinal Absorption Many orally administered drugs reduce absorption of foods from the GI tract. Some of these effects are predictable such as the decreased fat-soluble vitamin absorption caused by mineral oil and the decreased vitamin (folate) and mineral (iron, zinc) absorption caused by binding to cholestyramine. Presence of these two pharmacological agents shortens the contact time between the nutrient and the GI mucosa and thus reduces absorption. Prevention of micelle formation (mineral oil) and cationic binding of charged particles (by cholestyramine) prevent nutrients from reaching the villi, from which they can be transported across the GI tract. By increasing the pH in the intestine, any basic compound such as sodium bicarbonate can dramatically alter the absorption of folic acid and iron. Cimetidine also increases the pH of the intestine by preventing the secretion of hydrochloric acid in the stomach; therefore the uptake of some water-soluble vitamins such as vitamin B_2 is inhibited.

Drug Effects on Vitamin and Mineral Status / Antivitamins The majority of drug effects of nutrients involve the vitamins or minerals. The role of vitamins and minerals in the body is to activate or facilitate particular biochemical reactions. Such reactions are subject to specific interference by drugs. Drugs affect vitamins and minerals as follows:

1. Binding in the intestine and / or inhibition of absorption
2. Competition with nutrients for transport
3. Direct competition at the site of action
4. Destruction or deactivation of the nutrient
5. Overuse of the nutrient, resulting in depletion of stores
6. Alteration of the metabolic half-lives of nutrients by increasing the rate of removal from the blood or promoting loss of the nutrient from the body by increasing tissue loss via increased excretion

A drug may effect changes in different nutrients by one or more of these mechanisms (see individual drugs for specific examples).

REFERENCES

American Heart Association: A joint statement of the Nutrition Committee and Council on Artherosclerosis: recommendations for the treatment of hyperlipidemia in adults, Dallas, 1982, The Association.

Dubick MA and Rucker RB: Dietary supplements and health aids: a critical evaluation, part I, vitamins and minerals, J Nutr Educ 15:47, 1983.

Grundy SM: Comparison of monounsaturated fatty acids and carbohydrates for lowering plasma cholesterol, N Engl J Med 314:745, 1986.

Phillipson BE, Rothrock DW, Conner WE et al: Reduction of plasma lipids, lipoproteins, and apoproteins by dietary fish oils in patients with hypertriglyceridemia, N Engl J Med 312:121B, 1985.

Roe DA: Diet and drug interactions, New York, 1989, Van Nostrand Reinhold.

Shils ME and Young VR, eds: Modern nutrition in health and disease, Philadelphia, 1988, Lea & Febiger.

Trowell HC and Burkitt DP: In Burkitt DP and Trowell HC, eds: Refined carbohydrate foods and disease, London, 1975, Academic Press.

CHAPTER 62 Toxicology

ABBREVIATIONS

LD_{50}	dose of chemical that kills 50% of animals receiving it
IgG, IgM	immunoglobulins
TCDD	tetrachlorodibenzo-p-dioxin
FSH	follicle-stimulating hormone
LH	luteinizing hormone
ATP	adenosine triphosphate
CO	carbon monoxide
IQ	intelligence quotient
BAL	British anti-Lewisite
EDTA	ethylenediaminetetraacetic acid

WHAT IS TOXICOLOGY?

Industrial chemical and pharmaceutical development, environmental contamination, and illicit drug use present significant health hazards to the general population.

Each year in the United States it is estimated that approximately 8 million people suffer acute poisoning. About 20,000 patients die from illicit drug overdose per year. Acute toxicity from drug or poison ingestion accounts for as much as 10% to 20% of hospital admissions. Trends suggest that the number of toxic exposures will increase in the future.

Principles of Toxicology

Any substance injurious to humans may be classified as poison. Substances such as NaCl, oxygen, and many others generally considered nontoxic can be deleterious to human health under certain conditions. The terms poison, toxic substance, toxic chemical, and toxicant are synonymous. Toxicity or toxic response refers to the effects manifested by an organism in response to a toxic substance.

A common test, the LD_{50} was originally developed to quantify lethality in animals. However, LD_{50} is inappropriate in the assessment of toxicity in man. The LD_{50} is defined as the dose of a chemical that kills 50% of animals receiving it.

A toxic response can occur within minutes or after a delay of hours, days, months, or years, or any time interval between. These responses are often referred to as acute, subacute, subchronic, or chronic toxicities. Most acutely toxic agents rapidly interfere with critical cellular processes. For example, cyanide causes immediate injury by inhibiting cellular respiration. Acetaminophen is an example of subacute injury, since hepatic necrosis is not evident for 1 to 3 days after ingestion. Acetaminophen produces reactive intermediates that injure liver cells within a few hours. However, time is required (2 to 3 days) for this injury to become clinically manifest. Organophosphate insecticides cause an early cholinergic syndrome, which resolves before the development of peripheral neuropathy several days later.

A poison causing direct toxicity implies that direct contact and injury develops after interaction of the toxicant and the injured cell. Poisons causing indirect toxicity do so by injuring one group of cells, the injury of which precipitates injury in other cells. Similarly, interference with a normal physiological process may injure cells dependent on that process. For example, alterations of neuroendocrine function with reserpine or chlorpromazine alter sexual organ function.

Some substances such as strong acids of bases act locally. Most other toxic substances produce systemic effects or a combination of local and systemic effects. Hydrofluoric acid, a common industrial chemical, produces an extremely painful local penetrating injury at the site of skin exposure. In larger exposures, enough fluoride ions enter the blood to bind calcium and produce hypocalcemia. Most therapeutic drugs and toxicants other than strong acids or bases do not produce clinically significant local injury.

Many toxic substances are known to affect a particular target organ. The liver, nervous system, kidneys and lungs are examples in which toxicity can be related to altered physiological and biochemical functions. The liver receives a dual blood supply from the hepatic artery and the portal vein. It can be exposed to toxicants entering from the systemic circulation (as after inhalation) or from the splanchnic circulation (toxicants absorbed from the gastrointestinal [GI] tract). The leaky capillary system of the hepatic sinusoids is designed to promote the extraction of toxicants from the blood into the liver. This process exposes the liver to high concentrations of chemicals. The liver contains a high concentration of enzymes to metabolize (biotransform) many endogenous and exogenous chemicals. In some cases, the chemical modification produced by biotransformation results in bioactivation, i.e., the production of toxic/reactive metabolites that detrimentally react within the liver. For example, acetaminophen causes hepatic necrosis. This occurs because the liver is rich in cytochrome P-450—the enzyme system that metabolizes acetaminophen to its reactive intermediates, chiefly glutathione adducts. Other examples of compounds in which hepatic toxicity is caused by hepatic metabolism include solvents (carbon tetrachloride, halogenated benzenes), therapeutic drugs (isoniazid), and carcinogens (aflatoxin B, aromatic amines). When the rate of formation of reactive metabolites exceeds the liver's detoxification capacity, toxicity occurs.

The integrative role of the highly complex nervous system means that toxic injury to one part can result in adverse effects in other sites of the nervous system. Similarly, toxic injury in other organs and tissues can result in neuronal lesions. For example, chemicals that cause severe hypotension or hypoglycemia may result in neuronal cell death. Neurons have a high metabolic rate that requires a sustained delivery of oxygen and nutrients. Therefore sustained reductions in oxygen and glucose result in central nervous system (CNS)

damage. Similarly, chemicals (i.e., cyanide or dinitrophenol) that interfere with oxidative metabolism can also compromise neuronal viability.

Neurons are unique among cells because the cell body must provide support for dendrites and axons. The axon is devoid of any metabolic functions (i.e., protein synthesis) and thus must rely on transport, often over long distances, of materials from the cell body to the distal axon. Acrylamide and n-hexane are thought to produce peripheral neuropathies by interfering with axonal transport. Diketone metabolites of n-hexane can derivatize and cross-link neurofilaments. As these cross-links accumulate with repeated exposure to n-hexane, axonal transport is retarded, ultimately causing axonal atrophy.

Another key feature of the CNS is the lack of regenerative repair mechanisms for mature neurons. Lack of repair results in the accumulation of lesions within the nervous system (Figure 62-1). Because of plasticity within the CNS, expression of these lesions as neurotoxic events is often delayed. However, the accumulation of lesions after repeated chemical exposure eventually reaches a critical concentration, and the normal neuronal reserve can no longer compensate for the chemical lesions. There is also a normal, age-related attrition of neurons. Thus chemical exposure to neurotoxicants may reduce the age at which neurological and behavioral deficits appear. If exposure to the chemical occurred in the past, a causal relationship between chemical exposure and neurotoxicity will not be apparent.

Pulmonary toxicity is primarily mediated by respiratory exposure, although blood-borne toxicants may also cause pulmonary injury. The pulmonary system is composed of the nasopharyngeal and tracheobronchial airways and the pulmonary parenchyma (alveoli). The airways are directly exposed to many gaseous or particulate toxicants. Gases may react with airway mucosal cells or penetrate to the alveoli. Chlorine gas reacts with upper airway fluids and produces hydrochloric acid (HCl), causing mucosal injury. Cyanide and chloroform penetrate to the alveoli, are well absorbed, and cause systemic, not pulmonary, toxicity. Particulates impact in the airway or, if small enough, reach the alveoli. If trapped in the airway they may be cleared by the mucociliary apparatus. Substances reaching the alveoli can only be eliminated by absorption into the blood, by macrophage phagocytosis, or by biotransformation. Macrophages phagocytize toxicants in particulate form

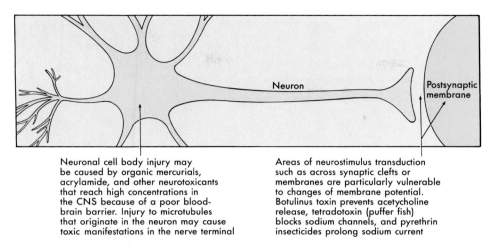

Neuronal cell body injury may be caused by organic mercurials, acrylamide, and other neurotoxicants that reach high concentrations in the CNS because of a poor blood-brain barrier. Injury to microtubules that originate in the neuron may cause toxic manifestations in the nerve terminal

Areas of neurostimulus transduction such as across synaptic clefts or membranes are particularly vulnerable to changes of membrane potential. Botulinus toxin prevents acetycholine release, tetradotoxin (puffer fish) blocks sodium channels, and pyrethrin insecticides prolong sodium current

FIGURE 62-1   Summary of some toxicant actions on the CNS.

and then enzymatically degrade them or simply carry them out of the alveolus. When asbestos is involved, this function may actually produce toxicity. Macrophages engulf but cannot degrade asbestos particles. Ultimately, macrophages die, releasing degradative enzymes into the interstitium, which damages adjacent cells. Repetition of this process eventually leads to progressive fibrosis and restrictive respiratory dysfunction. Pulmonary biotransformation of chemicals may also lead to toxicity. Specific cells, located in the terminal bronchioles, possess cytochrome P-450 activity that produces toxic metabolites associated with development of pulmonary injury. Inhalation of benzo(a)pyrene and other polycyclic aromatic hydrocarbons causes lung cancer as a result of reactive intermediates produced by pulmonary cytochrome P-450.

Blood-borne toxicants may affect the lung. Paraquat is a herbicide taken up by type II pneumocytes in the lung. Biotransformation of paraquat produces a reactive intermediate that undergoes redox cycling, a process that produces reactive oxygen species that injure the cell. Thus, although exposure to paraquat usually occurs after ingestion or skin contamination, death is caused by pulmonary injury. Similarly, certain pyrrolizidine alkaloids are metabolized in the liver to metabolites that circulate in the blood and produce toxicity in the lung (see Figure 62-2 for summary).

The kidney is also susceptible to specific toxicants. The mechanisms of renal injury include those similar to other organs, as well as mechanisms unique to the kidney. Delivery of blood-borne toxic substances to the kidney is high because (1) the kidney receives 25% of cardiac output and (2) its functions include filtering, concentrating, and eliminating toxicants. As water is reabsorbed, the concentration of chemicals in the tubule can increase to toxic levels. In some cases, the concentration may exceed the solubility of a chemical and lead to precipitation and obstruction of the affected area (see Figure 62-3 for summary).

Although to a lesser extent than the liver, the kidney also biotransforms chemicals. Cytochrome P-450 is located in the proximal tubule. This may explain the susceptibility of this region to chemical injury. For example, carbon tetrachloride and chloroform, two halogenated hydrocarbons that injure the proximal tubule, require biotransformation by the cytochrome P-450 system to form the toxic species. Many heavy metals damage the proximal tubules. Because heavy metals are not metabolized by cytochrome P-450, other mechanisms must be involved in this specificity. Heavy metals may concentrate in renal tubular cells. Heavy metals may also injure the blood vessels supplying the proximal tubule cells. Thus renal injury from heavy metals may be a combination of direct and indirect toxicity.

The kidney can compensate for excessive chemical exposure. Like many organs it has a reserve mass. Thus tissue injury equal to one entire kidney must be lost before loss of function is clinically apparent. The

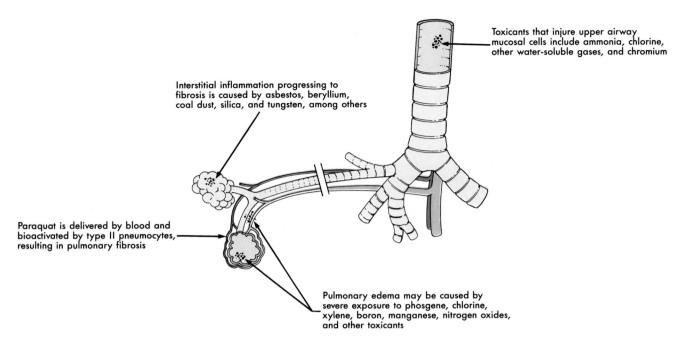

Toxicants that injure upper airway mucosal cells include ammonia, chlorine, other water-soluble gases, and chromium

Interstitial inflammation progressing to fibrosis is caused by asbestos, beryllium, coal dust, silica, and tungsten, among others

Paraquat is delivered by blood and bioactivated by type II pneumocytes, resulting in pulmonary fibrosis

Pulmonary edema may be caused by severe exposure to phosgene, chlorine, xylene, boron, manganese, nitrogen oxides, and other toxicants

FIGURE 62-2   Summary of some toxicant actions on pulmonary tissues.

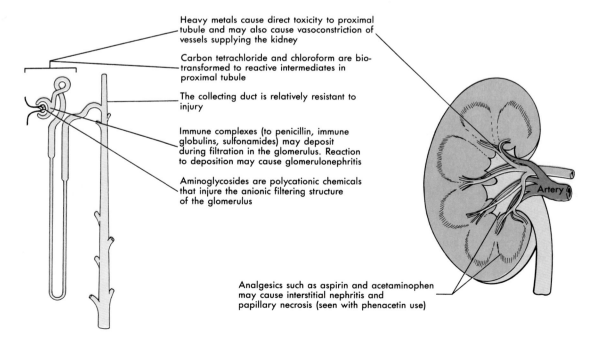

Heavy metals cause direct toxicity to proximal tubule and may also cause vasoconstriction of vessels supplying the kidney

Carbon tetrachloride and chloroform are bio-transformed to reactive intermediates in proximal tubule

The collecting duct is relatively resistant to injury

Immune complexes (to penicillin, immune globulins, sulfonamides) may deposit during filtration in the glomerulus. Reaction to deposition may cause glomerulonephritis

Aminoglycosides are polycationic chemicals that injure the anionic filtering structure of the glomerulus

Artery

Analgesics such as aspirin and acetaminophen may cause interstitial nephritis and papillary necrosis (seen with phenacetin use)

FIGURE 62-3   Summary of some toxicant actions on the kidney.

kidney also replaces lost functional capacity by hypertrophy. Perhaps because of its frequent exposure to metals, the kidney has developed binding proteins to remove heavy metals. Metallothioneins, a unique protein class, avidly bind cadmium, protecting the kidney and other organs from toxicity. However, if exposure exceeds binding capacity or a significant amount of the cadmium-metallothionein complex accumulates, renal toxicity will develop.

Although anatomical or functional characteristics predispose many organs to injury, designation of chemicals as specific organ toxicants (neurotoxic, cardiotoxic, etc.) is misleading for several reasons. First, toxic substances may have effects throughout the body. Although a chemical may primarily affect one organ, other organs probably concurrently experience less notable degrees of injury. Second, a toxic response in one tissue will undoubtedly have serious consequences for other tissues. A toxic response represents a spectrum influenced by the characteristics of the chemical (physical state, site of exposure, dose, and duration of exposure) and of the patient (general health, nutritional state, age, sex, enzyme induction, immune response, antioxidant concentrations). Thus a minor insult to an organ already compromised by disease may cause unexpected injury to organs other than the primary organ.

DETERMINANTS OF THE TOXIC RESPONSE

Generally the ability of a toxicant to reach the target organ embodies the same pharmacokinetic principles described for therapeutic agents (see Chapters 4 and 5). These pharmacokinetic principles suggest methods for reducing, reversing, or preventing the toxicity of many substances.

Poison may be absorbed by an organism via dermal, gastrointestinal (GI), or pulmonary routes. Measures to prevent absorption may reduce the concentration of toxicant at the site of the toxic action. Washing the skin, stomach lavage, and oral administration of charcoal are examples for reducing dermal or GI absorption of toxic substances. After absorption, toxic substances are distributed via blood to the tissues. In some cases it is possible to intercept the toxicant before it is absorbed or reaches its target. This can be accomplished by the following mechanisms:

1. Hemodialysis may be used to remove the toxic compound by filtration
2. Hemoperfusion may be used to remove toxicants from the blood by circulating blood through an activated charcoal filter
3. Oral administration of activated charcoal with subsequent gastric lavage may be used to remove toxicants from the stomach, thereby reducing the amount available for absorption into the bloodstream

It is generally too late to prevent cell or organ damage after the toxicant reaches the target cell. However, the effects of many toxicants may still be minimized at this stage. Compounds metabolized to reactive intermediates are good examples. An antidote to prevent biotransformation of the toxicant prevents injury produced by the reactive intermediate. Competitive antagonism of methanol by ethanol is based on this principle (see Chapter 31).

Toxic metabolites produced by biotransformation may injure the cell in which they are produced, or they may diffuse into the bloodstream and affect other areas. For a few toxic substances, this offers a final opportunity to eliminate toxic metabolites by measures (i.e., hemodialysis) that clear the bloodstream.

Another strategy for reducing injury is to allow the reactive intermediate to interact with an exogenously administered substance instead of interacting with an important cell constituent. Treatment of acetaminophen toxicity with N-acetylcysteine is based on this principle (see Chapter 29).

THE IMMUNE SYSTEM

The immune system can be affected by a wide variety of toxicants. These agents often cause immunosuppression by interfering with cell growth or proliferation, resulting in a reduction of capacity. Other compounds may directly destroy immune system components. A further mechanism is the ability of toxicants to inhibit or modify cell division. Finally, some chemicals distort normal signaling mechanisms that ultimately reduce the immune response. For example, benzene causes lymphocytopenia but also affects other bone marrow elements. The functional result is a deficiency in cell-mediated immunity. Workers exposed to benzene show decreased humoral immunity, as evidenced by depressed complement and immunoglobulin concentrations.

In humans, the effect of immunosuppression may be an increased incidence of bacterial, viral, and parasitic infections. For example, polychlorinated biphenyl exposure results in an increased incidence of respiratory infections, whereas lead exposure may produce a bacterial diarrhea in children. Theoretically, immunosuppression may also interfere with the immune system's surveillance function, resulting in an increased incidence of cancer. This consequence of immunosuppression is now being investigated.

In addition to being a target for chemical-mediated injury, the immune system may mediate injury by producing hypersensitivity reactions (see Chapter 60). Hypersensitivity reactions are adverse events caused by an immune response to foreign antigens. A type I hypersensitivity reaction (anaphylaxis) is an immediate reaction mediated by IgG bound to mast cells and basophils. Binding of antigen causes release of histamine and other mediators. Acute life-threatening responses to penicillin are an example of anaphylaxis. Type II (cytolytic) reactions involve IgG or IgM produced against a foreign compound. In some cases these immunoglobulins bind to other cells and produce destruction of that cell by stimulation of complement-mediated or other cell killing mechanisms. Several drugs, including penicillins, sulfonamides, and quinine can stimulate antibody formation, producing red cell hemolysis using a type II mechanism. Type III (serum sickness) reactions involve deposition of antibody-antigen complexes in the skin and membranes. Immune reaction to these complexes can cause inflammation of the skin, joints, kidney, and other organs. Serum sickness after antivenin administration is an example of drug toxicity mediated by this mechanism. Finally, type IV (cell-mediated) hypersensitivity is caused by T lymphocytes. T lymphocytes recognize the antigen and then recruit other cells to mount an inflammatory response to the antigen. Contact dermatitis to nickel, several industrial chemicals, and poison ivy is caused by this response.

TERATOGENESIS

The term *teratogen* refers to a drug or other agent that causes abnormal fetal development. Thalidomide is a notorious example of a teratogen. However, teratogens are only one form of toxicity occurring in utero. Any known type of toxic effect caused in adults can occur in the fetus, although there are certain special considerations. An extensive treatment of teratogenesis is discussed in Chapter 63.

CARCINOGENESIS

Cancer cells are cells that escape from the fine-control mechanisms that govern growth, development, and division of normal cells (see Chapter 43). Some cancers in humans are of environmental origin, having been caused by radiation, viral infection, or chemical exposure. In 1775, scrotal cancer was associated with chimney sweeps because they were exposed to soot; subsequent studies associate cancer with chemicals in the workplace.

Because animals develop cancer when exposed to large doses of chemicals over their lifetime, a significant portion of the public believes that synthetic chemicals are a primary cause of cancer. These chemicals could be drugs, pesticides, or industrial chemicals that contaminate the environment. However, it is probably life-style choices that result in the greatest exposure of humans to chemical carcinogens. Cigarette smoke contains many potent cancer-causing chemicals and is a causative factor of lung cancer. Similarly, chronic consumption of large amounts of ethanol is associated with an increased risk of esophageal and liver cancer. Charcoal broiling contaminates meats and fish with polycyclic aromatic hydrocarbons, which are the carcinogens in coal tars and soot. Many "natural" foods are known to contain potent carcinogens. A major percentage of cancers in humans could be prevented or delayed by reducing these "life-style" exposures to carcinogens.

Carcinogenic Process

A number of steps are involved in the process by which chemicals cause cancer. Duration, dose, and frequency of exposure are important variables. Because of cancer development may take 20 years or more, cause and effect relationships between chemical exposure and cancer incidents are difficult to establish.

Induction of cancer by chemicals is divided into three major steps: initiation, promotion, and progression. Initiation is the conversion of a normal cell into a neoplastic cell. Chemicals that cause this conversion are called *initiating agents.* The molecular target for these agents is deoxyribonucleic acid (DNA).

Within the past 20 years, significant advances in knowledge of the mechanisms of chemical carcinogenesis has led to the development of systems to test for the carcinogenic potential of a chemical. Such tests include structural comparison to known carcinogens, in vitro mutagenesis and cell transformation assays, and cancer bioassays in rodents. Some chemicals interact directly with DNA, but many require metabolic transformation to reactive species before covalent interaction with DNA can occur. If cell division occurs before enzymatic repair of the damaged DNA, then a permanent mutation is encoded in the genome. Because cellular damage undoubtedly kills some cells in the target tissue, the stimulus for division of adjacent cells is high. The result is a new cell type with altered genotypic and phenotypic properties.

In animal studies, some chemicals, referred to as *promoters*, increase the incidence of cancers and/or decrease the latency period for tumor development without interaction with DNA or production of mutations. These chemicals are effective only when administered repeatedly after an initial insult. For example, a cytosolic receptor has been identified in animals that promotes liver carcinogenesis in the presence of 2,3,7,8-tetrachlorodibenzo-p-dioxin (TCDD). This chemical triggers a pleiotropic response that results in enhanced gene expression. Initiated cells proliferate under the influence of the promoter and undergo clonal expansion into phenotypically altered foci, nodules, or papillomas. Endogenous substances such as growth factors and hormones may also act as promoters. For example, follicle-stimulating hormone (FSH) and leuteinizing hormone (LH) may promote chemical-induced ovarian cancers because of their trophic effect on the ovary. Carcinogens (i.e., initiating agents) also promote tumor development. They create the environment for selected proliferation of initiated cells and/or produce other cellular changes that provide a selective advantage for autonomous division and growth.

During tumor promotion, most foci and nodules regress. They do not become selective for the advantageous properties that distinguish between benign and malignant cells. The growth and division of malignant cells are not related to the growth and division of other cells within a tissue. An important property of malignant cells is metastasis (discussed in Chapter 43), but the sequence of events leading to the metastatic stage of carcinogenesis is largely unknown.

TOXIC GASES

The two most dangerous toxic gases are carbon monoxide (CO) and volatile cyanides. Both compounds are toxic because they deprive the cell of oxygen.

Carbon Monoxide

CO is the leading cause of death by poisoning. It also inflicts sublethal injuries, including myocardial infarction and cerebral atrophy.

The primary effects of CO are displacement of oxygen from hemoglobin and impairment of oxygen release from hemoglobin. CO displaces oxygen from hemoglobin because it has a >200 times higher affinity for hemoglobin than does oxygen. Even at a concentration of only 0.5%, CO displaces oxygen to produce 50% carboxyhemoglobin. However, CO produces more injury than simply replacing oxygen. Normally, hemoglobin binding of oxygen shows cooperativity: binding of one oxygen molecule promotes binding of subsequent oxygen molecules to a hemoglobin molecule. Similarly, hemoglobin shows cooperativity in releasing oxygen. However, carboxyhemoglobin does not release oxygen normally. CO shifts the oxyhemoglobin dissociation curve to the left and reduces oxygen release to the cell. The result of oxygen displacement and decreased release of oxygen from hemoglobin is anaerobic metabolism and cell death if not reversed.

The symptoms of CO poisoning are a reflection of oxygen deprivation to each organ. Early symptoms of nervous system dysfunction resemble the flu, including nausea, headache, malaise, lightheadedness, and dizziness. Later symptoms are more ominous: depressed sensorium, loss of consciousness, seizures, and death. The histopathology of nervous system injury includes necrosis of the globus pallidus, substantia nigra, hippocampus, cerebral cortex and cerebellum, typical of all anoxic injuries.

The heart is particularly susceptible to CO poisoning. The heart has high oxygen requirements and, because it normally extracts more oxygen from the blood than other organs, compensates poorly for decreased oxygen delivery. When CO decreases oxygen delivery, severe myocardial ischemia may develop. Symptoms are the same as other types of myocardial ischemia, although the usual cardiac risk factors may be absent. Histopathology shows patchy myocardial necrosis rather than regional necrosis found in typical myocardial infarctions.

As CO dissociates from the hemoglobin it is expired. However, because of its high affinity for hemoglobin, this is a slow process. The half-life of carboxyhemoglobin without treatment is 3 to 4 hours, depending on the patient's ventilation. Administration of 100% oxygen by face mask shortens the time to 90 minutes. Hyperbaric oxygen reduces the half-life to 20 minutes. The patient's outcome depends on the duration and the severity of hypoxic episode.

Cyanide

The common route of exposure to cyanide is through inhalation of smoke produced by burning of plastics. Certain paints may be an additional source. Other sources are ingestion of fruit seeds (e.g., apricots and cherries) containing toxic amounts of soluble cyanide. These seeds must be crushed and then metabolized by intestinal bacteria to release the cyanide. Potassium cyanide (in solution or solid form) has been used in suicide or homicide poisoning attempts.

Cyanide produces toxicity by avidly binding to ferric iron (Fe^{3+}) to prevent reduction to the ferrous (Fe^{2+}) form involved in the cytochrome oxidase electron transport system. The transfer of electrons from cytochromes to molecular oxygen is prevented, inhibiting ATP production and forcing the cell to produce energy by anaerobic metabolism. As in all cases of hypoxia, anaerobic glycolysis produces only small amounts of ATP and large quantities of lactic acid.

Thus victims of cyanide poisoning show symptoms and signs of hypoxia. Similar to CO, cyanide toxicity first affects organs that have high oxygen use. However, the onset of these symptoms, which depends on the route of exposure, is often faster. Inhalation may produce rapid demise, whereas ingestion delays symptoms for 30 minutes or more. CNS dysfunction causes loss of consciousness and respiratory arrest. Laboratory findings are typical of cellular hypoxia and include severe anion gap acidosis produced by lactic acid.

Treatment is based on preventing cyanide from reaching its target, cytochrome oxidase. Because cyanide has high affinity for ferric iron, ferric iron can be provided in the form of oxidized hemoglobin. This is accomplished by the administration of nitrate, which converts hemoglobin to methemoglobin, the ferric form. The latter effectively competes for the cyanide with cytochrome C by mass action, forming cyanmethemoglobin. Cyanide is removed from the body following metabolism to thiocyanate by rhodanase and is ultimately excreted in the urine. Sodium thiosulfate is administered to facilitate thiocyanate formation. An alternative is administration of hydroxocobalamin, which reacts with cyanide to produce cyanocobalamin. Because hydroxocobalamin and cyanocobalamin have little toxicity, this is a promising treatment of cyanide poisoning.

HEAVY METALS

The widespread occurrence of metals in the environment and their numerous industrial and medical uses makes them important potential toxicants.

The rate of absorption of heavy metals is dependent on their physical state. Metals may exist in their elemental state or bind to inorganic or organic ligands. The elemental and inorganic forms of metals may be well absorbed as a result of physical similarity to nutritionally essential metals. For example, lead is well absorbed by the normal transport protein for iron located in the GI mucosa. Organs containing these transport systems are predisposed to injury from these metals. Commonly injured organs include liver, kidney, and GI mucosa. Organic forms of metals are more lipid soluble than inorganic forms and may be well absorbed without specific transport systems.

Physical state also affects distribution of metals. Lipid soluble forms achieve higher concentrations in areas of high lipid content such as the CNS. For example, inorganic and elemental forms of mercury primarily injure the kidney, whereas organic forms such as methyl mercury injure the brain.

The body has developed specific defense mechanisms against certain metals. The kidney has a binding protein for cadmium called *metallothionein*. The strong cadmium binding of this protein concentrates cadmium in the kidney and reduces its excretion. The

Table 62-1   Mechanisms of Heavy Metal Toxicity

Metal	Mechanism	Target Organs
Arsenic	Reacts with sulfhydryl groups; interferes with oxidative phosphorylation	Peripheral neurons GI tract Hepatic necrosis Cardiovascular system
Lead	Reacts with sulfhydryl groups; interferes with heme synthesis; direct toxic effect to CNS	Hematopoietic system Central and peripheral nervous system Kidney
Mercury	Reacts with sulfhydryl groups; some forms have direct cytotoxic effect	Central and peripheral nervous system Kidney GI tract Respiratory system

Table 62-2   Metals Chelated by Therapeutic Drugs

Chelator	Metal
British anti-Lewisite (BAL)	Lead, arsenic, mercury
EDTA	Lead
penicillamine	Copper, lead
deferoxamine	Iron
dimercaptosuccinic acid (DMSA)	Lead, arsenic, mercury

binding prevents toxicity until the protein is saturated, at which time subsequent cadmium accumulation causes injury. The mechanism of heavy metal toxicity is poorly understood. Many metals function as essential cofactors of enzymes. Substitution by a similar but toxic metal may produce enzymatic dysfunction. Metals are generally very reactive and may bind to key sulfhydryl groups in active centers of enzymes, again producing dysfunction in many organ systems. Besides direct metal toxicity, metals produce hypersensitivity reactions. Nickel, chromium, gold, and others cause cell-mediated (type IV) hypersensitivity reactions (see Table 62-1 for summary).

Metal Chelation

Treatment for metal toxicity focuses on increasing excretion of the metal from the body. The term *chelator* drug stems from the root "chele", meaning claw. These drugs bind the metal between two or more functional groups to form a metal-drug complex that is excreted in urine. Certain chelators work best for certain metals. The uses of chelators are summarized in Table 62-2.

Lead

Lead is one of the oldest known poisons, its toxicity was described in Roman times. Lead continues to pose a significant health problem. Industrialization, mining, and leaded gasoline dramatically increase the amount of lead in the environment and consequently in humans. Lead is present in some ceramic glazes and paints. In older homes, paint containing lead flakes off or is present in dust, and may be ingested or inhaled by children, producing chronic lead toxicity. Adults are exposed to toxic concentrations in certain work environments.

Lead binds to sulfhydryl and other active sites in many enzyme systems, leading to enzyme inactivation. Although its effects are diffuse, certain manifestations predominate. Heme synthesis is sensitive to lead poisoning, with two enzymes in the heme biosynthetic pathway inhibited by lead, producing anemia. Impairment of enzyme activity is detectable before anemia develops.

Lead is particularly toxic to the nervous system, producing deleterious effects especially in children. In adults, lead exposure produces a peripheral neuropathy. Early symptoms in children include anorexia, colicky abdominal pain, lethargy, and vomiting. If lead exposure continues, children are more likely than adults to develop encephalopathy manifested by irritability progressing to seizures and coma, with approximately 30% having permanent neurological sequelae.

Low-concentration lead exposure may pose special risks for children. Subtle neurological injury from low lead exposure, detected by depressed IQ scores and learning disorders, is reported. Lead may accumulate in the immature nervous system because it may cross the blood-brain barrier more easily in children, and the CNS may be less capable of removing lead than in adults.

Adults exposed to lead generally develop vague complaints of headache and lightheadedness. With

Table 62-3   Physical Findings with Exposure to Toxic Agents

Agent	Signs of Toxicity
Narcotic	Miotic pupils, CNS and respiratory depression, hypotension, may have needle track marks
Anticholinergic	Dry, flushed appearance; mydriasis; decreased bowel motility; tachycardia; hallucinations
Cholinergic	Muscarinic—salivation, lacrimation, urination, defecation
	Nicotinic-muscle fasciculations, weakness, paralysis
Stimulants (cocaine, amphetamines)	Tachycardia, hypertension, hyperthermia, mydriasis, agitation, psychosis
Tricyclic antidepressants	Anticholinergic findings and electrocardiogram abnormalities (QRS widening, QT prolongation)

Table 62-4   Contraindications and Complications of Emesis and Lavage

Contraindications	Complications
EMESIS	**EMESIS**
Altered mental status	Aspiration
Age less than 6 months	Prolonged vomiting
Inability to protect airway	Esophageal tearing
Ingestion of agents causing rapid deterioration of mental status	
Convulsants	
Tricyclic antidepressants	
Camphor	
Ingestion of	
Acid	
Alkali	
Hydrocarbons	
Sharp objects	
Pregnancy	
LAVAGE	**LAVAGE**
Strong acid or alkali ingestion	Aspiration
Petroleum product ingestion	Esophageal perforation
Unconscious patients without endotracheal intubation	Intratracheal insertion

Table 62-5   Common Antidotes

Toxicant	Antidote	Mechanism
venoms—snake, black widow	antivenin	Immunological binding to toxicant
cholinesterase inhibitors	atropine	Blocks muscarinic receptors
cyanide	cyanide kit (Na nitrate, Na thiosulfate)	Induction of methemoglobinemia; cyanide binds preferentially to methemoglobin
digoxin	digoxin antibodies	Immunological binding to toxicant
metals	chelators	Binding of metal with subsequent urinary excretion
iron	deferoxamine	
lead	British anti-Lewisite	
mercury	EDTA	
arsenic	penicillamine	
methanol, ethylene glycol	ethanol	Competition for alcohol dehydrogenase (enzyme-producing reactive metabolites)
acetaminophen	N-acetylcysteine	Provides sulfhydryl groups to detoxify reactive metabolite
opiates	naloxone	Receptor blockade
carbon monoxide	oxygen	Oxygen in high concentration displaces CO molecules from carboxyhemoglobin
isoniazid	pyridoxine HCl	Competitively reverses isoniazid effect by providing substitute for pyridoxine kinase enzyme inhibited by isoniazid

increased exposure, a peripheral neuropathy is manifest.

In the patient with lead poisoning symptoms, whole blood lead concentrations are the best indicator of recent exposure. As concentrations rise, the danger of encephalopathy increases, although symptoms do not usually occur until lead concentrations approach 50 μg/dl. In adults, acceptable lead concentrations are under 40 μg/dl, with symptoms developing above 80 μg/dl.

Lead is slowly excreted from the body. Excretion is hastened by the use of chelators such as British anti-Lewisite (BAL). Unfortunately, BAL is an oily liquid that is painful when injected. Orally administered analogs of BAL are being developed to reduce patient discomfort. Other chemicals may bind metals using other functional groups.

OTHER TOXICANTS

Toxicities resulting from organophosphates or to drugs of abuse are discussed in Chapters 9 and 32, respectively.

CLINICAL MANAGEMENT OF TOXIC PATIENTS

The clinical diagnosis and management of patients subject to chemical toxicity is an extensive subject that is beyond the scope of this book. However, some overview guidelines are presented here to summarize the variety of symptoms (Table 62-3), to point out the contraindications and problems associated with emesis and gastric lavage (Table 62-4), and to provide a list of antidotes for common types of chemical toxicants (Table 62-5).

REFERENCES

Casarett LJ, Doull J, Klassen CD et al, eds: Casarett and Doull's Toxicology, New York, 1986, Macmillan.

Goldfrank LR, ed: Goldfrank's toxicologic emergencies, ed 2, East Norwalk, 1982, Appleton-Century-Crofts.

Roitt I, Brostoff J, Hale D: Immunology, ed 2, New York, 1989, Gower Medical Publishing.

Sax NI and Lewis RJ: Dangerous properties of industrial materials, ed 7, New York, 1989, Van Nostrand Reinhold.

CHAPTER 63

Perinatal / Neonatal Pharmacology

<table>
<tr><td colspan="2" align="center">ABBREVIATIONS</td></tr>
<tr><td align="right">Y protein</td><td>ligandin</td></tr>
<tr><td align="right">GFR</td><td>glomerular filtration rate</td></tr>
</table>

 ## THERAPEUTIC OVERVIEW

Limited understanding of the clinical pharmacology of specific drugs in pediatric patients emphasizes problems of the therapeutic pharmacological intervention in younger subjects such as newborn infants. Reliance on pharmacological data derived primarily from adults to determine appropriate efficacy and dosage guidelines for therapeutic use in children is risky. The problem of establishing efficacy and dosing guidelines for use in infants is further complicated, since the pharmacokinetics of many drugs change appreciably as the subject ages from a few weeks preceding birth to several months after birth—the dose-response relationships of some drugs may change between the weeks before and after birth.

In this chapter, perinatal refers to the period from the onset of labor through the first 4 weeks after birth and neonatal refers to the first 4 weeks after birth (for a premature or term birth (Figure 63-1). Newborn also designates the first few days or weeks after birth, after which the term *infant* applies. The changes in drug responses and drug disposition as the patient progresses from fetus to newborn to infant are mentioned briefly in Chapter 7 but are the primary topic for this chapter.

MATERNAL-PLACENTAL-FETAL UNIT

Maternal Pharmacokinetic Variables

Maternal physiological changes occur during pregnancy that result in differences in maternal pharmacokinetics of drugs administered during pregnancy compared to the nonpregnant state. These modified pharmacokinetic variables ultimately determine fetal therapeutic and toxic responses to drugs, drug metabolites, or toxic compounds in the maternal circulation that are capable of crossing the placenta.

Maternal drug absorption may be enhanced or decreased from the combination of delayed gastric emptying and decreased motility. Absorption from sites other than the gastrointestinal (GI) tract also may be affected, for example, increased pulmonary absorption may result from greater minute ventilation and increased cutaneous absorption as a result of greater surface area and blood flow.

Substantial changes in body mass and fluid distribution also accompany pregnancy. The apparent volume of distribution for some drugs (see Chapter 4) is expected to increase during pregnancy as a result of the dramatic increases in maternal aqueous and fatty tissue spaces (Table 63-1). Much of this gain in fat occurs between the 10th and 30th weeks of gestation (noted in Chapter 4).

Consistent with the gradual transient increase in maternal glomerular filtration rate that occurs during the first 8 months of pregnancy, the rate of elimination of renally excreted drugs increases more rapidly during this portion of pregnancy. Maternal hepatic en-

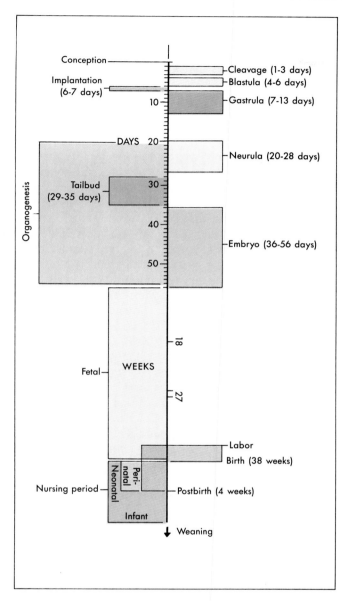

FIGURE 63-1   Sequence of normal human development.

Table 63-1   Change in Apparent Volume of Distribution of Some Drugs During Pregnancy

Agent	Gestation* (weeks)			
	10	20	30	40
ampicillin	36	45	57	68
caffeine	2	8	16	32
furosemide	1	9	20	29
meperidine	32	27	21	16

*Values represent % of control (prepregnancy values).

in the second trimester. The result of these changes on overall clearance and dose requirement is difficult to predict and varies among patients. Because changes in clearance cannot be predicted, it is important to titrate dosing to desired clinical effect.

The Placenta

The functions of the placenta during gestation are protection of the conceptus, maintenance of pregnancy, prevention of maternal rejection of the pregnancy as foreign tissue, transportation of nutrients and wastes, metabolism of endogenous and xenobiotic substances, and endocrine activity. *However, any drug or environmental agent that gains access to the maternal bloodstream should be considered capable of crossing the placenta and reaching the fetus unless demonstrated otherwise.*

Implantation of the fertilized ovum in the endometrial lining of the uterus is the beginning of placental development. Actually, two placentas form. The first is the yolk sac placenta, present until the fourth month of gestation. Its functions are red blood cell and embryonic midgut formation. The yolk sac is thus an important interim structure, present during the most sensitive time of development, but little is understood regarding its chemical transfer functions. The classical requirements for placental transfer, studied in late gestation mature placentas, may not apply.

Second, the chorioallantoic placenta begins to form at implantation. It gradually invades the maternal endometrial glands, stroma, and arterial walls to access the maternal blood supply in a villous structure that maximizes the surface area for maternal-fetal exchange. The structure allows the high-resistance maternal arterial system to become a low-resistance sys-

zyme activity, however, appears to decrease during pregnancy. For theophylline, a drug that normally undergoes considerable metabolism, the reduced intrinsic hepatic clearance resulting from slower metabolism is offset by reduced plasma protein bindings. The net effect is no significant change in nonrenal clearance during pregnancy. Concomitantly, renal theophylline clearance may be increased, particularly

tem in the spiral arteries. Maternal and fetal blood circulate in proximity by the third week of gestation. Until 12 weeks gestation, there are four tissue layers separating the maternal and fetal circulations: syncytiotrophoblast (the outer layer of the trophoblast), cytotrophoblast, villous connective tissue cores, and fetal capillary endothelium. By the third trimester, the cytotrophoblast is discontinuous, and only three layers separate the circulations.

At term, blood enters the spaces between the villi from over 100 spiral arteries; over 150 ml of blood may be contained in these spaces at a given time. The rate of blood flow increases during gestation from 50 ml/min at 10 weeks to 600 ml/min at term. Thus at term, the circulation replaces the blood volume in this space three to four times each minute.

Placental Processes

The basic process by which substances cross the placenta and gain access to the fetus are similar to those that occur in adults. The Fick equation describes the transfer of substances only by simple diffusion. The other processes require energy or special carriers.

The human placenta contains multiple enzyme systems, including those responsible for drug oxidation, reduction, hydrolysis, and conjugation. These systems are primarily involved with endogenous steroid metabolism; however, the activities of these enzymes are usually minor compared with those of maternal or fetal organs (including liver, kidney, and adrenal gland). Thus the presence of xenobiotic metabolizing systems in the placenta does not contribute markedly to overall drug clearance from the maternal-placental-fetal unit.

In general, lipophilic, unionized, low molecular weight drugs in their free nonprotein bound state tend to cross the placenta. Some of these agents, such as barbiturates, narcotic analgesics, and local anesthetics, are "flow-limited" in their placental transfer because a decrease in maternal blood flow to the placenta may reduce the placental passage of these agents. Normal uterine contractions during labor, oxytocic drugs, exogenously administered sympathomimetics, or β-adrenergic blocking agents all affect maternal and fetal hemodynamics and therefore may modify maternal drug distribution and placental transfer.

Fetal Development

Human development may be divided into three periods: preimplantation, embryonic, and fetal. During the preimplantation period, rapid cell division occurs, followed by embryonic differentiation and organogenesis. Because organ development includes structural formation and functional maturation, such development may continue through the perinatal period into infancy or later. For example, the lung does not mature fully until well after the end of gestation. The human brain is immature at birth and myelination of the brain and maturation of its function continues for many years. Thus the period of organogenesis bridges the late embryonic and early fetal periods and may extend into the first several years of life.

Most drugs pass freely to the postimplantation embryo. In animal model systems, embryonic tissue concentrations are generally lower than those measured concomitantly in the mother. Substances such as salicylic acid, diethylstilbestrol, and the herbicide (2,4, 5-T) may be present in increasing amounts in fetal tissues as gestation advances. Even some substances that are not well-transferred to the embryo (such as phenothiazines) may be found in higher concentrations in the fetus than the embryo.

The patterns of drug distribution in prenatal tissues also shows ontogeny. Early in embryonic development, exogenous substances accumulate in the neuroepithelium. The blood-brain barrier to diffusion is not developed until the last half of pregnancy, and the susceptibility of the central nervous system (CNS) to developmental toxins may be partly related to this preferential distribution.

After an agent traverses the placenta, it is first available to the fetal liver. If fetal liver metabolism is active, a substantial reduction in fetal plasma concentrations may occur rapidly, as a fetal "first-pass" effect.

The biotransforming enzyme systems of the fetus are first detectable at 5 to 8 weeks gestation, and their activity increases until 12 to 14 weeks, when it reaches only a fraction of adult activity. It is not until approximately 1 year after birth that liver enzymatic activity is comparable to that of the adult. The first system expressed is the cytochrome P-450 (or microsomal mixed-function oxidase) group of enzymes. These enzymes are detectable when the smooth endoplasmic reticulum develops (40 to 60 days in human gestation). It is most active in the fetal adrenal gland

and less active in the fetal liver. The fetal kidney and gut systems also have detectable activity.

The monooxygenases are composed of a number of inducible forms. This enzyme system may be divided into two major groups that are based on the substances that induce their activity, phenobarbital or polycyclic aromatic hydrocarbons. The latter group includes enzymes such as the aryl hydrocarbon hydroxylases, which metabolize benzo(a)pyrene, and other polycyclic aromatic hydrocarbon molecules. Aryl hydrocarbon hydroxylase activity is measurable in the blastocyst. The concentration of aryl hydrocarbon hydroxylase activity in the fetus is very low, approximately 2% to 4% of adult activity, but may be induced by maternal smoking. It appears that fetal induction of this enzyme shows ontogeny, in that a given level of maturity must be achieved before the system is inducible. There also appear to be genetic factors that govern inducibility of these hydroxylases. The phenobarbital-inducible monooxygenases appear early in development and gradually increase in activity until midgestation, when 20% to 40% of adult activity is attained. Hydrolytic enzymes, particularly epoxide hydrolases that convert stable or reactive epoxides to dihydrodiols, are also present in the fetus by 5 weeks gestation. The activity of the epoxide hydrolases is inducible and does not appear to show inter-individual variability on a genetic basis, in contrast to the mixed-function oxidases.

Alcohol dehydrogenase is expressed during the first 6 weeks of gestation. It is not certain when the reducing enzymes for subsequent detoxification of the aldehyde products are active in the fetus.

Human fetuses generally have well developed conjugating enzyme activities except for glucuronidation, which remains low until shortly before term. The early presence of the other conjugating systems in the human fetus may indicate a role in the modulation of activity of endogenous steroids. For endogenous compounds, conjugation may enhance activity. For example, certain steroid glucuronides and sulfates have greater potency than the parent compound.

Considering the limited protection afforded by the placenta, the ability of the fetus to metabolize xenobiotics may appear fortuitous. However, it can sometimes be detrimental. Fetal metabolism can result in the generation of reactive intermediates that lead to fetotoxicity, suggesting that the fetus and its genetic make-up may be major factors contributing

to developmental toxicity. A further effect of induction of metabolism in utero is that postnatal xenobiotic metabolism may be changed after prenatal exposures. Such exposures may enhance metabolism of the same or unrelated agents; for example, the ability of the newborn infant to metabolize bilirubin by conjugation may be induced by prenatal maternal phenobarbital therapy.

TERATOLOGY

Teratology is the study of birth defects, deviations from normal development resulting from prenatal or perinatal influences. Birth defects, comprising not only congenital malformations, but also prenatal infections, chromosomal abnormalities, and genetic diseases, are the leading cause of infant mortality. Chronic illness as a result of congenital anomalies account for one-half of all patient-hospital days (for patients of all ages). The medical costs of the care of children with birth defects are in excess of $13 billion annually in the United States. Currently, the overwhelming majority of birth defects are not preventable. Only a small fraction of birth defects are known to occur as a result of avoidable causes. Some toxic developmental influences include: uncontrolled maternal diseases (e.g., diabetes mellitus and phenylketonuria); infections (including rubella); and, to a lesser extent, environmental exposures (drugs, chemicals, radiation).

To be considered a teratogen, an agent must have little effect on the mother, since the presence of maternal toxicity precludes ascribing effects on the conceptus directly to the agent. The substance must cause transient or permanent, physical, or functional disorders in the fetus in the absence of toxic effects in the mother.

Not all adverse effects on prenatal development are malforming. Some agents result in death of the developing organism, whereas others produce only mild growth retardation. Death and growth retardation are not considered as teratogenic events per se. The term *developmental toxicity* is proposed as a broader categorization of outcomes. Developmental toxicity comprises four possible manifestations of abnormal development: altered growth (growth retardation), death, malformations (terata), and functional deficits or impairments.

The concept of a behavioral teratogen is described as an agent that disrupts normal behavioral development after prenatal exposure. Because some agents clearly produce mental but not physical disturbances, it is a useful subdivision of the concept of teratogens.

Mutagens are substances that cause permanent change in germ cell lines secondary to changes in deoxyribonucleic acid (DNA). All mutagens are teratogens, but not all teratogens are mutagens.

By examining known teratogens and the factors common to their production of malformations, seven general factors on the development of teratogenesis can be described (see box).

Vitamin A and its congeners are examples of how these principles can be applied to specific agents, as well as their shortcomings in characterizing all teratogens. Vitamin A is recognized as a teratogen in animals since 1953. Dietary vitamin A as carotene

FACTORS IN DEVELOPMENT OF TERATOGENESIS

The conceptus passes through an orderly succession of developmental stages. Each stage represents a different susceptibility to teratogens.

Pharmacokinetic characteristics of: absorption, disposition, biotransformation, and elimination influence the ultimate amount of teratogen to reach the embryo/fetus.

The higher the dose the more likely an adverse effect will be seen and the more severe it is likely to be. A threshold dose may exist below which defects are absent and above which defects are demonstrable.

Teratogenesis depends on the genotype of the conceptus and the manner in which it reacts with environmental factors.

The same defect may be produced by agents acting via different mechanisms. Conversely, one agent may produce different developmental toxicities by the same initiating mechanism.

Certain agents produce developmental toxicity; other substances are associated with developmental toxicity only at doses high enough to cause signs and symptoms of toxicity in the mother.

The type of response is determined by the individual characteristics of the exposure, particularly dosage and timing, and the organism's susceptibility to it.

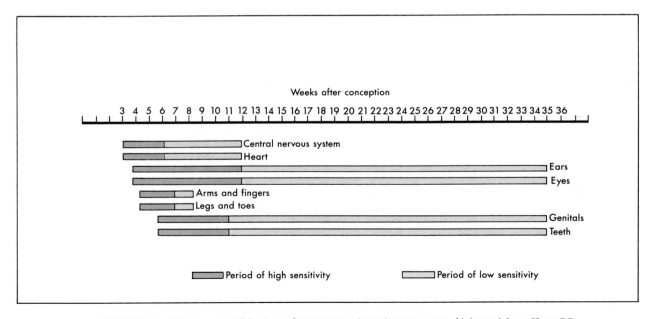

FIGURE 63-2   Most susceptible times for teratogenic actions to occur. (Adapted from Hays DP and Pagliaro LA: Human teratogens. In Pagliaro LA and Pagliaro AM, eds: Problems in pediatric drug therapy, Hamilton, Ill, 1987, Drug Intelligence Publications.)

(beta-carotene) is not associated with developmental toxicity in animals or humans. However, high-potency vitamin A prepared as retinol or retinyl esters is implicated as an animal teratogen, at dosages of 15 to 75 mg/kg/day and higher, producing cranial, brain, cardiovascular, limb, and/or genitourinary malformations. Human malformations are associated with daily doses of 25,000 international units of vitamin A or more, but no epidemiological studies are available to quantify the risk to humans. Isotretinoin, an agent used for the treatment of cystic acne, is an isomer of retinoic acid that may produce craniofacial, cardiac, thymic, and CNS abnormalities in humans. Etretinate, a vitamin A congener used in the treatment of psoriasis, is also a documented animal teratogen with similar potential in humans.

Direct teratogenic effects depend on the achievement of drug or active metabolite concentrations in the conceptus at a critical time period, especially during gestation weeks 3 to 12 (Figure 63-2). Thus the changes in maternal pharmacokinetic parameters and dosing requirements during pregnancy may be expected to influence the risk of malformations.

By recognizing and compensating for controllable variables, the dose-response relationships for individual anomalies or toxic effects may become clear. Because few agents appear to demonstrate a minimum teratogenic concentration for production of defects, it is a difficult task to determine the concentration at which a specific drug is safe in humans.

NEONATAL PHARMACOLOGY

Basic pharmacological principles (Chapters 1 thru 7) apply to neonates, as well as to children and adults. Only those processes that differ in the fetus, perinate, or neonate are discussed in this section.

Drug Absorption

At birth, gastric pH is usually between 6 and 8, but falls rapidly to 1.5 to 3.0 within several hours; however, this fall is variable and appears independent of birth weight and gestational age. In the premature infant, hydrochloric acid is rarely present before 32 weeks of gestational age, and the time course of acid production may be related to the initiations of enteral feedings.

The rate of gastric emptying is an important determinant of the overall rate and extent of drug absorption. The rate of gastric emptying is variable during the neonatal period and is affected by gestational maturity, postnatal age, and type of feeding. In addition, neonatal conditions of gastroesophageal reflux, respiratory distress syndrome, and congenital heart disease delay gastric emptying.

The ontogeny of bile salt formation and the colonization of bacterial flora in the GI tract may be a determinant in the absorption of drugs and nutrients. The absorption of some drugs may be affected by disease states in neonates (see box).

Chemical agents applied to the skin of a premature infant may result in inadvertent poisoning. For example, drug toxicities in neonates are reported for percutaneous absorption of such agents as hexachlorophene, pentachlorophenol-containing laundry detergents, hydrocortisone, and aniline-containing disinfectant solutions. Extreme caution should be exercised in using topical therapy on newborn infants.

Drug Distribution

The affinity of albumin for acidic drugs and total plasma protein concentration increases from birth into early infancy. These do not reach normal adult values until 10 to 12 months of age. In addition, although plasma albumin concentrations may reach

---

DISEASE STATES THAT MAY AFFECT DRUG ABSORPTION IN THE FIRST YEAR OF LIFE

Gastric acid secretion
  Proximal small bowel resection
Delayed gastric emptying and modified drug absorption
  Pyloric stenosis
  Congestive heart failure
  Protein calorie malnutrition
Intestinal transit time
  Protein calorie malnutrition
  Thyroid disease
  Diarrheal disease
Reduced bile salt excretion
  Cholestatic liver disease
  Extrahepatic biliary obstruction
Decreased GI surface area for drug absorption
  Short bowel syndrome
  Protein calorie malnutrition

adult values shortly after birth, the concentration of albumin in blood is directly proportional to gestational age, reflecting placental transport and fetal synthesis.

Different degrees of drug-protein binding may be observed between newborns and adults. The following four mechanisms are proposed to explain the differences in the protein binding of drugs between newborns and adults:

1. Displacement of drugs from binding sites by bilirubin in cord plasma
2. Different binding properties of cord and adult albumin
3. Different binding properties of globulins
4. Decreased binding properties of albumin as a result of interaction with globulins in newborns

Basic drugs bind to plasma α_1-acid glycoprotein. A three-fold reduction in plasma α_1-acid glycoprotein concentration exists in healthy term neonates compared to maternal plasma. When the α_1-acid glycoprotein concentration in cord blood becomes increased to adult values, the protein binding of lidocaine and propranolol approaches adult values, implicating the reduced plasma concentration of α_1-acid glycoprotein as the reason for the decreased protein binding.

Bilirubin noncovalently binds to albumin, and this association is reversible. The bilirubin-binding affinity of albumin at birth is independent of gestational age and is less for the newborn compared to the adult. The binding affinity of albumin for bilirubin increases with age and reaches that of adult serum by approximately 5 months of age. The lower bilirubin-binding affinity of albumin in neonates is believed to be a contributing factor in their susceptibility to kernicterus. Other factors such as the effect of hypothermia, acidosis, hypoglycemia, hypoxia, sepsis, birth asphyxia, and hypercapnea on the permeability of the blood-brain barrier and on bilirubin-albumin binding, must also be considered.

In summary, there appears to be a reduction in binding of drugs to plasma proteins during the neonatal period.

Drug Metabolism

The first step in drug metabolism is uptake of drug by the metabolizing cell. Ligandin, or Y protein, is a basic protein that binds bilirubin and organic anions, including some drugs. It is present in hepatocytes, as well as in proximal renal tubular cells and non-goblet, small intestinal mucosal cells. The concentration of ligandin in the fetus and newborn is low but appears to mature during the first 5 to 10 days of postnatal life. Thus it is likely that the hepatic clearance of capacity limited drugs is lower in neonates than in older infants and children.

During fetal life, drug metabolizing enzymes are present at 30% to 50% of adult activity in vitro. However, after correcting for differences in liver weight, the specific activity in vitro for many drug-metabolizing enzymes approaches adult activities. The appearance of these enzymes correlates with the development of rough endoplasmic reticulum and suggests that these enzyme systems increase in activity when smooth endoplasmic reticulum develops. The increase in monooxygenase activity observed in the first trimester plateaus during the second trimester.

Postnatally, the hepatic cytochrome P-450 monooxygenase system appears to mature rapidly. Phenytoin and its metabolites appear in the urine of newborns and adults in similar proportions. Furthermore, the decline in serum drug concentration parallels the rate of urinary metabolite excretion, suggesting that the rate of excretion reflects the rate of hepatic metabolism of phenytoin.

Glucuronide conjugations require the coordinated activity of UDP-glucose dehydrogenase and UDP-glucuronyl transferase. The first enzyme is present at 25% of adult activity in fetal liver at 8 to 18 weeks gestation, and the second enzyme is barely detectable by 20 weeks gestation. As a result, at birth, compounds that rely on glucuronidation for elimination have markedly prolonged half-lives or are conjugated via different pathways compared to children and adults.

Conjugation with glycine appears to occur as rapidly in fetal liver as in adult; whereas certain methylation reactions, which do not occur in adults, appear to be functional in the fetus and newborn. Theophyline is methylated to form caffeine in fetal livers that are 12 to 20 weeks old. Caffeine, discussed below, has therapeutic implications in the treatment of apnea of prematurity.

Renal Drug Elimination

Renal blood flow increases with age as a result of increased cardiac output and reduced peripheral vascular resistance. Kidneys in newborn infants receive only 5% to 6% of cardiac output compared to 15% to 25% for adults. Renal blood flow averages 12 ml/min at birth, increasing to 140 ml/min by 1 year of age, and, when based on body surface area, reaches adult values before 30 weeks of extrauterine age. Renal blood flow appears to increase in proportion to the development of the renal tubules.

At birth, the glomerular filtration rate (GFR) is directly proportional to gestational age. This linear relationship is not evident before 34 weeks gestation. In contrast, GFR, as measured by creatinine or inulin clearance, remains relatively constant at low rates of 1 ml/min before 34 weeks gestation. The reason for this is not clear but may relate to the ontogeny and functional organization of the glomerulus. The GFR for full-term infants at birth ranges from 2 to 4 ml/min. In the first 2 to 3 days of postnatal life, there is a marked increase in the GFR of full-term babies to 8 to 20 ml/min compared to increases in neonates less than 34 weeks gestation to 2 to 3 ml/min. The increase in GFR after birth is dependent on postconceptual age and not postnatal age. Adult values for GFR are reached by 2½ to 5 months of age. An example of the clinical implications of the maturation of GFR is the decreasing half-life for gentamicin with increasing gestational age in infants less than 7 days of age. Gentamicin is eliminated almost entirely by glomerular filtration (Chapter 45).

Proximal convoluted tubules in the normal kidney of a full-term infant are small in relation to their corresponding glomeruli. This glomerulotubular imbalance in size is reflected by functional differences in the secretory capacity of the proximal tubular cells. A tenfold increase in para-aminohippuric acid secretion (Chapter 5) occurs in the first year of life, with adult values (based on body surface area) attained by 30 weeks of age. Therefore tubular drug secretion matures at a slower rate than glomerular drug filtration function.

Penicillins, which undergo renal elimination, show high variability in elimination half-life in infants, but the range generally decreases to 1 to 2 hours by 2 weeks postnatal age. The capacity of the secretory pathways responsible for penicillin elimination appear to undergo substrate stimulation in animals, and such a process may also exist in humans. A reduction in elimination half-life for ampicillin in preterm and term infants occurs after multiple doses compared to single dose administration.

Clinical Factors

As a result of the often compromised cardiac output and peripheral perfusion of seriously ill infants,

IV drug administration is generally used to assure adequate systemic availability. Problems can be serious and include dilution and timed administration of small dosage volumes, maintenance of fluid balance, and the effect of the specific drug administration technique on resultant serum concentrations. In addition, mistiming of peak or trough serum drug determinations can result in clinical decisions to inappropriately adjust dosing regimens that result in increased risk of drug toxicity or of ineffective concentrations.

Certain drugs pose unusual therapeutic challenges when used in neonates or during the perinatal period because of the unique character of their distribution and/or elimination in these patients or because of the unusual side effects they may cause. These drugs include the antibiotics, digoxin, methylxanthines, and indomethacin.

Antibiotics Antibiotics are commonly used drugs in infants and newborns. Bacterial sepsis, pneumonia, necrotizing enterocolitis, and meningitis, as primary or secondary diseases, are frequent infections in these patients and are effectively treated with β-lactams, aminoglycosides, and glycopeptides. Because these drugs are primarily eliminated from the body unchanged via the kidneys, the renal function of the patient is an important variable in establishing doses and dosage intervals.

Another type of antibiotic, chloramphenicol (Chapter 45), is associated with the "gray baby" and "gray toddler" syndromes of drug-induced toxicities that are a direct result of excessively high and prolonged chloramphenicol serum concentrations (usually above 50 to 75 mg/L). These substantially elevated serum chloramphenicol concentrations usually arise from doses >75 mg/kg/day combined with an immature capacity for conjugation by the newborn liver.

Digoxin Digoxin is a commonly used cardiac glycoside in the treatment of myocardial disturbances in neonates, infants, and children. Extensive clinical experience shows that available data describing digoxin biodisposition in neonates and infants requires cautious interpretation. This caution is based on recent identification of a digoxin-like immunoreactive substance in the serum of human neonates who had no recorded exposure to digoxin in utero or after birth.

Methylxanthines The methylxanthine, theophylline, remains a frequently used bronchodilating drug in the United States. During the neonatal period, theophylline is used in the treatment of apnea of prematurity. However, the efficacy of theophylline in this syndrome may be related to the additive or synergistic action of caffeine, a metabolite of theophylline, which accumulates in the serum of infants receiving theophylline. The N-methylation of theophylline to caffeine does not appear totally unique to preterm

---

XENOBIOTIC EXPOSURES THAT MAY CONTRAINDICATE BREAST FEEDING

DRUGS THOUGHT TO HAVE A TOXIC EFFECT ON THE INFANT

antimetabolites: amethopterin, cyclophosphamide, doxorubicin, methotrexate
gold salts
cyclosporin
iodides
lithium
metronidazole
nalidixic acid
nitrofurantoin
radiopharmaceuticals
sulfonamides (in the first month of life)

DRUGS FOR WHICH SAFER ALTERNATIVES ARE AVAILABLE

bromides   indomethacin
chloramphenicol   methimazole
cimetidine   phenindione
clemastine   thiouracil

AGENTS FOR WHICH MILK SHOULD BE TESTED IF EXPOSURE OCCURS (infant effects not well known)

lead
mercury; methylmercury
pesticides
polyhalogenated hydrocarbons
strontium isotopes
tetrachloroethanol

DRUGS OF ABUSE

alcohol   heroin
amphetamines   marijuana
caffeine   nicotine
cocaine   phencyclidine
ergot alkaloids

DRUGS THAT MAY INTERFERE WITH LACTATION

bromocriptine
phenelzine

---

and newborn infants but is clinically important because of its prolonged elimination half-life. Caffeine is rarely detectable in the serum of older infants, children, or adults receiving theophylline alone.

The pharmacokinetics of theophylline in neonates are markedly different from those for older infants, children, and adults. These differences are likely due to different body water compartmentalization and decreased plasma protein binding of theophylline in neonates (averages 36% in neonates and 56% in adults). Although neonates can methylate theophylline, it is excreted largely unchanged in newborn urine as compared to only ~10% as unchanged drug in older children and adults.

Indomethacin The use of indomethacin in neonates to stimulate ductus arteriosus closure is associated with potentially serious drug-induced complications and thus is not without risk.

ENVIRONMENTAL AND THERAPEUTIC EXPOSURE IN THE NURSING MOTHER

A considerable number of agents are transferred from mother to neonate by breast milk, and the agents, some of which are listed in the box, should be avoided.

REFERENCES

Hays DP and Pagliaro LA: Human teratogens. In Pagliaro LA and Pagliaro AM, eds: Problems in pediatric drug therapy, Hamilton, Ill, 1987, Drug Intelligence Publications.

Johnson EM and Kochhar DM: Teratogenesis and reproductive toxicology in handbook of experimental pharmacology, vol 65, New York, 1983, Springer-Verlag.

Koren G: Maternal-fetal toxicology: a clinician's guide, New York, 1990, Marcel Dekker, Inc.

MacLeod SM and Radde IC: Textbook of pediatric clinical pharmacology, Littleton, Mass, 1985, PSG Publishing Co, Inc.

Mirkin BL: Pharmacodynamics and drug disposition in pregnant women, in neonates, and in children. In Melmon ML and Morrelli HF, eds: Clinical pharmacology: basic principles in therapeutics, ed 2, New York, 1978, MacMillan Publishing Co.

Roberts RJ: Drug therapy in infants: pharmacologic principles and clinical experience, Philadelphia, 1984, WB Saunders Co.

Yaffe SJ: Pediatric pharmacology: therapeutic principles in practice, New York, 1980, Grune and Stratton.

64

Gerontological Pharmacology

The rational use of drugs by the elderly is challenging to patient and physician. Decline in physiological functions as part of the normal aging process can lead to altered drug disposition and sensitivity to drug effects (see box). Increased chronic illness, multiple diseases, hospitalization, and long-term institutionalization contribute to increased drug usage and, in turn, more adverse reactions in the elderly than in younger people. In addition, inadequate nutrition, decreased financial resources, or poor compliance for various reasons may contribute to inadequate drug therapy.

Decisions about drug selection and dosage in the elderly are largely based on trial and error, anecdotal data, and clinical impression. Sound information on drug disposition and tissue or cellular responses to drugs in the elderly has been obtained only recently.

The objectives of this chapter are (1) to relate the normal physiological changes of aging to alterations in drug pharmacokinetics and to tissue or cellular responses and (2) to describe the geriatric pharmacology of some commonly used drugs.

PHYSIOLOGICAL CHANGES AND AGING

Several physiological functions in the human body decline linearly, beginning between 30 and 45 years of age, and have important influences on pharma-

FACTORS CONTRIBUTING TO ALTERED DRUG EFFECTS
Altered drug disposition and pharmacokinetics
Decreased lean body mass
Increased percentage body fat
Decreased liver mass and blood flow
Reduced renal function
Altered response to drug
Altered receptor and/or postreceptor properties
Impaired sensitivity of homeostatic mechanisms
Common diseases: glaucoma, diabetes, arthritis, hypertension, coronary artery disease, cancer
Social and economic factors
Inadequate nutrition
Multiple drug therapy
Noncompliance

cokinetic processes (see box, p. 852). For example, cardiac output decreases about 1% a year beginning at age 30. In the elderly, this is associated with redistribution of blood flow favoring brain, heart, and kidney and a reduction in hepatic blood flow. The percentage of lean body mass declines with age, such that body fat increases from 18% to 35% in men and from 33% to 48% in women between the ages of 18 and 55 years. Total body water decreases by 10% to 15% between the ages of 20 and 80 years.

Plasma albumin concentrations are lower in the elderly, particularly in the chronically ill or poorly nourished. The concentrations of α_1-acid glycoprotein increase, but more sharply in response to acute illness than simply to aging. Glomerular filtration rate and

PHYSIOLOGICAL CHANGES WITH AGING THAT AFFECT DRUG ABSORPTION, DISTRIBUTION, AND METABOLISM

DRUG ABSORPTION

Physiological Changes	Effect on Drug Absorption
Increased gastric pH	can be ↑ or ↓
Slowed gastric emptying rate	usually ↓
Reduced splanchnic flow	↓
Slowed GI motility	can be ↑ or ↓
Thinning and reductions of absorptive surface	↓

DRUG DISTRIBUTION AND METABOLISM

Decline in body weight with advanced age
Decrease in lean body mass
Increase in body fat
Decrease in total body water
Reduction in plasma albumin
Slight and variable reduction in α_1-acid glycoprotein
Redistribution of regional blood flow from liver and kidney
Reduction in hepatic microsomal enzyme activity

effective renal plasma flow decline steadily with advancing age. Note that serum creatinine does not increase as a function of aging as a result of smaller lean body mass. Tubular secretory capacity declines in parallel with glomerular filtration rate.

PHARMACOKINETIC CHANGES ASSOCIATED WITH AGING

Drug Absorption

Several physiological alterations in gastrointestinal (GI) function occur with aging: (1) decreased gastric parietal cell function with (2) a corresponding rise in gastric pH, (3) a slowed rate of gastric emptying, and (4) decreased active transport of glucose, vitamin B_{12}, and other nutrients. The rate and extent of absorption of most drugs are determined by passive diffusion in the proximal small bowel. This likely accounts for the general lack of clinically significant alterations in drug absorption in the elderly. An exception is a threefold increase in the bioavailability of levodopa as a result

of reduced activity of dopa decarboxylase activity in the stomach wall.

Drug Distribution

Reduced lean body mass, reduced total body water, increased fat, and decreased plasma albumin in the elderly can contribute to alterations in drug distribution. The effect of body composition on drug distribution depends largely on the physiochemical properties of individual drugs. Lipid-soluble drugs such as diazepam and lidocaine have a larger volume of distribution in the elderly; water-soluble drugs such as acetaminophen or substances of abuse such as ethyl alcohol have a smaller volume of distribution. Digoxin has a lower volume of distribution in the elderly, and therefore doses of digoxin must be reduced.

There is a slight trend to lower plasma albumin concentrations in the healthy elderly patient, whereas the hospitalized or poorly nourished elderly may have 10% to 20% decreased plasma albumin concentrations. This can result in increased unbound or free concentration of drug, the consequences of which can be complex. There are no guidelines available based on objective data for dosage modification to compensate for decreased protein binding.

Much of the pharmacokinetic data available for elderly patients reports only elimination half-life. Without corresponding measures of volume of distribution (V_d) and clearance, interpretation of half-life changes is not possible, as is clear from the equation (see also Chapter 4):

$$t_{1/2} = \frac{0.693 \times V_d}{\text{Clearance}} \qquad (1)$$

Drug Metabolism

The decline in the ability of the elderly to metabolize most drugs is relatively small but difficult to predict. In general, hydroxylation and N-dealkylation reactions catalyzed by hepatic microsomal mixed-function oxidase enzymes decrease slightly with aging. Conjugation reactions such as glucuronidation are not greatly affected by aging. Effects of change in cigarette smoking, diet, or alcohol consumption may be more important than physiological hepatic changes. For example, decreased dietary protein intake or reduction in cigarette consumption may lead to decreased liver microsomal enzyme activity. Studies in aging animals are not predictive in humans because of marked gender and species differences.

In the elderly, first-pass metabolism may be of clinical importance requiring decreased dosages. Total liver blood flow declines 40% to 45% with aging, partly as a result of reduced cardiac output, and diseases such as congestive heart failure may further compromise hepatic blood flow. Thus as hepatic blood flow declines, clearance of flow-dependent drugs will usually decrease and blood concentrations will rise.

The ability of hepatic mixed-function oxidases to respond to inducers is retained, although there are exceptions. Cigarette smoking and phenytoin induce hepatic theophylline metabolism to a similar degree in young and old. In contrast, the clearance of antipyrine is not increased by cigarette smoking in elderly subjects. The ability of cimetidine to inhibit microsomal drug metabolism is the same in young and old.

In summary, the rate of hepatic metabolism of a drug is not a predictable consequence of well understood alterations in hepatic function. Normal values of liver function tests do not predict normal drug metabolism. Nearly all of the available data is obtained in healthy, not sick, elderly subjects.

Drug Elimination

Consistent with the physiological decline of renal function with normal aging, the rate of elimination of those drugs dependent on the kidney is reduced in the elderly. Such drugs include the aminoglycosides, lithium carbonate, chlorpropamide, and digoxin. To avoid drug toxicity, renal function must be estimated and downward adjustments in dosage made accordingly.

As discussed in Chapter 5, drug clearance is often directly proportional to creatinine clearance whether elimination is by tubular secretion or glomerular filtration. Because of difficulties in obtaining accurate 24-hour urine collections to measure creatinine clearance directly (see Chapter 5, equation 10), it is usually estimated using nomograms or equation 2, which accounts for differences in age and body weight.

$$(CL)_{Cr} = \frac{[140 - age]\,[weight]}{[72]\,[S_{Cr}]} \qquad (2)$$

where $(CL)_{Cr}$ is creatinine clearance in ml/min, age is in years, weight in kg, and S_{Cr} is serum creatinine in mg/dl. The formula is multiplied by 85% for females. Interpretation of serum creatinine concentration in the elderly requires caution. Because creati-

nine is a product of muscle metabolism, less is produced as lean body mass declines. Thus an 80-year-old man with a serum creatinine concentration of 1 mg/dL may have a creatinine clearance of 60 ml/min, only one half that of a 40-year-old man with the same serum creatinine.

There are no absolute guidelines, but two general principles apply. First, most elderly patients do not have "normal" renal function when serum creatinine appears "normal." Second, most elderly patients require dosage adjustments for drugs that are eliminated primarily by the kidneys.

The decreased rate of elimination of inhalation anesthetics resulting from declining pulmonary function with aging is an important consideration regarding general anesthesia in the elderly.

DRUG RESPONSE CHANGES ASSOCIATED WITH AGING

Changes in drug responses in the elderly have received less study than have pharmacokinetic changes (see box). This is based on the relative difficulty of direct assessment of target organ responses. Nevertheless, clearly, drug responses are altered with aging. In general, an enhanced response can be expected (Table 64-1), although reduced responses occur to some drugs such as the β-adrenergic agonist isoproterenol, and a reduced dosage schedule is recommended to prevent serious side effects (Table 64-2).

Table 64-1   Altered Drug Responses in the Elderly

Drugs	Direction of Change
barbiturates	Increased
benzodiazepines	Increased
chlordiazepoxide	
diazepam	
flurazepam	
morphine	Increased
pentazocine	Increased
anticoagulants	Increased
warfarin	
heparin	
isoproterenol	Decreased
tolbutamide	Decreased

Table 64-2 Drugs Given in Reduced Dosage in the Elderly

Drug	Possible Effects of Usual Dosage
aminoglycosides	Nephrotoxicity and ototoxicity
carbamazepine	Drowsiness, ataxia
cimetidine	Confusion
digoxin	Toxicity more likely
levodopa	Hypotension
meperidine	Respiratory depression
metaclopramide	Confusion
thioridazine	Confusion
thyroxine	Myocardial infarction
vitamin D	Renal toxicity

Modified from the Report of the WHO Technical Group on the Use of Medicaments in the Elderly, World Health Organization, 1981.

Factors that affect the sensitivity or intensity of responses at target organs include the following:

1. Age-related changes in receptors and other postreceptor molecular mechanisms
2. Age-related changes in homeostatic control
3. Disease-induced changes
4. Drug-drug and drug-nutrient interactions

Age-related Changes in Receptors and Postreceptor Mechanisms

Age-related changes may occur at receptor and postreceptor levels. In general, there is little evidence for specific alterations causing altered sensitivity or intensity in responses. Possible mechanisms include the following:

1. Changes in receptor density or affinity
2. Altered second messenger (cAMP or cGMP) activity
3. Alteration in a biochemical response such as glycogenolysis
4. A mechanical effect such as vascular relaxation

The β-adrenergic system of the heart has been extensively studied. The sensitivity of the heart is decreased with aging in elderly subjects. For example, a higher dose of isoproterenol is required in the elderly to cause a 25 beat per minute increase in heart rate. This reduced sensitivity to isoproterenol is not caused by alterations in β-receptors but to changes in the cAMP system or in other postreceptor events proximal to calcium-troponin interaction.

The magnitude of the increased responses to benzodiazepines, diazepam, flurazepam, and nitrazepam in the elderly cannot be totally explained by pharmacokinetic differences. The occurrence of flurazepam induced adverse effects increases dramatically with aging.

Impaired Homeostatic Mechanisms

With advancing age, a number of critical physiological control mechanisms become increasingly inefficient. These include decreased activity of aortic and carotid body chemoreceptors, reduced baroreceptor reflexes, impaired thermoregulation, inappropriate response of blood glucose and insulin to an oral glucose load, and altered neurological control of bowel and bladder. Drug toxicity may therefore result.

Decreased baroreflex sensitivity may lead to increased risk of postural or orthostatic hypotension. In the elderly, this is a common problem with some phenothiazines and antidepressants (those with significant α_1-adrenergic antagonist properties), nitrates, and antihypertensives such as prazosin and α-methyldopa.

The normal homeostatic response of the aortic and carotid body chemoreceptors to morphine-induced respiratory depression is to increase respiratory stimulation. Impaired chemoreceptor activity may lead to greater than expected respiratory depressant effects of morphine.

Multiple mechanisms are implicated in the impaired patient. Thermoregulation may be seen in a significant number of elderly individuals and includes absence of shivering, failure of metabolic rate to rise, poor vasoconstriction, and insensitivity to a low body temperature. Chlorpromazine and many other psychoactive drugs may cause hypothermia. Alcohol tends to augment this effect.

Disease-Induced Changes

Multiple chronic diseases are common in the elderly. One third have three or more chronic diseases such as diabetes, glaucoma, hypertension, coronary artery disease, and arthritis. Multiple diseases may lead to multiple medications, an increased frequency of drug-drug interactions, and adverse drug reactions. Moreover, a disease may increase the risk of adverse drug reactions or preclude the use of the otherwise most effective or safest drug for another problem. For example, anticholinergic drugs (see box) may cause urinary retention in men with enlarged prostate glands or precipitate glaucoma, and drug-induced hypotension may cause ischemic events in persons with vascular disease.

Drug-Drug and Drug-Nutrient Interactions

Multiple drug therapies may lead to confusion, medication errors, and further drug-drug interactions. An often overlooked factor is the common use among the elderly of over-the-counter antacids, laxatives, analgesics, antihistamines, sleeping pills, and vitamins. Inadequate dietary potassium increases the likelihood of diuretic-induced hypokalemia, whereas excessive sodium chloride ingestion may attenuate the effect of an antihypertensive drug. Most drug-nutrient problems, however, are pharmacokinetic in nature.

EXAMPLES OF DRUG PROBLEMS AND PRESCRIBING IN THE ELDERLY

A number of drugs require dosage modifications for use in the elderly. Two examples of problematic drug use in the elderly are described.

Anticholinergic Drug Toxicity

Anticholinergic drug toxicity illustrates some of the inherent problems of drug treatment in the elderly. Some of the large number of drugs with atropine-like activity are listed in the box, above right. For some of those drugs, the anticholinergic response is the desired useful pharmacological effect, but for others, this may be an unwanted side effect. It is often common for elderly patients to concurrently receive several of these atropine-like drugs. Recently, a so-called anticholinergic syndrome (see box, right) has been recognized, particularly in the elderly, in whom the additive effects of these drugs lead to toxicity. Some elderly patients will be more susceptible than others to anticholinergic toxicity caused by impaired autonomic bowel or bladder innervation, glaucoma, benign prostatic hypertrophy, or impaired cognitive capacity. Some elderly patients are especially sensitive to cognitive disruption caused by anticholinergic drugs. Thus in the elderly, great care must be taken to avoid excessive antimuscarinic effects and to be observant for potential toxicity.

DRUGS WITH ANTICHOLINERGIC PROPERTIES

Antipsychotics, thioridazine
Antidepressants; amitryptiline, doxepin
Antidysrhythmics; disopyramide, quinidine
Anti-Parkinson drugs; benztropine, trihexyphenidyl
Antispasmodics; belladonna alkaloids, atropine, propantheline, clidinium
Antihistamines; diphenhydramine, chlorpheniramine
Ophthalmic preparations; tropicamide, cyclopentolate
Proprietary hypnotics, cold preparations

SIGNS AND SYMPTOMS OF ANTICHOLINERGIC SYNDROME

Systemic
  Tachycardia
  Warm, dry, flushed skin
  Decreased secretions
  Decreased bowel motility
  Urinary retention
  Mydriasis, loss of accommodation
  Hyperpyrexia
  Cardiac conduction problems
Neuropsychiatric
  Anxiety
  Agitation
  Confusion
  Delirium
  Increased forgetfulness
  Hallucinations
  Seizures

Benzodiazepine-based Depression

Benzodiazepines are more likely to cause greater CNS depression in elderly than in younger patients. Altered pharmacokinetics and increased tissue sensitivities are involved. Benzodiazepines, such as diazepam, which undergo oxidative hepatic metabolism, show a decline in metabolic clearance but a disproportionately longer plasma half-life and increase in volume of distribution. This is attributed to the relative increase in body fat and small decline in plasma albumin with aging. Oxazepam, lorazepam, and temazepam, which are all metabolized by conjugation, exhibit little alteration in metabolism and clearance with aging. Yet these latter drugs are associated with an increased sensitivity in response. The best evidence for altered tissue sensitivity is that at equal plasma concentrations of diazepam or nitrazepam, greater CNS depression occurs in the elderly. The molecular basis for this altered sensitivity remains unknown, but in the elderly, smaller doses should be employed and drugs with extremely long half-lives should be avoided if possible.

GUIDELINES FOR DRUG PRESCRIBING IN THE ELDERLY

Drug prescribing in the elderly can be safe and effective by adherence to the following principles:
1. Know all of the patient's medical problems
2. Ascertain all drugs being taken, including over-the-counter preparations
3. Know the pharmacology of the drugs
4. Start with small doses and titrate the drug based on response
5. Keep dosage regimens simple
6. Be sure that visual, motor, or cognitive impairments will not result in errors or noncompliance
7. Review treatment plan and response regularly
8. Regularly consider that new symptoms or problems may be drug-induced

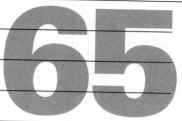

CHAPTER 65 Drugs to Treat Anemia

ABBREVIATIONS

BFU-E	burst erythroid colony forming unit
cAMP	cyclic adenosine monophosphate
CFU-E	erythroid colony forming unit
DHF	dihydrofolate
DOCB	deoxyadenosylcobalamin
Epo	erythropoietin
ESRD	end-stage renal disease
G-CSF	granulocyte–colony stimulating factor
G6PD	glucose 6-phosphate dehydrogenase
IF	intrinsic factor
IL-3	interleukin-3
LDH	lactic dehydrogenase
MCB	methylcobalamin
MCHC	mean corpuscular hemoglobin concentration
M-CSF	macrophage–colony stimulating factor
MCV	mean corpuscular volume
MTHF	methyltetrahydrofolate
PMN	polymorphonuclear neutrophil
RBC	red blood cell
rHuEpo	recombinant human erythropoietin
THF	tetrahydrofolate
TIBC	total iron-binding capacity

THERAPEUTIC OVERVIEW

Agents discussed in this chapter include iron, vitamin B_{12}, folate, and erythropoietin. All are used therapeutically to treat certain types of anemias.

Anemia is defined as a decrease in the number of circulating red blood cells (RBCs). A decrease in RBC production caused by cytoplasmic or nuclear maturation defects, or by an increase in destruction from intrinsic RBC abnormalities or extrinsic mechanisms, results in anemia. Regardless of etiology, clinical signs and symptoms are similar and occur because of reduced oxygen-carrying capacity. Anemias are usually classified according to the appearance of the RBC on microscopic examination.

THERAPEUTIC OVERVIEW

IRON AND IRON SALTS

Used to treat hypochromic, microcytic anemias associated with iron deficiency

VITAMIN B_{12} AND FOLATE

Used to treat megaloblastic anemia

ERYTHROPOIETIN

Used to treat anemia of end-stage renal disease

Anemias associated with cytoplasmic maturation defects exhibit peripheral blood smears that are usually hypochromic and microcytic. This category includes iron deficiency, sideroblastic anemias, thalassemia, and anemia of chronic disease. All are due to abnormal hemoglobin synthesis. Adequate iron, globin, and porphyrin are essential for hemoglobin synthesis. Iron deficiency, which may be caused by inadequate iron ingestion, absorption, or transport or by excessive blood loss, leads to abnormal heme synthesis. Sideroblastic anemia (characterized by cells having a perinuclear ring of iron granules) has multiple etiologies but primarily results from a defect in incorporation of iron into the porphyrin ring. Abnormal globin synthesis occurs in the genetic disease thalassemia. Anemia of chronic disease is caused by inability to transport iron from the body's storage sites to the RBC.

Anemias associated with immature RBC nuclear maturation defects have peripheral blood smears that appear normochromic and macrocytic. This category includes megaloblastic anemias caused by vitamin B_{12} (commonly called *pernicious anemia*) and/or folate deficiency. Both vitamins are essential for DNA synthesis, and a lack of either results in a decrease in DNA as well as protein synthesis.

Anemias from increased destruction (hemolysis) result from RBC abnormalities evolving from genetic defects such as sickle cell anemia, hereditary spherocytosis, and glucose 6-phosphate dehydrogenase (G6PD) deficiency. Other causes of increased destruction occur from external factors such as drug-induced antibodies. Diseases such as septic shock may result in RBC destruction associated with disseminated intravascular coagulation, where the RBC membrane is directly damaged by mechanical forces. The peripheral blood smear in these anemias exhibits spherocytes and fragmented RBCs.

Therapy of anemia must be tailored to the specific cause of the anemia. For example, iron is reserved solely for iron deficiency states and vitamin B_{12} for megaloblastic anemias related to B_{12} deficiency. Recently developed, human recombinant erythropoietin has been useful in diseases where inadequate erythropoietin is present because of renal disease.

MECHANISMS OF ACTION

Iron

Anemia caused by red-cell iron deficiency is treated by iron replacement therapy until hemoglobin concentrations are normal and iron stores have been repleted. Absorption, distribution, elimination, and regulation of body concentrations of iron and management of iron-deficiency anemia are discussed in the following sections.

Vitamin B_{12} and Folic Acid

Vitamin B_{12} and folic acid are both required for normal DNA and protein synthesis. Deficiency of one or the other results in defective nuclear maturation of rapidly and continuously replicating cells in bone marrow, with development of megaloblastic, macrocytic anemia. The roles of B_{12} and folic acid in the normal economy of the cell is illustrated in Figure 65-1. Vitamin B_{12} (cyanocobalamin) exists as two coenzymes,

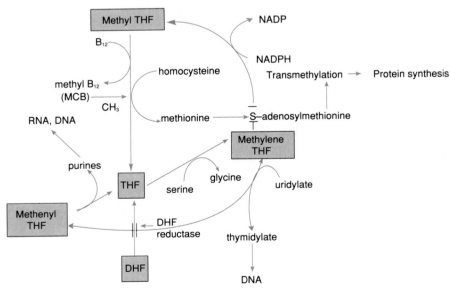

FIGURE 65-1   Folate metabolism; role of B_{12} (see text for explanation).

methylcobalamin (MCB,methyl B_{12}) and deoxyadenosylcobalamin (DOCB,deoxyadenosyl B_{12}). While both coenzymes are important in lipid and carbohydrate metabolism, MCB promotes methionine synthesis by transmethylation from homocysteine, important for normal folate metabolism. Methyl groups contributed by methyltetrahydrofolate (MTHF) form MCB, the latter acting as the methyl donor for the homocysteine-methionine conversion. Methionine is converted to S-adenosylmethionine, important in transmethylation and protein biosynthesis. With either a folic acid or B_{12} deficiency, the cell increases its MTHF pool and maintains methylation reactions at the expense of nucleic acid biosynthesis. A B_{12} deficiency prevents formation of tetrahydrofolate (THF) from MTHF, blocking folate metabolism. The cyanocobalaminfolate system thus plays a key role in synthesis of purines and pyrimidines, necessary constituents of DNA, leading to hematologic dysfunction (i.e., the development of megaloblastic anemia). Management of this type of anemia is achieved by the appropriate use of several preparations of vitamin B_{12} and folic acid.

Erythropoietin

Growth factors have been identified that stimulate proliferation, differentiation, and maturation of the bone marrow pluripotent stem cell to both lymphopoietic and hematopoietic cell lines. (Lymphopoiesis is discussed extensively in Chapter 60.) Several humoral and cellular factors are involved in erythropoiesis, the major one being erythropoietin (Epo). Others that may act synergistically with Epo are granulocyte- and macrophage-colony simulating factors (G-CSF and M-CSF) and interleukin-3 (IL-3).

Epo is a heavily glycosylated 36,000 dalton glycoprotein comprising 166 amino acids. The amino acid sequence of human Epo has been determined, and the gene has been cloned. Four cysteines are present, two joined by a disulfide bond. The polypeptide chain can be digested by trypsin and chymotrypsin to inactive products, and enzymatically deglycosylated Epo is not active in vivo. The carbohydrate moiety of Epo protects it from clearance by liver. Antibody studies have demonstrated that functional activity of Epo resides primarily in the 99-118 and 11-129 amino acid regions of the molecule.

About 90% of Epo is synthesized in renal cortical cells and the remainder in extrarenal sites, primarily

liver. Hypoxia is the stimulus for initiating production/secretion of Epo by kidney and extrarenal tissues. Thus any condition that results in hypoxia (anemia, hypobaria, or ischemia, with a subsequent decrease in renal blood flow) will promote production of Epo. A sequence of events leading from hypoxia to Epo production/secretion has recently been developed (Figure 65-2). The primary sensor of the renal target cell is thought to be the adenosine A_2-receptor. Adenosine production in the kidney is significantly increased early in ischemia. A_2-receptors are coupled to and stimulate a G protein that increases adenylate cyclase, leading to generation of cyclic adenosine monophosphate (cAMP), the activation of protein kinase A, and protein phosphorylation. The phosphoproteins produced may be involved in transcription/translation of the 166 amino acid Epo molecule. Several other stimuli of Epo secretion that may also act through an increase in adenylate cyclase are the prostanoids, (PGE_2, PGI_2, and 6-keto PGE), and H_2O_2 and

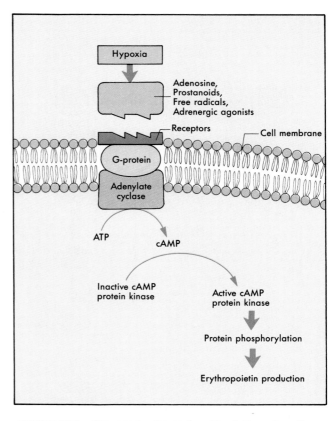

FIGURE 65-2 Proposed scheme for stimulation of erythropoietin production by hypoxia.

superoxide free radicals, generated during hypoxia. Epo production following hypoxia can be blocked by cyclooxygenase inhibitors. β-Adrenergic agonists also apparently promote Epo production/secretion, since β-blocking agents are inhibitory. Agents that increase or decrease Epo production are shown in Table 65-1.

Table 65-1   Agents That Increase or Decrease Epo Production

Increase	Decrease
Thyroxin	Estrogens
Growth hormone	Alkylating agents
Prolactin	Adrenergic β_2-blockers
Serotonin	Calcium channel blockers
Vasopressin	Diacylglycerol
Prostanoids	
Free radicals	
Adenosine A_2 agonists	
Adrenergic β_2 agonists	

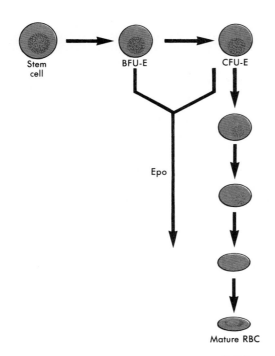

FIGURE 65-3   Stimulation by erythropoietin of RBC production (see text).

In end-stage renal disease (ESRD), there is no physiological mechanism for Epo production, since the kidney cells are largely destroyed. Epo must therefore be provided exogenously. Targets for exogenous Epo in marrow are the early erythroid colony forming unit cell (CFU-E), and the late burst erythroid colony forming unit (BFU-E). Epo expands the BFU-E compartment and stimulates CFU-E proliferation. This promotes a series of proliferation, differentiation, and maturation events from primitive stem cell to reticulocyte (Figure 65-3). Other regulatory glycoprotein factors act synergistically with Epo, including IL-3, G-CSF, and M-CSF. Epo apparently binds to saturable high-affinity sites on the erythroid cell to bring about its effects. Maturity of the progenitor cell determines the degree of differentiation and proliferation produced by Epo.

PHARMACOKINETICS

The pharmacokinetic characteristics of drugs used are shown in Table 65-2.

Iron and Iron Salts

The rate of absorption of iron reflects the total body burden of iron. Two forms of iron are available for absorption: heme and nonheme iron. Heme iron, a minor constituent of the normal diet, is readily absorbed from the gastrointestinal (GI) tract; its absorption is relatively independent of other dietary components. In contrast, nonheme iron accounts for the largest fraction of iron presented to the GI tract but is poorly absorbed and highly dependent on other components in the diet. Ascorbate, for example, facilitates nonheme iron absorption by reducing iron from ferric to the ferrous form. Meat promotes nonheme iron absorption by stimulating production of gastric acid.

Iron in the body exists in two compartments: a functional one as part of hemoglobin and myoglobin and other essential protein structures and the nonfunctional storage form of ferritin. Ferritin is present either as a monomer termed *apoferritin* or as aggregates referred to as *hemosiderin*. Apoferritin has a molecular weight of 450,000 daltons and is made up of 24 polypeptide subunits. Distribution of iron between functional and storage compartments is accomplished by the plasma protein transferrin, a glycoprotein of molecular weight of 76,000 daltons,

Table 65-2 Pharmacokinetic Parameters

Drug	Routes of Administration	Remarks
rHuEpo	IV, SC	SC may be as effective as IV; $t_{1/2}$ is 8 hours
iron	Oral, IM, IV	Oral absorption of ferrous good; ferric poor but enhanced by ascorbate; enteric-coated preparations unreliable
vitamin B_{12}	Oral, SC, IM	Oral route ineffective in malabsorption disease; enterohepatic cycling
folic acid	Oral, IM, IV	Oral absorption good; enterohepatic cycling

which binds ferric iron and controls iron movement to various transferrin binding sites located on cell plasma membranes. The iron-transferrin complex is taken up into the cell by endocytosis. The complexed iron is released intracellularly, and transferrin is extruded and returned to the extracellular compartment. The number of transferrin binding sites and the intracellular ferritin concentration are determined by the total body burden of iron. With adequate iron, fewer transferrin binding sites are synthesized and ferritin increases to promote iron storage. When the iron content is low, more transferrin binding sites are expressed by the cell and ferritin concentrations are reduced to minimize storage and maximize iron absorption. Remarkably, there is very little physiological iron loss; most iron is conserved. In men, loss is about 10% of total iron per year. Menstruating females may lose up to 20%. In pregnancy, higher iron intake is required, as in conditions associated with significant blood loss. Thus iron absorption is the most important factor determining total iron content.

Vitamin B_{12}

Deficiency of this vitamin is generally not dietary in origin. Vitamin B_{12} is available in animal products and in legumes and is readily absorbed from the GI tract with the aid of the intrinsic factor (IF). In pernicious anemia, there is a loss of gastric parietal cell function, resulting in failure to produce the IF, a glycoprotein with a molecular weight of 59,000 daltons, which complexes vitamin B_{12} under acid conditions in the stomach and is important for its absorption. The complex of IF-vitamin B_{12} reaches the ileum where it interacts with an ileal binding site, is absorbed, and enters the circulation. In the circulation, vitamin B_{12} binds to a plasma β-globulin (transcobalamin II) and is transported to tissues including liver,

where it is stored as active coenzyme. About 90% of the body's stores of this vitamin are in hepatic parenchymal cells. Cobalamin is also secreted into bile and reabsorbed from the intestine. Thus enterohepatic cycling plays a key role in maintenance of vitamin B_{12} concentrations. Tissue availability is related to the amount stored and also to the amount bound to transcobalamin II.

Folic Acid

Folates in the diet present as polyglutamates, are hydrolyzed by a carboxypeptidase, reduced by DHF reductase in the small intestine, and methylated to MTHF during GI transport. Once absorbed, MTHF is transported to body tissues. As with vitamin B_{12}, enterohepatic cycling plays an important role in maintaining folate concentrations. Liver reduces and methylates folates and transports the methylated product (MTHF) to the bile, where it is reabsorbed from the intestine.

Erythropoietin

Recombinant human erythropoietin (rHuEpo) is administered either by the IV (during hemodialysis) or SC route. The plasma half-life of IV Epo is approximately 8 hours (ranges from 6 to 10 hours) in hemodialysis patients or in those undergoing continuous ambulatory peritoneal dialysis. Following SC injection of rHuEpo, peak serum concentrations are observed within 8 to 12 hours and maintained for an additional 12 to 16 hours. Whether the SC is as effective as the IV route has not been established. rHuEpo distributes in a single body compartment after IV injection, with a mean apparent volume of distribution of approximately 10 liters in a 70 kg individual. Epo is metabolized primarily by liver.

RELATION OF MECHANISMS OF ACTION TO CLINICAL RESPONSE

Iron Deficiency

Iron deficiency is the most common cause of anemia and results from a negative iron balance in which chronic iron loss exceeds iron intake. Iron requirements depend on the amount of iron lost and the amount needed for growth. In the United States the most common cause of iron deficiency in men and postmenopausal women is GI blood loss. This may be due to the effects of alcohol or aspirin or to GI tract malignancies. GI bleeding is often intermittent and may be difficult to detect. In postmenopausal women, uterine bleeding is an additional common cause. Infants and pregnant women require an increase in iron intake for development; however, routine iron supplementation in these groups has lessened this cause of iron deficiency. In underdeveloped countries, decreased nutritional intake is an important cause. There has been a significant decline in iron deficiency anemia in developed countries, and pathologic blood loss should be pursued in evaluation of most clinical cases.

Specific signs and symptoms of iron deficiency are few and are generally those associated with any chronic anemia, including pallor, fatigue, lightheadedness, and in severe cases, palpitations, dyspnea, and angina pectoris. An interesting specific symptom of iron deficiency anemia is pica, a craving for nonfood substances including ice, clay, and laundry starch.

The most common laboratory manifestation of iron deficiency is a hypochromic and microcytic anemia. Microcytosis is measured by a decrease in mean corpuscular volume (MCV), hypochromia by a reduction in mean corpuscular hemoglobin concentration (MCHC).

Various tests are useful in measuring body iron stores. The most sensitive and specific method is by detection of iron on bone marrow examination. Apart from this invasive procedure, serum ferritin best reflects body iron stores and is the preferred method for determining iron depletion. Patients with chronic inflammatory and liver disease may have disproportionately elevated serum ferritin concentrations. Measurements of total serum iron, total iron-binding capacity (TIBC), and transferrin are additional laboratory procedures for detecting iron deficiency but are diagnostic only after total body iron stores are fully depleted.

Iron deficiency occurs in multiple stages. Initially, storage iron is depleted while serum iron concentration and hemoglobin remains normal. As iron deficiency progresses, there is a decrease in the serum concentration without anemia. With further progression to the most advanced stage, iron deficiency with anemia occurs.

Iron replacement therapy is generally administered orally as ferrous sulfate. In adults, 100 to 150 mg of elemental iron should be provided daily to treat anemia. In infants, 10 to 20 mg of elemental iron may be given prophylactically to prevent iron deficiency. Iron is best absorbed in the fasting state. It should be taken 1 hour before meals and at bedtime to maximize absorption. Adverse GI effects (nausea, heartburn, abdominal cramping, vomiting, diarrhea, and constipation, resulting from effects of unbound iron acting on the stomach and intestine) may require that it be ingested with food. These conditions can reduce iron absorption by 50%. The use of ferrous gluconate, liquid iron, or enteric forms does not always significantly reduce GI effects but should be tried. Because preparations vary in content of elemental iron, dosage adjustments must be made when changing preparations.

After initiation of iron therapy, it is essential to demonstrate an increase in immature RBCs (reticulocytes), which should occur within 7 days. Hemoglobin and ferritin concentrations should begin to increase within the first month of therapy. Iron should be continued for 6 months after correction of anemia to ensure that total body iron stores are repleted.

Parenteral iron should be used with caution and reserved for those patients with well-documented iron deficiency anemia, unable to absorb iron because of a pathological disorder of the small intestine, or unable to tolerate oral iron.

Megaloblastic Anemias

Both folate deficiency and vitamin B_{12} deficiency cause megaloblastic anemia. This anemia, which results in abnormal nuclear maturation of immature stem cells, is also observed with drugs such as DHF reductase inhibitors, antimetabolites, inhibitors of deoxynucleotide synthesis, anticonvulsants, and oral contraceptives.

Folate deficiency may be caused by inadequate nutritional intake, malabsorption, or an increase in folate requirement. Dietary sources of folate are critical because folate storage is limited in the body.

Inadequate nutritional intake, which is often associated with alcoholism, is the most common cause of this deficiency. Alcohol may also affect the enterohepatic cycling of the vitamin, leading to a decrease in absorption. Increased requirements for folate occur during pregnancy and in patients with acute or chronic hemolysis. Patients with sickle cell anemia and thalassemia have rapid RBC turnover and require folate supplementation to their normal diet. Occasionally, folate deficiency may occur from malabsorption associated with diseases of the small intestine, including nontropical and tropical sprue. Deficiency also may occur concurrent with vitamin B_{12} deficiency.

Many clinical features that occur in folate deficiency are also found with vitamin B_{12} deficiency. These include the nonspecific signs and symptoms of anemia. In addition, patients with folate deficiency may have diarrhea, anorexia, and sore tongue and may exhibit irritability and forgetfulness. Physical findings associated with severe deficiency include jaundice from ineffective hematopoiesis, petechiae from thrombocytopenia, glossitis, fever, splenomegaly, weight loss, and impaired mentation.

The most common laboratory manifestation of folate deficiency is megaloblastic anemia. The peripheral blood smear shows macrocytic RBCs and hypersegmented polymorphonuclear neutrophils (PMNs). The blood cell count will reveal an increased MCV. Additionally, thrombocytopenia and neutropenia may be present. If a bone marrow examination is performed, a hypercellular marrow is seen with abnormal nuclear maturation occurring in all cell lines. Low serum folate concentration is an early indicator of folate deficiency; however, serum folate concentrations reflect recent folate intake and may be low due to recent inadequate intake. Similarly, the concentration may appear normal when recent intake has improved, but tissue folate concentrations remain depressed. A better indicator of tissue folate status is the RBC folate concentration, which remains constant during the life span of the RBC and reflects folate turnover during the preceding 2 to 3 months. Decreased RBC folate concentrations may also be observed in vitamin B_{12} deficiency. Other findings that may be abnormal include elevated serum lactic dehydrogenase (LDH), serum bilirubin, and urine formiminoglutamate concentrations.

Before folate deficiency can be treated, it is important to exclude vitamin B_{12} deficiency, since folate therapy will correct the hematological abnormalities associated with vitamin B_{12} deficiency without correcting the vitamin B_{12}-related neurological abnormalities. Folate may be given orally or IV. For mild cases of folate deficiency or prophylaxis, the oral route is preferred. In more severe cases, such as in problems of malabsorption, intravenous folate should be given. The folate preparation is given until the deficiency is corrected and blood counts are normal. A rapid increase in reticulocytes normally occurs during the first week. The hematocrit should return to normal in 1 to 2 months.

Vitamin B_{12} Deficiency

Vitamin B_{12} (cobalamin) deficiency most commonly results from intestinal malabsorption. This is unlike folate deficiency, which results from poor nutritional intake and rarely from intestinal problems. Other etiologies of vitamin B_{12} deficiency include gastrectomy, which removes the source of IF, and Zollinger-Ellison syndrome, a gastrin-producing tumor that increases gastric and duodenal acid and prevents transfer of cobalamin to IF. Intestinal disorders such as extensive resection of the ileum, regional ileitis, and sprue lead to malabsorption of IF-vitamin B_{12} complex. Other causes include malabsorption due to pancreatic disease; fish tapeworm infestation in which the worm competes with the host for ingested cobalamin; and blind loop syndrome resulting from intestinal stasis, which leads to bacterial overgrowth and bacterial utilization of cobalamin before it can be absorbed in the intestine.

Many clinical features of vitamin B_{12} deficiency are similar to those found with folate, including nonspecific symptoms such as constipation, anorexia, and fainting. Unlike folate deficiency, vitamin B_{12} deficiency results in neurological disease. Signs and symptoms include paresthesias in distal extremities, disturbances in vibratory and position sense, and memory loss. If vitamin B_{12} deficiency progresses, a spastic ataxia, called *subacute combined system disease*, may occur. This disorder is caused by degenerative changes in dorsolateral columns of the spinal cord, manifested by nerve fiber demyelination.

The findings in the peripheral smear and bone marrow examination in vitamin B_{12} deficiency are indistinguishable from those in folate deficiency. Serum B_{12} concentrations are usually low but may be normal in 10% to 20% of deficient patients. The presence of increases in urinary methylmalonic acid is the most reliable evidence for vitamin B_{12} deficiency.

Schilling's test (a radiolabeled cobalt isotope test) can be performed to determine the cause of vitamin B_{12} deficiency.

In mild cases of megaloblastic anemia the underlying vitamin B_{12} deficiency should be demonstrated before instituting therapy. Since the cause of deficiency is usually malabsorption, the preferred route of administration of vitamin B_{12} is IM. In the majority of cases, maintenance therapy with monthly injections of vitamin B_{12} must be given for life.

Shortly after therapy is begun, the changes in bone marrow revert to normal morphology. Reticulocytosis begins within the first week of instituting therapy and peaks around day 7. Hypersegmented PMNs will also disappear from the circulation in the first week of therapy.

Erythropoietin

Epo is the most important growth factor responsible for the proliferation and further differentiation of the early erythroid colony forming units, and it is also instrumental in the release of reticuloctyes from the bone marrow. Recently, human Epo gene has been cloned. Due to recombinant techniques, large amounts of human Epo have been made available for therapeutic use. Initial clinical trials with rHuEpo in patients with ESRD anemia have shown an excellent response, and it has been recently licensed by the FDA for this use. Over 2000 patients have been treated since the clinical trials began in 1985, and all have shown increases in their hematocrits to a target range of 33% to 38%. Some patients have been treated for 3 years without any decrease in response or generation of an antibody to Epo. Recombinant human Epo has been recommended for patients with ESRD and a hematocrit less than 30%. The recommended starting dose is 150 U/kg IV given 3 times a week until the hematocrit reaches 30% without blood transfusions. The dose may then be reduced and adjusted to maintain the hematocrit in the target range. Increasing the hematocrit too rapidly in these patients, who have adjusted their blood volume to the chronic anemia, may result in hypertension. Patients with ESRD are especially vulnerable because they cannot regulate blood volume. Decreasing the dose may eliminate this side effect.

Other uses for rHuEpo have been studied. Although not presently licensed for these uses, rHuEpo has been found to be effective in treatment of anemias associated with rheumatoid arthritis and may be useful in the treatment of anemia of malignancy in bone marrow failure, or after the use of chemotherapy. Additional use may be in patients with acquired immunodeficiency syndrome (AIDS) treated with zidovudine and in patients undergoing preoperative autologous blood collection.

SIDE EFFECTS, CLINICAL PROBLEMS, AND TOXICITY

Iron and Iron Salts

Iron overdose most often occurs in children ingesting iron-containing products. There are four distinct phases that classically occur following the ingestion of greater than 20 mg per kg of elemental iron. Initially, vomiting and hemorrhagic gastritis are seen. Hypotension and lethargy develop early in severe intoxication. A quiescent period of up to 12 hours follows, during which deceptive improvement occurs. Life-threatening signs, including coma, seizures, cardiovascular collapse, pulmonary edema, hypoglycemia, and metabolic acidosis, predominate 12 to 24 hours after ingestion. Gastric scarring and pyloric stenosis appear in the late phase, at 1 month. The ingestion of 200 to 300 mg per kg is lethal.

Patients with serum iron concentrations greater than TIBC are at highest risk for serious toxicity. Treatment includes gastric lavage with sodium bicarbonate to treat the acidosis and chelation therapy parenterally with deferoxamine. Intravenous iron administration has been associated with life-threatening anaphylaxis and hypersensitivity reactions, which may occur in up to 10% of patients.

Vitamin B_{12}

Adverse effects of vitamin B_{12} therapy are rare. Transient hypokalemia from a massive increase in its use for cell production may occur when correcting severe deficiencies.

Folic Acid

Folate therapy should be restricted to replacement and prophylaxis of deficient states. Adverse effects of

CLINICAL PROBLEMS

IRON AND IRON SALTS

GI irritation, vomiting; overdose in children can be life threatening

VITAMIN B$_{12}$

Transient hypokalemia

ERYTHROPOIETIN

Hypertension; clotting; very expensive

TRADENAMES

In addition to generic and fixed combination preparations, the following tradenamed materials are available in the United States.

ERYTHROPOIETIN

Epogen, Eprex; rHuEpo, epoetin alfa

ORAL IRON AND IRON SALTS

Feosol, ferrous sulfate
Fergon, ferrous gluconate

PARENTERAL IRON

Imferon, iron dextran injection

VITAMIN B$_{12}$

Many oral preparations, combined with other vitamins
Redisol, cyanocobalamin injection

FOLIC ACID

Folvite, oral or parenteral use

IRON ANTIDOTE

Desferal, deferoxamine

folate are uncommon. A rare reaction to parenteral preparation has been noted. In large doses, folate has been reported to interfere with anticonvulsant therapy.

Erythropoietin

ESRD patients receiving rHuEpo should be monitored closely. Weekly hematocrits should be obtained until the target hematocrit is reached. Because iron deficiency is a common cause of anemia of ESRD and is a common adverse effect of rHuEpo therapy, serum iron, TIBC, and serum ferritin concentrations should be measured monthly to assess iron stores, and iron therapy should be instituted as needed. Approximately 50% of patients treated with rHuEpo will require supplemental iron therapy. Blood pressures and serum chemistries should be monitored monthly. If blood pressure cannot be controlled by medication or dialysis ultrafiltration, the rHuEpo may need to be discontinued until the blood pressure is within reasonable limits. In a European clinical trial, an increase in blood clotting in hollow-fiber dialyzers was also noted in some patients treated with rHuEpo. This may be secondary to an increased blood viscosity occuring with an increase in red cell mass or because of an increase in platelet count occuring with therapy. Minor adjustments in the heparin dose used during dialysis easily correct the problem.

REFERENCES

Babior BW: The megaloblastic anemias. In Williams WJ, Beutler E, Erslev AJ, et al: Hematology, ed 4, New York, 1990, McGraw-Hill, Inc.

Dallman PR: Manifestations of iron deficiency, Semin Hematol 19:19, 1982.

Finch CA and Heubers H: Perspectives in iron metabolism, N Eng J Med 306: 1520, 1982.

Fisher JW: Pharmacologic modulation of erythropoietin production, Ann Rev Pharmacol Toxicol 28:101, 1988.

Fisher JW, Bommer J, Eschbach J, et al: Statement on the clinical use of recombinant erythropoietin in amemia of end-stage renal disease, Am J Kidney Dis XIV:163, 1989.

66

Regulated Drug Development and Usage

OVERVIEW

Discovery, development, and clinical introduction of new drugs is a process involving close cooperation between researchers, medical practitioners, the pharmaceutical industry, and the U.S. government Food and Drug Administration (FDA). The drug development process begins with the synthesis or isolation of a new compound with biological activity and potential therapeutic use. This entity must then pass through preclinical, clinical, and regulatory review stages before availability as a therapeutically safe and effective drug. About 20 to 30 new chemical compounds and numerous new formulations are approved for use each year in the United States.

The FDA authority over drug review and approval began with the Federal Pure Food and Drug Act of 1906. This first drug law established standards for drug strength and purity. This legislation was fol-

lowed by the Federal Food, Drug and Cosmetic Act of 1938, which prohibited marketing of new drugs unless adequately tested to demonstrate safety under conditions indicated on their labels. The 1938 Act was amended by Congress in 1962 to state that pharmaceutical manufacturers must provide scientific proof that new products are efficacious and safe before marketing. The amendment also required that the FDA be notified before testing of drugs in humans. More recent legislation includes controls on the manufacture and prescribing of habit-forming drugs, drug development for treating rare diseases, and new drug applications for generic drug products.

CLINICAL TESTING AND INTRODUCTION OF NEW DRUGS

Potential new drugs or biological products must first be tested in animals for their acute and chronic toxicity, influence on reproductive performance, carcinogenic and mutagenic potential, and safe dosing range. Preclinical testing often requires 2 to 5 years at a cost of millions of dollars. Chronic safety testing in animals continues during subsequent trials in humans.

After successful preclinical pharmacological and toxicological studies, the sponsor files an Investigational New Drug (IND) Application with the FDA. In addition to animal data, the IND contains protocols for clinical testing in humans. Approximately 2000 INDs are received each year by the FDA. If the IND passes FDA review, clinical trials in humans are initiated. These studies are generally conducted in three phases:

Phase 1: Conducted on a small number of normal volunteers to determine safe dosage range and pharmacokinetic parameters

Phase 2: Conducted on several hundred patients to determine short-term safety and effectiveness of the drug in patients with specific diseases

Phase 3: Conducted on several thousand patients with specific diseases to determine overall risk-benefit relationships in specific populations of patients

These studies provide the basis for drug labeling. The completion of these clinical studies may take 3 to 10 years and may cost up to 100 million dollars.

Before initiating study of an investigational drug in humans, an investigator must also obtain approval from the local Institutional Review Board (IRB) of the hospital, university, or other institution where the planned study will be conducted. The IRB is responsible for ensuring the ethical acceptability of the proposed research and approves, requires modification, or disapproves the research protocol. To approve a clinical research study, the IRB must determine that the research design and procedures are sound and that the risk to subjects is minimized. In addition, the IRB must also approve the Informed Consent document that must be signed by each prospective subject or the subject's legally authorized representative. IRB approval is usually valid for 1 year (Figure 66-1).

The basic elements of informed consent include the following:

1. Explanation of the purposes and procedures of the research
2. Description of foreseeable risks
3. Description of expected benefits
4. Statement of available alternative procedures or courses of treatment
5. Statement on confidentiality of records
6. Explanation of compensation or available medical treatments if injury occurs
7. Description of whom to contact about the research and the subject's rights and the procedure to follow in the event of injury to the subject
8. Statement that participation is voluntary and refusal to participate does not involve penalty to the subject

If suitable preclinical and clinical findings demonstrate efficacy with minimal toxicity, the sponsors can submit a New Drug Application (NDA) to the FDA (see Figure 66-1). In approving an NDA, the FDA ensures the drug's safety and effectiveness for each use. Usually the sponsor and the FDA review the data and negotiate on the detailed information to accompany the drug for its use. This includes contraindications, precautions, side effects, dosages, routes of administration, and frequency of administration. The NDA approval process usually takes 2 to 3 years with drugs having the greatest potential benefit given priority. Postapproval research may be requested by the FDA as a condition of new drug approval. Such research may be used to speed drug approval, uncover unexpected adverse drug reactions, and define the incidence of known drug reactions under actual clinical use.

After NDA approval, the manufacturer promotes the new drug for approved uses described on the label. Post NDA–approval or marketing period (phase 4) requires monitoring of new drug safety during clinical use. The label information does not include all conditions in which a released drug is safe and effective; however, the FDA does not restrict use of released drugs to those conditions described on the label; the physician is allowed to determine its most appropriate use. There should be compelling scientific evidence before using a drug for an unapproved indication. Examples are β-blockers, which often are used interchangeably for various indications, although not all have identical FDA-approved indications (Table 66-1).

Early clinical testing of new drugs does not provide absolute assurance of safety, as evidenced by later discoveries of adverse effects after drugs are used clinically. In some instances, released drugs are withdrawn from the market after toxic or fatal adverse effects are discovered during large-scale clinical use. There are instances in which lack of efficacy of a new drug is not discovered until the drug is in large-scale clinical use with selected patient populations. The goal of postmarketing surveillance (PMS) is also important to define the true side-effect profile of a new drug.

New safety information obtained during large-scale clinical testing is used to update the current NDA and provide changes in the drug label. Side effect profiles in patients with multiple diseases are often imcomplete during early studies, and such in-

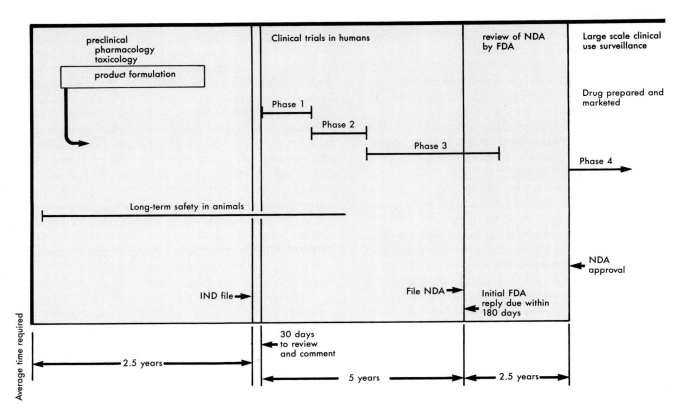

FIGURE 66-1   Stages of new drug development.

Table 66-1   Varied Uses of Several β-Adrenergic Blocking Agents

	acebutolol	atenolol	labetolol	metoprolol	nadolol	propranolol
LABEL INDICATIONS						
Hypertension	X	X	X	X	X	X
Angina	—	X	—	X	X	X
Dysrhythmia	X	—	—	—	—	X
Postmyocardial infarction	—	X	—	X	—	X
Pheochromocytoma	—	—	—	—	—	X
Hypertrophic subaortic stenosis	—	—	—	—	—	X
Essential tremor	—	—	—	—	—	X
Migraine prophylaxis	—	—	—	—	—	X

formation is vitally important for improving subsequent use. Reporting of rare and unexpected side effects not listed on the drug label is an important responsibility for prescribers; information is supplied to the FDA on the Drug Experience Form (FDA form 1639).

There are several sources of information available to physicians concerning the safety of new drugs. These include the Medical Letter on Drugs and Therapeutics, Facts and Comparisons, AMA Drug Evaluation, and the Physician's Desk Reference (PDR), a compilation of FDA-approved drug package inserts.

ORPHAN DRUGS AND TREATMENT INDs

New drugs that may benefit only a small number of patients with rare diseases, defined in the United States as fewer than 200,000 individuals, provide little economic incentive to pharmaceutical manufacturers for development and filing of an IND or NDA. The Orphan Drug Act of 1983 provides special incentives such as tax advantages and marketing exclusiveness to compensate companies for developmental costs of such agents. The National Institutes of Health also participates in development of orphan drugs, and more than 300 drugs have been given orphan status. These include human growth hormone, erythropoietin, and α_1-antitrypsin.

The FDA established guidelines to make promising investigational drugs available for treatment of patients with immediate life-threatening diseases, such as AIDS. These drugs receive highest priority at all stages of the drug-review process. The Treatment IND application enables patients not qualified for participation in ongoing studies to be treated with investigational drugs outside controlled clinical trials. The FDA generally considers Treatment INDs for drugs in later stages of clinical testing. The initial criteria include the following:

1. The drug is intended to treat a serious life-threatening disease
2. There is no comparable or satisfactory alternative to treat the disease
3. The drug is under investigation in a controlled clinical trial under an IND
4. The sponsor is actively pursuing marketing approval of the investigational drug

When no Treatment IND is in effect for an investigational drug, a physician may obtain the drug for "compassionate use." In such cases, the physician submits a Treatment IND to the FDA requesting authorization of an investigational drug for such use.

PRESCRIPTION WRITING

Prescriptions are written by the prescriber to instruct the pharmacist to dispense a specific medication for a specific patient. These include precompounded medications (prepared by the pharmaceutical manufacturer) and extemporaneously prepared medications. It is vitally important that a prescription communicate clearly to the pharmacist the exact medication needed and how this medication is to be used by the patient. Patient compliance is often related to the clarity of the directions on the prescription, and terms such as "take as directed" should be avoided. Equally important is the necessity for clarity when using proprietary drug names because of their similarities. In these instances the physician should designate the generic name, as well as the brand name, to avoid confusion.

Prescriptions contain the following elements to facilitate interpretation by the pharmacist:

1. Physician's name, address, telephone number
2. Date
3. Patient's name and address
4. Superscription (Rx how drug is to be taken)
5. Inscription (name and dosage of drug)

Prescriber's Name, Address, and Telephone Number

Date _____   Patient _____

Address _____

Rx

Drug name and strength
Quantity to be dispensed

Patient Instructions

Refill_____ times   Dr. Signature_____

No safety cap ☐   DEA No. _____

FIGURE 66-2   Typical prescription form.

6. Subscription (directions to the pharmacist)
7. Signature or transcription (directions to the patient)
8. Refill and safety cap information
9. Prescriber's (physician's) signature
10. DEA number of physician (for controlled substances)

A typical prescription blank is shown in Figure 66-2. Because both apothecary and metric systems are in use, it is important that prescribers become familiar with conversion units. Commonly used weights and measures are listed below:

2.2 pounds (lb) = 1 kilogram (kg)
1 grain (gr) = 65 milligrams (mg)
1 ounce (oz) = 30 milliliters (ml)
1 tablespoonful (tbsp) = 15 ml
1 teaspoonful (tsp) = 5 ml
20 drops (gtt) = 1 ml

Patient instructions (Signature) on a prescription are sometimes written with Latin abbreviations as shorthand for prescribers giving concise directions to the pharmacist on how and when a patient takes the medication. Although instructions written in English are preferred, some common Latin abbreviations are as follows:

po: by mouth
ac: before meals
pc: after meals
qd: every day
bid: twice daily
tid: three times a day
qid: four times a day
hs: at bedtime
prn: as needed
c̄: with
s̄: without
ss: one-half

Additional instructions may be added to the prescription to instruct the pharmacist to place an additional label on the prescription container (e.g., Take With Food).

In the United States a large number of drugs require a prescription from a licensed practitioner (e.g., physician, dentist, veterinarian, podiatrist) before being dispensed by a pharmacist. In addition, use of specific drugs, called *schedule drugs,* with high abuse potential are further restricted by the FDA, and special requirements are met when these drugs are prescribed. These controlled drugs (Table 66-2) are clas-

Table 66-2   Controlled Substances

Schedule	Symbol	Abuse Potential	Example
I	C-I	No accepted medical use in the United States	heroin
II	C-II	High abuse potential	morphine
III	C-III	Moderate potential for dependence	glutethimide
IV	C-IV	Low potential for dependence	diazepam
V	C-V	Lowest abuse potential	diphenoxylate

sified according to potential for abuse and include opioids, stimulants, and depressants. Schedule I drugs have no currently accepted medical use in the United States and may not be prescribed. Schedule II drugs have a high potential for abuse and cannot be refilled. In addition, Schedule II drugs may not be prescribed via telephone, and several states (e.g., Texas, Michigan, New York) require a special triplicate prescription blank. Other schedule drugs (III and V) can be refilled, but there is a 5-refill maximum and the prescription is invalid 6 months from date of issue. An exception to these regulations involves drugs in schedule V, which may be dispensed without a prescription if the patient is 18 years old, distribution is by a pharmacist, and only a limited quantity of a drug is purchased (refer to the Controlled Substance Act of 1970).

Many prescribed proprietary (brand name) drugs are available from multiple pharmaceutical manufacturers as brand name (tradename) or as less costly generic (nonproprietary) preparations. Pharmacists receiving prescriptions for brand name products may dispense a generically equivalent drug, if available (except as noted below), without prescriber approval and pass on potential savings to the patient. Some states have mandatory substitution laws, and the brand name product is dispensed only when "Dispense as Written" (D.A.W.) is stated on the prescription. Generic drugs are pharmaceutical equivalents to brand name products (except as indicated in Chapter 4).

Pharmaceutical manufacturers submit an Abbreviated New Drug Application (ANDA) to market products previously marketed by another manufacturer. Documentation of safety and efficacy is not required. Generic products tested by the FDA and determined to be therapeutic equivalents are listed by the FDA in Approved Drug Products with Therapeutic Equivalence Evaluations (Orange Book). These products contain the same active ingredients as their brand name counterparts and also meet bioequivalence standards (see Chapter 4). The FDA recommends substitution only among products listed as therapeutically equivalent. Not all generic drugs listed in the Orange Book are therapeutic equivalents of the pioneer or brand name products. Brand name products such as Lanoxin (digoxin), Dilantin (phenytoin), Premarin (conjugated estrogens), and Theo-Dur (slow-release theophylline) exhibit unique bioavailability characteristics and should not be substituted without physician supervision.

REFERENCES

Bosso JA: The role of the institutional review board in research involving human subjects, Drug Intell Clin Pharm 17:828, 1983.

Edlavitch SA: Postmarketing surveillance methodologies, Drug Intell Clin Pharm 22:68, 1988.

Kessler DA: The regulation of investigational drugs, N Engl J Med 320:281, 1989.

Myers AM and Moore SR: The drug approval process and the information it provides, Drug Intell Clin Pharm 21:821, 1987.

Steinbrook RS and Lo B: Informing physicians about promising new treatments for severe illnesses, JAMA 263:2078, 1990.

Strom BL: Generic drug substitution revisited, N Engl J Med 316:1456, 1987.

Strom BL, Melmon KL, and Miettinen OS: Post-marketing studies of drug efficacy: Why? Am J Med 78:475, 1985.

Young FE, Norris JA, Levitt JA et al.: The FDA's new procedures for the use of investigational drugs in treatment, JAMA 259:2267, 1988.

Index

A